ADVANCES IN PAIN RESEARCH AND THERAPY
VOLUME 1

Advances in
Pain Research and Therapy
Volume 1

Proceedings of the First World Congress on Pain

Editors

John J. Bonica, M.D.,
F.F.A.R.C.S., D.Sc.
President-Elect of IASP
Professor and Chairman
Department of Anesthesiology
Director of Anesthesia Research Center
Director of Pain Clinic
University of Washington
School of Medicine
Seattle, Washington

Denise G. Albe-Fessard, D.Sc.
President of IASP
Professor
Université Pierre et Marie Curie
Laboratoire de Physiologie
des Centres Nerveux
Paris, France

Associate Editors

B. Raymond Fink, M.D.
Secretary of IASP
Professor
Department of Anesthesiology
University of Washington
School of Medicine
Seattle, Washington

Louisa E. Jones, B.S.
Treasurer of IASP
Editor, Research Publications
Department of Anesthesiology
University of Washington
School of Medicine
Seattle, Washington

Raven Press ▪ New York

Raven Press, 1140 Avenue of the Americas, New York, New York 10036

Made in the United States of America

International Standard Book Number 0-89004-0907
Library of Congress Catalog Card Number 75-32095

Preface

This monograph contains the most important scientific papers presented at the First World Congress on Pain held September 5–8, 1975, in Florence, Italy. The Congress, sponsored by the International Association for the Study of Pain, was attended by over 1,100 scientists, physicians and other health professionals, and guests. The registrants, most of whom are members of the Association, represented 75 different disciplines from 35 countries. This is the largest and most extensive multidisciplinary and interdisciplinary meeting of professional people who have special interest and expertise in pain research or pain therapy, or both, that has ever been assembled anywhere.

The scientific session of the Congress was opened by the keynote lecture on "Modulation" by Professor Patrick D. Wall of the University of London. During the ensuing 3½ days, 18 special lectures, 250 papers, and six motion pictures pertinent to pain were presented and four workshops were held. In addition, three symposia were held in conjunction with the Congress that were not part of its Scientific Program. The lectures were presented at the single plenary sessions which were attended by all Registrants, while the papers and other activities were given at one of the section meetings.

Each special lecture was presented by an international authority in a specific field at the invitation of the Scientific Program Committee. These lectures were intended to provide a comprehensive overview of the specific topic, including new data from personal research and review of new and at times older data published by others. In addition to presenting information for the benefit of the extraordinarily diverse audience, each lecture was used to introduce shorter papers given at one of the 44 sectional meetings, two to five of which were held at the same time. One or more sections were devoted to 14 major areas of pain research or therapy, or both, which are listed in the Table of Contents.

In order to keep the size of this monograph to a manageable size, it was necessary to exclude two lectures and 112 papers out of an overall total of 264. Selection for inclusion in the monograph was made by the editors on the basis of the evaluation and rating given each paper by at least two, and in many instances three or more, members of the Editorial Board whose names appear on page ii, and each of whom has expertise in a particular field.

Most of the papers included in this volume had a rating of excellent or good previously unpublished data, or excellent previously published data. A few were included because of their special significance to readers and a very few to represent geographic regions. We regret that we were forced to omit many other informative papers to meet the page limitations. We express our thanks and appreciation to the authors of these submitted papers for their efforts and their appreciation of the editors' problem.

The first part of the book contains sections dealing primarily with research on pain mechanisms; the second part contains those sections dealing with research or therapy, or both; and the last portion contains papers on pain syndromes and a summary of two of the four workshops and of two mini-symposia. (The one-day symposium on Cancer Pain is being published by the National Institutes of Health of HEW for general distribution to the profession.) We have arranged the papers in each section in scientifically logical sequence. For example, papers in the first section start with basic issues and progress to those involving more complex or advanced aspects of the topic, papers dealing with the same subjects have been placed together, while those papers in the middle and last part of the book begin with research reports and progress to those dealing with therapy.

We believe that this volume will be of interest to basic and clinical scientists, medical and dental practitioners, nurses, sociologists, and other health professionals who have interest in the field of pain research or pain therapy. The importance of pain as a subject for serious scientific investigation and proper therapy needs no elaboration. As stressed by Bonica in the Introduction to the Congress, while acute pain serves a useful biological function, in its chronic form pain is a malefic force that imposes severe emotional, physical, and economic stresses on the patient and the patient's family, taxes the diagnostic acumen and therapeutic skills of all health professionals, and imposes severe economic and sociologic responsibilities on society. Because chronic pain is one of the most disabling disease states, it constitutes a serious world health and economic problem. The reasons for current deficiencies in managing patients with chronic pain and the recommendation for diminishing their magnitude are summarized in the Introduction to the volume.

We believe that these proceedings will help to fulfill some of the goals and purposes of the International Association for the Study of Pain, which, although barely 2 years old, has a membership of 1,600 scientists and practitioners from 55 countries and representing 81 different fields of research or practice. By providing readers with the most important papers of its first Congress, the monograph should promote and facilitate the dissemination of new information and thereby enhance communication and crossfertilization, stimulate greater research efforts, and promote education. In these and other ways, it should help improve the care of patients suffering from pain, a responsibility that remains one of the most important obligations and laudable objectives of all the health professionals.

John J. Bonica
Denise Albe-Fessard
July, 1976

Contents

Acupuncture

Contributors

Introduction to the First World Congress on Pain

Goals of IASP and the World Congress

It is now my privilege to give an overview of the background, development, current status, and future objectives of the International Association for the Study of Pain (IASP) and this First World Congress.

In addition to informing members who have recently joined the Association, it will serve as a framework for this, our First World Congress.

BACKGROUND

Although some of you have heard me mention some of these points before, I think they deserve retelling because many of these aspects remain unappreciated by the public and many scientists and health professionals.

We fully appreciate the biologic usefulness of acute transient pain, for it is the most common symptom of disease, compelling patients to seek help, and a useful diagnostic aid to the practitioner.

In contrast, in its chronic persistent pathologic form, pain is a malefic force that often imposes severe emotional, physical, economic, and sociologic stresses on the patient and his family as well as on society. When pain caused by disease or injury persists, the immediate autonomic reflex responses characteristic of acute pain become progressively less and within a short period of time, they disappear. Many patients with chronic pain undergo a progressive physical deterioration caused by disturbance of sleep, decrease or loss of appetite, and often by excess medication. Moreover, many patients with chronic pain undergo serious emotional, affective, and behavioral changes. The anxiety of acute pain is replaced by reactive depression and hypochondriasis—two important characteristics of chronic pain, whether attributable to somatogenic or to psychogenic processes. Many of these patients gradually lose interest in social activities and the pain becomes their central focus, dominating their life. Many of these patients are exposed to a high risk of iatrogenic complications: others give up medical care and consult quacks, who not only provide no relief, but may do harm; and some become so desperate as to commit suicide.

Why do these deficiencies exist which seriously detract from our other biomedical scientific achievements? The many reasons can be grouped into three major categories: voids in our knowledge of chronic pain syndromes, inadequate application of the knowledge currently available, and problems in communication. Although these are interrelated, they will be briefly considered separately.

Lack of Knowledge

There still exist great voids in our knowledge of the mechanisms and pathophysiology of chronic pain syndromes. It is true, of course, that in the one and one-half centuries, since the reports of Bell, Magendie, and Mueller stimulated the first truly scientific study of pain, a great mass of information has been adduced from the hundreds of studies that have been carried out. It is also true that these data, derived mostly from animal laboratory experiments or studies on human volunteers with artificially induced pain, have proved useful to a better understanding of the physiologic and psychologic responses to acute pain. Moreover, these data have spurred the introduction of various therapeutic modalities, which, although crude and nonspecific, have permitted the control of acute pain.

Unfortunately, most of this information has not been as beneficial to patients with chronic pain as one might anticipate or as many people believe. This less-than-optimal payoff from the many research efforts, in turn, resulted because until recently little attention was paid to the application of new knowledge and technology to the study of pain syndromes. Basic scientists, working in the isolation of the animal laboratory, the traditional "ivory tower," were not concerned with clinical pain. As a result of these fragmented, independent research efforts on artificially induced pain with little regard to the clinical problems, hypotheses and concepts were developed, which, although reasonable for the times and the scientific data available, were not relevant to chronic pain. Moreover, as pointed out by Melzack, pain research and theory remained conceptually stagnant for more than a century. Therefore, we have had little or no scientific information on the *exact* mechanisms by which headache, arthritis, herniated disc, postherpetic neuralgia, and causalgia, to name a few, produced chronic pain. To be sure, many speculations were proposed, but hard scientific data were lacking.

The few clinicians interested in the study of clinical pain have consistently faced the frustrating problem of the inability to quantify the pain, let alone study its mechanisms. The fact that pain is a subjective and very personal experience that cannot be seen, touched, or measured presents almost insurmountable problems to the study of its phenomena in patients. Consequently, clinicians borrowed the hypotheses of the basic scientists developed from acute pain experiments to explain chronic pain, which is now recognized as a totally different phenomenon. Moreover, on the basis of these hypotheses, therapeutic modalities were developed and applied, many of which were not only ineffective but produced serious complications of their own.

Another reason for the voids in our knowledge of clinical or chronic pain has been the lack of a sufficient scientifically trained workforce working on this problem. Related to this has been the meager amount or total lack of funds for research or research training in this field. In most countries, scientific research support by the government is nonexistent, and even in the so-called developed and affluent countries, the amount of money devoted to pain research is meager compared to expenditures for research of other diseases. In my own country, the National Institutes of Health (NIH), the federal agency responsible for supporting biomedical research, spends about $2.2 billion per year on research. Of this amount, only $34 million, or 1.5% of the total, are spent on "pain-related research." The NIH "pain-related research" programs are summarized in a news release prepared by Ms. Helen Neal, Chairperson of the Public Information Committee for this Congress. Although I commend Ms. Neal for her efforts, I would be less than candid if I did not point out that most of the funds are actually being spent on studies pertaining to anesthesia, pharmacology, cardiology, and other areas intended to prevent pathologic processes associated with pain or to define and correct problems somewhat peripheral to pain. Analysis of the records suggests that the research specifically directed to pain as a disease entity amounts to less than $3 million. This represents less than 10% of the pain-related research budget and about 0.014% of the total biomedical research budget. Finally, in this regard let me cite another statistic (which I will elaborate on at the Cancer Pain Symposium): Currently the National Cancer Institute (NCI) of the United States spends more than $0.5 billion per year for cancer research, but until recently, very little attention was being paid to research on cancer pain, which from the viewpoint of the patient is one of the most important aspects of this dreadful disease.

Another interrelated factor has been the lack of funds or opportunities, or both, for research training in this field. Hence, there has existed a vicious circle of inadequate scientific workforce → inadequate number of grant applications submitted to the NIH → inadequate amount of funds budgeted for pain research and research training → discouragement of scientists to pursue pain research. Which of these has been the initiating factor is clear, but the important thing is that we must break the vicious circle by activating the multipronged programs mentioned later.

Teaching

The second major reason for the deficiencies in managing patients with chronic pain has been the improper or inadequate application of knowledge currently available. The reasons for this include the lack of organized teaching of medical students and physicians and other health professionals in managing patients with chronic pain, the progressive trend toward specialization, and the inability or unwillingness of some practitioners to devote the necessary time and efforts to care for these patients.

I know of no medical, dental, or other health professional school that teaches the basic principles for managing patients with chronic pain. I believe that this is because of the total lack of appreciation by teachers of the marked differences between acute and chronic pain as a disease entity. Consequently, students are taught how to use pain diagnostically as well as how to apply the same methods used for treating acute pain to the management of patients with chronic pain. This invariably results in failures, drug toxicity, useless and at times mutilating operations, and other iatrogenic disorders mentioned earlier.

The current progressive trend toward specialization is conducive to each specialist viewing pain in a very narrow tubular fashion. Thus, the anesthesiologist attempts to treat all patients with nerve blocks, the neurosurgeon by cutting so-called pain pathways, the psychiatrist by traditional psychotherapy, and so forth. This type of tubular vision is particularly likely to occur when a specialist practices alone and sees these patients in isolation. These factors preclude viewing the pain problem within the perspective of the many diagnostic and therapeutic strategies that may be applicable to the particular problem and choosing which are best for that patient.

Communications

A matrix common to all of these causative factors has been the poor and indeed at times total lack of communication among investigators and between this group and clinicians. The usual mechanism of disseminating new information—publications in highly specialized journals limited to specific fields and meetings generally limited to a specific group—has precluded cross-fertilization and dissemination of information among the various basic science groups and clinicians. The poor interaction among basic scientists of different disciplines has impaired the application of vitally important new information acquired by neurophysiologists, for example, to the research programs of other scientific disciplines. Moreover, it has impaired cooperation among various basic scientists and clinical investigators—a condition necessary to solve clinical problems. This has also resulted in a great lag in the clinical application of new information useful and pertinent to the care of patients with chronic pain. Other major communication problems include lack of an international standard terminology for pain syndromes, no epidemilogic data on pain as a disease state, and the lack of national and international pain data banks or data pools—essential requisites to optimal communication and evaluation of old as well as new methods of therapy.

RECENT TRENDS AND DEVELOPMENTS

During the past two decades there have been various serious efforts to help rectify some of these deficiencies. For one thing, there has been an impressive surge of interest among some basic scientists in studying mechanisms of chronic pain syndromes and in collaborating with clinical investigators and practitioners to solve some of the major problems. Consequently, the field of pain research and theory has become alive—full of renewed fascination and great controversies that promise to spur greater research efforts. For example, the hypothesis of Melzack and Wall, which attempted to explain clinical pain syndromes within the framework of newly acquired knowledge, has indeed provoked controversies and many new investigations. Moreover, as a result of recent collaborative efforts between scientists and clinicians, animal models have been developed to simulate and study such important syndromes as trigeminal neuralgia, denervation hypersensitivity, and postamputation neuroma among others.

Other scientists have collaborated with clinicians to study patients with chronic pain problems in the course of neurosurgical operations, which permit the recording of neural activity in the central nervous system. Equally important have been the contributions of psychologists, who have helped to define the differences in the characteristics of acute and chronic pain and the importance of cultural, psychologic, and environmental factors to chronic pain behavior. Many of these investigators are attending this Congress.

Another development, especially gratifying to me, is that after some two decades of advocating it without any visible response, in recent years there has been a great surge of interest in a multidisciplinary pain clinic approach to complex chronic pain problems which F. A. D. Alexander and I, independently, first proposed in 1948. In addition to providing more efficient patient care, this team approach is an effective mechanism for teaching and for encouraging collaborative research by affording psychologists and other basic scientists insight into the problem of pain.

A development of the past year or two in the United States is the surge of interest by the NIH to significantly increase its support for research specifically targeted to pain. Through the efforts and leadership of Dr. Ganz, Dr. Dubner, and Dr. Driscoll of the National Institute of Dental Research (NIDR), Dr. Emilie Black of the National Institute of General Medical Sciences (NIGMS), and Dr. K. M. Nelson of the NCI, plans are being formulated to encourage the development of major pain research projects. All these individuals are participating in this Congress and are members of IASP. Moreover, as I will emphasize later, these agencies have provided support for this Congress.

Finally, another important trend intended to eliminate some of the problems of communication has been the publication of numerous books during the past two decades and the various international symposia on pain held during the past 10 years. The last of these, held in Seattle 3 years ago, was attended by over 350 scientists, physicians, and other health professionals from 13 countries and representing many disciplines. It was at that meeting that a proposal to found an international multidisciplinary society was made. Then, as now, my introductory remarks were devoted primarily to emphasizing deficiencies of past independent efforts as bases for the proposal. During the subsequent days, the question I posed at the beginning of this presentation—Do we need a new society and a new journal?—was thoroughly discussed by the working groups appointed to consider the proposal. After these discussions, it was the concensus that whereas much had been achieved through past efforts, much more needed to be done in research, teaching, and patient care related to pain. After some of these needs were defined, the group agreed that a multidisciplinary society would be useful, suggested the name International Association for the Study of Pain, and formulated its objectives. The proposal was unanimously endorsed, and four committees were appointed to carry out preliminary plans. Let me briefly summarize the activities of these committees during the past 28 months.

Organizing Committee

The Organizing Committee promptly began to review the organization and the articles of incorporation and bylaws of various existing international and national organizations including the International Association of Physiological Sciences, The World Federation of Societies of Anesthesiologists, and The Society for Neurosciences. The Committee also consulted some of the officers of these organizations and obtained legal advice about procedures for drafting the articles of incorporation and bylaws of IASP.

Very serious consideration was given to the matter of the country in which the Association should be incorporated. Although it was anticipated that the largest number of IASP members would be Americans, as Chairman of the Committee initially, I contended that it would best serve the cause of making the Association truly international, if it were incorporated in a country other than the United States. A relevant point that came up was the need to solicit funds to support the Association. Investigation showed that because many of the major pharmaceutical companies had their headquarters in the United States, and because it was known that they usually donate funds for this purpose, and further since U.S. law required that donations would be considered tax exempt only if given to associations incorporated in the United States, the Organizing Committee and all other key members of IASP whose opinion was solicited unanimously agreed it would be best to incorporate in the United States.

The IASP was officially incorporated on May 9, 1974. The official purposes or goals of the Association are listed in the Articles of Incorporation and Bylaws. I urge all of you to read and know them well. In compliance with the bylaws, a Council and Officers Pro Tem were designated to carry out the activities of the Association until this First World Congress. Once

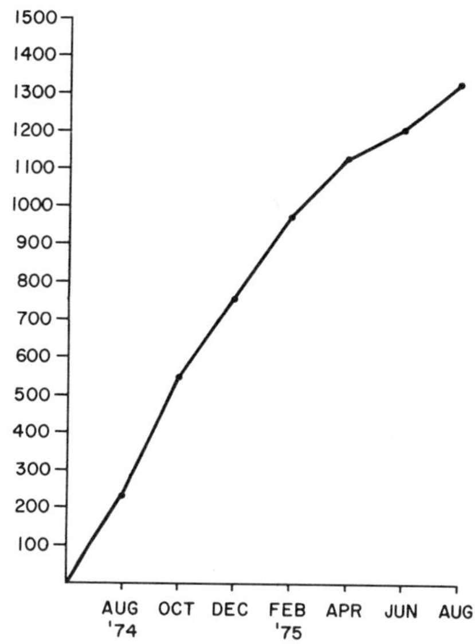

FIG. 1. Growth of IASP membership.

this was accomplished, a membership drive was begun by sending news releases announcing the founding of IASP to hundreds of scientific and professional journals and newsletters throughout the world.

The response was so rapid and so large that, although very gratifying, it created logistic problems in getting the applications recorded, reviewed, and approved by the Council Pro Tem. Figure 1 shows the number of members elected at monthly intervals. As of today, IASP has 1,325 active members from 50 different countries and representing 81 different fields of research and clinical interest.[1] Table 1 is a list of primary scientific and/or health professional disciplines, whereas Table 2 lists the membership according to distribution of countries and regions.

The Council decided to set the admission fee at $15.00 and the annual dues for 1975 at $25.00. These extremely low fees in these times of inflationary prices were adopted to encourage young basic scientists to join the Association. As you will learn from the Treasurer's report, these figures barely cover the $20.00 subscription price for the journal *Pain* for each member, in addition to the running of the Society. Realizing that these would be insufficient funds to run a vigorous society, early last year I began to solicit nonspecific grants from those industrial companies that had primarily supported the Seattle Pain Symposium. Although the response was not at the same level as in 1973, because of the recent economic recession, the Association has been given a total of $25,000 to date.

[1] At press time, these numbers have increased to 1,575; 55; 81, respectively.

TABLE 1. *Specialty areas represented in IASP*

Behavioral sciences

- Hypnosis
- Neuropsychiatry
- Neuropsychology
- Neuropsychopharmacology
- Physiological Psychology
- Psychiatry
- Psychoanalysis
- Psychobiology
- Psychology
- Psychopharmacology
- Psychophysiology
- Psychosocial Rehabilitation
- Psychosomatic Medicine
- Psychotherapy
- Sociology

Neural sciences

- Neuroanatomy
- Neurobiochemistry
- Neurobiology
- Neurochemistry
- Neurocytology
- Neuroendocrinology
- Neuropathology
- Neuropharmacology
- Neurophysiology

Other basic sciences

- Anatomy
- Biochemistry
- Bioengineering
- Biology
- Biometry
- Comparative Physiology
- Cytology
- Electrophysiology
- Oral Biology/Physiology
- Physiology
- Toxicology

Other

- History of Medicine
- Research Administration
- Public Information Specialist
- Science Editor
- Affiliates

Clinical sciences

- Acupunture
- Allergy
- Anesthesiology
- Community Health Education
- Dentistry
- Dental Prosthesis
- Electromyography
- Electroencephalography
- Emergency Medicine
- Endodontics
- Family Practice
- Gastroenterology
- Haemorrhageology
- Internal Medicine
- Intensive Care
- Neurology
- Neuroprosthesis
- Neuroradiology
- Neurosurgery
- Nursing
- Obstetrics & Gynecology
- Occupational Therapy
- Oncology
- Ophthalmology
- Oral & Maxillofacial Surgery
- Orthopedic Surgery
- Pain
- Periodontics
- Perioral Pain
- Pharmacology
- Physiotherapy
- Prostodontics
- Radiation Therapy
- Rehabilitation Medicine
- Rheumatology
- Spinal Cord Injury
- Stereoencephalotomy
- Surgery
- TMJ Dysfunction
- Traumatology
- Urology

TABLE 2. *IASP membership by region*[a]

Region	No.	Region	No.
Western Europe	399	Pacific	53
Austria	6	Australia	40
Belgium	12	New Zealand	11
Denmark	5	The Philippines	2
Finland	10		
France	51	North America	909
Germany (West)	60	Canada	82
Ireland	5	United States	827
Italy	73		
The Netherlands	38	Central and South America	50
Norway	2	Argentina	26
Portugal	1	Bolivia	1
Spain	14	Brazil	5
Sweden	34	Chile	3
Switzerland	12	El Salvador	1
United Kingdom	76	Mexico	4
		Netherlands Antilles	1
Eastern Europe	26	Nicaragua	1
Bulgaria	3	Puerto Rico	4
Czechoslovakia	3	Uruguay	2
Hungary	3	Venezuela	2
Poland	7		
Rumania	4	Asia	131
Russia	2	Hong Kong	5
Yugoslavia	4	India	6
		Iran	1
Africa	7	Israel	6
Algeria	1	Japan	99
Egypt	1	Lebanon	1
Nigeria	2	Pakistan	1
Republic of South Africa	2	Republic of China	2
Zambia	1	Saudi Arabia	1
		Thailand	1
		Turkey	4
		Viet-Nam (South)	4

[a] Total number of members, August 1976: 1,575

Editorial Committee

The Editorial Committee, chaired by Professor Patrick Wall, promptly began to explore the possibility of publishing a journal on pain. After several months negotiation with three publishers, the Editorial Committee selected Elsevier. The first issue of the journal was published in record time. I hope you agree with me that on the basis of the first two issues, the journal promises to be a high-quality and prestigious publication, which should help rectify one of the major deficiencies of communication. By publishing original communications, review articles, and abstracts containing clinical and basic science information of multidisciplinary interest as well as the selected bibliography, the journal should enhance communication and cross-fertilization among the members of such diversified background and research and clinical interests. Professor Wall will make a report on the journal at the first General Assembly.

Committee on Scientific Program

The Committee on Scientific Program, under the leadership of Professor Denise Albe-Fessard, began to plan for this Congress nearly a year and a half ago. At the initial meeting, it was decided that the central theme of the Congress would be "Modulation"—a most appropriate title at this time. Subsequently, an outline for the various subtopics under the theme of modulation was published in the first issue of the IASP Newsletter. The Committee had planned to have single sessions for the major part of each day and to have five or six simultaneous sessions devoted to communications on related topics for the remainder. This would have permitted about 170 papers for the program. The response to solicitation of papers was overwhelming. The Committee received more than 300 titles and, subsequently, over 275 abstracts. During a two-day meeting, the Committee reviewed the titles and abstracts and, after eliminating those of poor quality, still had 250 presentations. To fit all of these into the four days of the Congress, the final program which you have includes 18 special lectures intended to give an overview on specific topics and 252 10-minute presentations followed by 5-minute discussions. This is obviously a jam-packed Congress, which requires that each lecture and presentation, and the discussion period, be strictly limited to the alloted time.

The Scientific Program promises to be very informative and stimulating. I wish to publicly express the appreciation and gratitude of IASP to Professor Albe-Fessard and the other committee members for the outstanding job they have done in putting this program together.

Committee on Local Arrangements

The Committee on Local Arrangements, chaired by Professor Paolo Procacci, began its task two years ago with the selection of this beautiful Palazzo dei Congressi as the site of the meeting. Subsequently, they formulated many preliminary plans which were finalized during the two days I spent here the early part of the year. With the help of the Organizzazione Congressi Internationale, under the leadership of Dr. Bonamici, and the spouses of the committee members, they have been able to overcome the obstacle of shortness of time to take care of every minor detail to assure the success of the Congress. On behalf of IASP, I thank Professor Procacci, Professor Pagni, and the other members of the Committee for their very outstanding work.

Committee on Public Information

The Committee on Public Information has been given the very important responsibility of providing the news media and the public with information about the objectives and goals of IASP and the Scientific Program at this World Congress.

I hope you will agree with me that providing the public with accurate information about IASP and this Congress is one of our most important obligations. I would therefore ask those who will be contacted by this Committee to cooperate with them to the fullest extent.

On behalf of the Council and the membership, I wish to thank Ms. Helen Danforth, Ms. Helen Neal, Dr. Elie Cass, and the other members of this Committee who have offered to devote their time and energy gratis for the benefit of the Association.

Publication of Proceedings

Publication of the proceedings of this Congress is an extremely important responsibility of IASP. The information presented here should be made available to those IASP members who were unable to attend the Congress as well as to the rest of the biomedical scientific community and health professions. Raven Press of New York, who published the proceedings of the Seattle Symposium on Pain in record time and in a very high-quality volume, was selected among several companies to publish these proceedings. Selections of papers will be made by the Editorial Board, especially appointed for this task.

Co-Sponsors

Finally, I wish to express thanks and appreciation to the Co-Sponsors of the Congress, each of whom is listed in the Program. In addition to funds for running the Association, I solicited funds from various companies to help defray the expenses of the Congress. Dr. Dieter Gross and Professors Frey and Gerbershagen joined in this solicitation. The responses were somewhat disappointing because many companies did not contribute, allegedly owing to the current economic conditions. Of the eight companies listed in the program, Astra (Sweden and U.S.), Pfizer, Burroughs Wellcome Co., and Sterling Drug deserve special thanks for the sizable amounts they contributed to the Congress.

Through the efforts of Professor Procacci and certain members of the Local Arrangement Committee, the Congress has received funds from the City of Florence and the Italian Agency for Tourism, and from the Italian National Research Council. In view of the very serious economic conditions, these are very meaningful and very much appreciated.

In the early part of this year, I submitted applications to NIDR and NIGMS requesting funds to support this World Congress, and one to NCI to support the Symposium on Cancer Pain. I am extremely pleased to report that the three applications were approved. This also has special meaning because it not only provides funds to help defray the cost of the Congress as well as publication of the proceedings, but is an impressive indication of the interest of these three Institutes to nurture pain research. In these times of budgetary restrictions, it is especially significant that these Institutes have provided funds for this Congress.

CONCLUSIONS

In conclusion, I believe it is fair to state that the Association has made an impressive beginning in achieving its goals and objectives. The large membership achieved in only 15 months and the unexpectedly large attendance of this Congress confirms the conviction of many that this type of multidisciplinary society and meeting are very much needed. Through the Scientific Program of this Congress, the IASP has started to fulfill the obligations implied in the several purposes of the Articles of Incorporation. By bringing together such large numbers of people representing virtually every biomedical science and health profession from throughout the world, IASP will surely help to promote and facilitate dissemination of new information and thereby enhance communication and cross-fertilization, stimulate greater research efforts, and promote education, and thus eventually help improve the care of patients suffering from pain.

The publication of the journal *Pain* and the Congress Proceedings will also do much to enhance dissemination of basic science and clinical information of multidisciplinary interest and thus further improve communication.

IASP has already stimulated the formation of a number of national and regional groups with similar purposes. This should do much to further another objective of the Association.

It is hoped that our workshops prove successful in coming to grips with the difficult tasks of the sixth and seventh purposes—the adoption of a uniform classification, nomenclature, and definition of pain and pain syndromes, and the development of national and international data banks, uniform records, and effective systems for retrieval of such information. These are critically needed and should be among our first tasks.

It is also hoped that the activities of the Committee on Public Relations will help IASP achieve the ninth objective.

All of these initial achievements should encourage and spur all of us to vigorously pursue our goals and objectives. These are but the first steps in what I believe will be a long journey. IASP has now made the important commitment and assumed the obligation to help the rest of the biomedical scientific community, health professions, and societies as a whole to mount the multipronged program of much greater research effort, more effective teaching, and better patient care essential to the solution of the serious problem of pain.

We must provide the leadership in making the many changes necessary to achieve these goals. In research, we must encourage the exploitation of the vast amount of scientific knowledge and technology in all the scientific disciplines and bring them to bear on the problem of pain in a collective and collaborative fashion. In addition to continuing experimental laboratory studies, we must encourage investigations of pathologic pain states in patients. These objectives require a multidisciplinary approach to pain research, teaching, and patient care—a need I suggested a quarter of a century ago, which was reemphasized by Professor Wall at the Seattle Symposium two years ago.

These then, are the goals and objectives of, and the challenges to, the International Association for the Study of Pain and constitute its *raison d'être*.

John J. Bonica

Address from the Rector (President) of the University of Florence

I am happy to bring the greetings of the University of Florence to the First World Congress on Pain organized by the International Association for the Study of Pain. The greetings I bring to each of the nearly 800 scholars gathered here from all over the world, representing virtually every branch of the biomedical sciences, is on behalf of all the Faculty of the University and the people of Florence.

I do not belong to any of the fields represented here—I am a Professor of Statistics on the Faculty of Economics—and therefore I look with newly aroused interest at the Scientific Program of this Congress. I appreciate and admire the humanistic and scientific objectives of this Congress—to stimulate the study of the mechanism of pain and to reappraise all the therapies and suggest new modalities of treatment. It is a most impressively full and comprehensive program dealing with virtually all aspects of pain research and therapy.

It is especially gratifying to note that the program includes participation by many respected Florentine scholars worthy of the old tradition of our Medical School who represent research groups headed by Drs. Teodori, Arcangeli, Pepeu, Galletti, Sicuteri, and Procacci whom I would like to compliment and congratulate for the excellent job they have done in making the local arrangements for the Congress.

Leonardo da Vinci, the great example of the Renaissance Man, symbolized pain and pleasure and pain and joy in a drawing as two human figures rising from one body, undoubtedly inspired by the Neoplatonic conceptions popular in Florence at that time. Florence has been called "The Pain Capital of Italy." I ask myself if the definition is right for the city, especially because of the scientific contributions of the faculty of medicine whom I have just mentioned. The definition does not satisfy or even please me as a Florentine, even if correct from a technical and scientific point of view. I honestly believe that it is not applicable to this extraordinary city, which in its history, monuments, art treasures, and culture and its period of continued creative zeal, is trying always to overcome its torments.

This city, which even in the gray moments of its history has averted a vocation to universality, is happy to welcome scientists from all over the world. Our University has always enjoyed the honorific experiences it has acquired in the numerous international congresses that have met here. The University aspires to maintain its role worthy of its tradition.

In this spirit, I express the best wishes for the great success of your Scientific and Related Programs. I am confident that this World Congress on Pain will prove a very important step in the progress of all the disciplines that meet here to nurture the further study of the social, humanistic, and scientific aspects of pain.

Professor Giuseppe Parenti
President, University of Florence,
Official Representation of the Minister of Education of Rome

Welcoming Remarks

On behalf of the Local Arrangements Committee, I have the pleasure to welcome the participants to this Congress whom I see in a great number in this auditorium.

As you know, it was decided two years ago in Seattle that the First World Congress of the International Association for the Study of Pain (IASP) would be held in Florence. At that time, we were in the throes of founding our Association, and consequently we could not predict the number of members in IASP and how many would attend the Congress. When we began to formulate final plans for this Congress, IASP already had a membership of 850, and it was predicted that it would have a membership of 1,200 by the time of this Congress. Professional organizers of medical congresses informed us that usually about 25 to 30% of the total membership of the society attends their most important meeting. On this basis, we predicted that 350 would attend the Congress. I have just been informed that as of this morning the registration exceeded 700, and it is likely that this number will increase before the Congress terminates.[1]

This is an impressive number, far beyond our expectations, and provides further evidence of the validity and importance of the original idea to found IASP.

A well-known German proverb says: *Alles Angang ist schwer* (every beginning is difficult). Some difficulties, in fact, were met in the organization of this Congress, but most, if not all, were solved. For this, I wish to thank all the members of the various committees and particularly Dr. Bonamici and her staff of the Organizzazione Internazionale Congressi for the high professionalism, special interest, and enthusiasm they have shown in their work.

Particular attention has been devoted to the Social Program in order to offer time for relaxation and an opportunity for all participants to interact socially after hours of hard scientific work. The ladies will have an opportunity to see both the great art of the Renaissance and the latest creations of Italian fashion.

Some remarks about this building are in order here. In 1821, the French poet Alphonse Lamartine transformed some fields into the present park. It was here that the poet completed his work *Harmonies poetiques et religieuses.* At a later date, the entire property passed into the hands of the Strozzi family who built a villa in neoclassical style.

---

[1] The final total registration was 759, which included scientists and health professionals and about 250 guests of registrants.

About 10 years ago, the local Azienda di Turismo purchased the villa and the park. A major work was undertaken. A massive excavation produced an artificial depression, and in this shell, surrounded by grass and plants, nestles this Auditorium. On the second floor, a large hall, the Sala Verde, was remodeled, but in all the other rooms the original structures (roofs and ceilings) were preserved. In some rooms marvelous pieces of furniture still remain as in former times. We have in this building one of the best examples of how modern structures can harmonize with old works of art.

Some words on the graphic symbol of this Congress, the Laocoon: This marble group, now in the Vatican Museum, represents the Trojan priest Laocoon with his sons entangled in the coils of two serpents. It is one of the most famous classic sculptures, a Greek original of the first century B.C., signed Agesandros, Polidoros, and Athenodoros of Rhodes. The statue was discovered in Rome in 1506. It was one of the most admired statues during the Renaissance. Here in Florence, in the Uffizi Gallery, we have a famous copy, or better, a reinterpretation, by Baccio Bandinelli.

It is interesting to notice that famous artists and philosophers of the Renaissance, as Vasari and Adriani, considered this statue to be the most perfect expression of physical pain. The statue of Niobe, another famous Greek masterpiece, now in the Uffizi, was considered the best expression of psychic pain.

I conclude with an image of happiness, the "Primavera" by Botticelli, which we adopted as a cover of the Social Program, with the wish that this Congress on Pain can bring Pleasure to the participants.

Paolo Procacci
Chairman, Local Arrangements Committee

Advances in Pain Research and Therapy, Vol. 1,
edited by J. J. Bonica and D. Albe-Fessard.
Raven Press, New York © 1976.

Modulation of Pain by Nonpainful Events

Patrick D. Wall

Department of Anatomy, Cerebral Functions Research Group, University College, London WC1E 6BT, England

The classic view of pain mechanisms was one of great simplicity, and we should work to retain as much as possible of this simplicity. Injury is followed by pain, and pain implies injury. Classically, any deviation from this strong inevitable link between tissue damage and pain was assigned to the vagaries of the mind. These mental processes could exaggerate or ignore the report delivered to the brain. The only exception allowed by classic theory was the possibility of generating false signals so that disease of peripheral nerve or transmission pathways might produce pain in the absence of tissue damage. This approach to pain proposed a two-stage system, the first specialized mechanistic part resulted in sensation, a pure report on the nature of the event. This report triggered perception with its concomitants of emotion, learning, and memory.

Tasks were assigned to specialists. The neurologist and basic scientists must locate and examine the sensory mechanism leaving perception to psychiatrists, psychologists, and philosophers. The result of the work of those who looked for a specialized sensory mechanism was the proposal that there is a direct projection mechanism. It begins in the periphery where injury detectors are connected to small myelinated and unmyelinated afferents that terminate on cells in spinal cord, which decussate and project in ventrolateral white matter toward the brain. The end station of this reporting system was generally assumed to be in the thalamus.

Until recently, this entire superstructure was based on only two facts: (a) the reporting of injury to the CNS requires the presence of small-diameter peripheral nerve fibers; and (b) section of ventrolateral white matter in spinal cord produces analgesia. All the rest was speculation, implication, and guesswork. The theory was so simple that it remained the basis of most work in spite of many well-known phenomena.

The most obvious of the facts that challenge the concept of a straight specialized and insulated pathway is the existence of referred pain. Not only is the pain mislocated by the patient, but light pressure to the apparently painful zone increases the pain and local anesthesia decreases the pain. These simple observations immediately tell us that convergence from uninjured tissue modulates the injury message. These phenomena abolish the isolation of the specialized pain mechanism. These facts did not escape the notice of some clinicians and scientists such as Sherrington, Head, Zotterman, Livingston, and Noordenbos. Nevertheless, most clinicians and scientists continued to attempt to defend the classic view partly by proposing special pain mechanisms for each exception and partly by doubting the patients' sanity if they failed to report the expected degree of pain.

GATE CONTROL: A RESTATEMENT

In 1965 Melzack and I examined what was known at the time about pain mechanisms (33). A general restatement of the hypothesis is in order in the light of subsequent developments.

1. *Injury* produces nerve impulses in small-diameter myelinated afferent nerve fibers and in unmyelinated fibers.
2. These impulses excite *central transmission cells.*
3. Central transmission cells also receive *convergence* of excitatory and inhibitory influences, directly and indirectly, from other afferent fibers which are not necessarily high-threshold afferents. The existence of this convergence means that the cells' transmission is controlled not simply by the presence or absence of injury but also by the state of activity of other afferents.
4. Furthermore, *descending controls* from brainstem and cortex also strongly influence the excitability of the transmission cells. Consequently, the message transmitted toward the brain is not a simple message of the existence of nerve impulses in injury-detection fibers but is dependent for its strength on activity in other afferents and on activity in descending systems. The reception of this message in sufficient strength may trigger pain.
5. *Pain,* a state of perception in which the organism as a whole reacts to apparent injury, is triggered if the initial gate and subsequent stages of the transmission pathway are favorably set for the exhibition of this state.

Reaction to the Gate Control Hypothesis

We had issued a clear challenge to the traditional specificity theory and claimed that the facts better fitted the existence of a controlled dependent pathway in which the link between injury and pain included peripheral effects other than injury and included central factors. There was one immediate prediction of the theory. If low-threshold afferents as well as injury signals converged onto the transmission system, it was possible that inhibitory effects would predominate and the strength of the injury signal would be diminished by selective stimulation of large-diameter sensory fibers. Sweet and I immediately tested this on ourselves (with some trepidation) and then on patients (54). The observation of the temporary abolition of pain in men with electrical counterstimulation of low-threshold afferents obviously gave considerable impetus to the gate control theory.

There is no doubt that the publication of these two papers aroused considerable interest as can be judged by looking at the "Citation Index" or at the thumb-marked stain on the edge of volume 150 of *Science* in university libraries. The idea was incorporated in a number of explanations of different phenomena. Some took it and expanded it (9,31). Some took it as a challenge to question and to experiment. As was to be expected, there was a somewhat vehement reaction from those who understandably wished to preserve the purity and simplicity of the classic view. A welcome 19th century virulence appeared in the literature. "The gate control theory of pain: an unlikely hypothesis" was the title of one paper (41). In another we find the sentence, "I think therefore that one ought at this stage to strongly support Schmidt in his attempt to prevent the Gate Hypothesis from taking root in the field of neurology" (25). These responses were modified when this school of careful experimenters reported on their own examination of the facts of transmission from injury-detecting afferents (7,20), although it would be too much to hope that they would refer to their previous publications.

Spirited defenses by the "Old Believers" still appear in textbooks (37), but the facts are available in the literature for those who prefer them to propaganda. It is perhaps a little tedious that one must refer to the original papers or to the phenomena themselves. In a lyrical review, Dykes (16) attacked the gate control theory: "In addition to its dubious veracity, the theory is incomplete." To prove his point, he quoted Denny-Brown et al. (12) twice as arguing that "the input of both large and small fibers to the dorsal horn regulate relay through the region without requiring a gate mechanism." A glance at the three papers in the series (11,12,28) shows that the authors in fact are quite specific in using the exact gating mechanism Melzack and I adopted. One may hope that this period of vituperation will pass into a more mundane but constructive time.

We formulated a hypothesis that seemed to us to bring together all the facts available in 1965. Since that time much has changed. Some of the "facts" were wrong. Much more is now known. Therefore I would like to review the data, modify the details of the original statement, and justify the general statement.

INJURY

The facts available in 1965 about injury-detecting peripheral nerve fibers were wrong and positively misleading. In extensive searches, few examples had been detected of fibers that reacted specifically to injury. This seemed a definite conclusion because evidence had been presented that an adequate sample had been examined of all diameters of myelinated fibers (24). For the unmyelinated fibers, it was claimed that light pressure stimuli produced activity in the full range of C fibers (15). In both myelinated and unmyelinated fibers, important groups of fibers had been missed. They were revealed by the more careful dissection and recording techniques particularly developed to examine small fibers. The work was primarily that of the schools of Perl and Burgess (4) and Iggo (26). They discovered two groups of fibers, one in the A-delta group and one in the C group, which responded only to tissue-damaging high-intensity pressure. Does this mean that the problem of how we sense the presence of injury is now settled? Far from it.

A glance at the actual data shows that every one of the other eight categories of fibers also responds to the crushing of tissue. We must carefully reconsider the way in which the word *specificity* has been used for peripheral nerve fibers. One way of using the word is in a backward-looking sense. If nerve impulses are observed in a particular fiber, it might be claimed that a specific statement can be made about the nature of the events at its terminals. Even for the so-called specific nociceptive fibers in the A-delta and C group, this can no longer be claimed to be the case. Elsewhere in this book, Perl shows that once these fibers have been damaged or heated and are tested after the evoked discharge has died down, they have become sensitized so that light pressure or mild warming evokes firing. Moreover, Besson shows that repeated stimulation of the fibers with bradykinin sensitizes them to subsequent responses. If we try to make similar statements about the specific cause of nerve impulses in fibers that respond to light touch or to warming or cooling, we are in a worse quandary because crushing of the tissue also produces impulses in these fibers.

The second use of the word *specificity* is a forward-looking one in which it is proposed that impulses in a specific type of fiber inevitably lead to a specific sensory response. How can this be? When tissue is injured, every one of the 10 identified types of cutaneous afferent fibers delivers impulses to the spinal cord. The specificity chain requires one to believe that the sensory consequences of this barrage depend only on the small fraction of active fibers originating from nociceptors, while the great bulk of the barrage is in some way ignored.

We can now be satisfied that it is technically possible to examine the reactions of the full spectrum of nerve fibers in animals, and using the Vallbo and Hagbarth (46) technique, we can also examine single units in human nerves. In animals a nearly complete knowledge seems now available of reactions to pressure and temperature in cutaneous nerves. Far more needs to be known about reactions to tissue breakdown products, some of which, such as bradykinin, appear to be capable of powerful excitation, whereas others, such as the prostaglandins, only modulate the excitability of endings.

Ease of experimental approach has understandably led to an almost exclusive concentration on cutaneous afferents, and it is urgent that we now use these techniques for understanding the origin of impulses from deep structures particularly from joints and viscera. Thus the work of the past 10 years on afferents has led to the discovery of high-threshold afferents whose sensitivity is modulated by previous stimuli and by their chemical environment. Against the apparent simplification introduced by the long-sought discovery of high-threshold afferents, we must match the complication that low-threshold afferents also contribute to the overall barrage in the presence of injury.

Neuropathies

Any adequate theory of pain mechanisms clearly must include an explanation of the painful neuropathies. The gate control theory introduced two ways in which pain might appear in peripheral nerve damage, other than the generation of impulses in high-threshold afferents. One was the disappearance of the normal inhibition, and the other was the variation of the ongoing tonic barrage in afferent fibers. Postherpetic neuralgia was proposed as an example of pain and hyperesthesia because of a preferential loss of large-diameter afferents and the consequent loss of the central inhibitory effect of these fibers (39).

This explanation was encouraged by the discovery that electrical stimulation of the affected nerve would remove the hyperesthesia (38). It was further suggested that those cases with ongoing deep pain uninfluenced by peripheral stimulation were suffering the consequence of central deafferentation where transmission cells, stripped of their afferents, increased their ongoing discharge. During the past 10 years, detailed anatomical studies have been completed with electron microscopy to establish the complete fiber spectrum in a wide variety of neuropathies. The work has been done mainly in London and at the Mayo Clinic and is reviewed by Thomas (45). Only one positive statement emerges: pain is not felt if small fibers are missing. However, no generalization can be made about the histological picture associated with pain. A preferential loss of large-diameter fibers is not necessarily associated with pain. In trigeminal neuralgia where it is known that a specific type of low-threshold afferent evokes pain, there is no agreement that any morphological change at all occurs in the peripheral fibers.

The conclusion from these studies is that one cannot make functional predictions from morphological observations, for two obvious reasons. First, small fibers may be regenerated large fibers and may be functioning perfectly normally as large fibers. Second, fibers may appear completely intact morphologically but their physiology may be disturbed at the receptors, in their transmission properties, or at their central endings. We now have the possibility of resolving this problem because the Vallbo and

Hagbarth (46) technique allows a sampling of fibers to examine their actual functioning state. With this information, it should be possible to determine the nature and location of the disorders.

Neuromas

Neuromas are a special example of injury or neuropathy sometimes associated with pain. We set up an experimental model by cutting rat sciatic nerves, allowing the cut ends to regenerate into a sealed polythene tube and then studied the physiology and pharmacology of the fine sprouts (52,53). This preparation produced a reaction in the animals' behavior since they attacked their own anesthetic feet. Subsequent work showed that the large-diameter afferents completely failed to penetrate the neuroma, which is a pure culture of sprouts originating in small-diameter myelinated and in unmyelinated fibers (13). It is therefore not surprising that this structure was a potential source of pain, particularly when it was found that these normally silent fibers generated an ongoing barrage in the absence of stimulation.

The generators of these impulses showed abnormal characteristics. The most surprising of these was that if the nerve central to the lesion was electrically stimulated at high frequency so that antidromic impulses penetrated the neuroma, the discharge of the terminals was silenced and remained silent for long periods of time after the stimulation. This immediately suggested a new explanation for some of the effectiveness of electrical counterstimulation. Dykes (16), in his enthusiasm to demolish us, had missed the fact that we too knew that our theory was incomplete in not explaining the occasional slow onset and prolonged relief produced by electrical counterstimulation. Abrahams (1) and Melzack and Melinkoff (32) had discussed this issue and had introduced new central mechanisms. For the neuroma, Gutnick and I showed that some of the modulation produced by stimulation of peripheral nerves might have nothing to do with a central gate mechanism but was in fact the turn off of abnormal peripheral nerve impulse generators. We stressed that central factors must also be present. A further abnormality of the nerve fibers in the neuroma was that they were excited by norepinephrine. This new finding immediately suggested an explanation for the role of the sympathetics in certain types of pain.

Sympathetic Discharge and Pain

Clinical observation and therapy show quite clearly that the sympathetic system plays a crucial role in some painful syndromes. There are four theories discussed below.

Afferents in the Sympathetic System

Afferents course along with sympathetic nerves and pass through the sympathetic ganglia on their way to the spinal cord. Removal of sympathetic ganglia either by injection or by surgery interrupts both the efferents and the afferents. However, there are two reasons to reject the suggestion that the afferents cause pain. Walker and Nulsen (47) stimulated the efferents after removing the ganglia. In pain patients, this stimulation reproduced the pain they had suffered. In non-pain patients, the stimulation failed to induce any sensory changes. Evidently, the sympathetic efferents produce pain, and they do this only in patients who already have some peripheral disorder. This conclusion is confirmed by Hannington-Kiff (21), who has shown that local application of guanethidine limited to one limb abolishes pain. This drug blocks the transmitter release from the sympathetic terminals.

Ephaptic Jumping of Impulses from Efferents to Afferents

This theory became popular after Granit et al. (18) claimed that ephaptic transmission appeared after injury. However, Wall and co-workers (56) showed that their findings had an alternative explanation and on direct examination could find no ephapses. In neuromas, no signs of interaction between fibers have been discovered (52,53), but unmyelinated fibers have not yet been studied.

Pain Owing to Inadequate Blood Flow

It is quite obvious that ischemia produces pain in Raynaud's disease or intermittent claudication, for example. In Sudeck's atrophy, the role of ischemia is doubtful. In causalgia, vasodilation increases pain. It is also clear that there can be no vascular explanation for the troublesome post-sympathectomy pain that begins days after full vasodilation and lasts for long periods.

Pain Owing to Stimulation of Afferents by Norepinephrine

This now seems the most likely theory. In the normal intact sensory nerve, sympathetic transmitters do not evoke obvious injury signals, although they may modulate sensitivity. Partially damaged nerve membrane and the sprouts within a neuroma become sensitive to norepinephrine (53).

Summary of Modulation of Discharge from Peripheral Injury Detectors

The firing of normal peripheral nerve fibers when tissue is injured is influenced by the temperature, the vasculature, sympathetic efferents, the chemical environment, and previous stimuli. The firing of damaged or *regenerating* afferent nerve fibers is also influenced by these factors, as well as by the arrival at their endings of high-frequency antidromic impulses and by the presence of sympathetic transmitters.

CENTRAL TRANSMISSION CELLS

With intentional caution, we labeled the cells responsible for transmitting information about injury as T cells without identifying where they were. At that time there were a number of candidates, and in the past 10 years their number has multiplied. How can we choose between the candidates? It seems reasonable to require that the cells respond to some or all of the stimuli known to evoke pain. Such cells exist in laminae I and IV through VII (27,51). A more stringent requirement would be needed by those who wished to maintain the specificity theory where cells would have to respond to nociceptive inputs and to no others.

It has been claimed that one such set of specialized cells exists in lamina I (8). Let us examine the claim. The cells were found in extraordinarily small numbers, 110 in 52 animals, whereas most cells in this lamina respond to low-threshold stimuli (50). They do not respond to bradykinin and they do not discharge tonically. At least some of these cells are normally held inhibited by the ongoing afferent barrage arriving over neighboring roots since, if these roots are cut, the cells begin to respond to nonnoxious stimuli (3). These facts do not mean that the cells do not play an important role in signaling the presence of injury; the cells simply cannot be the only system.

The most commonly used candidates are the lamina V cells, which clearly respond to all known types of nociceptive afferents, both from skin and from deep structures (18,55). However, it is equally clear that most of these cells also respond to low-threshold afferents. Although not fulfilling the dreams of a specificity theorist, these cells cannot be excluded as possible triggers of pain because of their broad-range responsiveness. On the basis of simple response to injury, there is no reason to accept or reject any of the candidates.

A second selection procedure is to ask if the cells project to the brain by way of the contralateral ventrolateral white matter. Cutting this pathway leads to analgesia in man. However, this statement needs two reservations. The operation does not completely abolish pain; it raises the threshold. Postischemic pain, for example, can still be evoked. Furthermore, in a high percentage of patients who have survived the operation for more than a few months, the pain returns (58). Obviously, other pathways are capable of triggering pain. These are not necessarily direct long tracts. Basbaum (2) has recently confirmed Schiff's observation that a complete hemisection of the cord on one side with a complete hemisection of the other side two segments rostrally still allows the animal to react to noxious stimuli. Consequently, we cannot exclude a cell type if it does not have long running axons and if its axon does not run in ventrolateral white matter.

The cells of origin of the spinothalamic tract have been identified in rats and cats (14) and in monkey (59). Even these are not necessarily the important cells for injury reporting in the intact cord since many project into the ventral posterior lateral nucleus of the thalamus, and surgical destruction of this nucleus has been uniformly disappointing in pain control (27). There is positive evidence that other thalamic and brainstem structures play a much more crucial role in pain behavior (6), and therefore cells projecting directly or indirectly to these structures are at least as good candidates as those involved in the direct spinothalamic pathway.

We have no way of excluding any cord cell that responds to peripheral injury from playing some role in triggering pain. Several types of cells may combine to evoke the different types of pain. The answer or answers will come not from searching for the fulfillment of an ancient myth but from the patient matching of central cell responses to many types of known pain and non-pain situations. This is being done. Cells whose injury discharge is turned off by known analgesics, anesthetics, and narcotics and by stimulation of central structures which produce analgesia obviously become more interesting. It will be necessary to describe the firing of cells in the full range of circumstances under which pain actually does or does not occur before we can crack the code of what is the message which triggers the brain to evoke the behavior of pain. The ultimate test will be to induce this pattern of activity in cells to see if the correct message has in fact been discovered.

CONVERGENCE

It is a *sine qua non* that information about injury must be transmitted. It is equally obvious to anyone, except a psychophysicist, that somewhere in the brain this information must be brought together with other information and that the organism will react in consequence of the combination. The major issues are where and how the combination of different inputs occurs.

With some satisfaction, I can quote here work that comes entirely from a school previously opposed to the gate control theory rather than from my own work. This group of workers divides dorsal horn neurons into three classes: 1, those excited by sensitive cutaneous mechanoreceptors; 2, those excited by both sensitive mechanoreceptors and nociceptors; and 3, those excited only by nociceptors (4). (I have already given reasons above for doubting the purity of these classes, particularly 3, but for the moment we can accept their version which applies in their limited experimental conditions.) Handwerker et al. (20) showed that the responses of the class 2 cells were suppressed by stimulation of the largest cutaneous afferent fibers originating in the sensitive mechanoreceptors. So far this sounds remarkably reminiscent of our paper published 10 years ago. The main issue is the class 3 cells which had been heralded as the truly specific cells signaling only nociceptive information. The first investigator to describe them (8) did not mention inhibitory convergences. Willis et al. (59) were unable to inhibit the response of class 3 cells to noxious stimuli. Welcome as this report may have been to specifists, its relevance was limited by the fact that their animals were under chloralose, an excellent compound for the abolition of inhibition. Now two groups (7,26) have investigated the cells under the conditions of our original reports, and they find that class 3 (nociceptor) cells are inhibited by large myelinated afferent fibers. Finally, it appears that we are all in agreement that the firing of spinal cord cells depends on the balance of excitatory inputs counteracted by inhibitory inputs.

What is the Biological Meaning of the Inhibitory Convergence on Cells That Transmit Information About Injury?

No teleological meaning was apparent in our original paper. We had simply observed that stimulation of large-diameter fibers produced excitation plus a predominant inhibition. It is safe to predict that no biological system is driven by excitation alone and is unmatched by the checks and balances of counteracting forces. There is no reason why the injury-reporting system should be different from other biological control systems. But this is a general principle. What is the specific meaning of this particular interaction? It was a stroke of good fortune for us that large-diameter fibers happened to have a predominant effect. This was particularly fortunate because the large fibers were the easiest to stimulate by natural or electrical means. We wrote of the conflicting effect of large versus small fibers because that was the way our experiments were designed and that is the way the results came out. However, we were well aware that these two groups were each composed of many functionally different types of fibers. Electrical stimulation produces an artificial jumble of messages which the nervous system was not evolved to handle. We knew that it was highly likely that within these crude anatomical groups of large- versus small-diameter fibers, there were functional subdivisions, some fractions of which might have quite the opposite effect from the majority. We therefore turned away from the crudity of electrical stimulation of whole nerves to study single cells with natural stimuli (22,49). The answer was soon quite clear. To understand the biological meaning of this convergence, we had to consider not only the specialized nature of the different fibers but also their spatial origin.

When we examined lamina V cells with natural stimuli (22), we found that the cells had two modes of operation, one for low-intensity stimuli and the other for high. As everyone now agrees, a wide range of different types of fibers converges directly and indirectly onto these cells. The cells respond to low-level pressure stimuli, hair movement, and light touch. For low-intensity stimuli, the cell has a relatively small excitatory receptive field with an extensive inhibitory surround. With these stimuli the cell signals its information at a relatively low frequency. An increase of firing means touch in the central part of its receptive field. A decrease of ongoing firing means touch in its inhibitory surround. This type of organization is familiar in retinal ganglion cells with on centers and off surrounds.

This feature is common to all sensitive sensory systems and provides an improvement of discrimination of the spatial distribution of stimuli. The presence of an associated inhibitory mechanism is also seen in the excitatory center of the receptive field since the initial excitation is followed by a profound inhibition which terminates the initial burst of impulses. This postexcitatory inhibition improves the temporal discrimination ability of the cell just as the inhibitory surround improves the spatial discrimination. However, if the strength of the stimulus is raised to bring in the smaller diameter afferent fibers, a new mode of operational organization appears and the rate of firing of the cell increases. The area of the excitatory receptive field is larger for the intense stimuli than for small ones. As a stimulus is gradually increased in the outer zone, it first activates the inhibitory surround and then activates the excitation produced by the higher threshold fibers.

A final difference between the low- and high-threshold effects is that excitation of the latter is followed by a long period of increased excitability of the cell. This produces the "wind up" phenomenon first described by Mendell (34), in which stimuli repeated at 1-sec intervals produce a gradually increasing response of the cell. We can now see that the conflict of large and small fibers makes some sense. The large fibers produce excitation followed by inhibition in the center of the receptive field and inhibition in the periphery. This receptive field overlays a second receptive field where high-threshold fibers produce excitation followed by facilitation. Obviously, in normal circumstances it is not possible to fire the high-threshold mechanism without also activating the low-threshold one; therefore the end result is a balance between the various excitations, facilitations, and inhibitions.

What Is the Mechanism of the Convergences?

I now regret that in the original gate control paper the diagram showed only a presynaptic mechanism of control. In the text we clearly stated that postsynaptic mechanisms could also do the job. This led some to state incorrectly that presynaptic control was an essential feature of the gate and to attack the whole concept accordingly. In 1965 nothing was known of postsynaptic inhibition in dorsal horn interneurons, but evidence for exactly the required postsynaptic inhibition rapidly appeared (23). We had shown that large fibers produced a depolarizing shift of the membrane potential of primary afferent fibers, whereas the particular small fibers we stimulated produced the opposite effect (36). The result was denied by others but we were able to confirm it with newer techniques (10). However, it became quite clear that we had overgeneralized and that not all high-threshold fibers produced a hyperpolarizing change (42). Finally, it was shown that the hyperpolarizing change was produced by a special category of small afferents (35).

The whole discussion of presynaptic versus postsynaptic change may be specious because there remains no absolute evidence in the mammalian CNS that presynaptic changes are not always associated with postsynaptic ones (57). For the overall functioning of the systems, the important question is whether or not there are convergent inhibitions and facilitations. These are known to occur. The exact details of their mechanisms are secondary questions, and they continue to elude us. Similarly, the role of the substantia gelatinosa in modulating the transmission of injury signals by either pre- or postsynaptic mechanisms remains an open question. We knew that the Lissauer tract was involved in the spread of primary afferent depolarization from one segment to the other (48). Since that time it has been shown that this tract, a propriospinal system for substantia gelatinosa, controls the width and sensitivity of the dermatome (12). These facts point to the substantia as playing some role in modulation of transmission, but the details must await the development of techniques that allow us to examine single-unit activity within substantia.

Electrical Counterstimulation

The first test of predictions of the gate control hypothesis was the introduction of electrical stimulation (58), in which large-diameter nerve fibers supplying a painful region were stimulated. By now there are reports on many thousands of patients with intractable pain with a considerable percentage reporting prolonged adequate relief (30). Long-term follow-up studies show that the relief persists (38,43). Only one careful study of the sensory status of patients using counterstimulation has been published (29), and the results are particularly interesting in understanding the mechanism involved. The clinical pain of the patients was relieved and in particular hyperesthesia disappeared and was replaced by normal sensitivity. However, testing of the pain threshold by their particular method showed no change. This paradox is reminiscent of the effect of narcotics, which are obvious analgesics against clinical pain and yet do not shift the pain threshold as measured by most tests. It was proposed not that we were dealing with a mechanism that would switch off pain, but rather that a modulating mechanism would control the amplification factor at the first and subsequent synapses along the transmission pathway. The most striking success of counterstimulation occurs when there is a disorder of amplification rather than a simple excess of injury-generated signals. What are the proposed mechanisms by which electrical counterstimulation works?

Change of Sensitivity at the Terminals

We have shown that high-frequency antidromic nerve impulse invasion of a neuroma silences the ongoing abnormal firing of the fine sprouts (52,53). This explains some of the examples of relief after peripheral nerve stimulation, but a central gating mechanism would be necessary to explain how painless repetitive stimulation of peripheral nerves can be achieved with sufficient strength to fire the small-diameter afferents. Since the fine fibers that produce the sprouts which make up a neuroma (13) have to be stimulated to produce this effect and since these fibers do not run in the dorsal columns, dorsal column stimulation could not produce this antidromic effect in the periphery.

Electrical Block of Peripheral Nerve

It has been suggested that counterstimulation merely blocks the nerve which is stimulated (5). We have given reasons elsewhere why this is not so (53), the main reason being that the edge of such a block and the period of onset would be extremely painful themselves.

"Line Busy" Jamming

This could not be the explanation since the stimulus would replace the original cause of the pain with at least as severe pain-producing signals.

Suggestion

Placebo and suggestion effects undoubtedly occur in any therapy. However, on repeated application they fail to sustain their therapeutic effect. Psychogenic pain does not respond to electrical counterstimulation (30). Furthermore, suggestion is likely to be equally effective wherever the electrodes are placed, whereas it is constantly found that electrical counterstimulation must involve the dermatome in which the pain is generated.

Distraction

Distraction is likely to be involved in any therapy, particularly one in which the patient is actively involved. However, it might reasonably be argued that distraction would be most effective if the stimulus were far removed from the site of the pain, which is quite the opposite of the experience of those who have used electrical stimulation.

Activation of Brainstem Inhibitory Mechanisms

It was natural for some to suggest that the inhibitory effects were originating in the brainstem and perhaps descending from there into spinal cord. No clear evidence for this complication has been presented, although it is quite clear that inhibitory mechanisms are present in brainstem as well as spinal cord. It may be necessary to invoke these structures to explain slow onset and prolonged relief effects. We have shown that effects in the periphery can be prolonged (53), but there are also central descending slow-onset prolonged effect phenomena (1,32). It has been reported that dorsal column stimulation below the level of a complete cord transection in man will abolish flexor reflex spasms. This effect obviously cannot be because of brain stimulation.

Spinal Cord Inhibitory Mechanisms

This was the original suggestion, and all subsequent studies leave this as the simplest and most likely explanation to which must now be added the peripheral modulation. This statement does not exclude the other suggestions, which may play a role on occasions.

DESCENDING CONTROLS

The richest and most hopeful developments of the past 10 years have occurred in the area of descending controls. Brainstem stimulation was known to modulate the excitability of spinal cord cells (19,44). Even the pyramidal tract changes their excitability (17). In the decerebrate animal a powerful descending tonically active system activates the segmental inhibitory circuits (49). Reversible cold blocking of a segment of spinal cord allows one to study the response of transmitting cells with or without the presence of this descending inhibitory barrage.

Of the many powerful descending systems, the one which has received most attention is that discovered by Reynolds (40), where stimulation of a small area of the central gray produces a marked behavioral analgesia without other apparent disturbances of behavior. This observation has been rapidly extended and exploited particularly by Liebeskind and Besson, and the results are seen in a number of reports elsewhere in this book. Not only do these studies reveal the pathways and mechanisms of the electrically induced analgesia, but they suggest new therapies and furthermore they become involved in the probable explanation of why narcotics possess analgesic properties.

PAIN

Pain is not injury. It is a perceptual behavioral state of the whole animal. It may be triggered by the arrival of signals announcing the presence of injury. The gate control theory proposed a mechanism by which these injury signals were transmitted and were submitted to modulation by the concomitant effects of other afferent impulses and of the set of descending control systems. The facts of clinical medicine, anatomy, and physiology support this view.

REFERENCES

1. Abrahams, V. C. (1974): In: *Advances in Neurology, Vol. 4: International Symposium on Pain,* edited by J. J. Bonica, pp. 243–252. Raven Press, New York.
2. Basbaum, A. I. (1973): *Exp. Neurol.,* 40:699–716.
3. Basbaum, A. I., and Wall. P. D. (1976): *Brain Res.* (*in press*).
4. Burgess, P. R. (1974): In: *Advances in Neurology, Vol. 4: International Symposium on Pain,* edited by J. J. Bonica, pp. 11–18. Raven Press, New York.
5. Campbell, J. N., and Taub, A. (1973): *Arch. Neurol.,* 28:347–350.
6. Casey, K. L., Keene, J. J., and Morrow, T. (1974): In: *Advances in Neurology: Vol. 4, International Symposium on Pain,* edited by J. J. Bonica, pp. 197–206. Raven Press, New York.
7. Cervero, F., Iggo, A., and Ogawa, H. (1976): *Pain* (*in press*).
8. Christensen, B. N., and Perl, E. R. (1970): *J. Neurophysiol.,* 33:293–307.
9. Crue, B. L., Jr. (1975): *Pain—Research and Treatment.* Academic Press, New York.
10. Dawson, G. D., Merrill, E. G., and Wall, P. D. (1970): *Science,* 167:1385–1387.
11. Denny-Brown, D., and Yanagisawa, N. (1973): *Brain,* 96:783–814.
12. Denny-Brown, D., Kirk, E. J., and Yanagisawa, N. (1973): *J. Comp. Neurol.,* 151:175–200.
13. Devor, M., and Wall, P. D. (1976): *Nature* (*in press*).
14. Dilly, P. N., Wall, P. D., and Webster, K. E. (1968): *Exp. Neurol.,* 21:550–562.
15. Douglas, W. W., and Ritchie, J. M. (1957): *J. Physiol.* (*Lond.*), 139:385–399.
16. Dykes, R. W. (1975): *Brain Res.,* 99:229–245.
17. Fetz, E. E. (1968): *J. Neurophysiol.,* 31:68–80.
18. Granit, R., Leksell, L., and Skoglund, R. (1944): *Brain,* 67:124–140.
19. Hagbarth, K. E., and Kerr, D. I. B. (1954): *J. Neurophysiol.,* 17:295–307.
20. Handwerker, O., Iggo, A., and Zimmermann, M. (1975): *Pain,* 1:147–166.
21. Hannington-Kiff, J. G. (1975): *Pain Relief.* Heinemann, London.
22. Hillman, P., and Wall, P. D. (1969): *Exp. Brain Res.,* 9:284–306.
23. Hongo, T., Jankowska, E., and Lundberg, A. (1966): *Exp. Brain Res.,* 1:338–358.
24. Hunt, C. C., and McIntyre, A. K. (1960): *J. Physiol.* (*Lond.*), 153:99–112.
25. Iggo, A. (1972): In: *Pain,* edited by J. P. Payne and R. A. P. Bart. Churchill Livingstone, London.
26. Iggo, A. (1974): In: *Advances in Neurology, Vol. 4: International Symposium on Pain,* edited by J. J. Bonica, pp. 1–10. Raven Press, New York.
27. Kerr, F. W. L. (1975): *Pain,* 1:325–356.
28. Kirk, E. J., and Denny-Brown, D. (1970): *J. Comp. Neurol.,* 139:307–320.
29. Lindblom, W., and Meyerson, B. A. (1975): *Pain,* 1:257–270.
30. Long, D. M., and Hagfors, N. R. (1975): *Pain,* 1:109–124.
31. Melzack, R. (1973): *The Puzzle of Pain.* Penguin Books, Harmondsworth.
32. Melzack, R., and Melinkoff, D. F. (1974): *Exp. Neurol.,* 43:369–374.
33. Melzack, R., and Wall, P. D. (1965): *Science,* 150:971–979.
34. Mendell, L. M. (1966): *Exp. Neurol.,* 16:316–332.
35. Mendell, L. M. (1970): *Brain Res.,* 18:375–379.
36. Mendell, L. M., and Wall, P. D. (1964): *J. Physiol.* (*Lond.*), 172:274–294.
37. Mountcastle, V. B. (1974): In: *Medical Physiology,* 13th Ed., C. V. Mosby Co., St. Louis.
38. Nathan, P. W., and Wall, P. D. (1974): *Br. Med. J.,* 3:645–647.
39. Noordenbos, W. (1959): *Pain.* Elsevier, London.
40. Reynolds, D. V. (1969): *Science,* 164:444–445.
41. Schmidt, R. F. (1972): In: *Pain,* edited by J. P. Payne and R. A. P. Burt. Churchill Livingstone, London.

42. Schmidt, R. F. (1973): In: *Handbook of Sensory Physiology. VII. Somatosensory System,* edited by A. Iggo. Springer-Verlag, Heidelberg.
43. Sternbach, R. A., Ignelzi, R. J., Deems, L. M., and Timmermans, G. (1976): *Pain (in press).*
44. Taub, A. (1964): *Exp. Neurol.,* 10:357–374.
45. Thomas, P. K. (1974): *Can. J. Neurol.,* 5:92–97.
46. Vallbo, A. B., and Hagbarth, K. E. (1968): *Exp. Neurol.,* 21:270–278.
47. Walker, A. E., and Nulsen, F. (1948): *Arch. Neurol. Psychiat.,* 59:559–560.
48. Wall, P. D. (1962): *J. Physiol (Lond.),* 164:508–526.
49. Wall, P. D. (1967): *J. Physiol (Lond.),* 188:403–424.
50. Wall, P. D. (1968): In: *The Skin Senses,* edited by D. R. Kenshalo, pp. 512–533. Charles C Thomas, Publisher, Springfield, Illinois.
51. Wall, P. D. (1973): In: *Handbook of Sensory Physiology, Vol. 2,* pp. 253–270. Springer-Verlag, Heidelberg.
52. Wall, P. D., and Gutnick, M. (1974*a*): *Nature,* 248:740–743.
53. Wall, P. D., and Gutnick, M. (1974*b*): *Exp. Neurol.,* 43:580–593.
54. Wall, P. D., and Sweet, W. H. (1967): *Science,* 155:108–109.
55. Wall, P. D., Pomeranz, B., and Weber, W. V. (1968): *J. Physiol. (Lond.),* 199:511–532.
56. Wall, P. D., Waxman, S., and Basbaum, A. I. (1974): *Exp. Neurol.,* 45:576–598.
57. Werman, R. (1972): *Annu. Rev. Physiol.,* 34:337–374.
58. White, J. C., and Sweet, W. H. (1969): *Pain and the Neurosurgeon,* Charles C Thomas, Publisher, Springfield, Illinois.
59. Willis, W. D., Coulter, D. L., and Maunz, R. A. (1974): *J. Neurophysiol.,* 37:358–372.

Advances in Pain Research and Therapy, Vol. 1,
edited by J. J. Bonica and D. Albe-Fessard.
Raven Press, New York © 1976.

Sensitization of Nociceptors and Its Relation to Sensation

E. R. Perl

Department of Physiology, School of Medicine, University of North Carolina, Chapel Hill, North Carolina 27514

Nociceptors make up a large proportion of mammalian somatosensory receptors with fine afferent fibers. Two features distinguish them from other somatic sense organs: (a) a threshold elevated in comparison to other sensory receptors of the same tissue to all stimuli common in the organism's natural history; (b) a progressively augmenting response to progressively noxious, i.e., tissue-damaging, stimuli. As a consequence, such receptors provide signals to the central nervous system unequivocally differentiating noxious from nonnoxious events. Certain types of nociceptive sense organs differ from low-threshold receptors in still another way: their background activity and responsiveness increase rather than decrease after suprathreshold stimulation.

On repeated stimulation, most sense organs manifest fatigue by a period of depressed response after one or more suprathreshold stimuli. The degree and duration of fatigue vary considerably for different somatic receptors; however, both aspects are marked in the low-threshold mechanoreceptors with C (unmyelinated) fibers, which are common in nerves supplying the hairy skin of cat. Complete recovery of responsiveness lost in the fatigue of C mechanoreceptors takes many minutes; resting responsiveness to brief, weak mechanical distortion does not return for over 20 min (1,6). In contrast to the fatigue which dominates the postresponsive behavior of low-threshold receptors, cutaneous polymodal nociceptors (high-threshold receptors with C afferent fibers) typically show a long period of enhanced response and/or a lowering of threshold after activation by noxious heat (2). This is particularly significant in establishing the nature of sensory input from the skin because the C-fiber polymodal nociceptors make up a considerable fraction of unmyelinated afferent units in various mammals, including man (2,16,19). Figure 1 gives an example of the increased responsiveness on sequential stimulation for a primate C-fiber polymodal unit; its spot-like (ca. 1 mm diameter) receptive field was heated by a small electronically programmed thermode in the stepwise fashion illustrated by the bottom trace. The responses in the third and fifth trials (Fig. 1B and C) begin at lower temperatures (earlier in the sequence) and exhibit a higher frequency of discharge for a given temperature than in the first trial (Fig. 1A).

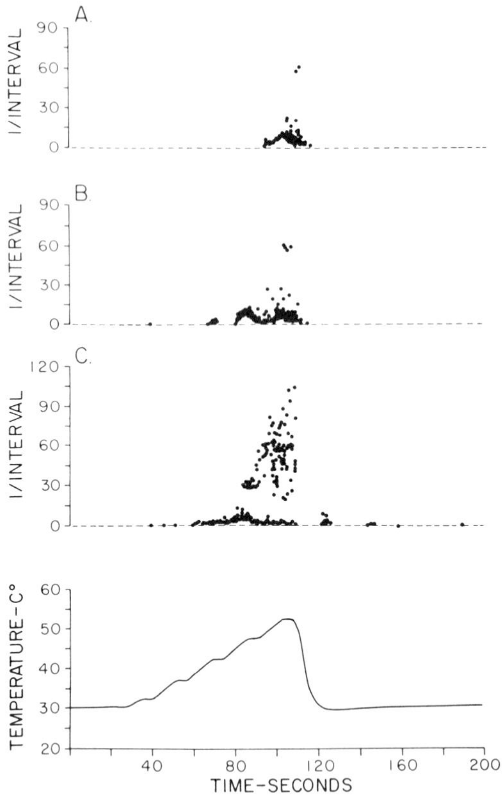

FIG. 1. Sensitization of a C-fiber polymodal nociceptor from monkey hairy skin. The receptive field was repeatedly heated by a small (3 mm^2) thermode undergoing the stepwise sequence shown by the bottom graph from about 32° to 52°C. At the end of the heating cycle, the thermode was rapidly cooled to approximately 30°C as indicated; the heating cycles were automatically repeated every 200 sec. Each discharge recorded from the afferent fiber is plotted against time in **A, B,** and **C** as a dot positioned vertically according to the reciprocal of the interval between it and the preceding impulse ("instantaneous frequency"). Time is shown from an arbitrary point on the heating-cooling cycle; **A, B,** and **C** are aligned according to the same points on the temperature cycle. **A:** First heating cycle; **B:** third heating cycle; **C:** fifth heating cycle. (From T. Kumazawa and E. R. Perl, *unpublished.*)

Polymodal nociceptors, as their name implies, respond also to strong mechanical stimuli and to irritation of the skin by chemical agents. Responsiveness of the polymodal receptors to mechanical and chemical stimuli is also enhanced, particularly in association with skin damage, but since it is less readily demonstrable and testable with such stimuli, their relation to it has not been thoroughly investigated. The increased responsiveness and lowering of polymodal nociceptors' threshold have been labeled *sensitiza-*

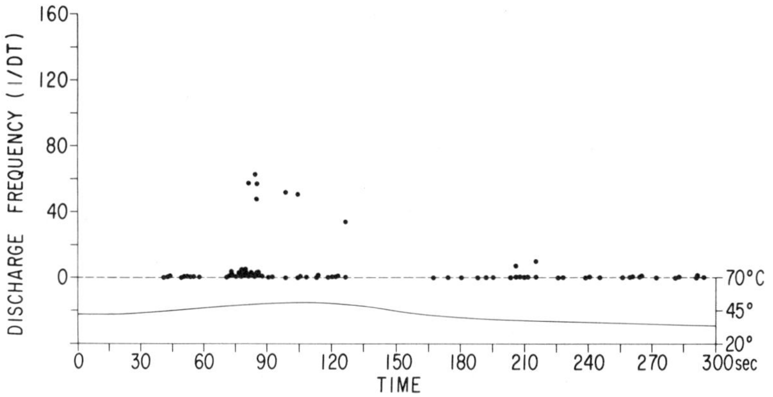

FIG. 2. Development of background discharge by a C-fiber polymodal nociceptor from cat hairy skin. Each discharge recorded from the fiber is plotted as a dot in the manner of Fig. 1. The continuous line below the "instantaneous frequency" zero level (*dashed line*) graphs the temperature of a small (3-mm²) contact thermode centered on the receptive field. The first heating of the receptive field is shown; no background discharge was recorded for 5 min before time shown. The first discharges were recorded at a thermode temperature of 42° to 43°C; the temperature at the peak of the heating was approximately 52°C. (Adapted from ref. 22.)

tion (2), and this phenomenon probably is similar to the situation reported for the injured frog's skin in 1937 by Echlin and Propper (4).

The conditions that lead to sensitization of polymodal units, noxious stimuli of suprathreshold stimuli, also initiate a low-frequency irregular background discharge that may continue for hours. The development of background discharge is illustrated by Fig. 2, which graphs discharge of a feline polymodal nociceptor as a function of time during a cycle of heating to noxious levels and subsequent passive cooling. The beginning of the ongoing discharge in Fig. 2 after the stimulating thermode had cooled to a previously subthreshold level is typical. The combination of increased responsiveness, lowering of threshold, and appearance of background discharge as a consequence of noxious stimulation is a regular feature of the cutaneous C-fiber polymodal nociceptors of cat, rabbit, and monkey; these changes differentiate them from not only the low-threshold mechanoreceptors with myelinated afferent fibers but also from other kinds of cutaneous C-fiber receptors.

Sensitivity is increased and background discharge appears in other types of mammalian cutaneous nociceptors, although these changes have not been extensively studied and documented. We know a great deal less about subcutaneous nociceptors than about those of the skin; however, high-threshold C-fiber receptors of skeletal muscle similarly develop long-lasting background discharge after mechanically or chemically caused tissue damage.

SOME CHARACTERISTICS OF SENSITIZATION

Duration and Magnitude of Sensitization

Study of sensitization requires careful control of stimulus parameters and, for practical reasons, has been confined to thermal stimulation. The time constant for cooling of the thermodes and, equally important, the skin itself, has made it impossible so far to determine the true latency of the sensitization effect. It is manifest within 1 min after threshold activation of a polymodal unit and may have a delay of onset shorter than this. It has a long duration compared to that of other neurophysiologically demonstrated changes in that it lasts for hours. Although temporal changes in the magnitude of the sensitization effect have not been established in detail, large changes in threshold and responsiveness are found 3 to 5 min after a stimulus, and if left quiescent for 20 to 40 min some elements exhibit decreases in the degree of increased responsiveness.

The magnitude of sensitization under similar conditions has varied considerably among individual polymodal nociceptors. Part of this variance may reside in the experimental technique, and part may reflect real differences in the characteristics of individual elements. Provided that heat stimulation does not exceed threshold by more than a few degrees, enhancement of response or a demonstrable lowering of threshold occurs in most elements with the mechanical and thermal characteristics of the C-fiber polymodal nociceptors. For some of the sensory units the effect is relatively small, representing less than a 30% increase in discharge for a given thermal stimulation or an apparent lowering of threshold by only a few degrees. On the other hand, a large number of the rabbit, cat, and monkey polymodal elements exhibit greater changes with threshold dropping by more than 5°C so that the liminal level falls to a temperature that would not be considered noxious (under 42°C). In some instances the response evoked at given temperatures can increase by factors of 10 or more. Moreover, lowering of threshold and increased responsiveness may be cumulative, progressing in repeated trials at least until the skin shows obvious signs of vasodilation and swelling.

Heretofore the emphasis has been on response enhancement; but the responsiveness of the polymodal nociceptors may also decrease. The nociceptors can be blocked, rendered inexcitable, by severe damage of the skin in which the terminals are situated. Thus repeated mechanical penetration of the receptive skin field with sharp objects can lead to deactivation of the receptor and cessation of the response to mechanical stimuli for long periods of time. Heating of the receptive region to temperatures over 55°C may cause loss of responsiveness in some cases and prevent or decrease the enhancement of response observed with more mildly damaging stimuli. Finally, repeated activation of the receptors mechanically or by heat does produce a type of fatigue similar to that observed with most sense organs which may be superimposed on a sensitized level of responsiveness.

Distribution of Peripheral Sensitization

The process leading to sensitization has a degree of localization. Polymodal nociceptors of the hairy skin of cat and monkey typically do not show background discharge before suprathreshold stimulation even though skin areas 1 to 2 cm away have been repeatedly subjected to localized noxious heat or mechanical stimuli. On the other hand, extensive trauma, such as surgical isolation of a skin flap, alters the responsive characteristics of the majority of C-fiber polymodal units of the flap so as to suggest sensitization even though their receptive fields have not been directly stimulated (14). The supposition of generalized sensitization in this instance was based on the presence of background activity in excess of 20 impulses per minute, excitation by heat on a first test at temperatures below those typical for units in more normal skin, larger-than-expected responses in the first suprathreshold heat stimulation, and relatively little enhancement of the response on repeated cycles of noxious heat stimulation. After more circumscribed trauma of the skin, a lesser extension of apparent sensitization has also been noted (1).

Relation of Background Activity to Enhanced Responsiveness

Several observations suggest that the mechanisms leading to background discharge, the evoked responses themselves, and increased responses with successive testing in part may differ. Heating the receptive skin field of polymodal units to temperatures above 60°C often is associated with a lesser response in a subsequent test, yet background activity appears and continues. Furthermore, some irritant chemicals initiate background activity but render the receptive field unresponsive to mechanical stimuli and less responsive to heat than would be expected. Unfortunately, the variation from unit to unit has made more detailed analysis of the interrelation between background and evoked response difficult.

STUDIES ON THE AGENCIES FOR PERIPHERAL SENSITIZATION

The results described above could be explained by one or more of the existing concepts for phenomena associated with pain. One possibility is that noxious stimulation induces changes in the damaged skin leading to the production of substances which in turn act on the receptive terminals of the polymodal nociceptors to change their responsiveness. The concept of a chemical mediator for pain and some of its related phenomena (*vide infra*) has an old currency [see reviews by Keele and Armstrong (7) and by Lim (13)]. Another possible explanation is Lewis' (12) "nocifensor" system, which was suggested to consist of branched, widely distributed axons forming a network in the skin. Lewis argued that "nocifensor" nerves were neither sympathetic nor afferent in origin and suggested that they might release a chemical agent which then acted on the true afferent nerves to change sensitivity. Although the nocifensor concept has not been conclusively disproven, it has lost favor because of the lack of morphological evidence for cutaneous nerve fibers other than those derived from the afferent or autonomic system.

We have attempted to study the mechanism of nociceptor sensitization using as a model the activity of primary afferent units recorded from isolated perfused rabbit's ear. In developing this preparation, Lynn (14) established that the kinds of cutaneous sensory units with C afferent fibers in nerves to the rabbit ear were similar in characteristics and proportion to those previously reported for the cat by Bessou and Perl (2). Polymodal nociceptor types of units are readily identifiable among the C-fiber population of the rabbit auricular nerve in ears perfused with an artificial serum; they sensitize in a fashion similar to that described for cat and primate polymodal units of skin with a normal circulation of blood.

Those of the artificially perfused ear differ from similar elements in rabbits with normal circulation only by the more frequent observation of background discharge at extremely low frequencies (2 to 10 per minute) before stimulation. Neither their responses nor the sensitization was markedly altered by the presence of epinephrine and serotonin in the perfusion fluid (8,16). Acidifying the perfusion fluid (to pH 6) or obtaining additional buffering capacity at normal pH also did not produce detectable changes in the response to the first stimulation, in the enhancement of response on repeated stimulation, or in the appearance of increased background activity after noxious stimulation (15). As could be expected from Fjällbrant and Iggo's (5) results, acetylcholine in moderate concentrations evoked responses, as did bradykinin and a variety of other chemical substances.

Many substances may alter nerve terminal permeability and transmembrane polarization; therefore, experiments in which chemical substances are added to either blood or an artificial solution perfusing the receptive field seemed discouragingly difficult to interpret from the standpoint of biological significance.

Recently we (9) have extended an earlier series of experiments from this laboratory (16) in which pharmacological agents, expected to interfere more or less specifically with the action of naturally occurring substances, have been added to fluid (modified Kreb's solution) perfusing the rabbit ear preparations. Perfusion with a solution not containing a large molecule increased capillary permeability as evidenced by edema of the ear; this arrangement was used to increase the probability of the added chemicals crossing the capillary walls. Unitary discharges of afferent fibers conducting at C velocity were isolated from the nerve bundle and tentatively classified by their response to mechanical stimuli and innocuous cooling. After selection of the afferent unit for study, we then switched the perfusion fluid to one containing one or more of the antagonist chemicals.

Figure 3 summarizes the results from some of these experiments obtained by using a standardized sequence of thermode heating; each graph represents pooled results for a number of fibers studied under similar conditions. The upper plot (1) or each pair in Fig. 3 gives the results from the first heating sequence, whereas the lower (2) represents the observations for the second cycle of heating; the difference between the upper and lower graphs thus is a measure of the degree of sensitization. Figure 3A shows control values. The perfusion fluid contained carboxypeptidase B (a bradykinin deactivator) for the data of Fig. 3B; indomethacin (an inhibitor of prostaglandin production) plus carboxypeptidase B for the observations of Fig. 3C; and mepyramine maleate (an antihistamine), methysergide (a serotonin antagonist), carboxypeptidase B, and indomethacin for the results shown in Fig. 3D. The graphs illustrate a trend toward progressive decrease in the response to the second stimulus sequence paralleling the number of added "blocking" substances. In spite of the considerable variance in the responsiveness of individual polymodal fibers, the trend toward lesser sensitization with the progressive addition of agents expected to destroy or antagonize the action of particular substances is suggestive of a progressive interference with the mechanisms underlying the enhanced responsiveness.

One interpretation of these observations is that the sensitization of polymodal fibers is related to the production of several substances known to appear in tissue fluids after tissue damage of the type which leads to inflammation. Even if this interpretation were correct, many questions remain unanswered such as possible synergism between compounds and the importance of a sequence of steps as has been postulated for inflammation (21). There are, of course, other explanations for our observations, including one which would argue that the action of the potent substances employed was not specific in antagonizing the action of a particular target substance. However, one other observation in our recent experiments is indicative of a link between sensitization and inflammatory processes. In several preparations of ears from rabbits pretreated with a synthetic adrenocortical steroid (dexamethasone), C-fiber polymodal elements appeared to have depressed static responses to heat at levels above those usually provoking vigorous discharge in untreated animals, and showed less background. We feel that the experimental evidence, taken together, suggests that a common mechanism for inflammation and the sensitization of the C-fiber polymodal nociceptors is deserving of further exploration.

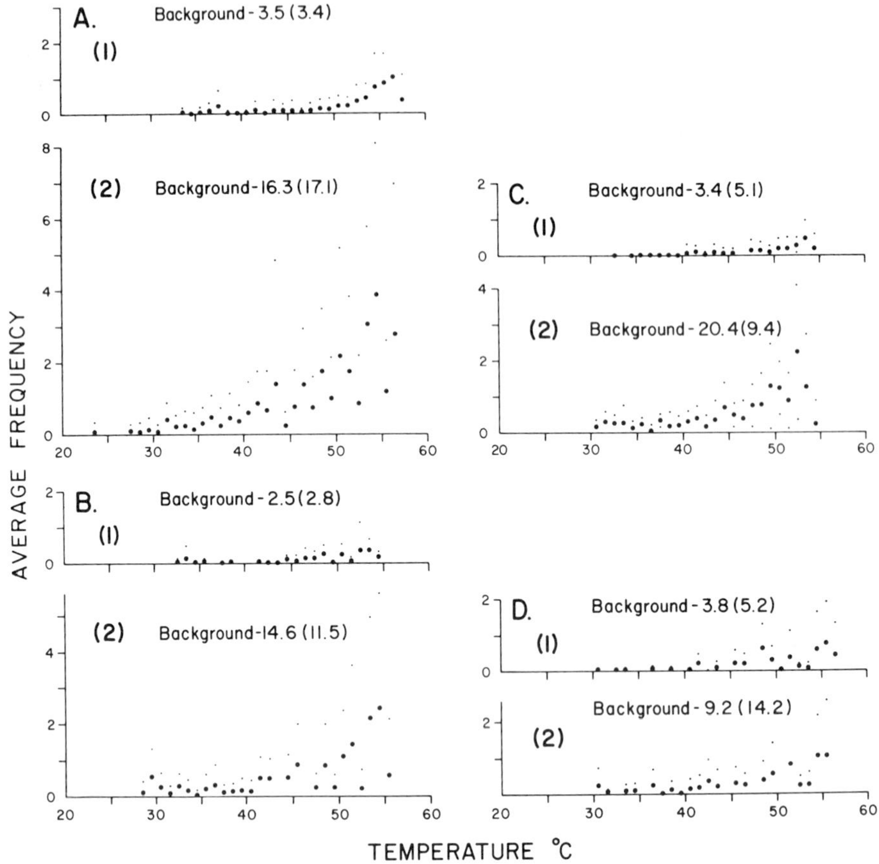

FIG. 3. Effect of chemical antagonists on the response of C-fiber polymodal nociceptors from the perfused rabbit ear. Each pair of graphs (1,2) was obtained from the same sensory units studied under similar conditions. Graph (1) is results from the first heating cycle, and graph (2) from the second. The larger dots plot the average discharge frequency recorded from a number of receptors as a function of temperature (abscissa) during a standardized heat stimulation cycle (3°C steps, 10 sec at each temperature, 5 min between cycles) using a 3 mm^2 contact thermode. The small dots above (and below if greater than zero) indicate the SE of the indicated mean average frequency (in sec); this value was obtained by averaging figures from each element obtained during 1-sec periods at the indicated temperatures. Figures indicated as background represent the average discharge frequency in min measured 5 min after the heat cycle. Perfusion fluid was a modified Kreb's solution containing the indicated additions. Perfusions with added chemicals were begun 20 min before cycle (1). **A:** Control group, 10 receptors. **B:** Carboxypeptidase B (2,000 U/l, 8 receptors). **C:** Carboxypeptidase B (2,000 U/l) + indomethacin (10 mg/l), 9 receptors. **D:** Carboxypeptidase B (2,000 U/l) + indomethacin (10 mg/l) + methysergide (40 mg/l) + mepyramine maleate (40 mg/l), 5 receptors. (From J. S. King, P. Gallant, V. Myerson, and E. R. Perl, ref. 9.)

EFFECT OF SENSITIZATION ON CENTRAL ACTIVITY

Does the enhanced responsiveness exhibited by individual high-threshold receptors, exemplified by the C-fiber polymodal group, have a correlation with the central neural activity associated with pain or other sensations? The fragmentary but intriguing present evidence on this point comes from a limited series of neurophysiological observations on the one side, and from a substantial body of common experience, clinical data, and psychophysical studies on the other.

My colleagues and I (3,10,11) have used information on the receptive characteristics of polymodal and other nociceptors and knowledge of the conduction velocity of their afferent fibers to analyze the nociceptor projection to the spinal dorsal horn. Within the substantia gelatinosa Rolandi (lamina II), certain neuronal units—presumably the larger ones—receive suprathreshold excitation only from unmyelinated afferent fibers. Certain of such lamina II cells respond as if the principal excitatory input comes from the C-polymodal nociceptors: they are not excited by innocuous mechanical and thermal stimuli but do respond to noxious heat (over 45°C) and to noxious mechanical stimulation. The responses of a spinal neuron of this type are illustrated by Fig. 4. Figure 4A shows the discharge evoked in the second of a series of similar cutaneous heat stimulation sequences. Figures 4B, C, and D plot a measure of discharge frequency as a function of temperature for the first, second, and third heating sequences, respectively. Note that the response to the first heating run was a single impulse at about 59°C, whereas the second cycle showed a number of impulses at 45°C and vigorous activity at 50°C. Decreased threshold and enhancement of response have been seen in a number of elements of the superficial lamina of the spinal dorsal horn which receive dominant excitation from high-threshold C-fiber receptors. We do not know if such central cells are part of rostrally projecting pathways, so it is premature to connect such activity to sensory experience. It is clear, however, that the sensitization of polymodal nociceptors is reflected in the activity of at least some spinal cord neurons.

The link between receptor sensitization and clinical and behavioral data may be less direct, but comparing these elements is instructive. After injury of the skin, the injured area and immediate surroundings have a lowered threshold for pain production. In this hyperalgesic state, stimuli not painful to normal skin cause pain. Moreover, stimuli of an intensity that might produce mild pain in the normal provoke from a hyperalgesic area an intense discomfort often reported to have a particularly unpleasant quality. An example of hyperalgesia which seems comparable to the sensitization of C-fiber polymodal nociceptors is that associated with burns produced by excessive ultraviolet exposure or heat; the reddened skin associated with burns is exceptionally sensitive to heat and other stimulation.

Circumstances that might be expected to produce hyperalgesia are those

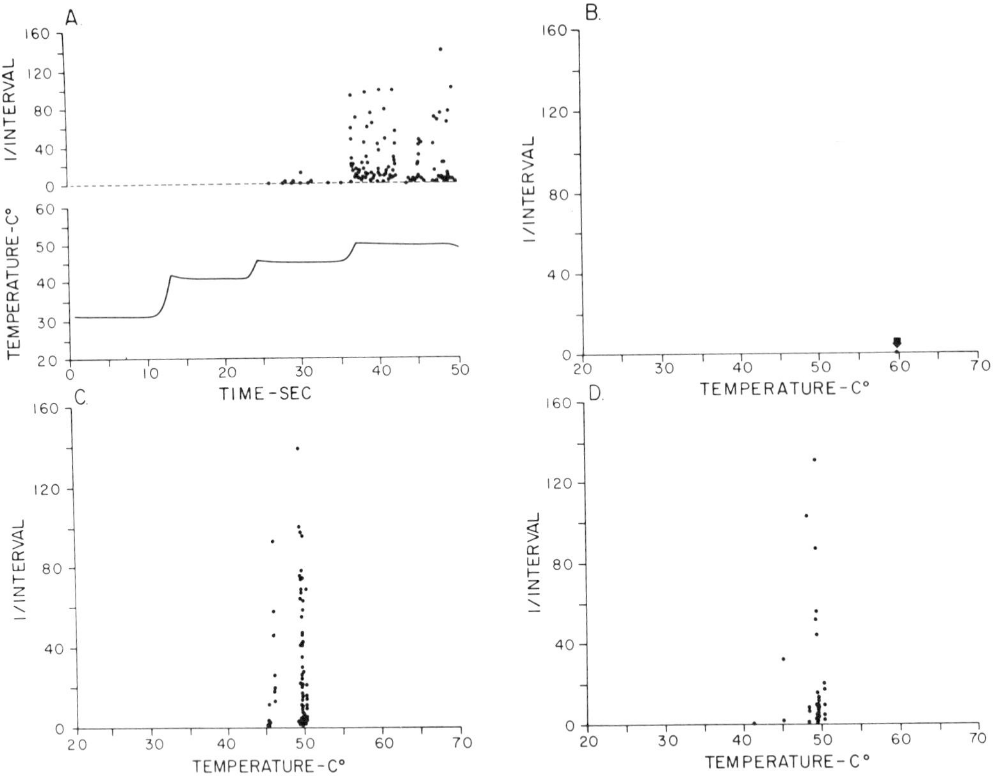

FIG. 4. Response of substantia gelatinosa (lamina II) neuron of monkey to repeated cutaneous heating. Discharge of a single neuron was recorded with a dye-filled microelectrode; the cell responded to electrically evoked single volleys only when they contained C-fiber activity. The unit responded to strong mechanical stimulation of the receptive skin field but not to marked skin cooling or to skin warming up to 40°C. Unitary discharge and thermode temperature to skin warming to 40°C are plotted as in Figs. 1 and 2. **A:** Data from the second cycle of skin heating (initial step to approximately 40°C and then to approximately 5° steps). **B, C,** and **D:** Results from the first, second, and third heat stimulation cycles, respectively, plotted as discharge (ordinate) against temperature (abscissa). (From T. Kumazawa and E. R. Perl, *unpublished.*)

that can be demonstrated to: (a) lower the threshold of the polymodal receptors, (b) increase their response to suprathreshold stimuli, and (c) initiate a background discharge in a previously quiescent sensory fiber. Although the definitive proof is lacking that polymodal nociceptors are sense organs whose activity leads to pain, work on the activity of afferent units recorded from the intact nerves of man strongly supports such a contention (17–20). These studies have shown that noxious skin heating evokes discharges in C fibers associated with receptive units that have the characteristics of the ubiquitous polymodal nociceptors. Conversely, noxious skin heating does not provoke activity in many other receptive units of the same nerves.

Therefore, it seems reasonable to hypothesize tentatively a connection between sensitization of the C-fiber polymodal (and possibly other) nociceptors and hyperalgesia.

Traditionally, inflammation is characterized by redness, swelling, and pain. The regular association of pain with inflammation has long led to the speculation that the mechanisms leading to inflammation also initiate activity in the peripheral sensory apparatus responsible for causing the painful sensation. This supposition led us to attempt to interfere with suspected chemical intermediaries of the inflammatory process while observing the sensitization and background discharge of the C-fiber polymodal receptors. On the basis of the preliminary results, it appears likely that one or more of the substances known to be released from cutaneous tissue when it is damaged (a polypeptide, a prostaglandin, serotonin, and histamine) play a part in making the polymodal terminals more sensitive and productive of ongoing activity. Details on the manner in which this occurs and the exact agents responsible await further study.

COMMENT

Direct evidence for increased sensitivity of a class of cutaneous sense organs as a consequence of tissue-damaging stimuli makes it important to consider this factor when dealing with alteration of sensation associated with pathology. Because sensitization occurs in sensory units capable of discriminately signaling tissue-damaging events rather than occurring universally in all somatic receptors, the phenomenon appears particularly relevant to the sensation of pain. At the clinical level, this argument suggests that in cases of persisting pain of peripheral origin, persisting increase in the responsiveness of normally high-threshold sense organs should be a first consideration. An increase in sensitivity of a receptor specialized to detect pain-causing stimuli could cause weak and ordinarily harmless stimuli to be signaled as if they were noxious. The concomitant of polymodal receptor sensitization, background activity in the absence of stimulation, would also produce a sensory message equivalent to that initiated by noxious events in the physiological or unsensitized state.

Obviously, sensitization of somatic receptors cannot explain all instances of long-lasting pain. It cannot be argued to serve as a basis for all types of enduring pain of peripheral origin. For example, a mechanism assuming sensitization does not deal adequately with the situation in which altered geometry of tissue—caused by tumors, skeletal malformation, degeneration, or some other defect—could lead to stress by normally innocuous events sufficient for activation of high-threshold receptors. Sensitization of nociceptors certainly is not a suitable explanation for pain of central origin. Furthermore, peripheral sensitization has no direct reference to questions that fascinate students of sensation, such as the interaction between different afferent systems and place of inhibition in ascending afferent transmission. In spite of these limitations, peripheral sensitization—specifically, a decrease of nociceptors' threshold and a concomitant increase of their background activity—appears to account partially for a frequent source of persisting physically caused pain, that which results from tissue injury and other circumstances related to inflammation.

ACKNOWLEDGMENT

Preparation of this manuscript and the experimental work it describes was supported by a grant from the National Institutes of Health (U.S. Public Health Service NS 10321). Support for computer facilities was also provided by a U.S. Public Health Service grant (NS 11132) and by the Alfred P. Sloan Foundation.

REFERENCES

1. Bessou, P., Burgess, P. R., Perl, E. R., and Taylor, C. B. (1971): *J. Neurophysiol.,* 34: 116–131.
2. Bessou, P., and Perl, E. R. (1969): *J. Neurophysiol.,* 32:1025–1043.
3. Christensen, B. N., and Perl, E. R. (1970): *J. Neurophysiol.,* 33:293–307.
4. Echlin, F., and Propper, N. (1937): *J. Physiol. (Lond.),* 88:388–400.
5. Fjällbrant, N., and Iggo, A. (1961): *J. Physiol. (Lond.),* 156:578–590.
6. Iggo, A., and Kornhuber, H. H. (1968): *J. Physiol. (Lond.),* 198:113P.
7. Keele, C. A., and Armstrong, D. (1964): *Substances Producing Pain and Itch.* Edward Arnold Ltd., London.
8. Kenins, P., and Perl, E. R.: *Unpublished.*
9. King, J. S., Gallant, P., Myerson, V., and Perl, E. R. (1976): In: *Sensory Functions of the Skin in Primates with Special Reference to Man, Vol. 28,* edited by Y. Zotterman. Pergamon Press, Oxford.
10. Kumazawa, T., and Perl, E. R.: *Unpublished.*
11. Kumazawa, T., Perl, E. R., Burgess, P. R., and Whitehorn, D. (1975): *J. Comp. Neurol.,* 162:1–11.
12. Lewis, T. (1935): *Clin. Sci.,* 2:373–423.
13. Lim, R. K. S. (1970): *Annu. Rev. Physiol.,* 32:269–288.
14. Lynn, B.: *Unpublished.*
15. Lynn, B., Kenins, P., and Perl, E. R.: *Unpublished.*
16. Perl, E. R., Kumazawa, T., Lynn, B., and Kenins, P. (1976): In: *Somatosensory and Visceral Receptor Mechanisms, Progress in Brain Research, Vol. 43,* edited by A. Iggo. Elsevier, Amsterdam.
17. Torebjörk, H. E., and Hallin, R. G. (1973): *Exp. Brain Res.,* 16(3): 321–32.
18. Torebjörk, H. E., and Hallin, R. G. (1974): *J. Neurol. Neurosurg. Psychiatry,* 37(6): 653–664.
19. Van Hees, J., and Gybels, J. M. (1972): *Brain Res.,* 48:397–400.
20. Van Hees, J., and Gybels, J. M. (1973): *Acta Neurol. Belg.,* 73(1):39–43.
21. Wilhelm, D. L. (1973): In: *Chemical Mediators in the Inflammatory Process, Vol. II,* edited by B. W. Zweifach, L. Grant, and R. T. McCluskey. Academic Press, New York.
22. Perl, E. R. (1972): In: *Cervical Pain,* edited by C. Hirsch and Y. Zotterman, pp. 157–164. Pergamon Press, Oxford.

Advances in Pain Research and Therapy, Vol. 1,
edited by J. J. Bonica and D. Albe-Fessard.

A New Method for Classification of C-Unit Activity in Intact Human Skin Nerves

H. Erik Torebjörk and Rolf G. Hallin

Department of Clinical Neurophysiology, University Hospital, Uppsala, Sweden

As recently shown, impulse activity from the entire nerve fiber spectrum can be recorded with microelectrodes from intact human skin nerves (5,7). Multifiber activity in large and thin myelinated (A) fibers was regularly encountered in responses to electrical or various natural stimuli in the skin. The recordings often permitted identification of single-unit discharges in myelinated fibers. Multifiber activity in afferent or efferent (sympathetic) unmyelinated (C) fibers was sometimes discernible, and single-unit impulses in unmyelinated fibers were occasionally identified by their amplitude, shape, and conduction velocity (6,12,14).

In recordings from intact nerves it is sometimes difficult to determine by mere inspection of the original neurogram if receptors with myelinated or unmyelinated fibers respond to a natural skin stimulus. In particular, single C-unit discharges may be difficult to identify, especially when the potentials of different units have similar amplitudes and interfere with each other. In addition, afferent impulses in fibers with slow conduction velocities might be confused with reflex responses in sympathetic fibers (11).

The purpose of this report is to describe a new method to classify discharges in afferent and sympathetic C units in neural responses recorded from intact human skin nerves.

METHODS

This chapter is based on illustrative experiments that have been published previously (9,11,13,15). Technical details concerning the experimental procedure, the lacquer-insulated tungsten microelectrodes, and the recording and display system were described in detail in previous reports (4,14,16).

Painful electric test shocks were delivered through small needles inserted intradermally within the innervation zone of the impaled nerve fascicle. Von Frey's hairs, sharp needles, or radiant heat were used to induce afferent C-unit discharges from the skin. Sympathetic reflex responses were evoked by arousal stimuli such as sudden loud noises (3,6,8).

In studying the C responses to combined electrical and natural stimuli, we used a dot display analysis to present changes in latency in a compact form (15).

RESULTS

Slowing of Impulse Conduction in C Fibers During Repetitive Firing

The averaged C response to single painful electric skin shocks in Fig. 1A was considerably reduced and delayed on repetitive stimulation (Fig. 1B). This is because of postactivation decrease of excitability and slowing of conduction in unmyelinated fibers (2), and the effects are pronounced in the thin nerve terminals in the skin even at low stimulation frequencies (15). As shown in Fig. 1C, small increases in stimulation frequency were accompanied by increases in latency of individual C-unit responses. A decrease in stimulation frequency was followed by a slow recovery of conduction.

Impulse conduction was slowed in both afferent and sympathetic C fibers as a consequence of repetitive firing, induced either by electrical or by various natural stimuli. With constant electrical stimulation at low frequency in the skin, transient increases in latency of the C-fiber responses

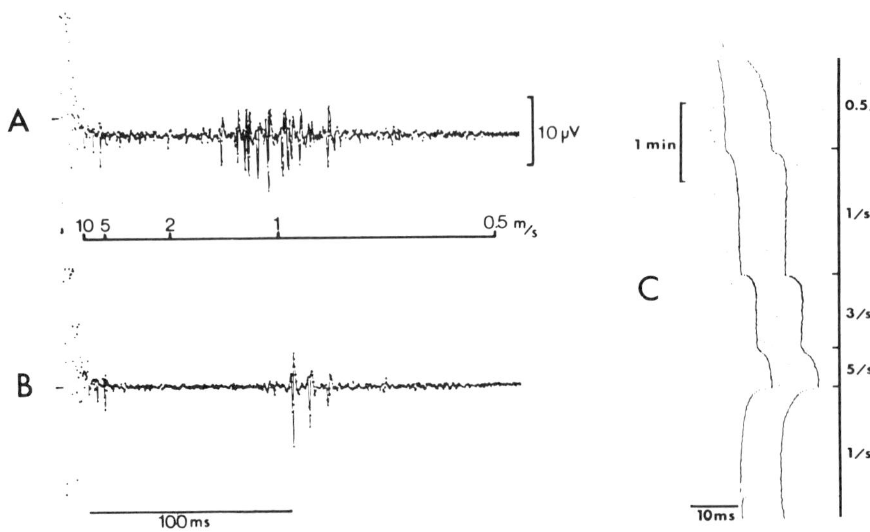

FIG. 1. Changes in the C response accompanying variations in stimulus frequency. **A,B:** Multiunit recording from the radial nerve. Each computer record is based on the averaging of 100 responses to electric intradermal stimuli of constant intensity. Because of the long time base, most of the A-fiber responses are hidden in the stimulus artifact. **A:** Pronounced C-fiber response to painful stimulation at a frequency of 0.5 Hz. **B:** Note the decrease and delay of the C-fiber response when the stimulation frequency was increased to 5 Hz (13). **C:** Single-unit recording from the median nerve. Centripetally conducted responses to electric intradermal stimuli of constant intensity in 2 sympathetic C units represented by dots in the compact display. First 130 ms after stimulus artifacts omitted. Note changes in latency of the C-unit responses at varying stimulation frequencies (indicated to the right) (9).

served as an index of increased firing in the C units under study (9,15). These observations were used to classify afferent and sympathetic C units activated by a combination of electrical and natural stimuli.

Identification of Afferent C-Unit Activity

The C-unit responses in Fig. 2A–C were elicited by electric test shocks delivered through stimulation needles in the skin. As the stimulation was continued at a constant low frequency (0.3 Hz), unitary activity was also induced by a needle prick near the stimulating electrodes (Fig. 2A). The increase in neural activity was accompanied by a marked transient increase in latency for one of the unitary components in the electrically induced C-

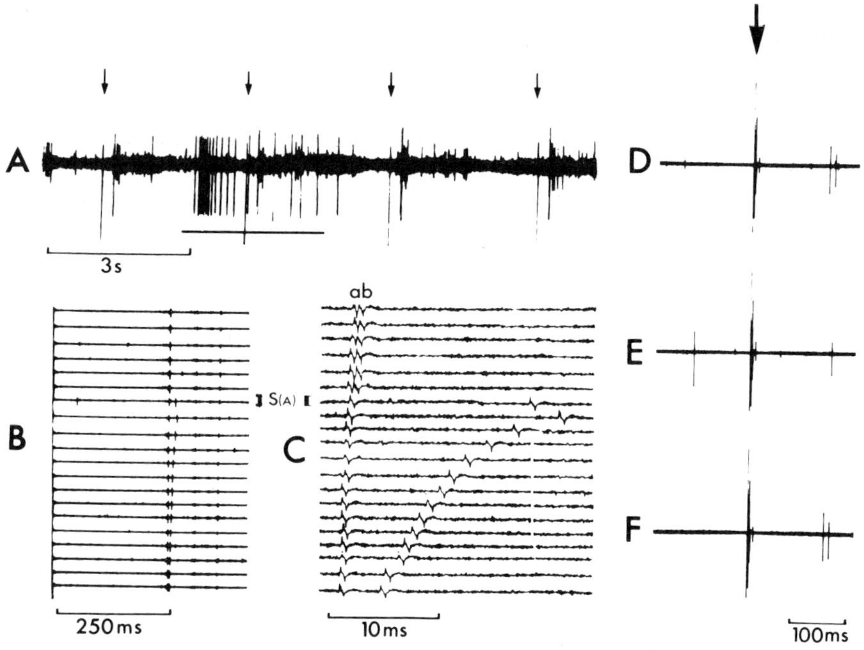

FIG. 2. Identification of afferent and sympathetic C units. **A–C:** Afferent C-unit activity recorded in the peroneal nerve. Intradermal electric shocks (*arrows*) delivered at a frequency of 0.3 Hz in the innervation zone of the impaled fascicle. **A:** Unitary responses to a combination of electrical stimulation and a pinprick (*bar*) near the stimulating electrodes. **B:** Successive C responses to electrical stimulation. Note changes in latency for one component in the responses associated with the unit activity evoked by natural stimulation in **A,** S(A). **C:** Same sequence as in **B** at a shorter time base with the first 245 ms after stimulus artifacts omitted; *a* and *b* indicate 2 different C units. **D–F:** Efferent C-unit activity recorded in the median nerve. Arrow indicates stimulus artifact and A-fiber response to intradermal electric stimulation. Centripetally conducted responses in two C units are seen at a latency exceeding 100 ms in control situations (**D, F**). One of the unit responses is missing in E due to collision with induced sympathetic reflex activity (9).

fiber responses (Fig. 2C). The change in latency was not caused by mechanical displacement of the stimulating electrodes, nor could it be provoked by maneuvers known to induce sympathetic reflex responses in human skin nerves. Only when neural activity was elicited by natural stimuli within a small defined skin area near the stimulating electrodes could the latency changes be reproduced. It was concluded that the neural activity induced by the needle prick in the skin was associated with repetitive firing and transient slowing of conduction in an afferent C unit. The impulse conduction velocity in this C fiber was approximately 1 m/sec.

Identification of Efferent Sympathetic C-Unit Activity

Electrical stimulation in the skin evoked not only orthodromic impulses in afferent fibers but also antidromic impulses in efferent sympathetic unmyelinated fibers (9). Sympathetic units in the centripetally conducted C-fiber responses to electric skin shocks were identified by slowing of impulse conduction associated with maneuvers that increased the sympathetic outflow.

The collision technique, which is based on the fact that impulses traveling in opposite directions in a nerve fiber extinguish each other if they collide (1,10), was also used to identify sympathetic C units. Signs of collisions between antidromic and orthodromic impulses in sympathetic fibers were observed in the centripetally conducted C response if the impulses collided between the stimulating and recording sites (Fig. 2D); or they were observed in the sympathetic reflex responses to the electric test shocks if the impulses collided between the recording site and the ganglion (9).

COMMENT

Application of the Identification Method

The electric test shocks in the skin should be delivered at a low frequency, 0.3 Hz or less, in order to minimize (a) depression of the excitability of afferent C endings and (b) interference with the sympathetic outflow by collision effects. Identification depends on proper activation of the C units, either by natural stimuli within well-defined receptive fields for excitation of afferent units, or by suitable maneuvers for inducing sympathetic activity. C units that respond only to electrical stimuli and not to other means of activation cannot be classified.

The characteristic changes in latency induced by a combination of electrical and natural stimuli serve as a "marking" of those C units that respond to the natural stimuli, whereas elements not activated by the natural stimuli remain uninfluenced in the electrically induced C responses. The testing procedure is simple and rapid and can be used "on line" during the experiments for classification and qualitative analysis of C-unit activity in multifiber recordings. An example is shown in Fig. 3. It is difficult to judge from the original neurogram if the skin heating in Fig. 3A induced activity in A or C fibers, or if the neural activity represents a sympathetic reflex response. An analysis of the responses to the electric test shocks revealed that at least three C units were activated since their latencies increased during heating (Fig. 3C). A fourth C unit was probably not activated, and the decrease in latency was caused by a temperature-dependent increase in conduction velocity. Further tests established that the first three C units were afferent, with polymodal receptive properties, whereas the fourth C unit was of efferent, sympathetic origin (11).

In our first studies of single-unit activity in intact nerves in man, only C units with large and characteristic potentials could be identified and analyzed among interfering multifiber activity. Such selective recordings were difficult to obtain, and only a few C units could be studied. With the described technique several C units can be quickly classified and individually analyzed in one recording site. This opens up the possibility of collecting large C-unit materials, which will provide a basis for a better understanding of the physiological role of afferent and sympathetic C fibers in man.

ACKNOWLEDGMENTS

This investigation was supported by the Swedish Medical Research Council, grant No. B74-04X-2881-05C, and AB Förenade Liv, Stockholm.

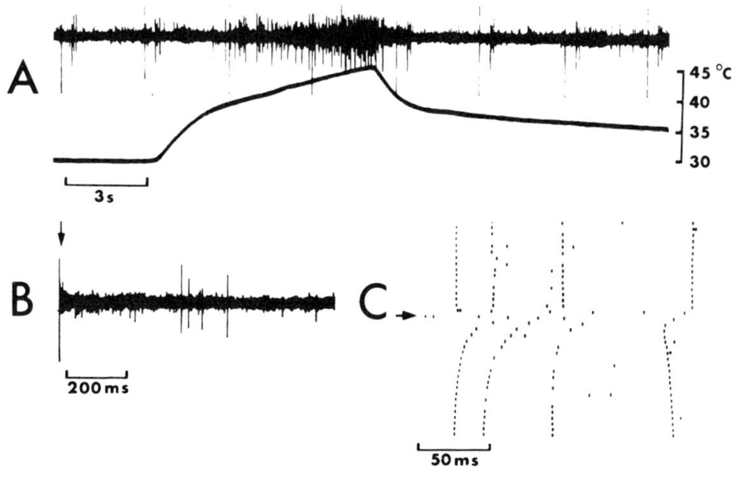

FIG. 3. Identification of active C units in a multifiber recording from the peroneal nerve. **A:** Upper trace shows neural responses to electrical stimulation in the skin every 3rd s and to an increase in skin temperature (indicated below). **B:** Each electric test shock induced responses in 4 C units. Vertical arrow indicates stimulation artifact. **C:** Compact dot display of successive C-unit responses at an expanded time scale with the first 375 ms after stimulus artifacts omitted. Skin heating in A (*horizontal arrow*) caused a transient increase in latency of the responses in 3 units and the reverse effect for 1 unit (11).

REFERENCES

1. Douglas, W. W., and Ritchie, J. M. (1957): *J. Physiol. (Lond.)*, 138:19–30.
2. Gasser, H. S. (1935): *Am. J. Physiol.*, 111:35–50.
3. Hagbarth, K.-E., Hallin, R. G., Hongell, A., Torebjörk, H. E., and Wallin, B. G. (1972): *Acta Physiol. Scand.*, 84:164–176.
4. Hagbarth, K.-E., Hongell, A., Hallin, R. G., and Torebjörk, H. E. (1970): *Brain Res.*, 24:423–442.
5. Hallin, R. G., and Torebjörk, H. E. (1970): *Acta Soc. Med. Upsal.*, 75:77–80.
6. Hallin, R. G., and Torebjörk, H. E. (1970): *Acta Soc. Med. Upsal.*, 75:277–281.
7. Hallin, R. G., and Torebjörk, H. E. (1973): *Exp. Brain Res.*, 16:309–320.
8. Hallin, R. G., and Torebjörk, H. E. (1974): *Acta Physiol. Scand.*, 92:303–317.
9. Hallin, R. G., and Torebjörk, H. E. (1974): *Acta Physiol. Scand.*, 92:318–331.
10. Iggo, A. (1958): *J. Physiol. (Lond.)*, 142:110–126.
11. Torebjörk, H. E. (1974): *Acta Physiol. Scand.*, 92:374–390.
12. Torebjörk, H. E., and Hallin, R. G. (1970): *Acta Soc. Med. Upsal.*, 75:81–84.
13. Torebjörk, H. E., and Hallin, R. G. (1973): *Exp. Brain Res.*, 16:321–332.
14. Torebjörk, H. E., and Hallin, R. G. (1974): *Brain Res.*, 67:387–403.
15. Torebjörk, H. E., and Hallin, R. G. (1974): *J. Neurol. Neurosurg. Psychiatry*, 37:653–664.
16. Vallbo, Å. B., and Hagbarth, K.-E. (1968): *Exp. Neurol.*, 21:270–289.

Advances in Pain Research and Therapy, Vol. 1,
edited by J. J. Bonica and D. Albe-Fessard.
Raven Press, New York © 1976.

Human C-Fiber Input During Painful and Nonpainful Skin Stimulation with Radiant Heat

J. Van Hees

Department of Neurology and Neurosurgery, K.U.L., Kapucijnenvoer 35, B-3000 Leuven, Belgium

INTRODUCTION

During recent years direct data have been obtained about the activity of afferent C fibers in the intact human nerve by percutaneously introduced tungsten microelectrodes (4–6). So far all afferent C fibers studied in this way show the characteristics of nociceptors (elevated threshold for mechanical and thermal stimuli and responsiveness to chemical substances). In the cat the discharges of "C-heat receptors" are linearly related to the level of skin temperature, and their thresholds are related to the human pain threshold for radiant heat (1).

It was our purpose to study in conscious man during radiant heat stimulation the relation between skin temperature, unitary C-fiber discharge, and the evoked sensation. The results of four C-fiber units in 4 subjects are presented.

METHODS

For registration of single C-fiber activity, we used the same technique as mentioned previously (6). All records were taken in the superficial branch of the radial nerve and the receptive areas were on the back of the hand. The skin (without blackening) was irradiated by a focused bulb, the heating current being controlled by the output voltage of a small thermistor fixed on the skin surface near the receptive center.

The subject was asked to say "yes" at the first moment of pain and to say "stop" when the pain became strong; he was asked to avoid burning lesions; when he said "stop," the stimulation was interrupted. Different skin temperatures between 40°C and 55°C were administered in repeated series. The intended temperature level was maintained for about 15 sec if tolerated. Between each stimulus the skin was allowed to cool to 35°C.

The C-fiber activity was counted as "mean frequency per second" during the stimulus plateau (number of spikes divided by plateau duration). Reliable data were obtained from C fibers in 4 subjects with a total of 148 stimulations. Except for slight reddening, there were no visible signs of skin damage.

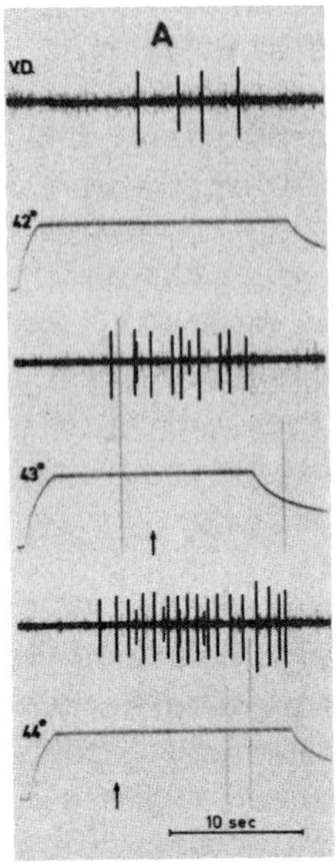

FIG. 1. Discharges of human afferent C-fiber unit activity at different skin temperatures. **A:** Specimen records at 3 different temperatures; arrow indicates the subject's report of beginning pain. **B:** Relation between skin temperature and neural response (mean spike frequency during stimulus plateau) of an afferent C fiber during 3 successive stimulation series. Thickness of the horizontal bars is proportional to the number of "yes" (beginning pain) and "stop" (strong pain) responses of the subject at the given temperature.

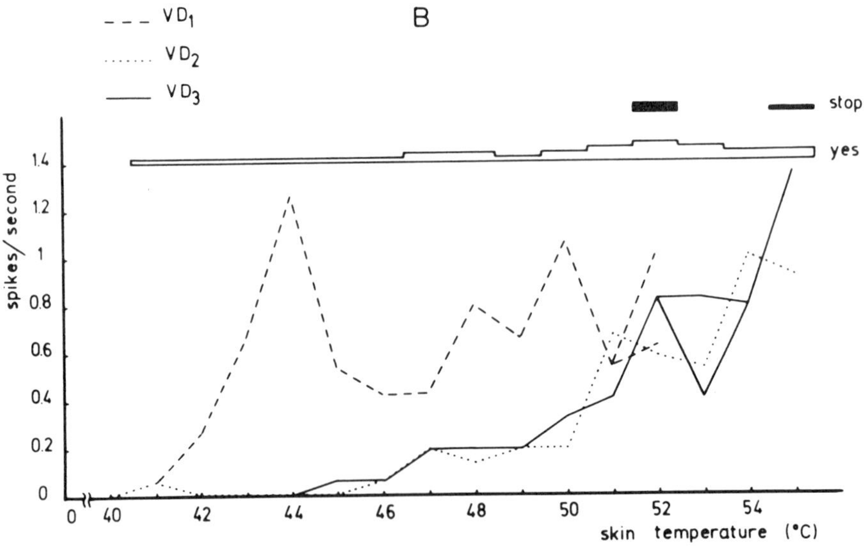

RESULTS

Figure 1 shows the results of the experiment in 1 subject. Three successive series of stimulations were done between 40°C and 55°C. The "yes" and "stop" responses are represented at the top of the diagram by horizontal bars the thickness of which is proportional to the number of responses at each temperature. It is obvious that on an average the mean firing frequency of the C fiber increases with increasing skin temperature, but also that there is some variability in neural responses to repeated stimuli of the same intensity. The rather weak correlation between skin temperature and afferent C-fiber discharge can be expressed by the correlation coefficients of the linear regression lines calculated in the 4 subjects: 0.91, 0.44, 0.70, and 0.50.

Figure 2 represents the results of the total of 148 stimulations in four different C units (in 4 subjects). The afferent discharge is of rather low frequency and does not as a rule exceed 2 spikes/sec even at stimuli reported as strongly painful.

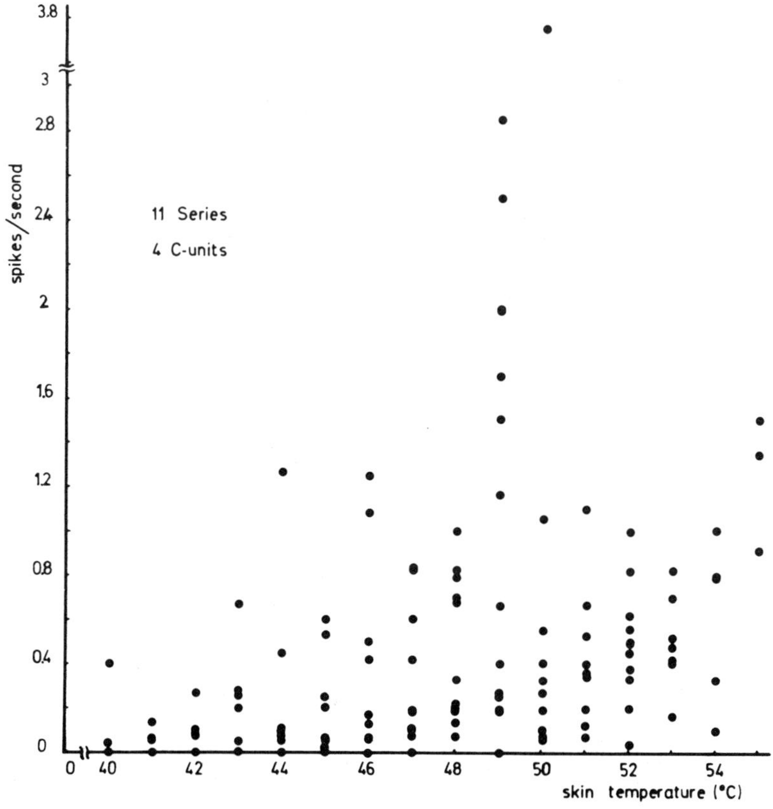

FIG. 2. Relation between skin temperature and neural response (mean spike frequency during stimulus plateau) of 4 different C fibers in 4 subjects.

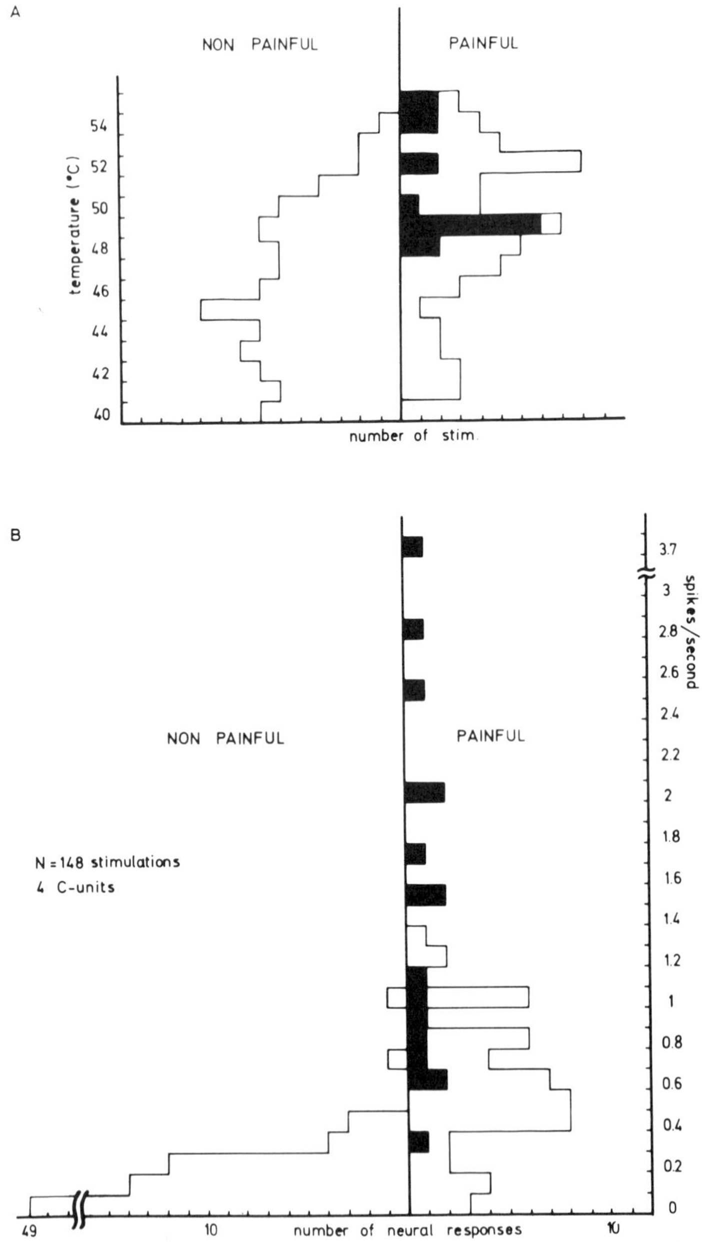

FIG. 3. A: Classification of the stimulations according to the subject's judgment. Black squares represent stimuli reported as strongly painful. **B:** Idem for neural responses.

A classification of the stimulations as painful or nonpainful as judged by the subjects is represented in Fig. 3A. All stimulations at 55°C were reported as painful, and all those at 40°C as nonpainful. The stimulations between these extreme values show a weak tendency to shift into the painful compartment with higher temperature values. Strong pain (*black squares*) was reported from 48° to 55°C. Similarly, the neural responses are plotted in the two classes of the subjects' judgment in Fig. 3B. Almost all stimulations evoking discharge frequencies exceeding 0.4/sec are reported as painful, whereas most of those evoking frequencies below 0.3/sec are classified as nonpainful.

DISCUSSION

The behavior of this small sample of human afferent C fibers in response to radiant heat differs from that of the cat "C-heat receptors" (1) only by the rather weak correlation between their discharge and the skin temperature. Considering at the same time the variability of judgments by the subjects at the same skin temperature, one could evoke some instability of stimulation conditions as responsible for both phenomena. In spite of the rigorous care taken about these conditions, such factors as variability of caloric conductance between the skin and the thermistor escape our control.

On the other hand, our results indicate that the C-fiber response is useful to make a fair prediction about the subjects' sensations: discharges exceeding 0.4/sec were mostly accompanied by a report of pain sensation, discharges exceeding 1.5/sec (although few in number) were invariability accompanied by a report of strong pain (Fig. 3B). Thus the contribution of this C-fiber group to the pain sensation is quite possible. These results also demonstrate that C-fiber activity of low frequency (below 0.3/sec) does not elicit pain sensation. This is in agreement with the observation that afferent C-fiber activity can be evoked by nonpainful electrical skin stimulation (5).

Compared with the maximal instantaneous frequency of 50 to 60 per second produced by intense heat stimulation of brief duration (5), the presented values obtained by controlled stimuli of longer duration are rather low, suggesting that only a lower fraction of the range of painful stimuli is explored in our experiments.

Psychophysiological experiments evidenced the absense of spatial summation in cutaneous pain (2). This would designate the discharge frequency in nociceptive fibers as most important in determining the intensity of pain sensation. If the human C fiber is really involved in eliciting cutaneous pain, its discharge frequency of about 0.3/sec could be equated with the heat pain threshold.

However, in the human nerve elements other than the C-fiber group also are activated or influenced by radiant heat stimulation.

We studied one delta afferent fiber (conduction velocity of 10 m/sec) that was activated by painful radiant heat stimulation with a relatively high discharge frequency.

Our experience is also in agreement with the observation made by Hensel and Boman (3) that the spontaneous activity of slowly adapting myelinated mechanoreceptors is inhibited by heat stimulation.

ACKNOWLEDGMENTS

The author is grateful to Mrs. Feytons-Heeren and Mr. P. De Sutter for their technical assistance. This investigation was supported by the F.W.G.O. (grant 20492) of Belgium.

REFERENCES

1. Beck, P. W., Handwerker, H. O., and Zimmermann, M. (1974): *Brain Res.*, 67:373–386.
2. Hardy, J. D., Wolff, H. G., and Goodell, H. (1952): *Pain Sensations and Reactions*, Williams & Wilkins, Baltimore.
3. Hensel, H., and Boman, K. K. A. (1960): *J. Neurophysiol.*, 23:564–578.
4. Torebjörk, H. E., and Hallin, R. G. (1973): *Exp. Brain Res.*, 16:321–332.
5. Torebjörk, H. E., and Hallin, R. G. (1974): *Brain Res.*, 67:387–403.
6. Van Hees, J., and Gybels, J. M. (1972): *Brain Res.*, 48:397–400.

Advances in Pain Research and Therapy, Vol. 1,
edited by J. J. Bonica and D. Albe-Fessard.
Raven Press, New York © 1976.

Influences of Algogenic Substances and Prostaglandins on the Discharges of Unmyelinated Cutaneous Nerve Fibers Identified as Nociceptors

Hermann O. Handwerker

Physiologisches Institut der Universität Heidelberg, Heidelberg, Germany

All stimuli able to elicit pain reactions in man or animals, when applied to the skin, also initiate the processes of inflammation, e.g., the production of vasoactive substances. Some of these substances, e.g., bradykinin, evoke pain reactions themselves when introduced into the skin, even in low concentrations.

In a previous study we showed (2) that bradykinin (BKN) or serotonin (5-HT) given by close arterial injection (single doses, 5 μg of BKN and 30 μg 5-HT) evokes spike responses in most cutaneous afferent C fibers that respond to noxious radiant heat. Although sensitive mechanoreceptors are excited as well, excitation of these nociceptive afferent fibers is probably responsible for the pain produced by intra-arterial BKN injections.

The present study (6) was done to test the influence of prostaglandins E_1 and E_2 on the excitation of cutaneous C-heat fibers. Prostaglandins of the E group have been described as being synthesized in the skin during inflammatory reactions (1,9). Although prostaglandins are not as potent algogenic substances as plasmakinins, they have been found to enhance nocifensive reflex hypertension elicited by BKN in dogs (4,8). The suppression of the biosynthesis of prostaglandins might explain the analgesic action of "aspirin-like" drugs (4,8).

METHOD

To measure directly the effects of prostaglandins on nociceptive neurons, we recorded discharges of single cutaneous C fibers from the plantar nerves of cats anesthetized with pentobarbital sodium (Nembutal®, 40 mg/kg). Approximately 16% of these C fibers were activated by application of noxious radiant heat (e.g., 50°C) to the receptive field, and they were therefore classified as C-heat receptors. A detailed description of methods and a quantitative assessment of the responses of these fibers to radiant heat are given elsewhere (3).

RESULTS

The normal skin temperature of the hindpaw in these experiments was in the range of 28° to 32°C. At these temperatures C-heat fibers were silent provided that the skin was not damaged by preceding stimulation. However, when 5 μg BKN in the 0.5 ml tyrode solution was injected into the femoral artery through a small polyethylene tube inserted into the stump of a muscle branch (for details of method see 2), most units of this fiber type responded with a burst of action potentials. As shown in Fig. 1A, this response decreases during repetitive injections at 1-min intervals. Injection

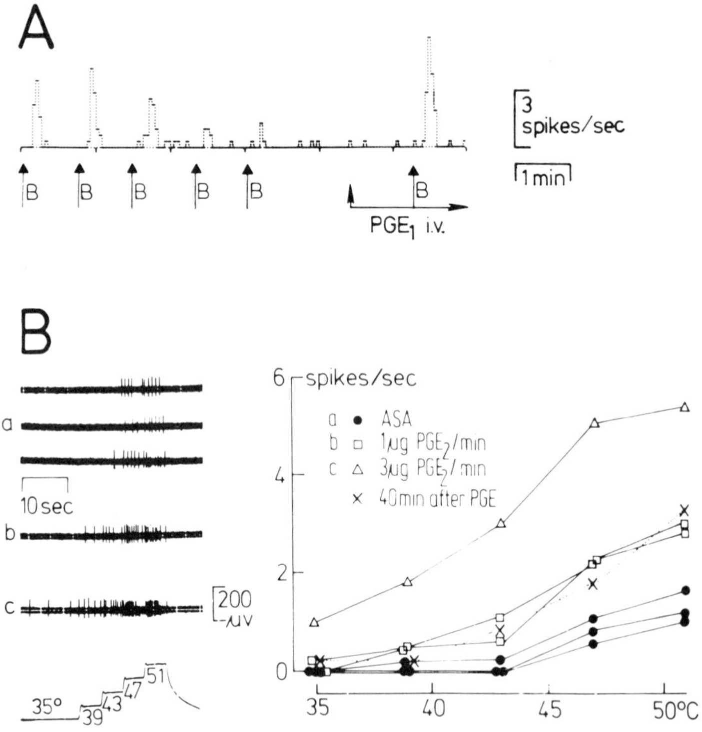

FIG. 1. Influence of prostaglandin (PGE) infusions on the discharges evoked by close arterial injection of bradykinin (B), and by heat, of single unmyelinated cutaneous nerve fibers from the cat's plantar region. **A:** At the times marked by arrows, 5 μg B was injected into the femoral artery. At the horizontal bar an additional continuous infusion of 5 μg/min PGE_1 was started into the radial vein. **B:** Recordings from a C fiber of the medial plantar nerve of another cat. Left: specimen records and time course of skin surface temperature during each radiant heat stimulus. Right: regression lines computed from integrated number of spikes at each temperature. **a** and ● : 3 control stimuli applied at 5-min intervals starting at 1 hr after injection of 180 mg lysine salicylate (equivalent to 100 mg aspirin) given to block endogenous PGE formation. **b** and □: Same heating stimuli applied with simultaneous infusion of 1 μg/min PGE_2. **c** and △: 3 μg/min E_2. **X** and **dotted line:** Control 40 min after arrest of PGE infusion.

of 5-HT elicited similar responses, but it was less potent. Since the tachyphylaxis to 5-HT does not influence responses to BKN and vice versa, it was concluded that both substances act on different pharmacological receptors in the membranes of the C fibers tested. However, an indirect action on tissue surrounding the receptive endings cannot be entirely excluded, e.g., via an action of both substances on different pharmacological receptors in the membrane of vascular smooth muscle.

In the experiments, as shown in Fig. 1A, continuous infusion of prostaglandin E_1 at 5 μg/min into the radial vein was started after approximately 5 min of BKN testing. This additional infusion led to an enhanced response to the same doses of BKN and the tachyphylaxis was abolished.

Because of this powerful potentiating action of prostaglandins on the BKN responses of C-heat fibers, I tried also to evaluate the effect of these substances on the responses to radiant heat stimulation. As described previously (3), heat was produced by radiation of a halogen bulb focused by a lens on the receptive field. A thermocouple was placed on the skin surface in the center of the focal spot. The current of the bulb was controlled by feedback from the thermocouple, and in this way the temperature could be clamped to preselected levels. To obtain information on the momentary excitability of C-heat fibers without time-consuming repetitive stimulations that might have changed the experimental conditions by exceeding noxious thresholds too often, we chose a stimulus program for the present experiments. The skin temperature was preadapted to a subnoxious level for 30 sec (to 35°C in the experiment shown in Fig. 1B) and was then raised in four steps of 5-sec duration and of 4°C height to noxious levels.

To obviate the formation of endogenous prostaglandins as a consequence of these stimuli, we administered 180 mg lysine acetylsalicylate (equivalent to 100 mg acetylsalicylic acid) intravenously before testing. Control experiments revealed that this substance had no effect on the responsiveness of the heat receptors.

In Fig. 1B specimen records and the integrated number of spikes at each temperature level are shown (*a* and *black dots*) of a C-heat fiber tested repetitively every 5 min. Continued testing during intravenous infusion of 1 μg/min prostaglandin E_2 produced a somewhat stronger response (*b* and *open squares*). Infusion of 3 μg/min prostaglandin E_2 led to a significant increase in responsiveness (*c* and *open triangles*). The effect of the prostaglandin infusion was not completely reversible as shown by a control test performed 40 min after stopping the infusion. A total of 15 identified C-heat receptors have been tested in this way in 9 cats with both prostaglandin E_1 and E_2. Of these, 7 were affected as shown in Fig. 1B, the others were not affected by intravenous infusion. Also, there was no significant difference in the actions of prostaglandins E_1 and E_2.

Since most of the prostaglandin (E group) infused into the systemic circulation is metabolized in the lungs (5), the sensitization described could be caused by a metabolite rather than by the prostaglandin itself. To test this alternative, we infused prostaglandins into the femoral artery in the same way as described for BKN injections. Doses of 0.5 to 1 μg E_1 or E_2 were found to lower thresholds to heating significantly in all units ($N = 9$) tested. Another feature of these experiments was an irregular discharge of the units at resting temperatures as a result of combined prostaglandin infusion and repetitive heating of the receptive field.

Another effective form of application was intracutaneous injection of 0.05 μg in 0.1 ml into the receptive field by means of a microliter syringe. This test reveals that the fibers are affected in their receptor region. Figure 2 shows an experiment in which prostaglandin E_2 was administered at first intravenously. This induced a slight increase in the responsiveness to radiant heat. However, a final test performed 10 min after intracutaneous injection of a single dose of 0.05 μg prostaglandin E_2 revealed a much stronger sensitization.

COMMENT

In a previous study (2) we showed that BKN applied by close arterial injection increased responsiveness of C-heat receptors in the cat's hindpaw

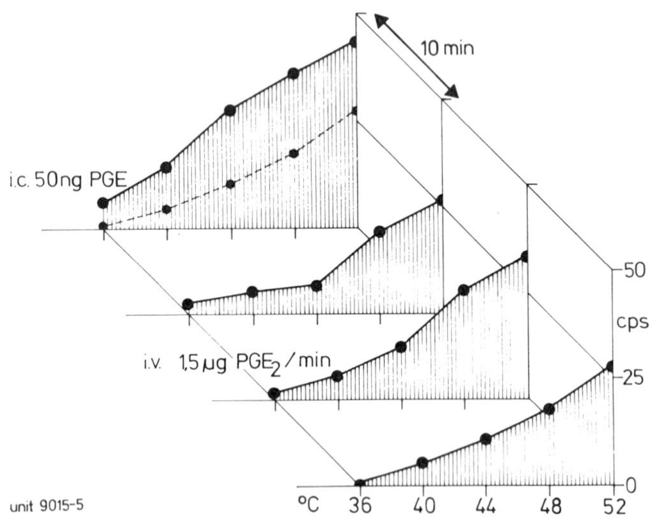

FIG. 2. Influence of different methods of application of prostaglandins on the discharges of a C fiber from the cat's plantar region. Time course of temperature stimulation as in Fig. 1, but preadaptation to 36°C and testing with 40, 44, 48, and 52°C. ●: Integrated number of spikes at each temperature level with 10-min intervals between 1st and 3rd control stimuli. 2nd stimulation during 1.5 μg/min PGE_2 given in radial vein. 4th stimulus was applied 10 min after intracutaneous injection of 50 ng PGE_2 into receptive field of the fiber. Response to the 1st control stimulus is projected for comparison with the last stimulus.

to radiant heat stimulation. In the present study prostaglandins of the E group have been shown to exert a similar effect. In addition, a new heating test program made it possible to assess the influence of these pharmacological agents more quantitatively at different temperatures. If regression lines, which have been computed from integrated numbers of spikes on thermal stimulation, are compared, a parallel shift to lower temperatures seems to be the main effect of prostaglandins (Figs. 1B and 2). There is a much less significant increase in steepness of the regression lines; i.e., under the influence of prostaglandins, C-heat fibers respond at much lower and previously nonnoxious temperatures. However, the relative increase in discharge rate with an increase in temperature is almost unchanged with this type of sensitization. This might be an experimental model of inflammatory hyperpathia.

It is not known whether the sensitizing effect of prostaglandins is exerted by a direct action on the nerve membranes or indirectly by influencing the surrounding tissue. All substances known to excite nociceptive nerve endings or to enhance their responsiveness to "natural" noxious stimulation also affect vascular smooth muscle. In the case of carotid baroreceptors and chemoreceptors, it has been shown that this vascular effect of prostaglandins is responsible for the changes in receptor responses these agents produce (7).

ACKNOWLEDGMENTS

I wish to thank H. Dickhaus who constructed the function generator for heat stimulation. I also thank K. D. Neher for his help in some of the experiments, K. Langenstein for his excellent technical assistance, and S. Fleminger for correcting the English.

Lysine acetylsalicylate was supplied by Bayer Leverkusen.

This work was supported by the Deutsche Forschungsgemeinschaft grant Ha 831/3.

REFERENCES

1. Arthurson, F., Hamberg, M., and Jonsson, C. E. (1973): *Acta Physiol. Scand.,* 87:270–276.
2. Beck, P. W., and Handwerker, H. O. (1974): *Pfluegers Arch.,* 347:209–222.
3. Beck, P. W., Handwerker, H. O., and Zimmermann, M. (1974): *Brain Res.,* 67:373–386.
4. Ferreira, S. H., Moncada, S., and Vane, J. R. (1973): *Br. J. Pharmacol.,* 49:86–97.
5. Ferreira, S. H., and Vane, J. R. (1967): *Nature,* 216:868–873.
6. Handwerker, H. O. (1975): *Pfluegers Arch.,* 355:R116.
7. McQueen, D. S., and Belmonte, C. (1974): *Q. J. Exp. Physiol.,* 59:63–71.
8. Moncada, S., Ferreira, S. H., and Vane, J. R. (1975): *Eur. J. Pharmacol.,* 31:250–260.
9. Willis, A. L. (1969): *J. Pharm. Pharmacol.,* 21:126–128.

Advances in Pain Research and Therapy, Vol. 1,
edited by J. J. Bonica and D. Albe-Fessard.
Raven Press, New York © 1976.

Human Skin Nociceptors and Their Chemical Response

M. S. Dash and S. S. Deshpande

Department of Physiology and Pharmacology, Vallabhbhai Patel Chest Institute, Delhi University, Delhi 7, India

The role of human subjects in a study of sensation is invaluable in neurophysiology. Objective signs, however direct—whether recorded from sensory cortex, tracts, fibers, or receptors—are poor substitutes for a verbal description by a human observer of the sensory experience. Numerous studies have been made on sensory mechanisms. Recording techniques have been vastly improved, but today neural discharges cannot be directly equated with evoked sensations. Lack of a reliable method for selective stimulation of one group of fibers or receptors with the exclusion of others seriously limits the interpretation of the results (even of the single-unit discharges recorded through microelectrodes from the peripheral nerves in conscious subjects). This is because contributions from other fibers and receptors, activated by the stimulus process toward the sensations evoked, remain unknown.

Alternatively, under such circumstances one may explore situations in which in otherwise healthy subjects, deafferentation has been caused pathologically. One such unique situation is seen in leprosy. Sensory dissociations with this disease are well documented. Often sensations of touch, pain, heat, and cold are lost separately in random order in various combinations, or they may be entirely absent in some areas of the skin with normal sensations preserved perfectly in others. Higher nervous functions appear unaffected, so such patients provide an excellent opportunity to study cutaneous sensations at certain stages of the disease.

In an earlier investigation, Dash (2) noted that some patients observed delayed pain and itching on completely anesthetic skin after mosquito bites. Others experienced itching and pain on the anesthetic skin when scabies or eczematous rashes were superadded. It was thought, therefore, that pain and itch sensations might be chemically induced from the anesthetic skin. If so, it would be technically possible to study pain and itch in isolation from other sensations.

MATERIAL AND METHODS

Of the several methods available for the study of pain and itch in man, the technique described by Keele and Armstrong (4) has a special advantage in that stimuli can be applied without mechanical or thermal excitation of the receptors under study. Aware that the technique provides only indirect information about the site of action of the chemicals and the nature of fibers and receptors stimulated, we used the above method in the present study. However, we limited the number of unknown variables by deliberately selecting as the site of study anesthetic skin where touch, pain (mechanical), heat, and cold receptive elements were absent or inactive, or their doubtful contributions—if any—could be neglected.

Experiments were conducted in 10 healthy volunteers and in 17 leprosy patients from the Leprosarium Shahadra. All 17 subjects gave informed consent for the study. Their ages ranged from 20 to 56 years, and the duration of illness from 3 to 23 years. All had received treatment in the past 3 to 4 years, and each had had complete anesthesia over his right forearm for several years. Some patients' entire forearms and hands were also anesthetic.

Usual clinical methods were employed in the examination with the leprosy patients. An area fully anesthetic to touch, heat, cold, and pain (pinprick) sensations and another area with all sensations intact were selected for raising two blisters. With the control subjects, only one blister was raised, on the right forearm, by applying cantharidin plaster (BPC 1949).

Effects of Chemicals on Blister Bases and Observations

The blister bases on the anesthetic skin were also found to be anesthetic to touch, mechanical pain, heat, and cold sensations. After confirming this, we applied various algogenic chemicals to the raw bases. The responses were recorded in the manner described by Keele and Armstrong (4). All solutions were isotonic with blood and had neutral pH, except when the effects of pH and hypertonicity were studied. The chemicals that were used included: pH_4 sodium acid phosphate 2.6%; pH_3 HCl; KCl 858 mEq/l; NaCl 855 mEq/l; histamine acid phosphate; phenyl diguanide; 5-HT creatinine sulfate; acetylcholine (ACh) and trypsin, each at a concentration of 10^{-3} g/ml, and capsaicin at two concentrations of 10^{-5} g/ml and 2×10^{-3} g/ml. In the beginning of the experiment, a standard dose of KCl solution known to produce severe pain in the volunteers was applied over the control blister on the normal skin of each patient. The intensity of pain was always severe and was used as a reference to grade pain later in the experiment.

The subjects could record the extent of pain on a rotating drum by pulling a mechanical writing device. The drum was kept out of sight of the subjects. There was no conversation with the subjects during application of the chemicals, nor did they know the nature of the chemicals applied. Verbal descriptions of the responses were recorded at the end of each application. The extent of pain was measured from the heights recorded over the drum for correlation with the verbal report. Each chemical was applied several times at random after a minimum interval of 15 to 20 min between two applications. The mean response was calculated at the end of the experiment.

RESULTS

In general, the intensity of responses was mild or moderate in the anesthetic skin. The character of pain was mostly described as burning. Two constant features in the production of pain were a long latency of onset often extending to 10 to 15 sec and sometimes a prolonged duration of pain for more than 2 min. The long duration of pain after a single chemical application cannot be explained entirely by afterdischarges or by assuming that the chemicals acted on nerve fibers which obey the all-or-none principle. Prolonged sensation depends on a continuous flow of impulses. Since a single application produced persistent pain, the site of action could have been the receptors.

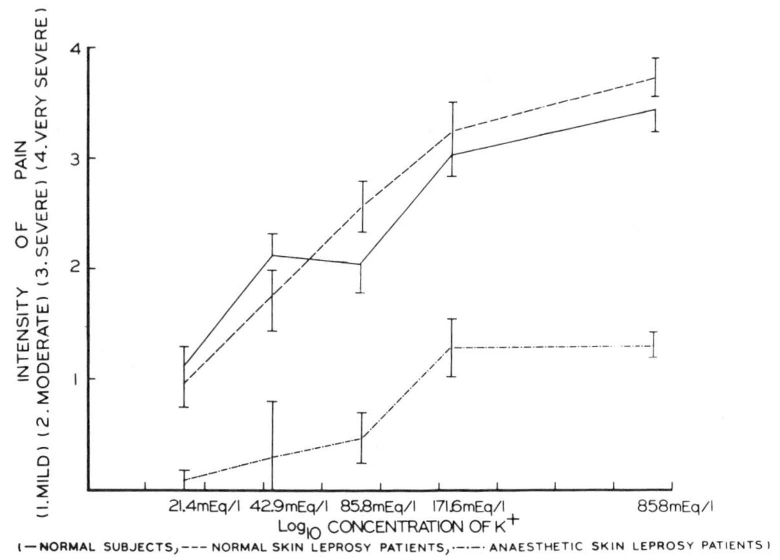

FIG. 1. Effects of potassium chloride on blister base. Dose-response relationship. Note the increasing pain responses with increasing concentrations of K^+.

KCl was found to be the most effective pain-producing agent in this study, whereas NaCl in almost equimolar concentration had no effect in the anesthetic base. (Figure 1 shows the dose-response relationship with KCl.) Application of histamine produced pain initially, followed by prolonged itching. There was a distinct time lag between the onset of pain and the onset of itching. Since one type of receptor normally signals one sensory modality, histamine probably acted at two different sites.

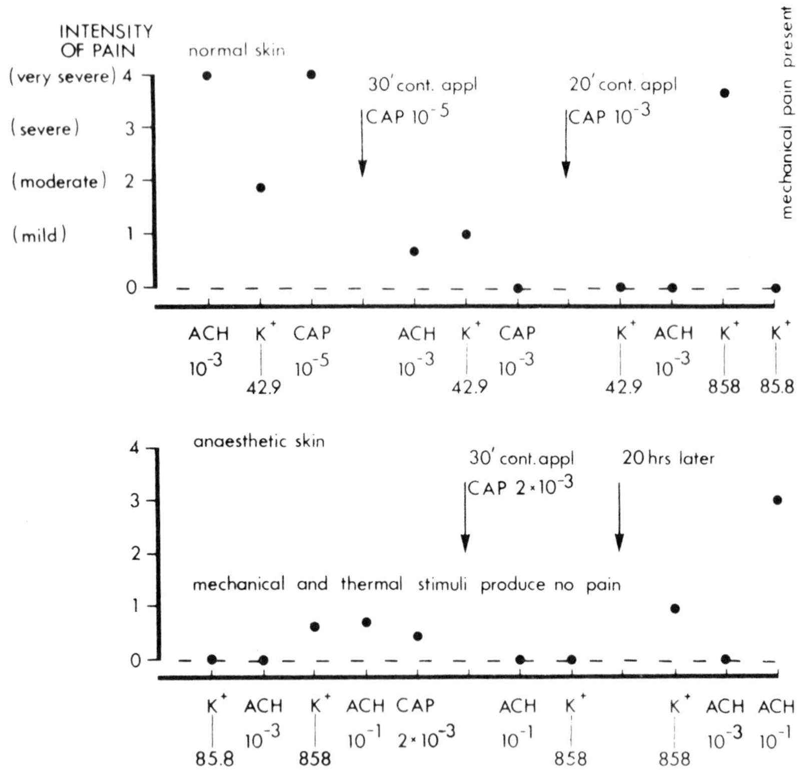

FIG. 2. Prolonged application of capsaicin (CAP) on blister base. Note the effects of capsaicin desensitization of the normal and anesthetic bases. Mechanical and thermal pain were present after desensitization in the normal base but completely absent in the anesthetic base. The desensitization was so complete in the latter that KCl elicited no response. But 20 hr later the base recovered remarkably and responded to acetylcholine (ACH) and KCl. Concentrations are expressed as g/ml for ACH and capsaicin and as mEq/l for K^+.

Janscó (3) observed that capsaicin applied to the skin produces burning pain (owing to the stimulation of pain receptors), but repeated application desensitizes these end organs with no pain produced on further application of capsaicin or other pain-producing chemicals. During the period of such desensitization, however, natural stimuli (mechanical) like touch and pin-prick remain unaffected.

The effect of capsaicin was, therefore, studied both in the normal and anesthetic bases. The intensity of pain was severe to very severe in the normal bases, but mild or moderate in the anesthetic bases. Mechanical and thermal stimuli were effective in the normal bases even during capsaicin desensitization, but the anesthetic bases remained as insensitive as before (see Fig. 2).

In the anesthetic skin, prolonged application for 30 min completely desensitized the neural elements, not only for capsaicin but also for acetylcholine. However, under conditions of capsaicin desensitization, KCl was still able to produce pain. Therefore, if capsaicin and KCl acted on the same neural elements, the site of action of KCl might be other than the one desensitized by capsaicin, or else KCl overcame the capsaicin desensitization.

COMMENT

Bessou and Perl (1) described a type of nociceptor (the so-called polymodal type) in the cat's skin, which responds to different types of nociceptive stimuli: mechanical, thermal, and chemical. More recently, similar receptors have been described in the human skin by Torebjörk (5). However, there was nothing to suggest their presence in the anesthetic base. Excessive thermal stimuli (60°C and 0° to 4°C) and pinprick with pressures up to 12 g produced no pain. Pain, although of mild or moderate intensity, could be induced from the anesthetic bases only by application of nociceptive chemicals. In these bases touch sensations were also absent. Any possible contribution by touch receptors to the pain observed could, therefore, be ruled out. The surviving receptive element in the anesthetic skin appeared to be specific for chemical stimulation, which produced pain, itching, or both. Based on the above observations, it may be suggested that specific chemosensory nociceptive elements may be present in the human skin.

ACKNOWLEDGMENTS

This investigation was conducted under the auspices of the Armed Forces Medical Research Committee, Ministry of Defence, New Delhi, India. The authors thank Prof. A. S. Paintal, the DG AFMS, the DMR, and the patients who took part in this study.

REFERENCES

1. Bessou, P., and Perl, E. R. (1969): *J. Neurophysiol.*, 32:1025–1043.
2. Dash, M. S. (1973): A study of the peripheral nerves in leprosy and later on nerve injuries. AFMRC, 306/68.
3. Janscó, N. (1968): In: *Proceedings of the 3rd International Pharmacological Meeting, Vol 9*. Pergamon Press, Oxford and New York.
4. Keele, C. A., and Armstrong, D. (1964): *Substances Producing Pain and Itch*. Edward Arnold Ltd., London.
5. Torebjörk, E. (1974): *Acta Physiol. Scand.*, 92:374–390.

Advances in Pain Research and Therapy, Vol. 1,
edited by J. J. Bonica and D. Albe-Fessard.
Raven Press, New York © 1976.

Irreversible Selective Blocking of Cutaneous Myelinated Fibers by Local Heating

M. Zimmermann

II. Physiologisches Institut der Universität Heidelberg, Heidelberg, Germany

Various methods have been reported previously for reversible selective blocking of myelinated (A) fibers, preserving the nonmyelinated (C) fibers (see 5). These methods have been applied to study the effects in the central nervous system of pure afferent C volleys. In this investigation local heating of the nerve was used to perform an irreversible selective block of myelinated fibers.

METHODS

In cats anesthetized by either pentobarbital sodium (initial dose 40 mg/kg) or N_2O/halothane-oxygen mixtures, the sural (SU), superficial peroneal (SP), and posterior tibial (PT) nerves of the hind leg were exposed. Two sections of each nerve, separated by approximately 60 mm, were prepared for bipolar electrical stimulation (distal) and recording (proximal) of the compound action potentials. Between these electrode pairs an additional section of nerve was separated from the underlying muscle and connective tissue, placed in the groove of a brass thermode, and covered with a brass lid. Between these three sites of dissection the nerve was left in its natural connective tissue environment to prevent the spread of stimulus current and to preserve the blood supply to the nerve. The latter was presumably essential for the success of a long-term differential block.

The length of nerve in contact with the thermode was 15 mm. Any space between the walls of the thermode groove and the nerve was filled by cotton wool soaked with saline. The temperature of the thermode was set by irrigation from thermostats; temperature could be raised from 37°C to higher levels (e.g., 50°C) by switching the irrigation from one thermostat to another. Consecutive 1- or 2-min periods of heating were applied until the A fibers were blocked completely. These periods were separated by intervals of approximately 10 min.

The temperature of the nerve was recorded by a fine thermocouple in contact with the nerve. The temperature gradient across the nerve did not exceed 1.5°C in the thickest nerves. The temperatures given in this investigation are those evaluated for the core of the nerve.

RESULTS

In Fig. 1 the compound action potentials of nonmyelinated (part A) and myelinated (part B) fibers of a PT nerve are displayed. The total time of heating to 50°C is indicated between the records. After 7.5 min the amplitude of the group II volley is diminished to 13% of the initial value; after 12.5 min of heating it has disappeared completely. The corresponding decrements of the C volley are to 97% and 67% after 7.5 and 12.5 min, respectively. This yields a selectivity coefficient of 0.67, which has been defined (5,6) as the C amplitude when the group II fibers were blocked totally, relative to the initial size of the C volley.

In six experiments a total of 12 irreversible nerve blocks were performed on the SU, SP, and PT nerves. The selectivity coefficients ranged from 0 (2 cases in which both A and C volleys declined in parallel) to 0.67. The highest values were obtained in PT nerves; the average from five experiments was 0.51. The mean value of all the 12 trials was 0.33. In the 12 experiments the total time necessary to achieve a complete block of the group II fibers ranged from 1 to 15 min, with an average of 8.3 min. The group III action potential, if discernible in the mass volley, disappeared with a time course similar to that of the group II fibers. The temperatures used ranged between 45° and 54°C, but in most experiments it was 50°C. The time required for a group II block to be obtained tended to be shorter at higher temperatures. Presumably, however, the selectivity of the block was impaired at higher temperature. More experiments are needed to clarify these details.

As was shown by an experiment performed under sterile conditions, the block persisted even after 2 weeks.

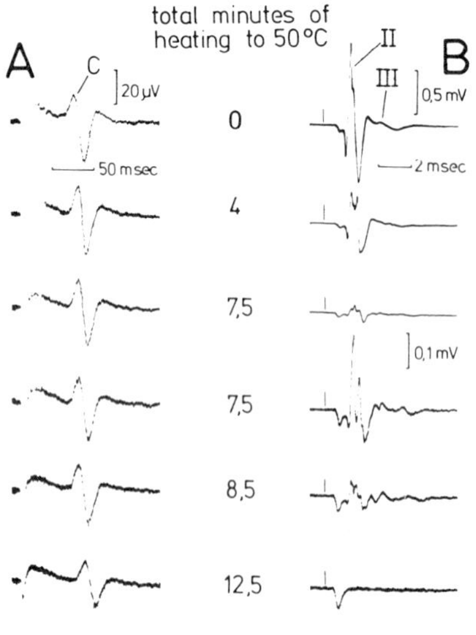

FIG. 1. Effect of local heating on A and C fibers. Recording of compound action potentials from the posterior tibial nerve; conduction distance, 58 mm. **A:** Display of C volleys, stimuli were 25 V, 0.5 msec in duration. **B:** Display of A volleys, stimuli were 1.5 V, 0.1 msec in duration. Numbers between columns indicate the total time of heating the nerve to 50°C for a length of 15 mm between stimulating and recording sites. Downward deflection persisting in bottom trace of **B** when the A volley had disappeared completely is an electrotonic spread of action current from a remote site of the nerve. Calibration above the 4th trace in **B** holds for the last 3 traces.

DISCUSSION

No mechanism can be offered to explain this preferential irreversible block of A fibers by local heating. A clue might be derived from the finding that heating depolarizes C fibers but not A fibers (1). This observation was fully confirmed in our experiments: during nerve heating vigorous ongoing discharges occurred in the C fibers but not in the A fibers, which indicates different influences of elevated temperatures on the excitable membranes.

Contrasting blocking effects have been obtained in excised saphenous nerves of the cat heated *in vitro* either by radiofrequency current or by conducted heat (3). In these preparations the vulnerability of nerve fiber groups increased in the sequence: II, C, III. Hence C fibers were blocked before II fibers in these *in vitro* studies. This effect might be caused by the absence of blood supply to the nerves: it is well established that C fibers are more vulnerable than thick myelinated fibers to changes in the extracellular fluid composition (2,4).

The irreversible differential block of A fibers obtained by our procedure is suitable for various experimental approaches to clarify the central connections of C fibers and their role in sensation. Since a large portion of C fibers are nociceptive afferents, such preparations might be used for studying the effects of predominant nociceptive input without a concomitant low-threshold input via A fibers. Thus the heat block, exempting part of the C fibers, possibly provides an experimental model for chronic pain.

ACKNOWLEDGMENT

This work was supported by the Deutsche Forschungsgemeinschaft, grant Zi 110.

REFERENCES

1. Euler, C. von (1947): *Acta Physiol. Scand.* [Suppl. 14], 45:1–75.
2. Jewett, D. L., and King, J. S. (1971): *Exp. Neurol.,* 33:225–237.
3. Letcher, F. S., and Goldring, S. (1968): *J. Neurosurg.,* 29:42–47.
4. Nathan, P. W., and Sears, T. A. (1962): *J. Physiol.,* 164:375–394.
5. Sassen, M., and Zimmermann, M. (1973): *Pfluegers Arch.,* 341:179–195.
6. Zimmermann, M. (1968): *Pfluegers Arch.,* 301:329–333.

Advances in Pain Research and Therapy, Vol. 1,
edited by J. J. Bonica and D. Albe-Fessard.
Raven Press, New York © 1976.

Differential Block of Cutaneous Nerve Fibers with Triangularly Shaped Stimulus Pulses

Neri Accornero, Giorgio Bini, and Mario Manfredi

I° Clinica delle Malattie Nervose e Mentali dell'Universita di Roma, Viale dell'Universita 30, Rome, Italy

Polarization of peripheral nerve by direct current blocks axonal conduction differentially, starting from larger fibers. The method operates by displacing the resting membrane potential of the axons to a level that inactivates spike propagation; conduction block is established in larger fibers first because of their greater internal conductance. Polarization is commonly accomplished with a couple of polarizing electrodes, independent of the stimulating ones, and placed on a separate portion of nerve (4–6,8–10). In our laboratory a new technique currently being used (1,2) allows the selective activation of fiber groups of different conduction velocities with a single pair of stimulating-polarizing electrodes.

METHODS

The method takes advantage of triangularly shaped stimulus pulses, with a steep rise front and a slow exponential decay, delivered through a couple of silver–silver chloride leads. The electrodes are placed on a restricted portion of nerve that is carefully dissected and distally sectioned. The recording site is a few centimeters away. The rising wave form of the triangular shock activates conducted spikes at the level of the cathodal lead, while the slowly decaying polarization blocks the fiber conduction under the anode without additional activation at the end of the pulse. By graduating the height and the duration of the triangular pulse it is possible in a cutaneous nerve to activate selectively: the largest myelinated beta or group 2 fibers with conduction velocity of 30 to 60 m/sec; the small myelinated delta or group 3 fibers with conduction velocity of 5 to 30 m/sec; or the unmyelinated C fibers or group 4 with conduction velocity of 0.5 to 2 m/sec. Triangular pulses of 5 to 30 V, 2 to 5 msec are generally used. The triangular shape is obtained by integration of a conventional square wave with a potentiometer and a condenser in parallel. The height and the decaying time of the triangular pulse can be adjusted by grading the strength of the incoming square wave or by varying the capacity of the condenser.

The method is currently applied on saphenous and sural nerves of the cat, but it has been used successfully to differentiate fast from slowly conducting fibers in somatic as well as in visceral nerves. A typical experiment is displayed in Fig. 1. On the left column, triangular pulses of progressively increasing strength are represented. The middle and right columns show the development of selective activation. The beta compound wave is activated initially (middle column, rows 1 and 2) and subsequently is progressively blocked (rows 3 to 7). The delta compound potentials develop at higher stimulus strength, coincident with failure of beta wave propagation, and in rows 7 to 9 an almost pure delta potential can be seen. Further raising the stimulus strength blocks the delta wave as well (rows 9 to 11). Next, the C wave is elicited and finally blocked. The right column shows an almost pure C wave (rows 10 to 12) at a slower time base. All myelinated components are blocked on traces simultaneously recorded at a faster time base in the middle column.

Plotting on the X-Y axis in another experiment (Fig. 2) shows that raising the stimulation strength makes the delta wave begin to appear when the beta wave is completely developed. This effect is still maximal when the beta inflection is blocked. The C elevation begins in the tail of the delta wave and reaches its 100% value when the delta wave is blocked. In this way pure beta, delta, and C potentials can be elicited by applying stimuli of appropriate strength (Fig. 2, *vertical bars*). The method also allows propagation of trains of selectively activated delta or C fibers without relevant decrement in subsequent volleys.

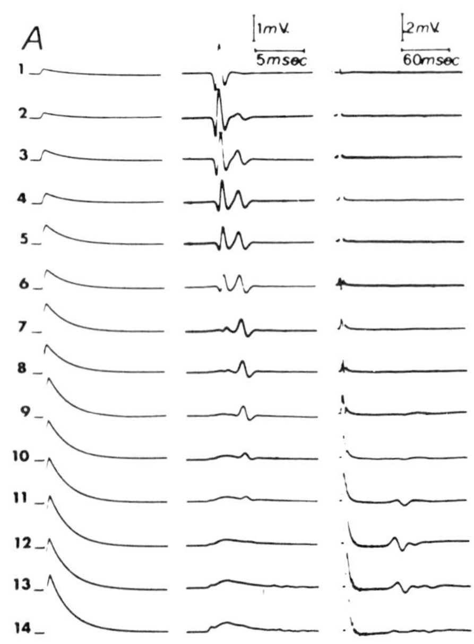

FIG. 1. Selective activation of peripheral nerve fiber groups. Left column: stimulating pulse. Middle and right columns: compound action potentials at different speeds and gains to show earlier components (*middle column*) and C wave (*right column*).

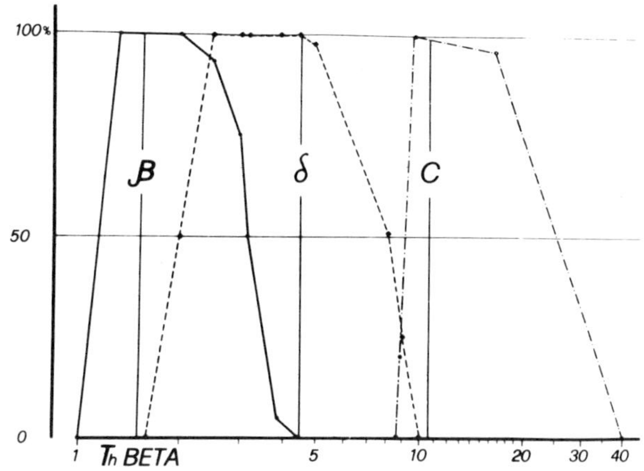

FIG. 2. Plot of the development of selective activation. Abscissa: stimulation strength as multiples of threshold activation of the beta wave. Ordinates: action potential amplitude as percent of maximum amplitude. Continuous line: beta wave. Dotted line: delta wave. Hatched line: C wave. Vertical bars: stimulus voltage evoking pure beta, delta, and C deflection.

Mode of Action of the Triangularly Shaped Stimulus

The separation among fiber groups by the triangularly shaped stimulus pulse can rely on two differential mechanisms. Polarization at the anodal site can block the conduction differentially by displacing the resting membrane potential to a level that inactivates the spike propagation. Since the flow of current in a fiber is proportional to the square of its diameter, larger fibers are blocked at lower current intensities. A second differential factor is caused by the different conduction velocities of the fibers. If the current pulse is removed at the anode before the slowly conducted waves arrive, only the fastest ones are subjected to polarization and consequently are blocked. A method of this kind has been employed by Kuffler and Vaughan-Williams (7) on the motor nerve of frog.

Selective activation of fiber groups by triangular pulses takes advantage of both these mechanisms. The relevance of different internal conductance has been demonstrated by testing the fiber excitability around the anodally polarized region during the delivery of a triangular pulse. Fiber excitability at the anodal site was depressed to a greater extent in larger fibers, and during the decaying phase of the triangular pulse it returned to its pre-polarization level more rapidly in smaller fibers. Bishop and Erlanger (3) discovered that the threshold of excitability is related to the level of polarization of the fiber membrane. This experiment therefore demonstrates that the membrane potential displacement at the anode is differential and is directly proportional to the fiber diameter.

The relevance of the second mechanism, namely, the conduction velocity, is demonstrated by the improvement of the selectivity of the activation which follows the increase of the conduction distance from the cathode to the anode of the stimulating = polarizing couple. As previously stated, propagated spikes are fired at the cathode and conduction is blocked under the anode. A quantum of current is required to block the beta spike. When the delta spike comes later, a larger quantum of current is required for hyperpolarization because of higher internal resistance of the delta fibers, and by that time the anodal polarizing voltage is significantly less because of pulse decay. At greater cathode = anode distance, the difference between the level of polarization encountered at the anodal site by beta and delta spikes increases, and the differential power is consequently improved.

Single-Fiber Recording

Selective activation of peripheral nerve fiber groups allows a satisfactory separation among compound potentials of different conduction velocities. However, compound waves are generally considered a rough method of estimation of conducted spikes. The selectivity of the differential effect has been therefore controlled by recording single myelinated units during selective activation of compound waves. A total of 238 beta and 41 delta units have been recorded from fine strands dissected from the nerve trunk or the corresponding dorsal roots; the compound potentials were concurrently recorded from the whole nerve.

In the experiments in which the compound waves indicated that the differential effect was satisfactory, practically all beta units (178 out of 179) were activated and subsequently were blocked together with the activation and block of the corresponding beta compound wave; only one unit survived the disappearance of the beta wave. The 22 delta units studied in these conditions showed the same behavior, as they were activated together with the delta wave and were still conducting when the beta wave was completely blocked. Failure of conduction in these fibers was accompanied by disappearance of the delta compound wave. A small number of units (59 beta and 19 delta) were recorded during three experiments in which the behavior of the mass potential indicated a poor differential effect. The behavior of these units corresponded to the indication of the gross neurogram, as half of beta units (33 out of 59) were blocked together with the beta compound wave, but in coincidence with a reduction of delta wave amplitude. Instead, the delta units continued to conduct within the strict response range of the delta compound potential.

CONCLUSION

In conclusion, selective activation with triangular pulses allows a satisfactory degree of separation between beta and delta fibers, i.e., complete beta block in the face of a 5% delta fiber loss. This result can be achieved in our hands in about 70% of experiments. Selective C activation has a greater safety margin and could be obtained in practically any experiment.

REFERENCES

1. Accornero, N., Bini, G., Lenzi, G. L., and Manfredi, M.: *In preparation.*
2. Accornero, N., Bini, G., and Manfredi, M.: *In preparation.*
3. Bishop, G. H., and Erlanger, J. (1926): *Am. J. Physiol.,* 78:630–657.
4. Brown, A. G., and Hamann, W. C. (1972): *J. Physiol.,* 222:66P.
5. Casey, K. L., and Blick, M. (1969): *Brain Res.,* 13:155–167.
6. Kuffler, S. W., and Gerard, R. W. (1947): *J. Neurophysiol.,* 10:383–394.
7. Kuffler, S. W., and Vaughan-Williams, E. M. (1953): *J. Physiol.,* 121:289–317.
8. Manfredi, M. (1970): *Arch. Ital. Biol.,* 108:52–71.
9. Mendell, L. M., and Wall, P. D. (1964): *J. Physiol.* (Lond.), 172:274–294.
10. Zimmermann, M. (1968): *Pfluegers Arch.,* 301:329–333.

Advances in Pain Research and Therapy, Vol. 1,
edited by J. J. Bonica and D. Albe-Fessard.
Raven Press, New York © 1976.

Neurophysiological Investigation of the Development of Heat Nociceptors in Regenerating Cutaneous Nerves of the Cat

H. Dickhaus, M. Zimmermann, and *Y. Zotterman

II. Physiologisches Institut der Universität Heidelberg, Heidelberg, Germany

In a cutaneous nerve regenerating after an experimentally produced lesion, all types of receptors of the hairy skin with myelinated afferents have been found with electrophysiological methods (4). The redevelopment of the receptor endings of nonmyelinated fibers, however, has not yet been reported. We have investigated this question with particular emphasis on cutaneous C heat receptors, which presumably are nociceptive in function (1).

METHOD

In 9 cats the medial and lateral plantar nerves, which innervate the skin and joints of the hind foot, were crushed over a length of 5 mm between 20 and 40 mm proximal to the center of the large footpad. The lesions were induced in a sterile operation under halothane/N_2O-O_2 anesthesia. In a separate experiment using recordings from single nerve fibers, it was shown that our crushing procedure interrupted conduction in quantitatively all myelinated (groups II and III) and nonmyelinated (C) fibers.

In subsequent experiments performed between 1 and 92 days after the nerve crush, single units were recorded from fine nerve strands dissected from the posterior tibial nerve, which contains the plantar nerves. All the fibers in a nerve filament that could be stimulated electrically from the plantar nerves at a site proximal to the previous crush were tested systematically for peripheral excitability by adequate mechanical and thermal stimulation. This chapter is concerned primarily with C heat receptors.

C heat receptor characteristics were studied quantitatively applying temperature-controlled radiant heat to the skin, as has been described previously (1).

RESULTS

Regenerating C fibers were not excitable by adequate skin stimulation before 28 days after the nerve lesions were induced. Afterward all three types

* Visiting Professor at Heidelberg University.

of C-fiber receptors described so far in the skin of the foot region reappeared in increasing numbers: low-threshold mechanoreceptors (2,7,9), mechanosensitive nociceptors (3), and heat receptors (1,6). At 40 days after crush and subsequently, C heat receptors accounted for approximately 18% of all C fibers in the plantar nerves. This value is practically the same as that found in normal nerves (1).

In all, 15 C heat receptors were found. Their thresholds to heating the skin of the receptive field ranged from 32° to 46°C. The cumulative probability distribution of the thermal thresholds is displayed in Fig. 1; the median value is 38.7°C. The broken line in Fig. 1 is the corresponding distribution of temperature thresholds of a control sample of 40 C heat receptors found in normal nerves (1); the median of these is 42.4°C. Thus the threshold distribution of our sample of C heat receptors in regenerating

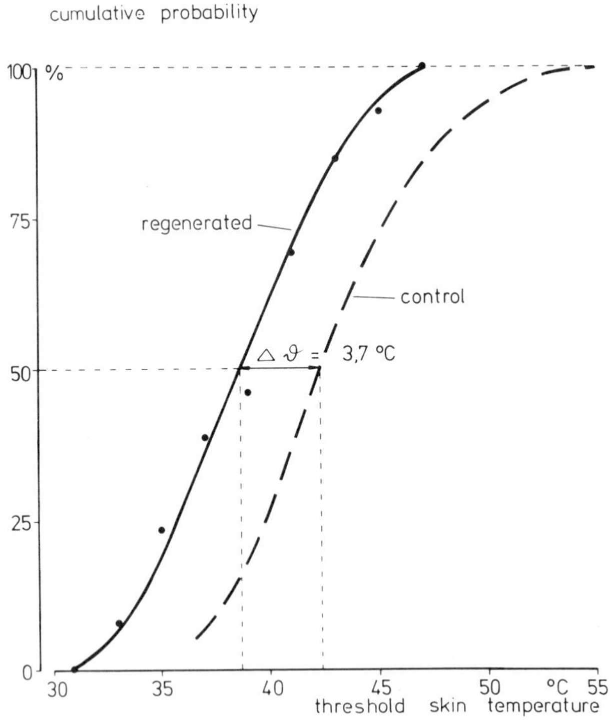

FIG. 1. Temperature thresholds of regenerated C heat receptors. Continuous curve plots the cumulative frequency of occurrence (*ordinate*) of temperature thresholds (*abscissa*) for a population of 13 regenerated C heat receptors; threshold criterion was the generation of at least 1 spike during a heat stimulus 10 sec in duration. Broken line shows the cumulative probability function of 40 C heat receptors sampled from normal nerves—results from Beck et al. (1). Indicated median values: 38.7°C and 42.4°C for the regenerated and control nerves, respectively.

nerves is shifted to lower temperatures by about 3.7°C relative to the thresholds of the C heat receptors of normal nerves.

In 11 of these regenerated C fibers, we measured intensity functions—i.e., the number of impulses discharged during 10 sec of heating—and plotted them against temperature. A linear correlation was found in most of these units between the temperature of the stimulus and the number of spikes per stimulus. The average intensity function calculated for these 11 receptors exhibited a shift to lower temperatures by about 3°C relative to the corresponding curve in normal animals. This shift of the intensity function is in agreement with the shift in threshold (Fig. 1).

DISCUSSION

The quantitative investigation of C heat receptors that develop in reinnervated skin reveals an increased sensitivity to radiant heat. By extrapolating this finding to the human nervous system, one might speculate that it represents a neurophysiological basis of hyperalgesia and hyperpathia, which are known to appear during nerve regeneration (5,8). Unfortunately, no measurements from psychophysical experiments are available for a quantitative evaluation of these reports of altered skin sensibility in man. Therefore, behavioral tests are going to be performed on cats after nerve lesions have been induced to correlate the escape reactions to graded heat stimuli with the neurophysiological data on C heat receptors.

ACKNOWLEDGMENT

This work was supported by the Deutsche Forschungsgemeinschaft, grant Zi 110.

REFERENCES

1. Beck, P. W., Handwerker, H. O., and Zimmermann, M. (1974) *Brain Res.*, 67:373–386.
2. Bessou, P., Burgess, P. R., Perl, E. R., and Taylor, C. B. (1971): *J. Neurophysiol.*, 34:116–131.
3. Bessou, P., and Perl, E. R. (1969): *J. Neurophysiol.*, 32:1025–1043.
4. Burgess, P. R., and Horch, K. W. (1973): *J. Neurophysiol.*, 36:101–114.
5. Head, H. (1920): *Studies in Neurology*. Oxford University Press, London.
6. Iggo, A. (1959): *Q. J. Exp. Physiol.*, 44:362–370.
7. Iggo, A. (1960): *J. Physiol.*, 152:337–353.
8. Trotter, W., and Davies, H. M. (1908): *J. Physiol.*, 38:134–246.
9. Zimmermann, M. (1976): In: *Somatosensory System*, edited by H. H. Kornhuber. Thieme Verlag, Stuttgart, pp. 45–53.

Advances in Pain Research and Therapy, Vol. 1,
edited by J. J. Bonica and D. Albe-Fessard.
Raven Press, New York © 1976.

Bradykinin as a Tool in Neurophysiological Studies of Pain Mechanisms

*G. Guilbaud, **D. Le Bars, and J. M. Besson

Laboratoire de Physiologie des Centres Nerveux, Université Pierre et Marie Curie, 4, Avenue Gordon-Bennet, 75016, Paris, France

It is well known that bradykinin (Bk), a nonapeptide that can be formed in plasma and inflammatory exudates, plays an important part in producing pain and the vascular responses of inflammation (18). As reported by Lim (21), the different Bk peptides have been found to be highly active in producing pain when injected intra-arterially or intraperitoneally in man and animals. As we initially mentioned (5), the intensity and relatively long duration of painful sensations and of nociceptive reactions induced by Bk in man and animals made it appear that its administration would be of great interest in the study of CNS structures involved in pain phenomena. By injecting Bk intra-arterially into the limbs, we have considered the role of spinal dorsal horn interneurons (2–4,20), of bulbar and mesencephalic reticular units (5,14,23), and of some thalamic units (10,13). The data obtained with this type of approach agree with those found by considering classic approaches, i.e., peripheral natural cutaneous stimulation or electrical stimulation of peripheral nerves. Moreover, we found that the latency and duration of unitary responses induced by Bk were of the same order as those of painful sensations in man and pseudoaffective reactions in animals.

However, several authors have objected to the method and conclusions. Beck and Handwerker (1) stated that the intra-arterial injection of Bk cannot be considered "specific noxious stimulation." Zimmermann (26) stated that "most of the activity measured in dorsal horn cells [as a result of Bk injection] arises in slowly adapting mechano-receptors." Lim et al. (22) showed that 75% of the splanchnic nerve fibers activated by Bk were in groups 3 and 4, whereas Mense and Schmidt (24) reported that group 4 afferent units from muscles were strongly activated by this substance. Moreover, studies performed on peripheral cutaneous fibers suggested that Bk has no specific effect on the fibers involved in pain processes. After applying Bk on "abraded skin" or injecting it into a "skin cut," Burgess and Perl (8) found no activation in thin fibers. Fjällbrant and Iggo (11), using

* Maitre de Recherche INSERM
** Atraché de Recherche INSERM

closed intra-arterial injections, showed that the tested slowly adapting pressure receptors with myelinated afferent fibers were all excited by Bk injection, whereas "unmyelinated fibres in the same strand were excited only very feebly if at all." More recently, Beck and Handwerker (1) found activation in unmyelinated fibers (group 4 or C) and also in myelinated afferent fibers (groups 2 and 3) of the slowly adapting mechanoreceptors.

Notwithstanding these authoritative reports, we feel that messages carried by different fiber types have to be integrated at one or more levels of the CNS before being recognized as noxious. Therefore, in our opinion, the major point is to consider the output of cells involved in transmitting and integrating nociceptive messages and to try to determine the relative influence of A and C inputs after intra-arterial administration of Bk into the limbs. This question is particularly pertinent for the lamina V–type cells of the dorsal horn, which receive both A and C inputs and are preferentially activated by the intra-arterial injection of Bk into the posterior limb (3,20) or into the mesenteric artery (2) of cat. Data derived from different studies performed by our group suggest that the excitatory effects observed at the central level after Bk administration are mainly caused by increase of the C-fiber input. This chapter reports some of these studies and summarizes both direct and indirect evidence that supports our thesis.

METHODS

In spinal cats, lumbar dorsal horn interneurons (located between 1,200 and 2,000 μm) receiving cutaneous ipsilateral afferents from the sural nerve were studied. All the other nerves of the limb had been sectioned previously. The electrical stimulation of the sural nerve and the recording of its evoked responses allowed the characterization of the afferent groups affecting the cells. Also, cells were characterized by considering peripheral natural cutaneous stimulation, and their peripheral excitatory fields (PEF) were delimited. The cells were then tested for their response to Bk injection into a small branch of the ipsilateral femoral artery. Additional injections were performed during a temporary cold block of A fibers using the technique of Franz and Iggo (12) and Iggo (17) (Fig. 1).

RESULTS

Direct Evidence

Direct evidence supporting our hypothesis has been obtained from studies of the activity of dorsal horn interneurons receiving input from: (a) A fibers; (b) A and C fibers with subsequent cold block of A fibers; and (c) only C fibers.

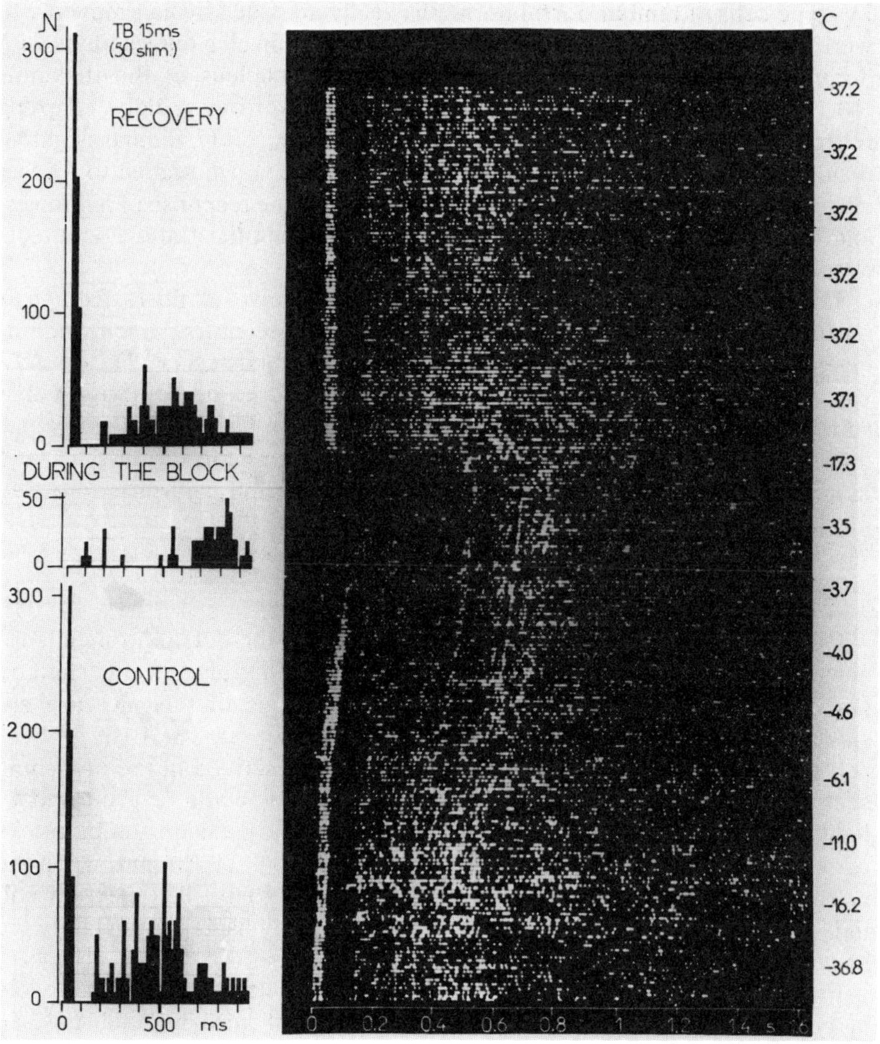

FIG. 1. Response of a dorsal horn cell to stimulation of the ipsilateral sural nerve. Each row of dot raster (*right*) shows spike activity for 1.6 sec after each stimulus; change in response from top to bottom shows the effects of cold block (temperatures at right) on conduction in the peripheral nerve. Histograms at left show density of spikes during first sec following stimulus before, during, and after cold block.

A-Afferent Fibers

Dorsal horn cells receiving sural input via A fibers only were activated by hair movement or light touch or light pressure applied in the PEF but were not modified by Bk administration. This observation is in agreement with the previous results of Besson et al. (3) who showed that the lamina

IV–type cells of lumbar dorsal horn, phasically activated by hair movement, were rarely affected by Bk injection. The observation also corresponds with our results obtained in the ventroposterolateral nucleus of the thalamus (10,13). These data indicate that afferent fibers from rapidly adapting receptors (groups 2 and 3) are never excited by Bk (1,11). Similar negative results were also reported by Smith and Creech (25), who failed to find an effect of many different pharmacological agents on the response of hair discs, and by Lim et al. (22), who found no effect of Bk on the Vater-Pacini corpuscle afferents.

The dorsal horn cells we have considered receive A fibers from hair receptors and also from slowly adapting mechanoreceptors, which, according to Fjällbrant and Iggo (11) and Beck and Handwerker (1), are activated by Bk. Moreover, electrical stimulation of the nerve showed that some of these dorsal horn cells were driven by A α fibers and also by A δ fibers, both of which are equally activated by Bk according to Beck and Handwerker (1). Nevertheless, in these cases the interneurons were also not affected by Bk.

A and C Fibers

Our data show that the spontaneous activity of the dorsal horn cells receiving sural afferents of both A and C fiber types was always enhanced by Bk injection. The latency, duration, and magnitude of this increase are similar to those that have been described previously (3). The PEF of these cells were usually wider than those of the cells described in the preceding section but were rarely larger than 1 cm^2. Excitation could be produced by light touch or hair movement, but pinches, strong pressure, or pinpricks evoked sustained tonic discharges. During cold block of A input, when the cell could receive only messages mediated by C fibers, Bk injection still induced strong activation of the cell. Evoked activity had approximately the same characteristics before and after cold block (Fig. 2).

From these experiments it appears that A fibers do not play a major role in bradykinin-induced cellular activation of dorsal horn interneurons. In contrast, the cold block technique clearly shows that the excitatory effects of Bk are mainly attributable to the activation of C fibers.

C Fibers

Three dorsal horn neurons receiving sural afferents via only C fibers were strongly activated by Bk administration.

Indirect Evidence

Using sural nerve stimulation, Le Bars et al. (19) found that the depressive effects of morphine on lamina V–type cells are particularly strong in blocking C-fiber input, with little effect on A δ input and practically none on A α

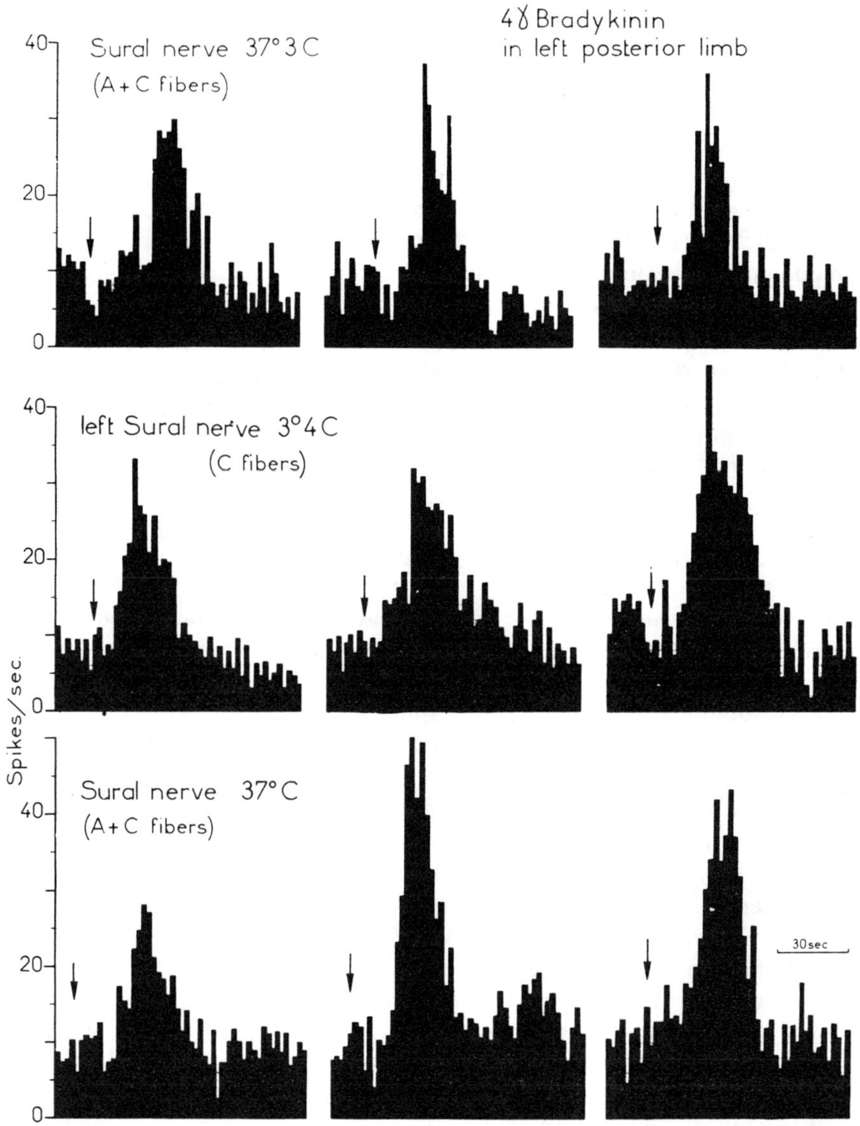

FIG. 2. Firing rates of a dorsal horn cell to 3 (*left, center, right*) injections of bradykinin (*arrows*). In the middle row, cold block of the peripheral nerve has eliminated conduction in large fibers, and the responses to bradykinin remain as large as when both large and small fibers were available for conduction. (Top row before, bottom row after cold block.)

input. In the same study, we simultaneously observed that activation of a dorsal horn cell by Bk was strongly depressed after morphine administration (2 mg/kg) i.v.; this depressive effect was reversed by the morphine antagonist naloxone. This experiment indirectly shows the important role of C fibers in mediating the effects of Bk.

In another series of experiments, we showed (4) that in the decerebrate cat, Bk injection did not strongly modify lamina V–type cells' activities. In contrast, the same cells were highly activated by this substance during temporary spinalization. The lack of action of Bk in the decerebrate preparation is due to the effects of descending inhibitory controls originating in the brainstem, which are strongly enhanced in this type of preparation. It has also been demonstrated that these controls are mainly acting on impulses driven by thin afferents (7,15,27). Moreover, our experiments have shown that late components of response of lamina V cells evoked by supramaximal electrical stimulation and present in the spinal state were dramatically reduced in the decerebrate state, although the first fast component was unchanged (4). In the decerebrate state, the reported activation by Bk of the persistent large-fiber input is not sufficient to produce a clear excitation of the cell. Cellular response modification is strongly revealed when messages driven by thin fibers are not inhibited.

CONCLUSION

All this direct and indirect evidence leads to the conclusion that at the dorsal horn level, peripheral A-fiber activation by Bk does not play an important role in cell excitation, whereas C-fiber activation always evokes a strong modification. So we can assert that when we are recording an excitation induced by Bk at central levels, this excitation is essentially caused by the activation of C fibers.

In cat C fibers are not responsible for noxious messages only. However, according to Bessou et al. (6), only 36% of C fibers of a peripheral nerve are excited by gentle mechanical stimulation. Furthermore, as Iggo (16) emphasized, C fibers are easier than the others to identify. Finally, the proportion of polymodal nociceptors in the C-fiber contingent is sometimes noted to be over 90% [see references in Burgess and Perl (9)], particulary in the distal part of the nerve. All the dorsal horn cells with C input recorded in these experiments always presented tonic discharges during sustained pinches or strong pressures applied in their PEF, and they were not driven by gentle prolonged mechanical stimulation. Moreover, these PEF were often located in the glabrous skin of the foot where Bessou et al. (6) found no low-threshold C mechanoreceptors. Therefore, we conclude that within the C fibers of the sural nerve excited by Bk, a large number of these C fibers could have been connected with nociceptors.

ACKNOWLEDGMENT

This work was supported by CNRS (ERA 237) and by UER de la Faculté de Médicine Paris-Ouest.

REFERENCES

1. Beck, P. W., and Handwerker, H. O. (1974): *Pfluegers Arch.*, 347:209–222.
2. Benelli, G., Besson, J. M., Guilbaud, G., and Lombard, M. C. (1974): *J. Physiol.* (*Paris*), 69:221-A.
3. Besson, J. M., Conseiller, C., Hamann, K. F., and Maillard, M. C. (1972): *J. Physiol.*, 221:189–205.
4. Besson, J. M., Guilbaud, G., and Le Bars, D. (1975): *J. Physiol.*, 248:725–739.
5. Besson, J. M., Guilbaud, G., and Lombard, M. C. (1974): In: *Advances in Neurology, Vol. 4, International Symposium on Pain,* edited by J. J. Bonica, pp. 207–215. Raven Press, New York.
6. Bessou, P., Burgess, P. R., Perl, E. R., and Taylor, C. B. (1971): *J. Neurophysiol.*, 34:116–131.
7. Brown, A. G. (1971): *J. Physiol.*, 219:103–125.
8. Burgess, P. R., and Perl, E. R. (1967): *J. Physiol.*, 190:541–562.
9. Burgess, P. R., and Perl, E. R. (1973): In: *Handbook of Sensory Physiology, Vol. II, Somato Sensory System,* edited by A. Iggo. Springer-Verlag, Berlin.
10. Conseiller, C., Wyon-Maillard, M. C., Hamann, K. F., and Besson, J. M. (1972): *C. R. Acad. Sci.* [*D*] (*Paris*), 274:3425–3427.
11. Fjällbrant, N., and Iggo, A. (1961): *J. Physiol.*, 156:578–590.
12. Franz, D. N., and Iggo, A. (1968): *J. Physiol.*, 199:319–345.
13. Guilbaud, G., Besson, J. M., Niederlander, D., Benelli, G., and Lombard, M. C. (1974): *Proceedings of the I.U.P.S., Vol. XI, XXVI International Congress.* New Delhi.
14. Guilbaud, G., Besson, J. M., Oliveras, J. L., and Wyon-Maillard, M. C. (1973): *Brain Res.*, 63:131–140.
15. Handwerker, H. O., Iggo, A., Zimmermann, M. (1975): *Pain,* I:147–165.
16. Iggo, A. (1960): *J. Physiol.*, 152:337–353.
17. Iggo, A. (1974): In: *Advances in Neurology, Vol. 4, International Symposium on Pain,* edited by J. J. Bonica, pp. 1–10. Raven Press, New York.
18. Keele, C. A., and Armstrong, D. (1964): *Substances Producing Pain and Itch.* Edward Arnold, Ltd., London.
19. Le Bars, D., Guilbaud, G., Jurna, H., and Besson, J. M.: *This volume.*
20. Levante, A., Lamour, Y., Guilbaud, G., and Besson, J. M. (1975): *Brain Res.*, 88:560–564.
21. Lim, R. K. S. (1968): In: *Pharmacology of Pain.* Pergamon Press, Oxford and New York.
22. Lim, R. K. S., Guzman, F., Rodgers, D. W., Goto, K., Braun, C., Dickerson, G. D., and Engle, R. J. (1964): *Arch. Int. Pharmacodyn. Ther.*, 152:25–58.
23. Lombard, M. C., Guilbaud, G., and Besson, J. M. (1975): *Eur. J. Pharmacol.*, 30:298–308.
24. Mense, S., and Schmidt, R. F. (1974): *Brain Res.*, 72:305–310.
25. Smith, K. R., and Creech, B. J. (1967): *Exp. Neurol.*, 19:477–482.
26. Zimmermann, M. (1974): In: *Advances in Neurology, Vol. 4, International Symposium on Pain,* edited by J. J. Bonica. Raven Press, New York.
27. Zimmermann, M., and Handwerker, H. O. (1974): In: *Advances in Neurology, Vol. 4, Pain,* edited by J. J. Bonica, pp. 29–34. Raven Press, New York.

Advances in Pain Research and Therapy, Vol. 1,
edited by J. J. Bonica and D. Albe-Fessard.
Raven Press, New York © 1976.

Segmental Circuitry and Spinal Cord Nociceptive Mechanisms

Frederick W. L. Kerr

Department of Neurological Surgery, Mayo Foundation, Rochester, Minnesota 55901

The manner in which nociceptive input to the spinal cord is distributed, the integrative processes it undergoes, and the subsequent relay of the modified input to higher levels encompass some of the major keys to the understanding and control of pain. No resolution of these issues is possible without precise information on the "wiring diagram" employed at the segmental level for such processing and transmission; however, although the structure of the spinal cord has been investigated for almost a century, the segmental circuitry has not been clarified, other than in general terms, and nothing approaching the hodology of cerebellar cortical circuits, as determined by Cajal (2), Eccles, Ito, and Szentagothai (8), and others, is available for the dorsal horn. However, the dorsal horn has a precisely organized although much less apparent pattern, as might be expected, and recognition of this began with the striking Golgi studies by Cajal (2) at the end of the last century. The application of electron microscopic techniques to both normal and experimental degeneration material has contributed to the resolution of a number of problems, but the picture remains far from complete.

This chapter summarizes current knowledge together with recent personal observations on the fine structural substrate of nociceptive pathways in the spinal cord and correlates these data, when possible, with neurophysiological and clinical findings.

DORSAL ROOTS

It is well established that nociceptive input to the cord is mediated by small myelinated (Aδ) and unmyelinated fibers; superimposed on this input are the modulating effects of large-calibered collaterals of primary afferents which enter the dorsal horn; their distribution and manner of interaction with the small-fiber input are of particular interest in view of much current work on electrical stimulation for control of pain.

Large and small fibers are randomly distributed in dorsal roots throughout much of their course but, as first reported by Lissauer (18) and by Bechterew (1), as the rootlets enter the cord a medial division composed of large fibers and a much smaller lateral division of small-calibered fibers are identifiable. Cajal (2), Ranson (27), Schimert (33), Szentagothai (39), and others confirmed this segregation of small axons, but doubts have been raised about it in recent years (7,38,40). This point has been reexamined in the cat, in which dorsal roots from both cervical and lumbar levels have been studied at selected levels 1 cm and 0.5 cm from the root entry zone and in serial sections from 1 mm down to their entrance into the dorsal horn (16). The roots were maintained under gentle traction in a position perpendicular to the root entry zone during and after perfusion. Large and small fibers were found to be randomly mixed until a point approximately 1 mm from the entry zone. At this level the small fibers were seen to be traveling toward the periphery, where they arranged themselves in a superficial ring. As more proximal sections were examined, these peripheral small fibers were seen to shift laterally, so that just as the arachnoid was penetrated they formed a conspicuous, although small, lateral division; shortly thereafter they joined the tract of Lissauer. Within the medial division, only occasional small myelinated fibers were seen. In man, Sindou et al. (37) have shown the same segregation of small fibers at the root entry zone.

Thus at the very first stage small fibers, in which the nociceptive input is included, are already separated from the large dorsal root afferents which, it is generally agreed, do not mediate nociception. As will be noted, this segregation tends to be maintained, even though there is "cross contact" between nonnoxious and nociceptive pathways at a number of levels.

TRACT OF LISSAUER

This system of fine fibers extends throughout the entire length of the spinal cord and merges with the spinal tract of the trigeminal nerve throughout the C_2 and C_1 segments. Located superficially in the latter area and in the cervical and lumbar enlargements, at other levels the tract of Lissauer is represented by a small, deeply placed wedge capping the dorsal horn, surrounded by the dorsal column medially and the lateral column laterally. Approximately 25% of its fibers are said to be of primary afferent origin (7), whereas the remainder stem from gelatinosa neurons. Some of the fibers bifurcate into ascending and descending branches on reaching the tract; others appear to bend abruptly and run either up or down (2). Myelinated fibers are of fine caliber, ranging from slightly less than 1 μm to 5 μm, with occasional larger elements (Fig. 1). In addition, great numbers of unmyelinated fibers fill the interstices between the myelinated axons.

Extrinsic fibers travel for 1 to 2 segments in the tract and then give collaterals to and terminate in the underlying gray. The intrinsic fibers extend over considerably greater distances—according to Szentagothai (39) for as many as 5 or 6 segments—before returning to the substantia gelatinosa; they provide numerous collaterals to the superficial layers of the dorsal horn. A

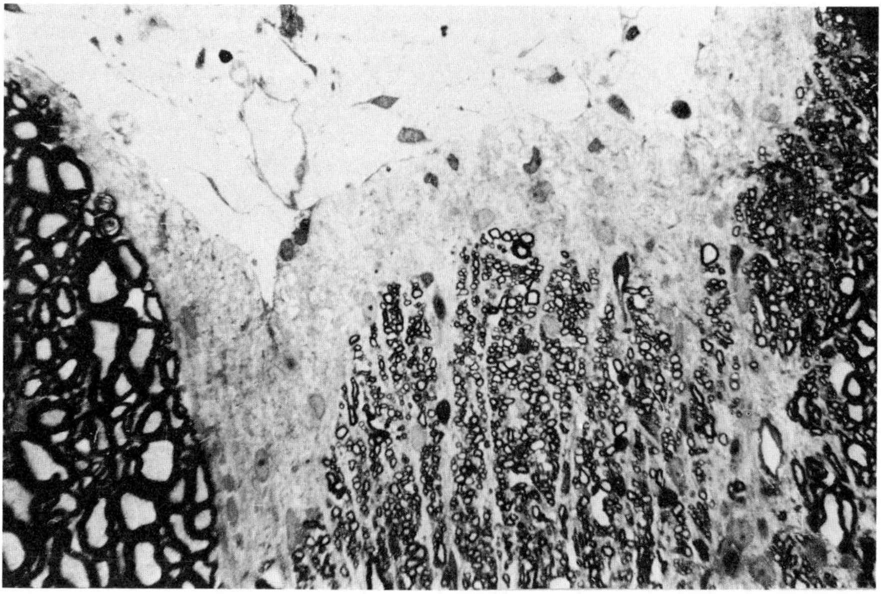

FIG. 1. The tract of Lissauer composed of fine-calibered myelinated fibers (compare with the large fibers of the dorsolateral funiculus on left); interstices between the fine fibers contain large numbers of unmyelinated axons, glial cells, and some neurons.

schematic representation of the course and some of the connections established by the above fibers is given in Fig. 2.

CYTOARCHITECTURE OF THE DORSAL HORN

Considerable differences in cytoarchitecture occur at various levels in the spinal cord, and the following descriptions refer to a prototype of the lumbar or cervical enlargement. Although the Rexed (30) laminar classification is followed, this too is only an approximation; cells in a given lamina have dendritic trees that extend for considerable distances beyond the lamina in which the soma is located, and the borders between laminae are often arbitrary and subjective.

Lamina I

Lamina I is a narrow strip of neurons and neuropil just beneath and partly within the tract of Lissauer. Its most characteristic cells are the large marginal or pericornual neurons, whose fusiform somata parallel the tract. From these cells, thick long dendrites emerge to branch repeatedly and extend broadly over the dorsal surface of the substantia gelatinosa, forming a

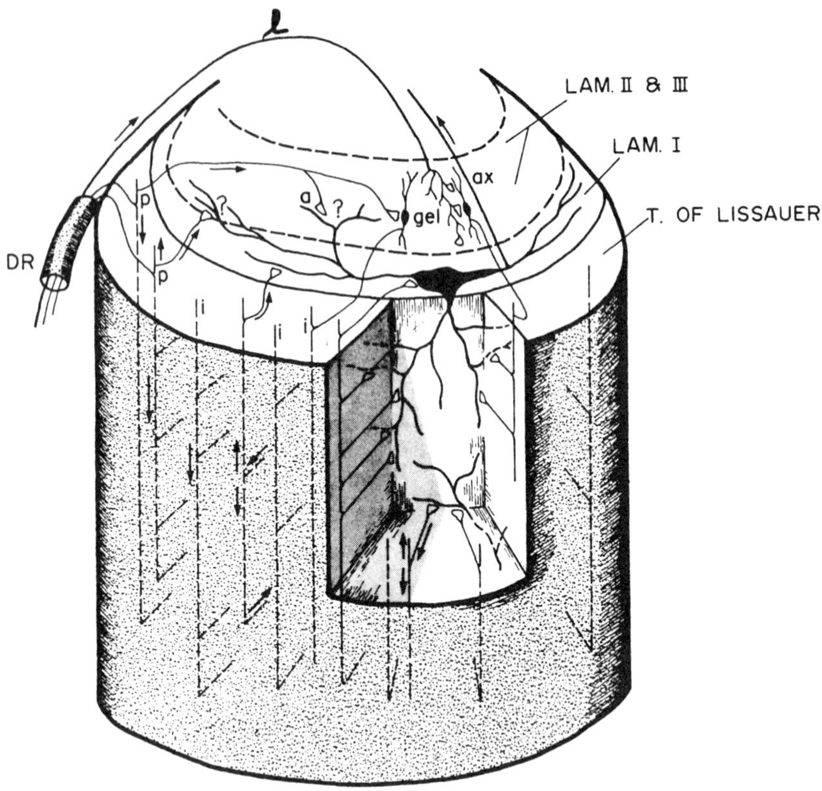

FIG. 2. Three-dimensional diagram of the dorsal horn to show the distribution of dorsal root (DR) fibers. Small primary afferents (p) enter the tract of Lissauer, ascend and descend and enter laminae I, II, and III; they make synaptic contacts with dendrites of marginal neurons and with gelatinosa cells (gel). The latter send their axons (ax) into the tract of Lissauer forming the intrinsic fibers (i), which return to synapse on marginal neurons and in laminae II and III. Cutaway illustrates the wide distribution of marginal neuron dendrites sandwiched between the tract of Lissauer and the substantia gelatinosa. Large primary afferents (l) follow an entirely different course. Further description in text.

widely distributed network between it and the tract of Lissauer; some of these dendrites penetrate deeply into the underlying substantia gelatinosa (2). Figure 2 shows that such a neuron is admirably arranged to intercept fibers passing between the tract of Lissauer and the substantia gelatinosa. The axons of these neurons have few or no collaterals and run either to the dorsolateral fasciculus proprius or to the anterior commissure (2), where they cross to reach the opposite anterolateral quadrant. At least two other cell types can be readily identified in this lamina; one of these resembles a gelatinosa neuron and can probably be regarded as such. The other is found on the border with the substantia gelatinosa and was named "limiting cell" by Cajal (2). It provides a prominent cluster of dendrites that penetrate almost vertically into the substantia gelatinosa; the axons extend to the dorsolateral fasciculus proprius.

The neuropil of lamina I has several characteristic features not present in the underlying substantia gelatinosa.

The first feature is a striking density of terminal boutons on the soma and on the large proximal dendrites of marginal neurons. As previously reported (13), great numbers of boutons accumulate at the base of these dendrites, establishing synaptic contacts with them and with their dendritic spines and forming occasional axo-axonic synapses among themselves. The origin and probable role of this input in terms of integration and modulation of activity of the important marginal neuron will be discussed later.

Second, a significantly larger proportion of boutons contain dense core vesicles than do those in other layers of the dorsal gray (13).

Third, a marginal plexus parallels the dorsal surface of the substantia gelatinosa (2,14,29). This plexus is composed in part of: primary afferents, since it undergoes partial degeneration after dorsal rhizotomy (14); initial portions of axons of marginal and limiting neurons (2); and other unidentified neurites.

Laminae II and III

Neuron Types

Laminae II and III correspond to the substantia gelatinosa and are characterized by the large number of small neurons surrounded by a complex neuropil containing few myelinated fibers, all of which are of fine caliber; this lack of myelin gives the area its translucent appearance.

The most common neurons are small cells less than 15 μm in diameter; in transverse sections they show a fairly dense dendritic tuft arising from their dorsal and ventral aspects, the cells being arranged parallel to the central axis of the dorsal horn. As pointed out by Cajal (2), who provided the most detailed description of these cells, the main dendritic expansions are seen only in oblique longitudinal sections in which they appear as prominent rostral and caudal tufts. Furthermore, gelatinosa cells are arranged in "lobules" (2,32), which can be envisioned as thin radial sheets of neurons separated from each other by the prominent brush-like expansions of large primary afferents which terminate in this area. Particularly noteworthy are the great numbers of dendritic spines, many with unusually long stems, which cover the processes (9,10,32) and whose participation in the glomeruli (see below) is of particular interest.

Axons

The axons of gelatinosa neurons usually arise from a dendrite at some distance from the soma and follow an extremely tortuous course in the neuropil of layers II and III, during which they provide numerous collaterals described in great detail by Matsushita (19). A single gelatinosa neuron may even have two separate axons (10). The final destination of most axons is the propriospinal tracts (or fasciculi proprii), which surround the dorsal horn; most of them enter the dorsolateral fasciculus proprius, large numbers course in the tract of Lissauer, and a few reach the small propriospinal tract in the dorsal column (2). On entering these tracts, either they bend fairly sharply and run rostrally or caudally or they bifurcate into ascending and descending branches, which, as already noted, extend up to 5 or 6 segments before returning to the substantia gelatinosa where they end (39). Less usual types of gelatinosa neurons are the transversely oriented variety, with dendrites spanning several lobules (2), and the rare large neuron, with at least some axons crossing the midline to ascend in the anterolateral quadrant (16).

Neuropil

The neuropil of the substantia gelatinosa is quite complex and contains vast numbers of unmyelinated axons running mainly longitudinally, as well as medium- and fine-calibered dendrites and innumerable terminal boutons, most of which establish axodendritic contacts.

A particularly noteworthy feature of the substantia gelatinosa is the presence of glomeruli (12,25,26,28), which are more frequent in lamina III than in other laminae. They consist of a large central irregular ending that Rethelyi and Szentagothai (28,29) have called the "dense sinuous axonal terminal." This terminal is presynaptic to a number of dendrites and dendritic spines and postsynaptic to a bouton containing flattened vesicles, and the complex is partially enveloped by glial lamellae. The organization of the glomeruli has been investigated in detail by Gobel (9), whose study together with data from the reports cited above have provided much of the information on which the diagram in Fig. 3 is based. In view of the multiplicity of contacts, the integrative possibilities offered by these structures appear to be great; their possible significance in terms of pain mechanisms will be discussed below.

Input

Afferent systems to the substantia gelatinosa include both large and small dorsal root fibers, axons of gelatinosa neurons as described above, axons ascending from cells at the junction between lamina III and lamina IV [pyramidal cells of Rethelyi and Szentagothai (29)], and no doubt other axons from as yet undetermined sources.

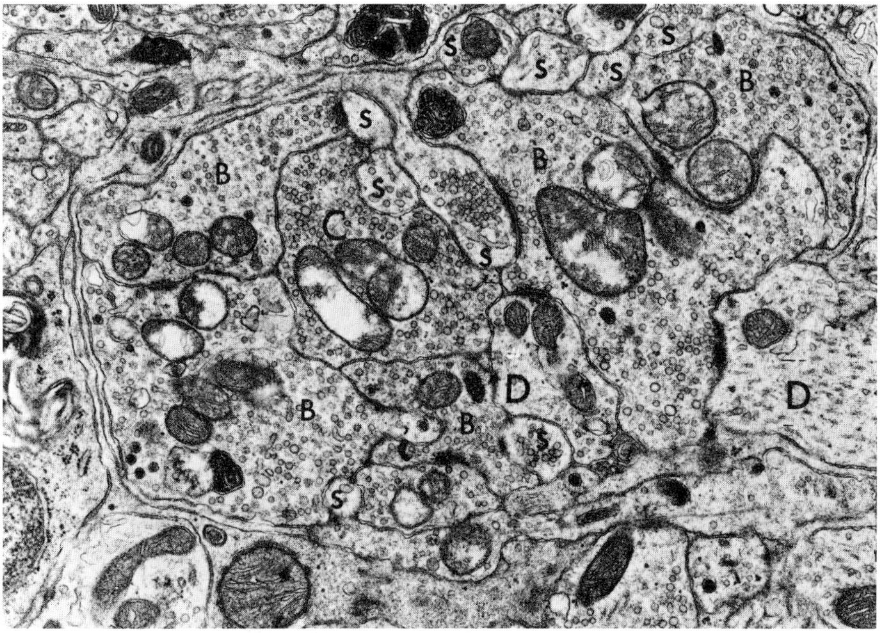

FIG. 3. A glomerulus in lamina II. Central bouton (C) of primary afferent origin has a darker matrix than the other boutons and is cut transversely. Five other boutons (B) of unknown source are present with specializations indicative of axo-axonic synapses. Two dendrites (D) receiving synaptic contacts and numerous dendritic spine heads (S) (9), some containing vesicles, are seen and the complex is almost completely enveloped by glial lamellae.

Primary Afferents

Both laminae II and III receive terminal boutons from primary afferent fibers, but such endings are denser in lamina III (2,4,11,14,26,28,29). The distribution of the fine fibers of the medial division is described above. The very different course of the large myelinated afferents to the dorsal horn has been extensively discussed by others (2,32,33,39); it is summarized briefly here and illustrated diagrammatically in Fig. 4. The incoming large primary fibers course along the medial aspect of the dorsal horn and, after giving a large collateral branch to the dorsal column, continue ventrally until, at the level of laminae IV and V, prominent branches enter the dorsal horn gray and reverse direction to sweep up into the substantia gelatinosa from its ventral aspect. In their course through laminae IV and V, branches are given to dendrites but no axosomatic boutons have been observed (14). On reaching the substantia gelatinosa, these axons bifurcate into ascending and descending branches, from which numerous profusely branching termi-

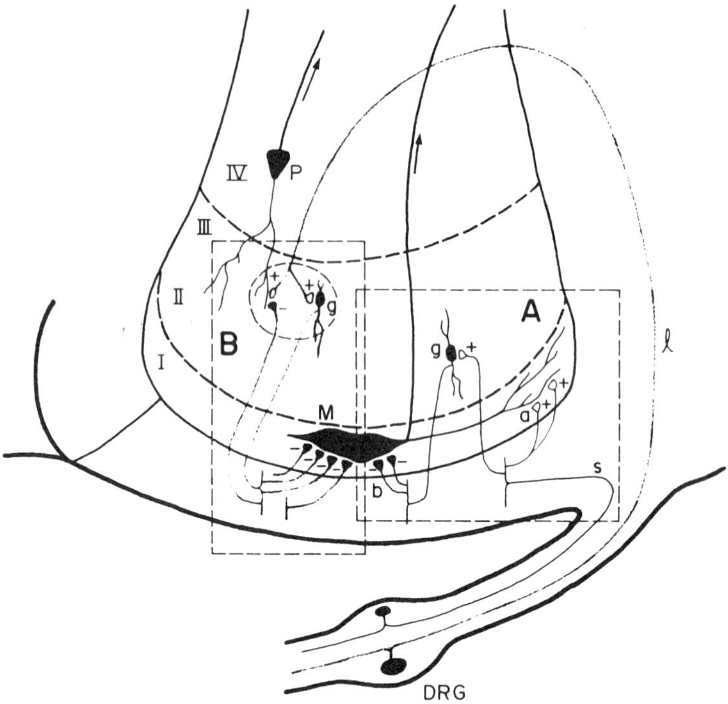

FIG. 4. Central relationships between the primarily nociceptive input from small fiber (s) to circuit A and from large (l) predominantly nonnociceptive fibers to circuit B. M, marginal neuron projecting to spinothalamic system; P, projection neuron of lamina IV; g, gelatinosa neurons; DRG, dorsal root ganglion. Further description in text.

nal brushes distribute to both laminae III and II (2,29,32,39). Since large numbers of primary fibers from the same and adjacent segments reach this area, the enormous density of endings can be appreciated. Axosomatic endings from dorsal roots have been observed on gelatinosa neurons (14), which indicates that these elements are monosynaptically excited by this route. There is indirect reason to believe that spine heads of gelatinosa dendrites are also activated in this way (see below), so that input from large primary afferents appears to be ideally organized to activate great numbers of gelatinosa neurons. Moreover, the terminal arbors of fine primary afferents are of exiguous proportions by comparison with the abundance of axonal endings of large fibers (2).

The manner in which boutons of afferents to the substantia gelatinosa terminate is only partially resolved. The large fibers provide the large central terminal of the glomerulus (4,9). In addition, many primary afferents do not contribute to glomeruli but end as axodendritic terminals in the general neuropil (14). Because the latter boutons are much smaller than those ending in the glomeruli, it seems likely that they are also functionally different; these smaller boutons may be the endings of fine afferents of the lateral division.

Primary afferents, however, constitute only a minor portion of the input to substantia gelatinosa, and the source of most boutons remains obscure. In recent studies I have produced degeneration of axons of gelatinosa neurons by transecting the tract of Lissauer since this tract is composed primarily of gelatinosa cell axons (2,7,39). Electron microscopic findings following this procedure have provided new data that appear to clarify some of the complex issues; only a brief summary is possible here.

Termination of Axons of Gelatinosa Neurons

Degenerating terminals were observed in laminae I, II, and III when the tract of Lissauer was transected and survival times of 24 to 48 hr employed.

In lamina I, numerous boutons making synaptic contacts with soma and proximal dendrites of marginal neurons showed degenerative changes consisting of markedly decreased density of the matrix with pronounced reduction and clumping of the synaptic vesicles. As noted earlier, none of the somatic and proximal dendritic boutons ever show degenerative changes after dorsal rhizotomy. Those terminals appear to end on the more distal portions of their dendritic trees; supporting evidence for this conclusion also comes from Cajal's observation that collaterals of unmyelinated fibers from the adjacent white matter end on dendrites of marginal neurons (see Fig. 110, ref. 2).

The distribution pattern of gelatinosa terminals in laminae II and III is currently under investigation. Whether or not any of the axons from the tract of Lissauer contribute to the glomeruli is uncertain at this time.

Laminae IV, V, and VI or Nucleus Proprius

Laminae IV, V, and VI or nucleus proprius are characterized structurally by having much larger neurons than the substantia gelatinosa and large numbers of myelinated fibers. The neurons increase in size from lamina IV to VI, but this is a trend and not a consistent feature. The myelinated fibers are arranged both longitudinally and radially. The longitudinally oriented fibers are of finer caliber near the apex of the nucleus proprius, and the system forms an important pathway I call the dorsal intracornual tract (DIT). The DIT is composed of ascending and descending branches of primary afferents (Cajal felt that they were all primary afferent collaterals) and of intrinsic association fibers.

The radially organized fibers are mainly primary afferent collaterals that enter from the dorsal column area and extend to the substantia gelatinosa as described earlier. The structural details of synaptic connections in this area (laminae IV, V, and VI) have not yet been determined. The large primary afferents that course through it do not provide axosomatic input to the neurons, but some axodendritic contacts are established (14) although the source of these dendrites is not known.

The neurons of lamina IV are activated via a number of inputs. The apical dendrites extend well into laminae III and II (2,32), where they probably receive synapses from the large primary afferents. Lateral basal dendrites receive input from the corticospinal tract (31); the input to medial basal dendrites is not known, but the system of fibers entering from the cornucommissural area of the dorsal column may establish contact with them (2,32).

Neurons of laminae V and VI probably receive similar contacts, and collaterals of lamina IV axons appear to converge on them (41). Some neurons in each lamina give rise to projection axons to the spinothalamic tract, although a larger number send their neurites to the dorsolateral fasciculus proprius (2).

The correlation between laminar organization and functional characteristics of neurons in these three laminae has been studied extensively by Wall and others, and Wall's review (41) should be consulted for details. Summarized briefly, there appears to be good evidence for progressive convergence from laminae IV through VI of receptive field as well as modality input; as a result, the size of the former increases while the variety of modalities subserved by a given neuron likewise increases in the deeper layers.

Functional Correlation

The organization of input may now be looked at from an overall standpoint and a pattern for the nociceptive segmental connections proposed. The input from the lateral small-fiber division of dorsal roots is distributed predominantly to the distal dendrites of marginal neurons (2) and to the substantia gelatinosa, where again some marginal neuron dendrites receive input (21,22); it appears probable that gelatinosa cells are also monosynaptically activated (14). The small volume of the terminal expansion of the fine fibers should be kept in mind. The large primary fibers have vast numbers of terminals in laminae II and III, many or all of which form the core ending of the glomerulus and activate dendrites of lamina IV and probably V neurons, with resultant relay up the spinothalamic tract. En route to the substantia gelatinosa, they provide collaterals to dendrites in the nucleus proprius. The details of the latter connection are still obscure, but the dendrites may activate neurons of these laminae without the integrative activity provided by the glomeruli in the gelatinosa. The other important action of large fibers is the activation of spine heads of gelatinosa neurons; Gobel (9) has shown in serial electron microscopic sections that many of the small profiles in glomeruli in the subnucleus caudalis of the spinal nucleus of V are connected via a relatively long stalk to dendrites; the subnucleus caudalis is structurally indistinguishable from the dorsal horn at C_1 and C_2 with which it blends. Furthermore, gelatinosa cell dendrites are characterized by having spines of precisely this type in Golgi-stained material (32); thus the correlation appears to be reasonable. The connections described above are briefly summarized in the diagram in Fig. 4.

Figure 4 shows two circuits, A and B. The large fibers, which are predominantly concerned with nonnoxious modalities, establish the connections illustrated in B. The main points to note are their abundant terminal distribution to laminae III and II and their role as the central element in the glomerulus leading to: (a) activation of dendrites of those neurons in laminae V and VI which project to the spinothalamic tract, and (b) activation of gelatinosa neurons via spines and thus a feedback to the same and other levels. This feedback appears to be inhibitory in nature (6) and reaches the soma and proximal dendrites of marginal neurons. Most of the boutons of this circuit contain flattened vesicles. In this way a powerful inhibitory circuit is established which projects onto marginal neurons; the circuit is powerful because of the great volume of terminals of the large afferents to the spine heads of dendrites of gelatinosa neurons. Finally, there is some structural evidence that primary afferents are not under presynaptic inhibitory influences via gelatinosa neurons since in investigations to date, with two doubtful exceptions, I have not seen boutons degenerating in tandem when both dorsal roots and the tract of Lissauer were severed.

The other circuit (A) is provided by small, mainly nociceptive fibers of the lateral division. The significant features of this input are (a) activation of marginal neurons via their distal dendrites; (b) activation of gelatinosa neurons, but in extremely small numbers compared to those discharged by the profuse terminal endings of large fibers; and (c) inhibitory feedback from (b) via the tract of Lissauer to marginal neurons (a). This inhibitory circuit is relatively weak because of the small number of gelatinosa neurons activated by the comparatively meager terminal arborization of the fine fibers.

Central (Postsynaptic) Inhibitory Balance and Pain

The preceding circuitry provides a basis for interpreting segmental pain mechanisms as follows. Stimulation of high-threshold receptors results in activity in small-caliber fibers which enter circuit A. This leads to firing of large marginal neurons, many of which are well known to be involved in nociceptive relay (3,5,7), as well as of neurons in lamina V. Inhibitory feedback to marginal neurons from small fibers is weak for reasons outlined above. Thus noxious input results in relatively uninhibited firing of marginal neurons.

Stimulation of low-threshold mechanoreceptors leads to activation predominantly of the large fibers in the medial division of the dorsal root (circuit B). The central effects are activation of dendrites of laminae IV, V, and VI neurons and discharge of nonnoxious activity up the spinothalamic tract. Also, great numbers of gelatinosa neurons are activated [via the glomerulus and by the occasional axosomatic contents of primary afferents in these neurons (14)] with a resultant heavy inhibitory discharge via the tract of Lissauer onto marginal neurons; evidence that gelatinosa neurons produce inhibition has been provided by Denny-Brown et al. (6), who showed that strychnine application resulted in constriction of cutaneous sensory fibers, whereas transection of the tract of Lissauer led to their enlargement.

Noxious, i.e., small-fiber, stimulation appears to result in relatively little inhibition at the segmental level. Furthermore, descending inhibition from the cerebral cortex does not affect the marginal neurons (5). The result would thus be a relatively uninhibited influx of noxious signals.

On the other hand, if large fibers are activated, a relatively massive discharge of gelatinosa neurons would occur, resulting in a heavy inhibitory barage onto marginal neurons. This theory would account for the sustained characteristics of pain and also for the modulating effects on pain of stimulation of large fibers because of their comparatively overwhelming inhibitory feedback.

Such a circuitry provides a basis for modulation of lamina I cells but leaves open the questions of the role of presynaptic inhibition and modulation of other dorsal horn nociceptive neurons.

With regard to presynaptic inhibition, as noted earlier, in unpublished observations (Pena and Kerr) in which combined dorsal root and Lissauer tractotomies were carried out, no convincing evidence for degeneration of both boutons in axo-axonic complexes was found; this suggests that gelatinosa neurons are not responsible for presynaptic depolarization.

The electrophysiological evidence for presynaptic control of nociceptive input has been the subject of considerable controversy; this has been reviewed in detail by Schmidt (34,35). The weight of evidence from a number of laboratories now indicates that there is no satisfactory support for a presynaptic gate mechanism in which nonnociceptive afferents modulate nociceptive afferents. Whitehorn and Burgess (43), on electrophysiological grounds, have indicated that presynaptic inhibition (PI) for pain is modality specific; thus modulation of nociceptive input would require a noxious or near noxious level of counterirritant stimulation which, to be effective, would have to be delivered within the same segment and close to the pain input area. However, pain in the human can be modulated by electrical activation of peripheral nerve without reaching nociceptive levels of stimulation.

Pharmacological observations on presynaptic inhibition also cast doubt on this mechanism in pain modulation. If in fact PI plays a role in pain modulation, drugs that potentiate and prolong PI would be expected to have analgesic properties. However, the tranquilizer diazepam, which is especially effective in this regard (36), does not produce analgesia. Similarly, drugs that decrease PI or primary afferent depolarization (PAD) do not produce hyperalgesia. If the electrophysiological, clinical stimulation, and pharmacological observations are taken together, there is little to suggest that presynaptic effects are of significance in pain modulation.

In addition to lamina I neurons, neurons in lamina V have been shown to respond to nociceptive stimulation (17,23,24,44), and smaller numbers of neurons in other laminae (IV, VI, VII, and VIII) in the monkey have been shown by antidromic stimulation to project to the thalamus (44). Whether all nociceptive neurons are subject to primary afferent modulation remains to be determined. In neurons in laminae IV and V, it is possible that inhibitory effects from gelatinosa neurons may reach their apical dendrites in the glomerular complexes of lamina III.

Clinical Correlation

Stimulation of large fibers in peripheral nerves was first demonstrated to be an effective means of blocking pain sensation by Wall and Sweet (42). The central inhibitory balance theory would account for this effect by postsynaptic inhibition in lamina I, as described above.

Stimulation of the dorsal columns has also been used with some success to control pain. In this situation the effect may also be accounted for by antidromic activation down the dorsal column fibers—which are the ascending branch of primary afferents—and continuation of this activity via the other branches that separate from them to enter the dorsal horn and reach the substantia gelatinosa, where they activate circuit A.

Certain problems are associated with stimulation for pain control, and among these is the distressing fact that in time it usually loses its effectiveness. This may be because of some type of progressive adaptation, but how and at what level this occurs cannot be suggested with the present data. An alternative explanation is that with repeated and prolonged stimulation, the electrical coupling between stimulator and nerve tissue changes, rendering the stimulus less effective.

Ascending Nociceptive Pathways

Ascending nociceptive pathways arise mainly from cells located in laminae I, V, and VI, and they cross in the anterior commissure and ascend in the spinothalamic tract. This system has been extensively studied and is dealt with in detail elsewhere (16). Although this is the main nociceptive relay, it is not the only one, yet the location of other pathways has until recently been mainly speculative. The spinocervical tract has been suggested as a possible supplementary or even main route for pain sensation. This system is extremely well developed in the cat, in which all the reported electrophysiologic studies have been carried out, but in the monkey it is markedly reduced [for discussion and references see Nijensohn and Kerr (20)]. In man only an occasional neuron representative of the lateral cervical nucleus, in which the system relays, can be found. Evidently, it is a system of decreasing significance as one progresses up the phylogenetic scale. Furthermore, its electrophysiological characteristics are not convincing in terms of its potential for nociceptive relay, as discussed elsewhere (16). Recently, a ventral spinothalamic tract has been demonstrated (15), which is relatively widely distributed in the anterior funiculus. Because its supraspinal connections include all the areas regarded as significant in nociception, it provides a potentially important supplementary pathway which is rarely transected in cordotomy procedures in human patients. Additional possibilities to be considered, although with considerably less likelihood, are the intrinsic ascending systems of the dorsal horn (the dorsal intracornual tract), the fasciculi proprii, and the tract of Lissauer. These possibilities have been discussed elsewhere (16).

REFERENCES

1. Bechterew, W. (1887): *Arch. Anat. Physiol. Anat. Abt.,* 126–136.
2. Cajal, S. R. (1909): *Histologie du Système Nerveux de L'Homme et des Vertébrés, Vol. 1.* Maloine et Cie, Paris.
3. Christensen, B. N., and Perl, E. R. (1970): *J. Neurophysiol.,* 33:293–307.
4. Coimbra, A., Sodre-Borges, B. P., and Magalhaes, M. M. (1974): *J. Neurocytol.,* 3:199–217.
5. Coulter, J. D., Maunz, R. A., and Willis, W. D. (1974): *Brain Res.,* 65:351–356.
6. Denny-Brown, D., Kirk, E. J., and Yanagisawa, N. (1973): *J. Comp. Neurol.,* 151:175–200.
7. Earle, K. M. (1952): *J. Comp. Neurol.,* 96:93–111.
8. Eccles, J. C., Ito, M., and Szentagothai, J. (1967): *The Cerebellum As a Neuronal Machine.* Springer-Verlag, New York.
9. Gobel, S. (1974): *J. Neurocytol.,* 3:219–243.
10. Gobel, S. (1975): *Brain Res.,* 88:333–338.
11. Heimer, L., and Wall, P. D. (1968): *Exp. Brain Res.,* 6:89–99.
12. Kerr, F. W. L. (1966): *Exp. Neurol.,* 16:359–376.
13. Kerr, F. W. L. (1970*a*): *Brain Res.,* 23:124–145.
14. Kerr, F. W. L. (1970*b*): *Brain Res.,* 23:147–165.
15. Kerr, F. W. L. (1975*a*): *J. Comp. Neurol.,* 159:335–355.
16. Kerr, F. W. L. (1975*b*): *Pain,* 1:325–356.
17. Levante, A., Lamour, Y., and Albe-Fessard, D. (1973): *C. R. Acad. Sci. [D] (Paris),* 276:1589–1592.
18. Lissauer, H. (1885): *Arch. Psychiat. Nervhlkd.,* 17:377–438.
19. Matsushita, M. (1969): *J. Comp. Neurol.,* 136:57–80.
20. Nijensohn, D. E., and Kerr, F. W. L. (1975): *J. Comp. Neurol.,* 161:459–470.
21. Pearson, A. A. (1952): *Arch. Neurol. Psychiatry,* 68:515–529.
22. Petras, J. M. (1968): *Experientia,* 24:1045–1047.
23. Price, D. D., and Browe, A. C. (1973): *Brain Res.,* 64:425–429.
24. Price, D. D., and Mayer, D. J. (1974): *Brain Res.,* 79:321–325.
25. Ralston, H. J. (1965): *Z. Zellforsch.,* 67:1–23.
26. Ralston, H. J. (1968): *J. Comp. Neurol.,* 132:303–329.
27. Ranson, S. W. (1912): *J. Comp. Neurol.,* 22:159–175.
28. Rethelyi, M., and Szentagothai, J. (1969): *Exp. Brain Res.,* 7:258–274.

29. Rethelyi, M., and Szentagothai, J. (1973): In: *Handbook of Sensory Physiology, Vol. 2, Somatosensory System,* edited by A. Iggo. Springer-Verlag, Berlin, New York.
30. Rexed, B. (1954): *J. Comp. Neurol.,* 100:297–379.
31. Scheibel, M. E., and Scheibel, A. B. (1966): *Brain Res.,* 2:333–350.
32. Scheibel, M. E., and Scheibel, A. B. (1968): *Brain Res.,* 9:32–58.
33. Schimert, J. (1939): *Z. Anat. Entw. Gesch.,* 109:665–687.
34. Schmidt, R. F. (1971): *Ergeb. Physiol.,* 63:20–101.
35. Schmidt, R. F. (1973): In: *Handbook of Sensory Physiology,* edited by A. Iggo, Springer-Verlag, Berlin, New York.
36. Schmidt, R. F., Vogel, M. E., and Zimmerman, M. (1967): *Nauyn Schmiedebergs Arch. Pharmacol.,* 258:69–82.
37. Sindou, M., Quoex, C., and Baleydier, C. (1974): *J. Comp. Neurol.,* 153:15–26.
38. Snyder, R. L. (1975): *Anat. Rec.,* 181:485.
39. Szentagothai, J. (1964): *J. Comp. Neurol.,* 122:219–240.
40. Wall, P. D. (1958): *J. Physiol. (Lond.),* 142:1–21.
41. Wall, P. D. (1973): In: *Handbook of Sensory Physiology, Vol. 2, Somatosensory System,* edited by A. Iggo, Springer-Verlag, Berlin, New York.
42. Wall, P. D., and Sweet, W. H. (1967): *Science,* 155:108–109.
43. Whitehorn, D., and Burgess, P. R. (1973): *J. Neurophysiol.,* 36:226–237.
44. Willis, W. D., Trevino, D. L., Coulter, J. D., and Maunz, R. A. (1974): *J. Neurophysiol.,* 37:358–378.

Advances in Pain Research and Therapy, Vol. 1,
edited by J. J. Bonica and D. Albe-Fessard.
Raven Press, New York © 1976.

Retrograde Cell Changes in Human Spinal Cord After Anterolateral Cordotomies. Location and Identification After Different Periods of Survival

Marion C. Smith

The National Hospital for Nervous Diseases, Queen Square, London, WC1N 3BG, England

Hundreds, if not thousands, of papers have been written about the course of nerve fibers degenerating as a result of spinal cord lesions, but only a handful of papers have been concerned with the retrograde cell changes in the parent nuclei of these degenerating fibers. Such papers are scarce because of the unsatisfactory and fragmentary nature of the evidence that can be obtained from such studies. Unfortunately, this also applies to the material in this chapter; the infrequency and inconstancy of cell changes do not allow one to draw definite conclusions regarding the cells of origin of some of the transected tracts.

MATERIAL

This report is based on the study of the spinal cords from 23 patients who had had anterolateral cordotomies for the relief of intractable pain. In 7 patients the operation was unilateral, in 16 bilateral. The survival period varied from 5 to 390 days. The level of operation ranged from the second cervical to the first lumbar segment. In 5 cases the operation was in the cervical cord, in 16 in the thoracic, and in 1 in the lumbar. Although the purpose of the operation was the transection of spinothalamic fibers, there was inevitable involvement also of other fibers including the spinoreticular, spinocerebellar, propriospinal, and descending fibers.

When the axon of a cell is injured, certain reactive changes may appear in the cell body. It may become chromatolytic; it may recover and return to its normal state; it may atrophy, becoming shrunken and pyknotic; or it may become a pale ghost without nucleus or nissl substance. The cell body may disappear completely, with or without an increase in glial cells. On the other hand, we have no grounds for assuming that all cells react to lesions of their axons. The preservation of a strong collateral system may prevent or diminish the cellular reaction, and other factors may play a part. Some cells may be more sensitive than others to axonal damage, and some may never react to trauma.

Large or medium-sized cells showing chromatolysis can usually be found easily, whereas atrophic cells are often found only with difficulty and the loss of cells may not be recognized at all. All changes are more easily detected when the affected cells are in a well-defined group; but the changes, other than chromatolysis, may escape notice when they are present in only a few cells of a nucleus with a small and scattered cell population.

When this general problem of cell changes after axonal division is applied to the present material, it is found that all forms of cell reactions are easily seen in the nucleus dorsalis and are harder to find elsewhere. It has been found in this study that certain retrograde cell changes occur at different times in different nuclei. Chromatolysis, the most convincing cell change, is always found in the nucleus dorsalis when the survival period after the cordotomy is less than 40 days and seldom is found when it is longer. Chromatolysis is found in other cells when the survival period is as varied as 5 to 390 days, being most marked when the survival period is approximately 150 days. Clearly, different groups of cells have different temporal patterns of reaction.

These observations and the location of the lesions will now be illustrated. The laminae of Rexed (8) are indicated as shown for man in Truex and Carpenter (13).

OBSERVATIONS

Nucleus Dorsalis (Clarke's Column): Lamina VII

The nucleus dorsalis is discussed first because it is the only group of neurons showing marked changes in all cases. Figure 1 illustrates the changes in the nucleus dorsalis. These cells were particularly sensitive to axonal damage. Five days after a lesion, or possibly sooner, marked chromatolysis of many of these cells occurred (Fig. 1a). Loss of cells was clearly recognizable by 39 days (Fig. 1c). Some cells appeared to persist indefinitely in a pale-staining ghost form, although others were shrunken and dark stained and gliosis (Fig. 1e) was evident. Retrograde changes in Clarke's column were most frequent ipsilateral to the lesion, but a few cells on the contralateral side also showed changes (Fig. 1a,b,e, showing both sides in unilateral cases). Retrograde changes were present after lesions of the anterolateral sector (Fig. 1b,e) or of the posterolateral sector (Fig. 1d) and after lesions destroying only the peripheral zone of the cord (Fig. 1c).

Evidence from all the cases supports the conclusion that cells of Clarke's column give rise to fibers that ascend the cord in both the posterolateral and anterolateral sectors. At least some of these fibers reach the periphery of the cord in the same segment as their cells of origin. The course of most of the fibers in the cord is ipsilateral to these cells, but a few have a contralateral course. Some of the contralateral fibers run in the anterolateral

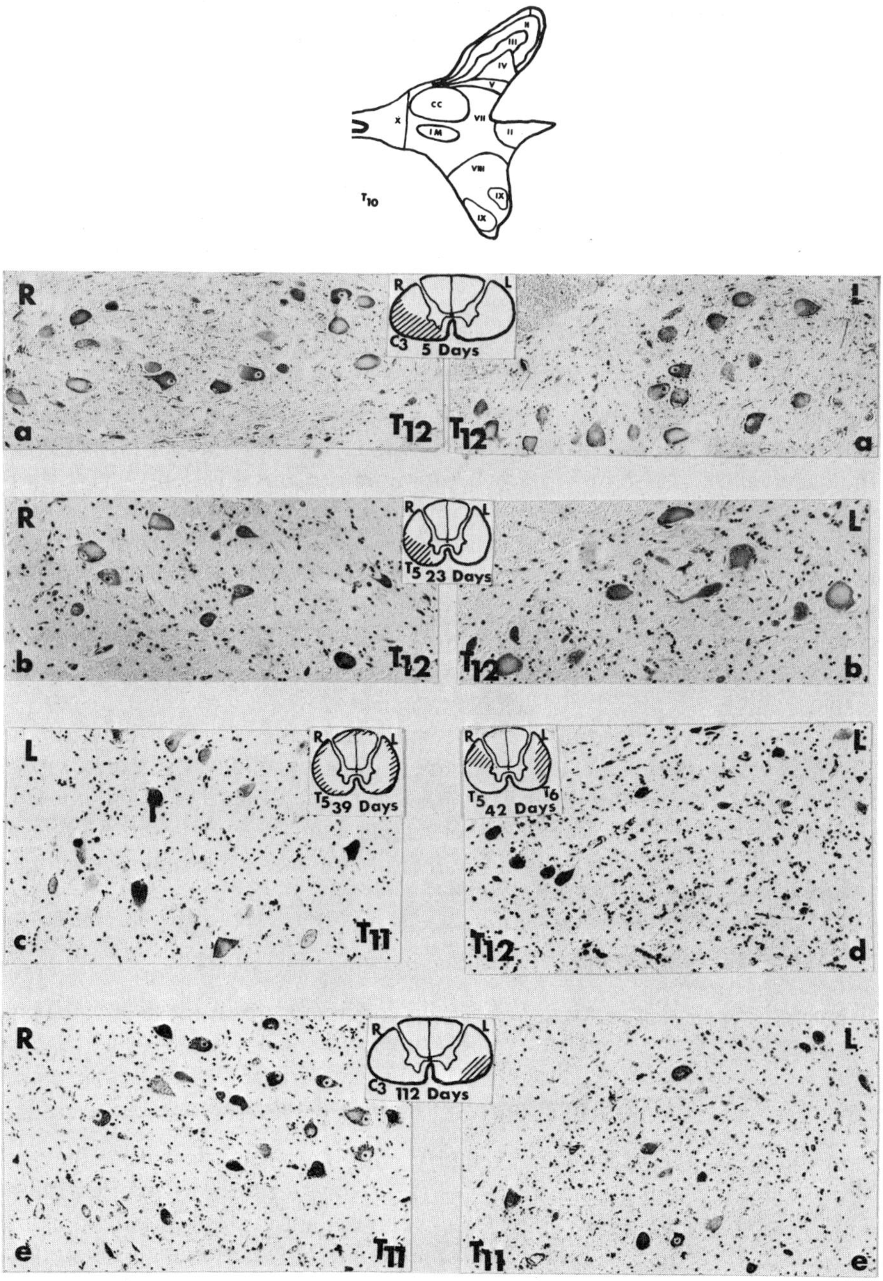

FIG. 1. Retrograde changes in nucleus dorsalis (CC) (lamina VII) after varying lesions and survival periods.

sector. No correlation was found between the location of the fibers on the periphery and the distribution of cell changes in either a rostrocaudal or posteroanterior direction.

Apical and Pericornual Cells: Lamina I

Figure 2a–c illustrates the retrograde changes in the apical and pericornual cells. As these cells are larger and more numerous in the lumbosacral cord, the changes were more easily recognized in these segments. In most cases changes were present in only a few cells, regardless of how extensive the lesion was; cell loss was difficult to detect. Chromatolysis occurred over longer periods of survival than in the nucleus dorsalis. In Fig. 2a the survival was 53 days. In this case, with extensive bilateral lesions, fairly numerous chromatolytic cells were present in lumbosacral segments, but no changes were seen in the apical or pericornual cells in the thoracic cord. In Fig. 2b the survival was 91 days after a bilateral anterolateral lesion. A few chromatolytic cells were present on both sides in all segments caudal to the lesions. In Fig. 2c the survival was 154 days after a bilateral posterolateral lesion. A few chromatolytic cells were present on both sides of the lumbosacral cord. In only 1 case in which the lesion was in the upper cervical level were any changes seen in the cervical segments. In the unilateral cases, retrograde changes were usually seen contralateral to the lesion; a few were ipsilateral.

All the material indicates that at least some of the fibers arising from the lamina I cells run in the anterolateral and posterolateral sectors, with a larger proportion in the anterolateral sector. The course of these fibers is mainly contralateral to their cells of origin, but a few have an ipsilateral course. Some of the fibers reach the lateral column in the same segment as their cells of origin.

Substantia Gelatinosa: Laminae II and III

No definite evidence of changes in the small neurons of these laminae has been found.

Nucleus Proprius: Laminae IV and V

In the large cells of laminae IV and V, chromatolysis is easily recognized after varied periods of survival—5 to 313 days—as shown in Fig. 2d–h. The abnormal cells in Fig. 2h (313 days) do not show classic chromatolysis, but possibly a form of "chronic" chromatolysis. The scattered chromatolytic cells seen in segments caudal to the lesion occurred in cases with lesions of the anterolateral sector (Fig. 2e,f,h) and in cases with lesions almost restricted to the posterolateral sector. The chromatolytic cells were found bilaterally in unilateral cases. In the cervical segments chromatolytic cells

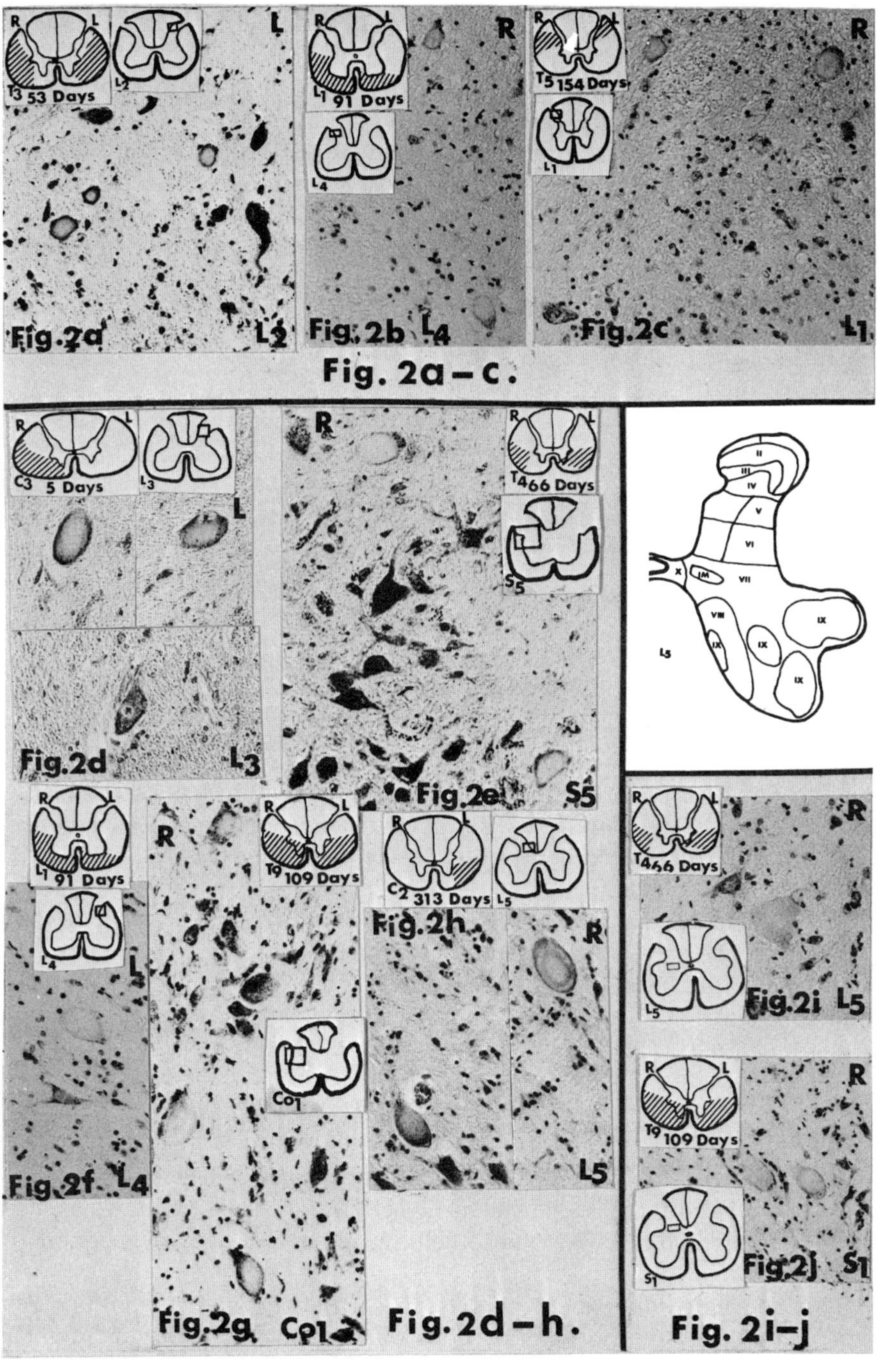

FIG. 2. a–c: Chromatolysis in apical and pericornual cells (lamina I) after varying lesions and survival periods. **d–h:** Chromatolysis in cells of nucleus proprius (laminae IV and V) after varying lesions and survival periods. **i–j:** Chromatolysis in cells at base of posterior horn and intermediate zone (laminae VI and VII).

were extremely rare. In no case were many chromatolytic cells seen, and in some cases no changes at all were found in the laminae. Cell loss could not be identified. The absence of retrograde degeneration in those cases is definite, for changes were looked for in serial sections throughout many segments in all cases.

The material indicates that some fibers ascending in the posterolateral and anterolateral sectors originate from the proprius cells in laminae IV and V. The course of these fibers is both ipsilateral and contralateral to their cells of origin.

Cells at Base of Posterior Horn and in Intermediate Gray Matter: Laminae V, VI, and VII

There are numerous cell groups in this region apart from the nucleus dorsalis and nucleus proprius already discussed. Many of these groups consist of small cells in which retrograde changes cannot be recognized. Chromatolytic larger cells were seen in only 8 of the 23 cases with survival periods varying between 23 and 170 days. Chromatolytic cells occurred in only a few sections in small numbers and from different areas (Fig. 2i,j). Chromatolytic cells were seen in cases with extensive lesions of the postero- and anterolateral sectors, and in cases with lesions of the anterolateral sector only. In neither case with lesions confined to the posterolateral sector were cell changes seen. Chromatolytic cells were seen after lesions confined to the periphery of the cord. In unilateral cases a few abnormal cells were seen on both sides of the cord. In only 1 case were any changes seen in the cervical cord.

It is concluded that fibers ascending in the anterolateral column, possibly only in its peripheral part, originate from cells at the base of the posterior horn and in the intermediate gray matter. These fibers are both ipsilateral and contralateral. It has not been proved whether or not any fibers arising from these cells ascend in the posterolateral column.

Anterior Horn Cells: Laminae VIII and IX

A few chromatolytic cells were seen in the anterior horn of the lumbosacral cord in both the lateral and medial groups of cells, most of which were contralateral to the lesion. These cells were seen after varied periods of survival.

It is concluded that some fibers ascending the cord in the lateral column arise from cells of the anterior horn of the lumbosacral segments. The majority of the fibers have a contralateral course. Some run in the anterolateral column, but it has not been ascertained if any run in the posterolateral column.

SUMMARY AND DISCUSSION

The evidence presented here shows that some fibers arising from all laminae of the cord, except laminae II and III, ascend the cord in the lateral column. A larger proportion of fibers arise from laminae I, IV, V, and VII than from the other laminae. The majority of those from lamina I have a course contralateral to that of their cells of origin, but a few have an ipsilateral course. More of the fibers run in the anterolateral than in the posterolateral sector. The fibers arising from laminae IV and V run in both the anterolateral and the posterolateral sectors, both contralateral and ipsilateral to their cells of origin. The major contribution of fibers from lamina VII arises from the nucleus dorsalis. The fibers are in both the posterolateral and the anterolateral columns. Most of them are ipsilateral to their cells of origin. Some fibers in the anterolateral column are contralateral to their cells of origin.

Some fibers arise from cells other than the nucleus proprius and the nucleus dorsalis in laminae V and VII, as well as from cells of lamina VI, and ascend both ipsilaterally and contralaterally in the anterolateral column. It has not been shown if any of these fibers also run in the posterolateral column. Some fibers arise from cells in laminae VIII and IX, mainly contralaterally. Some at least run in the anterolateral column. It has not been shown that any run in the posterolateral column.

Because the lesion made by anterolateral cordotomy transects a number of tracts, it is not possible to determine which cells give rise to which fibers. Nevertheless, the relationship between the nucleus dorsalis and the spinocerebellar fibers is well established. In my view, most of the spinocerebellar fibers, whether posterolateral or anterolateral, arise from the nucleus dorsalis in man (9,10). Some of the more anterior spinocerebellar fibers may arise from anterior or posterior horn cells. This could not be determined in the present material.

The question of greatest interest to us is which cells give rise to spinothalamic fibers. From earlier histological studies in man after anterolateral cordotomies, investigators deduced that the spinothalamic fibers arise only from the large cells of the posterior horn (1–3). In my material there are changes not only in these cells of the posterior horn, but also in cells at the base of the horn, in the intermediate gray matter, and in the anterior horn.

Current neurophysiological studies—especially those of Trevino and colleagues (11,12,14) and of Price, Mayer, and colleagues (4,6,7)—show that the origin of spinothalamic fibers in the monkey is very extensive. Neurons giving rise to these fibers have been found in all parts of the gray matter, except for the lateral part of the anterior horn occupied by the motor nuclei, most of the cells being in the lateral part of laminae IV and V (11,12,14). In view of this evidence, the possibility that the spinothalamic fibers in man also have a more extensive origin than that previously deduced must be considered.

The most surprising feature of the human material is that the number of cells showing retrograde changes is so small. This was noted also by Morin et al. (5) in the monkey. It is especially surprising in view of their presence after varied survival periods. One explanation for this might be the existence of collaterals of the spinothalamic fibers in the spinal cord. This conception, however, would not explain evidence of loss of pain after cordotomy if the collaterals arose in the distal part of the fibers. But if the collaterals arose in the first part of the spinothalamic fiber, this difficulty would not arise. This seems to be the most likely theory for the infrequency of retrograde cell changes after cordotomy.

ACKNOWLEDGMENT

I wish to express my sincere thanks to all the technicians who have contributed to this study.

REFERENCES

1. Foerster, O., and Gagel, O. (1931): *Z. Ges. Neurol. Psychiat.*, 138:1–92.
2. Kuru, M. (1938): *Gann*, 32:1–25.
3. Kuru, M. (1949): *Sensory Paths in the Spinal Cord and Brain Stem of Man.* Sogensya, Tokyo.
4. Mayer, D. J., Price, D. D., and Becker, D. P. (1975): *Pain*, 1:51–58.
5. Morin, F., Schwartz, H. G., and O'Leary, J. L. (1951): *Acta Psychiatr. Neurol. Scand.*, 26:371–396.
6. Price, D. D., and Mayer, D. J. (1974): *Brain Res.*, 79:321–325.
7. Price, D. D., and Mayer, D. J. (1975): *Pain*, 1:59–72.
8. Rexed, B. (1952): *J. Comp. Neurol.*, 96:415–496.
9. Smith, M. C. (1957): *J. Comp. Neurol.*, 108:285–352.
10. Smith, M. C. (1961): *J. Comp. Neurol.*, 117:329–354.
11. Trevino, D. L., Coulter, J. D., Maunz, R. A., and Willis, W. D. (1974): In: *Advances in Neurology, Vol. 4: International Symposium on Pain,* edited by J. J. Bonica, pp. 167–170. Raven Press, New York.
12. Trevino, D. L., Coulter, J. D., and Willis, W. D. (1973): *J. Neurophysiol.*, 36:750–761.
13. Truex, R. C., and Carpenter, M. B. (1969): *Human Neuroanatomy.* Williams & Wilkins, Baltimore.
14. Willis, W. D., Trevino, D. L., Coulter, J. D., and Maunz, R. A. (1974): *J. Neurophysiol.*, 37:358–372.

Advances in Pain Research and Therapy, Vol. 1,
edited by J. J. Bonica and D. Albe-Fessard.
Raven Press, New York © 1976.

Inhibition of Nociceptor-Driven Dorsal Horn Neurons in the Cat

A. Iggo, H. Ogawa, and *F. Cervero

SRC Somatosensory Research Group, Department of Physiology, Faculty of Veterinary Medicine, University of Edinburgh, Edinburgh EH9 1QH, United Kingdom

The existence of nerve cells in the dorsal horn that can be excited by an input in nociceptor (or at least small) sensory fibers has been known or suspected for 40 years. Successive investigations have refined the techniques from the early nerve stimulation work so that it is now feasible to record from individual dorsal horn cells; to mark their location in the cord and even fill them with dyes (e.g., procion yellow) or enzymes (e.g., horseradish peroxidase); to establish any central projections; and to explore their receptivity to controlled natural stimuli mediated by specified kinds of receptors.

Handwerker et al. (6) reported that class 2 dorsal horn neurons, which are excited by both sensitive mechanoreceptors and nociceptors, are selectively inhibited by an input from sensitive mechanoreceptors or by volleys of impulses electrically initiated in afferent fibers from the sensitive mechanoreceptors. This segmental inhibition could almost completely suppress the vigorous discharge of a class 2 cell caused by an input from thermal nociceptors. Subsequently, Guilbaud et al. (4) established that the C-thermal nociceptors were an effective input. The class 2 cells were also selectively inhibited by supraspinal mechanisms that are tonically active in anesthetized cats with intact spinal cords. These results are of considerable interest from the point of view of pain, but the ready excitation of the cells by an input from the mechanoreceptors together with the selective suppression of inputs from the nociceptors by both tonically active supraspinal and segmentally active inputs from the mechanoreceptors must raise serious doubts as to their primary importance as a pain pathway.

The report by Christensen and Perl (2) of superficially located cells in the dorsal horn that were exclusively activated by an input from cutaneous nociceptors (with myelinated and nonmyelinated afferent fibers) raised exciting new prospects for an advance in understanding of the mechanisms involved in pain. The present study is an extension of the kinds of experiments reported by Handwerker et al. (6).

* Wellcome Research Fellow

METHODS

We have used chloralose-anesthetized, gallamine-paralyzed, and artificially ventilated cats and examined the functional characteristics of 30 marked laminar I, II, and III neurons. Of these, 22 were class 3 (i.e., driven by nociceptors) in the lumbar spinal cord and had receptive fields on the leg or foot (Fig. 1). While recording extracellularly with glass microelectrodes from cells in the dorsal horn at L_{5-7}, it was possible to: (a) control the input from the skin from sensitive mechanoreceptors or from nociceptors; (b) control the intensity and rate of stimulation of the peripheral nerves connected to the skin explored with natural stimuli; (c) record from the cord surface; and (d) block the spinal cord reversibly at about T_{12}-L_1. In some experiments the nerve to lateral gastrocnemius was also used.

The marginal zone of the superficial dorsal horn (lamina I of Rexed) contains a variety of dorsal horn cells and class 2 (mechanoreceptor and nociceptor input), class 3 (nociceptor input), and cold (thermoreceptor in-

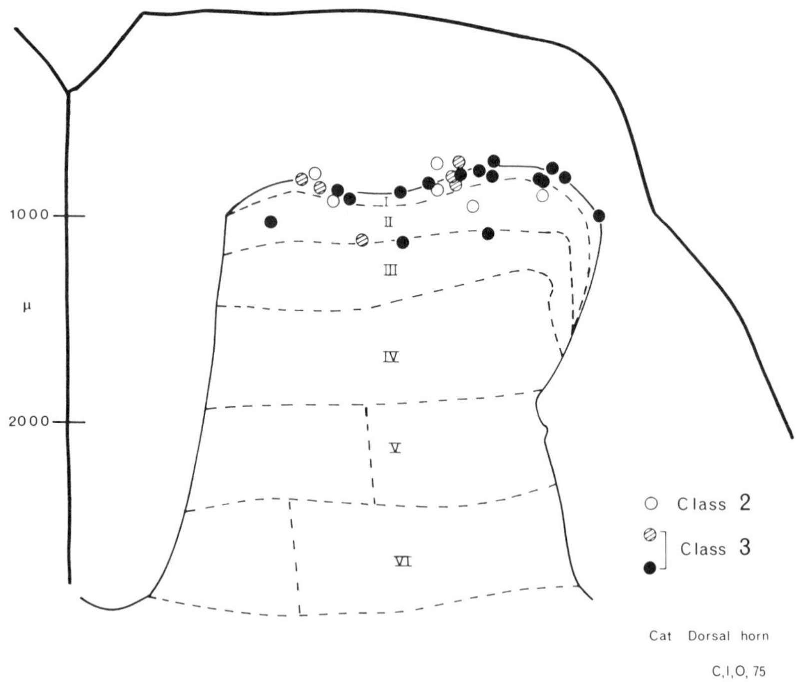

FIG. 1. Location of sites of recording from dorsal horn neurons at L_6 that were examined and marked by electrophoretic deposition of pontamine sky blue in 14 cats. All were in the superficial or marginal cell zone of the dorsal horn (lamina I of Rexed) or in the superficial substantia gelatinosa (lamina II). Most of the units were class 3 cells, but there was an admixture with class 2 cells. The sample is, however, biased since special attention was given to class 3 cells.

put) units. The class 3 cells correspond to the lamina I cells (2) in that they are excited by Aδ afferent fibers from mechanical nociceptors (9 cells in our total sample of 35 class 3 cells) or by both Aδ and C fibers (26 cells in our sample) (Fig. 2) in cutaneous nerves. Four of eight units tested were also excited by afferent volleys in small-muscle afferent axons.

RESULTS

The C nociceptors usually had a more potent excitatory effect in spinal cats than the Aδ fibers; in addition, when electrical stimulation of the tibial nerve was used to drive the cell, a conspicuous enhancement of the effect with successive volleys was seen—the "windup" of Mendell (7). The rate of firing in the class 3 cells was, however, generally lower than for the class 2 cells in spinal cats in identical conditions. Noxious stimuli were delivered to the skin using serrated forceps, sharp pins, or a radiant heater. The last mechanism has the advantage that there is no physical contact of the heat source with the skin, hence the afferent input is restricted almost entirely to C-thermal nociceptors, and there is no contamination by a discharge from sensitive mechanoreceptors as are associated with pinching and pricking the skin.

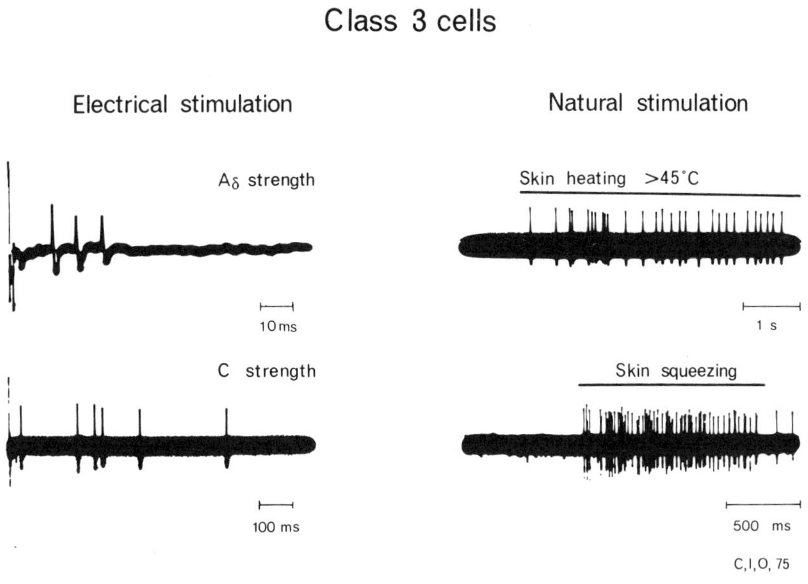

FIG. 2. Typical responses of class 3 neurons in a spinalized cat to electrical stimulation of the tibial nerve, at Aδ and C strengths (note difference in time scales), and to "natural" stimulation of the skin by radiant heating and by squeezing the skin with serrated forceps. The latter stimulus was more effective, probably because the neurons are converged on by both Aδ and C fibers.

A sustained discharge in the class 3 cells could be evoked by radiant heat which raised the skin temperature in the receptive field to more than 45°C, and the discharge continued for some time after the source of heat was removed. Several factors may contribute to the gradual buildup and sustained response, including sensitization of the receptor because of the release of algogenic agents in the skin by the heating (Iggo, *this volume*), and the progressive facilitation of the discharge of the class 3 neurons with continued afferent input ("windup"; 7), presumably attributable to interneuronal facilitation by the afferent input in the C nociceptors.

The class 3 cells, which project into long ascending spinal paths (5,8,9) and to the thalamus, would seem to be logical candidates for a pain pathway. Their sensitivity to inhibition of the kind reported for class 2 cells (6) was therefore tested in view of reports that pain can be suppressed by innocuous mechanical stimuli.

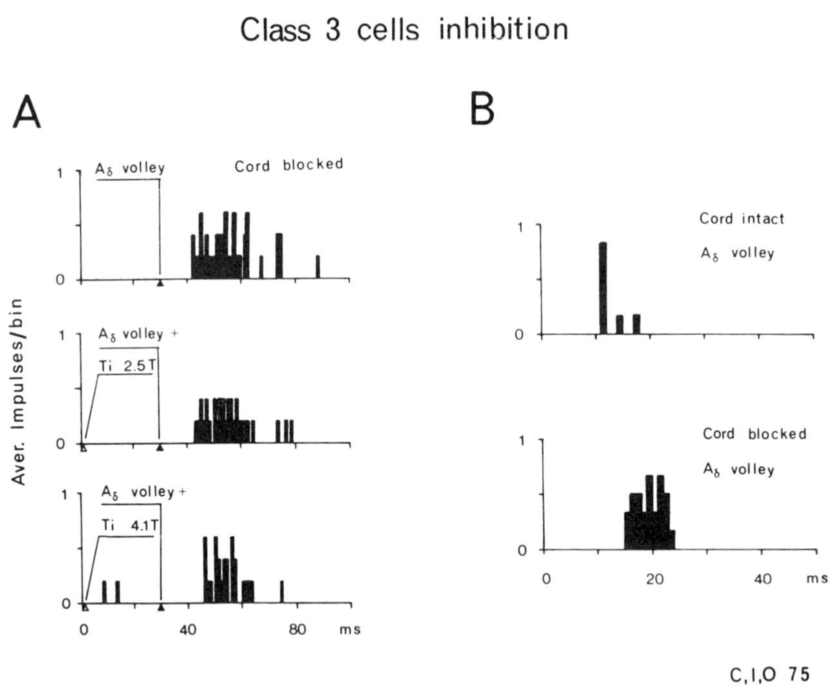

FIG. 3. Inhibition of Aδ volley–evoked discharges in class 3 (nociceptive) neurons by **A**, a single afferent volley in large mechanoreceptor afferent fibers in the tibial nerve (segmental inhibition) in a spinalized cat, and by **B**, tonic supraspinal inhibitory action. Each graph is prepared from averaged trials. In **A** the test volley in Aδ axons (indicated by ▲ on the base line) was preceded by the conditioning (△) volley in fast A fibers. The later part of the Aδ-evoked discharge is reduced. In **B** the response to an Aδ volley in the tibial nerve is much greater when the spinal cord is blocked at T_{12} (spinal state of the preparation).

In preparations in the spinal state, the response of class 3 cells to volleys of impulses restricted to the large mechanoreceptor afferent fibers was a reduction in the discharge evoked by a nociceptor input (Fig. 2). This inhibitory action was rapid in onset, could totally suppress the discharge in the class 3 cells, persisted during continued mechanoreceptor afferent input, and did not continue when this input was stopped. It was effective against an excitatory drive from the C-thermal nociceptors as well as from electrical stimulation of the nociceptor afferent fibers (Fig. 3). More exact information on the time course of the inhibition was obtained in experiments in which the nerves were electrically stimulated to control the inputs and several responses were averaged (Fig. 3). When the conditioning stimuli were timed appropriately, there was a reduction particularly of the later components of Aδ or C-volley evoked discharges. This late inhibition according to Game and Lodge (3) is probably mediated by gamma-aminobutyric acid (or a structural analogue).

DISCUSSION

The results leave no doubt that the excitability of the class 3 (nociceptor-driven) dorsal horn neurons can be depressed in the spinal cat by an input from the sensitive cutaneous mechanoreceptors, even though these neurons are not excited by the mechanoreceptors. The mechanism remains to be elucidated.

In cats with unblocked spinal cords, the class 3 neurons can still be excited by the nociceptors (Fig. 3), although to a lesser degree, and are still inhibited by the sensitive mechanoreceptors. They appear to be less sensitive to tonic supraspinal inhibition than the class 2 cells. They do not switch their sensibility to peripheral inputs, although there is a distinct reduction in the rate of firing to noxious stimuli. The inhibitory effect of peripheral inputs was reduced in the intact state of the cord when compared with the spinal preparation, as has previously been reported by Brown et al. (1) for spinocervical tract units with a nociceptor input.

Current interest in acupuncture analgesia and the relief of pain by electrical stimulation of afferent pathways gives the results reported here a topical interest. The inhibition we report may be part of any mechanism that affords relief by the procedures involving electrical stimulation of peripheral nerves or their collaterals in the spinal cord. In any case, this inhibition raises questions on the functional roles of the class 2 and 3 dorsal horn neurons. The latter appear to be the most straightforward candidates for peripheral and spinal pain pathways and their modulation.

REFERENCES

1. Brown, A. G., Hamann, W. C., and Martin, H. F., III (1974): *Adv. Neurol.,* 4:253.
2. Christensen, B. N., and Perl, E. R. (1970): *J. Neurophysiol.,* 33:293.

3. Game, C. J. A., and Lodge, D. (1975): *Exp. Brain Res.,* 23:75.
4. Guilbaud, G., Iggo, A., and Ramsey, R. L.: *In preparation.*
5. Handwerker, H. O., Iggo, A., Ogawa, H., and Ramsey, R. L. (1975): *J. Physiol. (Lond.),* 244:76P.
6. Handwerker, H. O., Iggo, A., and Zimmermann, M. (1975): *Pain,* 1:147.
7. Mendell, L. M. (1966): *Exp. Neurol.,* 16:316.
8. Price, D. D., and Browe, A. C. (1973): *Brain Res.,* 64:425.
9. Trevino, D. L., Coulter, J. D., and Willis, W. D. (1973): *J. Neurophysiol.,* 36:750.

Advances in Pain Research and Therapy, Vol. 1,
edited by J. J. Bonica and D. Albe-Fessard.
Raven Press, New York © 1976.

Response Properties of Dorsal Horn Neurons to Noxious and Nonnoxious Stimuli in the Spinal Rat

*Glenn J. Giesler, Jr., Daniel Menetrey, and Jean-Marie Besson

Laboratoire de Physiologie des Centres Nerveux, Université Pierre et Marie Curie, 4 Av. Gordon-Bennett, 75016-Paris, France

The rat has been a primary animal in neuropharmacological, neurochemical, and behavioral investigations of pain-related phenomena. However, this species has not received an equivalent amount of study by neurophysiologists who are interested in this field. One area that appears to be highly relevant but which has received little attention is the spinal cord dorsal horn. Indeed, with the exception of a brief description by Wall et al. (15), little work has appeared on the cellular responses of this area to cutaneous stimuli.

Therefore, as an initial study on the rat, we have performed a detailed analysis of unitary responses to noxious and nonnoxious stimuli. Because most neurophysiological investigations of the dorsal horn have been performed on the cat and to a lesser extent on the monkey, we have paid particular attention to the possible similarities and differences between these two species and the rat.

METHODS

Experiments were performed on unanesthetized decerebrate spinal rats. The animals were paralyzed with gallamine triethiodide (Flaxedil®) and maintained with artificial respiration. All unitary recordings were performed in the lumbar cord through glass micropipette electrodes filled with pontamine sky blue, which was iontophoretically applied at the conclusion of each tract. Standard techniques for recording, amplifying, analyzing, and storing data were used in these experiments. Natural cutaneous stimuli were delivered to the peripheral receptive field with a camel's hair brush (touch); a wooden probe (pressure); a serrated arterial clamp judged to be noxious when applied to human skin (pinch); and a 25-gauge needle (skin puncture). Transcutaneous electrical stimulation was given through a pair of needles inserted into the receptive field.

* Present address: Department of Psychology, University of California, Los Angeles, California, 90024

A total of 131 cells were recorded and analyzed in this study. According to the nature of the stimuli which were effective in driving these cells, they have been classified in four basic types.

Type 1: Cells Activated Only by Nonnoxious Cutaneous Stimuli (41 Cells)

We found 29 cells to be activated only by touch and/or hair movement, and these are referred to as type 1A cells. These cells were activated from relatively small receptive fields that often occupied less than the area of a single toe. Touch or hair movement gave short-duration bursts of activity (2 to 15 spikes) which were rapidly adapting. Additional increases of stimulus intensity never induced an additional increase in the evoked activity. The remaining 12 type 1 cells responded to increased stimulus strengths within the nonnoxious range and are referred to as type 1B cells. These cells either responded only to light pressure or clearly showed a greater response to light pressure than to brush strokes. Here again, noxious stimuli were without effect. For type 1A and 1B cells receptive fields on the proximal hindquarter were up to 40 times as large as those on the distal extremity. Within the dorsal horn, cells with the smallest receptive fields were located medial and dorsal to the other type 1 cells. For all type 1A and 1B cells tested, transcutaneous electrical stimulation produced short-latency and short-duration responses. Large increases in current strength had no effect on evoked responses.

Type 2: Cells Activated by Nonnoxious and Noxious Stimuli (41 Cells)

We found 28 cells to be activated by touch, hair movement, or both; when a continuous light pressure was applied to the receptive field, these cells showed a long-duration increase in firing rate. In addition, when the stimulus strength was increased to a noxious level by applying a serrated arterial clamp or by puncturing the skin with a needle, a corresponding increase in firing rate was produced. These cells are referred to as type 2A cells. In contrast to type 2A cells, 2B cells could not be excited by brush strokes or hair movement but required light pressure for threshold stimulation. Like type 2A cells, type 2B cells were powerfully activated by noxious stimuli. In general, these cells were driven from medium (area greater than that of one toe but less than the area of a paw) and large (equal to or greater than the area of a paw) receptive fields. We tested 28 type 2 cells for responses to transcutaneous electrical stimulation. All of these cells responded with short-latency and short-duration bursts of activity to low stimulation intensities. However, unlike type 1 cells, 67% of these cells showed additional long-latency (150 to 300 msec) responses to increased intensities of electrical stimulation (Fig. 1A).

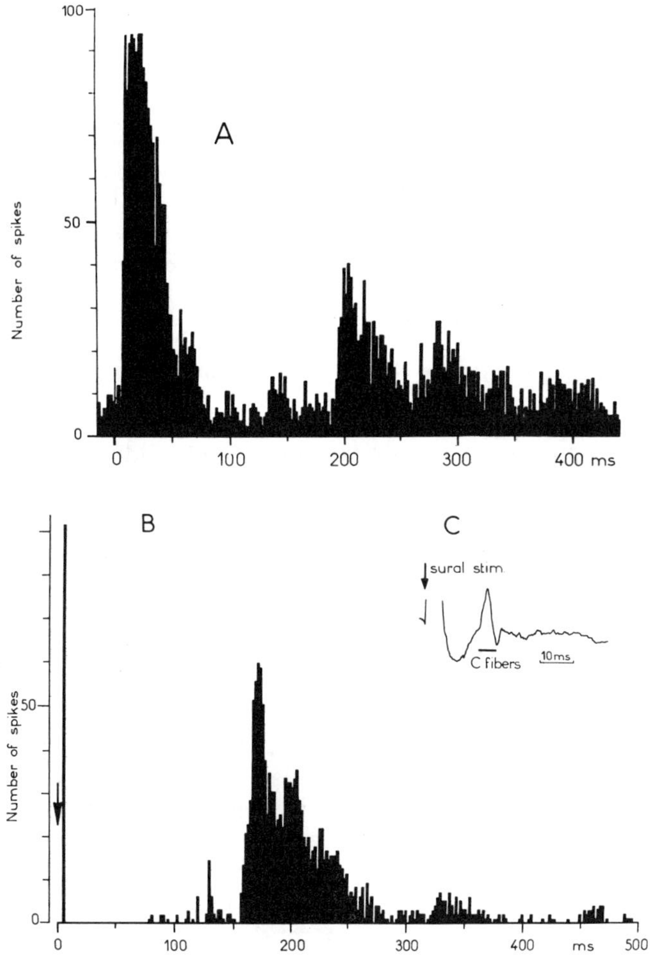

FIG. 1. Poststimulus histograms of 50 responses to high-intensity transcutaneous electrical stimulation **(A)** and to A- and C-fiber **(C)** activation in the sural nerve. **B:** Cellular responses resembling those produced by intense transcutaneous electrical stimulation.

Type 3: Cells Activated Only by Noxious Stimuli (11 Cells)

Eleven cells could be activated only by pinch and puncture of the skin. Six cells located deep within the dorsal horn could be excited from medium and large receptive fields, whereas the remaining cells located in the marginal zone (lamina 1) were driven only from small and medium receptive fields. Four of the five cells tested with transcutaneous electrical stimulation responded with long-latency bursts of activity to intense stimulation.

Type 4: Cells Activated by Joint Movement and Stimulation of Deep Tissue (23 Cells)

We found 11 cells to be activated by movement of the ankle or toes. Most units gave a phasic response during limb movement and maintained a frequency that was related to the position of the limb or toe. Twelve cells could be activated only by deep pressure. Because of the nature of the stimulus, it was impossible to delimit the cells' receptive fields accurately. In general, these cells were located in the same area of the spinal gray matter as joint movement cells.

Cellular Responses to Graded Stimulation of the Sural Nerve

Because the latency of the late components we have described is consistent with C-fiber activation of dorsal horn cells and the patterns of spike discharges are similar to those found in other species for a known C-fiber input (3,11), it appears likely that late components result from C-fiber activation. Therefore, in additional experiments we stimulated and recorded responses of the sural nerve to compare the effects on dorsal horn cells of controlled A- and C-fiber input and high-intensity transcutaneous electrical stimulation. In these experiments 11 of 18 cells studied had both A- and C-fiber input. Levels of stimulation that produced a C wave within the nerve (Fig. 1C) produced cellular responses (Fig. 1B) reminiscent of those produced by intense transcutaneous electrical stimulation. In addition, it was possible to locate and electrically stimulate the peripheral receptive field of three cells that had A- and C-fiber input. With these cells, activities evoked by nerve and transcutaneous stimulation were strikingly similar. Therefore, it seems likely that transcutaneous stimulation produces responses in type 2 and 3 cells which are dependent on C fibers for their activation. Cells that respond with late components to electrical stimulation were found throughout a wide area of the dorsal horn. Wide distributions of A and C input have also been reported for the cat (4,5). The proportion of cells having both A- and C-fiber input (61%) found with sural nerve stimulation is similar to those found by other workers in the cat (4,5,10) and in the monkey (13).

Locations of Cell Types Within the Dorsal Horn

From Fig. 2 it appears that a great deal of overlap exists in the distributions of cellular locations for the various response types, especially types 1 and 2. However, before accepting this conclusion it seems useful to discuss the nature of the histological material presented in Fig. 2 in more detail. Because of a paucity of detailed anatomical work on the laminar organization of the rat dorsal horn, we were forced to pool our data on a common map

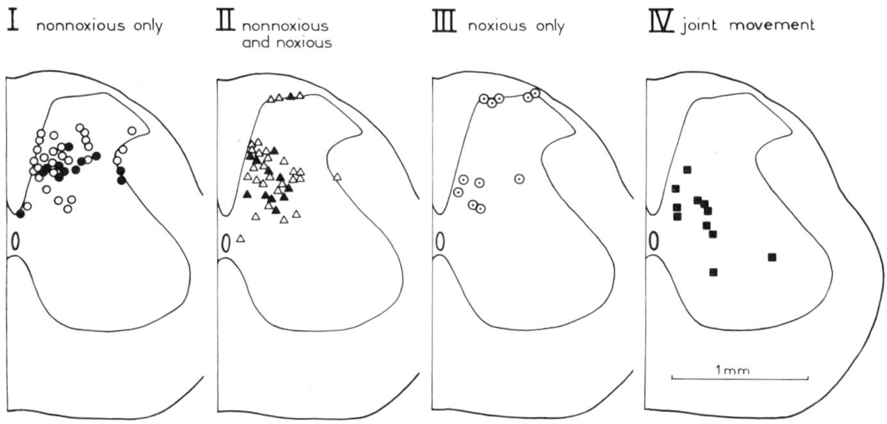

FIG. 2. Cellular locations of the 4 response types within the spinal cord. Type 1A cells, open circles; 1B, closed circles; 2A, open triangles; 2B, closed triangles.

in relation to their distances from gross features of the gray matter. That this procedure is hazardous and could lead to greater estimates of variability in cellular locations has been pointed out by Wall (14), who emphasized the variation in gross landmarks of the dorsal horn from one cat to another. We have seen similar variation in the rat. Therefore, in an effort to avoid these problems and determine the relative dorsal-ventral positions of the different cell types, we used a different approach. Individual microelectrode descents containing both types 1 and 2 neurons have been evaluated for the relative positions of the two types. Of the 27 descents in which type 1 and 2 cells were encountered, type 1 was dorsal to type 2 in 19 tracts. Therefore, it appears that generally type 1 is dorsal to type 2. Type 4 cells were typically found deeper within the dorsal horn than any of the other three types. Consequently, this work supports the laminar model of the dorsal horn as defined by Wall (14): that is, "zones of concentration rather than absolutely separate laminae of distinct specialization."

COMMENTS ON RESPONSE PROPERTIES

Response properties of dorsal horn cells of the rat spinal cord resemble those previously described in the cat and the monkey. Type 1 cells driven only by nonnoxious stimuli are comparable to the small dynamic-range cells of lamina 4 initially described in the cat by Wall (14). Cells with similar responses have been reported in the monkey (12). Type 2 cells, which received both nonnoxious and noxious input, were driven from larger receptive fields and correspond to the wide dynamic-range cells (lamina V–type cells) reported in the cat by Wall (14) and in the monkey by other authors (12,16).

Cells driven by only noxious stimuli were located in two areas; lamina 1 and in the lower part of the dorsal horn. Several authors have also reported high-threshold units in the deeper portions of the dorsal horn in the cat (1,6,8) and the monkey (16). Others have shown that lamina 1 neurons are also strongly activated by noxious stimuli and have a major role in the transmission of painful messages (2,7,9). Our results confirm these observations and expand them to the rat. Indeed, all nine of the lamina 1 cells we encountered responded powerfully to pinch. Furthermore, five of these cells could be activated only by such a stimulus. However, this area cannot be considered to receive only noxious input since four cells were also clearly activated by nonnoxious stimuli.

Finally, these initial experiments suggest that additional studies in the dorsal horn of the rat could provide a means to pool neurophysiological information with neurochemical, neuropharmacological, and behavioral data that are relevant to pain processes at the spinal cord level.

ACKNOWLEDGMENT

This work was supported by the CNRS (ERA 237).

REFERENCES

1. Brown, A. G., and Franz, D. N. (1969): *Brain Res.,* 7:231–249.
2. Christensen, B. N., and Perl, E. R. (1970): *J. Neurophysiol.,* 33:293–307.
3. Foreman, R. D., Applebaum, A. E., Beall, J. E., Trevino, D. L., and Willis, W. D. (1975): *J. Neurophysiol.,* 38:132–145.
4. Gregor, M., and Zimmermann, M. (1972): *J. Physiol.,* 221:555–576.
5. Handwerker, H. O., Iggo, A., and Zimmermann, M. (1975): *Pain,* 1:147–165.
6. Heavner, J. E., and De Jong, R. H. (1973): *Exp. Neurol.,* 39:293–306.
7. Iggo, A. (1974): In: *Advances in Neurology, Vol. 4: International Symposium on Pain,* edited by J. J. Bonica. Raven Press, New York.
8. Kolmodin, G. M., and Skoglund, C. R. (1960): *Acta Physiol. Scand.,* 50:337–355.
9. Kumazawa, T., Perl, E. R., Burgess, P. R., and Whitehorn, D. (1975): *J. Comp. Neurol.,* 162:1–12.
10. Mendell, L. M., and Wall, P. D. (1965): *Nature,* 206:97–99.
11. Price, D. D., Hull, C. D., and Buchwald, N. A. (1971): *Exp. Neurol.,* 33:291–309.
12. Price, D. D., and Mayer, D. J. (1974): *Brain Res.,* 79:321–325.
13. Wagman, I. H., and Price, D. D. (1969): *J. Neurophysiol.,* 32:803–817.
14. Wall, P. D. (1967): *J. Physiol. (Lond.),* 188:403–423.
15. Wall, P. D., Freeman, J., and Major, D. (1967): *Exp. Neurol.,* 19:519–529.
16. Willis, W. D., Trevino, D. L., Coulter, J. D., and Maunz, R. A. (1974): *J. Neurophysiol.,* 37:358–372.

Advances in Pain Research and Therapy, Vol. 1,
edited by J. J. Bonica and D. Albe-Fessard.
Raven Press, New York © 1976.

Effects of Halothane on Single-Unit Activity of Cells in Rexed Lamina VII

Luke M. Kitahata, Mamoru Yamashita, Kobra Ghazi-Saidi, Arthur Taub, and Whei C. Chang

Yale University School of Medicine, 333 Cedar Street, New Haven, Connecticut 06510

In recent years several investigators have tried to determine the localization of the cells of origin of the spinothalamic pathway in the cat. Using a chromatolytic method, Morin et al. (6) found such cells in lamina I of Rexed and also in the "center of the dorsal horn." With the Golgi technique, Szentagothai (7) demonstrated that axons decussating in the ventral commissure of the spinal cord arise primarily from cells in laminae VI, VII, and VIII.

Dilly et al. (2) used an electrophysiologic technique. In order to activate spinothalamic neurons antidromically, they stimulated a site just caudal to the thalamus. Simultaneously the spinal cord was searched with a recording microelectrode. Fifty-six cells in laminae V and VI of the cervical enlargement and one cell in the "ventral horn" of the lumbar enlargement were found to respond to antidromic stimulation in this site. Trevino et al. (8), employing computer summation of the antidromic response, used a similar technique and identified 105 spinothalamic tract neurons in laminae VII and VIII in the lumbar enlargement. Levante and Albe-Fessard (5) similarly determined the origin of such cells in laminae VII and VIII in both the cervical and lumbar enlargements. Extending these studies, Fields et al. (3) indicated that cells in laminae VI, VII, and VIII projected to the brainstem reticular formation. Albe-Fessard et al. (1) found that in contrast to the ventral horn origin of the spinothalamic projection in the cat, the major spinothalamic projection in the monkey arose in lamina V.

Previous studies from this laboratory have demonstrated a lamina-specific suppression of activity in laminae I and V of the dorsal horn of the cat by injectable and volatile analgesic agents (4). Data analysis has progressed through straightforward averaging and determination of interval histograms. In the present study the effect of halothane on single units in lamina VII of the lumbar spinal cord of the spinal cat is analyzed with the aid of a digital computer program developed to display the average and standard error of the number of interval histograms.

METHODS

Twenty-one cats weighing 2.5 to 4.0 kg were used. We studied 21 cells. Under halothane, nitrous oxide, and oxygen anesthesia, the animals were prepared with tracheostomy and with arterial and venous cannulation. Bilateral radiofrequency lesions were placed in the mesencephalic reticular formation. The animals were immobilized with gallamine triethiodide and artificially ventilated. The spinal cord was transected at the upper lumbar level. The dura was opened and raised by pins to form a sling for the spinal cord, which was then covered with oil at 37°C. Blood pressure, cardiac rate, EKG, rectal and spinal cord temperatures, end-tidal P_{CO_2}, arterial P_{CO_2}, P_{O_2}, and pH were recorded and maintained within normal limits.

Single units were recorded with the aid of a platinum-covered glass rod Transidyne Microtrode® microelectrode and field effect transistor preamplifier system. Single-unit activity was recorded on magnetic tape. Single-unit data were processed off-line with the aid of a computer program written specifically for this purpose, which computed the bin-by-bin mean of a number of interval histograms and displayed this mean and the bin-by-bin standard error.

The dorsal horn lamination was identified by the spontaneous firing patterns and evoked activities recorded. When a cell in Rexed lamina VI was identified, the microelectrode was further advanced ventrally for approximately 500 to 1000 μm to sample cells responding to peripheral natural stimuli. After an on-line recording of impulse frequency during a control period of 5 to 10 min, we administered 0.5% halothane until a maximal effect was observed. Halothane was then discontinued and the recovery was observed for approximately one-half to 1 hr. The experiment was then repeated with 1% halothane. In 6 animals the latency of activation of cells in laminae V and VII after the arrival of an afferent volley derived from electrical stimulation of the tibial nerve (square wave pulse, 1 msec duration, intensity at a level sufficient to excite A-delta fibers maximally, and the rate of 1/min) was measured.

Thermal lesions were produced by the passage of a DC through the recording electrode. Positions of the lesions were determined histologically.

RESULTS

As a microelectrode penetrates the spinal cord ventral to lamina VI, the number of large-amplitude potentials decreases. These cells were difficult to isolate. The location of the units isolated is shown in Fig. 1. Most of these units were found in the pars intermedia at the dorsal portion of the ventral horn. The receptive fields of these neurons varied in size from several ipsilateral paw pads to the entire hind limb bilaterally. In this experiment, only those cells facilitated by high-threshold mechanical stimuli applied

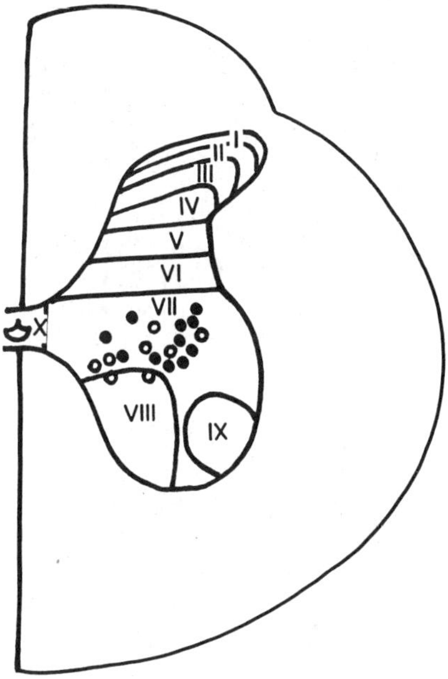

FIG. 1. Schematic representation of location of cells recorded in Rexed lamina VII. Filled circles, cells with burst activity; open circles, without burst activity as defined in text.

ipsilaterally were studied. Of the cells studied, 60% had contralateral excitatory fields and 40% had contralateral inhibitory fields. Cells in Rexed lamina VII respond to high-intensity cutaneous stimuli, deep squeezing, extreme deformation of joints, and application of ethyl chloride, but cells in this region do not respond to hair movement or light touch. The receptive field for response to ethyl chloride was larger than the receptive field for response to mechanical stimulation.

To evoke cells in lamina VII by stimulating ipsilateral tibial nerve with a square wave pulse of 1 msec duration, we needed intensity sufficient to excite A-delta fibers. Nerve conduction velocity following A-delta stimulation averaged 28.4 ± 1.8 msec (range 22.2 to 35.7 msec). A-delta fibers were excited at a threshold level of 0.25 V to a maximum of 2.5 V, at a pulse duration of 1 msec. Intraspinal cord latencies of cells in laminae V and VII were 2.0 ± 0.8 msec ($\bar{x} \pm$ SE; range 1.5 to 2 msec) and 3.9 ± 0.3 msec ($\bar{x} \pm$ SE; range 2.8 to 5.4 msec), respectively.

The spike interval histograms of these cells revealed two patterns of firing activity, one with burst activity (defined as potentials appearing within less than 10 msec of each other) and another without burst activity. Figure 2 displays the average spike interval histogram and its standard error during the control period and under 0.5% halothane anesthesia. During halothane anesthesia the peak mode shifted to the right, and the total area of the histogram decreased. Inhalation of 0.5% and 1.0% halothane has a significant depressive effect on the mean firing frequency of cells of both types.

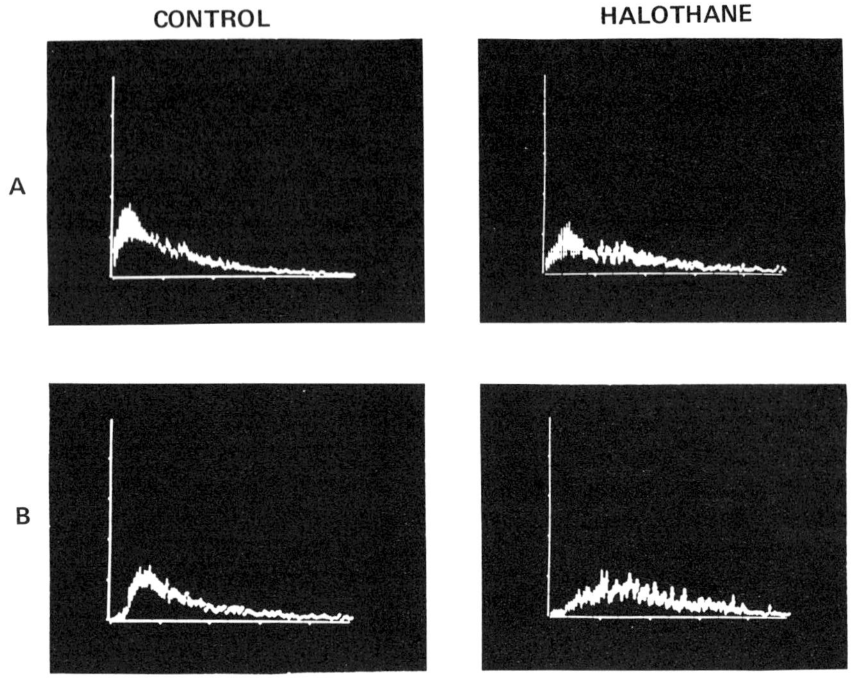

FIG. 2. Average spike interval histograms with the bin-by-bin mean of a number of interval histograms and the bin-by-bin SE during control period and during 0.5% halothane anesthesia. **A:** Single unit with burst activity. **B:** Single unit without burst as defined in text. Abscissa: one division is 20 msec; ordinate: one division is 25 spikes (total computation time, 1 min).

The cells with burst activity were depressed by 55.7 ± 8.3 ($\bar{x}$ ± SE) and 89.0 ± 2.7 ($\bar{x}$ ± SE) percent, respectively, and the cells without burst activity were depressed by 64.9 ± 8.1 ($\bar{x}$ ± SE) and 86.3 ± 5.7 ($\bar{x}$ ± SE) percent, respectively.

DISCUSSION

Previous studies in our laboratory suggest that the lamina-specific suppression of single-unit activity in laminae I and V may contribute in part to the analgesic effect of halothane at the spinal level. In this study the spontaneous activity of cells in lamina VII, which in the cat contributes to the spinothalamic pathway, were suppressed by halothane. Since cells in lamina VII respond to high-threshold mechanical stimuli with wide receptive field conversions and are suppressed by halothane, it appears likely that this may explain part of the analgesic effect of halothane at the spinal level. But this cannot be its entire effect since, in the cat at least, there is little evidence that unilateral or bilateral section of the spinothalamic pathway produces behaviorally observable analgesia. Halothane must act at least on cells in other Rexed laminae, as well as at central levels, for analgesia to be produced in the cat.

SUMMARY

Spontaneous and evoked single-unit activity in cells in Rexed lamina VII of otherwise unanesthetized, decerebrate, low spinal cats was studied with the aid of a specially written computer program for determining the average and standard error of spike interval histograms. Halothane 0.5% to 1.0% was found to suppress the spontaneous activity of cells in lamina VII. In the cat, cells in lamina VII have been shown to project within the spinothalamic pathway and to respond to high-intensity mechanical stimulation and not to low-intensity mechanical stimulation. The effects of halothane on cells in lamina VII may partially explain its analgesic effect with an action at the spinal level.

ACKNOWLEDGMENTS

This work was supported by National Institutes of Health Grant 09871 and in part by a grant from Ayerst Laboratories.

REFERENCES

1. Albe-Fessard, D., Levante, A., and Lamour, Y. (1974): *Brain Res.*, 65:503–509.
2. Dilly, P. N., Wall, P. D., and Webster, K. E. (1968): *Exp. Neurol.*, 21:550–562.
3. Fields, H. L., Wagner, G. M., and Anderson, S. D. (1975): *Exp. Neurol.*, 47:118–134.
4. Kitahata, L. M. (1975): *Int. Anesthesiol. Clin.*, 13:149–170.
5. Levante, A., and Albe-Fessard, D. (1972): *C. R. Acad. Sci.* [*D*] (*Paris*), 274:3007–3010.
6. Morin, F., Schwartz, H. G., and O'Leary, J. L. (1951): *Acta Psychiatr. Neurol. Scand.*, 26:371–396.
7. Szentagothai, J. (1964): *J. Comp. Neurol.*, 122:219–239.
8. Trevino, D. L., Maunz, R. A., Bryan, R. N., and Willis, W. D. (1972): *Exp. Neurol.*, 34:64–77.

Advances in Pain Research and Therapy, Vol. 1,
edited by J. J. Bonica and D. Albe-Fessard.

Extracellular K^+ Accumulation and Modulation of Sensory Transmission

M. E. Morris and K. Krnjević

Department of Research in Anaesthesia, McIntyre Medical Sciences Building, McGill University, 3655 Drummond Street, Montreal, Quebec, Canada

Significant numbers of potassium ions (K^+) accumulate in central synaptic regions such as the dorsal horn and dorsal column nuclei when activity is evoked in afferent fibers—either by weak electrical stimulation of peripheral nerves (2,5–7,12,14) or by natural stimulation of low-threshold mechanoreceptors (9). These changes in extracellular K^+ activity (a_K) appear to produce both prolonged depolarization of afferent fibers, which contributes to the mechanism of presynaptic inhibition, and secondary hyperpolarization.

Modulation of sensory information by the increased periterminal a_K, which is produced by preceding afferent fiber activity, therefore depends on both depolarizing and hyperpolarizing effects and any conditions that alter or influence them. In the present experiments we have studied the changes in extracellular a_K and associated slow potentials evoked in the synaptic regions of primary afferent fibers in the cuneate nucleus by peripheral nerve stimulation (1,6), the changes produced in them by interference with local tissue energy supplies, and the effects of raised K^+ levels on the efficiency of synaptic transmission.

METHODS

Experiments were performed in cats prepared during nitrous oxide and halothane anesthesia by exposure of the dorsal surface of the medulla and dissection of the nerves of one forelimb. After the animals were decerebrated at the midcollicular level, the anesthesia was discontinued. Breathing was spontaneous in many experiments; in others, we used muscle relaxants and artificial ventilation to reduce movements.

Liquid ion-exchanger K^+-sensitive microelectrodes were prepared according to previously described techniques (7,14). The reference electrode was attached so that its tip was $< 10\ \mu m$ from that of the K^+-sensing electrode. A high-input impedance electrometer (Keithley Model 604) was used for differential amplification of the potassium potential (E_K)—the potential difference between the K^+-selective and reference electrodes. At the same time, the voltage of the reference electrode with respect to ground reflected the focal tissue potential (V), which was amplified and recorded separately. In some experiments, a third microelectrode was attached to the twin K^+ electrode system; the cuneate afferent fiber terminals were stimulated through it with constant-current pulses according to the excitability testing technique of Wall (15), thus providing a means of studying the efficiency of synaptic transmission (11).

Bipolar platinum electrodes were used to stimulate or record from the superficial radial and median nerves of one forelimb and to record responses from the medial lemniscus at the transected midbrain.

OBSERVATIONS

Comparison of Changes in Extracellular K^+ and Associated Tissue Potentials During Afferent Fiber Activity

Stimulation of forelimb nerves at 20/sec evoked increases in the potassium potential recorded in the region of afferent fiber terminals of the cuneate nucleus, as shown in trace B of Fig. 1. A comparison can be made between this *in vivo* stimulation and the potential recorded when a similar rate of stimulation released K^+ into an agar gel from a KCl-filled electrode approximately 50 μm away from the K^+-recording electrode (trace A, Fig. 1). The *in vivo* accumulation of K^+ is not as sustained, decreases more rapidly at the end of the stimulation, and shows the additional feature of a late, prolonged undershoot below the resting level. These differences are attributable to active removal of the K^+ by the tissue in addition to the process of diffusion.

The slow tissue potential (ΔV) produced at the same time by the stimulation of afferent fibers is shown in trace C. An even more marked decline in this potential occurs during the stimulation, followed by a much more rapid decay and a large undershoot, which precedes that of the K^+ potential (see traces B and C). The early negative potential shift is presumed to represent depolarization of neuronal and glial elements, whereas the later decrease represents their hyperpolarization.

The increase in extracellular K^+ level can be assumed to be mainly responsible for the negative shift of the tissue potential. The decrease in a_K below the resting level during the poststimulation period, presumably because of active removal of K^+, also has a contributory effect—it hyperpolarizes cells and fibers. In addition, the presence of raised extracellular K^+, and presumably high intracellular Na^+, appears to stimulate markedly an electrogenic component of the active uptake process [cf. similar changes found in the cerebral cortex by Heinemann and Lux (4)]. This produces hyperpolarizing membrane shifts evidenced by the decline of V, even during the afferent fiber activity [an effect resembling the potential changes recorded inside primary afferent fibers by Eccles and Krnjević (3)], as well

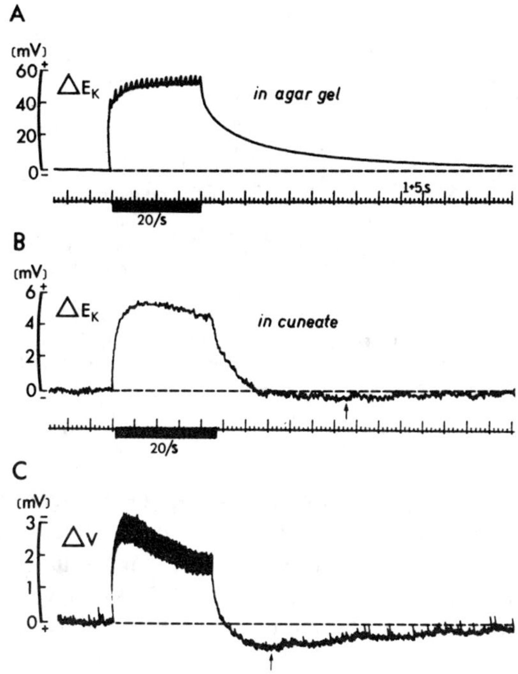

FIG. 1. A: Potassium potential change (ΔE_K) produced by ejection of K^+ by 2-ms iontophoretic pulses at a rate of 20/sec from microelectrode tip into 1% agar gel in 0.1 M NaCl. **B:** E_K recorded in cuneate in response to 20/sec stimulation (10 V, 0.1 ms pulses) of peripheral forelimb nerve. **C:** Tissue potential shift (ΔV) recorded at same time as E_K of trace **B.** Arrows indicate times of maximal undershoot. (Reproduced from Fig. 1 in Krnjević and Morris, ref. 10.)

as the rapid descent and positive undershoot which follow and are maximal while the K^+ level is still elevated.

Changes in Extracellular K^+ and Tissue Potentials During Interference with Local Availability of Energy Supplies

The accumulation of extracellular K^+ and the associated depolarization and hyperpolarization of neuronal and glial elements during afferent fiber activity are particularly sensitive to changes in local blood supply. Trace A of Fig. 2 shows how during a period of spontaneous hypotension, when mean arterial pressure fell from 75 to 60 mm Hg, the K^+ release (ΔE_K) was more sustained and showed no poststimulus undershoot, whereas the tissue potential became more negative with elimination or marked reduction of the phase of after-positivity (see traces labeled 2 with control traces labeled 1).

Similar changes were recorded in a more controlled situation (see B, Fig. 2) when a brief administration of 2% halothane lowered the pressure

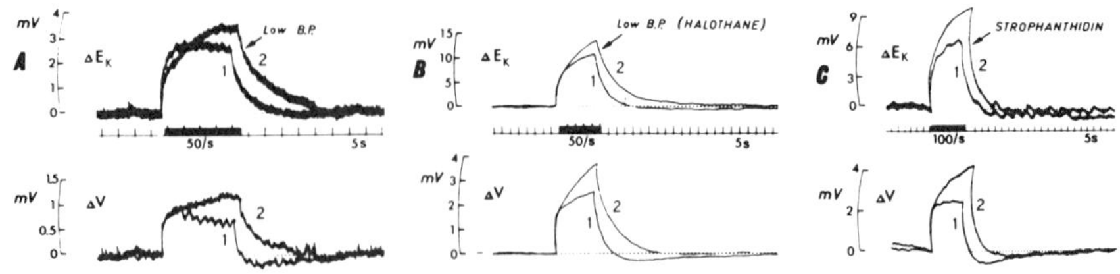

FIG. 2. Changes in potassium (ΔE_K) and tissue (ΔV) potentials evoked in cuneate by peripheral nerve stimulation (50 or 100/sec, 10 V, 0.1 ms). Traces labeled 1, control responses; traces labeled 2, superimposed responses. These responses were produced when **A:** mean arterial pressure fell spontaneously from 75 to 60 mm Hg; **B:** mean arterial pressure was lowered from 140 to 40 mm Hg by inhalation of 2% halothane; **C:** 10^{-4} M strophanthidin in Ringer was superfused over dorsal surface of medulla. (Reproduced in part from Fig. 6 in Krnjević and Morris, ref. 10.)

from a mean value of 140 to 40 mm Hg. That these changes may be attributed to lack of oxygen and interference with energy supplies of the Na-K pump is supported by the observation (8) that the same changes could be produced by superfusion over the cuneate a 10^{-4} M Ringer's solution of strophanthidin, a known blocker of membrane Na-K pumping.

Effects of Extracellular K^+ Accumulation on Synaptic Transmission

The above-described changes in extracellular K^+ levels and the concomitant depolarization and hyperpolarization of adjacent cellular elements may influence transmission across synapses in several different ways.

The effects of K^+ on synaptic transmission have been studied by directly exciting the afferent fibers near their terminals in the cuneate, while artificially raising a_K. The antidromically conducted potentials evoked by the stimulation and recorded from the peripheral nerves were used to estimate synaptic input, whereas the simultaneous postsynaptic responses to activated terminals, recorded as the orthodromically conducted potentials of the medial lemniscus, were used to estimate synaptic output. The input-output plots of Fig. 3 provide a computer-constructed display of integrals of these potentials, evoked with varying intensities of constant-current stimulation, and a superimposed stippled-line curve fitted to the points (see control values and curve of A).

When a K^+-enriched Ringer's solution was superfused over the medulla, the efficiency of synaptic transmission was progressively decreased as a_K increased (see B and C, Fig. 3, when extracellular a_K values near the stimulating microelectrode were 5.5 mM and 7.0 mM, respectively); this is shown by the shift in position of points and their fitted curve below the other curve (without points), which represents the control responses of A. Raising K^+ also caused input values to shift to the right (i.e., increase) indicating depolarization of the afferent fibers.

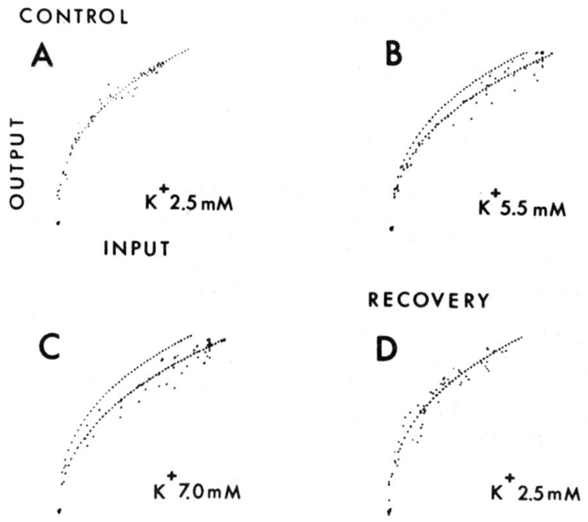

FIG. 3. Effect of increased extracellular K^+ on synaptic transmission. Input-output plots of integrals of antidromic nerve responses (input) and simultaneously recorded orthodromic lemniscal responses (output) to varying intensities of constant-current microelectrode stimulation of cuneate afferent fiber terminals (at a rate of 1/sec). **A:** Control values and a superimposed stippled line representing curve of best fit when extracellular K^+ activity (a_K) was 2.5 mM. **B** and **C:** When a_K was raised to 5.5 and 7.0 mM, respectively, output was decreased, as shown by lower distribution of scattered points and their curve. For comparison, control curve from **A** is also reproduced in **B, C,** and **D;** in **B** and **C** it is above plotted responses and their fitted curves, although in **D** it coincides with the recovery curve.

Depolarization of the afferent terminals is believed to decrease the amount of transmitter released with each successful impulse. However, when hyperpolarization occurs, transmitter release is increased and transmission facilitated. Furthermore, the degree of invasion of presynaptic terminals is probably variable and likely to be sensitive to these fluctuations in terminal excitability. The final effects of the changes produced by afferent activity will depend as well on changes in the excitability of postsynaptic structures and on the balance of both excitatory and inhibitory organization.

A significant role of K^+ release after afferent fiber activity may be in the suppression of high-threshold sensory inputs. Relatively large amounts of K^+ are released in synaptic areas by low intensities of stimulation (9). Therefore, activity in low-threshold, fast-conducting afferents may by this mechanism significantly depress transmission of high-threshold, slow-conducting inputs, especially if the latter have lower synaptic efficacy.

ACKNOWLEDGMENTS

We thank E. Leech and N. Schestakowich for technical and photographical work and the Medical Research Council of Canada for financial support.

REFERENCES

1. Andersen, P., Eccles, J. C., Schmidt, R. F., and Yokota, T. (1964): *J. Neurophysiol.*, 27: 78–91.
2. Bruggencate, G. ten, Lux, H. D., and Liebl, L. (1974): *Pfluegers Arch.*, 349:301–317.
3. Eccles, J. C., and Krnjević, K. (1959): *J. Physiol.*, 149:250–273.
4. Heinemann, U., and Lux, H. D. (1975): *Brain Res.*, 93:63–76.
5. Kříž, N., Sykova, E., Ujec, E., and Vycklický, L. (1974): *J. Physiol.*, 238:1–15.
6. Krnjević, K., and Morris, M. E. (1972): *Can. J. Physiol. Pharmacol.*, 50:1214–1217.
7. Krnjević, K., and Morris, M. E. (1974): *Can. J. Physiol. Pharmacol.*, 52:852–871.
8. Krnjević, K., and Morris, M. E. (1975): *J. Physiol. (Paris)*, 250:36–37.
9. Krnjević, K., and Morris, M. E. (1976*a*): *Can. J. Physiol. Pharmacol.*, 53:912–922.
10. Krnjević, K., and Morris, M. E. (1976*b*): *Can. J. Physiol. Pharmacol.*, 53:923–924.
11. Morris, M. E. (1971): *J. Physiol.*, 218:671–689.
12. Somjen, G. G., and Lothman, E. W. (1974): *Brain Res.*, 69:153–157.
13. Vyklický, L., Syková, E., Kříž, N., and Ujec, E. (1972): *Brain Res.*, 45:608–611.
14. Walker, J. L. (1971): *Anal. Chem.*, 43:89a–93a.
15. Wall, P. D. (1958): *J. Physiol. (Lond.)*, 142:1–21.

Advances in Pain Research and Therapy, Vol. 1,
edited by J. J. Bonica and D. Albe-Fessard.
Raven Press, New York © 1976.

Correlation Between the Inhibition of Impulse Transmission and the Increased Extracellular K^+ Produced by Peripheral Stimulation

L. Vyklický, Eva Syková, and N. Kříž

Institute of Physiology, Czechoslovak Academy of Sciences, Budějovická 1083, 142 20 Prague 4, Czechoslovakia

Peripheral stimulation is being used increasingly as a technique for producing local analgesia. Its mechanism is, however, still more a matter of speculation than of rational interpretation. It seems likely that more mechanisms are involved in this type of analgesia. One of these may result from the accumulation of K^+ in extracellular space after neuronal discharging.

In studies in which potassium-specific microelectrodes (7,8) were employed, investigators showed that the K^+ released during neuronal activity accumulates in the extracellular space of the spinal cord (1,3,5,6) and may account for, or at least contribute to, the primary afferent depolarization.

The aim of this study was to show whether or not some changes in impulse transmission correlate with increased extracellular K^+ that, in the spinal cord, accompanies peripheral stimulation.

METHOD

Experiments were performed on cats operated on under halothane anesthesia (Narcotan®). The spinal cord was exposed above the L_5-S_1 segments and peripheral nerves were dissected free on the left hindlimb. Animals were decerebrated at the intercollicular level and spinalized at the lower thoracic level. Anesthesia was then discontinued and the animal was immobilized with gallamine triethiodide (Flaxedil ®) and ventilated artificially with air. The expired CO_2 was maintained between 3.8% and 4.6%.

The recording system and the procedure of preparation of double-barrelled electrodes were the same as already described (3,7). In principle, the tip of one channel of a double-barrelled electrode was filled with K^+ liquid exchanger (Corning 477317) to a height of about 200 μm, and 0.5 M KCl was injected into the remaining part of this channel. The other channel of the electrode was filled with 0.15 M NaCl. Changes in potassium potential (K_e) were registered differentially between these two channels using a DC high-impedance amplifier, while field potentials were recorded between the NaCl channel and ground. Ventral root discharges were recorded by an RC coupled preamplifier.

RESULTS

Tetanic stimulation of peripheral nerves results in an increase of K_e in the corresponding spinal segment. The actual level of the increase depends on the frequency of stimulation, the position of the potassium-specific microelectrodes in the nucleus, and the anesthesia. The K_e was most increased in the intermediate region at the stimulation frequency of 100 Hz. A representative recording of transient changes in K_e in the intermediate region is demonstrated in Fig. 1A.

Tetanic stimulation of the posterior tibial nerve (100 Hz) resulted in an increase of K_e in the lumbar spinal cord from 3 mM to 7 mM. The increase in K_e was accompanied by a negativity, registered with the NaCl electrode against ground, as demonstrated in Fig. 1B. In other experiments extracellular K^+ increased from 3 mM to 9 mM.

K^+ accumulated after peripheral stimulation is redistributed not only by diffusion to inactive parts, but also by active transport. The active transport mechanism, which is electrogenic, does not stop its action after the original resting level of K_e is reached, and this results in a subnormal phase of K_e of 1- to 2-min duration. Partial hypoxia results in disappearance of the subnormal phase of K_e and in slowing of K^+ dissipation from extracellular space. The half-redistribution time of accumulated K^+, which follows the 30-sec peripheral stimulation, increases during hypoxia from 5 to 25 sec. Evidence was presented that the electrogenic transport mechanism is located in neurons that free the K^+ while discharging (3).

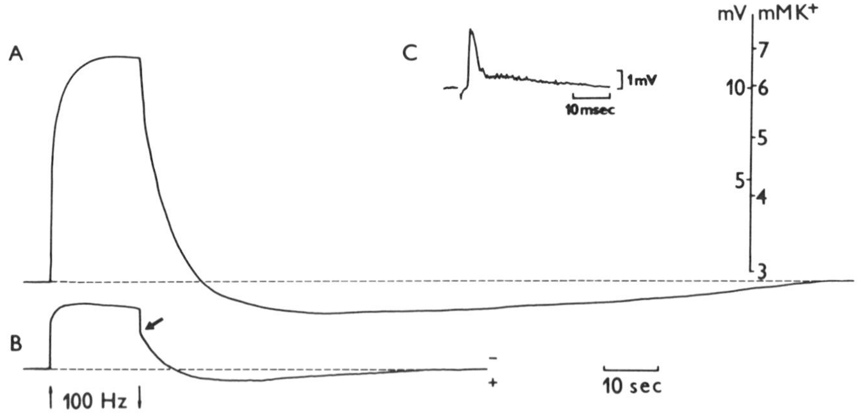

FIG. 1. Changes of K_e in the spinal cord and negative potentials produced by 100-Hz stimulation of the posterior tibial nerve. **A:** Differential record of K_e made with a double-barrelled potassium-specific microelectrode. **B:** Corresponding DC potential shifts recorded with NaCl-filled channel of the microelectrode against ground produced by 16-sec stimulation of posterior tibial nerve at 100 Hz. A highly sensitive linear recorder with the rise time of 0.5 sec for 10 mV was used. **C:** Field potential evoked by a single volley in the same nerve. Potassium-specific electrode was calibrated in solutions containing various K^+ concentrations with 150 mM NaCl background.

The efficacy of synaptic transmission has been shown to be decreased during depolarization of presynaptic terminals; this forms the essence on which the theory of presynaptic inhibition is based (2). On the other hand, the sudden increase in the K_e can also lower the membrane potential of the postsynaptic elements and in this way increase the probability of their firing. To determine whether changes in impulse transmission in the spinal cord correlate with the accumulation of K^+ in extracellular space, we examined the changes in the amplitude of the field potentials and ventral root discharges at various levels of K_e.

Figure 2A demonstrates an increase in K_e produced by stimulation of the posterior tibial nerve at 100 Hz. Examples of the field potentials evoked by a single volley in the same nerve, recorded with the NaCl channel at intervals, are indicated by dots on the curve of K_e. In B the amplitudes of the field potentials are expressed as percentages of the control and plotted against time during the K_e elevation. Two seconds after tetanic stimulation was discontinued, the amplitude of the field potential was reduced to approximately 50% of the control and the recovery of the amplitude closely correlated with the time course of the K_e changes. The amplitude of the field potentials did not recover completely after the K_e reached its original level, and it was still decreased by approximately 5% during the phase of subnormal K_e.

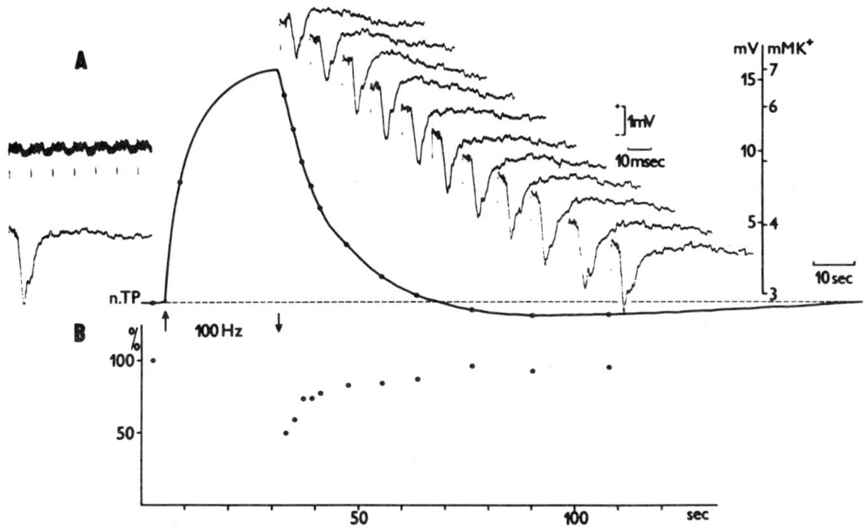

FIG. 2. Effect of accumulated K_e on the amplitude of the focal potentials. **A:** Record of K_e changes induced by stimulation of the posterior tibial nerve (n.TP) at 100 Hz. Focal potentials were evoked by a single volley in the same nerve at intervals shown by points on the curve of K_e. **B:** Amplitudes of focal potentials plotted as percentages of the control against time.

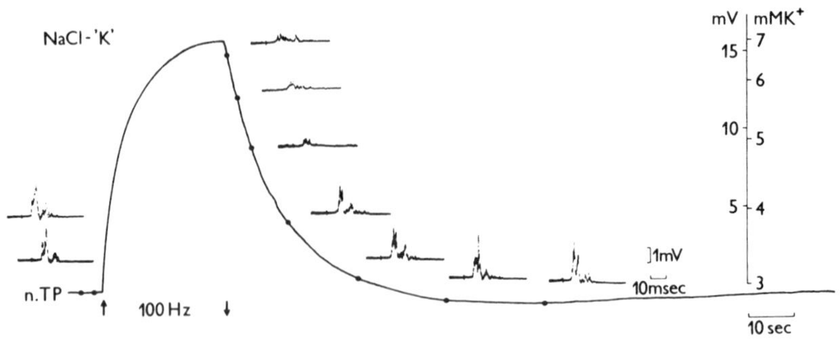

FIG. 3. Effect of accumulated K^+ on ventral root (VR) discharge. Curve represents the time course of K_e changes induced by 100-Hz stimulation of the posterior tibial nerve (n.TP). VR discharges were evoked by a single volley in the sural nerve at intervals indicated on the record of K_e.

Figure 3 demonstrates L_7 ventral root (VR) discharges elicited by a single stimulus applied to the sural nerve at various levels of increased K_e, induced by stimulation of the posterior tibial nerve at 100 Hz. The VR discharges were quite depressed during the phase of K_e elevation.

CONCLUSIONS

The correlation between the time course of elevated K_e which follows peripheral stimulation and the depression of field potentials and VR discharges suggests that elevated K_e results in decreased efficacy of synaptic transmission. Whether the depression occurs only at the presynaptic level or also at the postsynaptic elements must be clarified. It would be far-fetched to speculate on the possible participation of K_e in the processes resulting from the long-term plastic changes in the CNS. The well-known activation of metabolic processes combined with increased oxygen consumption that is induced by increased K_e would favor this idea.

REFERENCES

1. Bruggencate, G. ten, Lux, H. D., and Liebl, L. (1974): *Pfluegers Arch.*, 349:301–317.
2. Eccles, J. C. (1964): *The Physiology of Synapses.* Springer-Verlag, Berlin.
3. Kříž, N., Syková, E., Ujec, E., and Vyklický, L. (1974): *J. Physiol.*, 238:1–15.
4. Kříž, N., Syková, E., and Vyklický, L. (1975): *J. Physiol.*, 249:35–70.
5. Krnjević, K., and Morris, M. E. (1972): *Can. J. Physiol. Pharmacol.*, 50:1214–1217.
6. Vyklický, L., Syková, E., Kříž, N., and Ujec, E. (1972): *Brain Res.*, 45:608–611.
7. Vyskočil, F., and Kříž, N. (1972): *Pfluegers Arch.*, 337:265–276.
8. Walker, J. L. (1971): *Anal. Chem.*, 43:89A–92A.

Advances in Pain Research and Therapy, Vol. 1,
edited by J. J. Bonica and D. Albe-Fessard.
Raven Press, New York © 1976.

Differential Effects of Cutaneous Nerve Fibers (Myelinated and Unmyelinated) on Monosynaptic Flexor Reflex of the Cat

Neri Accornero, Giorgio Bini, Gian Luigi Lenzi, and Mario Manfredi

I Clinica delle Malattie Nervose e Mentali dell'Universita di Roma, Viale dell'Universita 30, 00185 Rome, Italy

This study was undertaken to define the conditioning effect of myelinated A beta and A delta and unmyelinated C volleys of cutaneous origin, obtained by selective activation of the sural nerve fiber groups, on spinal monosynaptic flexor reflex of the decerebrate cat.

METHODS

The monosynaptic reflex was evoked by electrical stimulation of the peroneus (P) nerve and posterior biceps semitendinosus (PBST) nerve and recorded from the corresponding ventral roots exposed by laminectomy. The conditioning afferent volley was monitored from the cutaneous nerve trunk. All ventral roots had been sectioned. The aim of the experiment was to determine if cutaneous volleys of different compositions act differentially on the spinal motoneuron pool subserving the reflex. Opposite effects of small and larger diameter fibers would be expected if the spinal gating mechanism proposed by Melzack and Wall (1) also acts at the level of the motoneuron pool. The conditioning testing curves were obtained by sampling the monosynaptic reflex at various intervals after afferent volleys segregated to various fiber groups. The amplitude of the conditioned response was compared to those of unconditioned ones.

RESULTS

When the monosynaptic flexor (peroneus) reflex was preceded by cutaneous beta volley (Fig. 1), a peak of facilitation became apparent as early as 5 to 10 msec after the conditioning stimulus, followed by a transient period of relative inhibition at 25 msec, and then by a late facilitation curve beginning at 50 msec. The facilitatory effect lasted for approximately 50 msec. Conditioning of the flexor reflex by a delta cutaneous volley determined a facilitation curve beginning at 25 msec, with a peak at 50 msec and a total

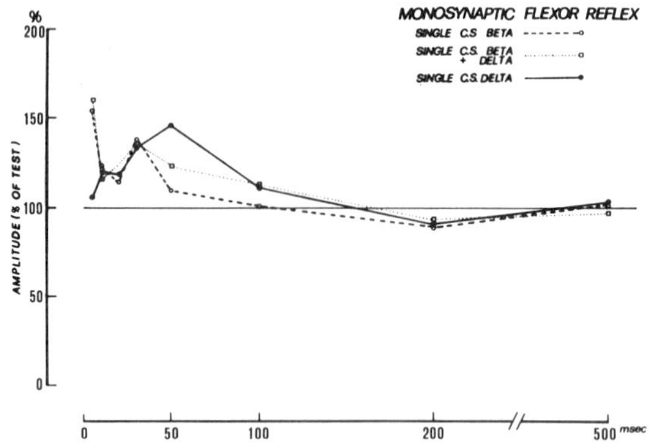

FIG. 1. Excitability cycle of the monosynaptic flexor reflex of the Peroneus muscle after a single conditioning volley in beta, beta-delta, and delta fibers of the sural nerve.

duration of 100 msec. Combined effects of beta and delta volleys are equal to the effect of each set of fibers fired separately. The main differential effect of large and small myelinated fibers was a time lag between the facilitatory peaks, the action of delta fibers becoming apparent later owing to the longer conduction time of the delta volley in the peripheral nerve.

The phase of relative inhibition which followed the beta volley at 20 msec was probably attributable to an occlusion phenomenon because it occurred at the peak of motoneuron discharge evoked polysynaptically by the cutaneous volley itself. This phenomenon has been extensively investigated on the monosynaptic flexor reflex of the PBST nerve, where the intermediate phase of inhibition after beta volleys was even more apparent and was strictly coincident in time with the afferent conditioning polysynaptic flexor discharge evoked by the afferent conditioning volley and mediating the avoidance reflex.

In the experiment shown in Fig. 2 a cutaneous beta volley evoked a polysynaptic flexor discharge which started approximately 2 to 3 msec after the stimulus and lasted up to 20 to 30 msec. The inhibition of the monosynaptic PBST twitch reached its peak at 12 msec, an interval coincident with the peak of the polysynaptic reflex (Fig. 2Ab). A beta-delta volley engendered a more prolonged motoneuron discharge, and the inhibitory phase of the PBST monosynaptic reflex was also prolonged (Fig. 2Ac). The polysynaptic reflex evoked by delta volleys started approximately 4 msec after the cutaneous nerve stimulation and reached its peak after 15 to 30 msec. The inhibitory phase of the monosynaptic PBST twitch was correspondingly delayed (Fig. 2Ad, 24 to 30 msec). Plotting of the early phase of the excitability cycle in Fig 2B shows clearly the different temporal patterns of the beta and delta conditioning effects and their summation when both myelinated groups of fibers are fired together.

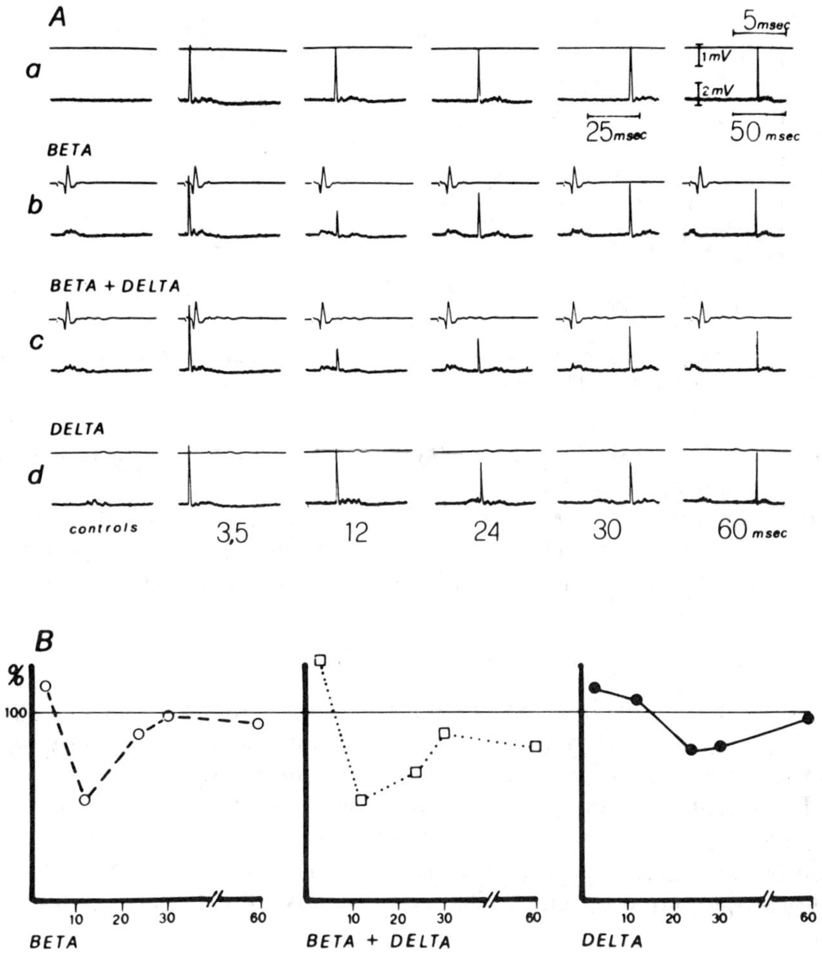

FIG. 2. Early phase of excitability cycle of the monosynaptic flexor reflex of the posterior biceps semitendinosus (PBST) muscle. **A:** Upper beam, afferent conditioning volley recorded from the sural nerve trunk; lower beam, monosynaptic and polysynaptic reflexes recorded from the corresponding ventral root. **a:** Unconditioned monosynaptic reflex; **b, c,** and **d:** monosynaptic reflex conditioned by beta, beta-delta, and delta single afferent volleys. First column shows effect of the conditioning stimulus without muscle nerve stimulation. Following columns show the monosynaptic reflex for conditioning testing intervals. **B:** Plot of excitability cycle of the monosynaptic reflex after beta, beta-delta, and delta single conditioning volleys.

Subsequently we studied the effect of unmyelinated volleys. Even in this case a facilitation of the monosynaptic (peroneus) reflex was constantly observed, and it was much more delayed in time: the facilitation began after 50 msec, was more evident at 100 msec, and faded away after 200 msec. The delayed action of C volleys is explained more simply by the late

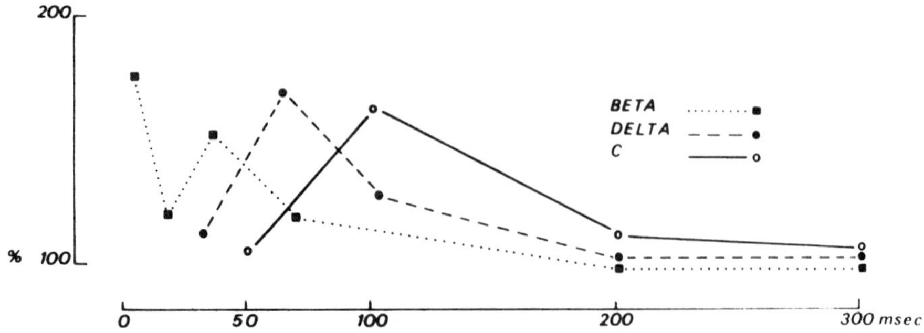

FIG. 3. Excitability cycles of the monosynaptic flexor reflex of the peroneus muscle after a single conditioning volley in beta, beta-delta, and C fibers of the sural nerve.

arrival of C impulses because of the slow conduction velocity of unmyelinated peripheral nerve fibers.

Plotting of the three beta, delta, and C conditioning curves of the peroneus reflex (Fig. 3) clearly demonstrates that the monosynaptic flexor reflex fundamentally is facilitated by all kinds of cutaneous afferents.

CONCLUSION

In conclusion, we have observed no substantial difference among effects of conditioning the motoneuron pool responding to the monosynaptic flexor reflex with different sets of peripheral nerve fibers.

The common result is a facilitatory phase interrupted by a period of relative or absolute inhibition. The facilitation is related to temporal summation of cutaneous and muscle afferents on the motoneuron pool of flexor muscle; the period of relative inhibition is caused by a phenomenon of occlusion.

The phases of facilitation and inhibition after conditioning by the different sets of cutaneous nerve fibers take place at different latencies related to conduction time of conditioning impulses in the peripheral nerve. Consequently, at a given delay cutaneous myelinated and unmyelinated fibers can act in opposite directions on the motoneuron pool activated by the monosynaptic flexor reflex, but the basic effect is fundamentally analogous for the various groups of different sizes. Therefore, these data do not support the existence of a gating system at the spinal level acting differentially after cutaneous volleys in fibers of different sizes.

REFERENCE

1. Melzack, R., and Wall, P. D. (1965): *Science,* 150:971.

Advances in Pain Research and Therapy, Vol. 1,
edited by J. J. Bonica and D. Albe-Fessard.
Raven Press, New York © 1976.

Evaluation of Central and Peripheral Pain Mechanisms by Nociceptive Flexion Reflex in Man

J. C. Willer, N. Bathien, and A. Hugelin

Laboratoire de Physiologie, Faculté de Médecine St-Antoine, Paris, France

Electrical stimulation of the sural (Su) nerve in man elicits a polysynaptic reflex response in the hindlimb flexor muscles (6,8,10). This response has two components: the first (RII) has a short latency and corresponds to the activation of low-threshold, large-diameter myelinated cutaneous (Cu) fibers (Lloyd's group AII) (12). The second (RIII) has a longer latency and a higher threshold and corresponds to the stimulation of small-diameter cutaneous fibers (group AIII).

In man (4,5) as well as in animals (1,9,13,18), group AII fibers transmit cutaneous tactile messages, whereas group AIII fibers convey painful sensations. Furthermore, a strict relationship links on the one hand the RII reflex of biceps femoris (BF) muscle and tactile sensation, and on the other hand the RIII reflex of the same muscle and pain sensation (7). Other authors (3) have confirmed these observations and have also shown that it is possible to modify selectively by pharmacological agents the threshold of both pain sensation and the RIII reflex. These results have shown that it is possible to ascertain the nature of the afferent volley while studying the corresponding sensation. However, this technique of stimulation of the sural nerve fibers does not test the cutaneous receptors from which the sensory messages and ensuing reflex activities normally originate.

Cutaneous innervation stems from two nervous plexuses parallel to the skin surface. The deep dermal plexus is composed of large-diameter fibers (AII), whereas the second, more superficial plexus is made of smaller diameter fibers (17). Some authors have suggested that the superficial network could contain pain receptors since it often terminates in complicated open loops and in endings that surround capillaries (11,15,16). According to this hypothesis, cutaneous stimulation activating the superficial plexus elicits pain sensation only.

In the present work, electrical cutaneous stimulation in the sural nerve sensory field was compared to stimulation of the sural nerve itself in a study of RIII reflex activity in BF and corresponding painful sensation. Following this, pharmacological agents (algogenics and analgesics) were used to test separately the excitability of cutaneous receptors and corresponding afferent fibers.

METHODS

Experiments were carried out on 15 young (20- to 30-year-old), healthy volunteers (10 men, 5 women) chosen among medical students and physiologists. All of them had participated previously in similar experimental series, and they were carefully briefed before each session. For the sessions, they were placed in an armchair specially designed to elicit satisfactory muscular relaxation.

Stimulations

The sural nerve was stimulated either percutaneously or transcutaneously. In the latter case, stimulation was achieved by two steel-needle electrodes insulated to the tip and inserted through the skin (2 cm apart) directly on the sural nerve at the retromalleolar level. Bipolar stimulation of the skin in the distal sural nerve sensory field was made by inserting two surface electrodes (2 cm apart) in the skin.

In each case, electrical stimulation consisted of a 20-msec wave (1 msec, 300 c/s) given by a constant-current stimulator every 5 sec. Intensity of stimulation varied from 0 to 15 mA and was measured by an intensity probe and CRO displayed. The intensity eliciting 60% to 70% of reflex responses was chosen as threshold.

Small-caliber fibers were electively activated by electric stimulation of sural nerve after ischemic block of group AII fibers of this nerve. The block was made by placing a pneumatic cuff above the ankle between stimulating and recording electrodes. The pressure in the cuff was maintained at a level that was twice the maximal blood pressure (approximately 300 mm Hg).

In 7 subjects the skin was rubbed with abrasive paste in the sensory field of the sural nerve to expose the dermis over an area of approximately 1 cm^2. Another maneuver was to apply on either the skin or the dermis a naphthalene solution (Napht) known to activate selectively small-diameter fibers (J. Gybels, *personal communication,* 1974).

Recordings

Recordings of the BF activity were made with bipolar surface electrodes currently used in electromyography (2,6). Sensations were measured in arbitrary units (AU) according to Gybels' method (*personal communication*).

In all subjects the actions of a local anesthetic (lidocaine 2%) and a peripheral analgesic (acetylsalicylic acid, ASA) were tested. In a few cases a central analgesic (pethidine, Peth) was also used. All these drugs were given at the low therapeutic dose currently used in patients complaining of pain. The effects of a placebo (dextrose) were also studied in 10 subjects.

Stimulation of the Sural Nerve

Percutaneous as well as transcutaneous sural nerve stimulation (Fig. 1A) elicits two types of reflex responses which correspond to two different types of sensations. The first response (RII) has a short latency (40 to 70 msec) and a low threshold (6 mA). A threshold stimulation of RII evokes a tactile sensation similar to that provoked by a superficial artery pulsation. The second response (RIII,Su) has a longer latency (90 to 150 msec) and a higher threshold (10 mA). The threshold stimulation of RIII,Su evokes at threshold a pricking pain (3.5 ± 0.2 AU) accurately localized at the level of the stimulating electrodes.

Skin Stimulation

A 10-mA stimulation applied on the skin in the sural nerve sensory field (Fig. 1B) elicits a supraliminal nociceptive reflex response (RIII,Cu), as well as a strong but short burning pain poorly localized in the area of stimulation. The threshold intensity provoking RIII,Cu is 5 mA and corresponds to the appearance of a painful sensation (3.7 ± 0.2 AU). In these conditions, no tactile RII response was ever observed.

These results suggest that: (a) an appropriate cutaneous stimulation activates only receptors from which small-caliber fibers originate, and (b) activation of group AII fibers during sural nerve stimulation inhibits both nociceptive reflex response (RIII) and pain sensation. Further experiments were then carried out to confirm this latter hypothesis: in 7 subjects a 10-mA stimulation was applied on the sural nerve during an ischemic block of group AII fibers. The tactile reflex response (RIII) decreases progressively and disappears between 10 and 12 min after the beginning compression. Concurrently, the amplitudes of both RIII,Su and corresponding pain increase and become supraliminal after the same delay; the threshold is then significantly lowered to 5 to 6 mA ($p < 0.001$).

The ratio of the thresholds RIII,Cu/RIII,Su was then studied to test the excitability of cutaneous receptors and afferent fibers, respectively. It has been observed that the value of this ratio is approximately 50% and that it stays constant for all subjects during successive recording sessions. How-

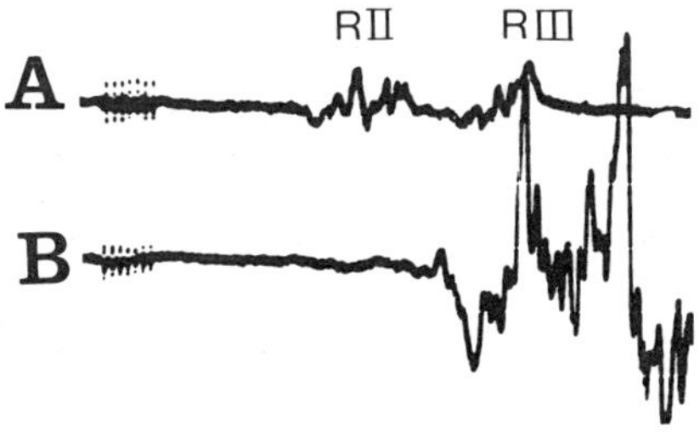

FIG. 1. Polysynaptic reflex responses recorded in biceps femoris muscle during a 10-mA stimulation of **A:** sural nerve, and **B:** skin in the distal sensory field of this nerve. Note an early RII reflex and a liminal RIII nociceptive response in **A.** However, no RII response is observed in **B,** whereas the nociceptive component (RIII) has a shorter latency and a greater amplitude than in **A.** Calibration: vertical, 100 μV; horizontal, 30 msec.

ever, this ratio is modified under the influence of pharmacological agents, as outlined in the following paragraphs.

1. Local application of Napht on the skin provokes after a 30- to 60-sec delay a painful burning sensation that lasts for 5 to 6 min. At the same time, the threshold of RIII,Cu is significantly lowered, whereas RIII,Su response is not modified. When the action of the drug is maximal, the ratio is reduced to 10%.

2. In contrast, application of a 2% lidocaine solution directly on the dermis provokes an increase of the threshold of RIII,Cu and corresponding pain. In this case also there is no modification of the respective RIII,Su threshold and corresponding pain. Identical observations were made on application of ASA (200 mg/ml). These thresholds are not changed when drugs are applied on undamaged skin. This effect was compared to the action of intravenous injection of ASA (1 g), which provokes after a 5- to 7-min delay an increase of RIII,Cu threshold and corresponding pain. As before, no changes can be observed on RIII,Su threshold.

3. In a few cases a central analgesic (Peth) was used. After i.m. injection of Peth (100 mg), the thresholds of RIII,Cu and pain sensation increased, whereas the threshold of RIII,Su decreased. A certain drowsiness was also observed in these subjects.

4. No changes in RIII,Cu or RIII,Su thresholds or in pain sensation were observed when a placebo (dextrose) was given per os. These results are summarized in Fig. 2.

	Control	Napht.	Lid.	A.S.A.	Peth.	Pbo.
RIII,Cu (mA)	5	↘	↗	↗	↗	→
RIII,Su (mA)	10	→	→	→	↘	→
RIII,Cu / RIII,Su %	50	↘ 10 •••	↗ 110 •••	↗ 90 •••	↗ 180 •••	→ 50

FIG. 2. Summary of changes in the RIII,Cu (mA) and RIII,Su (mA) thresholds, as well as the RIII,Cu/RIII,Su ratio (%) provoked by chemical or pharmacological agents, compared to control values. Napht., naphthalene; Lit., lidocaine; A.S.A., acetylsalicylic acid; Peth., pethidine; Pbo., placebo. Arrows indicate increase (↗), decrease (↘), or no change (→) in the RIII,Cu and RIII,Su thresholds and in the RIII,Cu/RIII,Su ratio. Numbers in the bottom line indicate RIII,Cu/RIII,Su values at the maximal drug effect. *** is significant at $p < 0.001$.

SUMMARY

A 10-mA stimulation of the sural nerve elicits in biceps femoris a tactile RII reflex response as well as a nociceptive liminal RIII,Su response corresponding to threshold of a painful sensation. However, a similar stimulation applied on the skin in the sural nerve sensory field evokes only an RIII,Cu nociceptive response of supraliminal amplitude as well as a strong painful sensation. These results confirm the existence of an inhibition exerted by AII on AIII fibers at the level of spinal cord. This is also supported by the observations made during selective ischemia of AII fibers on the sural nerve. The results are consistent with the gate control theory (14). On the other hand, they show a marked difference between the excitability of pain receptors and their corresponding fibers.

The study of the ratio of the thresholds of RIII,Cu/RIII,Su shows that its value is approximately 50% and that: (a) it stays constant for all subjects from one session to another; (b) it is lowered by algogenic chemical agents; (c) it is increased by local anesthetics, aspirin (i.v. or applied locally on the dermis), and central analgesics; and (d) it is not modified by placebos.

This ratio appears to be a reliable index of pain intensity since its stability contrasts with the marked variations observed in individual pain sensation. It should be useful in pharmacological as well as in clinical studies of pain.

REFERENCES

1. Adrian, E. D. (1931): *Proc. R. Soc. Lond.* [*Biol.*], 109:1–8.
2. Bathien, N., and Bourdarias, H. (1972): *Brain,* 95:447–456.
3. Bathien, N., and Willer, J. C. (1974): *Therapie,* 29:709–717.
4. Collins, W. F., Nulsen, F. E., and Randt, C. T. (1960): *Arch. Neurol.,* 3:381–385.
5. Henzel, H., and Boman, K. K. A. (1960): *J. Neurophysiol.,* 23:564–578.
6. Hugon, M. (1967): *Rèflexes Polysynaptiques Cutanés et Commande Volontaire,* Thése Sciences, Paris.
7. Hugon, M. (1973): In: *New Developments in Electromyography and Clinical Neurophysiology, Vol. III: Human Reflexes,* edited by J. E. Desmedt. S. Karger, Basel.
8. Hugon, M., Bathien, N., and Ducourthial, F. (1965): *J. Physiol.* (*Paris*), 57:631–632.
9. Hunt, C. C., and MacIntyre, A. K. (1961): *J. Physiol.* (*Lond.*), 143:195–212.
10. Kugelberg, E., Eklund, K., and Grimby, L. (1960): *Brain,* 83:394–410.
11. Lim, R. K. S. (1968): In: *Pharmacology of Pain,* edited by R. K. S. Lim, D. Armstrong, and E. G. Pardo. Pergamon Press, Oxford and New York.
12. Lloyd, D. P. C. (1943): *J. Neurophysiol.,* 6:293–315.
13. Maruhashi, J., Mizaguchi, K., and Tasaki, I. (1952): *J. Physiol.* (*Lond.*), 183:245–252.
14. Melzack, R., and Wall, P. D. (1965): *Science,* 150:971–979.
15. Weddell, G. (1945): *Br. Med. Bull.,* 3:167–172.
16. Weddell, G., and Sinclair, D. C. (1953): *Acta Neuroveg.* (*Wien*), 7:135–146.
17. Winkelman, R. K. (1960): *Nerve Endings in Normal and Pathologic Skin.* Charles C Thomas, Publisher, Springfield, Illinois.
18. Zotterman, Y. (1939): *J. Physiol.* (*Lond.*), 95:1–28.

Advances in Pain Research and Therapy, Vol. 1,
edited by J. J. Bonica and D. Albe-Fessard.
Raven Press, New York © 1976.

Peripheral and Central Trigeminal "Pain" Pathways

R. Dubner, S. Gobel, and D. D. Price

Neurobiology and Anesthesiology Branch, National Institute of Dental Research, National Institutes of Health, Bethesda, Maryland 20014

Sensory messages from the mouth and face travel along peripheral nerve fibers which project to a brainstem nuclear complex that extends from the pons to the upper cervical segments of the spinal cord. This core of neurons can be divided into subnuclei in the rostrocaudal direction, and each level consists of multiple neuronal cell types (24). Neurons that send direct projections to ventrobasal thalamus are found at all levels (4). Neurons with axons confined to the trigeminal brainstem nuclear complex and surrounding reticular formation also are numerous. Their intranuclear axonal projections ascend and descend throughout the body of the nucleus in distinct fiber bundles (13,35). In addition, there are projections to the trigeminal nuclei from the cerebral cortex (3,10), and physiological studies suggest that activity in the cerebral cortex and in other regions of the central nervous system can ultimately modify sensory transmission in these brainstem nuclei (4,23). This complex structural organization suggests that considerable modification of incoming sensory messages takes place at this level of the trigeminal system.

A trigeminal tractotomy procedure (Sjöqvist operation) which interrupts the trigeminal brainstem nuclear complex in its more caudal extent near the obex produces an almost complete loss of pain and temperature sensibility in the oral-facial region with minor effects on touch sensation (31,40,41). This sensory dissociation in humans has led to two major hypotheses about the role of the trigeminal brainstem nuclei in the transmission of nociceptive signals to other levels of the neuraxis. One general hypothesis states that the caudal region, nucleus caudalis, exerts a modulating influence on sensory transmission through the more rostral subdivisions of the nuclear complex via the intranuclear system. Mechanisms of summation, inhibition, and facilitation are critical determinants of the final output of trigeminothalamic projection neurons in the more rostral subdivisions. There is recent evidence in support of this hypothesis (6,34,43). The second general hypothesis considers nucleus caudalis to be the major component of the trigeminal nucleus concerned with nociception. It receives noxious input and conveys this information to the thalamus via a distinct primary afferent-projection neuron pathway, which does not include the more rostral subdivisions of the trigeminal brainstem nucleus. Recent anatomical and physiological studies in our laboratory have examined the organization of nucleus caudalis, and our data support this second hypothesis. This chapter describes some of these findings and our present ideas about the role of nucleus caudalis in pain mechanisms.[1]

PERIPHERAL NEURAL POPULATIONS RESPONSIVE TO NOXIOUS STIMULI

Several lines of evidence converge to indicate that the substantia gelatinosal (SG) layer of nucleus caudalis receives an exclusive projection of small myelinated and unmyelinated axons with receptor terminals activated primarily by noxious and thermal stimuli. Ramón y Cajal (30) showed that small-caliber axons terminated in the upper layers of nucleus caudalis. More recently, Gobel (11) reported that the trigeminal nerve endings in the SG layer differ morphologically from endings in other layers and in other subdivisions of the trigeminal nuclei. The inherent density of the axoplasm gives these endings a dark appearance when compared to trigeminal nerve endings in other areas. The long, thin, scalloped outline of these endings in the SG layer also distinguishes them from other trigeminal axonal endings.

The conclusion that these terminals arise from small-caliber axons is based on additional lines of evidence. Cell bodies in the trigeminal ganglion can be divided into pale and dark neurons with the smallest ones being dark (25,30). The perikaryl cytoplasm of these dark neurons (25) is similar in inherent density to that of the endings in SG (11). Ramón y Cajal (30) also showed that these small dark neurons have either unmyelinated or small myelinated axons. In addition, both the dark ganglion cells (25) and the trigeminal terminals in the SG layer (33) give a strong acid phosphatase reaction. A related finding in humans is that autopsied material from cases of congenital insensitivity to pain reveals an absence of small-caliber axons and small dorsal root ganglion neurons (37).

What are the physiological properties of small myelinated (A delta) and unmyelinated (C) trigeminal nerve fibers? Other than a small population of A-delta mechanosensitive fibers and approximately 10% of C fibers, these peripheral fiber populations in monkey respond to noxious or thermal stimuli or to both (ref. 8 and Beitel and Dubner, *this volume*). We have studied in detail the properties of trigeminal peripheral fibers responsive to noxious heat stimuli ($>45°C$) applied to the hairy skin of the monkey's face. Noxious heat is more easily quantified than noxious mechanical stimuli and

[1] Various aspects of the work were done in collaboration with R. Beitel, J. Hu, S. Starkman, and R. Sumino and have been published elsewhere (refs. 8,9,17,36 and Beitel and Dubner, *this volume*).

TABLE 1. *Summary of response properties of peripheral nerve fiber types activated by noxious heat*

Fiber Type	Cond. Vel. $\bar{X} \pm$ S.D. (m/sec)	R.F. Size	Thermal Response				
			Activity at 35°C	Cooling	Warming	Noxious Heat	Sensitization
Cold	9.0 ± 3.4 N = 94	<300μ spot	+	↑↑	↓↓	↑↑*	+
Warm	3.4 ± 1.7 N = 43	<300μ spot	+	↓↓	↑↑	↑↑	—
Heat Nociceptor	10.5 ± 7.6 N = 5	1-2mm spot	+*	—	↑ (above 38°C)	↑↑	+
Polymodal Nociceptor	0.82 ± 0.17 N = 20	1-2mm spot	+*	—	↑ (above 38°C)	↑↑	+

R. F., receptive field; *, after repeated exposure to noxious heat; +, response; −, no response; ↑, response increase; ↓, response decrease.

activates a more restricted group of peripheral fibers (8). In addition, extensive psychophysical experiments of pain sensitivity in humans to radiant heat (15) and recent behavioral experiments on escape performance in monkeys to noxious heat (7) can be correlated with peripheral neural activity to similar stimuli (Dubner and Beitel, *this volume*).

Table 1 illustrates some of the properties of the four major fiber types that were activated by noxious heat. Not included in Table 1 is a fifth fiber type, high-threshold mechanosensitive fibers, which sometimes responded after repeated exposure to heat (2,8,26). *Cold fibers* had conduction velocities in the A-delta range, and their firing rates were increased during cooling shifts and were suppressed during warming shifts. Their responses to innocuous temperature shifts were similar to those of cold fibers found on primate tongue (27) and digital skin (5). Initially they often responded to temperature shifts in the noxious heat range, but thresholds were very high—above 55°C. Repeated exposure to heat sensitized these fibers so that threshold responses were below 50°C and the magnitude of the response was increased at suprathreshold final temperatures (9). The initial high thresholds of these fibers rule out any significant role in the detection of noxious heat. However, after sensitization, their central effect may be more substantial.

Table 1 also shows that *small myelinated heat nociceptors* (R. E. Beitel and R. Dubner, *unpublished*) and *unmyelinated polymodal nociceptors* (Beitel and Dubner, *this volume*) also exhibited sensitization and showed threshold, latency, and sensitivity changes after repeated exposure to noxious heat. Observations of hyperalgesia in psychophysical studies (14) and after common experiences of excessive exposure to noxious heat (e.g., sunburn) may be related, in part, to the sensitization of these peripheral afferents.

Warm fibers had conduction velocities in the A-delta and C-fiber range, and their firing rates increased during warming shifts and were suppressed during cooling shifts (Table 1). Unmyelinated warm fibers with similar properties and receptive fields on primate limbs have been reported by others (16). Some warm fibers were activated by noxious heat stimuli and exhibited short-latency, high-frequency transient responses which increased in magnitude to final temperatures of 47° to 49°C (8,36). These sudden increases in activity may provide central activity related to the stinging, brief quality of heat-induced first pain (Price, *this volume*).

A-delta heat nociceptors and *C-polymodal nociceptors* have similar general properties (Table 1). Polymodal nociceptors have been studied in detail (Beitel and Dubner, *this volume*). Their thermal thresholds ranged from 38° to 49°C, and maximum discharge frequencies occurred in the noxious heat range (45° to 55°C). Over the range from threshold to 50° to 53°C, response magnitude increased as a monotonic function of stimulus intensity. Most of these nociceptors had intensity functions that were positively accelerating with the steep portion of the curve occurring in the 45° to 53°C range. Similar to polymodal nociceptors with receptive fields on the limbs of cat (1,2) and man (38), these nociceptors often had mechanical thresholds that were not considered noxious by human subjects.

A-delta heat nociceptors and C-polymodal nociceptors were the only fiber types that were sensitive over the range of skin temperatures to which humans scale radiant heat pain (15) and monkeys exhibit escape behavior (Dubner and Beitel, *this volume*). Clearly the activity of one or both of these fiber populations is essential for these discriminations. Aside from their conduction velocities, these fiber populations appear to have similar properties, although heat nociceptors are more sensitive to noxious heat stimuli in the 45° to 53°C range than polymodal nociceptors (Fig. 2 in Dubner and Beitel, *this volume*).

NEURONS IN NUCLEUS CAUDALIS RESPONSIVE TO NOXIOUS STIMULI

The next phase of our physiological studies involved a similar parametric analysis of the response characteristics of neurons in nucleus caudalis to noxious input. Trigeminothalamic neurons were identified by antidromic stimulation of their axon projections in the ventrobasal thalamus. This was a critical part of the analysis since it identified the presence of direct projections from nucleus caudalis to the thalamus which bypassed the more rostral subdivisions of the nucleus and provided additional support for the second hypothesis discussed above. Histological reconstruction of electrode tracks and small (25- to 50-μm) electrolytic lesions at the site of critical unit recordings enabled us to locate neurons in either the marginal (MAR) or magnocellular (MAG) layer of nucleus caudalis or in the contiguous lateral reticular formation (LRF).

TABLE 2. *Summary of response properties of trigeminothalamic projection neurons and interneurons in nucleus caudalis and contiguous lateral reticular formation*

Neuron Type	Antidromic Cond. Vel. X̄ ± S.D. (m/sec)	Orthodromic Latency X̄ ± S.D. (msec)	Location			R.F. Size			Thermal Response		
			Mar	Mag	LRF	S	M	L	Cooling	Warming	Noxious Heat
Touch	14.6 ± 6.4 N = 33	2.2 ± 1.0 (n = 11)	—	++	+	++	+	+	—	—	—
Touch-Pressure	14.0 ± 4.5 N = 24	2.2 ± 1.0 (n = 11)	—	++	+	++	+	+	+	—	—
Touch-Pressure-Pinch	11.6 ± 6.9 N = 27	3.1 ± 1.0 (n = 28)	+	++	++	+	++	++	+	+ (above 38°C)	++
Pressure-Pinch	7.0 ± 4.4 N = 14	9.6 ± 3.7 (n = 16)	++	+	++	++	+	+	—	+ (above 38°C)	+
Pinch	5.6 ± 4.4 N = 10	21.2 ± 8.2 (n = 9)	+	+	++	++	+	—	—	—	—

Mar, marginal layer, and Mag, magnocellular layer of nucleus caudalis; LRF, lateral reticular formation. S, small receptive fields (1–2 cm^2); M, medium receptive fields (>2 cm^2 but confined to 1 trigeminal major division); L, large receptive fields (>1 trigeminal major division); ++, many neurons; +, some neurons; –, no neurons.

Table 2 presents some of the general properties of the neuronal cell types studied (17). The analysis yielded five neuron types distinguished by the range of responses to mechanical stimuli. No trigeminothalamic neurons were found which were sensitive exclusively to noxious heat stimuli. A few projection neurons responded to warming or cooling in addition to noxious mechanical or thermal stimuli. The low yield of neurons responding to warming or cooling may be related to the anesthetic used (chloralose) or to the possibility that few such neurons are located in the region of nucleus caudalis sampled (0 to 4 mm below the obex). The distribution and types of neurons not antidromically activated by thalamic stimulation were similar to those of trigeminothalamic neurons with one exception. Most of the neurons responsive to low-threshold mechanical stimuli and located in the superficial part of the MAG layer were not antidromically activated.

Two neuron types ("*Touch*" and "*Touch-pressure*") exhibited either rapidly adapting or slowly adapting responses to light touch, pressure, or hair movement. They did not respond to noxious heat or discharge at higher rates than those at which they responded to noxious mechanical stimuli. They were located primarily in the MAG layer and usually had small (1 to 2 cm^2) receptive fields. They correspond to the types of neurons commonly found by others in this region (4,18). Orthodromic latencies to electrical stimulation of their receptive fields were very short (Table 2) and were indicative of exclusive input from large myelinated afferents sensitive to low-threshold mechanical stimuli (8,32). They were not studied in detail and no attempt was made to subdivide them according to input from distinct classes of mechanoreceptive afferents (21). These two types also had the fastest conducting axons of the trigeminothalamic neurons studied (Table 2). It is interesting to note that the conduction velocities of trigeminothalamic neurons are considerably slower than those of spinothalamic neurons (29,39).

Three neuron types did respond to noxious mechanical input, and many neurons in two of these categories also were activated by noxious heat (Table 2). *"Touch-pressure-pinch" neurons* responded maximally to pinch with serrated forceps but also were activated by hair movement and mechanical forces less than 1 g. They had larger receptive fields than the other neuron types and usually were located in the deep part of the MAG layer and the contiguous LRF. Neurons with similar general properties but not identified as trigeminothalamic neurons have been reported by Nord and Ross (22) in the adjacent LRF. Over 60% (27 of 44) of these neurons responded to noxious heat stimulation. Orthodromic latencies to electrical stimulation of the receptive fields were short, but stimulus intensities of 20 to 38 V evoked long-latency (> 100 msec) discharges characteristic of C-fiber activation (28). Presumably, Touch-pressure-pinch neurons receive primary afferent input from large myelinated, low-threshold mechanoreceptive afferents and C-polymodal nociceptors. Additional input from A-delta high-threshold mechanoreceptive afferents and A-delta heat nociceptors is likely, but it is not discernible from our present analysis.

"Pressure-pinch" neurons responded to firm pressure (force of 1 to 10 g with Von Frey filaments) and maximally to pinch with serrated forceps. Receptive field size was usually small, and most of these neurons were located in the MAR layer and the surrounding LRF. Approximately 20% (6 of 27) of these neurons responded to noxious heat stimulation. Orthodromic latencies to electrical stimulation of the receptive fields were always greater than 5 msec with a mean of 9.6 msec, suggesting that these neurons receive only A-delta and sometimes C-fiber input (late discharges were observed to 20- to 38-V electrical stimulation). "Pressure-pinch" neurons probably receive input from insensitive and high-threshold A-delta mechanoreceptors (8,26) and sometimes from A-delta heat nociceptors, C-polymodal nociceptors, or both.

The fifth type, called *"Pinch" neurons,* responded only to noxious mechanical forces exceeding 75 g (Von Frey filaments) or to pinch with serrated forceps. These neurons responded at stimulus intensities that were clearly noxious to human subjects. Their receptive fields usually were small, and they most often were located in the MAR layer and the LRF. With the exception of one equivocal response, none of them (20 neurons) were activated by noxious heat. Although orthodromic latencies to electrical stimulation were long, no late discharges suggestive of C-fiber input were found. These neurons probably receive input exclusively from high-threshold A-delta mechanoreceptive afferents, and many located in the LRF presumably are activated through polysynaptic pathways. Neurons with some of the general properties of Pressure-pinch and Pinch neurons have been reported previously in the cat nucleus caudalis (19,21), but none were identified as trigeminothalamic projection neurons.

The axonal conduction velocities of trigeminothalamic neurons classified as Pressure-pinch or Pinch were much slower than those of the Touch-pressure-pinch neurons (Table 2). Spinothalamic neurons activated almost exclusively by intense stimuli also have slowly conducting axons in comparison to other types of projection neurons (29,42). This difference permitted Price and Mayer (29) to compare refractory periods and antidromic activation thresholds of monkey dorsal horn neurons with parameters of stimulation required to produce pain evoked by cervical anterolateral quadrant stimulation in conscious humans (20). Their analysis indicates that the activation of wide dynamic range Touch-pressure-pinch neurons is sufficient to produce pain.

The summary data in Table 2 indicate that Touch-pressure-pinch and Pressure-pinch neurons can be distinguished further on the basis of orthodromic and antidromic latencies, receptive field size, and anatomical location. However, both neuron types have similar responses to noxious thermal stimuli. Thermal thresholds ranged from 38° to 50°C, and stimulus-response or intensity functions were monotonic to final temperatures of 48° to 52°C. Many of these intensity functions were positively accelerating with the steep portion of the curve occurring in the 45° to 52°C range (Fig. 1), and they were

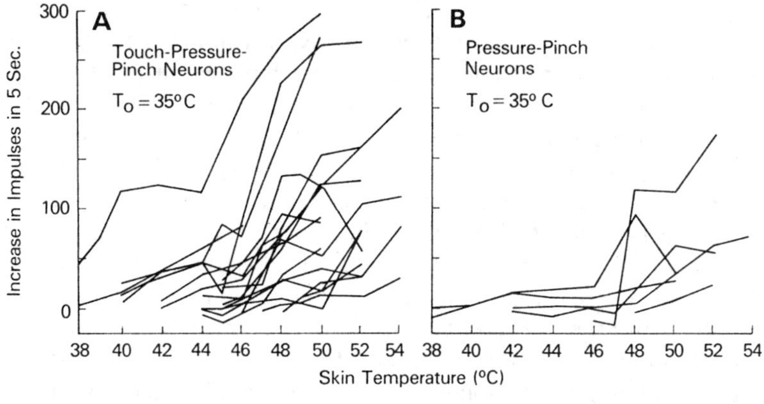

FIG. 1. Stimulus-response functions of Touch-pressure-pinch and Pressure-pinch neurons located in nucleus caudalis. The magnitude of the response expressed as the increase in impulses in the 5-sec period following the onset of the stimulus is plotted against final temperatures of individual trials. The base-line or adapting temperature was 35°C. **A:** Stimulus-response functions of 17 Touch-pressure-pinch neurons; **B:** 6 Pressure-pinch neurons.

similar in form to the intensity functions previously described for A-delta heat nociceptors and C-polymodal nociceptors.

Responses to noxious thermal stimuli could be divided into two groups based on neuron location. Neurons responsive to noxious heat and located in the MAR layer had little spontaneous activity and relatively flat intensity functions. On the other hand, neurons in the deeper part of the MAG layer and in the surrounding LRF exhibited higher levels of spontaneous activity and steeper intensity functions.

These results indicate that pain may be coded by the individual or combined output of three types of trigeminothalamic nociceptive neurons located in the MAR and MAG layers of nucleus caudalis and in the surrounding LRF. However, since we analyzed nucleus caudalis neurons in anesthetized monkeys, interpretations of the functional role of these neurons in pain sensation and reaction are partly dependent on future studies which correlate these neural events with behavior in awake animals.

ANATOMICAL ORGANIZATION OF NUCLEUS CAUDALIS

Many trigeminothalamic neurons in nucleus caudalis conveying noxious information appear to receive direct input from trigeminal primary afferent fibers based on orthodromic latencies to electrical stimulation and responses to natural stimuli (Table 2). This statement at first seems inconsistent with the previous conclusion that small-fiber input projects exclusively to the SG layer and with the observation that no SG neurons project beyond the limits of nucleus caudalis (12). However, Golgi preparations of the neuronal cell types, particularly in the MAR, SG, and MAG layers, provide a reasonable explanation of this apparent inconsistency (11,12). Not all of the dendrites in the SG layer are derived from SG neurons. Many MAR and some MAG neurons have dendrites that penetrate the SG layer and receive axodendritic synapses from small myelinated and unmyelinated primary afferent fibers. Many marginal neurons send some of their primary dendrites into the underlying SG layer where they undergo considerable secondary branching. Some dendrites actually penetrate the superficial layers of the MAG layer. The dendrites of MAR neurons which enter the SG layer emit large numbers of spines, whereas those which remain in the marginal layer exhibit relatively few spines. Dendrites of magnocellular neurons also enter the SG layer and divide into finer branches which become intertwined among the dendrites of the SG neurons. These fine MAG dendrites also emit numerous spines. Three types of SG neurons have been described in the SG layer (12), each with its distinctive dendritic branching pattern. In addition, the unmyelinated axons of SG neurons emit numerous collateral branches which also make a prolific contribution to the SG neuropil.

Figure 2 is a diagrammatic representation of how we envision primary

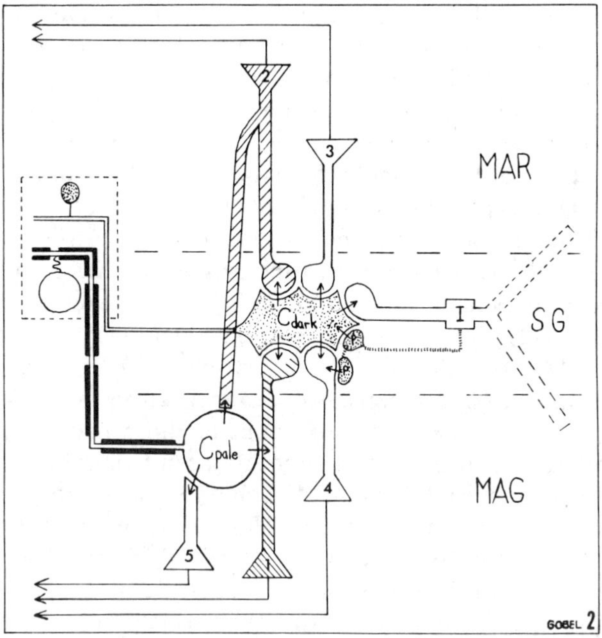

FIG. 2. Diagrammatic representation of the organization of trigeminal nucleus caudalis. Small-caliber trigeminal axons have small, electron-dense cell bodies in the trigeminal ganglion (*inset at left*) and dark (C dark) terminals in the SG layer. These terminals lie in the center of complex glomeruli and have synaptic connections with dendritic spines and shafts of MAR, SG, and MAG neurons. In addition, axonal endings arising mainly from SG neurons are presynaptic to this central axonal terminal. Large myelinated trigeminal axons have large, pale cell bodies in the trigeminal ganglion and pale (C pale) terminals in the MAG layer. These terminals synapse on the dendrites of MAG and MAR neurons. Cell 1 in the MAG layer receives both large myelinated afferent input in the MAG layer and A-delta and/or C fiber input in the SG layer and is the presumed morphological correlate of the "Touch-pressure-pinch" neuron. Cell 2 is a similar functional type located in the MAR layer. Cell 3 in the MAR layer receives only A-delta and/or C input via axodendritic synapses in the SG glomeruli; it is the presumed morphological correlate of "Pressure-pinch" or "Pinch" neurons. Cell 4 has similar functional properties but is located in the MAG layer. Cell 5 receives only large myelinated fiber input on dendrites restricted to the MAG layer and is the probable morphological correlate of "Touch" and "Touch-pressure" neurons. Cell I represents SG neurons, which are considered inhibitory interneurons. See text for further details.

afferent input is relayed to projection neurons and interneurons in nucleus caudalis. Small, dark trigeminal ganglion cells that respond to noxious input have small-caliber axons with dark terminals in the center of complex glomeruli in the SG layer. These primary axonal endings are surrounded by two kinds of dendritic spines, dendritic shafts and small axonal endings (ref. 11 and Gobel, *this volume*). Large, pale trigeminal ganglion cells that respond to low-threshold mechanical input have large myelinated axons, which leave the spinal trigeminal tract as cord-like rays that traverse the SG layer without emitting any collaterals and enter the MAG layer (13). Their terminals are the central endings of simpler glomeruli found in the MAG layer and at other levels of the trigeminal brainstem nuclei. Touch-pressure-pinch neurons in the MAG layer (Fig. 2, cell 1) or nearby LRF presumably have dendrites which penetrate the SG layer. They receive large myelinated afferent input via axodendritic synapses on dendritic spines and shafts located in the MAG layer, and A-delta and C-fiber input via axodendritic synapses on dendrites located in the SG layer. The few neurons with wide dynamic range responses in the MAR layer also may have dendritic arbors in the SG and MAG layers and receive similar afferent input (Fig. 2, cell 2). Pressure-pinch and Pinch neurons in the MAR (Fig. 2, cell 3) and MAG (Fig. 2, cell 4) layers receive A-delta input, C input, or both through axodendritic synapses on dendritic spines in the SG layer. The absence of large myelinated afferent input to those neurons in the MAG layer may indicate the lack of such connections or the presence of inhibitory synapses which suppress this input. Touch and Touch-pressure neurons in the MAG layer receive only large myelinated afferent input and have no dendritic arbors in the SG layer (Fig. 2, cell 5). Their absence from the MAR layer is explained by this simple model. Some SG neurons (Fig. 2, cell 1) are probably inhibitory interneurons which receive A-delta and/or C input through axodendritic synapses in the SG glomeruli. They are thought to inhibit transmission in the afferent axon-projection neuron pathway by axo-axonic synapses on trigeminal nerve endings and by axodendritic synapses on dendritic spines and shafts of projection neurons.

SUMMARY AND CONCLUSIONS

There is now considerable evidence to support the hypothesis that trigeminal nucleus caudalis is the major component of the trigeminal brainstem nuclear complex concerned with nociception. Peripheral fiber populations responsive to noxious input project exclusively to the substantia gelatinosal layer of nucleus caudalis. They form axodendritic synapses on projection neurons whose cell bodies lie in the marginal and magnocellular layers. Some of these neurons respond exclusively to intense or noxious stimuli. Others respond over a stimulus intensity range extending from light tactile input to intense stimuli that are painful to human observers. Many of these different types of nociceptive central neurons have direct projections to the ventral posterior region of the thalamus. These findings do not necessarily contradict the hypothesis that nucleus caudalis exerts a modulating influence on sensory transmission through the more rostral subdivisions of the trigeminal brainstem nuclei. However, this is clearly not the sole function of this nucleus. Noxious input is conveyed centrally by a primary afferent-projection neuron pathway through nucleus caudalis, which is separate from rostral parts of the trigeminal brainstem nuclear complex.

Neurons with a wide response range as well as those responsive exclusively to noxious stimuli are part of this pathway.

ACKNOWLEDGMENTS

We are extremely grateful to J. Binck, F. J. Brown, H. Burris, and M. Purvis for their assistance in various aspects of these studies.

REFERENCES

1. Beck, P. W., Handwerker, H. O., and Zimmermann, M. (1974): *Brain Res.*, 67:373–386.
2. Bessou, P., and Perl, E. R. (1969): *J. Neurophysiol.*, 32:1025–1043.
3. Brodal, A., Szabo, T., and Torvik, A. (1956): *J. Comp. Neurol.*, 106:527–555.
4. Darian-Smith, I. (1966): *Int. Rev. Neurobiol.*, 9:301–395.
5. Darian-Smith, I., Johnson, K. O., and Dykes, R. (1973): *J. Neurophysiol.*, 36:325–346.
6. Denny-Brown, D., and Yanagisawa, N. (1973): *Brain*, 96:783–814.
7. Dubner, R., Beitel, R. E., and Brown, F. J. (1976): In: *Pain: New Therapeutic Approaches and Frontiers for Immediate Research*, edited by M. Weisenberg and B. Tursky. Plenum Press, New York (*in press*).
8. Dubner, R., Sumino, R., and Starkman, S. (1974): In: *Advances in Neurology, Vol. 4: International Symposium on Pain*, edited by J. J. Bonica, pp. 61–71. Raven Press, New York.
9. Dubner, R., Sumino, R., and Wood, W. I. (1975): *J. Neurophysiol.*, 38:1373–1389.
10. Gobel, S. (1971): In: *Oral-Facial Sensory and Motor Mechanisms*, edited by R. Dubner and Y. Kawamura, pp. 183–204. Appleton-Century-Crofts, New York.
11. Gobel, S. (1974): *J. Neurocytol.*, 3:219–243.
12. Gobel, S. (1975): *J. Comp. Neurol.*, 162:397–415.
13. Gobel, S., and Purvis, M. B. (1972): *Brain Res.*, 48:27–44.
14. Greene, L. C., and Hardy, J. D. (1962): *J. Appl. Physiol.*, 17:693–696.
15. Hardy, J. D., Wolff, H. G., and Goodell, H. (1952): *Pain Sensations and Reactions*. Williams & Wilkins, Baltimore.
16. Hensel, H., and Iggo, A. (1971): *Arch. Ges. Physiol.*, 329:1–8.
17. Hu, J. W., Price, D. D., and Dubner, R. (1975): *Neurosci. Abstr.*, 1:149.
18. Kerr, F. W. L., Kruger, L., Schwassmann, H. O., and Stern, R. (1968): *J. Comp. Neurol.*, 134:127–144.
19. Kitahata, L. M., McAllister, R. G., and Taub, A. (1973): *Anesthesiology*, 38:12–19.
20. Mayer, D. J., Price, D. D., and Becker, D. P. (1974): *Pain*, 1:51–58.
21. Mosso, J. A., and Kruger, L. (1973): *J. Neurophysiol.*, 36:472–488.
22. Nord, S. G., and Ross, G. S. (1973): *Brain Res.*, 58:385–399.
23. Oliveras, J. L., Woda, A., Guilbaud, G., and Besson, J. M. (1974): *Brain Res.*, 72:328–331.
24. Olszewski, J. (1950): *J. Comp. Neurol.*, 92:401–413.
25. Peach, R. (1972): *J. Neurocytol.*, 1:151–160.
26. Perl, E. R. (1968): *J. Physiol.* (*Lond.*), 197:593–615.
27. Poulos, D. A. (1971): In: *Oral-Facial Sensory and Motor Mechanisms*, edited by R. Dubner and Y. Kawamura, pp. 47–72. Appleton-Century-Crofts, New York.
28. Price, D. D., and Browe, A. C. (1975): *Exp. Neurol.*, 48:201–221.
29. Price, D. D., and Mayer, D. J. (1975): *Pain*, 1:59–72.
30. Ramon y Cajal, S. (1909): *Histologie du Systeme Nerveux de l'homme et des Vertebres, Vol. 1.* Instituto Ramón y Cajal, Madrid (1952 reprint).
31. Raney, R., Raney, A. A., and Hunter, C. R. (1950): *Am. J. Surg.*, 80:11–17.
32. Rowe, M. J., and Sessle, B. J. (1972): *Brain Res.*, 42:367–384.
33. Rustioni, A., Sanyal, S., and Kuypers, H. G. J. M. (1971): *Brain Res.*, 32:45–52.
34. Sessle, B. J., and Greenwood, F. (1974): *Brain Res.*, 67:330–333.
35. Stewart, W. A., and King, R. B. (1963): *J. Comp. Neurol.*, 121:271–286.

36. Sumino, R., Dubner, R., and Starkman, S. (1973): *Brain Res.*, 62:260–263.
37. Swanson, A. G., Buchan, G. C., and Alvord, E. C., Jr. (1965): *Arch. Neurol.*, 12:12–18.
38. Torebjörk, H. E. (1974): *Acta Physiol. Scand.*, 92:374–390.
39. Trevino, D. L., Coulter, J. D., and Willis, W. D. (1973): *J. Neurophysiol.*, 36:750–761.
40. Walker, A. E. (1939): *J. Neurophysiol.*, 2:234–248.
41. Weinberger, L. M., and Grant, F. C. (1942): *Arch. Neurol. Psychiatr.*, 48:355–381.
42. Willis, W. D., Trevino, D. L., Coulter, J. D., and Maunz, R. A. (1974): *J. Neurophysiol.*, 37:358–372.
43. Young, R. F., and King, R. B. (1972): *J. Neurophysiol.*, 35:87–95.

Advances in Pain Research and Therapy, Vol. 1,
edited by J. J. Bonica and D. Albe-Fessard.
Raven Press, New York © 1976.

Sensitization and Depression of C-Polymodal Nociceptors by Noxious Heat Applied to the Monkey's Face

R. E. Beitel and R. Dubner

Neurobiology and Anesthesiology Branch, National Institute of Dental Research, National Institutes of Health, 9000 Rockville Pike, Bethesda, Maryland 20014

Polymodal nociceptors comprise an important group of unmyelinated or C-afferent fibers with high-threshold cutaneous receptors (2,6). They respond maximally to noxious thermal and mechanical stimuli and probably contribute to the delayed burning component of the double pain response produced by noxious heat (9, D. D. Price, *this volume*). Several workers also have shown that the response of polymodal nociceptors may be either enhanced (sensitization of the receptor) or depressed (partial inactivation of the receptor) by noxious heat (1,2,6,12,13). In the work reported here, trigeminal polymodal nociceptors in the rhesus monkey were stimulated with heat stimuli ranging from just suprathreshold to frankly damaging levels. To determine if these stimuli altered the sensitivity of the receptor, we examined units for signs of sensitized or depressed responses when heat stimuli were subsequently applied to the receptive field.

METHODS

The trigeminal ganglion was exposed by hemispherectomy, and single-unit activity was recorded extracellularly in rhesus monkeys anesthetized with sodium pentobarbital. Blood pressure, alveolar CO_2, and rectal temperature were maintained within physiological limits. Receptive field (RF) properties were investigated with hand-held thermal and mechanical stimulators. A unit's response to quantitative thermal stimuli was investigated by applying temperature shifts in the warming direction with a feedback-controlled contact thermode (1-cm diameter). The rate of thermal change was 8.5°C or 12.0°C/sec from a base-line temperature of 35°C. At least 3 min elapsed between stimulus presentations to minimize stimulus interactions. Conduction velocity was determined by electrical stimulation of the RF.

RESULTS

The sample of polymodal nociceptors had conduction velocities in the range for unmyelinated C fibers (mean = 0.82 m/sec; $N = 20$; SD = ±0.17).

Cutaneous RFs on the monkey's face were usually single spots (median diameter = 2 mm; $N = 37$) and were identical for thermal and mechanical stimuli. The one-impulse threshold temperature ranged from 38° to 49°C (median = 46°C; $N = 37$), and mechanical force thresholds ranged from 0.07 to 8.5 g (median = 1.2 g; $N = 39$). For a graded series of 5-sec duration thermal stimuli, the number of impulses usually increased as a monotonic function of stimulus intensity over the range from threshold to 50° to 55°C (see Fig. 2, curve 1). Most of the stimulus-response curves were positively accelerating over some portion of their monotonic range (Fig. 1A), and maximum discharge frequencies were obtained in the noxious heat range ($\geq$ 45°C).

When 5-sec duration temperature shifts into the noxious heat range were applied to the RF, the typical pattern of activity was a short accelerating burst of impulses followed by adaptation to a lower rate of discharge before termination of the stimulus (Fig. 1C). A similar pattern of discharge occurred in the initial portion of the response to 30-sec duration stimuli. If the final temperature was not more than 3° to 6°C above threshold temperature, the

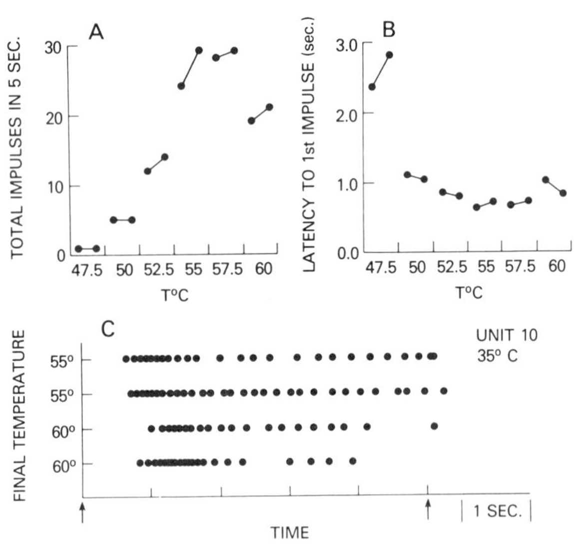

FIG. 1. Response sensitization and depression produced by noxious heat. **A:** Total number of impulses produced by two 5-sec duration temperature shifts to each of the final temperatures shown on the abscissa. Order of presentation was from left to right with a minimum interstimulus interval of 3 min. Points representing response to identical temperature shifts are connected by lines. **B:** Latency to the first impulse; same details as in **A. C:** Each row of dots depicts the occurrence of impulses as a function of time. Stimulus onset and termination are illustrated by arrows, and final temperature is indicated to the left of each row of dots. At each final temperature, the upper and lower rows correspond to the first and second temperature shifts, respectively. The 1-impulse threshold temperature for this unit was 47.5°C. Adapting temperature, 35°C; slope, 12.0°C/sec.

response during the final 25 sec was usually a low-frequency discharge (< 2 impulses/sec) which continued until the stimulus was terminated. However, units failed to respond throughout 30-sec duration stimuli if the final temperature exceeded 50°C.

When the responses of polymodal nociceptors to heat stimuli were examined for signs of altered sensitivity, it was found that stimuli 2° to 8°C above threshold temperature typically sensitized a unit, whereas more intense noxious heat produced a depressed response. Sensitization was manifested in one or more ways including: (a) an increase in impulse frequency to identical temperature shifts; (b) a decrease in first-impulse latency to identical temperature shifts; and (c) a decrease in threshold temperature. Several experimental paradigms were found useful for demonstrating sensitization, one of which is summarized in Fig. 1. Two identical 5-sec duration temperature shifts to the final temperatures shown on the abscissa in Fig. 1A were applied to the RF in ascending order of magnitude. The responses to these temperature shifts increased monotonically over a 10°C range from threshold to 57.5°C. The points connected by lines show that when final temperatures reached 52.5° to 57.5°C, the response to the second stimulus was larger than the response to the first stimulus. This sensitizing effect of the first stimulus on the response to the second stimulus was most pronounced at 55°C and was due to a higher rate of discharge during the first half of the response (Fig. 1C). Latency to the first impulse decreased monotonically over the range from threshold to 55°C (Fig. 1B), and a sensitizing effect on first-impulse latencies to temperature shifts to 50° and 52.5°C was produced by identical preceding temperature shifts.

We have found that one or two applications of a 5-sec duration temperature shift to 55°C frequently produce signs of response depression. These stimuli produce no observable changes in the skin other than a transient erythema. This suggests that the receptor is partially inactivated before either the skin or the receptor is irreversibly damaged by heat. Thus the increase in latencies to the second temperature shift to 55°C and to shifts to higher final temperatures shown in Fig. 1B may reflect an inactivation process. However, response depression is more vividly illustrated in Fig. 2. Curve 1 shows the average total impulses during the two 5-sec temperature shifts to each of the final temperatures shown on the abscissa. After the two 55°C final temperature trials, we repeated a series of single trials and extended them to a maximum temperature of 60°C (curve 2). Comparison of curves 1 and 2 shows a depressed response (curve 2) over the range of stimuli from threshold to 55°C. Although the unit remained maximally sensitive in the noxious heat range, curve 2 is nonmonotonic at 60°C.

The response to temperature shifts to 60°C is also nonmonotonic in Fig. 1A and, as illustrated by the dot patterns in Fig. 1C, is a result of the unit not discharging through the duration of these intense stimuli. The epidermis is irreversibly damaged when heat stimuli of 60°C are applied for longer

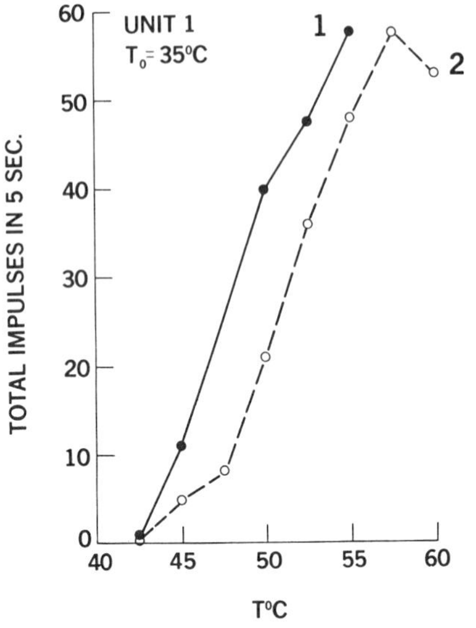

FIG. 2. Stimulus-response curves illustrating response depression. Average total number of impulses produced by two 5-sec duration temperature shifts to the final temperatures on the abscissa are shown by stimulus-response curve 1. Stimuli were presented in ascending order of magnitude, i.e., the 2 final trials were shifts to 55°C. Stimulus-response curve 2 shows the number of impulses produced subsequently by single 5-sec duration temperature shifts presented in ascending order of magnitude. The 1-impulse threshold temperature for this unit was 42.5°C. Adapting temperature, 35°C; slope, 12.0°C/sec. Minimum interstimulus interval was 3 min.

than approximately 3 sec (10); the response to temperature shifts to 60°C probably reflects direct heat damage to the receptor.

An afterdischarge frequently appeared when noxious heat stimuli, capable of altering the unit's responsivity without overt damage to the skin, were applied to the RF. Sometimes the afterdischarge appeared as a sign of sensitization, although on other occasions it followed the application of noxious heat which depressed the unit's response. Afterdischarges were irregular, low-frequency (0.2 to 5.0 impulses/sec) impulse patterns persisting for periods varying from approximately 1 min to several minutes after application of the stimulus. They usually did not persist long after their initial appearance, even when the RF was subsequently stimulated by temperature shifts to higher final temperatures.

DISCUSSION

The observations reported here are particularly interesting when compared to experimental and clinical observations on human subjects with either hyperalgesic or heat-damaged skin. Changes in threshold and sensitivity and the appearance of an afterdischarge frequently occur in polymodal nociceptors after heat stimuli a few degrees above threshold are applied. In a zone of primary hyperalgesia, the burning pain threshold is lowered (5), sensitivity to heat stimuli is enhanced, and subjects may report spontaneous burning pain soon after the skin becomes hyperalgesic (8). These observations suggest that sensitization of polymodal nociceptors may contribute to the enhanced sensitivity found in primary hyperalgesia.

When more intense noxious heat stimuli are applied to the RF, polymodal nociceptors are partially inactivated. Yet it is known both in common experience and experimentally that blistered or burned skin is more sensitive to heat stimuli than normal skin (8,11). These observations are not necessarily contradictory, however, since partially inactivated polymodal nociceptors may still be capable of vigorously exciting central neurons. It has been shown (4,7) that cells in the dorsal horn of the spinal cord which receive an excitatory input from polymodal nociceptors are inhibited by stimulation of cutaneous mechanoreceptors with myelinated afferent fibers. However, the response of these peripheral mechanosensitive fibers is depressed by noxious heat (1,3). Hence it seems reasonable to suggest that if the inhibitory influence of the mechanosensitive fibers is reduced or eliminated by noxious heat stimuli which damage their receptors, the level of excitability of central neurons which receive an input from polymodal nociceptors may be augmented when the RF is stimulated subsequently by heat.

REFERENCES

1. Beck, P. W., Handwerker, H. D., and Zimmermann, M. (1974): *Brain Res.*, 67:373–386.
2. Bessou, P., and Perl, E. R. (1969): *J. Neurophysiol.*, 32:1025–1043.
3. Dubner, R., Sumino, R., and Starkman, S. (1974): In: *Advances in Neurology, Vol. 4: International Symposium on Pain,* edited by J. J. Bonica, pp. 61–71. Raven Press, New York.
4. Handwerker, H. O., Iggo, A., and Zimmermann, M. (1975): *Pain,* 1:147–165.
5. Hardy, J. D., Wolff, H. G., and Goodell, H. (1952): *Pain Sensations and Reactions.* Williams & Wilkins, Baltimore.
6. Iggo, A. (1959): *Q. J. Exp. Physiol.*, 44:362–370.
7. Iggo, A. (1974): In: *Advances in Neurology, Vol. 4: International Symposium on Pain,* edited by J. J. Bonica, pp. 1–9. Raven Press, New York.
8. Lewis, T. (1942): *Pain.* Macmillan, New York.
9. Lewis, T., and Pochin, E. E. (1937): *Clin. Sci.*, 3:67–76.
10. Moritz, A. R., and Henriques, F. C., Jr. (1947): *Am. J. Pathol.*, 23:695–720.
11. Stone, L. J., and Dallenbach, K. M. (1934): *Am. J. Psychol.*, 46:229–242.
12. Witt, I. (1962): *Acta Neuroveg. (Wien)*, 24:208–219.
13. Witt, I., and Griffin, J. P. (1962): *Nature,* 194:776–777.

Advances in Pain Research and Therapy, Vol. 1,
edited by J. J. Bonica and D. Albe-Fessard.
Raven Press, New York © 1976.

Peripheral Neural Correlates of Escape Behavior in Rhesus Monkey to Noxious Heat Applied to the Face

R. Dubner and R. E. Beitel

Neurobiology and Anesthesiology Branch, National Institute of Dental Research, National Institutes of Health, Bethesda, Maryland 20014

A number of recent neurophysiological studies have identified neural populations in the spinal cord dorsal horn and in trigeminal nucleus caudalis which project directly to the thalamus and respond exclusively or maximally to noxious stimuli applied to the skin (7,9, and Dubner et al., *this volume*). However, all of these studies have been performed under general anesthesia or after surgical brain lesions, both of which alter central neuronal activity. Only tentative conclusions can be drawn from these experiments regarding the functional role of different neuronal populations in pain. A promising approach is one that correlates peripheral and central neural events with the behavioral assessment of pain sensation in awake animals (2). In this chapter we describe a behavioral model developed to study escape behavior to noxious heat in monkeys and compare these behavioral findings with results, obtained independently, on the response properties of peripheral nerve populations activated by the same stimuli.

Most previous behavioral animal models have used an operant escape response to electric shock as a measure of "pain" threshold. Such training procedures have a number of disadvantages if the behavior is to be related to nervous system events. First, they often measure absolute escape thresholds and neglect behavioral reactions to suprathreshold stimuli (6). Second, escape thresholds are difficult to establish in the presence of cues from innocuous stimuli, and animals learn to terminate and escape near-painful stimuli to avoid painful ones (1). Third, electric shock is an unnatural stimulus which activates in a synchronous fashion many types of peripheral nerve fibers responsive to innocuous as well as noxious stimuli. The functional role of central neuronal pathways activated by such stimulation in pain sensation and reaction is difficult to assess.

With these problems in mind, we have developed for monkeys a reaction time paradigm with the following attributes. A natural stimulus, noxious heat, is applied to the monkey's face. A considerable body of literature on pain thresholds to this stimulus in humans is available (5), and it is known to activate a restricted group of peripheral and central trigeminal neurons (4 and Dubner et al., *this volume*). The paradigm provides two measures, escape latency and escape probability, which can scale the range of behavior to innocuous and noxious heat stimuli. In addition, the training procedure uses positive and negative reinforcement and eliminates the tendency of animals to avoid rather than escape noxious stimuli.

Vigilance and activity are controlled by the need to respond to provide escape or positive reinforcement (reward). In brief, the animal is trained to detect the termination of an innocuous temperature increase (less than 45°C) in order to receive a reward on each trial. On trials in which the temperature increase reaches the noxious heat range (45° to 51°C), the monkey can escape the stimulus, but it receives no reward. Since the monkey initiates each trial, noxious stimuli cannot be avoided without eliminating opportunities for reward. Some details of the procedure are described below and have been published previously (3).

BEHAVIORAL OBSERVATIONS

The experimental situation is illustrated in Fig. 1A. A rhesus monkey was placed in a restraining chair and its head was fixed to the chair to reduce movements. A spring-loaded contact thermode was applied to the upper lip region, and a liquid reward could be provided in calibrated increments through a metal tube placed in the mouth (Fig. 1A, *upper left*). The thermode contacted a 1-cm diameter circular area of facial skin and was precisely controlled to present temperature changes of 9°C/sec in the range of 20° to 60°C.

The monkey initiated a trial by depressing a translucent panel button after the light behind it was turned on (Fig. 1A, *lower left*). At the same time the temperature at the surface of the thermode increased at a rate of 9°C/sec until it reached a predetermined final temperature. The monkey was rewarded with grape juice if the panel button was released within a fixed time period after the temperature shift terminated and began to return to the base-line level (a "correct" response). An "early" response occurred if the monkey released before the termination of the stimulus. This release terminated the temperature increase and the monkey received no grape juice reward. Temperature increases into the noxious heat range (45° to 51°C) occurred on one-sixth of the trials, and the monkey had the choice of either escaping the stimulus by releasing early and receiving no reward or waiting until the termination of the temperature shift and receiving a liquid reward.

Figure 1B summarizes data collected from two rhesus monkeys that received water *ad libitum* in the home-cage and were rewarded with 0.3 cc of grape juice for each correct response (CR) in the restraining chair. The

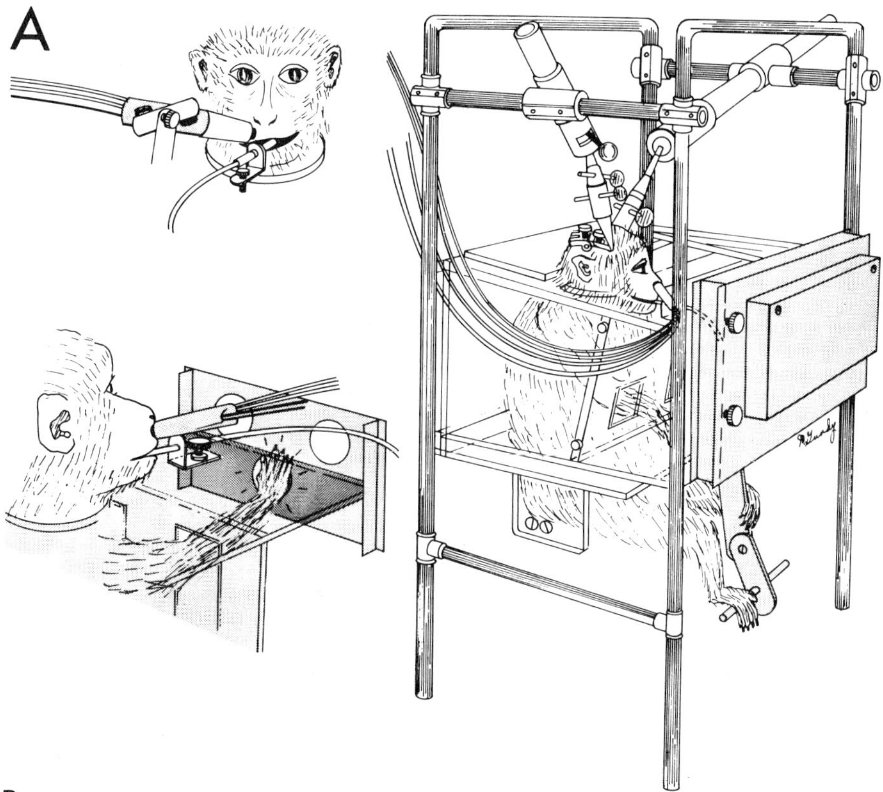

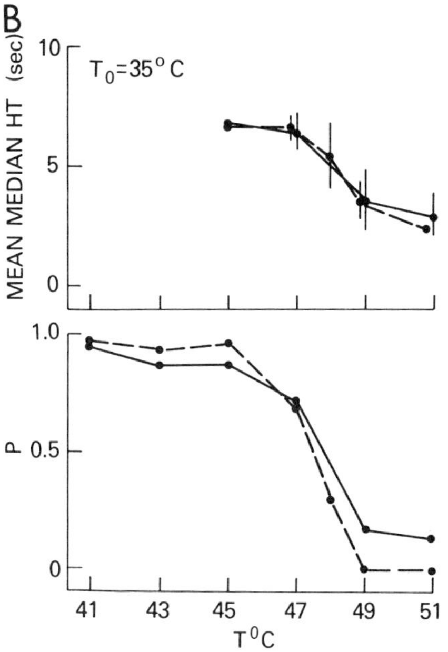

FIG. 1. A: Drawings of the experimental arrangement. See text for details. **B:** Summary data from 2 rhesus monkeys that received water *ad libitum* in the cage. The 2 curves in each graph represent data collected from 2 monkeys with a base-line temperature of 35°C. Upper curves show the hold times (HT; total time the button was depressed) for temperatures of 41° to 51°C. For 1 monkey (*dashed line*) medians were determined from 10 trials at each final temperature; for the other monkey (*solid line*), from 4 to 5 trials. Mean median values (*datum points*) and SDs of the median (*extent of vertical lines*) are shown and are based on at least 5 median values. Lower curves show probabilities of CRs for final temperatures of 41° to 51°C. Each data point is based on approximately 50 (*dashed line*) or 20 (*solid line*) trials.

two curves in the lower graph show the probabilities of CRs (depressing the button until termination of the temperature period and releasing during the reward period) for each monkey to final temperatures of 41° through 51°C, from a base-line temperature of 35°C. Each data point is based on the outcome of approximately 50 (*dashed line*) or 20 (*solid line*) trials. When final temperatures were 41° to 45°C, the monkeys had CRs on 85% to 95% of the trials. When the final temperature reached 47°C, the monkeys depressed the button until termination of the temperature period and received a reward on only 70% of trials. By final temperatures of 49°C or greater, the probability of a CR was 0 to 20%, and the monkeys escaped the stimulus on almost all the trials. For both monkeys the escape threshold (the 50% level) was between 47° and 48°C.

The curves in the upper graph of Fig. 1B show the mean median hold times (HT; the total time the button was depressed) and standard deviations of the median for the 45° to 51°C final temperature trials. Final temperatures above 47°C resulted in shorter HTs. From these data, hold time appears to depend on final temperature and to provide another measure of escape behavior to varying intensities of noxious heat.

Another measure of escape behavior was provided by lip movements monitored by a sensitive accelerometer attached to the thermode. Lip movements occurred before termination of the stimulus only when final temperatures were 48°C or greater. These movements probably represent a more reflexive motor act to escape the stimulus than does release of the panel button. The data indicate convergence of escape thresholds at 47° to 48°C when assessed by these two measures.

The outcome was different when the monkey's water needs during the experimental period were changed. Under water-restricted conditions (200 cc/day), escape thresholds were above 51°C, although lip movements continued to occur at temperatures of 48°C or higher (3). Thus the monkey's escape performance was sensitive to changes in motivational or drive state. However, sensitivity to the noxious stimulus appears unchanged when assessed by lip movements during the two conditions. The behavioral paradigm, therefore, provides a means of separating "pain sensitivity" from "pain response." The effect of analgesic agents on these behavioral measures in both of these drive conditions is of considerable interest. The differential responsiveness of neurons in central "pain pathways" during the above manipulations also warrants intense study.

PERIPHERAL NEURAL CORRELATES OF ESCAPE BEHAVIOR

We have found innervating the monkey's face only three peripheral nerve fiber populations that normally are sensitive to temperature changes in the 47° to 51°C range and are capable of initiating central neuronal activity involved in the monkey's ability to escape from noxious heat stimuli. These are unmyelinated or C-polymodal nociceptors, fine-myelinated or A-delta heat nociceptors, and A-delta or C-warm fibers (see Table 1, Chapter 19). Figure 2 shows stimulus-response functions of 4 A-delta heat nociceptors and a representative sample of 5 of 22 C-polymodal nociceptors (Beitel and Dubner, *this volume*). Maximum sensitivity of these two populations was in the 47° to 51°C range and over the range of threshold (38° to 44°C) to final temperatures of 51° to 53°C, response magnitude increased as a monotonic function of stimulus intensity. Heat nociceptors, however, exhibited higher discharge rates than polymodal nociceptors in the noxious heat range (Fig. 2).

We have found that the distribution of escape latencies to 49° and 51°C final temperatures cannot depend solely on the discharge of polymodal nociceptors. The temporal pattern of discharge of a representative population of polymodal nociceptors was indistinguishable at 49° and 51°C final temperatures within the first 3 sec of stimulation. However, within that same time period the proportion of escape responses for two monkeys at 51°C was almost 90%, whereas at final temperatures of 49°C it was less than 50%. Presently, we are increasing our sample of A-delta heat nociceptors so that a similar analysis of that fiber population can be made.

Some warm fibers also were sensitive to temperature changes in the noxious heat range (4,8). Few of these fibers, however, were maximally sensitive to noxious heat stimuli above 47°C, and none had monotonic stimulus-response functions beyond 49°C. Therefore, we conclude that

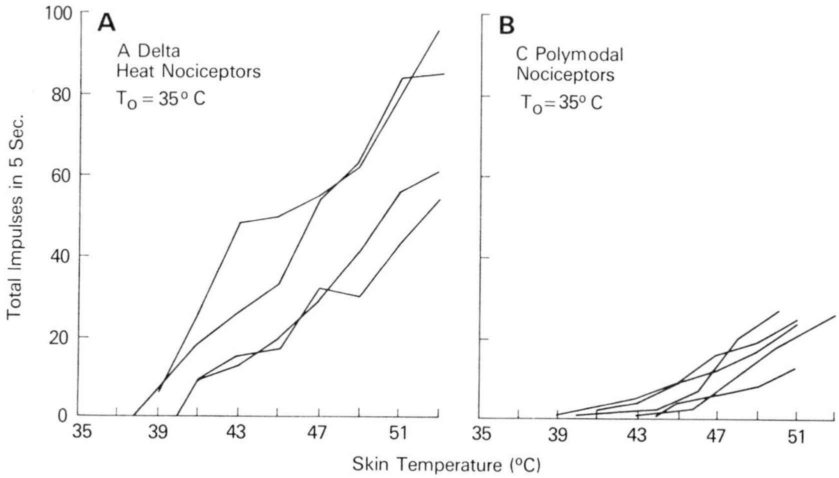

FIG. 2. Stimulus-response functions of A-delta heat nociceptors and C-polymodal nociceptors. Magnitude of the response expressed as total impulses in the 5-sec period after stimulus onset is plotted against final temperatures of individual trials. Base-line or adapting temperature was 35°C. **A:** Stimulus-response functions of 4 A-delta heat nociceptors; **B:** 5 C-polymodal nociceptors.

they alone cannot provide input essential for the monkey's escape behavior.

It appears, then, that neither warm fibers nor polymodal nociceptors alone can convey information centrally to account for the fast escape responses of the behaving monkeys. We suspect that the activity of A-delta heat nociceptors is essential for this behavior. However, the activity of polymodal nociceptors, warm fibers, or both may be important if central summation involving input from these fiber populations is a critical component of the behavior. Our studies in trigeminal nucleus caudalis of anesthetized monkeys suggest that convergent input from A-delta heat nociceptors and C-polymodal nociceptors on trigeminothalamic neurons provides the necessary information to the central nervous system (Dubner et al., *this volume*).

REFERENCES

1. Boren, J. J., and Malis, J. L. (1961): *Am. J. Physiol.*, 201:429–433.
2. Casey, K. L., Keene, J. J., and Morrow, T. (1974): In: *Advances in Neurology, Vol. 4: International Symposium on Pain,* edited by J. J. Bonica, pp. 197–205. Raven Press, New York.
3. Dubner, R., Beitel, R. E., and Brown, F. J. (1976): In: *Pain: New Therapeutic Approaches and Frontiers for Immediate Research,* edited by M. Weisenberg and B. Tursky. Plenum Press, New York (*in press*).
4. Dubner, R., Sumino, R., and Starkman, S. (1974): In: *Advances in Neurology, Vol. 4: International Symposium on Pain,* edited by J. J. Bonica, pp. 61–71. Raven Press, New York.
5. Hardy, J. D., Wolff, H. G., and Goodell, H. (1952): *Pain Sensations and Reactions.* Williams & Wilkins, Baltimore.
6. Manning, A. A., and Vierck, C. J., Jr. (1973): *J. Exp. Anal. Behav.*, 19:125–132.
7. Price, D. D., and Mayer, D. J. (1975): *Pain,* 1:59–72.
8. Sumino, R., Dubner, R., and Starkman, S. (1973): *Brain Res.*, 62:260–263.
9. Willis, W. D., Trevino, D. L., Coulter, J. D., and Maunz, R. A. (1974): *J. Neurophysiol.*, 37:358–372.

Advances in Pain Research and Therapy, Vol. 1,
edited by J. J. Bonica and D. Albe-Fessard.
Raven Press, New York © 1976.

Axonal Degeneration Patterns in the Cat Brainstem Spinal Trigeminal Nucleus after Tooth Pulp Removal

Lesnick E. Westrum, Robert C. Canfield, and Richard G. Black

Departments of Neurological Surgery, Biological Structure, Restorative Dentistry, and Anesthesiology, University of Washington, Schools of Medicine and Dentistry, Seattle, Washington 98195

Although evoked responses in the brainstem after tooth pulp stimulation are known to be distributed to the spinal trigeminal nucleus (2,3,7–9,13,16, 17,21), there is disagreement as to their exact localization within the complex. Pars oralis (2,7–9,16,17), pars caudalis (3,13), pars interpolaris (3), and the entire spinal trigeminal complex (7,8,21) all have been designated as the primary projection region of tooth pulp afferents.

The precise terminal distribution of the central processes of ganglion cells, whose peripheral processes innervate the teeth, apparently has not been shown anatomically. A recent report (5) describes the distribution of horseradish peroxidase (HRP) in the ganglion cells and the proximal parts of their central processes 2 days after injection of the tracer into tooth pulps. Also, there are a number of previous histological studies of trigeminal ganglion cells and of fibers in the peripheral trigeminal branches after tooth extractions or pulpectomies (1,14,20). These latter studies include no description of the central terminal distribution primarily because "transganglionic sensory degeneration" of central processes following damage to the peripheral processes is usually not considered a usable method for tracing pathways in the adult nervous system (6,11). The present study describes reproducible axonal and terminal degeneration patterns observed in a specific part of the spinal trigeminal nucleus at distinct times after pulpectomies. Parts of these observations were reported previously (19).

METHODS

Healthy mature cats without dental disease were used. Some of the animals were anesthetized and total pulp removals were performed on all of the teeth on one side, using aseptic root canal techniques. At several survival times between 7 and 100 days after the operation, the animals were reanesthetized and perfused via the left ventricle with a solution of 4% buffered formaldehyde (18). Transverse sections containing the three subnuclei of the spinal trigeminal nuclear complex were stained using either the Fink-Heimer (4) or the Nauta-Gygax (12) method. In addition, unoperated animals with healthy teeth were processed identically to serve as controls.

RESULTS

Degenerating axons and terminals are seen in each of the three subnuclei, but they are far more numerous in the pars interpolaris near and immediately

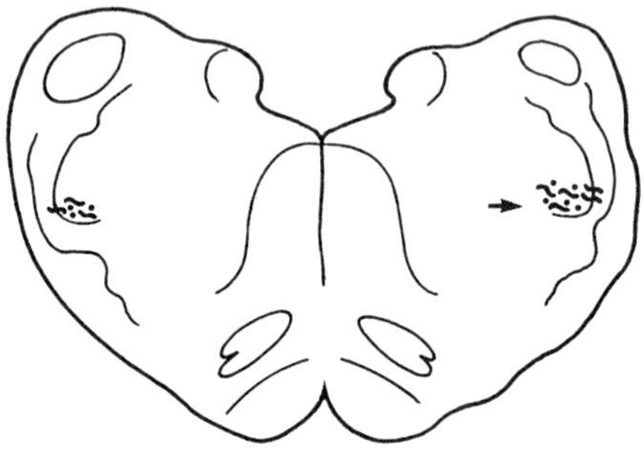

FIG. 1. Drawing from a silver-stained section of pars interpolaris showing the pattern and distribution in the area of maximum degeneration 11 days after unilateral tooth pulp removal. L and arrow indicate the operated side. R, control side; wavy lines, degenerating axons; dots, degenerating terminals.

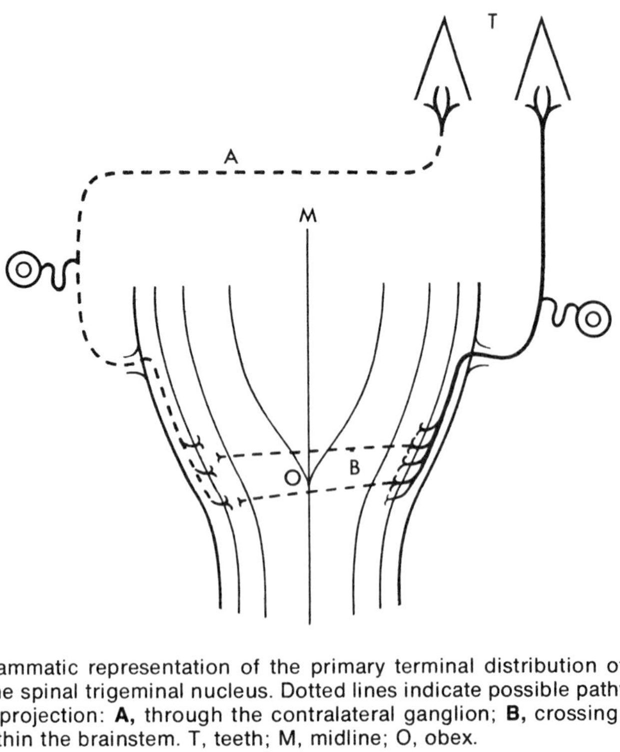

FIG. 2. Diagrammatic representation of the primary terminal distribution of tooth pulp afferents in the spinal trigeminal nucleus. Dotted lines indicate possible pathways for the contralateral projection: **A,** through the contralateral ganglion; **B,** crossing of fibers or collaterals within the brainstem. T, teeth; M, midline; O, obex.

rostral to the obex (Fig. 1) than in the adjacent pars caudalis or pars oralis. The degeneration is bilateral, but heavier on the operated side, and is concentrated in the ventral half to one-fourth of the nucleus (Fig. 1). Degeneration is heaviest at 11 to 14 days with less at shorter or longer survivals, but distribution of the degeneration is similar in all of the preparations. A few degenerating axons are seen in relation to the spinal tract (Fig. 1), but distinct fascicles of degenerating fibers crossing the midline have not been seen. No degeneration is seen in the unoperated animals with healthy teeth. Figure 2 summarizes the major anatomical distribution and possible pathways for tooth pulp afferents to the spinal trigeminal nucleus.

DISCUSSION

The observations reveal an anatomically precise region of termination of tooth pulp afferents in the spinal trigeminal nucleus. Although some degeneration is seen in all three subnuclei, the region of greatest degeneration is definitely within the pars interpolaris. Of the evoked potential studies this localization corresponds best with that reported by Dunker et al. (3), and less precisely with the study of Nord and Young (13). Other reports which suggest the pars oralis as the primary projection site for tooth pulp afferents (2,9,16,17) correlate least well with the present results. The distribution of degeneration within the ventral parts of the nucleus agrees with previous work (10,13), and this region may correspond to the specific cell aggregation described by Taber (15) in the same area.

A surprising observation is the homotopic distribution of degeneration contralateral to the pulpectomies. The electrophysiological reports usually indicate a principally ipsilateral distribution (3,13), although previous anatomical studies report increased numbers of chromatolytic cells in the Gasserian ganglion, contralateral as well as ipsilateral, after teeth extractions or pulpectomies (1,20). Although Furstman and associates (5) reported that there is apparently no HRP in the contralateral ganglion 2 days after injection of the pulp in rats, the precise types and numbers of teeth injected are not indicated for the ganglia described. Moreover, a different transport rate for this pathway is possible. Perhaps selective tooth pulp removals, rather than complete unilateral pulpectomies as done here, result in a different central distribution. In addition to the crossed projection possibly occurring through the contralateral ganglion (A in Fig. 2), fibers or collaterals crossing within the brainstem (B in Fig. 2) must be considered. The sections do not show a definite crossing pathway of degenerating fibers, but they may be sparsely distributed.

The dental surgery which causes degeneration of peripheral nerves and chromatolysis of ganglion cells (1,14,20) may also produce a "transganglionic degeneration" of the central processes and terminals. Although it is generally thought that mature nervous system does not respond in this fashion (6,11), studies of the type described here may reveal that it is not unique to the trigeminal system. Recovery of the ganglion cells after dental surgery (14) may also be accompanied by regeneration of the central terminals (11).

SUMMARY

Our results demonstrate an area of representation for tooth pulp afferents in the ventral aspects of pars interpolaris with some overlap into adjacent subnuclei, primarily near the obex. The projection is mostly ipsilateral but with a smaller contralateral component. The route of the latter is uncertain. The study also provides evidence of "transganglionic sensory degeneration" in a mature system as a means of anatomically tracing central projections of known peripheral receptors.

ACKNOWLEDGMENTS

This work was supported in part by National Institutes of Health Grants NS 09678 and NS 04053 from the National Institute of Neurological and Communicative Disorders and Stroke, and by Grant 11-0220 from the University of Washington. The authors gratefully acknowledge this support and wish to thank Mrs. J. Astafiev, William Congdon, Jerry Maddocks, and Zoltan Zelenak for technical assistance and Dr. Keith Webster for helpful suggestions on the manuscript.

REFERENCES

1. Brashear, A. D. (1936): *J. Comp. Neurol.,* 64:169–185.
2. Davies, W. I. R., Scott, D., Vesterstrom, K., and Vyklický, L. (1971): *J. Physiol. (Lond.),* 218:515–532.
3. Dunker, E., Grubel, G., and V. Rehren, D. (1967): *Pfluegers Arch.,* 296:289–307.
4. Fink, R. P., and Heimer, L. (1967): *Brain Res.,* 4:369–374.
5. Furstman, L., Saporta, S., and Kruger, L. (1975): *Brain Res.,* 84:320–324.
6. Grant, G., and Arvidsson, J. (1975): *Brain Res.,* 95:265–279.
7. Greenwood, F. (1973): *Arch. Oral Biol.,* 18:771–785.
8. Greenwood, L. F. (1971): *J. Physiol. (Lond.),* 218:72–73P.
9. Kawamura, Y., and Nishiyama, T. (1966): *Jap. J. Physiol.,* 16:584–597.
10. Kruger, L., and Michel, F. (1962): *Exp. Neurol.,* 5:139–156.
11. Lieberman, A. R. (1976): In: *The Peripheral Nerve,* edited by D. N. Landon. Chapman & Hall, London. pp. 187–278.
12. Nauta, W. J. H., and Gygax, P. A. (1954): *Stain Technol.,* 29:91–93.
13. Nord, S. G., and Young, R. F. (1975): *Brain Res.,* 90:195–204.
14. Strassburg, M. (1967): *J. Oral Surg.,* 25:107–114.
15. Taber, E. (1961): *J. Comp. Neurol.,* 116:27–69.
16. Tamarova, Z. A., Shapovalov, A. I., and Vyklicky, L. (1973): *Brain Res.,* 64:442–445.
17. Vyklický, L., and Keller, O. (1973): *Acta Neurobiol. Exp. (Warsz.),* 33:803–809.
18. Westrum, L. E., and Black, R. G. (1971): *Brain Res.,* 25:265–287.
19. Westrum, L. E., Canfield, R. C., and Black, R. G. (1976): *Brain Res.,* 101:137–140.
20. Windle, W. F. (1927): *J. Comp. Neurol.,* 43:347–356.
21. Young, R. F., and King, R. B. (1972): *J. Neurophysiol.,* 35:87–95.

Advances in Pain Research and Therapy, Vol. 1,
edited by J. J. Bonica and D. Albe-Fessard.
Raven Press, New York © 1976.

Principles of Organization in the Substantia Gelatinosa Layer of the Spinal Trigeminal Nucleus

Stephen Gobel

Neurobiology and Anesthesiology Branch, National Institute of Dental Research, National Institutes of Health, 9000 Rockville Pike, Bethesda, Maryland 20014

The substantia gelatinosa (SG) layer is a 120- to 150-μm wide C-shaped band sandwiched between the marginal and magnocellular layers of the caudal end of the spinal trigeminal nucleus (nucleus caudalis). In our laboratory we perform ongoing Golgi and electron microscopic (EM) studies in the adult cat to gain further insight into the role of the SG layer in processing information as it is relayed from first- to second-order neurons in trigeminal pain pathways. The complexity of the synaptic transformations taking place in the SG layer can be appreciated by considering the sheer number of neural elements that make up the SG neuropil. These include terminal axonal arbors of primary trigeminal neurons, axons and dendrites of three neuronal cell types indigenous to the SG layer (5), dendrites of marginal neurons, and dendrites of magnocellular neurons (Fig. 2). These neural elements establish synaptic contact in well-defined structural entities called glomeruli. Within the SG glomeruli the fundamental principles of structural as well as functional organization are to be found.

SG GLOMERULUS

Each SG glomerulus contains a primary afferent axonal ending which forms its core (Fig. 1). These endings have been identified as primary endings through EM degeneration studies of the SG layer after trigeminal nerve rhizotomy (3,5). The primary trigeminal endings in the SG glomeruli differ morphologically from the primary trigeminal endings in the rest of the trigeminal nuclei. They are distinguished by their darkened axoplasm and their thin scalloped outline (Fig. 1). In other parts of the trigeminal nuclei, the primary trigeminal endings are pale and bulbous (7,11). Several convergent lines of evidence suggest that the dark primary trigeminal endings in the SG glomeruli are derived from the dark, small, and medium-sized primary trigeminal neurons thought to respond to noxious and thermal stimuli (4 and Dubner et al., *this volume*).

The primary trigeminal afferents in the SG layer establish synaptic con-

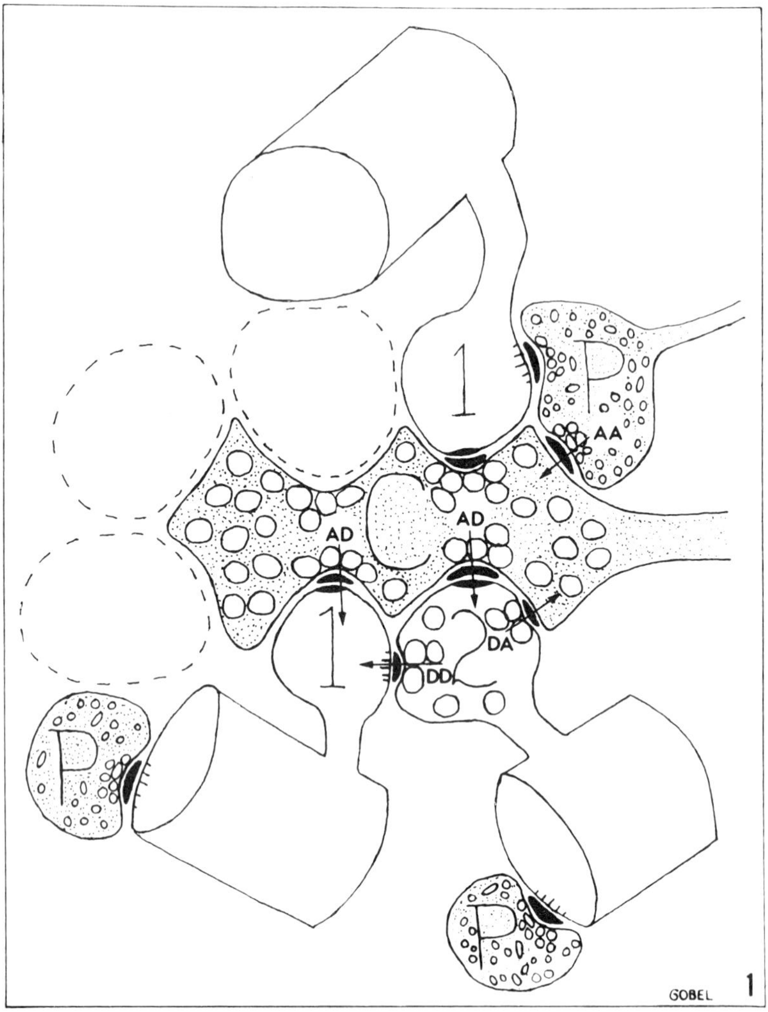

FIG. 1. Schematic diagram of some neuronal processes and synaptic connections in SG glomeruli. A dark primary trigeminal axonal ending (C) contains large, round synaptic vesicles and forms axodendritic (AD) synapses on 2 kinds of dendritic spines. One of these, the type 2 spine, also contains large, round synaptic vesicles and forms a dendrodendritic (DD) synapse on an adjacent type 1 spine and a dendroaxonic (DA) synapse on the primary ending. Small dark axonal (P) endings contain small, round, and flattened synaptic vesicles. P endings form axo-axonic (AA) synapses on the primary ending and axodendritic synapses on type 1 spines and on dendritic shafts.

tact with second-order neurons almost exclusively on dendritic spines (Fig. 1) and on small-caliber dendritic shafts. Three kinds of dendritic processes receive axodendritic synapses from the primary axons in the SG glomeruli. These include dendritic spines without synaptic vesicles (type 1 spines) and dendritic spines with large rounded synaptic vesicles loosely dispersed in their spine heads (type 2 spines; Fig. 1). Dendritic shafts containing small focal clusters of small rounded and flattened synaptic vesicles are also found in some SG glomeruli, and their presumed inhibitory dendrodendritic synaptic connections have been considered elsewhere (5).

AXO-AXONIC AND DENDROAXONIC SYNAPSES

Small axonal (P) endings with small rounded and flattened synaptic vesicles also are found in the SG glomeruli. These P endings are derived from unmyelinated axons and form axo-axonic synapses on the primary trigeminal endings in the SG glomeruli (Fig. 1). The primary endings in the SG glomeruli share this feature with other primary trigeminal endings in the main sensory (7) and spinal trigeminal (11) nuclei, as well as with all other somatosensory primary endings (see review in ref. 10). Many primary trigeminal endings in the SG glomeruli also are postsynaptic in a second kind of synapse, the dendroaxonic synapse (Fig. 1). In this respect they differ from other primary trigeminal endings as well as from the primary afferent endings in all other sensory pathways.

On receiving an axodendritic synapse from the primary ending, many type 2 spines in turn form a reciprocal dendroaxonic synapse back on the primary ending (Fig. 1). The dendroaxonic and axo-axonic synapses suggest that the primary ending is not only responsive to incoming action potentials, but that electrotonic potentials may be integrated on the axolemma of the primary ending. These synapses may play an active role in determining the amount and time course of transmitter release from the axodendritic synapses of the primary endings.

One hypothesis concerning the function of these synapses may be formulated on the basis of morphological considerations of synaptic vesicle size and shape (see review in ref. 4). The type 2 spines, like the primary ending, contain large rounded vesicles and are considered to be excitatory, i.e., they either increase or prolong transmitter release from the primary ending through their dendroaxonic synapses. The P axon with its mixture of small rounded and flattened vesicles (Fig. 1) might be expected to exert an opposite effect through its axo-axonic synapse by either inhibiting or decreasing transmitter release from the axodendritic synapses of the C ending. The axo-axonic synapses may diminish transmitter release from the primary ending by affecting the invasion of incoming action potentials (2).

SG INTERNEURONS

Three kinds of interneurons are found in the SG layer. Each of these neuronal cell types is considered a Golgi type II neuron in that its axons undergo numerous divisions near the dendritic arbors and do not project out of the nucleus caudalis. The three SG neurons are distinguished by their

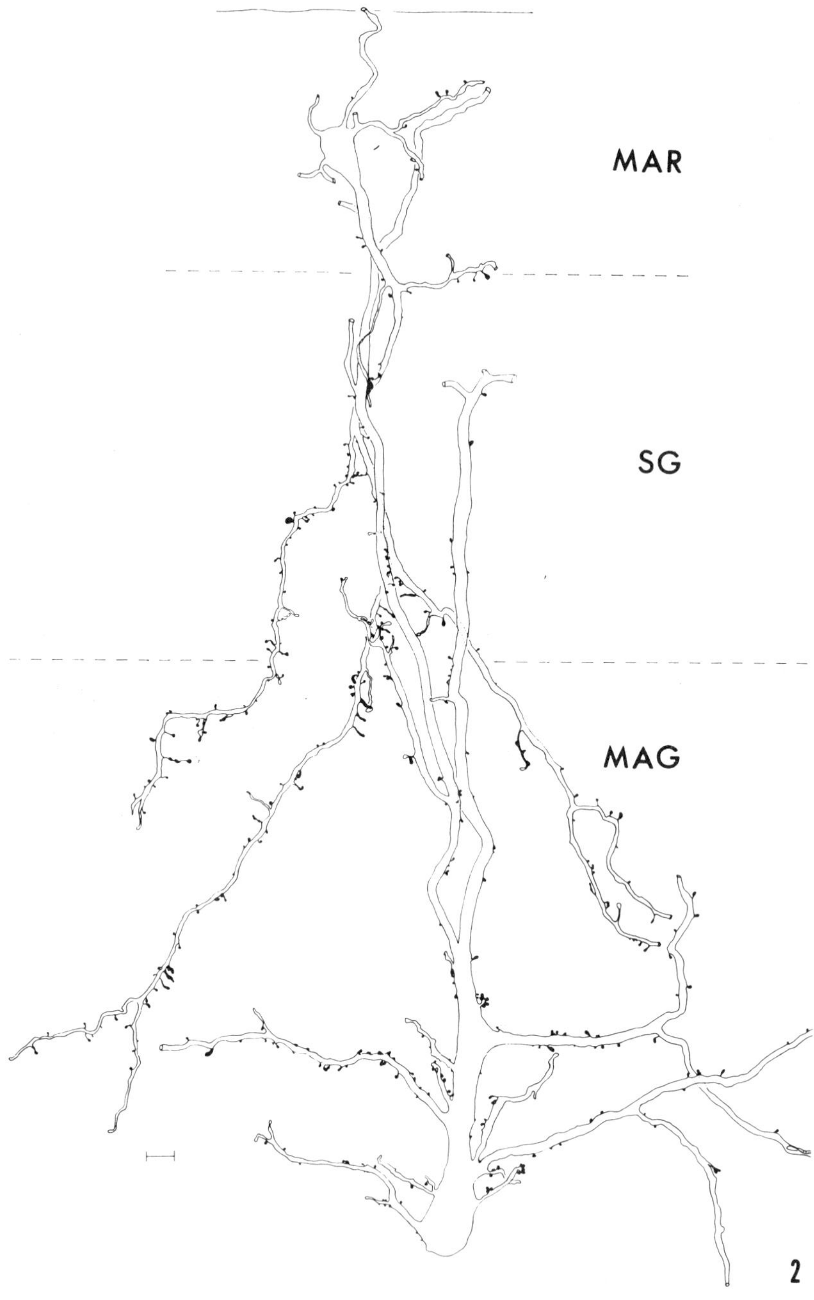

FIG. 2. Camera lucida drawing of a marginal neuron and a magnocellular neuron which send dendrites into the SG layer. The marginal neuron gives off a few thin dendritic branches in the marginal (MAR) layer and sends its thickest dendrite into the SG layer where it undergoes two divisions before descending into the magnocellular (MAG) layer. The number of dendritic spines increases on the branches of the descending dendrite as it passes through the SG and MAG layers. The magnocellular neuron gives off several small and medium-sized branches in the MAG layer and then sends 3 dendritic branches into the SG layer where they undergo further branching. Scale: 10μm.

dendritic branching pattern, spine distribution, geometric shape of the dendritic tree, axonal branching pattern, and laminar distribution of the axonal arbor (5).

The fine-caliber unmyelinated axons are the most numerous neural elements in the SG neuropil, and most of these are derived from the SG neurons. For example, the axon of the islet cell, the most common SG neuron, extends for at least 1 mm in the rostrocaudal axis of the layer. Each of its collaterals divides every 50 to 100 μm with one branch doubling back in the direction of the cell body and the other branch continuing on in the direction of its parent. In this manner each islet cell generates a profuse axonal plexus in the SG layer. Each axon collateral is characterized by numerous small boutons *en passant* and an occasional end bouton. Several islet cells have been found with two axons, each with an extensive, highly branched aborization (6). A second cell type, the stalked cell, sends axonal and dendritic branches into the SG and marginal layers, whereas the third cell type, the spiny cell, sends axonal and dendritic branches into all three layers of nucleus caudalis. The axons of the SG neurons are the major source of P endings. In addition to forming axo-axonic synapses in the SG glomeruli, P endings also form axodendritic synapses on large-caliber dendritic shafts and axosomatic synapses on SG neuronal cell bodies.

MARGINAL AND MAGNOCELLULAR NEURONS

Some neurons in both the marginal and magnocellular layers send their dendrites into the SG layer (Fig. 2) where they receive primary afferent input in the SG glomeruli. Among these neurons we can expect to find the second-order projection neurons in trigeminal pain pathways. Physiological studies have shown that both marginal neurons (Dubner et al., *this volume* and magnocellular neurons (1,8, Dubner et al., *this volume*) project to thalamic levels.

CONCLUSIONS

These anatomical studies suggest that three major synaptic circuits in the trigeminal pain pathway are located in the SG layer of nucleus caudalis. First, primary trigeminal axons which respond to noxious stimuli synapse on the dendrites of second-order projection neurons, the cell bodies of which are in the marginal and magnocellular layers. Second, these same primary afferents activate three kinds of interneurons with cell bodies in the SG layer. These interneurons in turn inhibit transmission in the primary axon-projection neuron circuit presynaptically through axo-axonic synapses on the primary endings and postsynaptically through axodendritic synapses. The third circuit concerns a neuron of unknown origin which sends dendrites containing synaptic vesicles into the SG glomeruli and which affects transmission in the primary axon-projection neuron circuit presynaptically through dendroaxonic synapses on the primary axon.

Two of the most provocative and perhaps related observations on trigeminal pain pathways concern (a) the general persistence of painful sensation long after the painful stimulus is removed, and (b) the presence in nucleus caudalis of second-order trigeminothalamic projection neurons which exhibit prolonged discharge after electrical stimulation of small-caliber primary trigeminal axons (9). The prolonged discharge outlasts the primary afferent barrage by more than 200 msec. A consideration of the synaptic connections between the primary ending and type 1 and type 2 spines (Fig. 1) suggests that one possible interpretation of these observations may lie in the dendroaxonic synapse of the type 2 spine. This interpretation is based on the hypothesis that has emerged from electron microscopic studies of afferent pathways in which processes containing large rounded synaptic vesicles are considered excitatory, whereas processes containing mixtures of small, rounded, and flattened synaptic vesicles are considered inhibitory. The type 2 spines receive their excitatory input through the axodendritic synapses of the primary endings. They in turn activate type 1 spines through their dendrodendritic synapses.

The following synaptic sequences (Fig. 1, *arrows*) illustrate how a type 1 spine might continue to be activated beyond the time of arrival of an action potential. First the type 1 spine would be activated directly by the primary ending (Fig. 1, C→1). Slightly later the type 1 spine would be activated in a disynaptic pathway through the dendrodendritic synapse of the type 2 spine (Fig. 1, C→2→1). The reciprocal pairing of the dendroaxonic and axodendritic synapses between the primary ending and the type 2 spine (Fig. 1, C⇄2) might allow transmitter release from the axodendritic synapses of the primary ending to persist for some time in the monosynaptic and disynaptic pathways from the primary ending to the type 1 spine (Fig. 1, 1←C⇄2→1). These excitatory circuits could be interrupted between the primary ending and the type 1 spine through either axo-axonic (Fig. 1, P→C) or axodendritic (Fig. 1, P→1) synapses of the small P endings.

REFERENCES

1. Darian-Smith, I., and Yokota, T. (1966): *J. Neurophysiol.,* 29:185–206.
2. Eccles, J. C. (1964): *The Physiology of Synapses.* Springer-Verlag, Berlin.
3. Gobel, S. (1971): In: *Oral-Facial Sensory and Motor Mechanisms,* edited by R. Dubner and Y. Kawamura. Appleton-Century-Crofts, New York.
4. Gobel, S. (1974): *J. Neurocytol.,* 3:219–243.
5. Gobel, S. (1975*a*): *J. Comp. Neurol.,* 162:397–415.
6. Gobel, S. (1975*b*): *Brain Res.,* 88:333–338.
7. Gobel, S., and Dubner, R. (1969): *J. Comp. Neurol.,* 137:459–494.
8. Gordon, G., Landren, S., and Seed, W. A. (1961): *J. Neurophysiol.,* 158:544–559.
9. Price, D. D., Hu, J., and Dubner, R.: *Unpublished observations.*
10. Schmidt, R. F. (1973): In: *Handbook of Sensory Physiology. Vol. II, Somatosensory System,* edited by A. Iggo. Springer-Verlag, Berlin.
11. Westrum, L. E., and Black, R. G. (1971): *Brain Res.,* 25:265–288.

Advances in Pain Research and Therapy, Vol. 1,
edited by J. J. Bonica and D. Albe-Fessard.
Raven Press, New York © 1976.

Trigeminal Subnucleus Caudalis Neurons Excited by Tooth Pulp Stimulation

Toshikatsu Yokota

Department of Physiology, Medical College of Shiga, Moriyama, Shiga Prefecture, 524, Japan

Clinical observations after spinal trigeminal tractotomy have attested to the role of the trigeminal subnucleus caudalis in the appreciation of pain (6). Some previous electrophysiological studies, however, revealed few, if any, single units in the subnucleus caudalis responding to electrical stimulation of the tooth pulp, even though pain is the only modality of sensation subserved by tooth pulp afferent fibers (1,2,7). The present study constitutes an attempt to examine this apparent paradox.

METHODS

Experiments were carried out in adult cats anesthetized with urethane-chloralose in an intravenous dose of 3.5 ml/kg (urethane 125 mg/ml and chloralose 10 mg/ml). The upper and lower canine teeth on both sides were prepared for electrical stimulation: in each canine tooth small cavities approximately 1 mm in diameter were drilled into the dentin at two sites approximately 3 mm apart on the labial side. The cavity floor was placed at or in the predentin, but pulp penetration was avoided. A silver wire 0.4 mm in diameter was applied to each cavity. Around the silver wire, an amalgam was firmly packed and dental cement was placed over the amalgam filling. Single-unit recordings were obtained using glass micropipette electrodes filled with fast green FCF in 1 M sodium acetate. During experiments, gallamine triethiodide was periodically administered to eliminate reflex activation of jaw muscles.

We analyzed 186 units that were histologically identified by recovering dye marks between 0.8 and 5.0 mm caudal to the obex. All units responded to tooth pulp stimulation and displayed stable discharges long enough for careful study, but they scarcely exhibited spontaneous discharges.

Populations of responsive units were located in two discrete sites: the dorsal marginal rim of the subnucleus caudalis and the lateral reticular formation.

Marginal Rim Units

Altogether 62 units were obtained from the dorsal marginal rim. They were most frequently encountered in the rostral part of the subnucleus caudalis. In most cases only one of the ipsilateral canines was effective in eliciting spike discharges: 20 units were fired by electrical stimulation of the ipsilateral upper canine, 30 units by that of the ipsilateral lower canine, and 9 units by both of them. In three units in the lateral half of the marginal rim, ipsilateral as well as contralateral canines were effective. All the units isolated from the medial one-third of the dorsal marginal rim were activated by either the upper or lower canine on the ipsilateral side except for one unit. An example of marginal rim is illustrated in Fig. 1.

The probability of response to single-shock stimulation was generally higher in units obtained from the medial one-third than in units from the lateral two-thirds. The minimum latency, which as a rule refers to the earliest reproducible discharges elicited by just supramaximal triple-shock stimulation, tended to be longer in the lateral direction. In Fig. 2, the histogram of minimum latency distribution of units in the medial one-third is given in A, while that of units in the lateral two-thirds is shown in B. The minimum latency ranges were from 4.1 to 11.8 msec in the former and from 7.1 to 28 msec in the latter. Monosynaptic excitation, if present, appears to take place in the medial one-third of the dorsal marginal rim.

When tested with low-intensity mechanical stimuli applied to the territory of the trigeminal nerve, none of the marginal rim units were activated. The

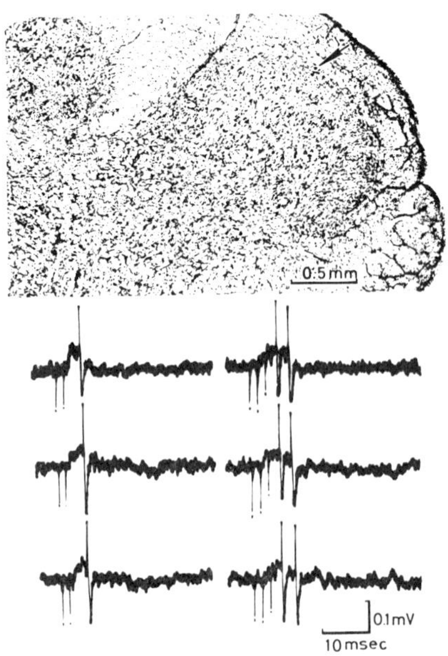

FIG. 1. Photomicrograph of a marginal rim unit showing the location of dye mark in the dorsal marginal rim. Consecutive records of responses to double- or triple-shock stimulation of the ipsilateral upper canine are given.

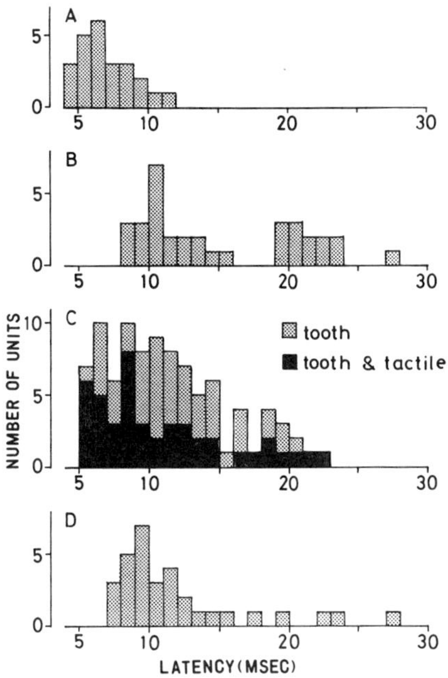

FIG. 2. Minimum latency distribution. **A:** Units in the medial one-third of the marginal rim. **B:** Units in the lateral two-thirds of the marginal rim. **C:** Ipsilateral lateral reticular formation (LRF) units. **D:** Bilateral LRF units. Ipsilateral LRF units are further divided into two groups: one responds to innocuous stimulation of trigeminal territory and the other does not.

marginal rim of the subnucleus caudalis probably contains units responding only to, or preponderantly to, noxious stimulation.

Lateral Reticular Formation Units

Altogether 124 units were obtained from the lateral reticular formation (LRF) ventromedially contiguous with the subnucleus caudalis. They were categorized in two groups: one responding to stimulation of the ipsilateral upper and/or lower canine tooth pulp (93 units), and the other responding to bilateral canines (31 units).

Ipsilateral LRF Units

Most units of this category were located in the subnucleus reticularis dorsalis medullae oblongatae of Meessen and Olszewski (4), particularly near the ventromedial border of the subnucleus caudalis. Of these, 41 units responded to the upper canine, 24 units to the lower canine, and the remaining 28 units to either canine. The minimum latency of the response ranged from 5.1 to 22.8 msec, as shown in the histogram of Fig. 2C.

Forty-eight of these units were also excited by light brushing of a restricted area in the ipsilateral face or oral cavity. When a conditioning electric shock was applied to the cutaneous receptive field, subsequent response to tooth pulp stimulation was usually suppressed. The results resemble those with lamina V units in the spinal cord (5). An example of ipsilateral LRF units is illustrated in Fig. 3.

Bilateral LRF Units

Bilateral LRF units were isolated from the subnucleus reticularis ventralis medullae oblongatae, which is ventral to the subnucleus reticularis dorsalis medullae oblongatae and the trigeminal subnucleus caudalis. In all cases, ipsilateral upper and lower canines were effective together with contralateral upper and/or lower canines. The probability of ipsilateral response to single-shock stimulation was larger than that of contralateral response. The number of spikes in each response was also larger in the ipsilateral response than in the contralateral one, as illustrated in Fig. 4. The minimum latency of ipsilateral response was always shorter than that of contralateral response and ranged from 7.1 to 28 msec, as shown in Fig. 2D. Monosynaptic excitation of bilateral LRF units by tooth pulp stimulation seems improbable.

Furthermore, all the bilateral LRF units obtained were also excited by mechanical stimulation of the ipsilateral cornea, which possesses unique unmyelinated innervation (8). In some cases light stroke of the cornea with a cotton wisp was sufficient, although light pressure was necessary in other cases. Some bilateral LRF units were also excited by light mechanical stimulation of the inside of the nose, which is innervated solely by free

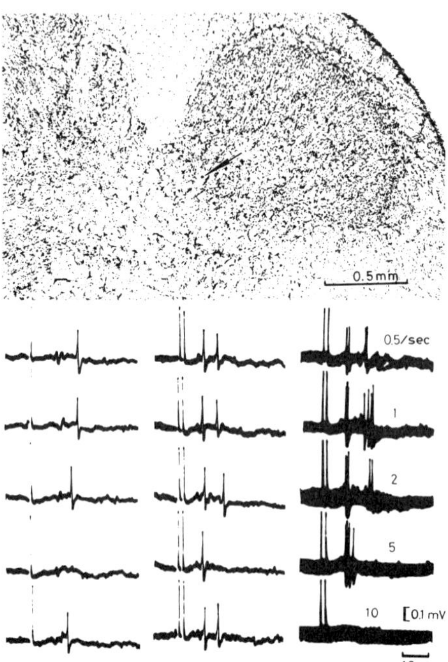

FIG. 3. Photomicrograph of an ipsilateral LRF unit showing the location of dye mark in the subnucleus reticularis dorsalis medullae oblongatae. **Left** and **middle:** 5 consecutive records of responses to single- or double-shock stimulation, respectively, of the ipsilateral upper canine once every 2 sec. **Right:** superimposed records of responses to double-shock stimulation at various frequencies.

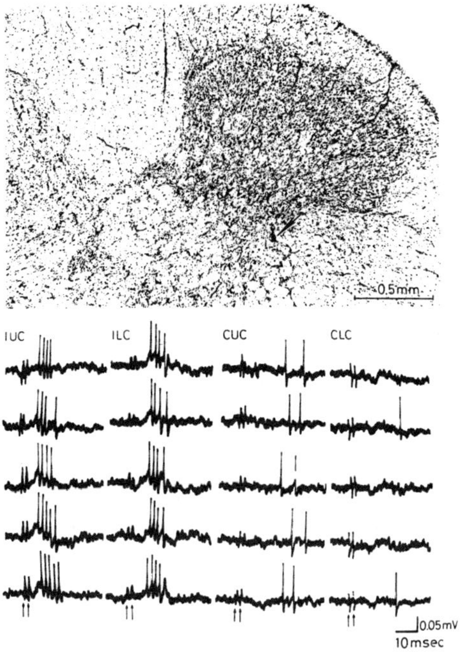

FIG. 4. A bilateral LRF unit. The dye mark was located in the subnucleus reticularis ventralis medullae oblongatae. Double-shock stimulation was successively applied to all canines. IUC, ipsilateral upper canine; ILC, ipsilateral lower canine; CUC, contralateral upper canine; CLC, contralateral lower canine.

nerve endings (3). In such cases gentle tapping on the dorsum of the ipsilateral nose elicited spike discharges, possibly because of transmission of mechanical distortion to the nasal cavity. In the remainder of the trigeminal nerve territory, however, innocuous stimulation was ineffective, although firm pressure to the ipsilateral or bilateral face was sometimes effective. The cutaneous receptive field was either quite extensive or rather restricted. These properties suggest that peripheral sensory inputs to bilateral LRF units are predominantly conveyed by small nerve fibers.

SUMMARY

In cats, single-unit activity was extracellularly recorded from the trigeminal subnucleus caudalis and its nearby structures after electrical stimulation of the canine tooth pulp.

Populations of responsive units have been identified in two discrete regions: the dorsal marginal rim of the subnucleus caudalis and the lateral reticular formation ventromedially contiguous with the subnucleus caudalis.

Marginal rim units were not fired when tested with innocuous stimulation of the trigeminal territory. These units appear to respond only to, or preponderantly to, noxious stimulation. Minimum latency measurement suggested that monosynaptic excitation may take place in the medial one-third of the marginal rim.

Lateral reticular formation units were categorized in two groups: ipsilateral LRF units and bilateral LRF units. Ipsilateral LRF units were isolated mainly from the subnucleus reticularis dorsalis, whereas bilateral LRF units were isolated primarily from the subnucleus reticularis ventralis. Most ipsilateral LRF units were excited by mechanical stimulation of the ipsilateral cornea and sometimes of the inside of the ipsilateral nose. Innocuous stimulation of the remainder of the trigeminal territory was ineffective. It was suggested that bilateral LRF units receive afferent inputs conveyed by small nerve fibers.

REFERENCES

1. Anderson, D. J., Hannam, A. G., and Matthews, B. (1970): *Physiol. Rev.,* 50:171–195.
2. Davies, W. I. R., Scott, D., Vesterstrøm, K., and Vyklický, L. (1971): *J. Physiol. (Lond.),* 218:515–532.
3. Harpman, J. A. (1951): *Br. Med. J.,* 2:497–498.
4. Meessen, H., and Olszewski, J. (1949): *A Cytoarchitectonic Atlas of the Rhombencephalon of the Rabbit.* S. Karger, Basel.
5. Pomeranz, B., Wall, P. D., and Weber, W. V. (1968): *J. Physiol. (Lond.),* 199:511–532.
6. Sjöqvist, O. (1938): *Acta Psychiatr. Scand. [Suppl.],* 17:1–38.
7. Tamarova, Z. A., Shaporalov, A. E., and Vyklický, L. (1973): *Brain Res.,* 64:442–445.
8. Zander, E., and Weddell, G. (1951): *J. Anat.,* 85:68–99.

Advances in Pain Research and Therapy, Vol. 1,
edited by J. J. Bonica and D. Albe-Fessard.
Raven Press, New York © 1976.

Trigeminal Neuron Subsets Excited by the Lingual Nerve: Response to Tactile and Noxious Stimulation

*M. A. Biedenbach and A. C. Brown

Department of Physiology and Biophysics,
University of Washington, Seattle, Washington 98195

INTRODUCTION

Several investigators have described neurons in the trigeminal nucleus and spinal cord responding either exclusively (2,3) or differentially (4,5) to noxious stimulation. However, because not all unit types driven by a peripheral nerve were sampled, a comprehensive picture of responses to tactile and noxious stimulation is not available. This study was designed to develop such a comprehensive picture by sampling all unit types activated by a single peripheral nerve, in this case the lingual nerve, and to compare and contrast responses to noxious and tactile stimuli.

EXPERIMENTAL PROCEDURE

In cats anesthetized with chloralose and paralyzed with gallamine triethiodide (Flaxedil®), the lingual nerve was exposed for stimulating with bipolar electrodes. The dorsal surface of the brainstem was exposed near the obex for unit recording. Unit potentials described in this study were obtained in the region extending 0 to 6 mm rostral from the obex and 4.2 to 6 mm lateral from the midline. An electrical stimulus was delivered to the lingual nerve every 4 sec while searching for unit potentials in the trigeminal area in order to identify neurons to which these peripheral fibers projected. When a driven unit was encountered, film records were made of responses to a range of electrical stimuli from threshold to supramaximal. The tongue, face, and head were explored manually to locate mechanosensory endings that excited this unit. When a receptive field was located, a series of mechanical stimuli ranging from tactile to noxious was applied, and the unit response was filmed. A schematic diagram of the experimental arrangement is illustrated in Fig. 1.

Quantitation of unit response to tactile-noxious inputs required the development of a special stimulator to apply a square wave of force, of

* Present address: Department of Physiology, University of Texas, Health Science Center, San Antonio, Texas 78284

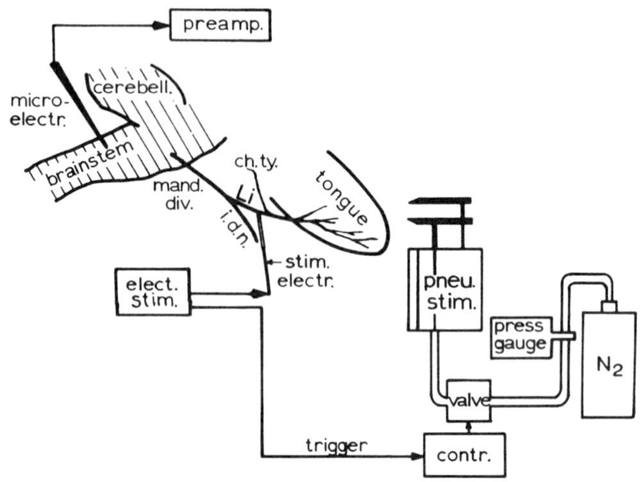

FIG. 1. Experimental arrangement for stimulation and recording.

controlled magnitude and duration, and with rapid onset and release. This stimulator was based on the small pneumatic cylinder in Fig. 1. When gas was admitted to the cylinder, a movable jaw attached to the piston was driven toward a fixed jaw, pinching the tissue under investigation. Admission of gas to the cylinder was controlled by a small solenoid valve powered by a solid-state driver. A second valve permitted exhausting gas from the cylinder at the termination of the stimulus. The applied force was determined by the gas pressure, which was controlled by a pressure regulator. The valve controller was activated by pressing a manual push button or by a pulse from the electrical stimulator.

Data were analyzed by projecting the film records onto a graphic digitizer tablet to generate a digital computer file for each unit at each of the various electrical and mechanical stimulus intensities (1). The digitized data were then used to construct latency histograms for response onset and displays of sequential spike intervals in long spike trains.

RESULTS

A total of 198 units driven by electrical stimulation of the lingual nerve were investigated. Based on their response properties, these units were divided into four main groups.

Unit Classification

Approximately 17% of the units had receptive fields on the tongue ("Tongue" units). Approximately 36% had receptive fields somewhere within the trigeminal nerve peripheral field (e.g., face, head, gingiva) but not on the tongue ("Face" units). Approximately 20% were not mechanosensitive ("Mute" units); that is, they could be excited by electrical stimulation of the lingual nerve but not by peripheral mechanical stimulation. The remaining 25% ("Tap-w" units) had several unusual properties. This group responded only to extremely abrupt mechanical taps. Generally they could be excited by peripheral electrical or mechanical stimulation from many parts of the body, but not by taps applied to the tongue or other very soft tissue.

Depth Distribution

The distribution of depth below the dorsal surface of the brainstem for the four groups of units is shown on the right of Fig. 2. The drawing on the left of Fig. 2 is a camera lucida tracing of a section taken 3 mm rostral to the obex. Deposition of dye by the microelectrode confirmed that at this brainstem level the dorsal border of the trigeminal nucleus lies at a depth of 2.4 mm, and the medial border begins at 4.2 mm lateral to the midline. Clearly, Tongue and Face units are concentrated in the trigeminal nucleus. Tap units are located dorsally in the region of the external cuneate nucleus or more rostrally in the vestibular nucleus. Mechanically Mute units were distributed over the whole depth of the region explored.

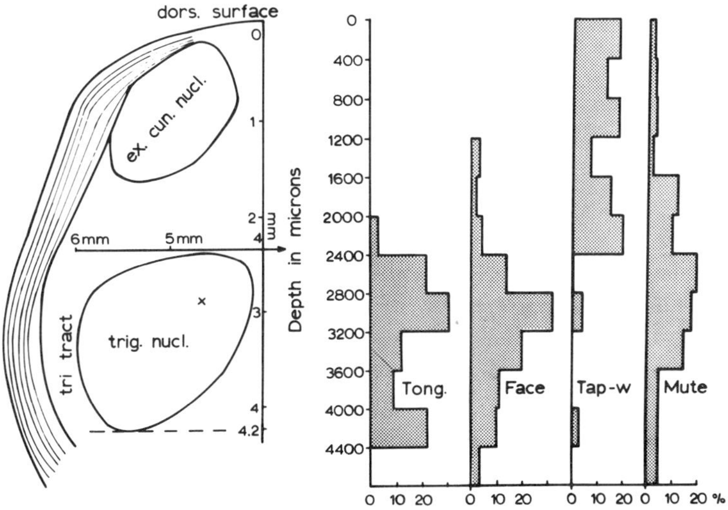

FIG. 2. Left: Cross section of brainstem 3 mm rostral to the obex, indicating area explored for unit potentials. **Right:** Depth distribution of the 4 neuron groups.

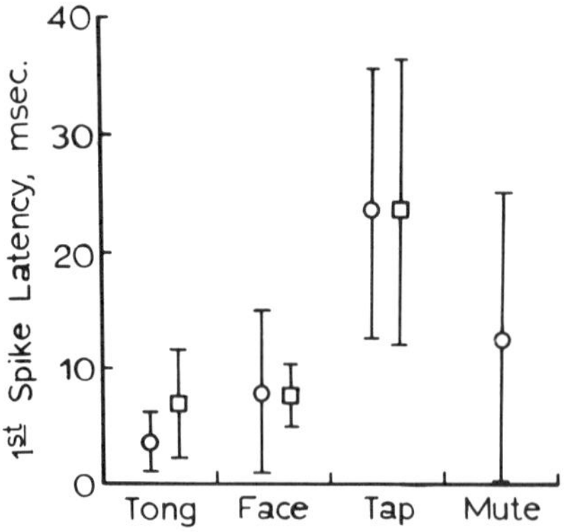

FIG. 3. Mean and standard deviation of the first spike latency for the 4 neuron groups. *Circles,* response to supramaximal electrical stimulation; *squares,* response to noxious mechanical stimulation.

Latency

Figure 3 illustrates the mean and standard deviation of the latency (interval between stimulus and first response) to electrical (*circle*) and mechanical (*square*) stimuli for each of the four groups. In response to electrical stimulation of the lingual nerve, Tongue units responded first, next Face units, followed by Mute units, and finally Tap units. In response to "pinching," the sequence of activation of the three mechanosensitive groups was the same as for electrical stimulation. Surprisingly, Face units appeared to show more latency variation on electrical stimulation than on mechanical stimulation. However, the electrical stimuli were applied to the lingual nerve, which probably has a less effective input on Face neurons than other branches of the trigeminal nerve which supply the cutaneous face region tested. In contrast, the lingual nerve has a very effective input for units with receptive fields on the tongue, as confirmed by the short latency and small standard deviation recorded from such electrically excited units.

Tactile-Noxious Response Patterns

Tap and rapidly adapting units in the Tongue and Face groups did not respond differentially to tactile versus noxious stimuli. These units produced only a few spikes or a short burst at the onset of the stimulus. But maintained or slowly applied pressure, even at noxious intensities, usually evoked no response. This was particularly true for Tap units which required the most rapid rate of change of stimulus. However, slowly adapting units in the Face and Tongue groups generated different responses to tactile and noxious stimulation. Tactile stimuli often evoked only a short response lasting a few hundred milliseconds, whereas noxious stimuli increased the response duration markedly; in most of these units discharge continued as long as the noxious pressure was applied. This change from a rather brief to a tonic response as stimulus intensity increased was especially pronounced for the Tongue units.

The sequence of spikes in the trains fell into two main patterns illustrated in Fig. 4. In this figure the logarithm of interspike interval is plotted as a function of the spike number in the train. The most common pattern, the "Cloud" or scatter pattern (Fig. 4B), was characterized by a brief burst of high frequency when the stimulus was first applied. This high frequency was followed by a silent period of several hundred milliseconds in some units, but most maintained firing with shorter and longer intervals randomly

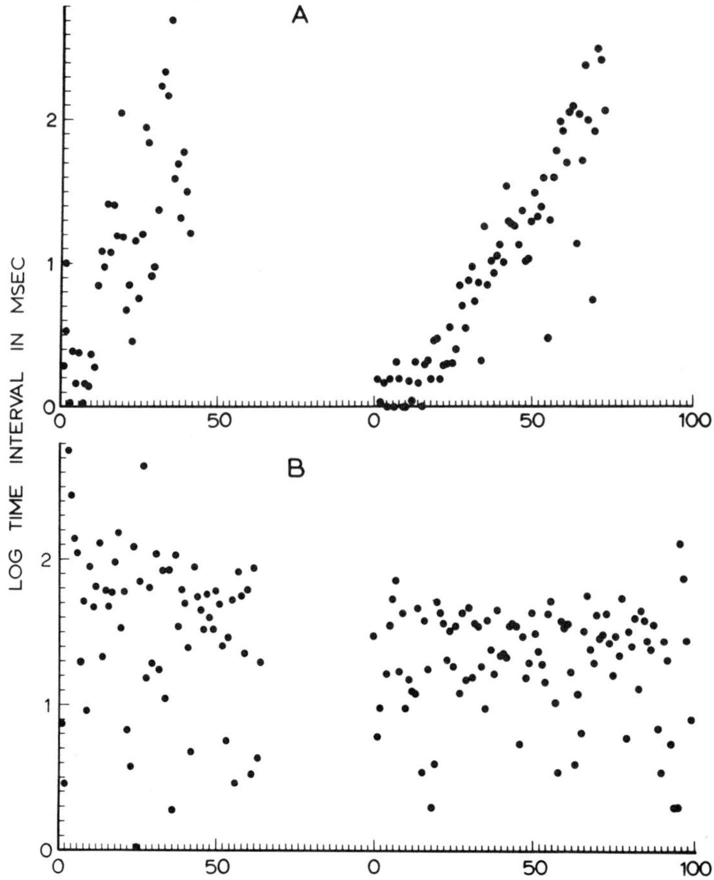

FIG. 4. Spike train patterns in response to mechanical stimuli. *Left,* response to 100 g (tactile) "pinch;" *right,* response to 500 g (noxious) "pinch." *Ordinate,* logarithm of the interspike interval; *abscissa,* spike number (up to 100 spikes). **A:** "Log-linear" patterns. **B:** Patterns of "Cloud" or scatter response.

mixed. Comparison of the left side of Fig. 4B, which represents the response to a light tactile stimulus, with the response to a noxious stimulus shown on the right, showed that the more intense stimulus evoked a somewhat more uniform firing pattern with fewer long interspike intervals. The second, less common, firing pattern among slowly adapting Tongue and Face units was the "Log-linear" pattern of Fig. 4A. Again, application of the stimulus evoked short bursts of spikes, but then the logarithm of the interval between successive spikes increased linearly with spike number; in other words, the interspike interval was directly proportional to $exp(n)$, where n is the sequence number of the spike in the train. Comparing the tactile (*left*) and noxious (*right*) unit response patterns in Fig. 4A reveals that the noxious response showed less scatter and smaller slope (less rapid decay of spike frequency) than did the tactile response.

CONCLUSION

Four groups of brainstem units—Tongue, Face, Tap, and Mute—were excited by electrical stimulation of the lingual nerve. Mapping the superficial receptive field of units activated by nerve stimulation demonstrated convergence in the trigeminal nucleus between trigeminal branches. Thus units discharged by tactile stimulation of the face could be activated also by electrical excitation of the lingual nerve. But since mechanical stimulation of the tongue could not activate Face units, this convergent input must be less effective (subthreshold) than the excitation via primary afferents in another trigeminal branch. Tap units showed greatest convergence and least topographical specificity since stimuli from many areas of the body surface appeared equally effective in evoking discharge. The long latency of Tap units indicates multisynaptic activation.

Applying mechanical steps of graded strength to the face or tongue evoked the following response patterns. A tactile force step caused an initial burst of spikes in both rapidly and slowly adapting units associated with the specific face or tongue area. Slightly later, Tap units discharged if the stimulus onset was sufficiently rapid. During the force plateau, only slowly adapting units continued to discharge, and most of these ceased firing within several seconds after force application. At the onset of a noxious pressure step, rapidly and slowly adapting units again produced a burst of spikes, but at a somewhat higher frequency compared with less intense stimulation. After a delay, Tap units discharged briefly. During the force plateau, slowly adapting units discharged for the full duration of the step, again at a higher mean frequency, with spike train patterns of the Cloud or Log-linear type. Since rapidly adapting Face and Tongue units and Tap units discharge only at the onset of the noxious stimulus, their role in signaling pain seems less important than that of slowly adapting units.

REFERENCES

1. Biedenbach, M. A., Beuerman, R. W., and Brown, A. C. (1975): *Cell Tissue Res.*, 157: 341–352.
2. Christensen, B. N., and Perl, E. R. (1970): *J. Neurophysiol.*, 33:293–307.
3. Mosso, J. A., and Kruger, L. (1972): *Brain Res.*, 38:206–210.
4. Nord, S. G., and Ross, G. S. (1973): *Brain Res.*, 58:385–399.
5. Wagman, I. H., and Price, D. D. (1969): *J. Neurophysiol.*, 32:803–817.

Advances in Pain Research and Therapy, Vol. 1,
edited by J. J. Bonica and D. Albe-Fessard.
Raven Press, New York © 1976.

Role of Trigeminal Nucleus Caudalis in the Modulation of Trigeminal Sensory and Motor Neuronal Activities

B. J. Sessle and L. F. Greenwood

Division of Biological Sciences, Faculty of Dentistry, University of Toronto, Toronto M5G 1G6, Canada

It is generally considered that trigeminal (V) nucleus caudalis is essential for oral-facial pain perception because it acts as the relay site of V nociceptive information to the thalamus and other higher centers. This view has been based largely on reports of numerous small-diameter fibers in the V spinal tract at the level of caudalis and of a morphology similar to that of the dorsal horn (5,19,22), and on clinical observations of the effectiveness of a V tractotomy operation in relieving V neuralgia and producing facial analgesia (4,5,19,21). However, recent anatomical evidence (6,10) indicates that most small-diameter axons in the tract are not V primary afferents but probably represent intranuclear connections within the V brainstem complex. Moreover, the clinical observations could be explained not only by an interruption of a nociceptive pathway relaying to the thalamus through caudalis but also by an interruption of one of these intranuclear connections that normally exert a tonic facilitatory influence on the relay of sensory information through more rostral components of the V complex. This possibility, investigated in this chapter, is suggested from recent findings of V primary afferent excitability changes (23) and sensory changes (4) after V tractotomy in cats and monkeys.

METHODS

The effects of V tractotomy and reversible cold block of synaptic transmission in nucleus caudalis (14,16,17) were noted on the responses of single rostral V neurons to oral-facial stimuli. Neuronal responses in decerebrate or anesthetized (chloralose) cats were recorded in stereotaxically located and histologically confirmed microelectrode penetrations of the V main sensory nucleus (MSN), nucleus oralis, and V motor nucleus region (16). Since the tooth pulp is generally considered to be a site from which the sensation of pain only can be elicited and which is innervated only by small-diameter nerve fibers (1,12), isolated bipolar electrical stimulation (7) of the ipsilateral maxillary and mandibular canines was used routinely as a test for nociceptive input to MSN-oralis sensory neurons and to motor neurons, but sometimes serrated forceps and radiant heat were also used. Mechanical innocuous stimulation of oral-facial tissues was achieved by hand-held probes or by an electronically controlled mechanical stimulator (15,16). The infraorbital (IO), glossopharyngeal (IX), and superior laryngeal (SLN) nerves were also isolated and electrically stimulated, and V-thalamic relay neurons were identified by their antidromic response to bipolar stimulation of the contralateral medial lemniscus or ventrobasal thalamus (16). Motor neurons were identified by their antidromic response to bipolar stimulation of the isolated masseter or digastric nerves that innervate jaw-closing and jaw-opening muscles, respectively. In some animals the effect of cooling caudalis was noted on the reflex electromyographic (EMG) response (18) in the digastric and perioral facial muscles to peripheral nerve stimulation.

RESULTS AND DISCUSSION

Over 350 single neurons were recorded in the MSN-oralis and motor nuclei and adjacent regions. In accordance with previous findings (3,15), restricted mechanoreceptive fields were typical of MSN-oralis neurons, although many had IX and SLN inputs; e.g., 12% of MSN-oralis neurons relaying to contralateral thalamus could be activated by IX and/or SLN stimulation.

Ten neurons that could be activated only by noxious stimulation of localized or widespread skin areas were located in or adjacent to MSN-oralis. A particularly striking feature was the large proportion (45%) of sensory neurons that could be activated by stimulation of one or both tooth pulps (17), and 20% of V-thalamic relay neurons had pulp input (Fig. 1A). Most could be activated with a short latency (2.5 to 4.5 msec) by low-intensity (< 1.0 mA, 0.1 msec, single pulses) pulp stimulation, and 20% had only a pulp input identified (none of these were antidromic). However, 80% could be activated by other inputs and had localized mechanoreceptive fields in the oral and perioral regions. A tooth pulp input to the MSN-oralis region has been reported by others (7,9,24), and a projection has also been found (7,13) to caudalis, classically considered to be the relay site of V nociceptive information. Nevertheless, the proportion of caudalis neurons activated by pulp stimulation is apparently much less (7,9), and in studies with R. Dubner and G. E. Lucier (*unpublished*) we recently found a much lower incidence of cells with pulp input in the caudalis region than in MSN-oralis in the same cats. Moreover, these caudalis cells generally have widespread peripheral inputs and variable and long latencies (5 to 30 msec) to pulp stimulation. They are located mainly deep in or to caudalis, and few can be activated antidromically from thalamus. Thus a role for these cells in pain perception as a direct relay to thalamus now seems unlikely; they may serve as interneurons in oral-facial reflex control (20) or in modulating MSN-oralis cells (13,16,24). The large pulp projection to and relay through MSN-

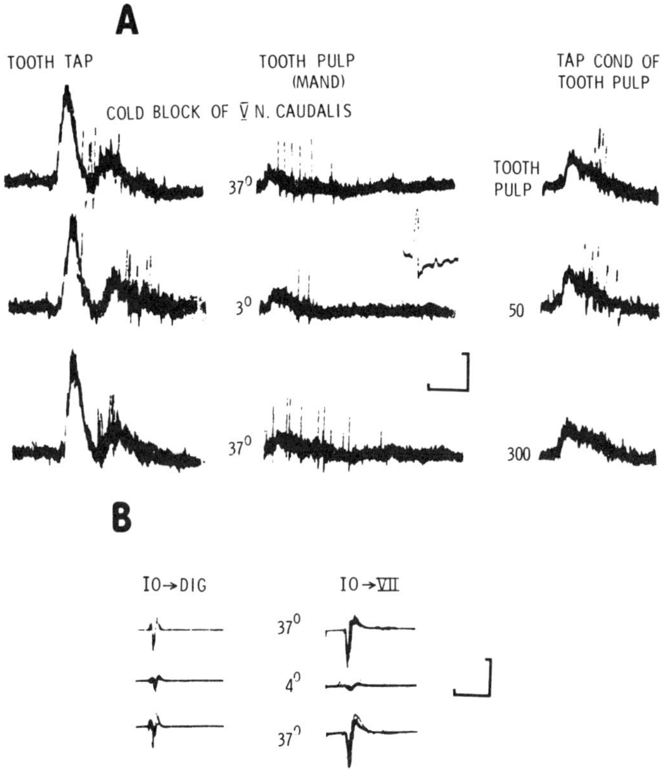

FIG. 1. A: Responses of a single V-thalamic relay neuron (from decerebrate cat) with localized intraoral receptive field including maxillary and mandibular (MAND) tooth pulp. Cooling caudalis from 37° to 3°C reversibly depressed the neuron's response to tooth pulp stimulation and to mechanical stimulation of the maxillary canine. Note neuron's antidromic response to contralateral medial lemniscus stimulation (*insert*), and effect on the neuron's response to maxillary pulp stimulation of a conditioning vibratory (50 Hz, 50 msec duration) stimulus applied to the mandibular canine (*right*). Neuron's response was facilitated at 50 msec and then inhibited for 400 msec; records show its control response to pulp stimulation (*top*) and its responses to the same stimulus when preceded by the conditioning mechanical stimulus at 50 msec (*middle*) and 300 msec (*bottom*). Voltage calibration: 0.2 mV; time calibration: 2 msec (antidromic response) and 4 msec (all other responses); some spikes retouched. **B:** Depressive effects of reversible cold block of caudalis on reflex responses to low-intensity (0.3 mA, 0.1 msec) infraorbital nerve (IO) stimulation in digastric (DIG) and facial (VII) muscles; in some cats depression of reflexes elicited by pulp stimulation was also often noted. Voltage calibration: 0.4 mV; time calibration: 10 msec. Each record in **A** and **B** represents 5 superimposed responses to 5 successive stimuli delivered at 1/sec.

oralis may in contrast be important in the central transmission of dental nociceptive information to higher perceptual levels (9,11). Our findings of a significant input to MSN as well as oralis disagree with the recent proposition (9) that a small part of oralis serves as the relay site for transmitting pulp information to thalamus.

In addition to its excitatory effects, pulp stimulation inhibited responses to IO, mechanical, or pulp stimuli. In no instance (70 cells) was a late period of facilitation (24) observed after pulp-induced inhibition in MSN-oralis, although this effect was seen in adjacent reticular formation. Prolonged inhibition of responses to pulp stimulation of relay and nonrelay cells was also noted with IO, IX, SLN, and oral-facial mechanical stimuli (Fig. 1A), and it might be involved in mechanisms of pain control such as in acupuncture analgesia of dental tissues (2).

Responses to pulp and noxious cutaneous stimuli could also be modulated by V tractotomy or reversible cold block or caudalis, and an example is shown in Fig. 1A. These procedures produced depression in about 25% of pulp responses tested, but 90% of IO or mechanically evoked responses were depressed (Fig. 1A). A marked reduction in mechanoreceptive field size was typically produced, and the dynamic mechanosensitivity of rapidly adapting cells and the stimulus-response relation of slowly adapting neurons (15) could also be depressed (16). Cold block of caudalis also was effective in depressing reversibly the effects of interacting pulp and mechanical stimuli, but it did not directly influence rostral neurons since no change occurred in MSN-oralis temperature or in the orthodromic response of V primary afferents and the antidromic response of relay neurons and motoneurons (16).

Since reversible interruption of caudalis predominantly depresses the responsiveness of MSN-oralis neurons to oral-facial innocuous and noxious stimuli, it indicates that caudalis exerts a net tonic facilitatory influence on the relay of sensory information through more rostral V regions. This is compatible with reports of anatomical connections between caudalis and these rostral regions (6), and with findings that caudalis has a tonic presynaptic hyperpolarizing influence on V primary afferent endings in MSN-oralis (23) and both facilitatory and inhibitory influences on the perception of V stimuli (4). The possibility of an inhibitory influence is also suggested from our studies since caudalis block led to facilitation of responsiveness to IO, pulp, or mechanical stimuli in 5% of cells tested. Our findings thus indicate that the classic view that caudalis is essential to pain perception by functioning as a relay site of V nociceptive information is simplistic. Although information related to mechanical, thermal, and noxious stimuli is relayed to thalamus (3,8,14,15), caudalis also exerts a modulating influence on rostral V cells. Depression of a tonic facilitatory influence from caudalis may in part explain the analgesia and partial loss of tactile sensibility seen in humans and animals after V tractotomy (4,5,19,21). The disruption of this complex interplay between caudalis and MSN-oralis and the depression of mechanosensitivity of MSN-oralis cells might also be implicated in the relief that this operation affords from V neuralgic attacks, which are usually triggered by a light tactile stimulus.

In addition to its essential role in the perception of oral-facial noxious stimuli, caudalis has recently been implicated in oral-facial motor control (20). Moreover, many of the nonrelay MSN-oralis cells reversibly depressed by caudalis block may also serve as interneurons for oral-facial reflexes (18,20). We have therefore tested the effects of V tractotomy and reversible cold block of caudalis on responses of single V motor neurons and on digastric and facial EMG activity. The antidromic response of V motor neurons was unaffected by these procedures, but the peripherally evoked responses in digastric motor neurons and in digastric and facial EMG could be reversibly depressed (Fig. 1B). This observation indicates that caudalis can also modulate oral-facial motor activity, an effect which might, for example, contribute to the reflex depression seen in animals and man after V tractotomy (4,5).

REFERENCES

1. Anderson, D. J., Hannam, A. G., and Matthews, B. (1970): *Physiol. Rev.,* 50:171–195.
2. Anderson, S. A., Ericson, T., Holmgren, E., and Lindqvist, G. (1973): *Brain Res.,* 63: 393–396.
3. Darian-Smith, I. (1966): *Int. Rev. Neurobiol.,* 9:301–395.
4. Denny-Brown, D., and Yanagisawa, N. (1973): *Brain,* 96:783–814.
5. Gerard, M. W. (1923): *Arch. Neurol. Psychiatr.,* 9:306–338.
6. Gobel, S. (1971): In: *Oral-Facial Sensory and Motor Mechanisms,* edited by R. Dubner and Y. Kawamura. Appleton-Century-Crofts, New York.
7. Greenwood, L. F. (1973): *Arch. Oral Biol.,* 18:771–785.
8. Hu, J. W., Price, D. D., and Dubner, R. (1975): *Proc. Soc. Neurosci.,* 133:9 (Abstr.).
9. Keller, O., Butkhuzi, S. M., Vyklický, L., and Brozek, G. (1974): *Physiol. Bohemoslov.,* 23:45–53.
10. Kerr, F. W. L. (1971): In: *Oral-Facial Sensory and Motor Mechanisms,* edited by R. Dubner and Y. Kawamura. Appleton-Century-Crofts, New York.
11. Lund, J. P., and Sessle, B. J. (1974): *Exp. Neurol.,* 45:314–331.
12. Mitchell, C. L. (1970): *Adv. Oral Biol.,* 4:131–149.
13. Nord, S. G., and Young, R. F. (1975): *Brain Res.,* 90:195–204.
14. Rowe, M. J., and Sessle, B. J. (1968): *J. Physiol. (Lond.),* 196:19–35.
15. Rowe, M. J., and Sessle, B. J. (1972): *Brain Res.,* 42:367–384.
16. Sessle, B. J., and Greenwood, L. F. (1974): *Brain Res.,* 67:330–333.
17. Sessle, B. J., and Greenwood, L. F. (1975): *J. Dent. Res.,* 54(B):B201–B206.
18. Sessle, B. J., and Kenny, D. J. (1973): In: *Fourth Symposium on Oral Sensation and Perception,* edited by J. F. Bosma, D.H.E.W., Bethesda, Maryland.
19. Sjöqvist, O. (1938): *Acta Psychiatr. Scand. [Suppl.]* 17:1–139.
20. Sumino, R. (1971): In: *Oral-Facial Sensory and Motor Mechanisms,* edited by R. Dubner and Y. Kawamura. Appleton-Century-Crofts, New York.
21. Walker, A. E. (1939): *J. Neurophysiol.,* 2:234–248.
22. Windle, W. F. (1926): *J. Comp. Neurol.,* 41:453–477.
23. Young, R. F., and King, R. B. (1972): *J. Neurophysiol.,* 35:87–95.
24. Yu, Y. J., and King, R. B. (1974): *Brain Res.,* 72:147–152.

Advances in Pain Research and Therapy, Vol. 1,
edited by J. J. Bonica and D. Albe-Fessard.
Raven Press, New York © 1976.

Modulation of Tooth Pulp Input into the Spinal Trigeminal Nucleus by Electrical Stimulation of Remote Cutaneous Areas in the Cat

Joseph W. Tamari and Suhayl J. Jabbur

Departments of Human Morphology and Physiology, School of Medicine, American University of Beirut, Beirut, Lebanon

The modulation of central nervous system function by externally applied electrical energy has been of scientific interest since the time of Galvani. Despite the continuing interest during the ensuing 2 centuries, little was accomplished before the last 20 years. Moreover, a good deal of this work, at basic and clinical levels, has centered on the problem of pain.

Electrical stimulation of virtually the entire cutaneous surface has been found to inhibit transmission of cutaneous input across the dorsal column nuclei (5) and the spinal trigeminal nucleus (3). The latter nucleus offers the unique advantage of receiving neural input from the tooth pulp, which may be exclusively engaged in the transmission of painful stimuli (1,6,10). The purpose of this chapter is to describe inhibitory influences from the entire cutaneous surface on neurons of the spinal trigeminal nucleus responding to tooth pulp stimulation (TPS).

METHODS

Cats were anesthetized with pentobarbital sodium (35 mg/kg) or α-chloralose (50 mg/kg), immobilized with a muscle relaxant (gallamine triethiodide), and artificially ventilated. End-tidal CO_2, femoral blood pressure, and rectal temperature were continuously monitored and maintained within physiological limits.

A special technique that confines the electrical stimulus to the tooth pulp was used (8). Test stimuli consisted of single-current pulses comparable to those that give pain perception from TPS in man (7). Conditioning stimuli consisted of single pulses or short trains of pulses applied through bipolar needle electrodes to "widespread cutaneous sources," which included the skin of all four paws, both sides of the face, and the end of the tail, with the understanding that each of these inputs was stimulated separately. After fixing the animal's head in a stereotaxic instrument, we placed recording electrodes in the spinal trigeminal nucleus either by locating stereotaxic coordinates (after drilling holes in the parietal bone) or by using the obex as a landmark (after surgical exposure of the posterior fossa). Three types of recordings were used: gross and single-unit potentials from the rostral part of the spinal trigeminal nucleus in response to TPS, and antidromic compound action potentials from the tooth pulp in response to single-pulse stimulation of primary afferents within the trigeminal nucleus. Stimulation and recording electrode positions were verified histologically.

RESULTS

Systematic tracking with large microelectrodes in the medulla oblongata revealed a negative (N) wave in response to TPS, with 2.5-msec latency and 10-msec duration, which was localized to the rostral part of the spinal trigeminal nucleus. Conditioning stimulation in "widespread cutaneous sources" depressed the test N wave evoked by TPS. This depression was maximal at conditioning-testing (C-T) interval of 55 to 60 msec and lasted approximately 200 msec (Fig. 1).

Reversal of the stimulation and recording positions allowed the measurement of excitability changes in the primary terminals of the tooth pulp afferents using a modification by Davies et al. (2) of Wall's (9) method. Cathodal rectangular pulses were applied to the microelectrode with sufficient intensity to give submaximal response recorded antidromically in the

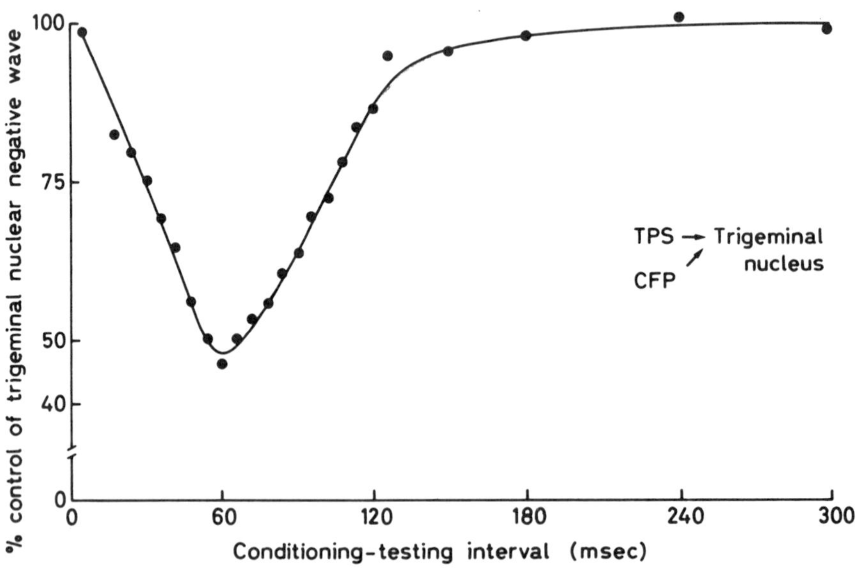

FIG. 1. Time course of the effect of conditioning contralateral forepaw (CFP) stimulation on the negative field potential evoked by test tooth pulp stimulation (TPS). The CFP stimulus consisted of single pulse (0.01 msec and 4 V). The area of the negative deflection measured from the base line was plotted against the conditioning-testing interval.

tooth pulp. Conditioning stimulation in "widespread cutaneous sources" caused an increase (up to 150% of the test response) in the antidromic potentials recorded from tooth electrodes. The increased excitability reached a maximum between 50 and 60 msec and lasted over 200 msec.

Extracellular recordings were made from 56 single units classified as postsynaptic elements, and all were located in the rostral part of the spinal trigeminal nucleus. In agreement with reports of Davies et al. (2) and Greenwood (4), some units were driven by facial stimulation as well, and a few units were evoked by "widespread cutaneous sources." These latter units behaved like reticular neurons. Units driven specifically by TPS had usually short (2.5 to 5 msec) latencies and little spontaneous firing. Conditioning stimulation in "widespread cutaneous sources" inhibited almost all the neurons driven by TPS stimulation. This inhibition took the form of a decrease in the probability of discharge, an increase in the initial spike latency, a decrease in the number of spikes per discharge, or, as often happened, a combination of some or all of these effects (Fig. 2). Although our unit sample was too small to allow any generalization on population behavior, inhibition was evident from "widespread cutaneous sources."

DISCUSSION

Inhibition from "widespread cutaneous sources" persisted in the midcollicular decerebrate preparation. The time course and the excitability

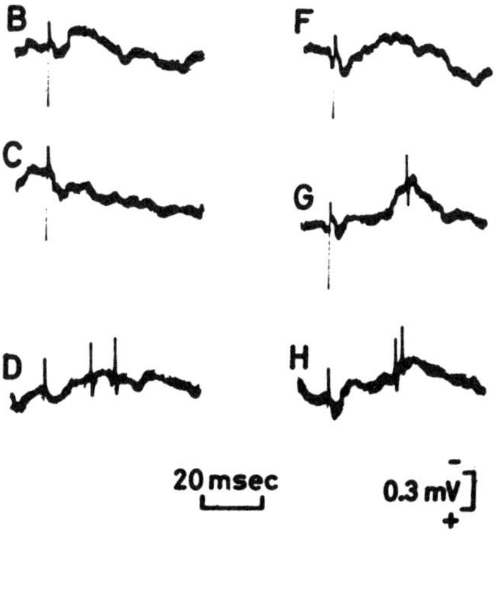

FIG. 2. Inhibition of a spinal trigeminal neuron by "widespread cutaneous sources." Sample records. **A:** Test control response of neuron to tooth pulp stimulation (TPS; single pulse, 0.01 msec, 3 V). **B-H:** TPS response of the same neuron preceded at 55 msec by conditioning cutaneous stimulations (2 shocks at 300 Hz, 0.1 msec, 7 V) at various remote sites: **B,** ipsilateral face; **C,** contralateral face; **D,** tail; **E,** ipsilateral forepaw; **F,** contralateral forepaw; **G,** ipsilateral hind paw; **H,** contralateral hind paw.

changes suggested that the inhibition was, at least in part, presynaptic. Inhibition was most effective from skin of either side of the face and diminished as the cutaneous conditioning stimulus was moved away from the head region. It was possible to demonstrate, however, that the entire cutaneous surface, although not routinely tested, had a similar inhibitory influence. Contrary to what would be expected from acupuncture charts, no localized areas were found which were particularly effective in inhibiting input into the spinal trigeminal nucleus from TPS.

ACKNOWLEDGMENT

This research was supported by a grant from the Lebanese National Council for Scientific Research.

REFERENCES

1. Brookhart, J. M., Livingston, W. K., and Haugen, F. P. (1953): *J. Neurophysiol.*, 16:634–642.
2. Davies, W. I. R., Scott, R., Jr., Vesterstrøm, K., and Vyklický, L. (1971): *J. Physiol. (Lond.)*, 218:515–532.
3. Erickson, R. P., King, R. L., and Pfaffmann, C. (1961): *J. Neurophysiol.*, 24:621–632.
4. Greenwood, F. (1973): *Arch. Oral Biol.*, 18:771–785.
5. Jabbur, S. J., and Banna, N. R. (1970): *J. Neurophysiol.*, 33:616–624.
6. Mahan, P. E., and Anderson, K. V. (1970): *Am. J. Anat.*, 128:235–238.
7. Mumford, J. M. (1968): In: *Pain*, edited by A. Soulairac, J. Cahn, and J. Charpentier. Academic Press, New York.
8. Tamari, J. W., Naccache, A., To'mey, G. F., and Jabbur, S. J. (1974): *Exp. Neurol.*, 45: 663–666.
9. Wall, P. D. (1958): *J. Physiol. (Lond.)*, 142:1–21.
10. Young, R. F., and King, R. B. (1972): *Arch. Oral Biol.*, 17:1649–1657.

Advances in Pain Research and Therapy, Vol. 1,
edited by J. J. Bonica and D. Albe-Fessard.

Effects of Sympathetic Stimulation on the Response of Intradental Nerves to Chemical Stimulation of Dentin

B. Matthews

Department of Physiology (Oral Biology), The Medical School, University Walk, Bristol BS8 1TD, England

In the course of experiments in our laboratory on the origin of impulses recorded from dentin in the cat (11,12), the cervical sympathetic trunk was stimulated on a few occasions to determine if some of the impulses recorded from the teeth might be of sympathetic origin. No impulses were recorded during this procedure, and it was concluded that the recording system was incapable of resolving action potentials in intradental sympathetic fibers. However, an incidental finding in those experiments was that sympathetic stimulation, although it produced no response on its own, sometimes increased the frequency of impulse discharge evoked by simultaneous chemical stimulation of the dentin. The object of the experiments described here was to investigate this effect in greater detail.

Edwall and Scott (9) reported that sympathetic stimulation produced an increase, followed by a decrease, in the frequency of spikes recorded from dentin during the application of isotonic sodium citrate to a cavity in the tooth.

METHODS

The experiments were carried out on 8 adult cats anesthetized with sodium pentobarbital. The general preparation of each animal and the methods used for recording from dentin were essentially the same as those described previously (12). Both common carotid arteries and the cervical sympathetic trunks were exposed and enclosed in a pool of warm liquid paraffin with the animal supine. Recordings were made from upper or lower left canine teeth. The dentin at the tip of the tooth was exposed for recording and was stimulated chemically by the application of 2.5 moles/l NaCl. Unlike previous experiments (12), these experiments did not incorporate simultaneous recordings from dissected nerve filaments because it proved impossible to dissect pulpal afferent fibers from the inferior dental nerve without blocking the effects of sympathetic stimulation. It appeared that the postganglionic sympathetic fibers were present in the same bundles as the afferent fibers.

The effects of stimulating the peripheral cut end of the left cervical sympathetic trunk on the discharge evoked by chemical stimulation of the dentin were determined. The right sympathetic trunk was stimulated as a control. Electrical stimuli were applied at frequencies of 1 to 20 per sec, for 30 sec, with at least 90 sec intervening between periods of stimulation. Individual stimuli were rectangular pulses of 10 V amplitude and 1 msec duration. The impulses recorded from dentin were counted electronically over successive periods of 1 to 4 sec, and an analogue signal representing the count was displayed on a pen recorder.

Control data on the adequacy of sympathetic stimulation were obtained by recording the flow of saliva from the left submandibular salivary gland and the contractions of the left nictitating membrane. A nylon cannula was inserted into the submandibular duct. Salivary flow rate was recorded using a modification of the technique described by Burgen (5). The resistance to air flow was a 1.25-in, 23-gauge needle through which a flow of 0.6 ml/min required a pressure difference of 1 mm H_2O. Contractions of the nictitating membrane were recorded with an isometric transducer connected to the membrane with a fine suture passed through its cartilaginous border. The resting tension was 1 to 5 g. The eyelids were held away from the nictitating membrane with sutures, and the eye was covered with liquid paraffin to prevent drying. Arterial blood pressure was recorded from either the left lingual artery or the femoral artery. All the records from the animal were displayed simultaneously on a four-channel pen recorder (Devices, Welwyn Garden City; type M 4).

In addition to determining the effects of sympathetic stimulation, I determined the effects of clamping both common carotids for 30 sec and of close-arterial injections of up to 5 μg/kg of epinephrine or norepinephrine. These drugs were given in volumes not exceeding 0.2 ml by retrograde injection into the left lingual artery. The effects of sympathetic blocking agents given intravenously were also determined. The alpha blocking agents phentolamine and phenoxybenzamine were given in doses up to 5 mg/kg, and the beta blocking agent propranolol in doses up to 1 mg/kg.

RESULTS

The characteristics of the responses recorded from dentin during stimulation with 2.5 M NaCl alone were similar to those obtained previously (12). With periods of chemical stimulation of up to 4 min, responses were obtained when the solution was applied to the inner but not to the outer dentin. As the thickness of the dentin was reduced, the latency of the response decreased, the mean frequency of the evoked discharge increased, and the period for which the discharge continued after the NaCl solution was washed away became shorter. Most of the observations in the present experiments were made when the amount of dentin removed from the tip of the canine was such that a continuous application of 2.5 M NaCl evoked a maintained, low-frequency discharge of 5 to 30 impulses per second, with impulses appearing with a latency of 2 to 3 min. In other experiments it has been found that about 0.5 mm of dentin remains over the pulp cornu when this response pattern is obtained. The sympathetic trunk was cut at different stages during the removal of dentin in different experiments, and at none of these stages was there any significant difference between the responses evoked by 2.5 M NaCl before or after section of the sympathetic trunk.

With stimulation of dentin at levels at which 2.5 M NaCl alone evoked no response, the addition of ipsilateral sympathetic stimulation for 30 sec had no effect. At deeper levels, in 6 of the 8 animals sympathetic stimulation caused a marked increase of up to 30-fold in the discharge evoked by 2.5 M NaCl (Fig. 1). In the other 2 animals there was no effect on the response, and in 1 of these the pulp was exposed. In those in which there was an effect, the frequency of stimulation affected the latency more than the magnitude of the increase in firing rate (Fig. 2). The response continued beyond the period of stimulation by up to 30 sec, and the peak firing rate sometimes occurred after stimulation ceased. As far as could be determined from examination of the wave forms, the increase in firing rate appeared to be caused by an increase in the discharge frequency of units already active before sympathetic stimulation, rather than by recruitment of units previously silent. None of the evoked potentials were synchronized to the electrical stimuli, and there was no other evidence that the recorded action potentials were from sympathetic fibers. With stimulation frequencies of up to 10/sec, the increase in firing rate could be maintained for 3 min—the longest stimulation period tested. With stimulation at 20/sec, the elevated

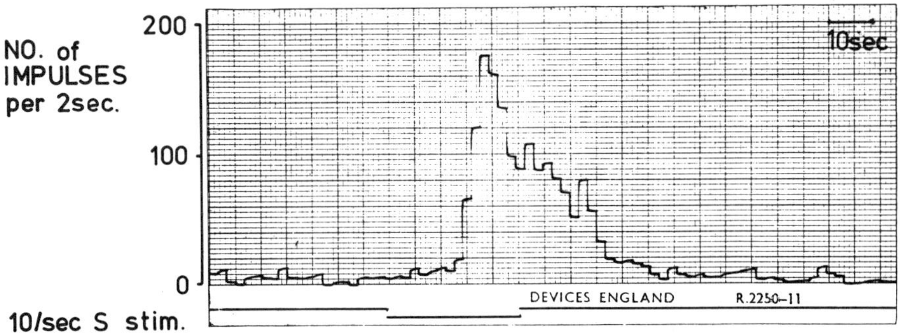

FIG. 1. Numbers of impulses recorded from dentin in successive 2-sec periods. Dentin was stimulated with 2.5 M NaCl throughout. During the period indicated by lower trace, ipsilateral cervical sympathetic trunk was stimulated at 10/sec. Records shown in Figs. 2 through 4 were obtained from the same preparation as this.

firing rate began to decrease after 1 min of stimulation. Contralateral sympathetic stimulation did not affect the discharge.

The effect of sympathetic stimulation appeared to be optimal with dentin removed to the level at which 2.5 M NaCl evoked a maintained discharge of 5 to 30 impulses per second. The effect was less marked with stimulation of more superficial and deeper levels in the dentin when the ongoing discharge rate was lower or higher than the optimal rate.

Sympathetic stimulation also produced the expected contraction of the nictitating membrane and secretion from the submandibular salivary gland in all the animals, and the magnitude and time course of these responses varied according to the frequency of stimulation (Fig. 2). The salivary response consisted of two components: an initial rapid flow not evident with stimulation below 10/sec, and a more delayed component that was maximal with stimulation between 10 and 20/sec.

A close arterial injection of epinephrine (2 to 5 μg/kg) or norepinephrine (2 to 5 μg/kg) during stimulation of the dentin with 2.5 M NaCl caused a transient increase in discharge rate of intradental nerves as well as con-

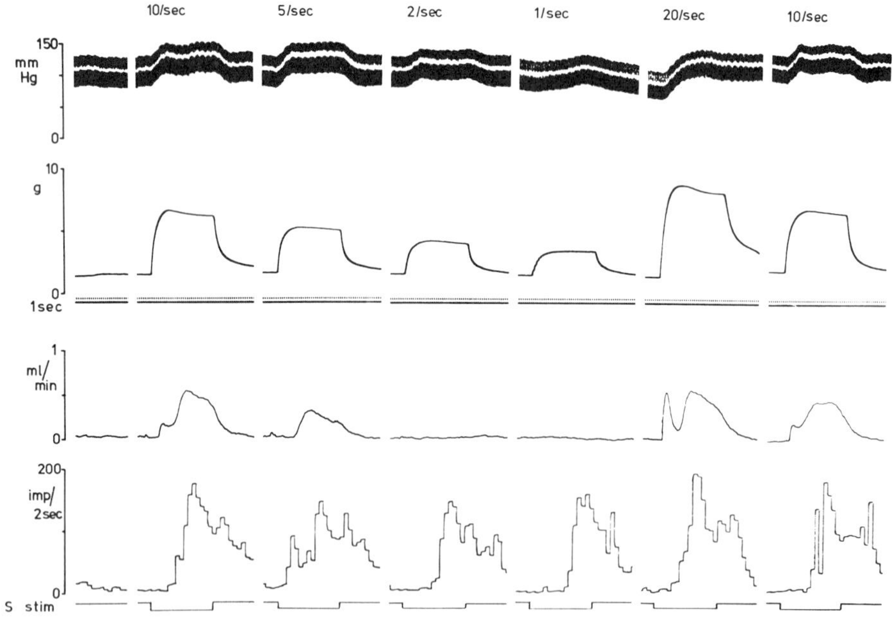

FIG. 2. Records (*top to bottom*) of femoral arterial blood pressure, isometric tension of left nictitating membrane, 1/sec time marker, flow rate of saliva from left submandibular salivary gland, and numbers of impulses recorded from lower left canine in successive 2-sec periods. Bottom trace is an event marker showing the 30-sec periods during which the left cervical sympathetic trunk was stimulated. Frequency of stimulation is shown over each group of records. The first group are control records. Stimuli were applied in the order shown and at 2-min intervals.

traction of the nictitating membrane and secretion of saliva. With norepinephrine the discharge rate was subsequently depressed during the large rise in arterial blood pressure.

Clamping the ipsilateral common carotid artery for 30 sec produced no significant change in the discharge rate of intradental nerves, but clamping both carotids produced an increase in impulse frequency (Fig. 3A). There was no response in the nictitating membrane or the salivary gland. The mean pressure in the left lingual artery fell by only 10 to 20 mm Hg when only the ipsilateral common carotid was clamped, whereas bilateral clamping caused an initial drop to near atmospheric pressure, which slowly increased over 15 sec to approximately 30 mm Hg.

The adrenergic blocking agent phentolamine, administered intravenously in a dose of 1 mg/kg, caused a transient increase in the ongoing activity of the intradental nerves in approximately 2 min, which corresponded with the period of hypotension. Phentolamine reduced by approximately 50% the

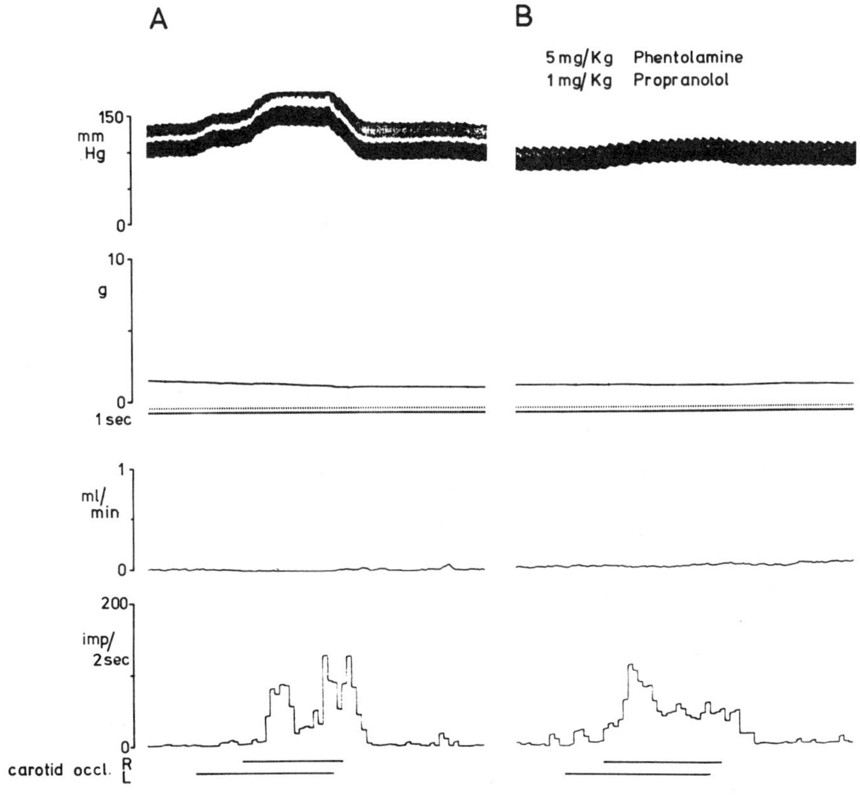

FIG. 3. Traces correspond with those in Fig. 2. **A:** Effects of bilateral occlusion of the common carotid arteries. **B:** Effects of carotid occlusion 24 min after i.v. administration of phentolamine and 12 min after that of propranolol.

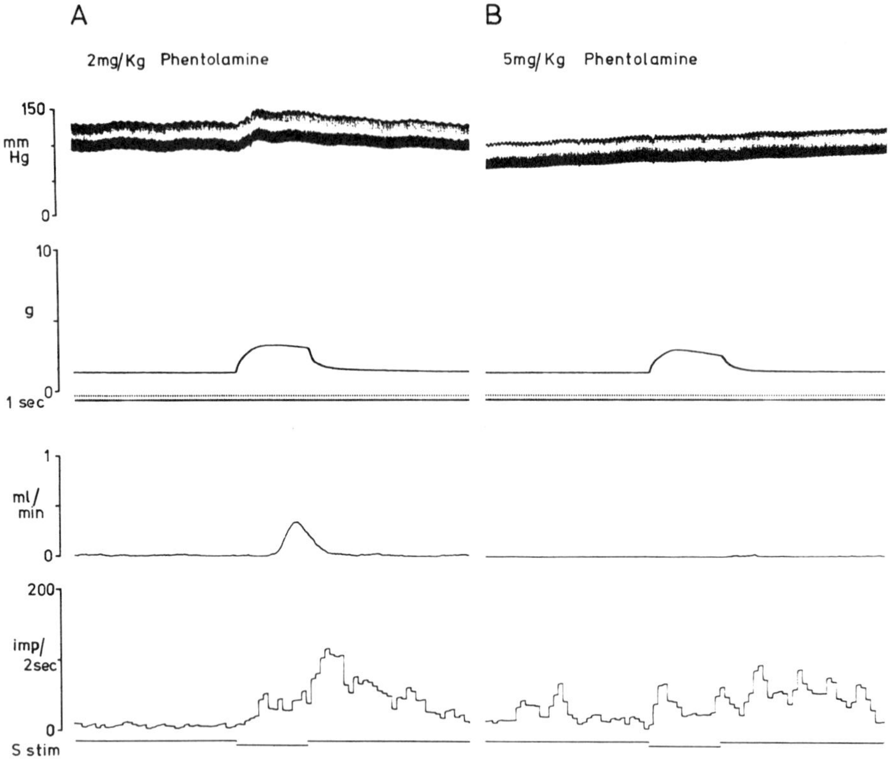

FIG. 4. Traces correspond with those in Fig. 2. Both show responses to sympathetic stimulation at 10/sec. **A:** Effects 5 min after i.v. phentolamine administration. **B:** Effects 10 min later and 5 min after the dose of phentolamine was increased.

increase in firing rate produced by sympathetic stimulation, the salivary response, and the tension developed by the nictitating membrane (Fig. 4A). Increasing the dose of phentolamine to 5 mg/kg caused a further increase in the ongoing discharge of the pulpal nerves and blocked completely the increase in firing rate previously produced by sympathetic stimulation (Fig. 4B). Thirty minutes after administration of the drug, the response of the nictitating membrane was reduced to only between 20% and 30% of control values. Phenoxybenzamine produced similar effects but over a longer time course. Phentolamine also blocked the effects of intra-arterial epinephrine and norepinephrine but did not block the increase in firing rate of intradental nerves which followed occlusion of both common carotid arteries (Fig. 3B).

The increased firing rate produced by sympathetic stimulation, the increased firing rate produced by carotid occlusion, and the increased ongoing activity that followed administration of an alpha blocking agent were not affected by the beta blocking agent propranolol (1 mg/kg).

DISCUSSION

Identity of Impulses Recorded from Dentin

Many, and possibly all, of the impulses recorded from dentin with the technique employed in the present experiments are associated with propagated action potentials in pulpal nerves (12). The method is capable of recording impulses from some of the larger diameter pulpal fibers with conduction velocities between 35 and 12 ms^{-1} and only rarely does it record those from smaller myelinated fibers. There is no evidence that action potentials can be recorded from single nonmyelinated fibers in the tooth. No response is recorded from dentin during sympathetic nerve stimulation in the absence of a chemical stimulus; and when sympathetic fibers are stimulated during a discharge produced by chemical stimulation, there is no detectable synchronization of the evoked response to the electrical stimuli. Also, the discharge recorded during chemical stimulation of a lower tooth is not affected by section of the inferior dental nerve (12). There is therefore no evidence that any of the impulses are efferent in origin.

Effects of Sympathetic Stimulation on the Discharge of Intradental Nerves

The results of the present experiments show that the discharge of sympathetic nerves, at frequencies within the range that is likely to occur physiologically, can increase markedly the response of intradental nerves to chemical stimulation of dentin. The test stimulus, 2.5 M NaCl, has been shown previously to evoke a discharge from intradental nerves (12) and would be expected to cause pain when applied to human dentin (2). Therefore, the sympathetic system could exert a similar modulating effect on the sensitivity of nerve endings involved in pain sensation in human teeth. In the pentobarbital-anesthetized cats, it appears that the sympathetic fibers responsible for the modulating effect were silent since cutting the cervical sympathetic trunk produced no effect on the discharge from the tooth.

Some of the results correspond with some of those obtained by Edwall and Scott (9) using isotonic sodium citrate as a dentin stimulus, although there was little evidence of the marked depression in impulse discharge which they observed with stimulation at 3 and 6 per second after 1 or 2 min.

The mechanism responsible for the increase in impulse discharge produced by sympathetic stimulation has not been established. Little is known of the identity and location of the receptors in teeth (1,16), and it is not known how chemical stimuli excite intradental nerves. Five possible mechanisms for the sympathetic effect have been considered:

1. An increase in receptor excitability occurs secondary to vasoconstriction and ischemia. There is evidence for sympathetic vasoconstrictor innervation of dental pulp (8,19,22) which is alpha mediated (7) and not tonically active in anesthetized cats (7).

2. Changes in pulpal tissue fluid pressure cause a change in the response of mechanosensitive endings (4,9), which respond to osmotic effects through dentin. Sympathetic stimulation causes an alpha-mediated fall in intrapulpal pressure in the dog (14).
3. A reduction in pulpal tissue fluid pressure results in a decrease in the rate of outward flow of fluid through dentinal tubules and hence a more rapid diffusion of ions from the exposed dentin surface.
4. A reduction in pulpal blood flow allows the chemical stimulus to produce a greater change in the composition of the extracellular fluid around the nerve endings.
5. A more specific mechanism exists whereby sympathetic fibers regulate receptor excitability. There is some evidence that the ondontoblast may function as a receptor (1,16,17) and adrenergic terminals have been identified histologically associated with ondontoblasts (6).

Sympathetic stimulation and injected epinephrine have been shown to modulate the excitability of various types of mechanoreceptors in different ways (3,10,13,15,18,20,21), and both direct and indirect mechanisms have been proposed to account for the effects. Whatever the mechanism in teeth, it appears to be alpha mediated. The effects of carotid occlusion favor a nonspecific mechanism. The increase in ongoing activity after administration of alpha blocking agents could have been secondary to the fall in arterial blood pressure and a consequent fall in pulpal tissue fluid pressure, although no data are available on the changes in pulpal tissue fluid pressure under these conditions.

The lack of response in 2 animals may have been because of variations in sympathetic innervation of the pulp between animals, although those to the submandibular salivary gland and nictitating membrane were unaffected. Edwall (7) found that evidence of sympathetically mediated pulpal vasoconstriction was sometimes absent when deep cavities were cut into dentin in cat's canines.

ACKNOWLEDGMENT

This work was supported by a grant from the Medical Research Council.

REFERENCES

1. Anderson, D. J., Hannam, A. G., and Matthews, B. (1970): *Physiol. Rev.,* 50:171–195.
2. Anderson, D. J., and Matthews, B. (1967): *Arch. Oral Biol.,* 12:417–426.
3. Bhoola, K. D., Diete-Spiff, K., and Webster, R. A. (1962): *J. Physiol. (Lond.),* 164:16–17P.
4. Brännström, M., and Åström, A. (1964): *J. Dent. Res.,* 43:619–625.
5. Burgen, A. S. V. (1964): In: *Salivary Glands and Their Secretions,* edited by L. M. Sreebny and J. Meyer, pp. 303–307. Pergamon Press, Oxford.
6. Cox, C. F., and Avery, J. K. (1975): *J. Dent. Res.,* 54 [Suppl. A]: L59 (Abs.).

7. Edwall, L. (1971): *Some Effects of Sympathetic Nerve Activation in Oral Tissues as Studied by Tracer Disappearance.* Kihlstrom & Soner Boktryckeri AB, Stockholm.
8. Edwall, L., and Kindlova, M. (1971): *Acta Odontol. Scand.,* 29:387–400.
9. Edwall, L., and Scott, D., Jr. (1971): *Acta Physiol. Scand.,* 82:555–566.
10. Eldred, E., Schnitzlein, H. N., and Buchwald, J. (1960): *Exp. Neurol.,* 2:13–25.
11. Horiuchi, H., and Matthews, B. (1972): In: *Oral Physiology,* edited by N. Emmelin and Y. Zotterman, pp. 297–302. Pergamon Press, Oxford.
12. Horiuchi, H., and Matthews, B. (1974): *J. Physiol. (Lond.),* 243:797–829.
13. Hunt, C. C. (1960): *J. Physiol. (Lond.),* 151:332–341.
14. Kroeger, D. C. (1968): In: *Biology of the Dental Pulp Organ,* edited by S. B. Finn, pp. 333–346. University of Alabama Press.
15. Loewenstein, W. R. (1956): *J. Physiol. (Lond.),* 132:40–60.
16. Matthews, B. (1972): *Proc. R. Soc. Med.,* 65:493–495.
17. Matthews, B., and Holland, G. R. (1976): *Brain Res. (in press).*
18. Nilsson, B. Y. (1972): *Acta Physiol. Scand.,* 85:390–397.
19. Ogilvie, R. W. (1967): *Anat. Rec.,* 157:379 (Abs.).
20. Paintal, A. (1959): *J. Physiol. (Lond.),* 148:252–266.
21. Schiff, J. D. (1974): *J. Gen. Physiol.,* 63:601–608.
22. Taylor, A. C. (1950): *Science,* 111:40.

Advances in Pain Research and Therapy, Vol. 1,
edited by J. J. Bonica and D. Albe-Fessard.
Raven Press, New York © 1976.

What Is the Most Unique Form of Stimulus to Evoke Dental Pain?

Donald Scott, Jr., and Richard Maziarz

Department of Physiology, University of Pennsylvania, Philadelphia, Pennsylvania 19174

For approximately 10 years we have investigated various factors that evoke tooth pain. Looking back on the results from our laboratory and others, we have been curious whether we could find any common characteristic among the several forms of noxious stimulation which might throw some light on a possible transducer mechanism. From this work certain common factors have become increasingly clear, and we will discuss these briefly.

Most authorities believe that only the sensation of pain is felt when any form of stimulation is applied to a human tooth, although some workers have also described a poorly defined form of "pre-pain." For the purposes of this chapter, we refer to two classes of factors that either increase or decrease pain in the tooth: factors that constitute a noxious insult and those that influence membrane excitability but may not be involved in the more common causes of pain. Only the factors in the first category are discussed here for reasons that will soon become apparent. Because each of these factors can interact with others, in experimental analysis all but one factor must be kept constant.

METHODS

The sensation of pain in the tooth is mediated in the tooth pulp via afferent axons, many of which have been shown to be directly related to sensory units in dentin. We have recorded afferent nerve impulses from human teeth and have shown an increase in frequency during brief periods of noxious stimulation when the subject reported a sensation of pain. However, it has proven much more convenient to record from the dentin of cat canine teeth during general anesthesia because of the higher impedance of the cat pulp. A schematic description of our preparation and the methods used in our procedures is shown in Fig. 1. Figure 2 contains a record from an oscilloscope during heat stimulus application.

Although we have studied the effects of 15 forms of increasing or decreasing the excitability of the receptors in dentin (10), we will discuss here

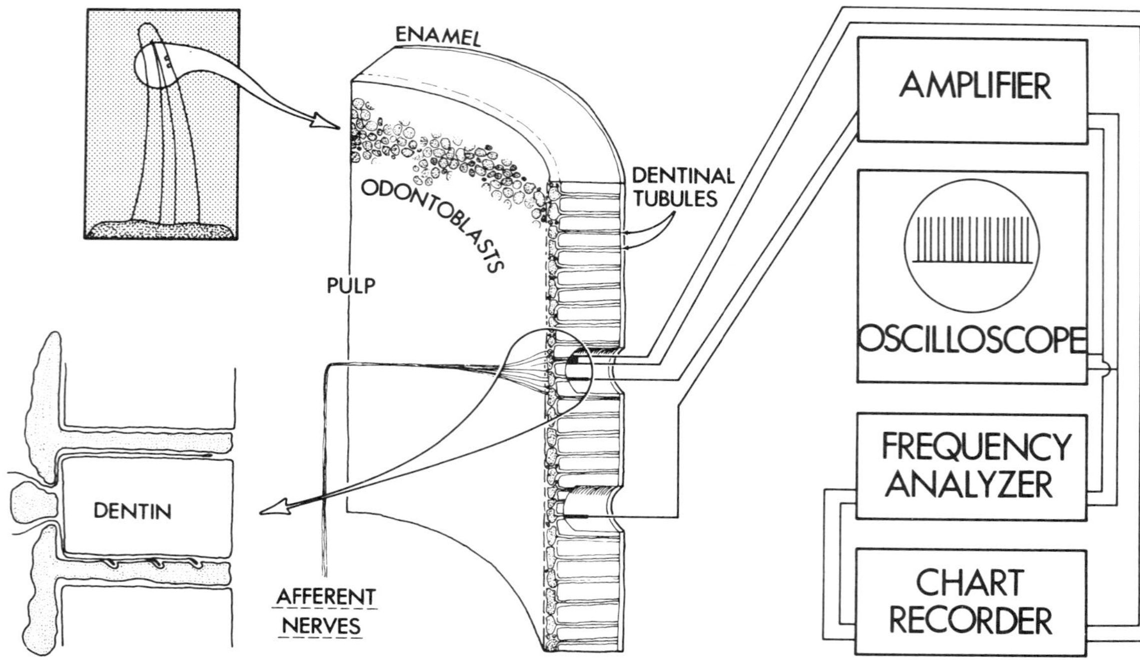

FIG. 1. Schematic diagram of pulp, dentin, and enamel of cat canine tooth. Sensory terminals shown in dentin as described by Arwill (1) and Frank (6). Recording electrodes placed in cavities in dentin and thermocouple also placed in one cavity. Records obtained from oscilloscope and frequency analyzer.

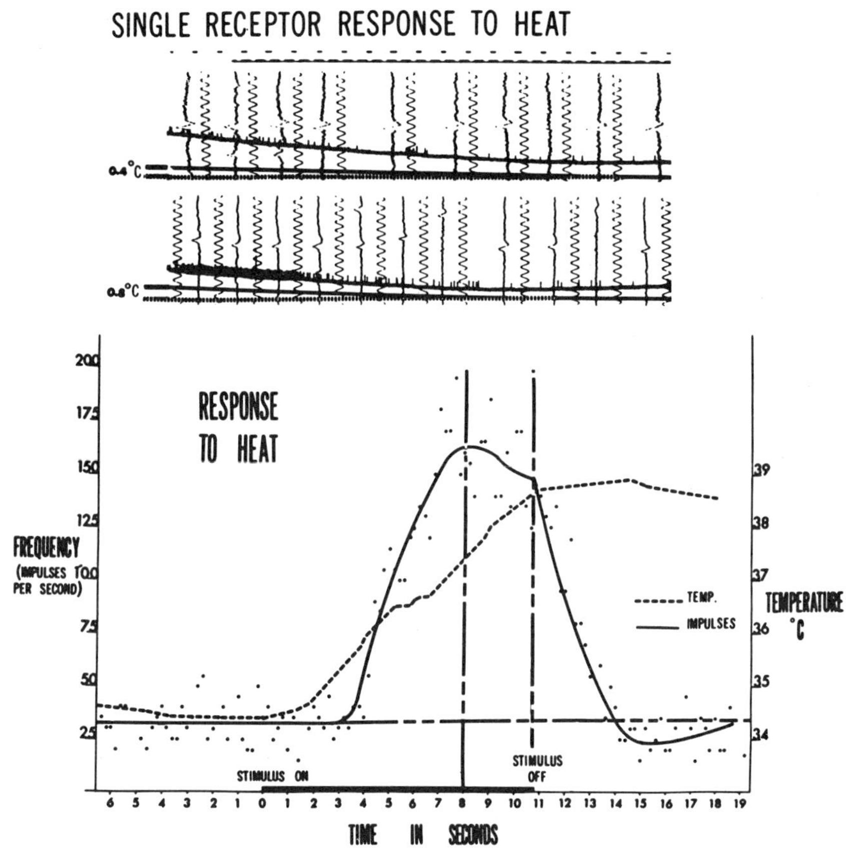

FIG. 2. Record from oscilloscope during heat stimulus. Top: photographic record of impulses from oscilloscope (*horizontal record*) and expanded trace of individual impulses (*vertical trace*) to show wave form. Bottom: frequency plot of recorded impulses during heat stimulation compared to temperature of dentin.

the seven forms of painful stimulation that are a common clinical experience. Most of these seven forms, listed in Table 1, have been reported by human subjects and have evoked afferent neural discharges in animal experiments. Since it has been possible to design more fully controlled experiments with animals, we will discuss these results from each form of stimulation briefly and then, in conclusion, compare the summary of each form of excitation.

RESULTS

Mechanical Stimulation

Simple mechanical stimulation was administered with a dental bur or a glass probe (11) (Fig. 3). Each touch of the instrument on the dentin evokes

TABLE 1. *Excitability modification of the sensory unit in dentin*

Type of modification	Response elicited: Experimental (cat)	Response elicited: Clinical (human)
Noxious insults		
Mechanical (dental bur or probe)	+	+
Heating (short duration; bur or hot application)	+	+
Hydraulic (applied to dentin)		
1. Internal pulp or systolic pulse pressure	+	+
2. Direct suction	+	
3. Osmotic solutions		+
4. Evaporative dehydration	+	+
5. Filter paper or air blast dehydration	+	+
Factors influencing membrane excitability		
Ions (potassium, sodium, etc.)	+	
Drugs (wide variety of effects on neural mechanisms, mitochondria, microcirculation, etc.)	+	
Metabolic factors		
1. Cold (axon membrane depolarizer; decreases circulation [effect blocked by TTX])	+	+
2. Microcirculatory decrease (depresses metabolism)	+	
3. Slow linear heating (probable mitochondrial activation)	+	

a short burst of potentials. Such stimulation distorts the microstructure of the tubular matrix in dentin. These potentials are not streaming potentials as defined by the Helmholtz-Smaluchowski equation [quoted by Mumford and Newton (8)]. Nor are they caused by the piezoelectric effect of hard tissue as shown by Liboff and Shamos (7) since in both cases the potentials that would be expected from the force we have found adequate to excite

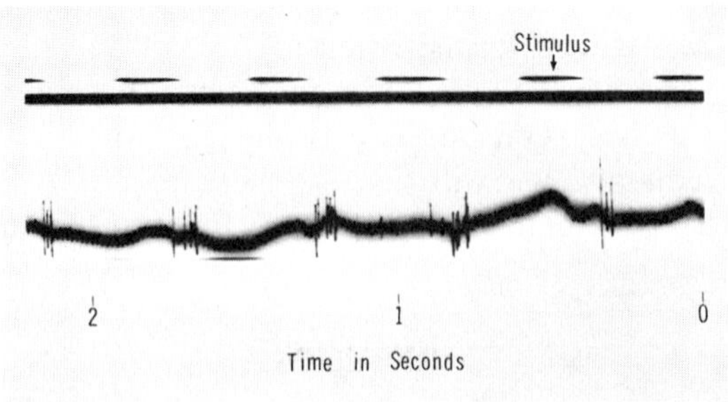

FIG. 3. Response of sensory unit in dentin to touch with fine glass probe. Touch applied at signals indicated on top line. Corresponding bursts of potentials shown on bottom line.

are orders of magnitude smaller than that necessary for excitation. Furthermore, the normal sensitivity of dentin to touch depends on a living subject with normal circulation having a normal ionic environment and normal tooth temperature. From these considerations it seems most likely that pain from mechanical stimulation of dentin is mediated through distortion of the matrix of dentinal tubules and the consequent changes in fluid flow within them.

Stimulation by Heat

Heating the tooth by friction of a dental bur or by a hot application (Fig. 4) refers to short periods of heating from 3 to 10 sec and increases of tooth temperature from 3° to 12°C. The latency of this effect was about 3 sec. The peak frequency response of the evoked potentials occurred before the maximum temperature was reached. Almost immediately after the end of heating, the frequency declined rapidly even though the tooth temperature might remain elevated for many times the stimulus duration. A period of postexcitation depression usually followed the end of heating.

The frequency increase resulting from a thermal pulse may be due to (a) a direct thermal effect on tissue, but this is not likely because slow heating produces an exact linear increase in frequency with temperature ($\Delta F \equiv \Delta T$); (b) the effect of increased microvascular flow, but Edwall and Scott (5) showed that 10°C heating produced a 15% microvascular increase but a 200% increase in impulse frequency; or (c) the effect of expansion of pulp fluids. The pulp volume of the cat canine is 20 mm^3, and a 15°C increase in temperature would cause an increase of 0.1% (assuming that the pulp is filled with water). From this the estimated movement of fluid in the dentinal tubules would be approximately 60 μm. All three of these factors must be taken into consideration, but the last appears to be the most probable major effect.

Hydraulic Stimulation

Circulatory Pulse Wave

One form of hydraulic stimulation results from increases in internal pulp pressure or the systolic pressure of the circulation. Although pain from various forms of pulp inflammation may involve the release of chemical irritants as well as increased intrapulpal pressure, the pulp pressure changes caused by systolic pulse changes are mirrored by the pressure changes of the dentinal fluid, which Beveridge and Brown (2) found to be 5 mm Hg (Fig. 5). On this record the systolic pulse was observed by impedance plethysmography, and synchronous with each systole a burst of 1 to 4

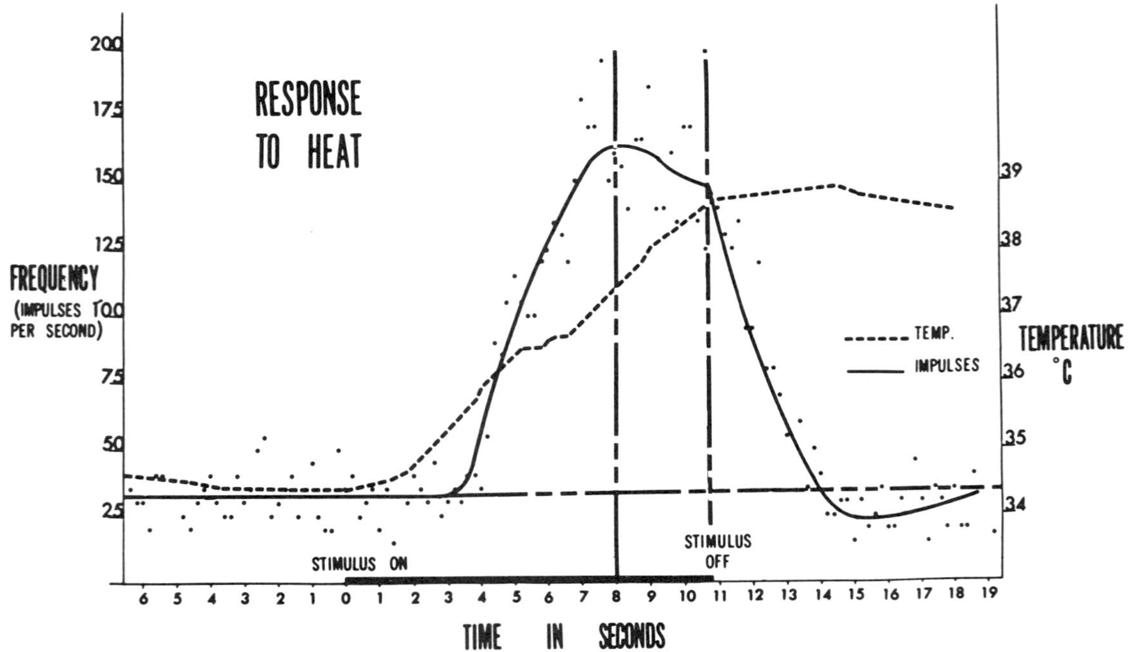

Fig. 4. Frequency plot of potentials evoked during 11-sec heating of tooth (as in Fig. 2, *bottom*). Note latency of response after start of heating. Maximum frequency recorded at maximum rate of temperature change. Frequency decreases abruptly when heat is terminated, although tooth temperature remains elevated.

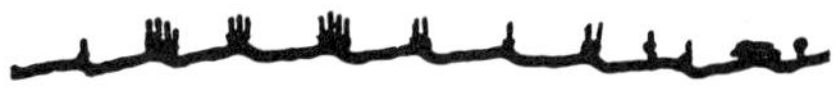

FIG. 5. Bursts of potentials from dentin correlated with systolic pulse. Base-line oscillations indicate pulse wave obtained by impedance plethysmography. Potentials from dentin superimposed by direct recording. (Individual spikes enlarged and retouched to show number in each burst.)

potentials can be seen (11) (potentials have been retouched slightly for better visibility).

From these records it is apparent that the receptor in dentin responds to pressure changes of 5 mm Hg and probably less. Because of the structure of dentin with 30,000 parallel tubules per square millimeter, it seems clear that the pressure measured by Beveridge and Brown would result in fluid movement in the dentinal tubules. Such periodic bursts of potentials would correspond to the throbbing pain often reported by patients.

Air Blast in Dental Cavity

Another example of hydraulic stimulation is the pain evoked when an air blast is applied to a dental cavity. Although this procedure is clinically useful to prepare for restorative treatment, the resulting dehydration inevitably causes the outward movement of fluid in the dentinal tubules as

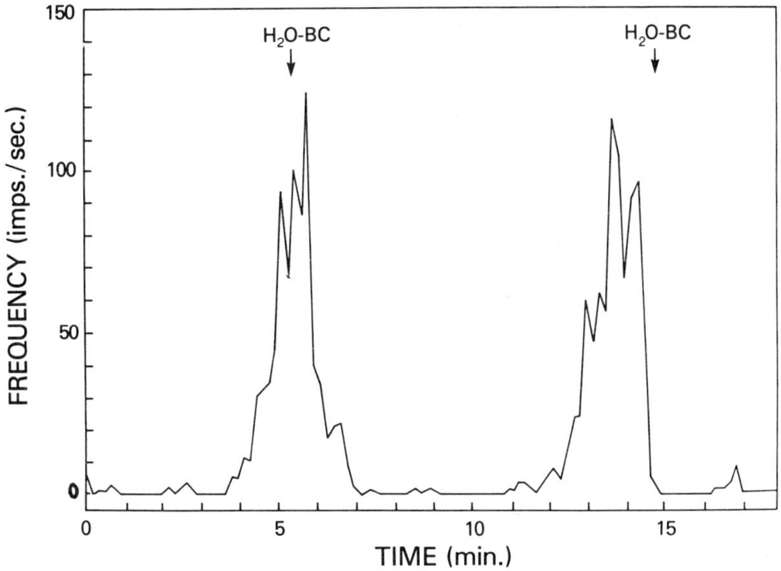

FIG. 6. Effect of dentinal dehydration on sensory excitation. One μl distilled water placed in each cavity of dentin as indicated by arrows above figure. Periods of enhanced excitability are caused by dehydration of dentin. BC, both cavities.

shown by Brännström (3) from histologic studies of dentin in teeth that had been treated with air blast and subsequently extracted. Thus the application of air blast to a dentinal cavity is known to cause pain, to evoke an active discharge of the sensory receptor, and to result in demonstrable outward flow of dentinal fluid in the tubules. We used this procedure when recording impulse frequency from human subjects during their report of pain sensation.

Other Forms

Other painful procedures that induce hydraulic stimulation include the application of hypertonic solutions (such as sucrose), the osmotic effect of which is well known to cause pain. Likewise, Brännström as well as our own group have shown that even simple evaporative dehydration or the application of filter paper to a cavity base produces both pain and a discharge of sensory impulses (Fig. 6). Finally, Edwall and I (4,9) have found that the direct application of hydraulic suction to a cavity is a potent stimulus for high-frequency impulse discharge.

DISCUSSION

What suggestions can be found in these observations from mechanical, thermal, and hydraulic forms of excitation? The examples chosen correspond to many forms of pain sensation in human teeth (Table 2). In each case we found that the noxious stimulation resulted in some distortion of the normal balance of physical forces in dentin, which are summarized in Table 2.

TABLE 2. *Primary and secondary effects of noxious stimulation of dentin*

Type of stimulus	Primary effect	Secondary effect
Mechanical (by bur or probe)	Deformation of dentinal matrix	Displacement of dentinal fluid in tubules
Heat Pulse (brief heating)	Expansion of fluids in pulp	Outward movement of fluid in dentinal tubules
Hydraulic		
1. Circulatory pulse wave	Corresponding pulse wave in dentinal fluid	Pulse pressure causes flow in tubules
2. Air blast in dental cavity	Rapid evaporation of fluids from dentin surface	Compensatory movement of fluids in dentinal tubules
3. Osmotic stim., evaporative dehydration, hydraulic suction	Excite sensory mechanisms in dentin	Outward flow of fluids in dentinal tubules

Finally, is it reasonable to suggest that fluid movement in the dentinal tubules could be the first step in the sensory mechanism? We do not yet have all the evidence to prove this, but it is very suggestive that terminals of the sensory axons are frequently elaborated in the tubules and that they are morphologically coupled with specialized areas of the odontoblast process in a manner that could be attributable to neither artifact nor chance. There is evidence pointing toward this two-cell interrelation as the heart of the sensory transducer, but that must wait for another presentation. For the moment we look toward the hydraulic distortion of the intimate relation of these specialized structures as the key to understanding the arousal of pain in the tooth.

REFERENCES

1. Arwill, T. (1967): *Odontol. Rev.,* 18:191–208.
2. Beveridge, E. E., and Brown, A. (1965): *Oral Surg.,* 19:655.
3. Brännström, M. (1961): *J. Dent. Res.,* 40:960–970.
4. Edwall, L.: *Personal communication.*
5. Edwall, L., and Scott, D., Jr. (1971): *Acta Physiol. Scand.,* 82:555–566.
6. Frank, R. M. (1966): *Arch. Oral Biol.,* 11:179–199.
7. Liboff, A. R., and Shamos, M. H. (1971): *J. Dent. Res.,* 50:516.
8. Mumford, J. M., and Newton, A. V. (1969): *J. Dent. Res.,* 48:226–229.
9. Scott, D., Jr.: *Unpublished results.*
10. Scott, D., Jr.: (1972): In: *Oral Physiology,* edited by N. Emmelin and Y. Zotterman. Pergamon Press, Oxford.
11. Scott, D., Jr., and Tempel, T. (1963): In: *Sensory Mechanisms in Dentin,* edited by D. Anderson. Pergamon Press, Oxford.

Advances in Pain Research and Therapy, Vol. 1,
edited by J. J. Bonica and D. Albe-Fessard.
Raven Press, New York © 1976.

Spinothalamic System: Physiological Aspects

W. D. Willis

Marine Biomedical Institute and Departments of Anatomy and Physiology and Biophysics, University of Texas Medical Branch, Galveston, Texas 77550

The spinothalamic tract is believed to be the principal pathway for nociception in man and in primates (7,13,15,16,22). Other ascending tracts such as the spinoreticular and spinotectal tracts may also play some role, and the spinocervical tract is likely to be especially important in some mammals such as the cat (4,5). It is now feasible to study the activity of single neurons of the primate spinothalamic tract through the use of antidromic activation of these cells by stimulation within the thalamus (1,20). This permits their identification so that the responses of spinothalamic tract cells can be studied separately from those of other spinal cord neurons. A sample of nearly 500 such cells has been investigated in our work, and the responses of many other cells belonging to or probably belonging to the spinothalamic tract have been reported by the laboratories of Albe-Fessard (1), Price (17,18), and Perl (12).

In general, it can be said that the responses of spinothalamic tract cells allow them to be classified in several groups (24). Many neurons respond to tactile stimulation. However, of these, most also respond to more intense mechanical stimulation, including intense pressure, pinch, and pinprick. Another category of spinothalamic tract cell requires intense stimulation for activation. Some of these cells are in lamina I, although others are in deeper layers of the dorsal horn, including lamina V in monkey and VII in cat. An additional class of spinothalamic tract cells is activated by proprioceptive stimuli. The peripheral fibers which activate spinothalamic tract neurons include Aβ, Aδ, and C fibers, but the tactile cells are more affected by large fibers than are the high-threshold cells (8).

This chapter is concerned with a review of some of our findings which are pertinent to an understanding of the role of spinothalamic tract neurons in nociception. The organization of the axons of the tract is described, and then the responses of the high-threshold class of spinothalamic tract neurons to noxious mechanical and thermal stimulation are considered. Some of the information has been published elsewhere (2,23).

METHODS

The experiments were done on young adult rhesus monkeys (*Macaca mulatta*) anesthetized with α-chloralose and maintained with small supplemental doses of sodium pentobarbital. A laminectomy exposed the lumbar spinal cord, and a craniotomy allowed the introduction of a concentric bipolar stimulating electrode into the thalamus. For cell recording stimulation was contralateral to the recording point in the spinal cord, whereas for axonal recording an ipsilateral stimulus was used. Stimuli were applied in the posterior region of the thalamus (ventral posterior nucleus or posterior nuclear zone) to activate spinothalamic tract neurons antidromically. The recognition of antidromic activation depended on a constant latency spike, high-frequency following (333 Hz), and collision with orthodromic activity. In many instances the critical collision interval was determined and found to equal twice the conduction time plus a refractory period.

Spinothalamic axons were recognized as belonging to an ascending rather than a descending tract on the basis of their response latencies to orthodromic activation. Recordings were made extracellularly from spinothalamic tract neurons or intracellularly from spinothalamic axons using glass microelectrodes filled with 4 M NaCl or with 3 M KCl. The spikes from gray matter had a prominent negative phase and could be recorded over distances of several hundred microns; therefore, they were judged to be from somatodendritic regions. The axonal spikes were positive and were recorded within the white matter.

Afferents in the hindlimb were stimulated in any of several ways. Natural mechanical stimulation included hair movement, gentle mechanical stimulation of the skin, pressure applied to folds of skin by fingers or by forceps, pinch using an arterial clip, insertion of a sharpened point into the skin, and application of a graded series of von Frey filaments to determine thresholds to mechanical stimuli. Controlled step or ramp identations of the skin were applied using a servo-controlled mechanical stimulator, which allowed monitoring of both the position of the probe and the force generated. Thermal stimulation has recently involved the use of a peltier device to apply servo-controlled changes in either the heating or the cooling direction and extending well into the noxious range. Electrical stimulation has also been used for particular experiments; such stimuli were applied either within the receptive field on the skin or to dissected peripheral nerves.

RESULTS

Organization of the Spinothalamic Tract

The locations of 83 spinothalamic tract axons in the ventrolateral white matter are shown in Fig. 1. The units are classified according to the weakest form of mechanical stimulation that activated them. Two tactile classes were hair activated and low threshold. Again, most of these units could also be discharged by intense stimuli. The high-threshold cells required pressure and noxious intensities of mechanical stimulation for their activation. The

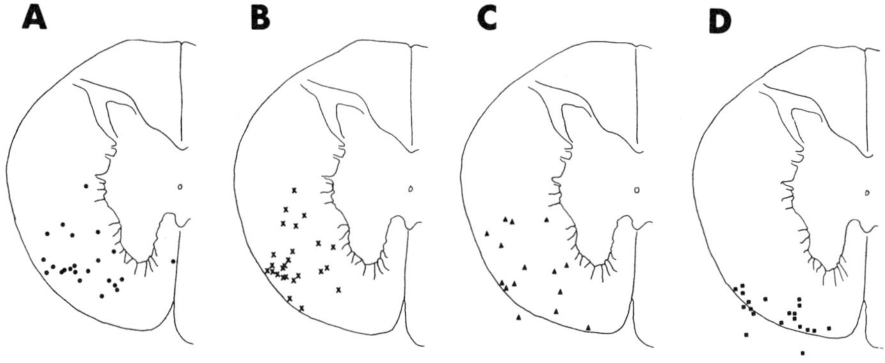

FIG. 1. Locations of 83 spinothalamic tract axons shown on representative drawing of the upper lumbar spinal cord. The 4 classes of cells are **(A),** hair activated; **(B),** low threshold; **(C),** high threshold; and **(D),** deep.

units labeled deep were excited by proprioceptive stimuli such as joint bending or manipulation of muscle. Some of these cells also had cutaneous receptive fields, although many did not. As Fig. 1 indicates, there was essentially a complete overlap in the distribution of axons belonging to the tactile and high-threshold classes of spinothalamic tract neurons. The only axons with a distinctly different location belonged to the class having deep receptive fields. These axons formed a band along the ventral margin of the white matter at an upper lumbar level.

There was at least a rough somatotopic organization of the spinothalamic axons. Receptive fields on the caudalmost segments of the body activated axons located dorsolaterally in the tract at an upper lumbar level, whereas receptive fields on more rostral dermatomes excited axons placed more ventromedially.

Responses to Noxious Mechanical Stimulation

Spinothalamic tract neurons typically had a spontaneous discharge rate of 10 to 15 Hz under the conditions of our experiments. (The rate was higher for cells connected with deep receptors.) Some of the cells tended to discharge in bursts, even during their spontaneous activity. However, most developed a pronounced bursting discharge in response to a noxious mechanical stimulus. The discharge rate during bursts occurring soon after the stimulus onset could exceed 600 Hz, although the mean firing rate might be 50 to 100 Hz over a 10-sec period of maintained noxious stimulation.

Figure 2A-E shows the graded response of a high-threshold spinothalamic tract cell to several intensities of mechanical stimulation using a servo-controlled vibrator. The displacement of the skin ranged up to 1,435 μm, and the pressure associated with the skin displacement ranged up to 380

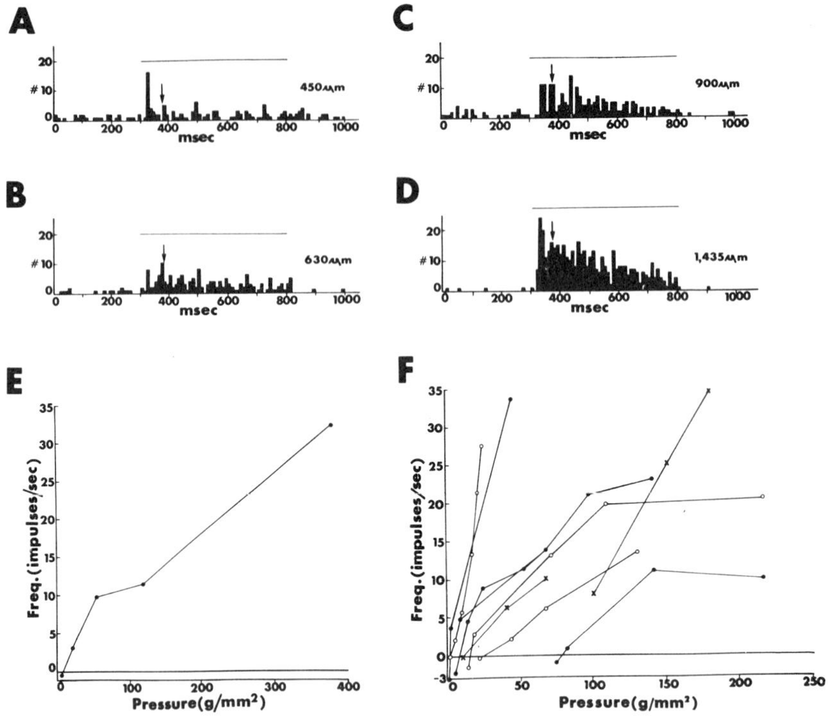

FIG. 2. Responses of spinothalamic tract cells to graded displacements of the skin using a servo-controlled vibrator. **A–D:** Peristimulus histograms of the activity of a high-threshold spinothalamic tract neuron. Durations of step displacements of the skin are indicated by the bars, and arrows show the beginnings of the maintained portions of the discharges; response measured was the mean discharge rate from the arrow until the stimulus was terminated. The amount of skin displacement for each record is indicated. Stimuli were repeated every 4 sec, and the histograms were sums of 25 responses. **E:** Relationship between cell response and skin pressure produced by the stimulator probe. **F:** Similar stimulus-response curves for 9 other spinothalamic tract cells. Open circles, hair activated; crosses, low-threshold neurons; filled circles, high-threshold neurons.

g/mm². The responses of other spinothalamic tract cells to graded stimuli are shown in Fig. 2F. Many of these showed continuous increments in discharge rate as the mechanical stimulus increased into the noxious range, which is presumably over 40 g/mm² (3). The thresholds of some of the neurons appeared to be in the noxious range.

Responses to Noxious Thermal Stimulation

Graded thermal stimuli were obtained by use of a servo-controlled peltier device. Since all of the spinothalamic tract neurons were activated by mechanical stimulation, the thermal stimuli were applied within the receptive field mapped by use of mechanical stimuli. Most spinothalamic tract cells responded to some level of thermal stimulation, most often to noxious heating. Figure 3A shows the response to graded thermal changes of three high-threshold spinothalamic tract neurons located in lamina I (Fig. 3D). All were antidromically activated from the region of the posterior thalamic nuclei (Fig. 3E). The temperatures were measured at the interface between the stimulator and the skin. The values for the firing rates of the cells were determined 15 sec after a new steady temperature was reached, and each value represents the mean discharge rate over a 10-sec period. The adapting temperature was 35°C. One of the cells responded to warming, noxious heating, and perhaps also to cooling (Fig. 3A, *filled circles*). The cell had a spontaneous discharge rate of approximately 17 Hz at the adapting temperature, and it had a large receptive field (Fig. 3F). In addition to its thermal response, the cell could also be discharged by application of pressure by a clip (Fig. 3B) or by a noxious mechanical stimulus (Fig. 3C). The average firing rate during noxious heating to 50°C was 69 Hz, and that during noxious mechanical stimulation was 68 Hz. The other two cells behaved quite differently. They responded to noxious heating and to cooling, but

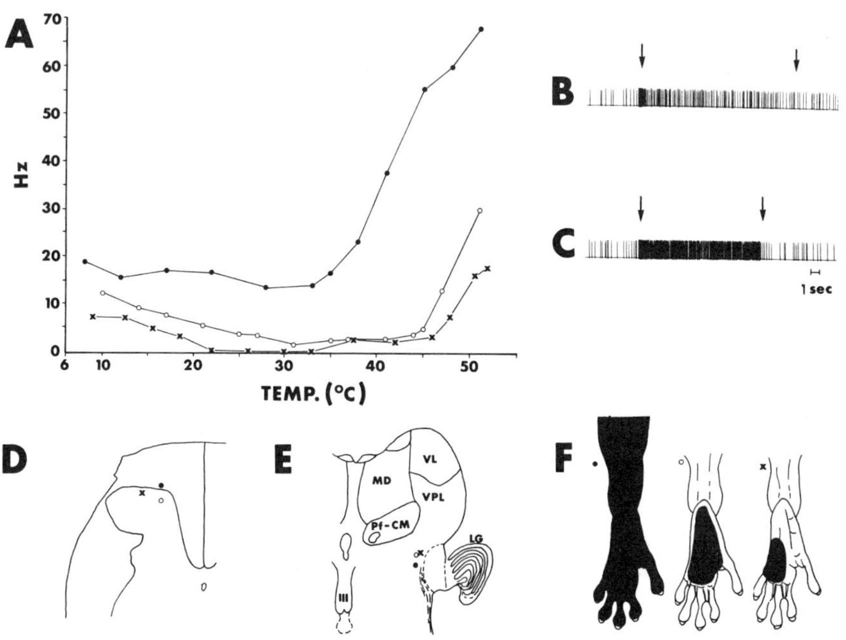

FIG. 3. Responses of lamina I cells to thermal stimuli. **A:** Average firing rate of 3 spinothalamic tract cells during maintained thermal stimulation at temperatures from less than 10° to 50°C or more. Responses of the cell in **A** (*filled circles*) to pressure and noxious mechanical stimulation are shown in **B** and **C,** respectively. Arrows indicate the times of attachment and removal of skin clips. **D:** Locations of the cells in lamina I. **E:** Points within the diencephalon from which cells were antidromically fired. **F:** Receptive fields for mechanical stimulation.

not to warming (Fig. 3A, *open circles and crosses*). They also responded to intense mechanical stimuli (not illustrated). The receptive fields to mechanical stimulation were small and restricted to the plantar glabrous skin (Fig. 3F). Neither cell had significant spontaneous activity (approximately 3 Hz). The conduction velocities of the axons of these neurons were 21 and 19 m/sec, whereas the conduction velocity of the unit that responded to warming was 40 m/sec. It is possible that lamina I cells can be subdivided into several populations depending on whether or not they respond to the input from specific thermoreceptors.

Possible Participation of Hair-Activated and Low-Threshold Cells in Nociception

It has been suggested that the spinothalamic tract neurons that respond to a wide range of mechanical stimulus strengths may be involved in pain transmission, although it was not excluded that the high-threshold spinothalamic tract neurons also participate (14,18). However, in our investigation of the responses of spinothalamic tract neurons to stimulation of the dorsal columns (8), we found that these cells were discharged by volleys descending in the dorsal column. Repetitive stimulation of the dorsal column could drive these cells at 50 Hz. Since dorsal column stimulation at 50 Hz does not cause pain, it can be questioned that spinothalamic tract cells of this type are importantly involved in pain transmission.

DISCUSSION

The organization of the spinothalamic tract of the monkey suggests that there is no separation into lateral and ventral subdivisions as has been suggested on the basis of clinical observations (7). The lateral spinothalamic tract has been considered to transmit pain and temperature information to the brain, whereas the ventral spinothalamic tract has been thought to relay tactile information. Our findings indicate that, at least in the monkey, tactile information is carried by axons that are intermingled with those of spinothalamic tract cells responding only to intense forms of stimulation. Few recordings were made from axons in the ventral funiculus, so little can be said at this time about the possibility that a specific kind of information is carried by axons in this location. However, the fact that the axons of the ventral funiculus distribute essentially to the same brain regions as do the axons in the ventral part of the lateral funiculus (11) argues against this. Segregation of the axons of spinothalamic tract cells with deep receptive fields into a ventrally placed band is of interest, and this finding warrants further investigation. The possibility of a separation of axons concerned with pain and with temperature sensation has been suggested on the basis of clinical evidence (7,19), but no conclusions can be drawn about this until more detailed information on the thermal responses of spinothalamic tract neurons is available. The rough somatotopic organization of the monkey spinothalamic tract is in keeping with clinical findings in man (10,21).

The responses of spinothalamic tract cells to noxious mechanical stimulation are in keeping with the probable role of the tract in nociception. However, it must be recognized that the animals studied were anesthetized, and it has been found that somatosensory neurons in the thalamus have different response patterns according to the presence or absence of anesthesia, and the responses vary also with state of consciousness of the animal (6). Therefore, it will be necessary to confirm the response properties of spinothalamic tract neurons in unanesthetized animals when a suitable technique becomes available. Nevertheless, cells with axons projecting to the cervical spinal cord have been studied in unanesthetized monkeys rendered insensitive to pain by carotid ligation, and the response properties of these neurons (17), which are probably spinothalamic, are similar to those reported by our group (24).

We have consistently found that high-threshold neurons, including those in lamina I, are activated by both intense mechanical and intense thermal stimulation. Others have found that some of these cells respond to activation of specific cold receptors and that such spinothalamic tract neurons are poorly activated by mechanical stimulation, indicating that they may form a specific pathway for thermoreception (9,12). We cannot disagree with this, although we have not found such units, since the sample of lamina I neurons in our study is small. However, one of our lamina I cells appeared to signal warming, although this cell was also activated by mechanical stimulation. In contrast to two other lamina I cells, it had a large receptive field and considerable spontaneous activity. These properties may be of significance to cells that participate in thermoreception.

From our observations using dorsal column stimulation to modify the activity of spinothalamic tract neurons, we conclude that nociception is more likely to be mediated by high-threshold spinothalamic tract cells than by the cells having a wide range of responsiveness. This opinion is in disagreement with that of Price's group (14,18). However, it is possible that the threshold and refractory period characteristics of the axons of human spinothalamic tract neurons are different than those of the axons of the pathway in the monkey or that dorsal column stimulation does not effectively activate wide dynamic range neurons in the human. Another possibility is that ascending volleys in the dorsal column or other sensory pathways interfere at a higher level with pain transmission.

SUMMARY

The spinothalamic tract in the ventrolateral white matter of the monkey spinal cord consists of intermingled axons of cells activated by tactile and by intense forms of mechanical stimulation. This suggests that the tract is not separated into lateral and ventral subdivisions. The only group of axons with a distinctly different location is from cells having proprioceptive inputs. The spinothalamic tract in the monkey does have a rough somatotopic organization, with caudal areas represented by axons in the dorsolateral part of the tract and rostral areas represented by more ventromedially situated axons.

The responses of many spinothalamic tract neurons to noxious levels of mechanical or thermal stimulation suggest a role for such neurons in nociception. However, the finding that dorsal column stimulation activates the cells responding to a wide range of stimulus strengths argues against an important involvement of these cells in nociception since dorsal column stimulation is not painful.

ACKNOWLEDGMENTS

The work described was supported by a research grant from the National Institutes of Health, U.S. Public Health Service (NS 09743), by training grants from the N.I.H. (NS 05743; GM 00459), and by a grant from the Moody Foundation of Galveston.

The author wishes to thank Gail Silver for her expert technical assistance.

REFERENCES

1. Albe-Fessard, D., Levante, A., and Lamour, Y. (1974): *Brain Res.,* 65:503–509.
2. Applebaum, A. E., Beall, J. E., Foreman, R. D., and Willis, W. D. (1975): *J. Neurophysiol.,* 38:572–586.
3. Bessou, P., and Perl, E. R. (1969): *J. Neurophysiol.,* 32:1025–1043.
4. Brown, A. G. (1970): *Brain Res.,* 17:152–155.
5. Brown, A. G., and Franz, D. N. (1969): *Exp. Brain Res.,* 7:231–249.
6. Casey, K. L. (1966): *J. Neurophysiol.,* 29:727–750.
7. Foerster, O., and Gagel, O. (1932): *Z. Ges. Neurol. Psychiatr.,* 138:1–92.
8. Foreman, R. D., Beall, J. E., Coulter, J. D., and Willis, W. D. (1975): *International Association for the Study of Pain.*
9. Handwerker, H. O., Iggo, A., Ogawa, H., and Ramsey, R. L. (1975): *J. Physiol.,* 244:76–77P.
10. Hyndman, O. R., and Van Epps, C. (1939): *Arch. Surg.,* 38:1036–1053.
11. Kerr, F. W. L. (1975): *J. Comp. Neurol.,* 159:335–356.
12. Kumazawa, T., Perl, E. R., Burgess, P. R., and Whitehorn, D. (1975): *J. Comp. Neurol.,* 162:1–12.
13. Kuru, M. (1949): In: *Sensory Paths in the Spinal Cord and Brain Stem of Man.* Sogensya, Tokyo.
14. Mayer, D. J., Price, D. D., and Becker, D. P. (1975): *Pain,* 1:51–58.
15. Mehler, W. R. (1974): *Adv. Neurol.,* 4:127–146.
16. Mehler, W. R., Feferman, M. E., and Nauta, W. J. H. (1960): *Brain,* 83:718–750.
17. Price, D. D., and Mayer, D. J. (1974): *Brain Res.,* 79:321–325.
18. Price, D. D., and Mayer, D. J. (1975): *Pain,* 1:59–72.
19. Sherman, I. C., and Arieff, A. J. (1948): *J. Nerv. Ment. Dis.,* 108:285–292.
20. Trevino, D. L., Coulter, J. D., and Willis, W. D. (1973): *J. Neurophysiol.,* 36:750–761.
21. White, J. C., Richardson, E. P., and Sweet, W. H. (1956): *Ann. Surg.,* 144:407–420.

22. White, J. C., and Sweet, W. H. (1955): In: *Pain, Its Mechanisms and Neurosurgical Control,* Charles C. Thomas, Publisher, Springfield, Illinois.
23. Willis, W. D., Maunz, R. A., Foreman, R. D., and Coulter, J. D. (1975): *J. Neurophysiol.,* 38:587–600.
24. Willis, W. D., Trevino, D. L., Coulter, J. D., and Maunz, R. A. (1974): *J. Neurophysiol.,* 37:358–372.

Advances in Pain Research and Therapy, Vol. 1,
edited by J. J. Bonica and D. Albe-Fessard.
Raven Press, New York © 1976.

Experimental Central Pain and Itch Syndromes: Modeling and General Theory

G. N. Kryzhanovsky

Institute of General Pathology and Pathological Physiology of AMS USSR, Moscow 125315, USSR

The basic theoretical premise for this investigation is the concept of the role of a determinant dispatch station (DDS) in the activity of the central nervous system (11–13). The DDS is the CNS structure that forms functional messages, modulates the subsequent parts to which these messages are addressed, and determines the pattern of their activity. Thus it determines the behavior of the whole physiological system it activates.

Under pathological conditions, which cause insufficiency of the inhibitory mechanisms in the neuron population constituting the DDS, the latter becomes hyperactive and acts as a generator of pathologically enhanced excitation. Such a hyperactive DDS generator produces abnormal function and gives the physiological system certain pathological qualities. The properties of the generator have been studied extensively by this writer (10,14).

The hyperactive DDS's generators underlie various neuropathological syndromes. Specificity of the latter depends on the system in which the hyperactive DDS develops. If the hyperactive DDS generator is formed in those parts of the CNS involved in nociception, central pain syndromes develop.

METHODS

To study this phenomenon of abnormal DDS, we have developed animal models in which the inhibitory mechanism in the neuron population was disturbed and consequently the hyperactive DDS generator was produced by applying certain agents to some part of the sensory (afferent) system in the neuraxis. For this purpose we have used purified tetanus toxin (TT), which blocks several kinds of postsynaptic and presynaptic inhibition (2,3,5,19,20); strychnine, which blocks the glycine postsynaptic inhibition (4,7); and penicillin, which blocks gamma-aminobutyric acid (GABA) inhibition (6–8). In these experiments the abnormal generator was formed as a direct consequence of primary disinhibition of the neuron population. For primary excitation of neurons, we used KCl and ouabain as depolarizing agents, which cause a secondary relative insufficiency of the inhibitory mechanisms. We have developed models and studied the phenomenon in the spinal cord, the trigeminal system, and the thalamus.

Spinal Cord

In the spinal cord we have produced the pathologic process by injecting TT stereotaxically while applying strychnine, penicillin, KCl, and ouabain (as well as TT in special experiments) to the dorsal surface of the spinal cord. To prolong the action of the toxins, we used a method of "agar plate," which we developed: the drug was deposited in 1% agar, and the plate was then gently applied to the dorsal surface of the lumbar spinal cord. Because the toxins diffuse slowly from the agar into the dorsal horn, this technique permits us to prolong the effect of the toxins and thus observe the pathologic syndrome under conditions of free behavior of the animal for a period of time.

Some time after TT was injected into the dorsal horns of the lumbar enlargement or after it was applied onto the dorsal surface of the lumbar cord segments, the animals (rats, cats) became agitated and aggressive and licked, scratched, and even bit the tissues of the corresponding hindlimb supplied by the affected spinal segments (Fig. 1). Subsequently these areas lost their hair, underwent injury, and became trigger zones: relatively weak stimulation provoked an attack. In addition to the evoked responses, abnormal spontaneous activity developed. Animals cried, ran away, rushed about the cage, and furiously gnawed surrounding objects. Sometimes they kept the paw in a half-bent position as if to avoid stimulation. At later stages the animals gnawed their limb tissues. The attacks were associated with alteration of respiration, hypertension, dilatation of the pupil, and bulging of the eyeball. After the spinal cord in the thoracic region was sectioned, the attacks disappeared.

A similar picture of severe pain and itch was observed in experiments in which strychnine, penicillin, KCl, and ouabain were used.

Thus the creation of the hyperactive DDS generator in the dorsal spinal horn by various methods resulted in the rise of severe pain and itch syndromes of spinal origin.

Trigeminal Nucleus

The creation of the hyperactive DDS generator in the caudal trigeminal nucleus induced trigeminal pain and itch syndromes (Fig. 2A1). The animals scratched the corresponding areas of the snout on the side of TT injection, sometimes tearing the tissues. These areas became trigger zones of facilitated provocation of the attacks. The paroxysmal attacks arose spontaneously, and scratching was alternated with vigorous attempts at escape.

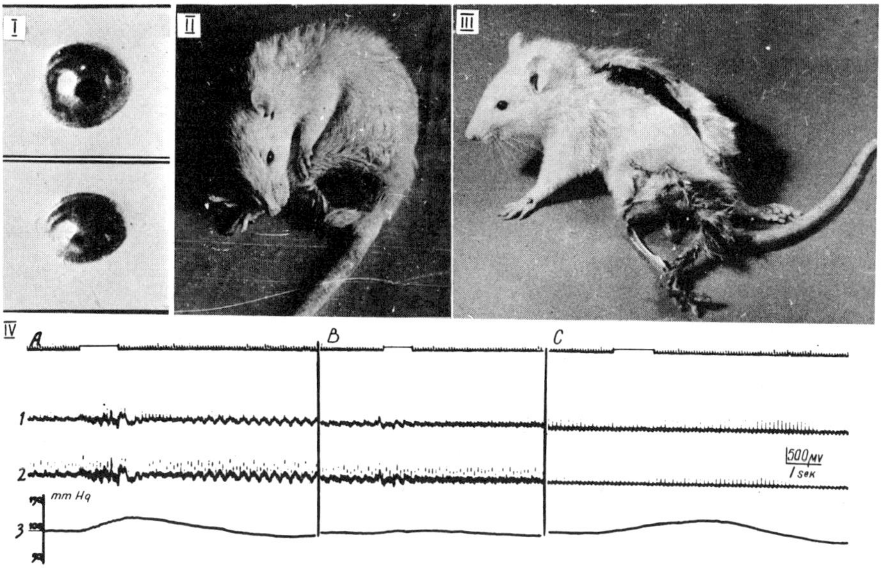

FIG. 1. Pain and itch of spinal origin. **I:** Dilatation of pupil and bulging of the eyeball during pain attack (*top*); eye of the same rat in a resting state (*bottom*). **II:** Area of licking on the left thigh (hairless, eroded). **III:** In one of the final stages of the syndrome, the animal has gnawed the soft tissues to the bone; **IVA:** Changes in respiration (1 and 2, electrical activity in respiratory muscles) and elevation of arterial pressure (3) in the attack produced by tactile stimulation of the trigger zone (left thigh). **B:** Absence of the effect at similar stimulation of the same area of contralateral limb. **C:** Elevation of arterial pressure during stimulation of the trigger zone under conditions of total curarization of the animal and artificial respiration.

Thalamus

The thalamic syndromes (Fig. 2B) were reproduced by creation of the excitation generator in the medial thalamic nuclei after TT injection into these nuclei (nuclei gelatinosi in rats). The animals became anxious and aggressive: they cried, jumped, ran away, rushed about the cage, furiously gnawed surrounding objects, and scratched and bit the skin areas at the scapulae, perineum, genitals, back, hindlimbs, and other areas.

Role of Inhibitory Transmitters

Inhibitory transmitters can suppress the activity of the generator (10,14). Injection of glycine into the affected dorsal horns or caudal trigeminal nucleus where the generators had previously been created abolished the whole spinal and trigeminal syndromes during the period of transmitter action (Fig. 2A2): the animals became quiet, the paroxysmal spontaneous

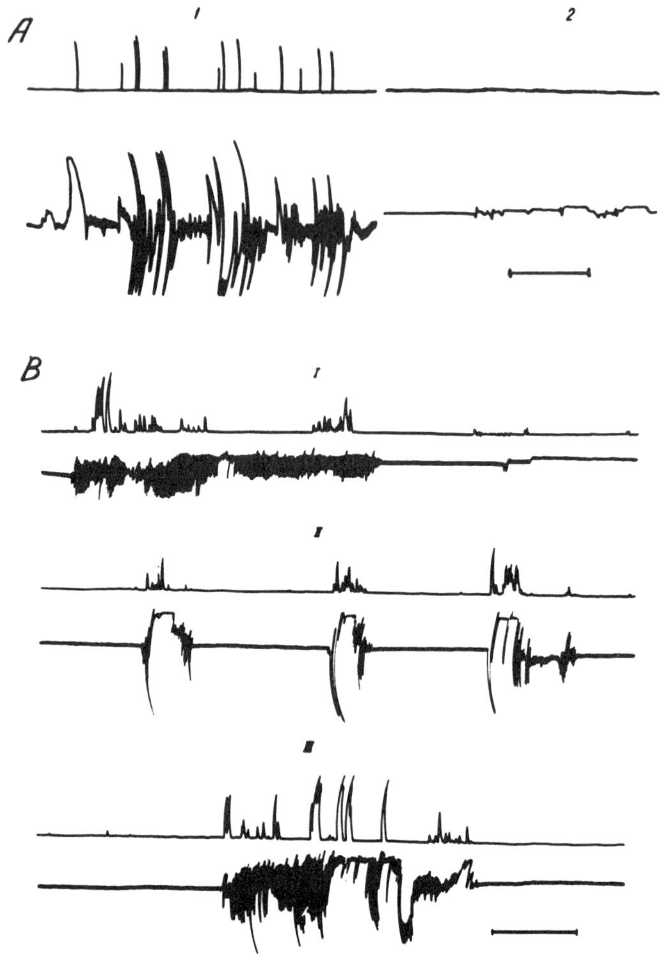

FIG. 2. Trigeminal and thalamic pain and itch syndromes. **A:** Trigeminal syndrome in rat after injection of purified tetanus toxin (1 DLM for rat) into caudate nucleus of spinal trigeminal tract before (1) and 30 min after (2) the injection of glycine (20% solution, 3×10^{-4} ml) in the same nucleus.
B: Thalamic syndrome in rat after injection of purified tetanus toxin (1 DLM for rat) into nucleus gelatinosus. Different variants (I, II, III) of spontaneous attack are presented. In all parts of the figure the upper traces are phonograms (records of cries) and the lower traces are actograms (records of running around the cage; attacks of scratching, licking, etc.).

attacks disappeared, and stimulation of the trigger zone did not provoke any attacks.

The suppressing effect of inhibitory transmitters on the generator of pathologically enhanced excitation depends on the pathogenetic specificity of the generator, that is, on the kind of inhibition disturbed in the generator.

As inhibitory transmitters, GABA and glycine revealed the specific suppressing effect when their receptors on the generator neurons were not blocked by disinhibitors.

DISCUSSION

We suggest that one method of producing relief in patients with pathological central pain is the activation of the inhibitory systems and the suppression of the generators. In regard to these effects, the pathogenetic specificity of the generator seems to be of great importance. The experiments showed that carbamazepine (Tegretol®) could abolish the spinal pain syndromes induced by "ouabain," "potassium," and "TT" generators but had only slight effect on the syndrome induced by the "strychnine" generator and was ineffective in the syndrome induced by the "penicillin" generator.

We suggest that trigger zones—which, when stimulated, produce an attack—are tissues or zones connected with the more excitable disinhibited generator neurons. In the model experiments on the spinal pain syndrome, it was shown that localization of the trigger zones corresponded to that of generator.

Formation of the generator of pathologically enhanced excitation is thought to underlie phantom pains. This is suggested by data from our experiments on spinal pain syndromes in which the nerves of the hindlimb or dorsal roots were cut before the injection of the TT into the dorsal horns. Under such conditions injection of the TT created the generator in dorsal horns of lumbar segments, which then produced the typical pain syndrome with projection of pain to the corresponding areas of the hindlimb deprived of sensitivity.

Analysis of the data reveals that several other peculiarities of central pain such as spontaneous rise, paroxysmal attacks, prolonged duration, refractory period after the attack, and failure or insufficient relief after section of the peripheral neural pathways can be explained by the theory of the generator mechanisms of central pain.

The proposed theory of generator mechanisms of central pain does not contradict but, on the contrary, in many points agrees with existing fruitful theories of physiological and pathological pain (1,9,15–18,21,22). It is a part of the more general conception of the basic role of the hyperactive determinant dispatch station in CNS pathology (11,12,23–25).

SUMMARY

The theory of the generator mechanisms of pain syndromes of central origin is stated. Modeling of pain and itch of spinal, trigeminal, and thalamic origin by creation of generators of pathologically enhanced excitation under conditions of disturbed inhibitory mechanisms in the respective parts of the

CNS is described. Pathogenetic and clinical characteristics of central pain syndromes in the plan of analysis of the formation and properties of the generators are considered. Suppression of the generators of excitation by inhibitory mediators involves liquidation of the whole pain syndrome during the mediators' action. Some aspects of treatment of pain syndromes on the basis of the theory of the generator mechanisms are analyzed. The theory of the generator mechanisms of central pain represents part of a more general concept of the role of generators of pathologically enhanced excitation as hyperactive determinative dispatch stations in inducing neuropathological syndromes.

REFERENCES

1. Albe-Fessard, D. (1968): *J. Psychol. Norm. Pathol.,* 1:1–45.
2. Brooks, V. B., Curtis, D. R., and Eccles, J. C. (1957): *J. Physiol. (Lond.),* 135:635–672.
3. Curtis, D. R., and De Groat, W. C. (1968): *Brain Res.,* 10:208–212.
4. Curtis, D. R., Duggan, A. W., and Johnston, G. A. R. (1971): *Exp. Brain Res.,* 12:547–565.
5. Curtis, D. R., Felix, D., Gane, C. J. A., and McCulloch, R. M. (1973): *Brain Res.,* 51:358–362.
6. Curtis, D. R., Game, C. J. A., Johnston, G. A. R., McCulloch, R. M., and MacLachlan, R. M. (1972): *Brain Res.,* 43:242–245.
7. Curtis, D. R., and Johnston, G. A. R. (1974): *Ergeb. Physiol.,* 69:97–188.
8. Davidoff, R. A. (1972): *Brain Res.,* 45:638–642.
9. Hassler, R. (1970): In: *Trigeminal Neuralgia,* edited by R. Hassler and A. E. Walker, pp. 123–138. George Thieme Verlag, Stuttgart.
10. Kryzhanovsky, G. N. (1973): In: *Convergence and Synapses.* Conference of Brain Institutes of AMS USSR, pp. 109–113. Moscow.
11. Kryzhanovsky, G. N. (1970): In: *General Neurophysiology and Experimental Pathology of Nervous System,* Vol. XIII, edited by the Institute of Normal and Pathological Physiology AMS USSR, pp. 43–46. Moscow.
12. Kryzhanovsky, G. N. (1973): *Patol. Fiziol. Eskp. Ter.,* 4:3–10.
13. Kryzhanovsky, G. N., and Lutsenko, V. K. (1975): *Neirofiziologiia,* 7:234–242.
14. Kryzhanovsky, G. N., Sheikhon, F. D., and Rekhtman, M. B. (1975): *Neirofiziologiia,* 7:608–617.
15. Melzack, R., and Wall, P. D. (1970): *Int. Anesthesiol. Clin.,* 8:3–33.
16. Melzack, R., and Wall, P. D. (1965): *Science,* 150:971–979.
17. Noordenbos, W. (1960): *Acta Neurochir.* (Wien), 8:113–120.
18. Noordenbos, W. (1959): *Pain.* Elsevier, Amsterdam.
19. Osborne, R. H., and Bradford, H. F. (1973): *Nature* [*New Biol.*], 244:157–158.
20. Sverdlov, Y. S. (1965): In: *Recent Advances in the Pharmacology of Toxins,* edited by H. W. Raudonat, pp. 113–120. Pergamon Press, Czechoslovak Medical Press, Prague.
21. Wall, P. D. (1974): In: *Proceedings of the International Union of Physiological Sciences,* Vol. X, p. 68. New Delhi.
22. Winther, K. (1973): *Eur. Neurol.,* 10:65–74.
23. Kryzhanovsky, G. N., Rekhtman, M. B., Konnikov, B. A., and Petljuk, V. K. (1976): *Biull. Eksp. Biol. Med.,* 81:22–25.
24. Kryzhanovsky, G. N., Rekhtman, M. B., Konnikov, B. A., and Sheikhon, F. D. (1976): *Biull. Eksp. Biol. Med.,* 81:147–150.
25. Kryzhanovsky, G. N., and Aliev, M. N. (1976): *Biull. Eksp. Biol. Med.,* 81:397–399.

Advances in Pain Research and Therapy, Vol. 1,
edited by J. J. Bonica and D. Albe-Fessard.
Raven Press, New York © 1976.

Prefrontal Cortex and Modulation of Response to Aversive Stimulation in the Rat

Steven J. Cooper

Department of Psychology, The Queen's University of Belfast, Belfast BT7 1NN, Northern Ireland

Melzack and Casey (12) have proposed that the central mechanisms which influence behavioral responses characteristic of pain include not only a sensory-discriminative system but also a motivational-affective system and a neocortical cognitive system. According to their model, the activation of reticular and limbic structures mediates the unpleasant motivational dimension of pain, although neocortical processes can exert a modulating control, taking account of such cognitive factors as previous experience and the anticipation of future outcome. Anatomically, the prefrontal cortex is particularly noteworthy in having considerable two-way connections with reticular and limbic structures, as well as with many other cortical regions (13). In this Chapter I describe some of our initial attempts in the rat to determine the parts played by the prefrontal cortex in the behavioral responses to aversive stimulation.

PREFRONTAL CORTEX—ANATOMY

The prefrontal cortex in the rat, defined as the cortical projection field of the mediodorsal nucleus (MD) of the thalamus, has been described by Leonard (9). The sulcal prefrontal cortex forms the dorsal bank of the rhinal sulcus. It is reciprocally connected with the medial division of the MD, and thus it may be homologous to the caudal orbitofrontal cortex of the monkey. The medial prefrontal cortex forms the medial wall of the hemisphere anterior and dorsal to the genu of the corpus callosum. It is reciprocally connected with the lateral division of the MD. The dorsal sector of this medial cortex may be comparable with the caudal prefrontal cortex (the frontal eye field) of the monkey, whereas the ventral region of the medial cortex may be homologous to the major part of the monkey's frontal convexity cortex (9).

ANESTHETIZATION OF SULCAL PREFRONTAL CORTEX

Applying a small volume of anesthetic solution directly to a brain site is a convenient method of producing a short-lasting and reversible blockade of neural function during behavioral tests. We have used this method to block the function of localized regions within the prefrontal cortex while measuring the thresholds of the rat's response to aversive footshock (4). Stainless steel guide cannulae, each fitted with an obturator, were implanted bilaterally in adult male hooded rats (300 to 350 g) as described previously (14). The steel cannulae were removed and replaced with injection cannulae before an injection experiment. Cannulae directed at the sulcal prefrontal cortex were implanted bilaterally in 10 rats (Fig. 1).

Responses to aversive footshock were determined using a modification of Evans' "jump-flinch" test (5) as follows. Each rat received six series of shocks, each series consisting of scrambled electrical shock (0.5 sec duration) delivered at 15-sec intervals to the floor of the test box. The shock intensities in each series were 10 consecutive values from the range 0.13 to 1.60 mA (Grason-Stadler shock generator, E1064GS). There was a 60-sec

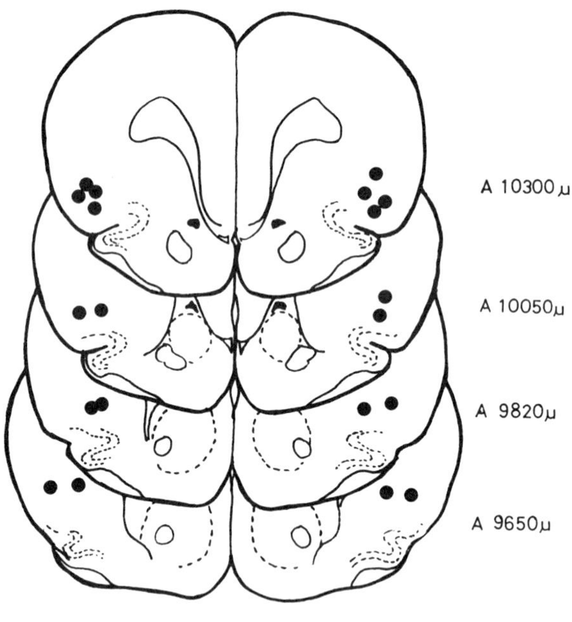

FIG. 1. Positions of termination of bilateral cannulae tracks in or near the sulcal prefrontal cortex for the 10 rats used in the anesthetization experiment. Stereotaxic coordinates for the cannula implantation were 2.3 mm anterior to the bregma, 3.5 mm lateral to the sagittal sinus, and 4.0 mm beneath the dorsal surface of the brain (+2.3:3.5:4.0 mm down), using a level-head position. Either 5% procaine hydrochloride in 0.9% saline or saline alone was injected bilaterally. At the end of the experiments, brains were perfused, removed, and mounted in paraffin. Ten-micron sections were stained with Luxol® blue and Pyronine® Y. Outline drawings in the figure were redrawn from Figs. 8b–11b of König and Klippel's stereotaxic atlas (8).

interval between each series. Shocks were delivered in ascending and descending order on alternate series. The rat's response to each shock was recorded as no response, a flinch, or a jump. The rat was removed, injected bilaterally with 1.0 μl 5% procaine hydrochloride, and immediately returned to the test box. Six more shock series were run to determine postinjection flinch and jump thresholds. After 30 min, the rat was reinjected with 2.0 μl 5% procaine, and a second set of six postinjection shock series was run. For statistical analysis, the mean flinch and jump threshold values over the six-shock series were calculated, and results for the pre- and postinjection series were compared using a correlated *t*-test (two-tailed).

After 1.0 μl 5% procaine hydrochloride was injected bilaterally, the preinjection jump threshold (averaged over the six-shock series) of 0.86 ± 0.22 mA (mean ± SD) was reduced to 0.77 ± 0.19 mA ($t = 6.2$; $p < 0.0001$), and after the bilateral injection of 2.0 μl procaine, the threshold was further reduced to 0.73 ± 0.21 mA ($t = 6.9$; $p < 0.0001$). Every animal exhibited a reduction in the jump threshold after either the 1.0 μl or 2.0 μl bilateral injections of procaine. In the saline control experiments, performed with the same animals, the mean preinjection jump threshold of 0.86 ± 0.22 mA did not differ significantly from the threshold value of 0.87 ± 0.22 mA after the injection of 2.0 μl saline bilaterally. Figure 2 compares the mean jump thresholds before and after the injection of either 5% procaine or saline. In contrast to the reduction in the jump threshold after the bilateral injection of procaine, the flinch threshold remained unchanged. The preinjection

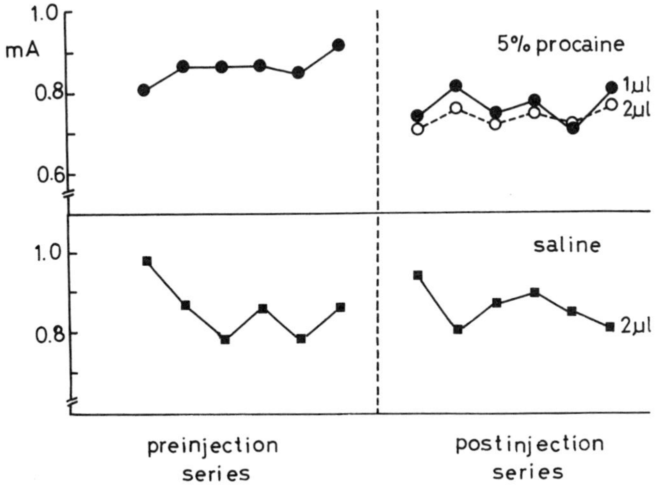

FIG. 2. Effect of bilateral injection of 5% procaine hydrochloride into the sulcal prefrontal cortex on the jump threshold (mA) in the "jump-flinch" test ($n = 10$). *Top left,* mean jump threshold for each preinjection series of shocks; *top right,* mean jump threshold for each postinjection series of shocks after injection of 1.0 and 2.0 μl procaine. *Lower panels,* results of injection of 2.0 μl 0.9% saline.

flinch threshold was 0.19 ± 0.05 mA, whereas after the bilateral injection of 1.0 μl procaine it was 0.18 ± 0.03 mA, and after 2.0 μl procaine it was 0.18 ± 0.03 mA (no significant difference).

The reduction in the jump threshold did not reflect a nonspecific reduction in response thresholds since, first, the flinch threshold remained unchanged and, second, bilateral anesthetization of the sulcal prefrontal cortex in the rat increases the threshold for intracranial electrical self-stimulation (14). Bilateral procaine injections seemed to be necessary since we failed to observe reliable reductions in the jump threshold after unilateral injections in the sulcal region. Bilateral anesthetization of the medial prefrontal cortex did not change the jump threshold (Fig. 3). The preinjection jump threshold of 0.78 ± 0.24 mA was not significantly different from the postinjection jump threshold of 0.79 ± 0.24 mA ($N = 4$). Hence the reduction in the jump threshold was produced by bilateral anesthetization of the sulcal but not of the medial prefrontal cortex. These results with procaine were confirmed in a further study with rats given small bilateral electrolytic lesions within the prefrontal cortex (S. J. Cooper, *unpublished results*). Jump and flinch thresholds were determined in rats before the lesion procedure. After recovery to at least presurgery body weights, rats with bilateral lesions limited to the sulcal prefrontal cortex had significantly lower jump thresholds than before but unchanged flinch thresholds. In contrast, sham-operated animals had closely similar pre- and postsurgery jump thresholds. The lesion effect was localized since lesions of a comparable size situated bilaterally in either the medial prefrontal cortex or the dorsal caudate nucleus did not change the

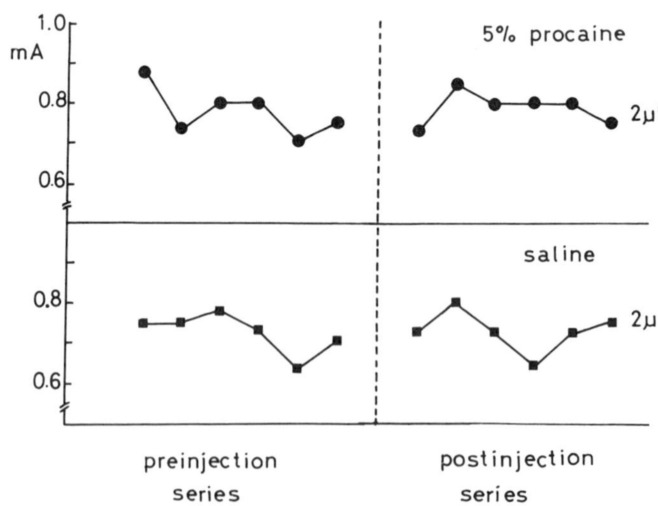

FIG. 3. Effect of bilateral injection of 5% procaine hydrochloride into the medial prefrontal cortex on the jump threshold (mA) in the "jump-flinch" test ($n = 4$). Conventions and procedures as for Fig. 2.

jump threshold. Hence either damage to or a functional blockade of the prefrontal cortex, localized within the sulcal region, has a relatively specific effect in reducing the jump threshold. Since the jump response but not the flinch response seems to be particularly related to the strongly aversive effects of footshock (5), I suggest that in the intact rat a region in or near the sulcal prefrontal cortex can function to limit the response to specifically aversive stimulation.

It is perhaps more than coincidence that the rhesus monkey displays a greater sensitivity to aversive stimuli after lesions of the orbitofrontal cortex (possibly analogous to the rat sulcal prefrontal cortex) but not of the dorsolateral frontal cortex (possibly comparable to the rat medial prefrontal cortex) (2). In the monkey too, therefore, there seems to be a localized structure within the frontal cortex which may normally serve to limit responses of aversion. There are also data for man which suggest the existence of an aversion-limiting system in the frontal region. Frontal lobotomy has been shown to reduce the threshold for pain elicited by thermal stimulation of the skin (3,7). These similarities are consistent with the possibility that localized within the prefrontal cortex, a neural system with a modulatory function can attenuate responses to noxious stimulation, and that such a system might operate in primates as well as in the rat. The hypothesis seems to merit further investigation.

DOPAMINE AND SULCAL PREFRONTAL CORTEX

The anesthetization technique is nonspecific in blocking neural function, and therefore our next step has been to inject more specifically acting drugs into the sulcal prefrontal cortex. Our recent work indicates that a dopaminergic system in or near the sulcal prefrontal cortex may be involved in the rat's response to aversive footshock (S. J. Cooper and M. C. Ostermeyer, *unpublished results*). Dopamine (0.5 μg) was injected bilaterally into the sulcal prefrontal cortex in 5 animals. The preinjection jump threshold (mean $\pm$ SD) of 0.71 ± 0.12 was raised to 0.85 ± 0.08 ($t = 8.22$; $p < 0.01$) after the injection of dopamine. The flinch threshold, in contrast, remained unchanged. In the same animals, the bilateral injection of 1 μl 0.9% saline had no effect on the jump threshold. In the procaine experiments, therefore, anesthetization of a dopamine system might have been responsible for the fall in the jump threshold. Such an explanation is supported by the findings that both haloperidol (20 μg) and chlorpromazine (20 μg), which are both potent dopamine-receptor blockers, also reduced the jump threshold when injected bilaterally into the sulcal prefrontal cortex. For example, the preinjection jump threshold of 0.76 ± 0.17 was reduced to 0.68 ± 0.15 ($t = 3.04$; $p < 0.05$) after the bilateral injection of haloperidol. Hence the threshold of the jump response can be raised by the injection of dopamine or lowered by the injection of dopamine antagonists into the sulcal prefrontal cortex.

An intense dopaminergic innervation of the frontal cortex has recently been described for the rat (1,10,11,15). Dopamine-containing neural fibers arise from cell bodies in the midbrain to terminate widely in the subcortex with a major branch ascending to give an extensive dopaminergic innervation in the frontal cortex (10). There is therefore a direct dopaminergic pathway from the midbrain to the frontal cortex. I suggest that this pathway, or some component of it, may modulate the rat's response to strongly aversive footshock. Affecting the activity of the dopamine input to the sulcal prefrontal cortex or the effects of its activity by the direct application of dopamine or dopamine antagonists may be sufficient to account for the increases and decreases in the jump threshold that we have observed. Specifically, we think that the activation of the ascending dopamine system to the frontal cortex may result in the attenuation of responses to at least some forms of aversive stimulation. Experiments have been begun to examine this possibility further.

MEDIAL PREFRONTAL CORTEX

We failed to find any effect of anesthetization of the medial prefrontal cortex on the rat's responses to aversive footshock in the "jump-flinch" test (Fig. 3). Nevertheless, we have observed that bilateral anesthetization of the medial prefrontal cortex produced a marked reduction in shock-elicited aggression in the rat (S. J. Cooper and R. J. Rodgers, *unpublished observations*). The reason for the reduction is not yet clear, but the results do suggest that the medial prefrontal cortex may be involved in at least some categories of responses elicited by aversive stimulation. Interestingly, Kelly (6) has shown that single units in the medial prefrontal cortex are activated in a specific way by aversive electrical stimulation at central gray sites. Hence certain neurons in the medial prefrontal cortex may help to facilitate or mediate certain categories of response elicited by aversive stimulation. Our results appear to point to a dissociation of function between the sulcal and medial prefrontal cortex in the rat in relation to the rat's responses to aversive footshock.

ACKNOWLEDGMENTS

Janssen Pharmaceutica generously donated the haloperidol. I thank M. C. Ostermeyer for his assistance and Mrs. Janet Curwell for performing the histological studies.

REFERENCES

1. Berger, B., Tassin, J. P., Blanc, G., Moyne, M. A., and Thierry, A. M. (1974): *Brain Res.*, 81:332–337.
2. Butter, C. M., and Snyder, D. R. (1972): *Acta Neurobiol. Exp.* (*Warsz*), 32:525–565.

3. Chapman, W. P., Rose, A. S., and Solomon, H. C. (1948): *Res. Publ. Assoc. Nerv. Ment. Dis.,* 27:754–762.
4. Cooper, S. J. (1975): *Nature,* 254:439–440.
5. Evans, W. O. (1961): *Psychopharmacologia,* 2:318–325.
6. Kelly, P. H. (1974): The physiological basis of reward and punishment. Thesis, University of Oxford.
7. King, H. E., Clausen, J., and Scarff, J. E. (1950): *J. Nerv. Ment. Dis.,* 112:93–96.
8. König, J. F. R., and Klippel, R. A. (1970): *The Rat Brain.* R. E. Krieger Pub. Co., Huntington, New York.
9. Leonard, C. M. (1969): *Brain Res.,* 12:321–343.
10. Lindvall, O., and Björklund, A. (1974): *Acta Physiol. Scand.* [*Suppl.*], 412:1–48.
11. Lindvall, O., Björklund, A., Moore, R. Y., and Stenevi, U. (1974): *Brain Res.,* 81:325–331.
12. Melzack, R., and Casey, K. L. (1968): In: *The Skin Senses,* edited by D. Kenshalo. Charles C Thomas, Publisher, Springfield, Illinois.
13. Nauta, W. J. H. (1972): *Acta Neurobiol. Exp.* (*Warsz*), 32:125–140.
14. Rolls, E. T., and Cooper, S. J. (1974): *Physiol. Behav.,* 12:563–571.
15. Thierry, A. M., Stinus, L., Blanc, G., and Glowinski, J. (1973): *Brain Res.,* 50:230–234.

Advances in Pain Research and Therapy, Vol. 1,
edited by J. J. Bonica and D. Albe-Fessard.
Raven Press, New York © 1976.

An Electrophysiological Investigation of the Dorsal Column System—Its Possible Role in Nociception

D. Angaut-Petit

*Centre d'Etudes de Physiologie Nerveuse du C.N.R.S.,
4 Avenue Gordon-Bennett, 75016 Paris, France*

The sensory functions of the dorsal column (DC) system have recently been discussed according to the impairment of various sensitivities resulting from selective damage to or stimulation of this ascending pathway. There is still some discrepancy between behavioral or clinical data and the specific properties of the long ascending fibers of this bundle or cells of their bulbar relay. Classically, no direct involvement in transmission of noxious impulses is attributed to the DC system, although its interaction with nociceptive mechanisms was long ago described (15–19). In 1936 Foerster (6) proposed three hypotheses to explain the reappearance of noxious sensations after anterolateral cordotomies; in one of them he considered the possible involvement of fibers located in the dorsal columns. Although no primary fibers conducting noxious impulses were reported to ascend in the DC, the suggestion that this bundle is involved in pain transmission could be explained either by connections of its fibers at the segmental level with other ascending systems (7,8) or by conduction of impulses to central structures (1) through long ascending fibers or spinospinal fibers. The properties of the fibers that ascend the DC pathway are not completely known, and transsynaptically activated fibers identified recently in the fasciculus gracilis (13) resembled those described by Uddenberg (17) in the cuneate tract. The contrast between the properties of these dorsal column postsynaptic (DCPS) fibers located in the fasciculus gracilis and the properties of the primary afferent fibers of the same bundle was striking since the former fibers conveyed information elicited by various stimuli, including those of noxious intensity. This chapter concerns the properties of these DCPS fibers, their comparison with the properties of a population of cells in the nucleus gracilis, and the possible involvement of these elements in pain transmission.

METHODS

Adult cats were anesthetized with intraperitoneal sodium pentobarbital (Nembutal®, 40 mg/kg) or chloralose (70 mg/kg) and paralyzed with gallamine triethiodide. Spinal cats were used in some experiments. The activity of single units was recorded from the fasciculus gracilis (fibers) at the 12th thoracic segment (T_{12}) and from the nucleus gracilis (cells) with micropipettes or tungsten microelectrodes, the latter being used to mark the recording sites. As the microelectrode was advanced through the structure, the sciatic nerve was regularly stimulated (2/sec) at a strength that was supramaximal for the myelinated fibers. Both gentle and noxious stimuli were applied for examination of receptive field properties: hair movement and light stroking of the skin were provided by a glass rod with a fire polished tip 2 mm in diameter. Long-lasting pressure or pinch of constant intensity was obtained using three forceps to grasp a fold of skin; the stimuli were roughly called nonnoxious, firm, and noxious according to the reactions of a freely moving cat to which they were applied. Noxious heating was produced with a radiant source or with a contact heating device.

RESULTS

Postsynaptic activity was identified according to the properties of the responses elicited by stimulation of the sciatic nerve. Three criteria were used to differentiate a postsynaptic activity from a primary afferent response associated with a dorsal root reflex (3): (a) the number of spikes evoked by a single sciatic shock; (b) the latency of the first impulse; and (c) the frequency of repetitive stimulation that the first spike was able to follow. In a postsynaptic element, a single shock to the sciatic nerve elicited a high-frequency multiple discharge, the duration of which increased with the intensity of the stimulus; the latency of the response fluctuated (up to 0.6 msec) with the repetition of a threshold electrical stimulus; the rate of frequency following did not exceed 200/sec even for the first spike of the discharge.

All but a few of the postsynaptic fibers studied in the fasciculus gracilis at T_{12} reached upper cervical levels. These long postsynaptic fibers were found to represent 9.3% of the total population of fibers studied in the fasciculus gracilis and 14.5% of those with receptors in the skin. They lay between the primary fibers of cutaneous and those of deep origin. The conduction velocities of the impulses in the DCPS axons measured between T_{12} and the first cervical segment indicated a very wide range in their diameters and a gross overlap with the diameters of the primary afferent fibers. The latencies of the responses evoked in the DCPS fibers by stimulation of the sciatic nerve implied that impulses conveyed by the fastest fibers of the cutaneous alpha group impinged on their cells of origin. The appearance and the latency of a second group of impulses when the peripheral stimulus was about 60 times threshold probably indicated that C fibers contributed also to the DCPS activation. Further, in many cases a stimulus became increasingly effective when regularly repeated (Fig. 1). This increasing activity could be compared to the "wind-up" phenomenon described by Mendell and Wall (11).

The DCPS fibers have been classified according to their responses to

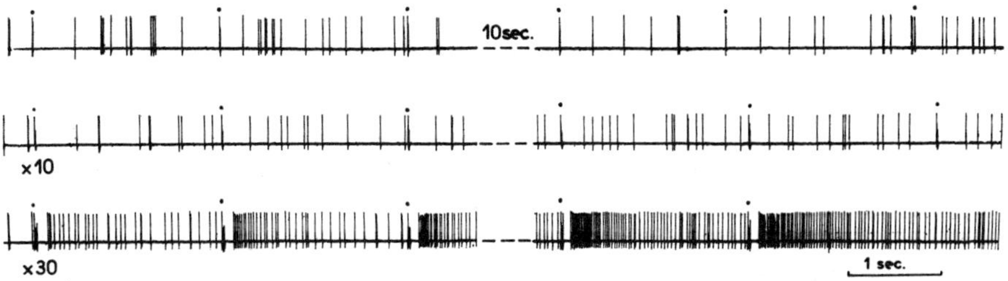

FIG. 1. DCPS fiber activity elicited by repetitive stimulation of the sciatic nerve with shocks of increasing intensity. Top, threshold; middle, 10 times threshold; bottom, 30 times threshold. This last stimulus intensity is very effective in producing the "wind-up" phenomenon. Dots indicate time of stimulation.

natural stimulations. Of the total number of DCPS fibers tested with natural stimuli, 77% showed convergent properties and were characterized by their sensitivity to both gentle and noxious stimuli. They were sensitive to hair movement and to gentle skin distortion. When a fold of skin was successively grasped by the three forceps, slowly adapting responses occurred. A postactivity response was usually present after removing the forceps. The frequency of these evoked tonic discharges increased with the strength of the mechanical stimulus applied (Fig. 2A). The frequency

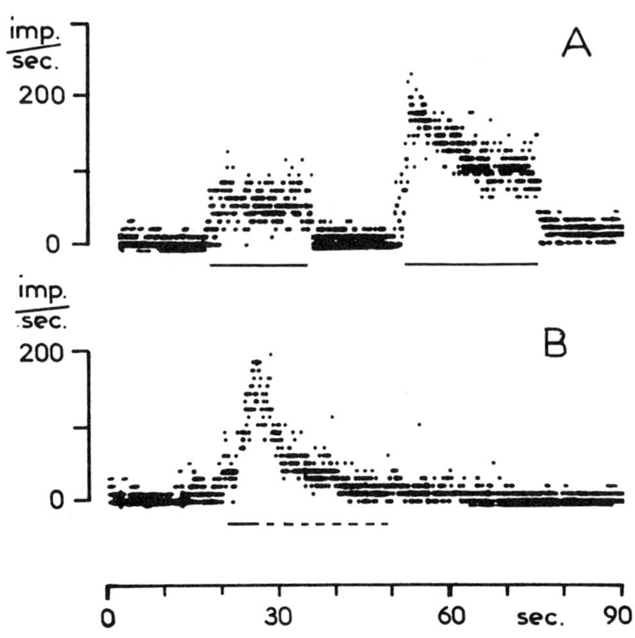

FIG. 2. Mean frequency of responses evoked in a DCPS fiber by noxious stimulation (*bars*). **A:** Noxious mechanical stimuli (*left,* firm clip; *right,* noxious clip). **B:** Noxious radiant heating. Impulses were counted during 100-msec time periods. (From ref. 4.)

reached 150 to 200/sec when the noxious clip was applied. The discharge evoked by the noxious stimulation tended to be both higher in frequency and more regular than the discharge evoked by a nonnoxious one (see ref. 4).

Noxious heating of the skin with radiant heat produced a vigorous discharge (up to 300/sec, Fig. 2B). Contact heating produced a slowly adapting discharge which occurred when the skin surface temperature exceeded 45°C. Properties of the nucleus gracilis cells were compared and contrasted with those of the DCPS axons. More than 30% of the total number of cells investigated were also characterized by a high degree of modality convergence and were sensitive to noxious mechanical and thermal stimuli; the frequency of the sustained discharge evoked by constant mechanical stimulation of the skin increased with the strength of the stimulation. Therefore, the DCPS fibers and the polymodal cells of the nucleus gracilis shared common properties as both of them were characterized by their multimodal input and their responsiveness to noxious stimuli. Further, their firing increased with the damaging quality of the stimulation. The location of the polymodal cells and their physiological properties, together with recent anatomical data (14), were taken to indicate that the polymodal cells were the relays of the impulses conveyed through the DCPS fibers.

DISCUSSION

Therapeutic stimulation of the DC (see refs. 12–16) has been used to produce analgesia according to the gate control theory of pain (9). Nevertheless, the inhibitory effect on pain transmission produced by either DC or cutaneous stimulation did not always occur. Further, a few authors have reported that DC as well as cutaneous stimulation could enhance the effect of pain-producing stimuli (10–16), suggesting a facilitatory role of DC impulses on pain transmission. This facilitatory effect of DC impulses occurred only in severe pain (10). Vierck et al. (18) corroborated this finding in monkey and showed that a DC lesion attenuated the escape-producing quality of a high-intensity stimulation but did not affect escape threshold. Perhaps the increased pain experienced after DC stimulation was directly caused by excitation of the DCPS fibers, i.e., direct influence of the impulses relaying in the polymodal cells on rostral structures involved in pain sensation. Another possible functional role for the DCPS fibers and their bulbar relay can be considered. Burgess (5) has proposed that nociceptor activity might inhibit systems activated by other cutaneous receptors. Such a possible role of the noxious impulses could occur through the discharges of the DCPS fibers and the polymodal cells since these cells would correspond to the small multipolar gracile interneurons (see ref. 4), which were reported to exert an inhibitory influence on transmission through the DC nuclei (2). If this is the function of the DCPS system, its activity would influence the pain experience by reducing the input of a major cutaneous somatosensory pathway to higher centers during noxious stimulation.

In conclusion, the controversy about the effects of a DC lesion or DC stimulation on pain transmission could be related to the intensity of pain considered, and the role played by the DC system might depend on the relative importance of the discharges transmitted by the two sets of DC units: those which are modality specific—the primary afferent fibers and their bulbar relay cells; and those which are modality convergent—the DCPS fibers and the polymodal cells.

ACKNOWLEDGMENTS

The author is indebted to Professor D. Albe-Fessard for all facilities provided during the experiments and for helpful discussion, and to Dr. P. R. Burgess for critical comments.

REFERENCES

1. Albe-Fessard, D. (1968): In: *Pharmacology of Pain, Vol. 9,* edited by R. K. S. Lim, pp. 131–168. Pergamon Press, Oxford and New York.
2. Andersen, P., Eccles, J. C., Schmidt, R. F., and Yokota, T. (1964): *J. Neurophysiol.,* 27:1080–1095.
3. Angaut-Petit, D. (1975*a*): *Exp. Brain Res.,* 22:457–470.
4. Angaut-Petit, D. (1975*b*): *Exp. Brain Res.,* 22:471–493.
5. Burgess, P. R. (1974): In: *Advances in Neurology, Vol. 4: International Symposium on Pain,* edited by J. J. Bonica, pp. 11–18. Raven Press, New York.
6. Foerster, O. (1936): In: *Handbook of Neurology, Vol. 5,* edited by O. Bumke and O. Foerster, pp. 1–403. Springer-Verlag, Berlin.
7. Hillman, P., and Wall, P. D. (1969): *Exp. Brain Res.,* 9:284–306.
8. Mallart, A., and Petit, D. (1963): *J. Physiol. (Paris),* 55:291–292.
9. Melzack, R., and Wall, P. D. (1965): *Science,* 150:971–979.
10. Melzack, R., Wall, P. D., and Weisz, A. Z. (1963): *Exp. Neurol.,* 8:35–46.
11. Mendell, L. M., and Wall, P. D. (1965): *Nature,* 206:97–99.
12. Nashold, B., Somjen, G., and Friedman, H. (1972): *Exp. Neurol.,* 36:273–287.
13. Petit, D. (1972): *Brain Res.,* 48:380–384.
14. Rustioni, A. (1973): *Brain Res.,* 51:81–95.
15. Schiff, J. M. (1858): In: *Lehrbuch der Physiologie des Menschen, Vol. 1, Muskel und Nervenphysiologie,* edited by M. Schöneberg, pp. 1–424. Lahr.
16. Shealy, C. N., Mortimer, J. T., and Hagfors, N. R. (1970): *J. Neurosurg.,* 32:560–564.
17. Uddenberg, N. (1968): *Exp. Brain Res.,* 4:377–382.
18. Vierck, C. J., Hamilton, D. M., and Thornby, J. I. (1971): *Exp. Brain Res.,* 13:140–158.
19. White, J. C., and Sweet, W. H. (1969): In: *Pain and the Neurosurgeon.* Charles C Thomas, Publisher, Springfield, Illinois.

Advances in Pain Research and Therapy, Vol. 1,
edited by J. J. Bonica and D. Albe-Fessard.
Raven Press, New York © 1976.

Collateralization of Reticulothalamic Projections and Its Possible Significance for Pain Sensation

David Bowsher

Neurobiology Laboratory, Department of Anatomy, University of Liverpool, Liverpool L69 3BX, England

It is known, on the basis of Golgi and degeneration studies (6,8,15,17) that there is a substantial input to ventral posterolateral thalamic nuclei (VPL) and other thalamic projection nuclei from the reticular formation. Convergent extralemniscal input to the ventrobasal complex has been physiologically demonstrated (7) and subsequently was quantified by Berkley (3), who found 29% of ventrobasal units showing various types of "unspecific" response in the intact barbiturized cat.

The activation of midbrain reticular formation (MRF) units from the centromedian thalamic nuclei (CM) and ventral posterolateral thalamic nuclei are discussed in this chapter in an attempt to explain the failure of intralaminar thalamotomy to bring about long-lasting changes in either pain sensation or EEG patterns.

MATERIAL AND METHODS

The data presented are taken from experiments performed on 5 adult cats, anesthetized with α-chloralose, immobilized with gallamine, and artificially ventilated. Body temperature was kept constant at 37°C and expiratory CO_2 was monitored and kept at 4%.

Concentric bipolar electrodes were inserted, under physiological control, into the forelimb area of VPL and the anterior plane A 10.0 or A 10.5 and into CM at A 7.0, L 3.0. MRF units were sought and recorded with metal microelectrodes between planes A 2.0 and A 4.0, L 3.0 and L 4.0. [The sensory properties of this area had previously been investigated (9).]

MRF units showing convergent responses to limb stimulation were tested for responses to stimulation of VPL and CM. When such responses were found, antidromicity was tested by (a) ability to follow high frequencies of stimulation without variations in latency (superimposed records on a storage oscilloscope), and (b) cancellation by collision with orthodromic impulses. No activity was considered antidromic unless it satisfied both these criteria.

At the end of every experiment the animal was sacrificed under anesthesia, and stimulating and recording sites subsequently were identified by histological examination.

RESULTS

Fifty midbrain reticular units responding to peripheral stimulation were found to be activated by stimulation of CM or VPL or both. The results are summarized in Table 1. One unit, antidromically activated from VPL, also showed antidromic cell response to CM stimulation. Moreover, two units transsynaptically activated from CM were also driven antidromically from CM. A unit showing antidromic response to stimulation of both CM and VPL is shown in Fig. 1.

TABLE 1. *MRF units with convergent responses to peripheral stimulation*

Site and type of stimulation	Number of units
Antidromically activated from:	
CM and VPL[a]	4
CM only	24
VPL only	1
VPL giving antidromic tract wave in central tegmental tract[b]	8
Transsynaptically activated from:	
CM	14[c]
VPL	1

[a] CM, centromedian thalamic nuclei; VPL, ventral posterolateral thalamic nuclei.
[b] One unit also showed antidromic cell response to CM stimulation.
[c] Two of these units were also driven antidromically from CM.

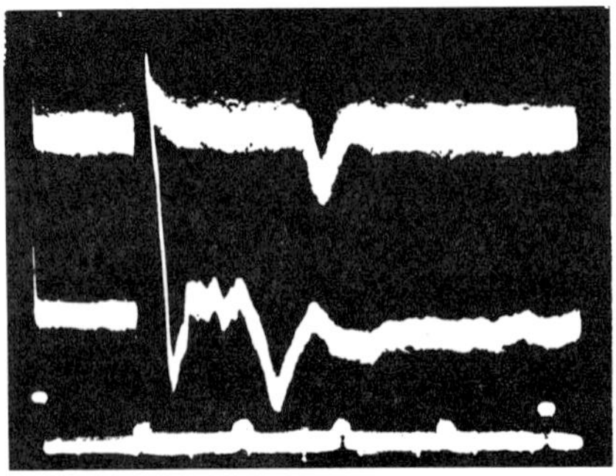

FIG. 1. Antidromic responses of a midbrain reticular unit at A 2.0, L 4.15, H − 1.775 to stimulation of ventral posterolateral thalamic nuclei (*upper trace*) at A 10.0, L 6.0, H + 2.5, and of centromedian thalamic nuclei (*lower trace*) at A 7.0, L 2.5, H + 0.5. Superimposed traces during stimulation at 500 Hz. Time marker, 1 ms.

DISCUSSION

With intracellular recordings in *encéphale isolé* cats, Mancia et al. (12) demonstrated antidromic invasion of both bulbopontine and mesencephalic reticular units from the intralaminar thalamus, as well as transsynaptic excitatory postsynaptic potentials (EPSPs). Fuller (10), using cats anesthetized with halothane and nitrous oxide, recorded the responses of reticular units between planes AP 0 and P 7.0 to stimulation of a large number of diencephalic sites and found that many units were excited from two or three sites; he also recorded a number of transsynaptic responses. Presumably, the antidromic waves found in the central tegmental tract (CTT) in the present study represented the projection to VPL of more caudally placed reticular neurons.

The results obtained by Fuller and the present small sample are consistent with the morphological finding, in Golgi material, of widespread branching of reticular axons (16,17). On the assumption that the ascending reticular system represents the anatomical substrate of second pain (4) as well as of EEG control, we can discuss the functional implication of the findings with reference to Fig. 2. The majority of ascending reticular units project to the intralaminar nuclei of the thalamus, and many send collaterals to other diencephalic nuclei, including one or more of the cortically projecting thalamic nuclei. Thus the telencephalic representation of pain involves most of the cerebral cortex, although not equally in all areas.

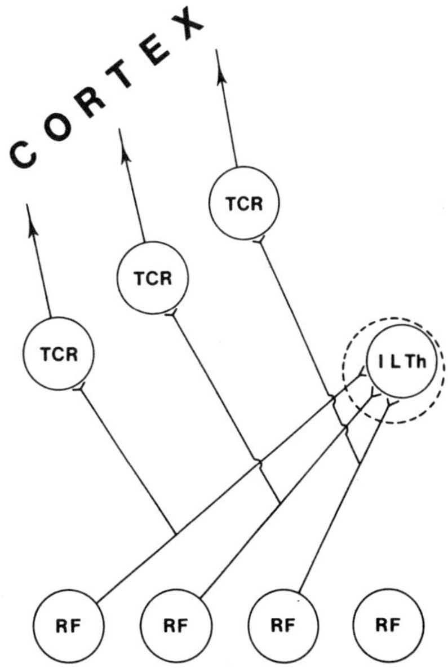

FIG. 2. Schema of projections from midbrain reticular formation (RF) to intralaminar thalamic nuclei (ILTh) and to various thalamocortical relay nuclei (TCR). For further explanation, see text.

A lesion placed within the interrupted circle of Fig. 2, involving the intralaminar nuclei, will also destroy reticulofugal terminations in this area. Such destruction leads to reversible inactivation of collateral axons in other thalamic nuclei, thus temporarily reducing or abolishing the sensation of second pain, which then recurs when the undamaged collateral endings start to function again. This is the usual sequence found after intralaminar thalamotomy.

The best results of thalamotomy appear to be obtained when a lesion involving CM and the adjacent part of VPM is made for facial pain (13). This is consistent with the hypothesis because in such a case reticulofugal endings in both the intralaminar nuclei and the appropriate specific nucleus are destroyed; and it raises the theoretical question as to whether or not double (specific and nonspecific) thalamic lesions are effective for pain at other sites—although of course there are serious drawbacks to such a procedure.

Although a widespread but not dense cortical projection from the intralaminar nuclei has been demonstrated by the methods of retrograde (1,14) and orthograde (5,18) degeneration, antidromic activation (2), retrograde transport of horseradish peroxidase (11), and orthograde transport of tritiated amino acid (D. Bowsher and A. J. Bower, *unpublished observations*), the failure of intralaminar thalamotomy to control pain shows that this projection alone cannot be responsible for painful sensation.

ACKNOWLEDGMENT

The work presented was supported by a grant to the author from the Medical Research Council.

REFERENCES

1. Adrianov, O. S. (1960): *Acta Neurol. Belg.*, 60:704–722.
2. Albe-Fessard, D., Levante, A., and Rokyta, R. (1971): *Int. J. Neurosci.*, 1:327–338.
3. Berkley, K. J. (1973): *J. Neurophysiol.*, 36:940–952.
4. Bowsher, D. (1957): *Brain*, 80:606–622.
5. Bowsher, D. (1966): In: *The Thalamus*, edited by D. P. Purpura and M. D. Yahr, pp. 99–108. Columbia University Press, New York.
6. Bowsher, D. (1967): *C. R. Acad. Sci.* [*D*] (*Paris*), 265:340–342.
7. Bowsher, D. (1971): *Arch. Ital. Biol.*, 109:59–74.
8. Bowsher, D. (1975): *Brain Res.*, 95:211–220.
9. Bowsher, D., and Petit, D. (1970): *J. Physiol.*, 206:663–675.
10. Fuller, J. H. (1974): *Brain Res.*, 83:349–368.
11. Jones, E. G., and Leavitt, R. Y. (1974): *J. Comp. Neurol.*, 154:349–378.
12. Mancia, M., Marginelli, M., Mariotti, M., Spreafico, R., and Broggi, G. (1974): *Brain Res.*, 69:297–314.
13. Mark, V. H., Ervin, F. R., and Yakovlev, P. I. (1962): *Confin. Neurol.*, 22:238–245.
14. Murray, M. (1966): *J. Comp. Neurol.*, 127:341–367.
15. Nauta, W. J. H., and Kuypers, H. G. J. M. (1958): In: *Reticular Formation of the Brain*, edited by H. H. Jasper, L. D. Proctor, R. S. Knighton, W. C. Noshay, and R. D. Costello, pp. 3–30. Little, Brown, and Co., Boston.

16. Scheibel, M. E., and Scheibel, A. B. (1958): In: *Reticular Formation of the Brain,* edited by H. H. Jasper et al., pp. 31–55. Little, Brown, and Co., Boston.
17. Scheibel, M. E., and Scheibel, A. B. (1966): In: *The Thalamus,* edited by D. P. Purpura and M. D. Yahr, pp. 13–46. Columbia University Press, New York.
18. Totibadze, N. K., and Moniava, E. S. (1969): *J. Comp. Neurol.,* 137:347–360.

Advances in Pain Research and Therapy, Vol. 1,
edited by J. J. Bonica and D. Albe-Fessard.
Raven Press, New York © 1976.

Human Spinothalamic Tract—Stimulation Mapping in the Spinal Cord and Brainstem

R. R. Tasker, L. W. Organ,* I. H. Rowe,** and P. Hawrylyshyn

*Department of Surgery, University of Toronto, Division of Neurosurgery, Toronto General Hospital, Toronto, Canada; and Departments of *Physiology and **Electrical Engineering, University of Toronto, Toronto, Canada*

The neospinothalamic tract has always been an elusive structure to study in the laboratory because of the impossibility of providing a pure pain stimulus or measuring a pure pain response. In 240 percutaneous cordotomies and 130 computer-plotted stereotactic procedures performed on conscious man in which electrical stimulation was used for physiological localization, we have attempted to take advantage of the ability to communicate with the patient in order to trace the course of the neospinothalamic tract in the spinal cord, midbrain, and thalamus.

METHODS

Percutaneous cordotomy is carried out by the lateral approach at the C_1-C_2 interspace by the method described by Tasker et al. (4). Threshold stimulation of the cord is performed with a sharpened 0.4-mm Teflon®-insulated stainless steel monopolar electrode at a depth of 2 mm beneath the pia using trains of 100-Hz negative 3-ms rectangular waves.

Stereotactic procedures for the relief of either involuntary movement or intractable pain are performed by the author's method (3). Threshold stimulation is carried out with a bipolar 1.1-mm concentric electrode with 0.5-mm pole separation using trains of 60- to 100-Hz biphasic 3-ms square waves, and the results are plotted graphically in the form of Woolsey-type figurine charts on line (6) by computer.

RESULTS

We traced the human neospinothalamic tract by observing: the quality of hallucinatory response induced by threshold stimulation, the somatotopographic organization of the body parts to which the hallucination is referred, the somatosensory deficit produced by a lesion, and autopsy studies of electrode tracts and lesion sites.

Observations in Spinal Cord

Experience in the anatomically less sophisticated spinal cord is reviewed first.

We recognize the induction by stimulation of a warm or cool tingling in some part of the contralateral body as evidence that the electrode lies within the spinothalamic tract. For ideal sites where lesions produced solid analgesia, the stimulation-induced hallucination was described as warm or hot tingling in 70% of cases, cool or cold tingling in 24%, burning or painful in 5%, and tingling in 1%. At such sites lesions invariably resulted in persistent dissociated analgesia of large parts of the body and in thermanalgesia in virtually the same area. Lesions at sites where stimulation resulted in responses other than temperature-coded tingling were much less successful. The effects of stimulation of the spinothalamic tract were always referred to the contralateral half of the body, but in 12% of cases they flowed over to a small portion of the ipsilateral side as well. Ipsilateral responses have never been seen alone, and analgesia induced by lesions has always been contralateral.

The somatotopographic organization of the spinothalamic tract is readily discernible during cordotomy. As the cordotomy electrode is systematically manipulated in a given patient from ventral to dorsal across the spinothalamic tract, the body region in which the stimulation-induced hallucination is felt and the region of lesion-induced analgesia progress systematically through the side of the neck, radial aspect of the shoulder, arm, forearm and hand, digits 1 through 5, ulnar aspect of the hand, forearm and arm, trunk, lower extremity, and perineum.

A similar conclusion is reached by reviewing pooled data from a series of patients, comparing the body sites to which stimulation-induced responses are referred when different cord sites are stimulated as shown in Table 1. Sites were deemed "too anterior" or "too posterior" when motor responses to stimulation indicated activation of ventral horn or pyramidal tract,

TABLE 1. *Body sites responsive to spinal cord stimulation*

Location of stimulation-induced response	Electrode position with respect to spinothalamic tract (% responses)			
	Too anterior	Central	Posterior	Too posterior
Neck	26	4	0	9
Upper extremity	19	38	24	7
Trunk	14	15	13	7
Lower extremity	9	17	21	34
Whole side of body	2	17	28	4
Other	30	9	14	49

respectively. "Central" and "posterior" locations within the spinothalamic tract were determined by the distribution of lesion-induced analgesia.

In conclusion, the spinothalamic tract can be identified by stimulation of the cord in conscious man by the induction of a contralateral sensation of cool or warm tingling. Clear-cut dorsoventral somatotopic organization of cord fibers is easily recognizable. The results of lesion making and autopsy studies support these conclusions.

Observations in the Midbrain

Stimulation of the brainstem in conscious man during stereotactic surgery permits the recognition of the primary sensory pathways (auditory, vestibular, visual, lemniscal, and spinothalamic) by means of the induction of stereotyped, specific, invariable responses similar to those reported from cerebral cortex. When stimulation data from the upper midbrain between 5 and 12 mm from the midline obtained in 32 stereotactic procedures performed for the relief of intractable pain are examined, a situation analogous to that reported in the cord is found. Between 9 and 12 mm from the midline, low-threshold stimulation induces a contralateral feeling of tingling, vibration, or electric shock at sites that coincide with the course of the medial lemniscus. In 1 patient a lesion made deliberately in this pathway induced the contralateral loss of all modalities of sensation, strongly suggesting that the pathway is indeed the medial lemniscus, and in 2 patients autopsy confirmation was possible (5).

Immediately contiguous dorsal and medial to these medial lemniscal responses stimulation almost invariably induces a response of a different character as shown in Fig. 1. It is not a feeling of vibration, electric shock, or tingling, but of cool or warm tingling, burning, or, rarely, pain. Although such responses are always referred to the contralateral half of the body, approximately 10% are also referred to a smaller portion of the ipsilateral body. Immediately dorsal to such responses, auditory and vestibular responses are readily identified just deep to the pial surface. When plotted by computer on an atlas diagram, these sites fall where the spinothalamic fibers have been located anatomically, sandwiched between the medial lemniscus ventrolaterally and the lateral lemniscus and brachium of inferior colliculus dorsally. That such responses arise from stimulation of the spinothalamic tract has been confirmed in 25 stereotactic procedures in which lesions made at sites generating such responses invariably produced dissociated analgesia and thermanalgesia. On one occasion autopsy confirmation was possible (5).

The somatotopographic organization of the mesencephalic spinothalamic tract is such that the closer a lesion lies to the medial lemniscus, the dermatomally higher the analgesia, suggesting a vertically upside-down arrangement.

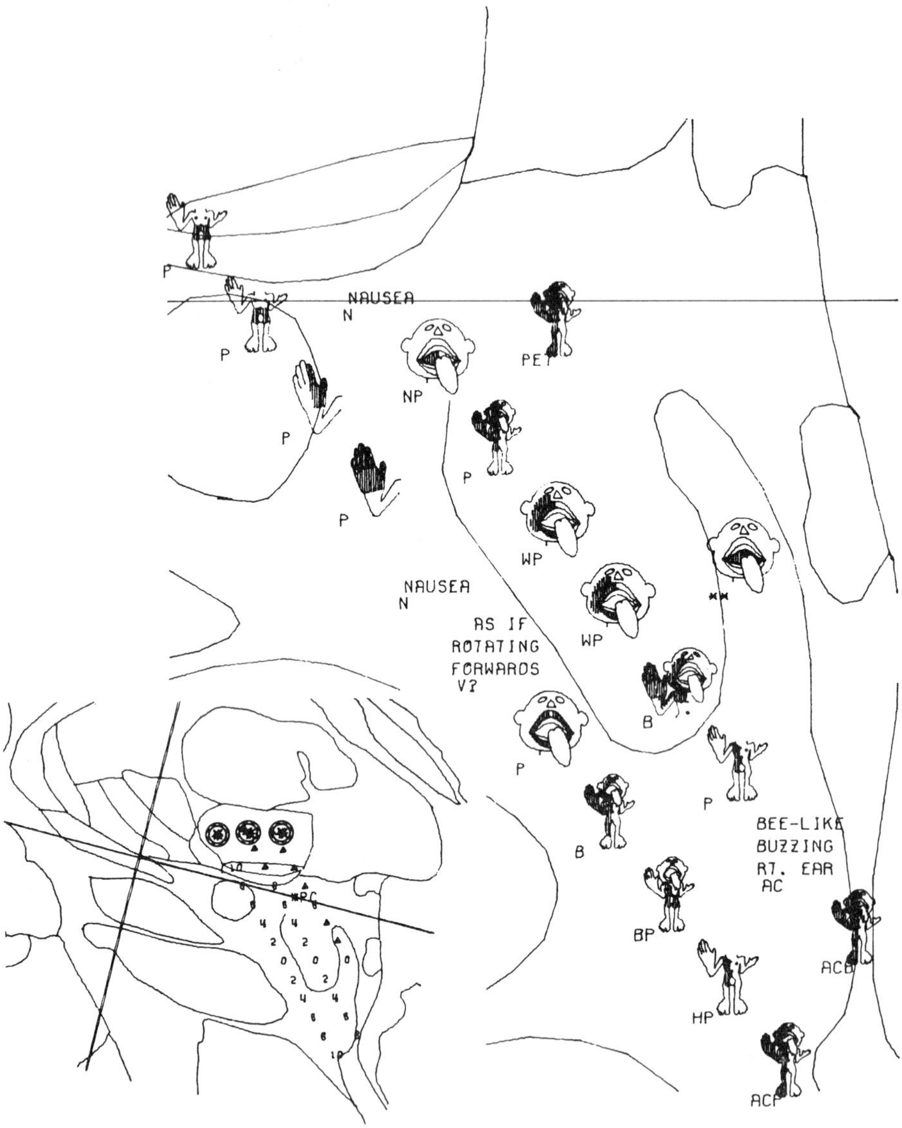

FIG. 1. Unedited computer plot of data obtained by stimulating left midbrain at 9 mm from the midline. Inset locates stimulation and lesion sites (*stars*) on the computer-fitted atlas diagram (2). Body sites to which stimulation-induced responses were referred are indicated by Woolsey-type figurine charts: P, paresthesia; N, nausea; V, vertigo; B, burning; H, hot; AC, contralateral auditory; W, warm; E, emotional sensations. All somatosensory responses were contralateral. Double asterisks indicate ipsilateral head pain caused by pial stimulation. Note the general dorsal position of the temperature-coded responses, representing spinothalamic sites and their interposition between medial lemniscal (paresthetic) and auditory sites at the dorsum of the midbrain.

Observations in Thalamus

The major portion of the electrically excitable somatosensory thalamus between 9 and 18 mm lateral gives rise to a feeling of tingling, vibration, or shock on the contralateral side of the body and constitutes the thalamic relay for the medial lemniscus, somatotopographically organized from medial to lateral. However, inferior and posterior to such responses between 14 and 17 mm from the midline, a different type of response (Fig. 2) is described as warm or cool tingling, and occasionally as burning or painful. Moreover, these responses, although always contralateral, may also involve a portion of the ipsilateral half of the body, unlike those of the medial lemniscal system. When these responses are plotted they occupy the thalamus between the more anterior lemniscal responses in the ventrobasal complex and the auditory and vestibular responses of the medial geniculate body located posteriorly, as seen in Fig. 2. On three occasions lesions made in this region of the thalamus induced dissociated analgesia and thermanalgesia as reported by Hassler (2). On one occasion autopsy studies localized such sites to the posterior thalamic nuclei (5). We believe they arise from the thalamic relay of the spinothalamic tract.

In contrast to the clear-cut mediolateral organization of the thalamic lemniscal relay, the somatotopy in this area is differently organized. As soon as a stimulating electrode enters this region, the homuncular continuity of the responses is disrupted, the change occurring coincident with that observed in the quality of the responses, as is shown in Fig. 2. A study of our data suggests that the somatotopographic organization here is dorsoventral, as if the spinothalamic homunculus were standing on the auditory portion of the medial geniculate body (1).

In summary, the spinothalamic tract may be recognized by stimulation of the human brainstem by the same features as those observed in the spinal cord.

SUMMARY

In 240 percutaneous cordotomies and 130 computer-plotted stereotactic procedures in which electrical stimulation of the central nervous system was the means of physiological localization, we traced the neospinothalamic tract through the spinal cord, midbrain, and thalamus. Its stimulation in conscious man gives rise to the hallucination of warm or cool tingling, and less often of burning or pain, referred to some portion of the contralateral half of the body, and in 10% to 15% bilaterally. The site of reference indicates a somatotopographic organization distinct from that of the lemniscal system. The course of the neospinothalamic tract passes through the ventrolateral quadrant of the spinal cord. In the dorsal midbrain it lies sandwiched between the medial lemniscus ventrolaterally and

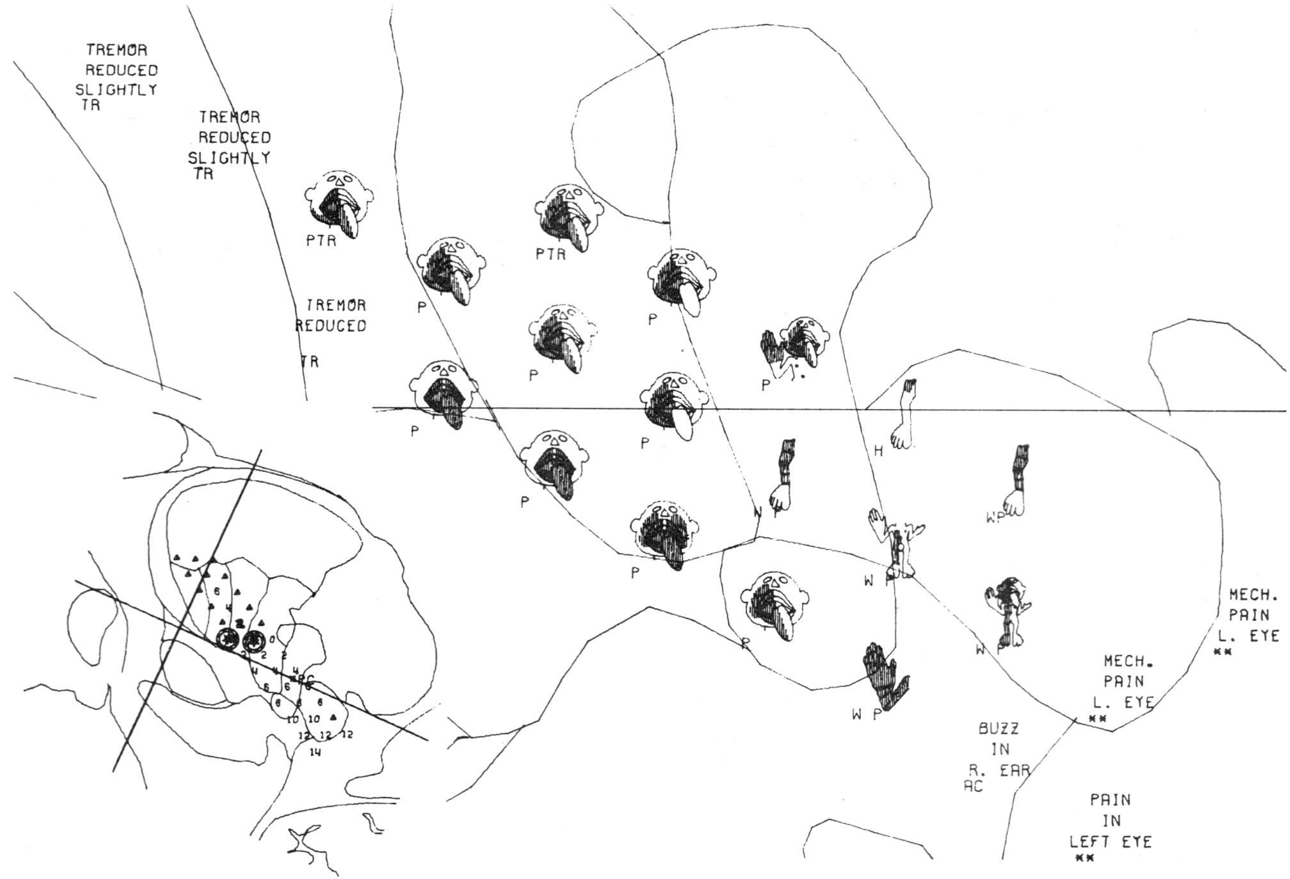

FIG. 2. Same format as in Fig. 1. Stimulation of left brainstem 14 mm from the midline. Note sharp break in continuity between the paresthetic face responses of the lemniscal relay superoanteriorly in thalamus and the temperature-coded trunk and leg responses of the spinothalamic relay posteroinferiorly, adjacent to auditory region of the medial geniculate near pial surface of the brainstem.

the auditory path in the lateral lemniscus dorsally, both readily identified by stimulation. In thalamus it lies posteroinferior to the lemniscal relay in the ventrobasal complex filling the structures between the latter and the auditory responses of the medial geniculate body. Its location has been further confirmed by the production of dissociated sensory loss by lesions along its course, and in a few cases by autopsy studies.

ACKNOWLEDGMENTS

This work was supported in part by grants from the Toronto General Hospital Foundation and the Ontario Ministry of Health.

REFERENCES

1. Emmers, R., and Tasker, R. R. (1975): *The Human Somesthetic Thalamus.* Raven Press, New York.
2. Hassler, R. (1959): In: *Introduction to Stereotaxis with an Atlas of the Human Brain, Vol. 1,* edited by G. Schaltenbrand and P. Bailey. Georg Thieme Verlag, Stuttgart.
3. Tasker, R. R., and Organ, L. W. (1972): In: *Neurophysiology Studied in Man,* edited by G. G. Somjen, pp. 169–187. Excerpta Medica, Amsterdam.
4. Tasker, R. R., Organ, L. W., and Smith, K. C. (1974): *Acta Neurochir.* (*Wien*), Suppl. 21:111–117.
5. Tasker, R. R., Richardson, P., Rewcastle, B., and Emmers, R. (1972): *Confin. Neurol.,* 34:184–196.
6. Tasker, R. R., Rowe, I. H., Hawrylyshyn, P., and Organ, L. W. (1976): *J. Neurosurg.,* 44:458–464.

Advances in Pain Research and Therapy, Vol. 1,
edited by J. J. Bonica and D. Albe-Fessard.
Raven Press, New York © 1976.

Effects of Nociceptive and Innocuous Stimuli on the Firing Patterns of Single Neurons in the Feline Nucleus Reticularis Gigantocellularis

Gary S. Pearl and Kenneth V. Anderson

Department of Anatomy, Emory University, Atlanta, Georgia 30322

In recent years, neurophysiological (5–7,10–12,14) and behavioral (3,8,13) evidence has been accumulated suggesting a role for nucleus reticularis gigantocellularis (NGC) in nociception. Anatomical studies (4,17) have shown that spinal afferents project primarily to the caudal half of this nucleus, and behavioral studies (3) clearly show that this is the area of NGC most intimately involved in nociception. Although some investigators have shown that neurons in caudal NGC respond either exclusively or maximally to nociceptive stimuli (6,7,11), systematic studies of firing patterns of NGC neurons to such stimuli have not been reported, and receptive fields of NGC neurons have not been delineated using nociceptive stimuli. Further, since NGC is involved in processing nociceptive information, it was considered important to determine the effect of clinical procedures used to alleviate pain in human patients, such as high-frequency dorsal column (16,19,20) and peripheral nerve (15,16,21) stimulation, on the neuronal responses in NGC to nociceptive stimuli.

MATERIALS AND METHODS

In the first phase of this research, single cells were isolated in the caudal NGC [P 7.0 to 10.0; L 1.0 to 2.0; H (−)6.0 to (−)9.0] of 31 cats anesthetized with pentobarbital sodium. The responses of 162 NGC neurons to stimulation of the ipsilateral and contralateral canine tooth pulp (0.10 to 0.40 mA, 0.5 to 0.8 Hz, 0.1 msec PD), superficial radial nerve (0.15 to 0.75 mA, 0.5 to 0.8 Hz, 0.1 msec PD), and sciatic nerve (0.15 to 0.75 mA, 0.5 to 0.8 Hz, 0.1 msec PD) were studied using computer analysis techniques. Post-stimulus-time histograms (PSTs) were computed from the data that resulted from 100 consecutive presentations of a particular type of stimulation. The tooth pulp was chosen as a primary stimulus site because stimulation of the tooth pulp elicits only pain and prepain sensations in humans (18) and selectively activates A-delta (1) and C (2) fibers in the cat. After PSTs had been computed for all of the test stimuli, receptive fields were delineated for each neuron using natural noxious (pinch and prick) and innocuous (light pressure and touch) stimuli.

In the second phase of this research, we studied responses of NGC neurons before, during, and for up to 1.5 hr after high-frequency stimulation of the dorsal columns (0.15 to 0.45 mA, 50 to 100 Hz, 0.1 msec PD), superficial radial or sciatic nerve (0.15 to 0.70 mA, 50 to 100 Hz, 0.1 msec PD), or tooth pulp (0.10 to 0.15 mA, 50 to 100 Hz, 0.1 msec PD). When high-frequency peripheral nerve stimulation served as the conditioning stimulus, two procedures were used. In the first procedure, the conditioning and test electrodes were both placed on either the sciatic or the superficial radial nerve, with the conditioning electrode either proximal or distal to the test electrode. In the second procedure, either the sciatic or the superficial radial nerve was split longitudinally, and the conditioning and test electrodes were placed on separate segments of the nerve. The purpose of this phase of the research was to determine the effects of high-frequency conditioning stimulation on neuronal responses in NGC to sensory stimulation.

RESULTS

Responses of NGC Neurons to Electrical Stimulation

Neurons in NGC responded to nociceptive stimuli in one of four ways: (a) 51% of the cells studied responded to stimuli with a short-latency, short-duration excitatory period followed by a prolonged period of suppressed activity, relative to control levels (E-S unit); (b) 25% of the cells studied responded only with a short-latency excitatory period (E unit); (c) 6% of the cells studied responded only with a prolonged period of suppressed activity (S unit); and (d) 18% of the cells studied had mixed responses (M unit), with the response depending on the type of stimulus presented. Of the M units studied, 67% had E and E-S responses, 6% had E and S responses, and 27% had E-S and S responses. Figure 1 shows the responses of an M unit with E (frame 4) and E-S (frames 2 and 3) responses, Fig. 2 shows the responses of an M unit with E (frame 1) and S (frames 3 and 4) responses, and Fig. 3 shows the responses of an E unit.

Responses of NGC Neurons to Natural Stimulation

Receptive fields were determined for 127 neurons in NGC. Of the units studied, all responded to noxious stimulation of the face, body, or both, although none responded only to innocuous stimulation. Of the neurons that responded to noxious stimulation, 17 (13%) also responded to innocuous stimulation of some part of the face or body from which a re-

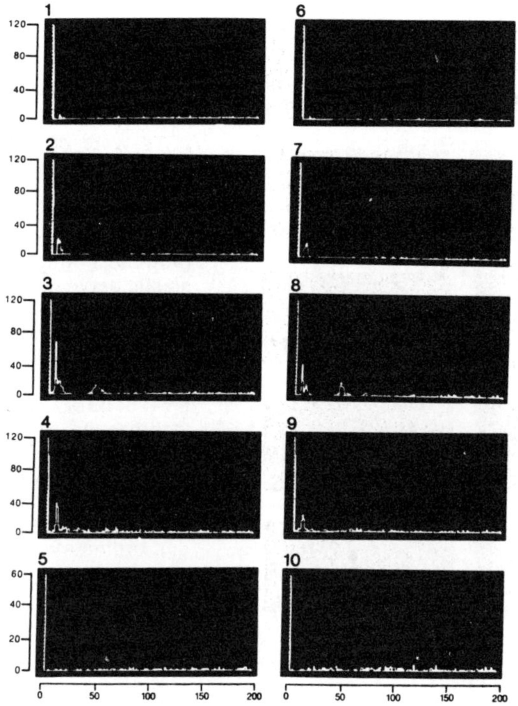

FIG. 1. Effect of high-frequency dorsal column stimulation on an M unit in nucleus reticularis gigantocellularis. Frames 1–4, post-stimulus-time histograms (PSTs) of this neuron without conditioning stimulation; frames 6–9, PSTs with conditioning stimulation. Frames 5 and 10 are control histograms without and with conditioning stimulation, respectively. PSTs were computed after stimulation of the ipsilateral upper canine tooth (frames 1 and 6), contralateral upper canine tooth (frames 2 and 7), contralateral superficial radial nerve (frames 3 and 8), and contralateral sciatic nerve (frames 4 and 9). The number of responses to stimulation of the superficial radial (frame 8) and sciatic (frame 9) nerves were reduced by conditioning stimulation. The abscissa is calibrated in bins, each with a 5.0-msec bin width, and the ordinate is calibrated in spikes per bin.

sponse to nociceptive stimulation could be elicited. In these latter units, however, the responses to nociceptive stimulation were always more vigorous than the responses to innocuous stimulation.

Most of the receptive fields for NGC neurons were large, discontinuous, and bilaterally symmetrical. Units with unilateral receptive fields responded more frequently to stimulation of contralateral body areas than to ipsilateral body areas. Further, more units responded to stimulation of the face (70%) and forelimbs (70% ipsilateral, 77% contralateral) than to the hind limbs (40% ipsilateral, 44% contralateral). Few neurons responded to stimulation of the trunk (9%) and tail (17%). Of the units studied, 77 (61%) responded to stimulation of the face, body, and teeth, and 103 (81%) responded to stimulation of two or more of these areas.

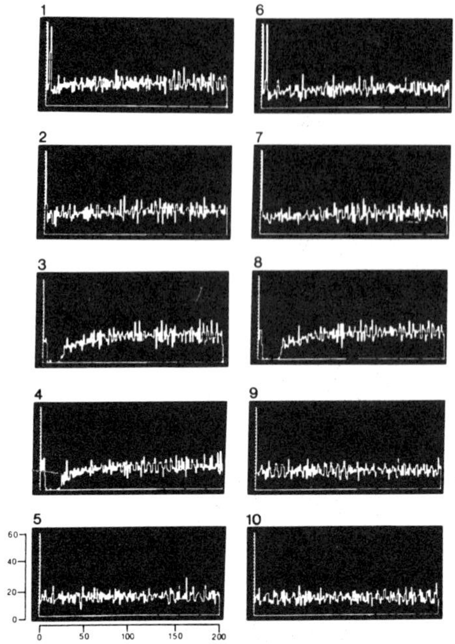

FIG. 2. Effect of high-frequency sciatic nerve stimulation on an M unit in NGC. PSTs were computed to stimulation of the ipsilateral lower canine tooth (frames 1 and 6), contralateral lower canine tooth (frames 2 and 7), contralateral superficial radial nerve (frames 3 and 8), and contralateral sciatic nerve (frames 4 and 9). PSTs in frames 1–4 were computed without conditioning stimulation, those in frames 6–9, with concomitant conditioning stimulation. Frames 5 and 10 are control histograms computed without and with conditioning stimulation, respectively. Response to sciatic nerve stimulation (frame 9) is blocked by conditioning stimulation applied to the sciatic nerve. Abscissa and ordinate as in Fig. 1.

Effects of High-Frequency Conditioning Stimulation on Neuronal Responses in NGC

The effects of dorsal column stimulation on neuronal responses in NGC were studied on 35 neurons. Dorsal column stimulation never completely blocked neuronal responses in NGC to sensory stimulation, although the amplitudes of PSTs to superficial radial and sciatic nerve stimulation were somewhat reduced in 10 of the units studied. The responses to tooth pulp stimulation were never altered by dorsal column stimulation. Figure 1 shows the responses of a neuron that was affected by dorsal column stimulation.

Two procedures were used to test the effect of high-frequency peripheral spinal nerve stimulation on neuronal responses in NGC. The first procedure, in which the test and conditioning electrodes were placed on the same nerve, was tested on 18 NGC neurons. In one case neuronal excitation after stimulation of the superficial radial nerve was reduced by conditioning stimulation of the superficial radial nerve when the conditioning electrode was proximal to the test electrode. In another case unit responsiveness was reduced when the conditioning electrode was distal to the test electrode. In the other 16 cases, high-frequency peripheral nerve stimulation had no effect on neuronal responses. The second procedure, in which the conditioning and test electrodes were placed on different divisions of a nerve,

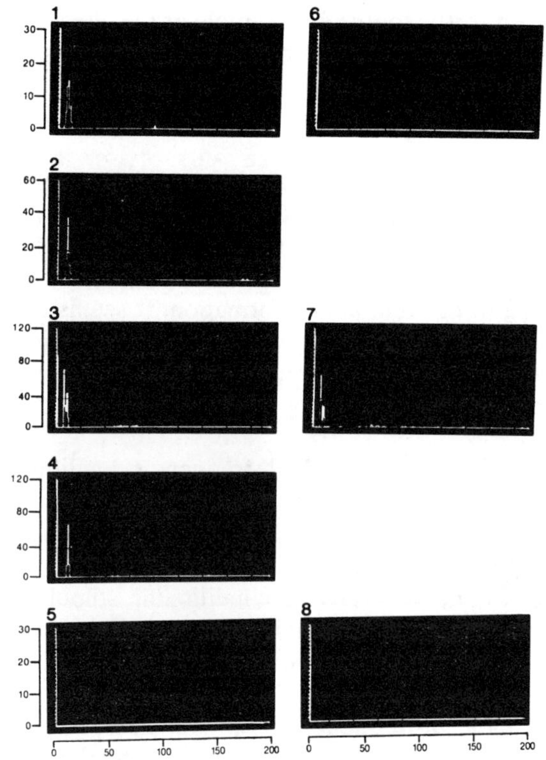

FIG. 3. Effect of high-frequency tooth pulp stimulation on an E unit in NGC. PSTs were computed to stimulation of the ipsilateral lower canine tooth (frames 1 and 6), contralateral lower canine tooth (frame 2), contralateral superficial radial nerve (frames 3 and 7), and contralateral sciatic nerve (frame 4). PSTs in frames 1–4 were computed without conditioning stimulation, and those in frames 6 and 7, with concomitant conditioning stimulation. Frames 5 and 8 are control histograms without and with conditioning stimulation, respectively. Response to stimulation of the ipsilateral canine tooth (frame 6) is blocked by conditioning stimulation. Abscissa and ordinate as in Fig. 1.

was tested on 30 NGC neurons. With this procedure neuronal responsivity to the test stimulus was consistently reduced (75% to 85%) or abolished during and for up to 1.5 hr after 10 min of conditioning stimulation. The responses to other sensory stimuli (tooth pulp and superficial radial or sciatic nerve) were never affected by the conditioning stimulation. An example of the effect of high-frequency sciatic nerve stimulation on neuronal responses in NGC to sensory stimulation is shown in Fig. 2.

High-frequency conditioning stimulation of the contralateral canine tooth was used as a conditioning stimulus on four NGC neurons. In each case the response to stimulation of the ipsilateral canine tooth was abolished during and for up to 1.5 hr after 10 min of conditioning stimulation. The responses to spinal nerve stimulation were not affected by conditioning stimulation applied to the tooth. An example of the effect of high-frequency tooth pulp stimulation on neuronal responses in NGC is shown in Fig. 3.

DISCUSSION

Caudal NGC neurons were activated primarily by nociceptive stimuli, and each neuron was responsive to stimulation of large discontinuous areas of the body, face, or both. These findings indicate that NGC may be intimately involved in nociception and that its primary role is probably not the processing of discrete pain information. It seems that NGC may be involved in one or more of the following: (a) the processing of diffuse pain sensations; (b) the elaboration of affective reactions to pain (9); (c) sensory-motor integration [NGC neurons are known to project to spinal cord motor neurons (22)].

The results of the studies on high-frequency conditioning stimulation indicate that conditioning procedures do not act directly on NGC neurons since dorsal column stimulation had no consistent effect on neuronal sensory excitability and peripheral nerve stimulation affected only the responses to stimulation of the nerve receiving conditioning stimulation. These findings, together with the fact that conditioning stimulation was most effective when the test and conditioning stimuli were not applied to the same nerve fibers, strongly suggest that a "gating" mechanism, somewhere in the CNS, is operative during high-frequency peripheral nerve stimulation. Further studies are necessary to determine where this "gating" occurs.

ACKNOWLEDGMENTS

This investigation was supported by Grant 5 F12 GM 56036, a Medical Scientist Award, to G.S.P., from N.I.G.M.S.

REFERENCES

1. Anderson, K. V., and Pearl, G. S. (1974): *Exp. Neurol.,* 43:281–283.
2. Anderson, K. V., and Pearl, G. S. (1975): *Exp. Neurol.,* 47:357–359.
3. Anderson, K. V., and Pearl, G. S.: *Unpublished observations.*
4. Bowsher, D. (1957): *Brain,* 80:606–623.
5. Bowsher, D., Mallart, A., Petit, D., and Albe-Fessard, D. (1968): *J. Neurophysiol.,* 31:288–300.
6. Casey, K. L. (1969): *Exp. Neurol.,* 25:35–56.
7. Casey, K. L. (1971*a*): *Int. J. Neurosci.,* 2:15–28.
8. Casey, K. L. (1971*b*): *Int. J. Neurosci.,* 2:29–34.
9. Casey, K. L. (1973): *Am. Sci.,* 61:194–200.
10. Casey, K. L., Keene, J. J., and Morrow, T. (1974): *Adv. Neurol.,* 4:197–205.
11. Goldman, P. L., Collins, W. F., Taub, A., and Fitzmartin, J. (1972): *Exp. Neurol.,* 37: 597–606.
12. Guilbaud, G., Besson, J. M., Oliveras, J. L., and Wyon-Maillard, M. C. (1973): *Brain Res.,* 63:131–140.
13. Keene, J. J., and Casey, K. L. (1970): *Exp. Neurol.,* 28:155–166.

14. LeBlanc, H. J., and Gatipon, G. B. (1974): *Exp. Neurol.,* 42:264–273.
15. Long, D. M. (1973): *J. Neurosurg.,* 39:718–722.
16. Long, D. M., and Hagfors, N. (1975): *Pain,* 1:109–123.
17. Mehler, W. R., Feferman, M. E., and Nauta, W. J. H. (1960): *Brain,* 83:718–750.
18. Mumford, J. M. (1965): *Arch. Oral Biol.,* 10:957–968.
19. Nashold, B. S., and Friedman, H. (1972): *J. Neurosurg.,* 36:590–597.
20. Shealy, C. N., Mortimer, J. T., and Hagfors, N. R. (1970): *J. Neurosurg.,* 32:560–564.
21. Wall, P. D., and Sweet, W. H. (1967): *Science,* 155:108–109.
22. Wolstencroft, J. H. (1964): *J. Physiol.* (*Lond.*), 174:91–108.

Advances in Pain Research and Therapy, Vol. 1,
edited by J. J. Bonica and D. Albe-Fessard.
Raven Press, New York © 1976.

Body Representation in the Anterolateral Funiculus as Reconstructed by Percutaneous Cordotomies for Benign Intractable Pain

*Richard J. Schneider and **Ronald L. Paul

**Division of Neurosurgery, University of Maryland Hospital, Baltimore, Maryland 21201; and **York Hospital, York, Pennsylvania 17403*

The anterolateral funiculus was established as an area of the spinal cord through which pain fibers ascended by Spiller (16) on the basis of a patient who had lost pain and temperature sensation in the lower half of his body and at postmortem examination was found to have bilateral anterolateral tuberculomas. According to White and Sweet (19), the anterolateral cordotomy for the relief of pain was employed experimentally by Schüller as a result of this discovery and was developed on a clinical basis by Martin, Beer, Foerster, Tietze, and Frazier.

Anatomical studies have traced the termination of the anterolateral pain pathway (spinothalamic tract) and differentiated two components. There is a pontine and mesencephalic converging component, the information of which is conducted to the nucleus centralis lateralis of the thalamus (paleospinothalamic tract) and a component (neospinothalamic tract) ending in the ventroposterior thalamic nuclei (2–6,8–12). Studies of the spinal distribution of the spinothalamic fibers have suggested a laminar arrangement with caudal dermatomes most lateral and rostral dermatomes most medial (14, 18). In addition, several authors have interpreted their results as suggesting a slight dorsal displacement of caudal dermatomes when compared with rostral dermatomes at rostral levels of the spinal cord (7,15,17).

METHODS

During percutaneous cordotomies, low-voltage (0.1 V) electrical stimulation was delivered via an electrode (100-μm tip) insulated to within 3 mm of the tip. The depth of the tip within the spinal cord was measured, and the patient's report as to the body area affected by this stimulation was recorded. Thus for each penetration the body position relative to depth could be compared. The position of each penetration was reconstructed on a C_2 spinal cord segment template from X-rays taken at the time of electrode insertion.

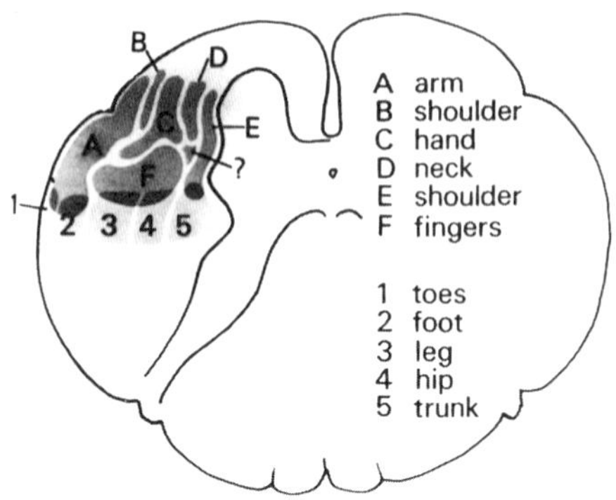

FIG. 1. A map of the representation of the spinothalamic tract in the cervical spinal cord at C_2. Note orderly arrangement of hindlimb dermatomes, split representation of some rostral dermatomes ("?" refers to several readings from the arm), and isolated, enlarged representation of distal forelimb body areas. Also note that readings occupy area of ventral spinocerebellar tract, and overlap between body areas occurs. Both of these findings may have resulted from the long exposure at the electrode tip, although the former finding may also have resulted from failure of afferent activity in the ventral spinocerebellar tract to reach consciousness.

RESULTS

A composite of penetrations from 10 patients was assembled from which a map of our findings was composed (Fig. 1). We wish to emphasize the following findings from the map. The caudal dermatomes were located dorsally in the anterolateral white matter; there they displayed an orderly arrangement progressing from apical body areas to proximal areas as one moves from the superficial to the deep white matter. As one moves anteriorly in the quadrant, some rostral body parts become superficial (arm), some tend to have split representations (shoulder), and some have uniquely separate representations (hand and fingers). The hand and fingers occupied relatively greater nervous system area than body surface area.

Radiofrequency lesions (60 to 100 mA) for 20 to 30 sec produced the most satisfactory analgesia. However, of 6 patients on whom satisfactory analgesia was produced at the time of operation, only 3 retained a satisfactory level after 6 months.

DISCUSSION

The results from these procedures in regard to the body representation must be regarded as fortuitous rather than systematic. With tip exposures of 3 mm and no certain means of localization, it is not surprising to find overlap of body areas as well as many debatable results. Thus it is reasonable to ask if there is any justification to our observations. Three grounds may be cited for such support.

First, the anatomical papers purporting to demonstrate lamination have done so only in the broadest sense, admitting that much segmental overlap existed. Weaver and Walker (18) qualified their statements by writing ". . . there is no absolute segmental lamination." Indeed, high cervical lesions to the spinothalamic tract when examined at cervical levels slightly above the lesion tend to show broad bands of degeneration from lateral to medial (14), and extreme caudal lesions are not used in demonstrating lamination in the cervical cord.

Second, Walker's (17) idea of the lamination in the cervical cord of monkeys and findings of no evidence for the customary somatotopy in the ventroposterior lateral thalamic nuclei (2,8) are difficult to reconcile. Anatomical studies involving selective lesions of the isolated spinothalamic tract are difficult to accomplish. Physiological studies of the body representation in experimental animals have been done in the lumbar, not the cervical, spinal cord (1) and thus the region we were exploring has not been probed.

Third, a rearrangement within as well as between the ascending dermatomal laminations may occur as fibers ascend to high cervical levels. When such a rearrangement occurs, all dermatomes relating to a body part (e.g., leg, foot, hip) are brought together. That this may not have yet happened for the rostral dermatomes may explain their disorder on the map as well as Mullan's difficulty in obtaining selective lesions of arm or trunk during percutaneous cordotomies performed at the same cervical segment (13). Such rearrangements have been shown to occur in the dorsal funiculi (20).

CONCLUSION

The segmental lamination of the spinothalamic tract does not appear in our observations of the human C_2 segment. We believe that reasons beyond our admitted experimental uncertainty may account for this.

REFERENCES

1. Applebaum, A. E., Beall, J. E., Foreman, R. D., and Willis, W. D. (1975): *J. Neurophysiol.,* 38:572–586.
2. Boivie, J. (1971): *Exp. Brain Res.,* 12:331–353.
3. Bowsher, D. (1957): *Brain,* 80:606–622.
4. Bowsher, D. (1960): *J. Neurol. Neurosurg. Psychiatry,* 23:351.
5. Bowsher, D. (1962): *Psychiatr. Neurol.,* 143:75–99.
6. Clark, W. E. Le Gros (1936): *J. Anat.,* 71:1–40.
7. Hyndman, O. R., and Van Epps, C. (1939): *Arch. Surg.,* 38:1036–1053.
8. Kerr, F. W. L., and Lippman, H. H. (1974): In: *Advances in Neurology, Vol. 4: International Symposium on Pain,* edited by J. J. Bonica. Raven Press, New York.
9. Mehler, W. R. (1957): *Anat. Rec.,* 127:332.
10. Mehler, W. R. (1962): In: *Basic Research in Paraplegia,* edited by J. D. French and R. W. Porter. Charles C Thomas, Publisher, Springfield, Illinois.
11. Mehler, W. R. (1969): *Ann. N.Y. Acad. Sci.,* 167:424–468.
12. Mehler, W. R., Feferman, M. E., and Nauta, W. J. H. (1960): *Brain,* 83:718–750.
13. Mullan, S. (1966): *Surg. Clin. North Am.,* 46:3–12.
14. Poirier, L. J., and Bertrand, C. (1955): *J. Comp. Neurol.,* 102:745–757.
15. Riley, H. A. (1943): *An Atlas of the Basal Ganglia, Brain Stem and Spinal Cord Based on Myelin-Stained Material.* Williams & Wilkins, Baltimore.
16. Spiller, W. G. (1905): *J. Nerv. Ment. Dis.,* 32:318–320.

17. Walker, A. E. (1940): *Arch. Neurol. Psychiatr.*, 43:284–298.
18. Weaver, J. A., and Walker, A. E. (1941): *Arch. Neurol. Psychiatr.*, 46:877–883.
19. White, J. C., and Sweet, W. H. (1969): *Pain and the Neurosurgeon.* Charles C Thomas, Publisher, Springfield, Illinois.
20. Whitsel, B. L., Petrucelli, L. M., Sapiro, G., and Ha, H. (1970): *Exp. Neurol.*, 29:227–242.

Advances in Pain Research and Therapy, Vol. 1,
edited by J. J. Bonica and D. Albe-Fessard.
Raven Press, New York © 1976.

Cerebral Cortical Modulation of Primate Spinothalamic Neurons

J. D. Coulter, R. D. Foreman, J. E. Beall, and W. D. Willis

Marine Biomedical Institute and Departments of Physiology and Biophysics, Psychiatry, and Anatomy, University of Texas Medical Branch, Galveston, Texas 77550

Transmission of sensory information through the spinothalamic tract is subject to descending control from the cerebral cortex (5). This finding is consistent with data showing that responses of various other ascending tracts can be modulated by descending influences from the cerebral cortex (4,6,7,9,17). The control by the cerebral cortex of the responsiveness of spinothalamic neurons is presumably relevant to pain perception. Certain aspects of the interaction between the cerebral cortex and the transmission of sensory input through the spinothalamic system may be related to motor feedback control.

As a continuation of previous work (5), this study was designed to determine more exactly the cortical origin of the descending modulation of spinothalamic tract neurons. Discrete localization of effective cortical regions was achieved by intracortical microstimulation. Furthermore, the primary sensorimotor cortex neurons, which project directly to the lumbar spinal cord dorsal horn, have been identified by retrograde labeling with the enzyme horseradish peroxidase (HRP).

METHODS

Anesthesia, surgical preparation, and other details of technique, as well as the methods of antidromic identification of spinothalamic neurons and characterization of their peripheral receptive fields, have been described previously (16,20). A bipolar stimulating electrode was positioned in the contralateral caudal diencephalon to activate spinothalamic neurons antidromically in the lumbosacral enlargement. The activity of individual spinothalamic neurons was recorded extracellularly with glass microelectrodes. Stimuli were applied to the receptive field on the hindlimb, using either a servo-controlled mechanical stimulator (19) or needle electrodes. A silver ball electrode was used to explore the cortical surface. Stimuli were trains of three pulses at 333 Hz. Pulse duration was 0.2 msec, and anodal or cathodal stimuli with strengths up to 2 mA were used.

For stimulation within the cortical gray matter, we used a grid of three parallel, glass-insulated tungsten microelectrodes (tip diameters 10 to 20 μm) constructed according to the technique of Stoney, Thompson, and Asanuma (15). The cathodal stimulating currents were 100 μA or less (monitored across a 100-Ω series resistor). Small lesions (5 μA for 5 to 10 sec) were made in the cortex to mark the positions of the electrode tips. The locations of the stimulating points within defined cytoarchitectonic areas (3,12,14) were mapped on drawings of nissl-stained frozen sections from the lesion sites and micromanipulator readings. For the identification of the cells of origin of corticospinal projections, we used retrograde labeling with HRP (11). A 50% solution of HRP (type VI, Sigma) in saline was slowly injected (0.2 μl), using a microsyringe fitted with a glass pipette having a tip diameter of 70 to 100 μm.

The animals were allowed to survive for 3 days, and then they were reanesthetized and perfused with fixative consisting of 0.4% paraformaldehyde and 2.4% glutaraldehyde in a 0.1 M phosphate buffer, pH 7.4. After fixation, 50-μm serial frozen sections were cut in the sagittal plane. The sections were incubated in the buffer solution containing 0.025% of 3,3-diaminobenzidine with the addition of 0.3 ml of 3% hydrogen peroxide per 100 ml of buffer for 30 min. The sections were then washed, dried, and stained for nissl substance.

RESULTS

Effects of Gross Stimulation

In 20 monkeys the effects of cortical stimulation have been studied on 29 spinothalamic tract neurons. Stimulation of the hindlimb area of the pre- or postcentral gyri with a short train of pulses affected the responses of 21 of these neurons. The cortical stimulation depressed the spontaneous or evoked activity of 7 cells, whereas it excited and then depressed the activity of 14 other cells. Most units showing just a depression were located in Rexed's lamina IV (13), although two units were in the intermediate region. The units that were excited and then depressed were scattered in laminae IV to VI. By contrast, five of the eight spinothalamic neurons not influenced by cortical stimulation were in lamina I. All the neurons affected by cortical stimulation had low thresholds to natural stimulation of the skin. Furthermore, cortical stimulation was much more effective in depressing the rapidly adapting discharges evoked in these cells by tactile stimulation than in changing the responses of the same neurons to intense mechanical or thermal stimulation. Depression could commence as early as 10 to 15 msec after cortical stimulation. Some neurons were depressed for as long as 200 msec, although others were depressed for a shorter period.

Effects of Microstimulation

In seven experiments intracortical microstimulation was used to identify the precise cortical region(s) from which the descending influences on the spinothalamic tract originate. Surface mapping suggested that the most effective area is near the central sulcus, so this region has been explored first. Figure 1 shows results from two experiments. Penetrations of the three stimulating microelectrodes are plotted in Fig. 1C on a drawing of a sagittal section of the hindlimb sensorimotor cortex. The most effective stimulating points in this experiment, using a constant stimulus current of 50 μA, were in cytoarchitectonic field 3a. The caudal electrode, which passed through area 3b, had little effect until it reached the white matter. The histograms show the depression of the activity evoked in the cell by an

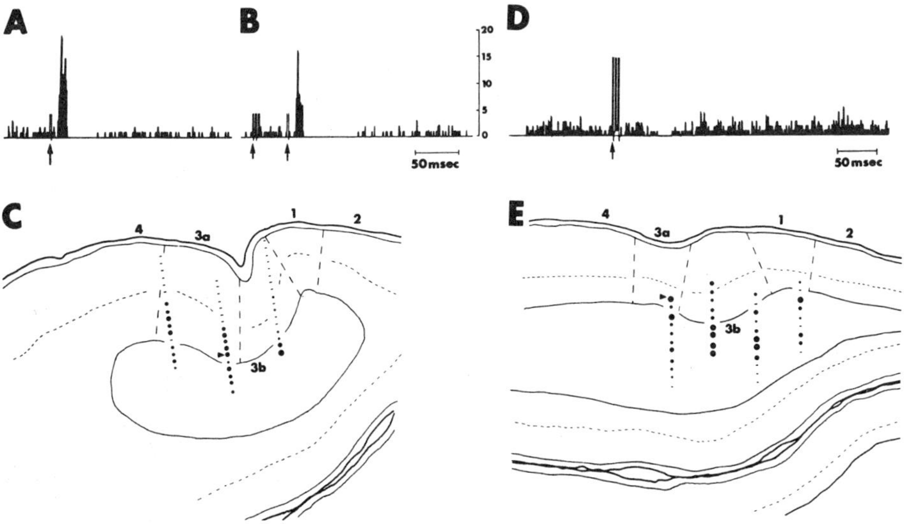

FIG. 1. Effects of cortical microstimulation on spinothalamic tract neuron. **A:** Poststimulus histogram showing response of a hair-activated spinothalamic tract neuron to electrical stimulation of the skin within the receptive field; arrow indicates time of the stimulus. **B:** Depression of the response of cerebral cortical microstimulation consisting of a train of 3 shocks at 333 Hz; the first stimulus of the train preceded the test stimulus by 40 msec (*arrows*). Stimulus strength, 50 μA. **C:** Points stimulated within sensorimotor cortex. Cytoarchitectural areas are labeled and their approximate boundaries are shown (*dashed lines*). The dotted line parallel to the cortical surface is along layer V. The 3 electrode tracks are indicated by the following symbols: negative signs, points stimulated with no resultant change in spinothalamic neuron discharge; filled circles, points which produced a depression. Relative amount of depression is indicated by the size of the filled circles. Arrowhead shows the stimulation site for the depression illustrated by **B. D:** Peristimulus histogram showing effect of cortical microstimulation on the activity of a low-threshold spinothalamic tract neuron in another experiment. Spontaneous discharge level is seen before the cortical stimulation (*arrow*). A depression of activity occurs approximately 30 msec later and lasts for some 60 msec. **E:** Cortical points stimulated; arrow indicates the point stimulated for the response in **D** (stimulus strength, 100 μA).

electrical stimulus applied to the skin in the receptive field. A stimulus of 25 μA was almost as effective as the 50-μA pulse used for the record illustrated.

A second experiment showed that the spontaneous activity of a spinothalamic tract cell could be depressed by stimulation in cytoarchitectonic area 3a or 3b (Fig. 1E). The histogram in Fig. 1D shows the effect of a stimulus having an intensity of 100 μA. In these studies the effects of cortical stimulation were most evident when the electrode tip was near or deep to layer V. Stimulation within more superficial layers had little or no effect. These findings, taken in conjunction with the results of other studies (1,2) and the histologic observations in the next section, suggest that the effects of cortical stimulation are mediated by the pyramidal cells of layer V.

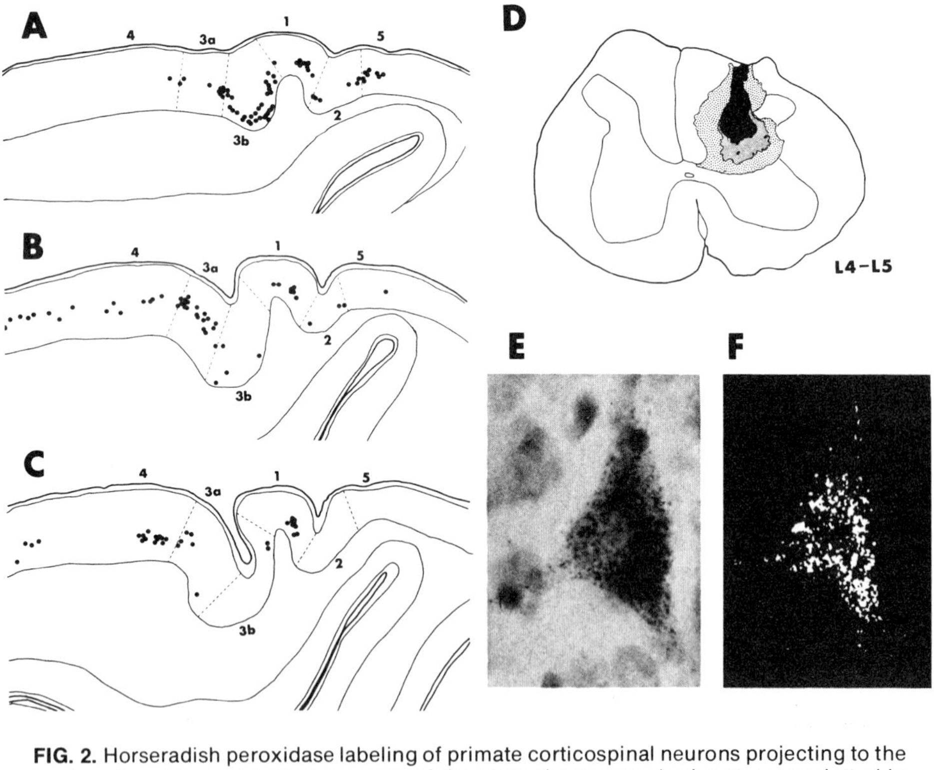

FIG. 2. Horseradish peroxidase labeling of primate corticospinal neurons projecting to the lumbar dorsal horn. Labeled neurons of the sensorimotor cerebral cortex are plotted in **A–C** on representative sagittal sections through the hindlimb area separated by 350 μm. An especially large number of labeled neurons were found medially **(A)** in cytoarchitectonic fields 3a and 3b. **D:** Maximum transverse distribution of the injected HRP within the dorsal horn of the contralateral L_4-L_5 spinal cord. Typical granular reaction product can be seen within a single large layer-V pyramidal cell, photographed with bright-field **(E)** and with dark-field **(F)** illumination.

Identification of Cortical Projection to Dorsal Horn by HRP

Anatomical studies using HRP labeling of cortical neurons projecting directly to the lumbar dorsal horn have been done to localize the cortical region(s) which may be involved in the descending control of sensory transmission. A small amount of the enzyme was injected (Fig. 2D), and the reaction product was identified in cortical neurons of the primary sensorimotor region. Labeled neurons contained small, dark brown granules which filled the cell body (exclusive of the nucleus) and the proximal dendrites (Fig. 2E and F). The locations of corticospinal neurons in one experiment are plotted in Fig. 2A–C on drawings of representative sagittal sections. The marked cells had a pyramidal shape and were found exclusively in layer V. Some large Betz cells in cortical areas 4 and 3a were labeled, along with many smaller neurons (diameters of 20 μm or less), which were particularly numerous in area 3b. More caudally, medium-sized pyramidal cells were found to be labeled in areas 1, 2, and 5.

With the exception of some isolated, weakly labeled cells in area 4, there was a tendency for labeled cells to occur in small clusters, separated by areas in which no labeled cells could be found. Each cytoarchitectonic area contained labeled cells, and the concentration was especially dense in areas 3a and 3b. Of the marked neurons, 22% were in area 4, 23% in area 3a, 25% in area 3b, 17% in area 1, 7% in area 2, and 6% in area 5. Ventral horn injections of HRP would be expected to produce a different distribution of labeled neurons. Similar results with respect to location in cortical laminae and distribution in the different cytoarchitectonic fields have been obtained in cats.

DISCUSSION

Spinothalamic tract neurons were found to be either depressed or excited and then depressed by stimulation within the cerebral cortex. The observations were similar to those of Fetz (7) for interneurons and ascending tract cells of the cat dorsal horn after stimulation of the pyramid. Gordon and Miller (10) found that the sensorimotor cortical zone in the cat which projects to the dorsal column nuclei is cytoarchitectonic area 3a, whereas spinothalamic tract cells in the monkey appear to be affected by several areas, including 3a and 3b. Although the results indicate that stimulation of the cortex in the region of the central sulcus modulates the activity of spinothalamic neurons, this does not rule out the participation of other cortical areas.

Microstimulation has little effect until the stimulating electrode reaches layer V, which suggests that the pyramidal cells of this layer are responsible for modulation of spinothalamic tract neuronal activity. This hypothesis is strengthened by the horseradish peroxidase labeling experiments showing that a large number of cortical neurons in layer V of areas 3a and 3b project to the dorsal horn of the lumbar spinal cord.

The role of cortical modulation of spinothalamic neurons in pain is probably significant. The cortical descending effects often interfere with the responsiveness of spinothalamic neurons to tactile stimuli. This might serve as a switching mechanism, changing the role of these neurons from a tactile to a nociceptive one. Evidence is presented in other papers from this laboratory which argues against the participation of tactile spinothalamic tract neurons in pain transmission (8,18), but this possibility should not be overlooked. Other cortical areas will be tested to see if the cortex can depress selectively the responses to intense stimulation.

SUMMARY

Stimulation of the cerebral cortex in the region of the central sulcus depresses or excites and depresses the activity of spinothalamic tract neurons. The neurons involved appear to be located in cortical areas 3a and 3b, although other areas are not excluded. Microstimulation becomes effective when the electrode reaches layer V, suggesting that the effects depend on activation of the pyramidal cells of this layer. Horseradish peroxidase labeling indicates that numerous corticospinal neurons in layer V of areas 3a and b could be responsible for the cortical effects on spinothalamic tract neurons.

ACKNOWLEDGMENTS

The work was supported by research grants from the National Institutes of Health (NS 12481; NS 09743), by N.I.H. training grants (NS 05743; GM 00459), and by a grant from the Moody Foundation of Galveston.

The authors wish to thank Gail Silver, Cindy Carter, Linda Ewing, and William Gross for their assistance.

REFERENCES

1. Asanuma, H., and Rosén, I. (1972): *Exp. Brain Res.,* 14:243–256.
2. Asanuma, H., and Ward, J. E. (1971): *Brain Res.,* 27:97–109.
3. Bonin, G. von, and Bailey, P. (1947): *The Neocortex of Macaca Mulatta.* University of Illinois Press, Urbana.
4. Brown, A. G., and Short, A. D. (1974): *Brain Res.,* 74:338–341.
5. Coulter, J. D., Maunz, R. A., and Willis, W. D. (1974): *Brain Res.,* 65:351–356.
6. Coulter, J. D., Mergner, T., and Pompeiano, O. (1976): *J. Neurophysiol.* (*in press*).
7. Fetz, E. E. (1968): *J. Neurophysiol.,* 31:69–80.
8. Foreman, R. D., Beall, J. E., Applebaum, A. E., Coulter, J. D., and Willis, W. D.: *This volume.*
9. Gordon, G., and Jukes, M. G. M. (1964): *J. Physiol.* (*Lond.*), 173:291–319.
10. Gordon, G., and Miller, R. (1969): *Q. J. Exp. Physiol.,* 54:85–98.
11. LaVail, J. H., and LaVail, M. M. (1974): *J. Comp. Neurol.,* 157:303–358.

12. Powell, T. P. S., and Mountcastle, V. B. (1959): *Johns Hopkins Med. J.*, 105:108–131.
13. Rexed, B. (1952): *J. Comp. Neurol.*, 96:415–496.
14. Roberts, T. S., and Akert, K. (1963): *Schweiz. Arch. Neurol., Neurochir. Psychiatr.*, 92:1–43.
15. Stoney, S. D., Thompson, W. D., and Asanuma, H. (1968): *J. Neurophysiol.*, 31:659–669.
16. Trevino, D. L., Coulter, J. D., and Willis, W. D. (1973): *J. Neurophysiol.*, 36:750–761.
17. Wall, P. D. (1967): *J. Physiol. (Lond.)*, 188:403–423.
18. Willis, W. D.: *This volume.*
19. Willis, W. D., Maunz, R. A., Foreman, R. D., and Coulter, J. D. (1975): *J. Neurophysiol.*, 38:587–600.
20. Willis, W. D., Trevino, D. L., Coulter, J. D., and Maunz, R. A. (1974): *J. Neurophysiol.*, 37:358–372.

Advances in Pain Research and Therapy, Vol. 1,
edited by J. J. Bonica and D. Albe-Fessard.
Raven Press, New York © 1976.

Comparison of Spinoreticular and Spinothalamic Projections in the Cat

H. L. Fields and S. D. Anderson

Departments of Neurology and Physiology, University of California, San Francisco, California 94143

Anatomical studies of the major ascending spinal pathways consistently reveal a large projection to the medial tegmental regions of the pons and medulla (2,4,13,15). Some of the projections are axon collaterals of fibers destined for more rostral sites (16), but most are derived from axons that end within the brainstem reticular formation (13,15).

Previous physiological studies (6,11) of spinal neurons antidromically activated from medial pontomedullary reticular formation (PMRF) did not distinguish between neurons projecting only to PMRF and those projecting to diencephalon. Electrodes in PMRF could activate medially located fibers of passage or collaterals of spinothalamic axons as well as direct spinoreticular projections.

The present experiments were designed to examine the function of the direct spinoreticular projection and, if possible, to distinguish true spinoreticular neurons from others with axons passing by or through the medial reticular formation to terminate in midbrain or thalamus.

METHODS

For details of the methods employed, see Fields, Wagner, and Anderson (6). Briefly, cats were anesthetized with sodium pentobarbital (35 mg/kg) or a mixture of halothane and nitrous oxide. Two sets of stimulating electrodes were stereotaxically implanted: an array of four concentric bipolar electrodes, two on each side at different rostrocaudal levels of the medial PMRF, and a second array of four monopolar electrodes of alternating polarity spanning the midbrain (MB) at the level of the superior colliculus.

A laminectomy was performed from L_4 to S_1, and the spinal cord was explored with glass micropipettes filled with 0.5 M K^+ acetate saturated with Niagara® sky blue. Units responding to brainstem stimulation with a fixed latency spike demonstrating collision with a spontaneous or peripherally evoked spike are said to be antidromically activated by, or to project to, the region of the effective electrode (Fig. 1). Units projecting to PMRF or MB were studied with respect to conduction velocity, receptive field, cell locus, and site of termination.

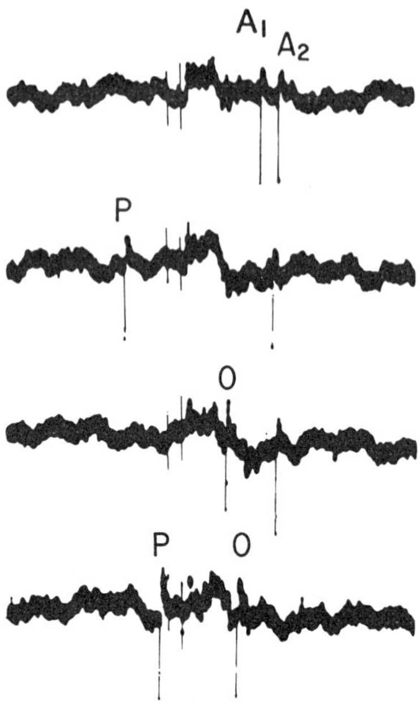

FIG. 1. A cell in the lumbosacral enlargement activated both antidromically and orthodromically from the ipsilateral pontomedullary reticular formation. Pairs of stimuli, S_1 and S_2, were delivered to the brainstem. The cell's receptive field on the ipsilateral hindlimb was manipulated. The commonest response (*top trace*), occurring in approximately 70% of the trials, is a pair of spikes, A_1 and A_2, the earlier of which is demonstrated in the second trace to be antidromic by the criterion of collision with a peripherally evoked spike, P. In a less common response (*third trace*), occurring approximately 20% of the time, a spike (O) follows the brainstem stimulus at shorter latency and collides with A_2. The spike occurring at O is probably produced by descending synaptic input from brainstem. In the bottom trace, a spike evoked by stimulation in the peripheral receptive field (P) and one evoked by descending synaptic input (O) collide with A_1 and A_2, respectively, demonstrating that A_1 and A_2 are both antidromic and that O is not.

RESULTS

A total of 52 antidromically activated neurons was found in 13 cats. Of these 52 neurons, 19 were antidromically activated by the MB electrode array. The remaining 33 represent a spinal projection terminating in PMRF; these will be referred to as direct spinoreticular fibers (Fig. 2).

Of the 19 neurons projecting to MB, 13 were also antidromically activated from PMRF. Four of this latter group were activated at the same or shorter

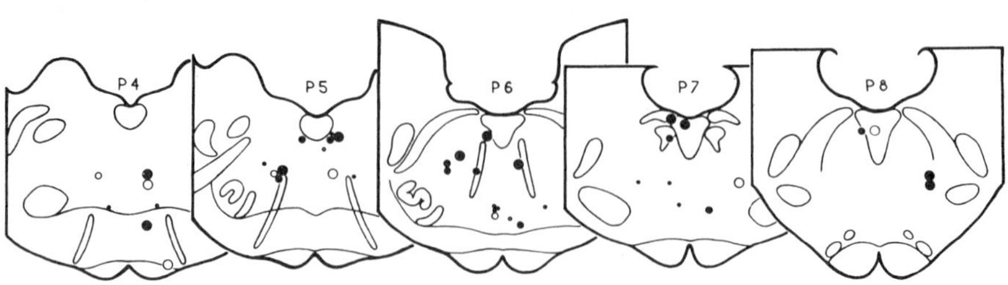

FIG. 2. The 42 sites in pontomedullary reticular formation from which spinal cord cells were antidromically activated. Histologically determined loci have been projected onto sections traced from Snider and Niemer's atlas (17). On the left of each section are those sites ipsilateral to the cell somata; on the right, those contralateral. Thresholds (T) are indicated by the size of the circle: largest circles, T ≤ 1 mA; smallest circles, T > 2 mA. An open circle indicates that the cell could, in addition, be antidromically activated from midbrain (MB); a filled circle, that the cell does not project to MB.

latency from MB than from PMRF, suggesting a slowly conducting, medially directed axon collateral to PMRF from a larger, laterally placed axon ascending to MB.

Of the 33 neurons terminating in PMRF, 18 projected ipsilaterally, 14 contralaterally, and 1 to both sides. Of 19 neurons reaching MB, 9 projected ipsilaterally, 5 contralaterally, and 5 were bilateral or midline projections. No difference in the location or physiological properties of cells is correlated with the laterality of their PMRF termination, except that neurons without detectable excitatory receptive fields were found to project only to the contralateral PMRF.

Figure 3 compares the cell locations of direct spinoreticular neurons with those of neurons projecting to MB. Neurons of both groups are distributed widely in the spinal gray, including a significant proportion in laminae IV and V of the dorsal horn. No qualitative differences in cell location are observed between direct spinoreticular and MB-projecting neurons.

The mean conduction velocity of neurons projecting to MB (59 m/s) is higher than that of direct spinoreticular neurons (36 m/s). This is the most striking difference in the properties of the two groups of neurons.

According to their receptive field properties, the neurons fall into three categories: superficial, deep, and complex. Superficial receptive fields consist of a single, restricted unilateral cutaneous region. Deep fields consist of similarly unilateral and restricted but subcutaneous structures believed to be tendons, muscles, or periosteum. Complex fields consist of multiple or extensive bilateral cutaneous regions or deep structures. Some neurons of each receptive field type were found to respond maximally to high-intensity

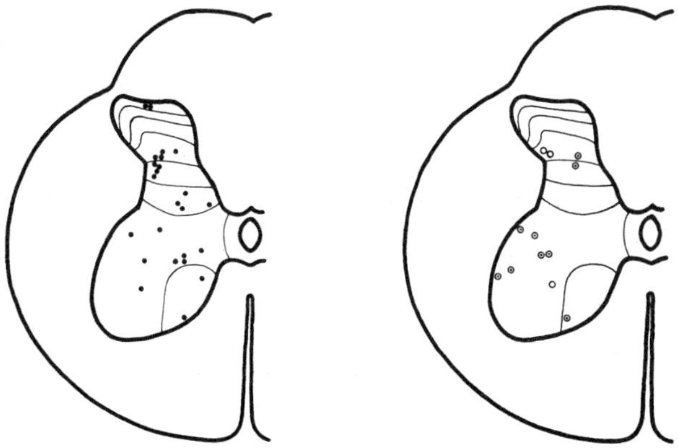

FIG. 3. Recording sites of 36 antidromically activated cells, projected on a typical lumbosacral cord cross section. Only well-localized cells are shown. Approximate boundaries of the Rexed laminae are indicated. Left: cells activated from pontomedullary reticular formation (PMRF) only; right, those from midbrain, either exclusively (*open circles*) or from PMRF as well (*dotted circles*).

TABLE 1. *Receptive fields of projecting spinal neurons*[a]

Field type	PMRF only	MB and PMRF	MB only	Total
Superficial	5	4	4	13
Deep	10	1	1	12
Complex	12	0	4	16
No excitatory	6	1	4	11
Total	33	6	13	52

[a] PMRF, pontomedullary reticular formation; MB, midbrain.

tissue-damaging stimuli or to injection of agents such as bradykinin and hypertonic saline, which are known to produce pain.

Although direct spinoreticular and MB-projecting neurons overlap in terms of their receptive field types, a direct spinoreticular neuron is more likely to have a deep or complex receptive field, whereas MB-projecting neurons are more likely to have superficial receptive fields (Table 1).

DISCUSSION

These experiments demonstrate that although some input to PMRF may arrive via collaterals from spinotectal and spinothalamic tracts, the majority of axons reaching PMRF terminate there and are neither fibers of passage nor collaterals of ascending tracts. Consistent with previous anatomical (2,4,13,15,16) and physiological (6) studies, this direct spinoreticular projection is bilateral.

Most spinoreticular neurons have somatosensory receptive fields, implying that the spinoreticular tract is a sensory pathway. The type of information relayed by this pathway is different from that relayed by other sensory pathways that have been investigated. Although some direct spinoreticular neurons have restricted cutaneous receptive fields, the majority have either deep or extensive complex receptive fields. The extent and complexity of the receptive fields of some spinoreticular neurons indicate a highly convergent, bilateral, and multisegmental input. This is in contrast to MB-projecting spinal neurons, a majority of which have more restricted cutaneous fields.

Our results on MB-projecting spinal neurons are consistent with those of recent anatomical studies of cat spinothalamic tract. Trevino and Carstens (18) have shown that in cat a bilateral projection to thalamus originates from cells in dorsal and ventral horns of cervical and lumbosacral cord. Their preliminary results also suggest a significant direct projection to midbrain regions as well as to thalamus. The present experiments do not distinguish between spinomesencephalic and spinothalamic neurons.

The receptive field properties of MB-projecting neurons are similar to those of spinothalamic tract neurons. Spinothalamic neurons with restricted cutaneous receptive fields having wide dynamic range have been found in cervical (5) and thoracic (7) cord of cat and in lumbosacral cord of primate and rat (1,5,19).

Assuming that some of the MB-projecting neurons are spinothalamic neurons, these experiments indicate that dorsal horn cells responding to a wide range of peripheral stimulus intensity project to both PMRF and thalamus in the cat. Since there is evidence in cat, primate, and man that such dorsal horn neurons mediate pain (3,8,9,12,14), these results support the hypothesis that both spinothalamic and spinoreticular pathways are involved in pain transmission.

The relationship of the spinothalamic and spinoreticular pathways remains unclear. To a large extent, the ascending axons of the two systems occupy the same region of the spinal cord (2,10,13), and physiological studies, including the present one, demonstrate overlap in the locations of their cells of origin (1,5–7,11,18,19). Our experiments indicate that in the cat, although there is a degree of functional overlap, the spinoreticular projection is a distinct pathway that appears to be concerned with input from deep receptors.

ACKNOWLEDGMENTS

The authors would like to thank Mr. Charles Clanton and Dr. Allan Basbaum for assistance in some of these experiments. This research was supported by P.H.S. Grants NS-11529 and NS-70777.

REFERENCES

1. Albe-Fessard, D., Levante, A., and Lamour, Y. (1974): *Brain Res.*, 65:503–509.
2. Anderson, F. D., and Berry, C. M. (1959): *J. Comp. Neurol.*, 111:195–229.
3. Besson, J. M., Consiller, C., Hamann, K.-F., and Maillard, M.-C. (1972): *J. Physiol. (Lond.)*, 221:189–205.
4. Bowsher, D. (1957): *Brain*, 80:606–622.
5. Dilly, P. N., Wall, P. D., and Webster, K. E. (1968): *Exp. Neurol.*, 21:550–562.
6. Fields, H. L., Wagner, G. M., and Anderson, S. D. (1975): *Exp. Neurol.*, 47:118–134.
7. Hancock, M. B., Foreman, R. D., and Willis, W. D. (1975): *Exp. Neurol.*, 47:240–248.
8. Handwerker, H. O., Iggo, A., and Zimmermann, M. (1975): *Pain*, 1:147–166.
9. Hillman, P., and Wall, P. D. (1968): *Exp. Brain Res.*, 9:284–306.
10. Kerr, F. W. L. (1975): *J. Comp. Neurol.*, 159:335–356.
11. Levante, A., and Albe-Fessard, D. (1972): *C. R. Acad. Sci.* [*D.*] (*Paris*), 274:3007–3010.
12. Mayer, D. J., Price, D. D., and Becker, D. P. (1975): *Pain*, 1:51–58.
13. Mehler, W. R., Feferman, M. E., and Nauta, W. J. H. (1960): *Brain*, 83:718–750.
14. Price, D. D., and Mayer, D. J. (1975): *Pain*, 1:59–72.
15. Rossi, G. F., and Brodal, A. (1957): *Arch. Neurol. Psychiatr.*, 78:439–453.
16. Scheibel, M. E., and Scheibel, A. B. (1958): In: *Reticular Formation of the Brain*, edited by H. H. Jasper. Little, Brown and Co., Boston.
17. Snider, R. S., and Niemer, W. T. (1961): *A Stereotaxic Atlas of the Cat Brain*. University of Chicago Press, Chicago.
18. Trevino, D. L., and Carstens, E. (1975): *Brain Res.*, 98:177–182.
19. Willis, W. D., Trevino, D. L., Coulter, J. D., and Maunz, R. A. (1974): *J. Neurophysiol.*, 37:358–372.

Advances in Pain Research and Therapy, Vol. 1,
edited by J. J. Bonica and D. Albe-Fessard.
Raven Press, New York © 1976.

Effect of Nitrous Oxide on Evoked Cellular Responses in the Cat Nucleus Reticularis Gigantocellularis

Dennis Spencer, Mamoru Yamashita, Luke M. Kitahata, W. F. Collins, Jr., and Robert Bradford Duckrow

Yale University School of Medicine, 333 Cedar Street, New Haven, Connecticut 06510

The nucleus reticularis gigantocellularis has been described as a relay center of the ascending pain pathways (1,2,10,11). It lies in the medial pontine reticular formation, and its caudal cells receive major afferents from the ventrolateral spinal cord. Electrophysiological experiments show that the majority of these cells respond to noxious physiological stimuli (12) and more precisely, to A-delta and C-fiber activity in the peripheral nerve (5,6,9). Casey demonstrated that stimulation of these cells correlated with escape behavior in the cat (3,4). The present experiment was undertaken to define better the role of the nucleus reticularis gigantocellularis in the appreciation of pain by a combined electrophysiological and pharmacological study using nitrous oxide (N_2O), a known analgesic agent in man and the cat (14). Cells were first defined and grouped according to their individual extracellular electrophysiological response patterns. N_2O was then administered and its effect on cellular activity carefully analyzed by computer methodology.

METHOD

We studied 22 cells in 22 cats weighing 2.5 to 5 kg. The animals were anesthetized with 2% halothane in a 75% N_2O = oxygen (O_2) mixture and were prepared with a tracheostomy and arterial and venous cannulation for anesthetic administration, respiratory control, blood pressure monitoring, and fluid and drug administration, respectively. The end-tidal CO_2 tension, arterial O_2, CO_2 tension and pH, blood pressure, and body temperature were monitored continuously and maintained within narrow physiological limits. Gallamine triethiodide was administered intravenously at 5 to 7 ml/kg/hr for muscular relaxation. The animal was placed in a stereotaxic apparatus and decerebration was accomplished by stereotaxically placed bilateral mesencephalic reticular formation lesions, the effect of which was monitored by EEG recordings. Bilateral superficial radial and sural nerves were isolated in the forelimbs and hindlimbs, respectively, immersed in mineral oil, and attached to bipolar silver electrodes for stimulation and recording. A suboccipital craniectomy was performed, and a region 1 to 3 mm lateral and up to 3 mm rostral to the obex was probed with a Transidyne Microtrode® platinum-covered glass microelectrode (tip diameter 1 to 2 μm). Single cells were isolated and studied by applying a train of ten 1-msec square wave pulses for a duration of 100 msec to the peripheral nerve at a voltage (1 to 2.5 V) sufficient to produce the A-delta wave in the peripheral nerve action potential. This stimulus train was repeated every 60 sec for 5 min for each portion of the study. The evoked activity was studied in the unanesthetized preparation before and after 25%, 50%, and 75% N_2O in O_2 were given. The single cell response was recorded on a Hewlett Packard four-channel tape recorder for off-line poststimulus time histogram (PSTH) analysis. An electrolytic lesion was then made at the recording site and verified histologically.

RESULTS

Included for study were only cells that increased their firing rate after stimulation of the peripheral nerve. The highest firing rate after stimulation was defined as the peak frequency, and the difference between the peak frequency and the base-line activity as the evoked response (ER). The time interval between stimulus onset and peak frequency was the ER latency, and the return of the response to tonic base-line firing the duration of the ER. The ER duration varied in different cells and was not further defined in the present experiment. Between stimuli the base-line was recomputed as the average firing rate in the first 12 sec after cessation of the ER (Fig. 1). The effect of N_2O on each component of cell activity was examined.

After administration of N_2O, two main cell groupings emerged. Averaging the ER and base-line together, we found that 17/22 cells showed suppression of average firing frequency with increasing N_2O doses, whereas 5/22 showed a dramatic increase in base-line activity and thus average firing frequency.

Using the PSTH, 16/17 cells suppressing with N_2O could be further analyzed. The control histograms before N_2O fell into three statistically significant groups according to the latency of the evoked response: short latency (830 msec), 7/16 cells; middle latency (6.4 sec), 4/16 cells; long latency (18.4 sec), 5/16 cells. Each of these latency groups had a different response pattern (Fig. 2). The short-latency unanesthetized ER frequency was 60 impulses per second (I/sec) and was not affected by 25% N_2O but was suppressed 73% by 50% and 75% N_2O (Fig. 2A). The middle-latency unanesthetized ER began at 50 I/sec, was completely suppressed by 25% N_2O, and then reappeared with increasing gas concentrations (Fig. 2B). The base-line frequency of both groups was around 30 I/sec and was diminished by approximately 30% at each N_2O concentration. The long-latency unanesthetized ER was 35 I/sec, and both the ER and base-line were

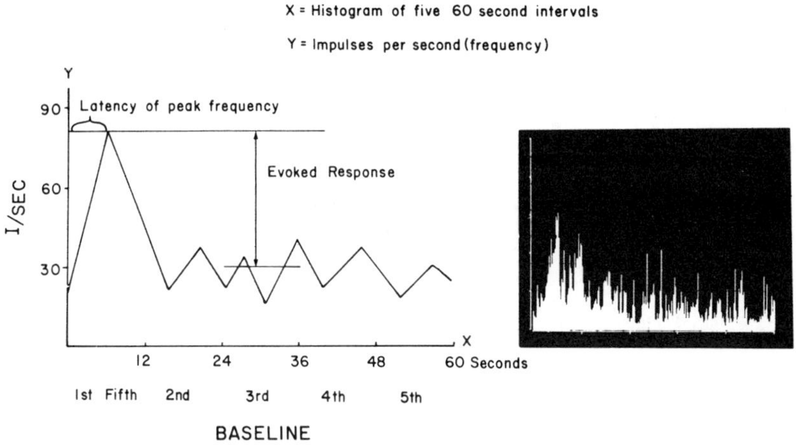

FIG. 1. Model histogram. Left: schematic model of the poststimulus time histogram shown on the right. One histogram represents the average of five 60-sec intervals. Evoked response (ER): peak frequency minus base-line activity. Base-line activity: average frequency of the first fifth (12 sec) after return of the response to tonic firing. ER latency: duration from stimulus at time zero to peak frequency firing.

increasingly suppressed, eventually by 90% at 75% N_2O (Fig. 2C). The latency of the ER was not significantly altered by any dose of N_2O.

The second main group of cells (5/22) with facilitating base lines after N_2O administration were distributed among all latency groups. Figure 3 demonstrates that the base-line activity rose with each dose of N_2O to three times control after 75% N_2O. The ER, however, was halved by 25% N_2O but recovered to control firing as the N_2O concentration increased.

Nineteen cells could be verified histologically. Cells with firing rates suppressed by N_2O were distributed throughout the caudal gigantocellularis. However, all cells with facilitating base-lines were grouped in the most dorsocaudal region of the nucleus reticularis gigantocellularis within 1.75 mm of the fourth ventricular floor and 2 mm lateral to the midline raphe (Fig. 4).

DISCUSSION

The effect of N_2O on the evoked activity of single cells in the brainstem reticular formation has been studied almost exclusively in the mesencephalon. Shimoji and Bickford noted that single units in the mesencephalic reticular formation responding to repetitive electrical stimulation of the skin decreased their firing rate when subjected to deep anesthesia with N_2O (13). They recorded two units, however, which increased in firing activity after administration of the agent, but they did not define these seemingly paradoxical units further by electrophysiological or histological means.

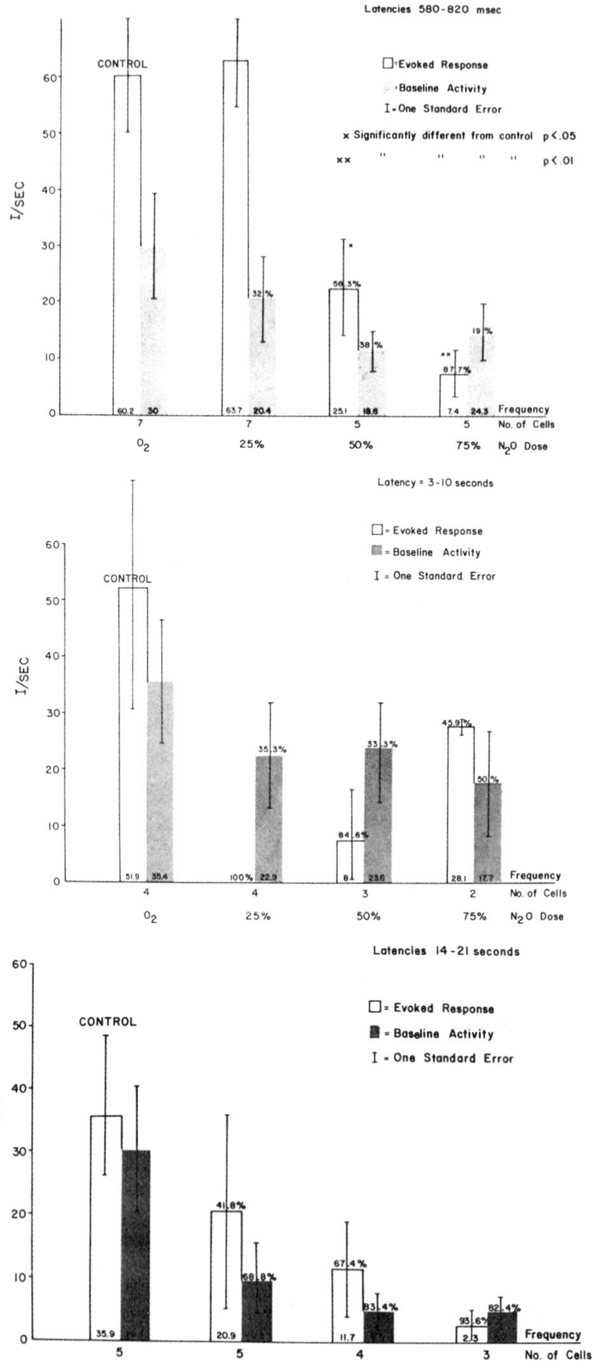

FIG. 2. Suppressed cells. Comparison of evoked response and base-line activity of all 3 latency groups (**top,** group A; **middle,** group B; **bottom,** group C) after administration of 25%, 50%, and 75% N_2O in O_2. Both ER and base-line activity were suppressed.

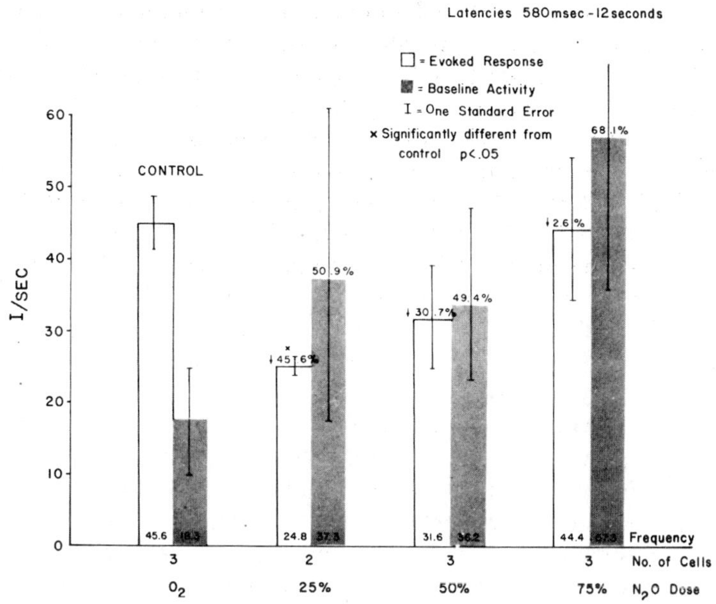

FIG. 3. Facilitated cells. Comparison of evoked response and base-line activity in cells showing facilitating base-line firing with N_2O. Note initial suppression of ER.

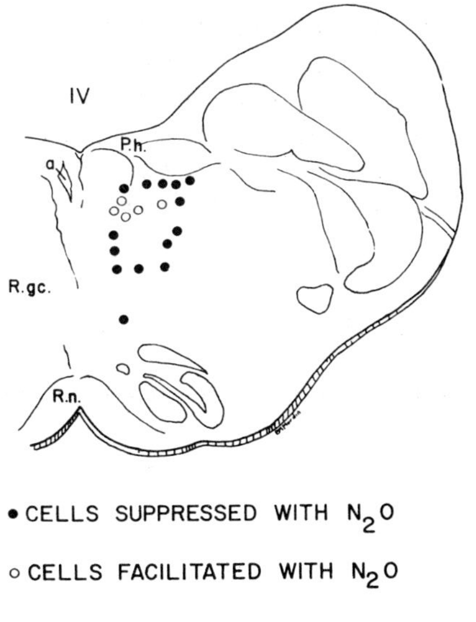

FIG. 4. Histology. Diagram of the cat nucleus reticularis gigantocellularis (R.gc.) showing the distribution of cells studied.

In 1971, while studying the effect of anesthetics on the Rexed laminae of the feline lumbar spinal cord, Kitahata et al. noted lamina-specific suppression by N_2O. They found that N_2O significantly suppressed spontaneous cellular activity of lamina V and slightly suppressed the activity of lamina I, both of which respond primarily to noxious peripheral stimuli. The cells in lamina IV responding only to nonnoxious stimuli were not affected by N_2O, and cells in lamina VI responding primarily to proprioceptive stimuli were slightly facilitated by N_2O (8). Again in 1973, Kitahata et al. found deep in the lamina propria of the trigeminal nucleus caudalis a group of high-threshold mechanoreceptors which decreased their spontaneous activity by N_2O, and in the most dorsorostral aspect of the nucleus caudalis a group of low-threshold mechanoreceptors which increased their spontaneous activity by N_2O (7).

The present experiment demonstrates a similar phenomenon as that found in the lumbar spinal cord and trigeminal nucleus, only within the reticular formation. This has two important connotations. First, the use of N_2O may provide one method for delineating structure within the reticular formation, perhaps even some form of laminar pattern may emerge. Second, the experiment shows a definite pattern in which tonic activity is markedly enhanced while the ER is suppressed or remains unchanged. This evidence suggests discrete cellular modulation during the analgesic state.

SUMMARY

Single cells in the caudal nucleus reticularis gigantocellularis were subjected to electrophysiological and pharmacological investigation. Using microelectrode extracellular single-cell recording techniques during noxious electrical stimulation of a peripheral nerve, we could group cells according to the latency of their evoked response and their activity pattern after nitrous oxide administration. Two main groups emerged; the majority of cells decreased in firing frequency following N_2O administration. However, a small number of cells lying dorsally in the nucleus showed increasing base-line tonic firing as the concentration of N_2O increased. The ramifications of this grouping are discussed in light of previous studies with N_2O on the central nervous system.

ACKNOWLEDGMENT

This work was supported by the National Institutes of Health Grant NS-09871.

REFERENCES

1. Bowsher, D. (1960): *J. Neurol. Neurosurg. Psychiatry*, 23:351–360.
2. Casey, K. L. (1969): *Exp. Neurol.*, 25:35–56.

3. Casey, K. L. (1971*a*): *Int. J. Neurosci.*, 2:29–34.
4. Casey, K. L. (1971*b*): *Science*, 173:77–80.
5. Collins, W. F., and Randt, C. T. (1958): *J. Neurophysiol.*, 21:345–352.
6. Goldman, P. L., Collins, W. F., Taub, A., and Fitzmartin, J. (1972): *Exp. Neurol*, 37: 397–606.
7. Kitahata, L. M., McAllister, R. G., and Taub, A. (1973): *Anesthesiology*, 38:12–31.
8. Kitahata, L. M., Taub, A., and Sato, R. (1971): *J. Pharmcol. Exp. Ther.*, 176:101–108.
9. LeBlanc, H. J., and Gatipon, G. B. (1974): *Exp. Neurol.*, 42:264–273.
10. Mehler, W. H., Feferman, M. E., and Nauta, W. J. H. (1956): *Anat. Rec.*, 124:332–333.
11. Rossi, G. F., and Brodal, A. (1957): *Arch. Neurol. Psychiatr.*, 78:439–453.
12. Segundo, J. P., Takenaka, T., and Encabo, H. (1967): *J. Neurophysiol.*, 30:1221–1238.
13. Shimoji, K., and Bickford, R. (1971): *Anesthesiology*, 35:76–80.
14. Venes, J. L., Collins, W. F., and Taub, A. (1971): *Am. J. Physiol.*, 220:2029–2031.

Advances in Pain Research and Therapy, Vol. 1,
edited by J. J. Bonica and D. Albe-Fessard.
Raven Press, New York © 1976.

Psychological Factors in Pain

Richard A. Sternbach

*Pain Treatment Center, Scripps Clinic Medical Group, Inc.,
La Jolla, California 92037*

Several volumes have been written about the psychological aspects of pain, from psychoanalytic (13), phenomenological (5), experimental (8), and clinical (7,10) viewpoints, among others. It is thus clearly impossible to do justice to this topic in a brief chapter. Nevertheless, certain concepts are sometimes unrecognized in discussions of pain and they deserve emphasis.

ACUTE PAIN

Pain of recent onset and of relatively short duration elicits a characteristic pattern of responses. Cardiac rate, blood pressure, respiration, peripheral blood flow, palmar sweating, pupillary diameter, and muscle tension are all increased. This pattern of autonomic responses shows a predominance of sympathetic nervous system activity, a mixed epinephrine-norepinephrine pattern (6).

The emotion most frequently associated with acute pain is anxiety. The autonomic patterns are virtually identical in pain and anxiety. Indeed, there is considerable evidence to suggest that anxiety is a set of responses that have been conditioned to an unconditioned pain stimulus.

Almost all experimental research on pain—certainly laboratory studies in humans—has dealt with acute pain. Similarly, we are only now beginning to see the development of an animal model of chronic pain (2,15).

The results of studies of experimental pain have been relatively consistent in showing that whatever reduces anxiety also reduces the subjective intensity of pain and the magnitude of pain responses, whether the anxiety is reduced by hypnosis, by explanations, or by giving the subject control of the pain stimuli (8).

This principle is well known in clinical situations, and most dentists and surgeons are alert to the need to reduce anxiety in their patients in order to minimize postoperative pain.

CHRONIC PAIN

It may be insufficiently recognized that the pattern of responses in acute pain does not persist when the pain continues. If the pain is relatively constant (not intermittent) and continues for weeks or months, there is a habituation of the autonomic responses. A pattern of vegetative signs emerges instead. Patients report sleep disturbance, appetite disturbance, decreased libido, irritability, withdrawal of interests, weakening of relationships, and an increased somatic preoccupation (9).

The affect most frequently associated with chronic pain is depression. (In some cases the patient is not aware of a depressed mood; this is then referred to as a "masked" depression because the focus is on a somatic symptom.)

There is virtually no experimental research on the relationship between chronic pain and depression, so we have had to rely on clinical studies. We have learned that chronic somatic pain usually results in a reactive depression (10), and that relieving the pain usually alleviates the depression (12). Similarly, treating the depression either reduces the pain or makes it more bearable (4).

Patients' estimates of the severity of pain is usually associated with their perception of the impact the pain has had on their daily activities. However, a more accurate measure of pain, the tourniquet pain test, shows that the intensity of the patients' pain is most highly correlated with their degree of depression (14).

The close relationship between chronic pain and depression suggests that some common mechanism may underlie the two phenomena. Preliminary studies with chronic pain patients suggest that increasing the activity of certain brain amines either decreases the intensity of clinical pain or increases pain tolerance. This seems true at least for brain serotonin and perhaps as well for brain dopamine (11). This finding supports both the aminergic hypothesis of depression and the work of Akil (1) on the interaction of these amines and electrical stimulation–produced analgesia in animals.

The Complaint of Pain

Turning now from psychophysiological considerations to more traditional psychological approaches, we note that when a patient comes to a physician with a pain complaint, this complaint is both the endpoint of a number of factors and the beginning of a series of complex transactions.

The patient's experience of pain is influenced not only by the somatic pain generator but also by his degree of neuroticism. The neuroticism usually features anxiety or depression and usually has little effect on the lower pain threshold but serves to diminish pain tolerance. Thus the degree of neuroticism is highly correlated with the amount of pain the patient experiences (7).

The way the patient presents his complaint of pain is less likely to be a function of his neuroticism than of his expressive style. Pain expression is influenced primarily by the degree of introversion or extraversion and by ethnic or sociocultural membership. Introverts are less expressive than extroverts of their pain experience. Members of demonstrative cultures easily complain of pain, and members of undemonstrative cultures are inhibited in pain expression. Pain expression apparently is not related to pain threshold or neuroticism, but it may influence pain tolerance (8).

The probability that a patient will present with a complaint of pain is also a function of certain socioeconomic vectors. When matched against other medical patients whose symptoms do not include pain, the pain patient tends to be older, to come from a lower socioeconomic (laboring) class, to come from a family with more siblings, to have had more relatives who had pain experiences, and to have had previous painful illnesses, injuries, or surgical procedures (7).

Thus it appears that the complaint of pain is likely to come from a patient with a unique combination of certain personality variables and a certain social exposure history. Therefore, it should not be surprising that the complaint of pain, by itself, is almost equally likely to indicate a psychological or a physical disturbance: that is, approximately half of the initial cases of pain complaints are diagnosed as psychogenic.

If we add to the psychogenic pain problems the number of cases of somatogenic pain in which there is some payoff or gain for the pain complaint, it seems that psychological factors can be significant in the majority of chronic pain patients. Consequently, simply attacking the somatic pain generator often fails to silence the complaint of pain, even though the therapy is technically successful.

For this reason, also, we can appreciate the recommendation by Bonica (3) that the successful pain clinic must be multidisciplinary. Psychodiagnostics, including the measurement of the patient's pain, and behavior therapy must parallel somatic work-up and somatic therapies, rather than being done in series (after all else has failed). This simultaneous approach can prevent the patient's unwitting sabotage of his treatment, and can also prevent the analgesist from unknowingly reinforcing the pain complaint.

Evaluation of the Pain Patient

The first step in evaluating a patient with pain is to determine the severity of pain and the patient's ability to describe it accurately. Patients who overstate the intensity of pain may be overtreated, whereas those who understate it may suffer needlessly.

The traditional methods of obtaining pain thresholds are of little help in this matter. Measures of pain thresholds, or upper limits of pain tolerance, simply give one a figure—in volts, for example—which at best can be compared with a distribution of scores from some sample. The individual patient may then be said to be more or less tolerant of pain than the average in the sample, but this tells us nothing of the intensity of the clinical pain experienced.

Our solution to this problem is to obtain the patient's estimate of the average severity of the pain, using a 0 to 100 scale. Then, using the submaximum effort tourniquet technique, we obtain the time required to match the average severity of the pain (clinical pain level) and the time to reach the upper limit of tolerance to the ischemic pain (maximum pain tolerance). When the clinical pain level is expressed as a percentage of the maximum pain tolerance, the resulting figure can then be compared with the patient's pain estimate (10).

Although we prefer to use ischemic pain, similar results may be obtained with a pressure algometer, electric shock, ice water, radiant heat, or other measures. The important point is to have the patient match his usual or average clinical pain and then determine his maximum tolerance level. The resulting percentage is a reliable approximation of the severity of the clinical pain, and when it is compared with the previously obtained pain estimate, one has some idea of how accurately the patient describes pain. Marked discrepancies require some explanation.

The next step in evaluating the patient is to obtain a clinically useful personality profile, or some assessment of the degree to which there may be an affective disturbance or a thought disorder. This may be done by psychological test, psychiatric interview (mental status examination), or, preferably, both. It should be emphasized, however, that unless the psychologist and/or psychiatrist has a specific interest in pain problems, his interpretations may be too general to be of much help in patient management.

From what was said earlier, we may expect to find clinically significant levels of anxiety in acute pain states and in cases of recurrent intermittent pain. Generally, there seems to be a rough correlation between the degree of anxiety and the severity of pain. Also from what was described earlier, we may expect to find clinically significant levels of depression in chronic pain states, with the degree of depression being roughly proportional to the severity of the pain. However, there are at least two complicating factors, and I must draw on clinical experience as well as on published works (see, for example, ref. 10).

First, depression seems to be related in part to the duration of pain as well as to its severity. Second, depression is frequently complicated or masked by a form of hypochondriasis that consists of somatic preoccupation. This hypochondriasis, in turn, seems to be inversely related to the degree to which the patient has satisfying relationships at home and at work.

Finally, in evaluating the patient, the physician must recognize the limits of psychological assessment. Nothing in the battery of pain tests and personality examinations can indicate whether a patient's pain is psychogenic or somatogenic. That determination can be made only by appropriate medical tests, i.e., whether or not there are relevant physical findings to account for the symptom of pain. Not even the use of placebo analgesics or placebo blocks can serve to distinguish psychogenic from somatogenic pain since placebo responses can be obtained from a large proportion of patients with clearly identifiable lesions.

TREATMENT OF THE PAIN PATIENT

Far more important than the question of whether pain is psychological or physical in origin is the issue of whether there are treatable psychological or physical findings. When a patient comes to a pain clinic, his or her usual expectation is that something will be done to relieve the pain. Of course, the staff of the clinic must have something to treat and will not merely attempt to silence the complaint of pain. Somatic therapists attempt to identify and correct underlying pathology, and similarly the psychological therapists identify and treat psychopathology. In cases of chronic intractable pain, both forms of pathology can usually be identified.

In these days of advances in psychophysiology, psychological therapy increasingly includes somatic manipulation and no longer is restricted to "talking" therapies. Furthermore, these psychophysiological approaches may have a direct effect on pain reduction and need not be considered as merely "teaching the patient to live with his pain."

Psychotropic Agents

Antianxiety agents have long been known to reduce acute pain; we now are beginning to obtain evidence that increasing the levels of brain serotonin may increase pain tolerance in chronic pain (11). Even when this is not the case, as with nonspecific antidepressants, patients report feeling more rested, more optimistic, and thus better able to tolerate pain.

Detoxification from Narcotics

Many chronic pain patients become heavily addicted to narcotic analgesics, which is partly an iatrogenic problem. Physicians tend to prescribe analgesics on an "as needed" (*prn*) basis. Patients usually fear becoming addicted, so they wait until pain is severe before taking the analgesic. Because severe pain is difficult to reduce, patients take several pills, thus increasing their physical dependence and necessitating still larger doses. In our experience, by detoxifying the patient and using "by the clock" dosage schedules (e.g., q.4 hr), pain levels are directly reduced and weaker analgesics are sufficient to make the pain bearable. Of course, patients must understand that pain abolition is not possible with analgesics alone.

Biofeedback

The form of operant conditioning by means of which a physiological system is detected, amplified, and displayed to the patient as a continuously varying visual or auditory display, biofeedback has been shown to have a directly useful effect on pain reduction as the patient acquires voluntary control of previously involuntary systems. For example, electromyographic feedback has been found useful for muscle tension (as in tension headaches) and muscle spasms (as in spasmodic torticollis). Skin temperature feedback is effective in migraine prevention and in certain sympathethic dystrophies. Other applications may also be found, e.g., bowel sounds in spastic colon.

Behavior Therapies

Many clinics are now using contingency management to teach patients to increase activity levels and to decrease pain behavior. The evidence thus far is that this is more than mere instruction in stoicism; patients' reported pain levels decrease, and this reduction is maintained on follow-up evaluation (10).

SUMMARY

It is a truism to note that psychological factors are significant in most clinical pain problems. We are beginning to see not only the kinds of social learning that influence pain behavior but also some of the neurochemical processes that may underlie both the psychological and physical models of pain. Consequently, the psychological treatment of pain patients is increasingly attending to both the modification of learned pain behavior and the use of agents that modify mood as well as pain levels.

REFERENCES

1. Akil, H. (1972): Monoaminergic mechanisms underlying stimulation-produced analgesia. Doctoral dissertation, University of California, Los Angeles.
2. Basbaum, A. I. (1974): *Exp. Neurol.,* 42:490–501.
3. Bonica, J. J. (ed.) (1974): *Advances in Neurology, Vol. 4: International Symposium on Pain.* Raven Press, New York.
4. Bradley, J. J. (1963): *Br. J. Psychiatry,* 109:741–745.
5. Buytendijk, F. J. J. (1962): *Pain: Its Modes and Functions,* translated by E. O'Shiel. University of Chicago Press, Chicago.
6. Engel, B. T. (1959): *J. Exp. Psychol.,* 57:389–396.
7. Merskey, H., and Spear, F. G. (1967): *Pain: Psychological and Psychiatric Aspects.* Bailliere, Tindall and Cassell, London.
8. Sternbach, R. A. (1968): *Pain: A Psychophysiological Analysis.* Academic Press, New York.
9. Sternbach, R. A. (1974*a*): In: *Somatic Manifestations of Depressive Disorders,* edited by A. Kiev. Excerpta Medica, Princeton, New Jersey.

10. Sternbach, R. A. (1974*b*): *Pain Patients: Traits and Treatment.* Academic Press, New York.
11. Sternbach, R. A., Janowsky, D. S., Huey, L. Y., and Segal, D. S.: *This volume.*
12. Sternbach, R. A., and Timmermans, G. (1975): *Pain,* 1:177–181.
13. Szasz, T. S. (1957): *Pain and Pleasure: A Study of Bodily Feelings.* Basic Books, New York.
14. Timmermans, G., and Sternbach, R. A.: *This volume.*
15. Wall, P. D., and Gutnick, M. (1974): *Nature,* 248:740–743.

Advances in Pain Research and Therapy, Vol. 1,
edited by J. J. Bonica and D. Albe-Fessard.
Raven Press, New York © 1976.

SAD Index for Clinical Assessment of Pain

Richard G. Black and C. Richard Chapman

Departments of Anesthesiology, Psychiatry and Behavioral Sciences, and Psychology; and University Hospital Pain Clinic, University of Washington School of Medicine, Seattle, Washington 98195

Lack of clear taxonomy for clinical pain complaints often leads to a wrong diagnosis and resultant inappropriate therapy. These errors can be serious enough that unnecessary and even harmful surgery may be performed, often repeatedly, in a desperate attempt to eliminate a "pain" that may have no surgically correctable cause. Alternate, yet still inappropriate, management with strong analgesic medications prescribed in ever-escalating doses may lead the patient into a vicious circle of depression, confusion, and increased expression of pain.

Experience gained at the University of Washington Pain Clinic has demonstrated that the usual descriptive terminology applied to pain problems is of little help and that a therapeutically meaningful taxonomy of pain does not exist. Not only is there no standard taxonomy of pain, but the terms used force the clinician to condense a constellation of problems related to human suffering into a single diagnostic category with a single therapy.

The pain complaint as an expression of suffering is a strong stimulus that can be relied on in our society to evoke attention, sympathy, and solicitude. Expressed feelings of despair, loneliness, or anxiety often repulse individuals who would have readily responded to a physically based pain complaint. Some individuals learn this rapidly so that the single complaint of pain, assumed to have a physical cause, can serve as the most acceptable, strongest, and most effective plea for help for many forms of suffering.

Harm can result when a pain complaint generated by emotional stress is taken at its face value. Unrecognized anxiety, depression, or even social problems may then be treated inappropriately by strong analgesics or surgery, as if these complaints were caused by a broken bone or pinched nerve. Unfortunately, the universal appeal and acceptability of the complaint of "physically based" pain results in its wide use by emotionally stressed patients and ready acceptance by physicians. This chapter offers an alternative scheme for evaluating pain complaints in patients whose suffering seems to greatly exceed their organic defect. Termed the SAD index, this frame of reference divides the patient's problem into three dimensions, each a well-known clinical entity with an accepted, effective therapy. In brief, each pain problem is defined in terms of *S*omatic input, *A*nxiety, and *D*epression.

For an easy understanding of the relation of the patient's pain complaint to these factors, it is useful to visualize the magnitude of the somatic, anxious, and depressive components of the patient's suffering scaled along the axes of a three-dimensional system of rectangular coordinates (Fig. 1). Each axis shows the magnitude of its component on a scale of 0 to 10. The vertical or "Somatic" axis indicates a measure of somatic input on this scale of 0 to 10 with 0 at the origin representing no somatic input. The horizontal axis to the viewer's left, or "Anxious" axis, indicates some measure of anxiety, while the horizontal axis to the right, the "Depression" axis, indicates in an analogous manner the patient's degree of depression.

Although we have not yet developed a formal diagnostic package, the magnitude of each component could be arrived at by a combination of information from a series of clinical tests and psychological questionnaires. However, the index may be used informally at the bedside by a skilled clinician who subjectively assesses his patient in terms of these three components. Adopting the basic concept of the SAD index, he views the patient's complaint as a composite of somatic, anxious, and depressive entities, assigning a subjective value to each dimension. This results in a more meaningful description of the patient's pain complaint and improves communication of his interpretation of the problems to other health care professionals.

The patient's total suffering is represented by the vector sum of the dimensions represented on the three axes. For the nonmathematically inclined reader, the vector sum is the line extending from the intersection of the axes to a point reached by moving up so many Somatic units, out to the left so many Anxious units, and out to the right to so many Depressive

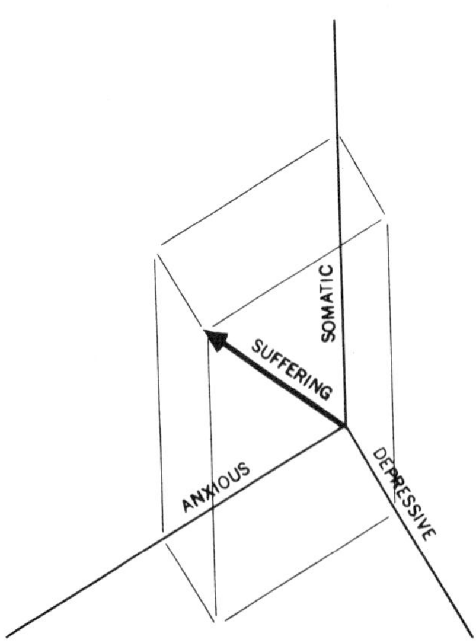

FIG. 1. Relationship among somatogenic signals, anxiety, and depression expressed in terms of rectangular coordinates. Evaluation of a patient along all 3 dimensions permits definition of a point in a 3-dimensional space. Vector connecting this point to the origin is defined as suffering.

units. The length of this vector increases with increases of any or all of the individual components.

The formal evaluation of the magnitude of the Somatic axis is a difficult problem involving quantification of clinical judgment as well as psychophysical assessment of the patient's subjective state. Variables that can be used for this evaluation include: history and functional inquiry, activity diary, clinician's subjective impression, experience with comparable disease, pain description questionnaires, and pain matching tests: ischemic, cold, and heat. The results from these assessments are then combined to yield a value between 0 and 10. Subjective physician and patient data as well as scale comparisons of similar diseases can be obtained by short, easily answered, one-page questionnaires. All or some of these items can be used in a formal evaluation.

The physician can assess the components of anxiety and depression by using several short questionnaires. The Anxiety axis can be quantified by any or all of the following indices: history and functional inquiry, clinician's response, State-Trait Anxiety Inventory (5), Taylor Manifest Anxiety Scale (6), Institute of Personality and Ability Testing Anxiety Scale (IPAT) (2), and secondary MMPI scales (4). The Depressive axis can be quantified by any or all of the following: history and functional inquiry, clinician's impression, Zung Depression Scale (7), Beck Depression Scale (1), Hamilton Depression Scale (3), and MMPI Depression Scale (4).

Within each dimension, information from two or more items should be combined to yield a score ranging from 0 to 10. Weights for combining information optimally to arrive at a single score for each dimension have not yet been defined.

The patient's total suffering is the vector sum of these three components and is calculated by the following formula:

$$\text{Suffering} = 0.58\sqrt{S^2 + A^2 + D^2},$$

where S = value of Somatic component, A = value of Anxious component, D = value of Depressive component, and 0.58 = scale correction factor limiting suffering to 10.

Actual calculation of the suffering vector is primarily of research interest. For most clinical and therapeutic applications of the SAD index, it is sufficient to generate only the component values. For example, an index of SAD = 1:4:8 may represent the chronically depressed low-back cripple with minimum physical disability. A very anxious but not depressed patient with mild incisional pain from a breast biopsy may have a SAD index = 3:7:0 (Fig. 2). Appropriate therapy for this patient is treatment of anxiety. If, however, her total vector of suffering, the behavior observed clinically, calculated as 4.41, is interpreted as all incisional or somatic pain and the patient is treated with strong analgesics with their side effect of depression, the somatic component will be reduced at the cost of increasing the de-

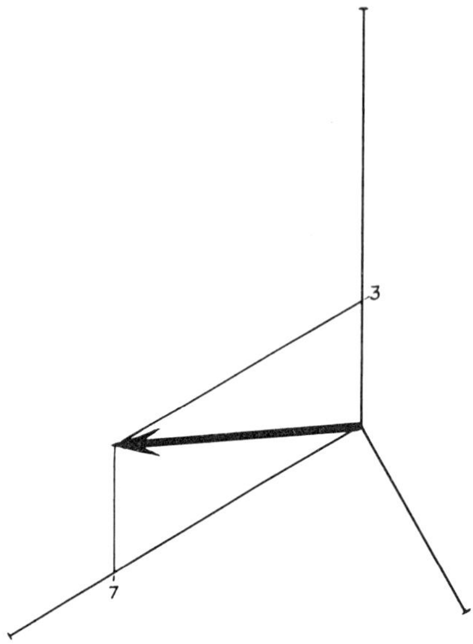

FIG. 2. Assessment of an anxious patient with minimal or no depression.

pressive component. The situation might now be changed to SAD = 1:7:6 (Fig. 3), which yields a total suffering vector of 5.35, indicating that this inappropriate therapy has increased the patient's apparent suffering. This patient now belongs to that group of patients shown by Sternbach (4) to have less pain after withdrawal of strong analgesic medications.

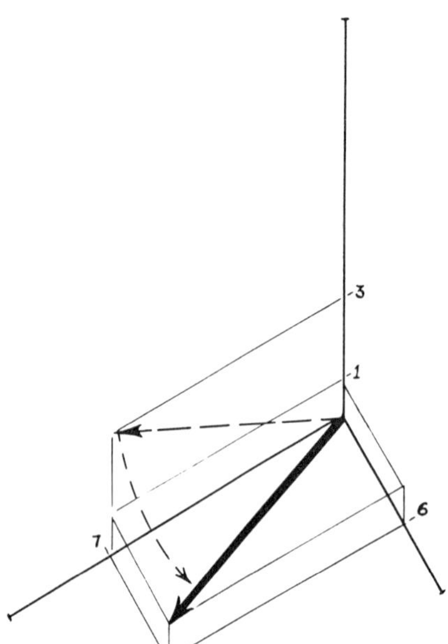

FIG. 3. Effects of inappropriate treatment on the suffering vector.

For the management of difficult chronic pain patients who have learned to express pain as a means of dealing with emotional stress, the SAD index may be extended into a Pain Profile which incorporates scales reflecting other factors affecting pain behavior. A list of factors currently under assessment for evaluation of the chronic pain patient is:

Somatic	S_c	Somatogenic chronic
	S_a	Somatogenic acute
Anxiety	A_s	State anxiety
	A_t	Trait anxiety
Depression	D_e	Endogenous depression
	D_r	Reactive depression
	D_m	Depression secondary to medications
Social	S'_w	Social situation at work
	S'_h	Social situation at home
Gains	G_c	Gains from compensation
	G_l	Gains expected from litigation
	G_p	Personal gains
Cultural	C	Cultural factors

The complaint of pain is complex and may invite well-intended, but inappropriate, and sometimes harmful, therapy. By dividing this complex complaint into simpler components, the SAD index permits more accurate diagnosis leading to appropriate and therefore effective therapy. The SAD index is primarily intended as an intuitive aid to diagnosis and secondarily, after more evaluation, as a pain research tool. It has proven useful in its application to patients both as an abstract model assisting clinicians in sorting out judgments and as a teaching tool for students as yet unfamiliar with the complexities of pain.

ACKNOWLEDGMENT

This work was carried out in part under the Anesthesia Research Center, Grant GM 15991-07, University of Washington School of Medicine, Seattle, Washington.

REFERENCES

1. Beck, A. T., Ward, C. H., Mendelson, M., Mock, J., and Erbaugh, J. (1961): *Arch. Gen. Psychiatry,* 4:53–63.
2. Cattell, R. B., and Scheier, I. H. (1963): *Handbook for the I.P.A.T. Anxiety Scale Questionnaire.* Institute for Personality and Ability Testing, Champaign, Illinois.
3. Hamilton, M. (1960): *J. Neurol. Neurosurg. Psychiatry,* 23:56–62.
4. Sternbach, R. A. (1974): *Pain Patients—Traits and Treatment.* Academic Press, New York.
5. Spielberger, C. D., Gorsuch, R. L., and Lushene, R. (1970): *Manual for the State-Trait Anxiety Inventory.* Consulting Psychologists Press, Palo Alto, California.
6. Taylor, J. A. (1953): *J. Abnorm. Psychol.,* 48:285–290.
7. Zung, W. W. K. (1965): *Arch. Gen. Psychiatry,* 12:63–70.

Advances in Pain Research and Therapy, Vol. 1,
edited by J. J. Bonica and D. Albe-Fessard.
Raven Press, New York © 1976.

Human Chronic Pain and Personality: a Canonical Correlation Analysis

Gretchen Timmermans and Richard A. Sternbach

Pain Unit, Veterans Administration Hospital, San Diego, California 92161

Earlier we reported (6) results of an analysis of personality and pain measures of patients with chronic benign pain (more than 6 months' duration) who were being evaluated for admission to the inpatient Pain Unit of this hospital. A principal-components factor analysis resulted in separate factors for the personality and pain measures. The first three factors were *interpersonal alienation and manipulativeness, clinical pain intensity,* and *pain endurance*. We concluded that if a patient with chronic pain were to be treated successfully, the treatment must not only deal with the reduction of pain but must also provide supportive social integration and increased responsible self-control by the patient over his own life.

This study elicited comments (1) suggesting that a canonical correlation analysis would be appropriate to identify the combination of pain variables that would have the maximum correlation with a combination of personality variables. That is, is there some set of pain variables that is strongly related with a set of personality variables? Canonical correlation analysis is designed to identify the overall relationship between personality and pain measures. Canonical correlation looks for the best linear combination of variables in each set (in the set of pain and in the set of personality measures) so that the resulting correlation between the two sets is maximum. In addition, canonical correlation can provide an estimate of the statistical significance of the relationship between the pain and personality measures.

METHODS

The results of the canonical correlation analysis are presented here as performed on an expanded group of chronic pain patients. The original sample of 119 patients was enlarged to 204 by adding 85 consecutive patients admitted to the Pain Unit. The expanded group of patients had the following diagnoses: degenerative spinal disease (136 patients), peripheral nerve injury (47 patients), central nerve injury (3 patients), cancer (5 patients), tension headache (5 patients), migraine headache (1 patient), and no physical findings (7 patients). Of the total patient group, 156 were men and 48 were women.

As in the previous analysis, the patients completed a Minnesota Multiphasic Personality Inventory (MMPI), a Health Index (5), gave a pain estimate rating the average intensity of their pain on a scale from 0 to 100 (4), and took a tourniquet pain test (4). This tourniquet pain test, which is our adaptation of the submaximum effort tourniquet technique (3), produces arm ischemic pain. In the current study, the measure used from the tourniquet test is the ratio score (computed by dividing the clinical pain level by the maximum pain tolerance level and multiplying the quotient by 100). This ratio score, the most useful measure derived from the tourniquet pain test, is interpreted as an indirect measure of the patient's physical pain intensity. In contrast, the pain estimate is interpreted as a measure of the patient's subjective feeling about the pain intensity, and it reflects his anxiety and emotional distress owing to the pain.

RESULTS

The first set of variables for the canonical correlation analysis (2) contains the pain estimate and the tourniquet test ratio. The second set is composed of the personality measures and the sex and age variables. The results of the analysis are presented in Table 1. The two pain measures

TABLE 1. *Results of canonical correlation analysis of pain and personality variables*

Response measures	Canonical variates	
	1	2
Set 1. Pain measures		
Pain estimate	1.01186	−0.41283
Tourniquet pain test	−0.03036	1.09241
Set 2. Personality measures		
Health Index subscales		
Invalidism	0.26700	0.44976
Manifest depression	−0.00841	0.81289
Pain preoccupation	0.82630	−0.51234
Pain games	0.02557	−0.06809
MMPI Scales		
Hs (hypochondriasis)	0.00213	−0.19232
D (depression)	0.08165	0.55842
Hy (hysteria)	−0.20815	0.13211
Pd (psychopathic deviate)	−0.26773	−0.07156
Mf (masculinity-femininity)	0.05166	−0.41490
Pa (paranoia)	0.12987	0.25684
Pt (psychasthenia)	−0.29392	−0.51709
Sc (schizophrenia)	0.42580	−0.61289
Ma (hypomania)	−0.02649	0.26266
Si (social introversion)	−0.33580	−0.12377
Sex (coded 0 = female, 1 = male)	−0.37316	0.50176
Age	−0.02757	−0.19550
Canonical correlations	0.37478[a]	0.27668

[a] Significant at 0.05 level with 32 df, as tested by chi square. See Table 2.

appear separately, the pain estimate on the first canonical variate, and the tourniquet pain test ratio on the second canonical variate.

The Health Index subscale pain preoccupation is the personality variable most highly correlated with the pain estimate and is the only such variable that is strongly related. This subscale contains items that refer to how much the pain interferes with normal daily activities, such as sleep, sex, or taking medicines. The higher the pain patient rates his pain on the 0 to 100 pain estimate scale, the more activities it seems to interfere with and the more he tends to focus his attention on it.

The second canonical variate, composed of the tourniquet pain test ratio, is most highly related to the manifest depression subscale of the Health Index, and to a lesser degree to the depression scale of the MMPI. Additionally, high correlations in a negative direction are found on the psychasthenia (Pt) and schizophrenia (Sc) scales of the MMPI. This combination seems to indicate that the depression, positively related to the pain intensity, is a reactive depression, and that lower levels of pain intensity may be associated with an agitated confusion.

CONCLUSIONS

These results seem to support the impressions of those who attempt to treat patients with chronic benign pain. As the pain is subjectively rated higher, the more the patient centers his life around the pain, and the more his estimate of its severity reflects the impact of the pain on his daily functioning. However, as the pain intensity (as measured by the tourniquet pain test) increases, the patient is more depressed, that depression being a reaction to the pain.

The measure of significance of linear association between the two sets of variables is tested by chi-square tests of significance. Table 2 presents the significance test data and indicates that the linear relation between the two sets of variables in the first canonical variate does, in fact, have a significant linear relationship at the 0.05 level of significance with 32 degrees of freedom. Although the second canonical variate does not reach statistical sig-

TABLE 2. *Significance of the canonical correlations*

Canonical variate sets	Corresponding canonical correlations	Chi square	Degrees of freedom	Significance level
1. Pain estimate and preoccupation with pain	0.37478	44.92917	32	0.05
2. Pain intensity and reactive depression	0.27668	15.48962	15	ns

nificance, the interrelationships between the depression measures and the measure of pain intensity do merit some tentative consideration as they support much clinical experience in working with pain patients.

ACKNOWLEDGMENTS

This work was supported by the Veterans Administration Hospital, San Diego, California 92161. We thank Karen Anderson, M.S., Computing Facility, University of California, Irvine, and Charles C. Berry, Ph.D., Department of Community Medicine, University of California, San Diego, for their help.

REFERENCES

1. Bookstein, F. L., Wolff, B. B., and Posavac, E. J. (1975): *Science,* 187:859–861.
2. Nie, N. H., Hull, C. H., et al. (1973): *SPSS Statistical Package for the Social Sciences: Update Manual,* National Opinion Research Center, University of Chicago, Modification Identifier A-003-244.
3. Smith, G. M., Egbert, L. D., Markowitz, R. A., Mosteller, F., and Beecher, H. K. (1966): *J. Pharmacol. Exp. Ther.,* 154:324–332.
4. Sternbach, R. A., Murphy, R. W., Timmermans, G., Greenhoot, J. H., and Akeson, W. H. (1974): In: *Advances in Neurology, Vol. 4: International Symposium on Pain,* edited by J. J. Bonica, pp. 281–288. Raven Press, New York.
5. Sternbach, R. A., Wolf, S. R., Murphy, R. W., and Akeson, W. H. (1973): *Psychosomatics,* 14:52–56.
6. Timmermans, G., and Sternbach, R. A. (1974): *Science,* 184:806–808.

Advances in Pain Research and Therapy, Vol. 1,
edited by J. J. Bonica and D. Albe-Fessard.
Raven Press, New York © 1976.

Pain and Personality in Cancer Patients

Michael R. Bond

Professor of Psychological Medicine, University of Glasgow, Southern General Hospital, Govan Road, Glasgow, G51 4TF., Scotland

In 1827 J. G. Guthrie commented on an observation all of us have made many times during our professional life when he said "in two persons apparently suffering from the same kind of injury and with the same detriment one will writhe with agony whilst the other will smile with contempt." In other words, for a physical disorder or injury of given severity, some experience pain but others do not, and of those in pain some complain whereas others remain silent about their discomfort. There are several reasons for variations in pain behavior among individuals, including the level of emotion pain evokes, personality differences, the significance of the pain in the light of past experience, and family and ethnic influences (9). This chapter presents evidence to support the hypothesis that one of the most fundamental reasons for variations in the pain experienced by people in similar circumstances is the presence of differences in the response of the central nervous system to the input of stressful stimuli, particularly those that are physically noxious. These differences are responsible for variation in both the ease with which pain is aroused and the behavior associated with its presence. It is concluded that a link between basic neurophysiological and psychophysiological mechanisms underlying pain and aspects of behavior associated with it may be demonstrated using data from work previously published by the author (2,3).

METHOD

Two groups of patients with cancer have been studied. The first were investigated to determine the incidence of pain in women with advanced cancer of the cervix and its relation to their personality structure (3). In the second, members of a group of patients with severe chronic pain were examined before and after successful cervical percutaneous cordotomy to assess the effects of pain relief on personality (2). In each experiment pain was assessed at 2-hr intervals between 8 A.M. and 8 P.M. each day throughout the period of study using an analogue scale as previously reported (4).

Personality was assessed by the Eysenck Personality Inventory (6), which measures two fundamental dimensions of personality: neuroticism and extraversion. Briefly, neuroticism is defined here as emotional lability or overresponsiveness and a liability to neurotic breakdown under stress; the higher the neuroticism score, the greater the level of emotionality. Extraversion is the presence of an outgoing personality with relatively uninhibited social tendencies that are increasingly noticeable as the extraversion score increases. Eysenck proposes that the neuroticism scale gives a quantitative measure of those elements of emotion determined principally by interaction between the reticular arousal system and the limbic system. Moreover, there is evidence that measures on the scale correlate significantly with physiological concomitants of emotionality, especially those associated with anxiety. He suggests that the extraversion scale measures aspects of behavior that are controlled by higher cortical centers (5).

RESULTS

First Experiment

A total of 52 women with advanced cancer of the cervix at the same clinical stage, with a mean age of 52 years (SD $\pm$ 5.29), and with illness of similar duration were examined. Of these patients, 13 were pain free (group 1), 17 had pain but did not require or request analgesic drugs (group 2), and 22 had pain for which they received treatment (group 3).

Extraversion Scores

Consideration of extraversion scores for the whole patient group reveals that their mean score was similar to that of a normal population (Table 1). Examination of the subgroups shows that pain-free patients were extroverts, as were those in pain who received drugs. Patients who had pain and yet did not request or receive drugs tended to be introverted, and their mean score is significantly lower than that of the other groups (Mann-Whitney U. $p < 0.05 > 0.02$.) (10). Because the extent and duration of illness were similar in all patients, the results so far suggest that complaints of pain are associated primarily with extraversion and that lack of complaint is related to introversion. Therefore, these aspects of personality seem to be important determinants of complaint behavior.

TABLE 1. *Mean extraversion and neuroticism scores*

		All patients	Group 1	Group 2	Group 3	Normal housewives
E	Mean	14.00	15.38	12.00	15.00	13.92
	SD	3.95	2.79	5.04	3.09	4.22
N	Mean	10.64	5.23	12.82	11.59	9.42
	SD	6.18	3.59	4.81	5.47	5.19

Neuroticism Scores

The neuroticism scores of the whole group did not differ significantly from those of a normal population of healthy women (Table 1). However, examination of the subgroup scores shows that patients without pain had very low scores, whereas those in pain had higher scores, and scores were highest for patients who did not receive drugs. The difference between the neuroticism scores of pain-free patients and scores of those with pain is statistically significant (Mann-Whitney U. $p < 0.02 > 0.01$.) (10).

The results for neuroticism suggest that the presence or absence of pain is associated with distinct differences in levels of emotionality. In the light of Eysenck's hypothesis that this dimension of personality is determined by activity within the reticulolimbic system, it is reasonable to assume that the latter may function differently in the two groups. Therefore, rather than postulating that pain leads solely to an increase in emotionality, which is the general belief (1,7,8,11), it could be argued that the susceptibility of an individual to increased emotionality is based on the response of an area of the brain that also plays a part in the modulation of the input of noxious stimuli to higher centers. Thus, on the one hand, facilitatory activity—perhaps in the reticulolimbic system—may be activated by noxious stimuli, in which case it is associated with pain and a general response leading to higher-than-normal levels of emotional activity. On the other hand, facilitatory activity may inhibit incoming information with the result that the patient remains pain free or has a low level of pain and exhibits low levels of emotional activity.

Second Experiment

This experiment concerns 30 patients with severe pain owing to carcinoma. All underwent successful cervical percutaneous cordotomy and were completely freed from pain. Personality assessments were carried out on every patient preoperatively and on 12 after surgery. All drugs, especially narcotics, were reduced to the minimum in the week before operation. The forms A and B of the Eysenck Personality Inventory (EPI) were used to overcome the effects of practice on the test results.

The mean neuroticism score for patients is higher preoperatively and lower after surgery than such a score for a normal population, but differences between the scores of the respective groups are not significant. Mean extraversion scores for patients before and after operation were lower than those of normal individuals, but the differences were not statistically significant (Table 2).

Before surgery the distribution of neuroticism scores was unusual, having a bimodal pattern (Fig. 1). Further examination of the levels of pain recorded by individuals in each of the two groups showed that the scores were significantly higher among those with high neuroticism scores. After

TABLE 2. *Mean neuroticism and extraversion scores before and after cervical percutaneous cordotomy*

		Preoperative scores		Postoperative scores	
		Patients	Normal population	Patients	Normal population
	N	30	2,000	12	2,000
E	Mean	11.20	12.10	13.80	14.10
	SD	4.20	4.37	3.75	3.92
N	Mean	10.20	9.10	8.83	10.50
	SD	5.40	4.78	3.59	4.71

operation the general pattern of neuroticism scores was unchanged, but the extreme values disappeared from each end of the scoring range, and further analysis of the data revealed that high scores had fallen and low scores had risen. This is clearly demonstrated in Fig. 2 where pre- and postoperative neuroticism scores have been converted to *t*-values to enable comparison.

Data for extraversion scores are not discussed further because they showed a normal distribution curve before and after surgery.

The results of this experiment indicate that the severe stress of chronic and unrelieved pain leads to changes in personality and, in particular, in the level of emotionality. Quite unexpectedly, the preoperative neuroticism scores showed a bipolar distribution, and after operation—which produced total pain relief—high scores were lowered and low ones were raised. It was also observed that before operation patients with higher levels of neuroticism had higher levels of pain.

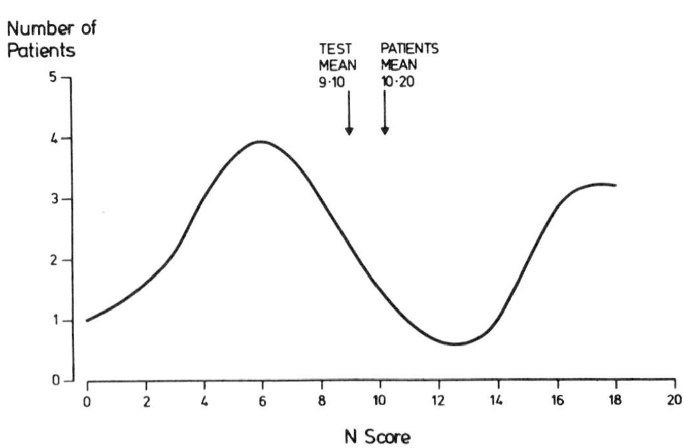

FIG. 1. Precordotomy distribution of neuroticism scores (*N*-30).

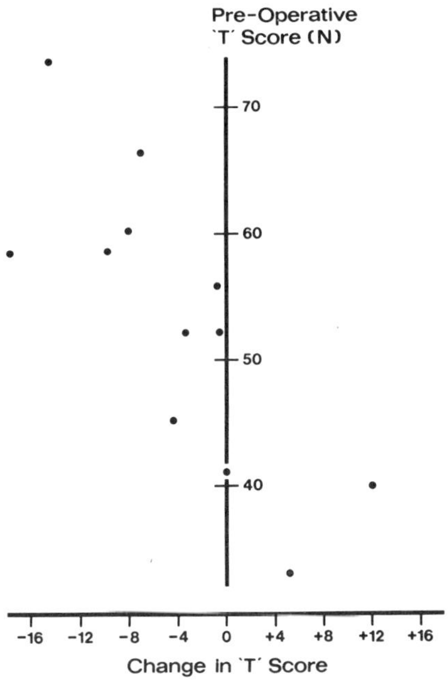

FIG. 2. Changes in neuroticism scores resulting from the complete relief of intractable pain.

CONCLUSIONS

The contention that the central nervous system varies in its response to noxious stimuli is supported by the results of the experiments described. It is also concluded that even in the absence of any other physical or environmental changes, cessation of noxious stimuli alone with an attendant reduction in activation of centers in the brain is associated with changes in the pattern of scoring on the EPI toward normal values, although the changes were not complete in the subjects studied. Comparable observations have been made by Sternbach and Timmermans (11) who concluded that, "the neuroticism associated with chronic pain is the result of it and may be reversible when pain is reduced or abolished." Kissen (7) reported similar findings with respect to postoperative pain several years ago, but our understanding of the problem can be extended now in the light of the results reported here. It appears that under normal circumstances each individual has a personality "setting or style" that changes in response to the stress of severe physical illness with a general trend toward introversion and either increased or decreased emotionality in one of several forms. Chronic pain appears to increase the emotional response beyond the level produced by other features of illness.

SUMMARY

Personality, as measured by the Eysenck Personality Inventory, is related to both the severity of pain experienced in physical illness and variations in complaint behavior. Emotionality, measured by the Neuroticism Scale of the EPI, may increase or decrease in patients with cancer, the change being determined by the individuals' preexisting personality setting. Further, emotionality appears to return toward a normal level with relief of pain. High levels of emotionality are associated with significantly more pain than low levels. The evidence presented supports the original hypothesis that the neurophysiological and psychophysiological mechanisms underlying pain and variations in behavior associated with it are linked in the brain through a modulating inhibitory/excitatory mechanism common to both.

REFERENCES

1. Bendien, J. (1963): *J. Psychosom. Res.*, 7:1–10.
2. Bond, M. R. (1973): *J. Psychosom. Res.*, 17:257–263.
3. Bond, M. R., and Pearson, I. B. (1969): *J. Psychosom. Res.*, 13:13–19.
4. Bond, M. R., and Pilowsky, I. (1966): *J. Psychosom. Res.*, 10:203–208.
5. Eysenck, H. J. *A Monograph in American Lectures in Living Chemistry,* edited by Kugelmass. Charles C Thomas, Publisher, Springfield, Illinois.
6. Eysenck, H. J. and Eysenck, S. G. B. (1964): *Manual of the Eysenck Personality Inventory.* University of London Press, London.
7. Kissen, D. M. (1964): *J. Psychosom. Res.*, 8:145–149.
8. Lovell, R. R. H., and Verghese, A. (1967): *Br. Med. J.*, 3:327–330.
9. Merskey, H., and Spear, F. G. (1967): *Pain: Psychological and Psychiatric Aspects.* Bailliere, Tindall and Cassell, London.
10. Siegal, S. (1956): *Non-Parametric Statistics for the Behavioral Sciences.* McGraw-Hill, New York.
11. Sternbach, R. A., and Timmermans, G. (1975): *Pain,* 1:177–181.

Advances in Pain Research and Therapy, Vol. 1,
edited by J. J. Bonica and D. Albe-Fessard.
Raven Press, New York © 1976.

Correlation of Personality Profile with Pain Syndrome

K. Jamison, *M. T. Ferrer-Brechner, *V. L. Brechner, and C. P. McCreary

*Departments of Psychiatry and * Anesthesiology, University of California School of Medicine, Los Angeles, California 90024*

The multifaceted and highly complex nature of pain and of chronic pain patients has been discussed many times (2–5) and will not be further elaborated on in this chapter. The purpose of the study outlined here was to: (a) describe a pain patient population with a battery of psychological tests—several of which had not been used on this kind of patient group before, and (b) investigate the relationship between certain personality variables and treatment outcome.

METHOD

Sample

The study sample included 51 patients who came to the UCLA Department of Anesthesiology Pain Management Clinic with chief complaints of chronic pain. The average age of the sample was 50.8 years (SD 11.1), with a range of 25 to 72 years. Approximately one-third of the sample (35.3%) was male, and there was a wide diversity and heterogeneity of physical diagnoses (low back pain, postherpetic neuralgia, causalgia, phantom limb pain, and so on). The average length of time from first admission to the Pain Management Clinic (PMC) and follow-up was 7.2 months (SD = 3.2) with a range of 3 to 13 months.

Procedure

All patients were seen and evaluated by either a faculty member or a house officer in the Department of Anesthesiology. The degree of objective physical findings was ascertained and rated by the admitting physician on a 0 to 8 point scale; ratings were based on radiologic findings, neurologic and general physical examination findings (including sensory change, absent reflexes, muscle wasting, and EMG of denervation), and clinical laboratory results. During the initial evaluation, patients were given a routine battery of psychological tests [Minnesota Multiphasic Personality Inventory

(MMPI), Eysenck Personality Inventory, Internal-External Locus of Control Scale, Aas Hypnotic Susceptibility Scale, and Questionnaire A, an inventory designed to measure assertiveness]. In order to avoid contaminating the physician's ratings of the degree of physical findings and the follow-up evaluations of response to therapy, we did not reveal the results of the psychological testing to the evaluating physician except in rare instances when MMPI results were necessary for a case conference.

Patients were treated with a variety of procedures including nerve blocks of different kinds, transcutaneous neural stimulation, surgery, and pharmacotherapy. Follow-up data were then obtained for each patient at least 3 months after admission to the Pain Management Clinic. The following rating scale was used as a gauge of response: 0, worsened during therapy; 1, no improvement; 2, minimal improvement during therapy but relapse to previous condition when therapy was discontinued; 3, definite improvement sustained for at least 1 month; 4, almost complete recovery; 5, complete relief of pain.

Data Analysis

The demographic, medical, personality, and outcome data were coded and analyzed; frequency distributions for all variables were then obtained. The sample was subdivided into those patients designated as having had an "unsuccessful" outcome (scores of 0 or 1 on the response to treatment rating scale described above) and those designated as having had a "successful" outcome (score of 3 or more). These groups were compared on mean scale scores on the various personality dimensions. Similar analyses were carried out comparing men and women. Two stepwise multiple-regression analyses were done: one using the variables with greatest predictive strength to predict to a continuous outcome criterion (categories 0 through 5 on outcome rating scale described above), and one using variables to predict to a dichotomous outcome criterion (i.e., the above-described "successful" versus "unsuccessful" dichotomy).

RESULTS

The results of the mean scale score analyses for the various divisions of our sample are summarized in Table 1. When the total sample was broken down into men and women, no significant differences were found in terms of response to treatment, degree of physical findings, or any personality variables except for the following MMPI scales (women scored significantly lower on all of these): Depression ($p < 0.01$), Psychopathic Deviate ($p < 0.01$), Masculinity-Femininity ($p < 0.01$), and Alcoholism ($p < 0.05$); clearly, T-scores rather than raw scores were used for all MMPI analyses except for subscales of the test. The only significant difference between patients in the "successful" group and those in the "unsuccessful" group

TABLE 1. *Characteristics of chronic pain patients*

Variable name	Total sample ($N = 51$) $\bar{X}$	SD	Men ($N = 18$) $\bar{X}$	SD	Women ($N = 33$) $\bar{X}$	SD	Successful outcome ($N = 16$) $\bar{X}$	SD	Unsuccessful outcome ($N = 21$) $\bar{X}$	SD
Extent of physical findings	2.0	1.6	2.4	1.9	1.8	1.4	2.0	1.1	2.0	1.8
Response to treatment	1.8	1.3	2.0	1.5	1.7	1.2				
Age	50.8	11.1	49.9	13.4	51.4	9.8	48.8	12.5	52.6	7.2
Time since admission to PMC	7.2	3.2	6.7	3.1	7.5	3.3	6.8	3.5	7.6	3.5
EPI—Extraversion	11.1	2.8	10.5	2.5	11.4	2.9	10.9	2.9	11.3	2.8
EPI—Neuroticism	10.7	5.6	9.1	5.8	11.5	5.4	8.5	5.5	10.6	5.4
EPI—Lie Scale	3.7	2.0	4.4	2.1	3.3	2.0	4.0	1.9	4.0	2.3
Assertion Questionnaire	17.6	4.3	17.8	3.5	17.6	4.7	17.1	3.2	17.9	4.4
Aas Hypnotic Susceptibility	3.3	1.7	2.8	1.5	3.6	1.7	2.6	1.8	3.4	1.7
Internal-External Scale	8.8	4.6	8.3	3.7	9.1	5.0	9.5	3.3	8.3	4.7
MMPI—Q (unanswered questions)	6.0	13.0	4.6	14.0	6.9	12.6	7.4	17.1	7.9	13.2
MMPI—L	52.6	9.4	51.8	7.6	53.1	10.5	51.0	7.5	51.5	10.8
MMPI—F	56.6	8.5	58.2	5.9	55.6	9.8	55.7	7.7	54.8	7.4
MMPI—K	55.5	8.4	54.9	9.4	55.8	7.9	59.4	7.5	53.2	8.3
MMPI—Hysteria	75.4	12.6	79.3	13.8	73.0	11.5	72.6	9.2	78.3	14.5
MMPI—Depression	71.9	11.4	78.5	9.2	67.8	10.8	70.9	9.1	72.2	12.6
MMPI—Hypochondriasis	74.0	10.5	75.0	11.6	73.3	10.0	73.3	10.0	76.1	10.7
MMPI—Psychopathic Deviate	62.0	10.4	66.9	11.8	58.9	8.3	63.6	12.2	61.5	10.2
MMPI—Masculinity-Femininity	49.8	12.4	60.4	8.5	43.1	9.5	52.5	12.0	51.3	14.2
MMPI—Paranoia	57.6	8.4	60.2	10.2	55.9	6.8	57.9	7.0	58.2	10.8
MMPI—Psychasthenia	60.2	10.1	61.2	12.3	59.5	8.5	59.0	10.0	59.1	9.2
MMPI—Schizophrenia	59.7	11.3	61.1	14.1	58.7	9.3	59.3	12.0	59.8	11.2
MMPI—Mania	55.8	9.8	56.5	11.4	55.3	8.8	54.6	8.1	58.2	9.3
MMPI—Social Introversion	52.0	8.5	51.8	6.9	52.1	9.4	49.5	5.7	50.5	7.8
MMPI—Ego Strength	47.5	10.7	48.1	9.6	47.1	11.5	47.4	10.5	47.2	10.2
MMPI—Alcoholism	22.1	3.8	23.6	4.0	21.1	3.5	23.1	4.2	22.1	3.2
MMPI—Overcontrolled Hostility	14.8	2.6	14.1	1.9	15.2	2.9	14.0	2.7	15.4	2.0
MMPI—Low Back Pain	13.0	2.7	13.5	2.8	12.7	2.7	12.9	3.3	13.3	2.3

is that the former had a significantly higher mean *t*-score on the MMPI K Scale.

In predicting to the continuous outcome criterion, we found that a five-variable model proved the most efficient. In decreasing order of predictive power the following variables were maximally effective in accounting for the variance ($R^2 = 0.65$): MMPI K Scale, amount of time since first seen at the Pain Management Clinic, MMPI Hypochondriasis Scale, MMPI Ego Strength subscale, and the number of unanswered questions (Q) from the MMPI.

A three-variable model was most efficient in predicting to a dichotomous outcome. Once again, in decreasing order of predictive power the following variables were maximally effective in accounting for the variance ($R^2 = 0.64$): the Overcontrolled Hostility (OH) subscale from the MMPI, the Internal-External Locus of Control Scale, and the number of unanswered questions (Q) from the MMPI.

DISCUSSION

Several interesting comments can be made about the results of the data analysis. First, it is clear that the pain patient population reported here shows a mean MMPI profile consistent with that found by several other investigators (2,5); i.e., elevations on the first three clinical scales: Hypochondriasis, Depression, and Hysteria. Likewise, there is a significant mean elevation on the Low Back Pain subscale. This finding indicates that, in general, these patients have a large emotional component to their pain disorders, and this is consistent with their history of lack of response to treatment for pain at other facilities. Furthermore, also in agreement with other researchers (1,6) is our finding that the pain patients scored relatively lower on extraversion, higher on neuroticism, and higher on the lie scale of the Eysenck Personality Inventory than a population of normal subjects. Our hypothesis that hypnotic susceptibility (as measured by the Aas Test, admittedly a less accurate measure than a more behavioral, or trial induction, technique) would be a good predictor of response to treatment did not prove to be true, nor did our hypothesis that degree of social assertiveness (as measured by Questionnaire A) would correlate with outcome.

The failure to find a pattern of personality differences between successfully and unsuccessfully treated groups (the later scoring higher on MMPI scales Hypochondriasis and Hysteria) reported by others (2) most likely resulted from the restricted range of our sample since our facility serves, for the most part, as a "last resort" clinic working with patients who were referred because other physicians could not understand or cure their pain problems.

Even though only one variable was significantly different for the successful versus the unsuccessful group (elevation on K Scale of the MMPI), a combination of variables proved effective in accounting for a significant proportion of the variance. Not only is a combination of scores clearly more powerful, but there is virtually no overlap between those variables that predict to a continuous outcome versus those that predict to a dichotomous one. This clearly raises issues of what exactly does one want to predict to and how does one go about maximizing the effectiveness of a predictive test battery. Obviously, the next step is to try to replicate the findings, ideally with a more homogeneous group of patients from a diagnostic point of view —including patients without long histories of treatment failure—and with more clearly controlled and systematically varied treatment procedures. Additionally, the use of behavioral variables for outcome criteria would add to the use of physician ratings of outcome only. Perhaps a sum score of physician rating, patient rating, and behavioral rating would be most potent.

ACKNOWLEDGMENTS

The authors would like to express their appreciation to Dr. Donald Guthrie for his time and help with the computer analysis. Computing assistance was obtained from the Health Sciences Computing Facility, UCLA, supported by N.I.H. Special Research Resources Grant RR-3.

REFERENCES

1. Bond, M. R. (1971): *Br. J. Psychiatry,* 119:671–678.
2. McCreary, C. P., and Jamison, K. (1976): In: *Consultation-Liaison Psychiatry,* edited by R. O. Pasnau. Grune & Stratton, New York.
3. Melzack, R. (1973): *The Puzzle of Pain.* Basic Books, New York.
4. Melzack, R., and Torgerson, W. S. (1971): *Anesthesiology,* 34:50–59.
5. Sternbach, R. A. (1974): *Pain Patients: Traits and Treatment.* Academic Press, New York.
6. Woodforde, J. M., and Merskey, H. (1972): *J. Psychosom. Res.,* 16:167–172.

Advances in Pain Research and Therapy, Vol. 1,
edited by J. J. Bonica and D. Albe-Fessard.
Raven Press, New York © 1976.

Psychological Predictors of Success or Failure of Surgical Intervention for Intractable Back Pain

Anthony E. Blumetti and Luciano M. Modesti

Upstate Medical Center, State University of New York, 750 East Adams Street, Syracuse, New York 13210

The complaint of chronic low back pain not only is extremely common in most large medical settings and pain clinics but many times remains a baffling, frustrating, and elusive problem to clinical practitioners. Despite recent advances in surgical and chemotherapeutic techniques, treatment failures are often prevalent. The reasons for failure with the patient manifesting symptoms of chronic low back pain are many and complex. However, as Sternbach et al. (7) have pointed out, treatment failure may be caused by a failure to recognize and treat low back pain as a psychosomatic illness with substantial psychological components. Probably because of the incidence of treatment failure, a good deal of energy has been put forth recently to investigate the psychological components of pain involved (3,4,6). The purpose of the present study is to expand on past investigations in hopes of predicting success or failure of surgical intervention for chronic low back pain.

METHODS

Psychometric evaluations consisting of the Wechsler Adult Intelligence Scale (WAIS), the Minnesota Multiphasic Personality Inventory (MMPI), and the Rorschach Ink Blot Test were performed on 24 female and 57 male patients referred for chronic low back pain to the Department of Neurological Surgery of a university hospital. All evaluations were completed by the senior author or by an advanced intern directly under his supervision. Of these patients, 42 – 8 women and 34 men – were independently selected for surgical intervention for relief of pain primarily on the basis of medical history, physical examination, radiographic studies, and degree of debilitation. Procedures varied but consisted of either placement of a dorsal column stimulator (DCS), rhizotomy, cordotomy, or, rarely, stereotaxic thalamotomy. All but 2 patients had undergone previous surgery for back pain which consisted of disc fusion, laminectomy, or both. The degree of chronicity ranged from 10 months to 12 years with a mean of 2.5 years.

On at least a 6-month follow-up, patients were rated as having the pain unchanged, slightly improved, significantly alleviated, or abolished; 19 patients were in the last two categories. These 19 improved cases were then compared to the remaining 23 unimproved cases on several variables consisting of age, sex, socioeconomic status, IQ, length of symptomatology, type of surgery performed, MMPI scales, and five structural and content scores in percentage form derived from the Rorschach Ink Blot Test. Form (F), the degree to which an individual's response is dictated only by the contour and articulation of the blot area chosen, was employed as an index of rigidity and constriction of psychological defense mechanisms. Anatomy responses (At) were used to assess the degree of preoccupation with bodily concerns. A Symbiosis (Sy) score recently developed by Moelis and Fisher (5) was used as a measure of extreme dependence on others. Fisher and Cleveland's (2) Barrier (Br) score was also used and developed primarily as an indicator of body boundary and level of integration of self-image. Finally, we used Elizur's (1) Hostility (H) scale, which taps overly antagonistic or overly submissive character traits.

RESULTS

Analysis of the findings showed no significant differences between the improved or unimproved cases on any of the descriptive variables of age, sex, socioeconomic status, IQ, length of symptomatology, or type of surgery performed. The unimproved group, however, scored significantly ($p < 0.05$) higher on the Hypochondriasis and Hysteria scales of the MMPI as well as on the Form and Symbiosis scores on the Rorschach. The Barrier score was significantly ($p < 0.05$) lower in the unimproved group than in the improved group. No significant differences were found on either the Hostility or Anatomy scores.

DISCUSSION

In terms of these findings, it would seem that in comparison to the "treatment failures," those patients who respond favorably to neurosurgical intervention for chronic low back pain are relatively less pathologically preoccupied with overall bodily concerns, less dependent, and more capable of a higher level of individuation. They are also less rigid and constricted in terms of defense mechanisms and can rely on more than just somatic complaints to deal and interact effectively with the world around them.

Using the five obtained significant indices, we established cutoff points for each index (Table 1) on the basis of means and standard deviations for each of the groups studied. Indices were then assigned as present or absent for each patient in terms of whether obtained scores were above the cutoff score for four of the variables and below the cutoff for the Barrier score.

Patients with three or more signs present were then classified as poor

TABLE 1. *Cutoff scores of significant variables*

Variable	Score
Hypochondriasis (MMPI Scale 1)	75[a]
Hysteria (MMPI Scale 3)	70[a]
Form (F)	80[b]
Symbiosis (Sy)	35[b]
Barrier (Br)	20[b]

[a] Presented in T-score form.
[b] Presented in percentage form.

surgical risks to give up pain symptomatology. With this method we classified 32 out of 42 patients correctly in terms of success or failure of surgery for a total hit rate of 76%.

REFERENCES

1. Elizur, A. (1949): *J. Proj. Tech.,* 13:247–284.
2. Fisher, S., and Cleveland, S. E. (1958): *Body Image and Personality.* D. Van Nostrand, New York.
3. Fordyce, W. E. (1973): *Postgrad. Med.,* 53:123–128.
4. Melzack, R., and Chapman, C. R. (1973): *Postgrad. Med.,* 53:69–75.
5. Moelis, I., and Fisher, S. (1975): Unpublished manuscript. Upstate Medical Center, Syracuse, New York.
6. Sternbach, R. A. (1973): *Clin. Neurosurg.,* 21:323–333.
7. Sternbach, R. A., Wolf, S. R., Murphy, R. W., and Akeson, W. H. (1973): *Psychosomatics,* 14:52–56.

Advances in Pain Research and Therapy, Vol. 1,
edited by J. J. Bonica and D. Albe-Fessard.
Raven Press, New York © 1976.

Behavioral Mechanisms of Human Pain: Effects of Expectancy, Magnitude, and Type of Cross-Modal Stimulation

B. Berthold Wolff, Patricia Cohen, and Cara T. Greene

Pain Research Group, New York University Medical Center, 550 First Avenue, New York, New York 10016

The human pain response is a complex reaction shaped by a multitude of physiological, psychosocial, and ethnocultural factors. There has been a tendency to classify these factors into two categories: namely, physiological (including anatomical, physiological, and chemical variables) and psychological (containing all other variables such as attitude, emotion, personality, and culture). In analgesic assays it is necessary to include a placebo and use a double-blind approach to control for these psychosocial-cultural factors. Wolff (6) has questioned whether these controls, although necessary, are sufficient or adequate. He has suggested that expectancy may be an important behavioral mechanism not properly controlled in the usual analgesic evaluations. Some investigators (1) have even suggested that the entire pain response is basically a placebo response and that the global psychosocial milieu rather than the specific drug or other treatment is more pertinent for study. The elegant experiment of Lyerly et al. (3) supports this notion. Consequently, we decided to study expectancy in some detail using the concept of certainty/uncertainty of stimulation as a dimension.

There has been a tendency to confuse aversion and pain, although these should be clearly differentiated (4). Thus we considered it important to include both pain-inducing and aversion-producing techniques in our study of expectancy, as the latter may be differentially affected by stimuli (2). Furthermore, the inclusion of distracting stimuli as controls seemed important. Finally, stimulus intensity was considered an additional interesting variable for study.

The purpose of this study, therefore, was to investigate the effects of expectancy and magnitude and type of aversive, noxious, and distracting stimuli on several experimentally induced cross-modal aversion and pain response parameters and on a timed visuomotor task. It was hypothesized that: (a) expectancy and magnitude and type of stimulation would significantly alter pain threshold, pain tolerance, aversion response parameters, and timed visuomotor tasks; and (b) the pain sensitivity range (PSR) would not be significantly changed by such aversive, noxious, or distracting stimuli.

METHOD

Subjects

We gave 25 paid, healthy college students or graduates (13 women and 12 men), from 21 to 35 years old (median age, 23.5 years), an initial screening interview and examination involving a confidential medical and personal history, a check of vital signs, and a semistructured psychological interview. The study was then explained in detail, and signed informed consent was obtained.

Procedure

Each subject participated in three experimental sessions, the first of which was always a 2-hr "Base-line Session." This was followed on 2 other days by a "Pain Response Session" and a "Digit Symbol Session," in balanced order, each lasting about 4 hr.

In each session, the subject undressed and put on pajama trousers (women were also given a halter) so that the back was exposed from the waist up. Then the subject was seated in a sound-attenuated and electrically shielded isolation chamber with a one-way window.

Base-Line Session

In the first session, three pain induction methods involving radiant heat, cold pressor, and electrical stimulation were administered. Three pain response parameters were measured: the pain threshold—the point at which pain is first perceived; pain tolerance—the point at which the subject terminates noxious stimulation; and the pain sensitivity range—the difference between pain tolerance and threshold. Details of these methods have been published previously (8). Briefly, our radiant heat method involved stimulating ten areas of the India ink–blackened back with a Hardy-Wolff-Goodell dolorimeter using Wertheimer's (5) single-trial technique at a constant radiant heat flux of 250 mcal/sec/cm^2. The experimenter was present in the isolation chamber for this method in order to place the radiant heat lamp on the subject's back. She was also present for the cold pressor method, which consisted of placing the subject's nondominant foot into an ice water bath at 0°C. The experimenter was not present for all other methods, such as electrical stimulation. This consisted of presenting trains of square wave pulses to two fingers, each placed in a 250-ml beaker filled with 10% saline serving as fluid electrodes and in series with a Grass stimulator, a specially constructed attenuator, and a stimulus isolation unit.

Two aversion-producing methods, white noise and brightness, were also administered. In the former, the subject wore two earphones, connected to a Grason-Stadler noise generator, measuring three aversion response parameters: (a) minimal aversion threshold (MAT), the point at which the white noise begins to be annoying or irritating; (b) aversion tolerance, the noise level at which the subject wishes to terminate stimulation; and (c) the aversion range (AR), the difference between tolerance and the MAT. For safety, noise above 130 dB was not presented. Aversion responses to brightness were similarly measured, using three floodlights, each with 200-W bulbs connected to a powerstat controlled by the experimenter.

Finally, a timed visuomotor task, Digit Symbol, was used with 20 different symbols per sheet. The subject was instructed to complete as many of the digit symbol boxes as he could. Two 5-min trials were given at 10-min intervals.

Pain Response Session

In the pain response session the subject held a pencil in his dominant hand with the digit symbol sheets in front of him; the nondominant fingers were placed in the saline beakers for the electrical stimulation technique; earphones were fitted over the ears, and the ice water bath was placed beside the subject's bare feet. There were three sets of dependent variables consisting of electrical, radiant heat, and white noise stimulation.

The complex experimental design consisted of three randomized presentations of each of eight independent variables (i.e., disruptive conditions). These were digit symbol, cold pressor, electrical, white noise, brightness, brightness plus electrical, brightness plus white noise, and white noise plus electrical stimulation. There were four blocks of time, each lasting about 30 min, three of which were "Experimenter Absent" conditions (electrical and white noise stimulation), and one "Experimenter Present" condition (radiant heat). Several rest periods were scheduled between blocks of time. Each of these independent stimuli was presented at several intensity levels and in various combinations with the three dependent variables, as illustrated in Table 1. Duration of presentation at each intensity level was 60 sec, except for digit symbols (5 min) and cold pressor (variable).

The three intensity levels of electrical and white noise stimulation were based on each subject's base-line scores. Thus for white noise low was at 10% below the subject's MAT, medium was at MAT + $\frac{1}{3}$ AR; and high was at MAT + $\frac{2}{3}$ AR. Similarly, for electrical stimulation low was at 10% below the pain threshold; medium was at pain threshold + $\frac{1}{3}$ PSR; and high was at pain threshold + $\frac{2}{3}$ PSR.

Brightness was presented at four levels: dark, dim, high, and maximum. Combined brightness and white noise or electrical was presented at two levels: low and high. The cold pressor had only one level, 0°C. The digit symbol task was presented for 5 min.

Finally, latency of onset of stimulation for the pain or aversion response

TABLE 1. *Experimental design indicating combinations of dependent and independent variables*

Dependent variables	Independent stimuli: Type	Independent stimuli: Magnitude levels
Electrical method		
Ascending pain threshold	White noise	3
Pain tolerance	Brightness	4
Descending pain threshold	White noise + brightness	2
Pain sensitivity range (PSR)	Digit symbol	—
Radiant heat method		
Pain threshold	Cold pressor	1
Pain tolerance	Electrical	3
PSR	White noise	3
	Electrical + white noise	2
	Digit symbol	—
White noise		
Minimal aversion threshold	Electrical	3
Aversion tolerance	Brightness	4
Aversion range	Electrical + brightness	2
	Digit symbol	—

parameters of the three dependent methods served as another factor. Three time intervals were used: (a) immediate, starting together with presentation of the independent stimulus; (b) intermediate, starting 15 sec after presentation of the independent stimulus; and (c) long, starting 30 sec after presentation of the independent stimulus. For digit symbol the time intervals were somewhat different: immediate; intermediate—2 min after start; and long—4 min after start. Some placebo stimulation was included when no actual stimulation was given. There were 42 independent stimuli, consisting of 30 actual stimuli as described above and 12 placebo stimuli.

Statistical Analysis

The dependent-response parameters for the three methods (electrical, radiant heat, and white noise) were each subjected to a three-way analysis of variance (ANOVA), with subjects (between subjects), stimulus (within subjects), and latency of onset (within subjects) as the three factors. Each of the dependent variables had ten conditions, e.g., three white noise levels, four brightness levels.

Digit Symbol Session

Forty digit symbol sheets were placed in front of the subject who was instructed to complete the task as quickly and accurately as possible so that he could receive $1 for each correctly completed sheet. As the task was devised, no subject was expected to complete a sheet in the time allowed

(3 min). However, one very bright subject was able to do so within the time limit.

Electrical and white noise stimulations were presented at three intensities (as described before), two durations (20 or 40 sec), and 3 latencies (0, 60, and 120 sec). There were 36 actual and 4 placebo presentations in a randomly balanced order, with 10-min rest periods every 30 min. The scores (completed boxes) were subjected to three-way ANOVAs as previously described.

RESULTS

Pain Response Session

Stimulus Intensity and Type

Table 2 clearly indicates that the independent (distracting) stimuli had highly significant ($p < 0.001$) effects on both the pain threshold and pain tolerance for the two pain induction methods. In contrast, no significant effects occurred with white noise. These results clearly differentiate between pain and aversion induction and suggest that pain but not aversion can be manipulated by external stimuli impinging on the organism.

The PSR was less significantly affected by the independent stimuli. This suggests that the PSR includes pain components other than pain threshold and pain tolerance (7).

Latency of Onset (Expectancy)

The latency of onset of aversive or noxious stimulation was our measure of expectancy, i.e., certainty/uncertainty. It was found that the pain thresh-

TABLE 2. *Effects of stimulus magnitude and type: summary of analyses of variance*

	Independent stimuli		
Dependent variables	df	F	Significance
Electrical ($N=25$)			
Pain threshold	9;216	3.39	<0.001
Pain tolerance	9;216	5.21	<0.001
Pain sensitivity range (PSR)	9;216	2.36	<0.025
Radiant heat ($N=23$)			
Pain threshold	9;198	7.55	<0.001
Pain tolerance	9;198	6.11	<0.001
PSR	9;198	1.17	ns
White noise ($N=22$)			
Minimal aversion threshold	9;189	0.55	ns
Tolerance	9;189	0.40	ns
Aversion range	9;189	0.62	ns

TABLE 3. *Effects of latency of stimulus onset: summary of analyses of variance*

Dependent variables	Independent stimuli		
	df	F	Significance
Electrical ($N=25$)			
Pain threshold	2;48	9.89	<0.001
Pain tolerance	2;48	5.34	<0.01
Pain sensitivity range (PSR)	2;48	1.13	ns
Radiant heat ($N=23$)			
Pain threshold	2;44	8.64	<0.001
Pain tolerance	2;44	6.06	<0.005
PSR	2;44	0.33	ns
White noise ($N=22$)			
Minimal aversion threshold	2;42	5.53	<0.01
Tolerance	2;42	6.92	<0.005
Aversion range	2;42	0.94	ns

old, pain tolerance, MAT, and aversion tolerance were significantly ($p <$ 0.01 and better) decreased as the latency increased (Table 3). No such effects were obtained for the PSR and AR. This suggests that as uncertainty of aversive and noxious stimulation grows, it leads to a lowering of tolerance and increased sensitivity to such stimuli. The lack of apparent effects on PSR and AR are related to our previous suggestion that these may measure different components (7). Furthermore, in contrast to stimulus magnitude, expectancy seems to affect both pain and aversion.

Digit Symbol Session

The results of the ANOVAs indicated that electrical stimulation and white noise had little effect on digit symbol performance. Occasionally, intensity of electrical stimulation decreased performance slightly, but in general, stimulus magnitude, duration, or latency of onset had no significant disturbing effects on this timed visuomotor task.

CONCLUSIONS

It is concluded that, first, manipulation of expectancy in terms of increasing uncertainty of the onset of pain or of aversion rapidly lowers tolerance and enhances sensitivity to pain or aversion. Second, pain responses are changed by some but not by all cross-modal stimuli in a complex fashion depending on both stimulus magnitude and modality. In contrast, aversive responses are less subject to such changes, supporting the notion that aversion and pain are different concepts and should be differentiated. Third, the PSR seems to be a relatively stable response for a given individual; it is not readily changed by external stimuli, which supports Wolff's (7) hypothesis that it may be an (indirect) measure of the pain endurance factor—a personality characteristic. Finally, motivated (e.g., financial incentive) simple task performance is not easily disrupted by the kind of stimuli used in this study.

ACKNOWLEDGMENTS

This work was supported in part by grant MH-16434, National Institute of Mental Health, Department of Health, Education and Welfare.

REFERENCES

1. Dinnerstein, A. J., Lowenthal, M., and Blitz, B. (1966): *Perspect. Biol. Med.,* 10:103–117.
2. Fellner, C. H. (1971): *Psychosomatics,* 12:313–315.
3. Lyerly, S. B., Ross, S., Krugman, A. D., and Clyde, D. J. (1964): *J. Abnorm. Soc. Psychol.,* 68:321–327.
4. Sullivan, R. T., and Freimark, N. (1969): *Psychon. Sci.,* 15:107–108.
5. Wertheimer, M. (1952): *Am. J. Psychol.,* 65:297–298.
6. Wolff, B. B. (1968): In: *Proceedings of the 3rd International Pharmacological Meeting, July 24–30, 1966, Vol. 9: Pharmacology of Pain,* edited by R. K. S. Lim. Pergamon Press, Oxford.
7. Wolff, B. B. (1971): *J. Abnorm. Psychol.,* 78:292–298.
8. Wolff, B. B., and Jarvik, M. E. (1964): *Am. J. Psychol.,* 77:589–599.

Advances in Pain Research and Therapy, Vol. 1,
edited by J. J. Bonica and D. Albe-Fessard.
Raven Press, New York © 1976.

Emotional and Psychological Factors Modifying the Pain Response of Animals

Dennis D. Kelly and Murray Glusman

New York State Psychiatric Institute, and Department of Psychiatry, College of Physicians and Surgeons, Columbia University, New York, New York 10032

The proposition that the human pain response can be influenced broadly by nonsensory factors seems so widely accepted today that it is difficult to recall that until recently scientific study of these variables, beyond anecdotal acknowledgment, was considered somewhat outside the mainstream of pain research. Among other advances, the application of signal detection theory to the psychophysics of pain has helped establish the scientific respectability of such important psychological modifiers of pain as anxiety, attention, and expectancy. It now seems well confirmed that the neural activity associated with pain is probably the most easily modified of any sensory system.

Signal detection theory conceptualizes the human pain report as a blend or product of both sensory information processing and decision making by the brain (4,6,9). Verbal acknowledgment of pain is viewed as depending only in part on sensory experience and in part, as well, on a collection of variables that affect response bias, or the person's willingness to report what he or she has experienced. For human subjects the nonsensory bias factor is considered particularly important for it reflects the action of such vital variables as social context, attitude, instructions, costs and payoffs, and expectancy (4). Although pain detection and pain tolerance thresholds were previously considered unique, valid, and impervious benchmarks of the subjective pain experience, they are now often revealed as simply two adjustable criteria exercised by a subject along the same graded continuum of sensory experience. For example, both Clark (5) and Feather et al. (8) have demonstrated with signal detection that the effects of suggestion caused by administering a placebo on subjects' judgments of radiant heat pain were reflected behaviorally not as a sensory change but as an attitudinal shift, a new bias. Such plasticity of the human pain experience suggests that neural activity, or previously coded experience, somewhere in the nervous system can act to modify activity induced elsewhere by noxious stimuli.

Although the human nervous system undoubtedly shares a common origin and many functional properties with those of other species, there has been a notable reluctance to acknowledge a comparable sensitivity of the pain responses of nonhuman animals to psychological and emotional modulation. Perhaps because of some species-typical response bias, we tend to regard the behavior of other species as more reflexive and automatic, less malleable than our own, in similar situations. For example, on purely theoretical grounds the placebo phenomenon has been proposed at times as evidence of man's virtually unique psychological overlay on the pain reflex. Yet practiced veterinarians know the value of stroking a dog's head before examining its injured limb.

In the scientific literature on aversive conditioning and learning, much experimental evidence argues that animals react to pain, and to anticipated pain, in a behaviorally complex manner controlled by variables qualitatively similar to those encompassed by the construct of human response bias. To cite several examples: The use of a painful shock as a signal for positive reward in a pavlovian counterconditioning paradigm has been shown to dampen the behaviorally disruptive properties of shock (17,18) and to hasten the extinction of "fear" responses (21). In a similar vein, moderately intense shocks have consistently produced less behavioral suppression of intermittently reinforced responding when presented immediately before the delivery of a positive reinforcement than when presented after nonreinforced responses (1,15,20). As with humans, the experimental pain thresholds of rats and monkeys have been found sensitive to nonnarcotic psychotropic agents (19), and those of cats to "anchoring" or stimulus-context cues (13). In fact, almost wherever probed, the pain responses of animals and humans have appeared differentially malleable not in kind, but in degree, which likely reflects our more complete understanding of methods for manipulating the human pain response.

AVERSIVE THRESHOLDS, ESCAPE LATENCIES, AND MESENCEPHALIC DAMAGE

The following two sets of observations concerning the stereotyped latencies with which individual cats escape from marginally aversive stimuli are related to each other and most likely to the issue of psychological determinants of pain in animals. Both experiments were performed with adult cats in which a pair of stimulating electrodes were implanted bilaterally in each flank (Fig. 1). Previous work in our laboratory (11) had shown that an electrical stimulus defined in terms of a constant alternating current would produce a constant behavioral effect (escape) provided current density and the site of stimulation were held constant, as in the subcutaneous preparation.

The first data appeared as a by-product of a larger experiment (12) that examined the effects of electrolytic destruction of selected mesencephalic structures on aversive thresholds as measured by a discrete-trial version of

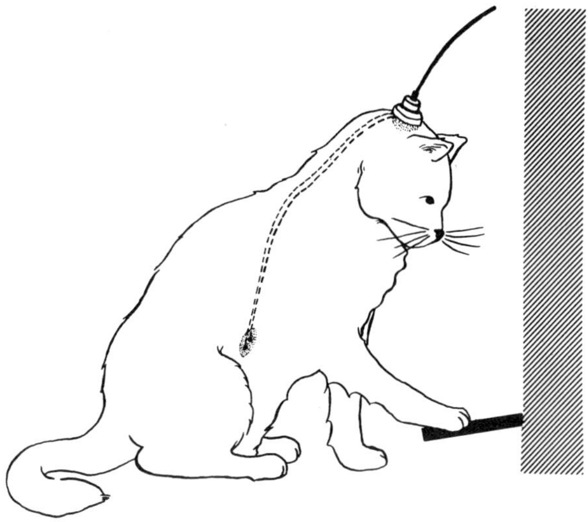

FIG. 1. Cat implanted with subcutaneous electrodes, 2 stainless steel screws imbedded 1.6 cm apart in a thin polyethylene disk. Subcutaneous wires (*dashed lines*) were run to a connector mounted on the skull.

the titration schedule of Weiss and Laties (19). On each trial, a cat received shock for 6 sec unless it pressed a lever that terminated shock immediately. If the cat chose to terminate the shock, the intensity programmed for the next trial was decreased. If the cat endured the full 6-sec trial without responding, shock was terminated automatically by a clock and the intensity of the next trial was increased. Thus the sequence of trial intensities was determined by the cat's own escape behavior, and the median of this intensity series was taken as the aversive threshold. Trials were separated by a variable interval (mean, 15 sec). Intertrial responding on the lever was ineffective.

Figure 2 presents the aversive thresholds and corresponding mean escape latencies for 16 individual cats, each represented by a pair of bars reflecting pre- and postoperative measurements. Comparing these bars in the lower graph reviews the effects on aversive thresholds of destroying various midbrain regions in the cat. Relevant to the present discussion is simply the overall observation that although some lesions proved effective in altering aversive thresholds (specifically, lateral tegmental lesions, either alone or in conjunction with tectal damage), others did not (tectum, periaqueductal gray, and central tegmental region ventral to the periaqueductal gray).

The more specific effects of these lesions have been described fully elsewhere (12), replicated (16), and need not concern us further, except perhaps to note their variance with some recent evidence concerning the possible role of the mesencephalic periaqueductal gray matter in pain and analgesia

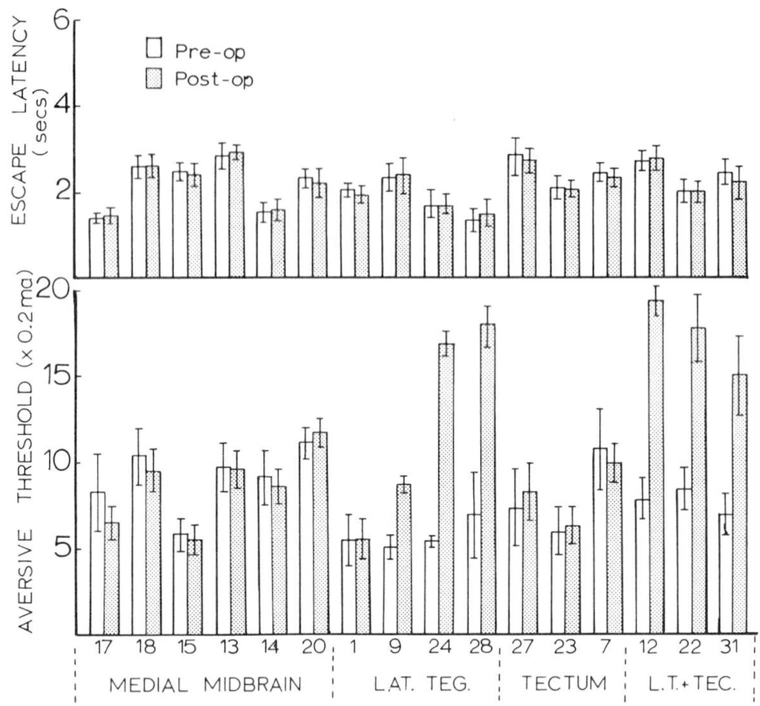

FIG. 2. Aversive thresholds **(bottom)** and mean escape latencies **(top)** for 16 cats before and after destruction of mesencephalic areas indicated along abscissa. Subject identification numbers correspond to those cited in Kelly and Glusman (12). Escape latencies were measured only on trials terminated by the subject. Open bars reflect mean ± 1 SD of the final ten 265-trial preoperative sessions; shaded data are derived from 18 sessions spaced over 5 weeks. LAT. TEG. and L.T., lateral tegmentum; TEC., tectum.

(10,14, but see also 2). Regardless of their effect on thresholds, if any, none of these lesions resulted in any alteration in the subjects' typical patterns of escape latencies. (An escape latency was defined as the time elapsed from the onset of shock to an escape response, given the occurrence of the latter.) Escape latencies remained stable postoperatively even for those subjects (e.g., nos. 24, 28, 12, 22, and 31) that showed two- to threefold increases in the shock intensity required to elicit escape responding.

Each cat established a characteristic escape latency early in training (note the varying preoperative, open-bar latencies), and this behavior proved independent of the shock intensity needed to evoke the response, brain lesion or none, high threshold or low. The idiosyncratic response latency of each cat in no way represented an inflexible minimum reaction time, for further increases in shock intensity beyond a liminally aversive level resulted in a shortening of these latencies, in accord with the common finding of escape conditioning (3,7,22). The possibility that escape latencies possessing these properties might reflect a decision process involving the relative aversiveness of mild shocks prompted a brief follow-up study.

PROBABILITY OF ESCAPE FROM LIMINALLY AVERSIVE STIMULI

The second experiment involved a liminal escape procedure identical to the titration schedule except for the elimination of the intensity-adjusting contingency. Otherwise, a cat was presented on each trial with a low-intensity shock and, as before, given the option of turning it off or allowing a clock to do so at some later time. Shock intensity was set constant at a

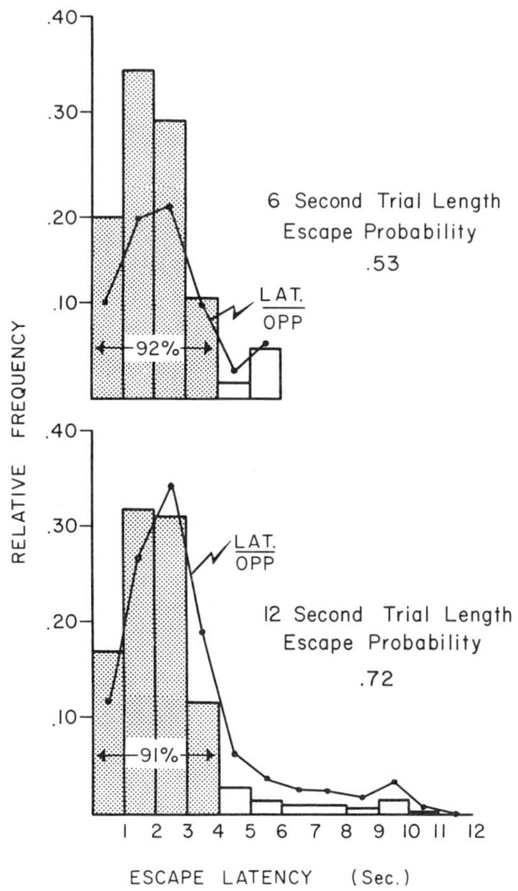

FIG. 3. Latencies to escape from 1.2-mA subcutaneous shocks presented for either 6 or 12 sec in the absence of a response. Each distribution is the average of 10 sessions of 400 trials each. Shaded bars represent 91%–92% of area under the distribution. LAT./OPP, latency per opportunity, is a conditional probability measure of likelihood of a response latency, *x*, given that subject has already waited at least *x* sec.

level that the subject chose to terminate on roughly half of the 6-sec trials. We then asked what would happen to the normal subject's characteristic escape latency, and to its likelihood of terminating the same intensity shock (escape probability), if the trial duration were simply lengthened from 6 to 12 sec. This maneuver involved no change in stimuli, no novel sensations, until shock exceeded 6 sec in length, the former trial duration. And yet, as Fig. 3 indicates, although this cat terminated 53% of the 6-sec trials, it chose to terminate 72% at the longer trial duration. Instead of half, the subject now terminated almost three of every four trials.

The higher escape probability was not due to the newly expanded opportunity to respond afforded by the additional trial length because latency distributions remained virtually unchanged. Were the cat to terminate either a projected 6-sec or a 12-sec trial, it normally did so early in the trial, almost always by 4 sec. Given an escape response, the likelihood of a latency equal to or less than 4 sec was $p = 0.92$ with the short trial length, and $p = 0.91$ with the longer. Thus even though the cat escaped from a greater proportion of the longer trials, its elective responses were distributed similarly in time, occurring as early in the shock period as before. The animal responded not as a reflexive automaton to the presence of painful shock but as a decision maker—able to include in its assessment of a stimulus some estimate of its future length.

DISCUSSION

The telling alteration in this second experiment was evidently the modified consequence to the subject of failing to respond, a new contingency that had to be weighed in coming to a decision early during the trial as to respond or not. In light of the earlier discussion of psychophysical thresholds, we might ask which of these functions in Fig. 3, 6 or 12 sec, more closely approximates the "true" pain detection threshold of the cat. The dilemma is unresolvable for there really is no unique negative reinforcement threshold. In fact, there are as many operationally valid behavioral thresholds of aversion as there are statistics to describe behavioral change, as there are procedures for aversively controlling behavior, and as there are parameters of those procedures. Perhaps the salient feature of an aversive threshold in animal psychophysics is its almost complete malleability. The absolute value it takes in any situation depends largely on the experimenter's selections from among the many known parameters of the subject's evaluation of when it becomes worth its while to engage in the experiment. Were similar considerations raised in the context of human psychophysical investigations, reference would likely be made to the role of psychological and motivational factors in the modification of the pain response.

ACKNOWLEDGMENTS

The authors express their deep appreciation to those associates who have contributed to the pain research project, particularly Drs. Lanny Fields, Wallace Orlowsky, and Cornelis Stokman. This work was supported by National Institutes of Health Grant MY-3660 and National Institute of Mental Health Grant MH-10315.

REFERENCES

1. Appel, J. B. (1968): *Psychol. Rep.,* 22:267–271.
2. Bevan, T., and Pert, A. (1975): *Fed. Proc.,* 34:713.
3. Boren, J. J., Sidman, M., and Herrnstein, R. J. (1959): *J. Comp. Physiol. Psychol.,* 52: 420–425.
4. Chapman, C. R. (1974): In: *Advances in Neurology, Vol. 4: International Symposium on Pain,* edited by J. J. Bonica, pp. 115–122. Raven Press, New York.
5. Clark, W. C. (1969): *J. Abnorm. Psychol.,* 74:363–371.
6. Clark, W. C., and Hunt, H. F. (1971): In: *Physiological Basis of Rehabilitation Medicine,* edited by J. Downey and R. Darling. W. B. Saunders Co., Philadelphia.
7. Dinsmoor, J. A. (1968): In: *Miami Symposium on the Prediction of Behavior 1967: Aversive Stimulation,* edited by M. R. Jones. University of Miami Press, Coral Gables.
8. Feather, B. W., Chapman, C. R., and Fisher, S. B. (1972): *Psychosom. Med.,* 34:290–294.
9. Green, D. M., and Swets, J. A. (1966): *Signal Detection Theory and Psychophysics.* John Wiley & Sons, New York.
10. Jaquet, Y. F., and Lajtha, A. (1974): *Science,* 185:1055–1057.
11. Kelly, D. D., and Glusman, M. (1964): *Psychonom. Sci.,* 1:207–208.
12. Kelly, D. D., and Glusman, M. (1968): *J. Comp. Physiol. Psychol.,* 66:25–34.
13. Kelly, D. D., and Glusman, M. (1971): *Physiol. Behav.,* 7:837–840.
14. Mayer, D. J., and Liebeskind, J. C. (1974): *Brain Res.,* 68:73–93.
15. Murray, M., and Nevin, J. A. (1967): *J. Exp. Anal. Behav.,* 10:301–309.
16. Orlowsky, W., and Glusman, M. (1969): *J. Comp. Physiol. Psychol.,* 67:245–251.
17. Pavlov, I. P. (1927): *Conditioned Reflexes.* International Publishers Co., New York.
18. Pearce, J. M., and Dickinson, A. (1975): *J. Exp. Psychol.,* 104:170–177.
19. Weiss, B., and Laties, V. (1970): In: *Animal Psychophysics,* edited by W. C. Stebbins. Appleton-Century-Crofts, New York.
20. Williams, D. R., and Barry, J., III (1966): *J. Comp. Physiol. Psychol.,* 61:154–156.
21. Wilson, G. T., and Davison, G. C. (1971): *Psychol. Bull.,* 76:1–14.
22. Winograd, E. (1965): *J. Exp. Anal. Behav.,* 8:117–124.

Advances in Pain Research and Therapy, Vol. 1,
edited by J. J. Bonica and D. Albe-Fessard.
Raven Press, New York © 1976.

The Pain Control Unit Nursing Program

Ronald M. Lawrence and Eleanor B. Lawrence

7535 Laurel Canyon Boulevard, North Hollywood, California 91605

At the April 1972 conference, Bonica (1), in discussing the organization of a pain clinic, alluded to the role of nurse specialists, stating: "it is preferable that the beds available to the pain clinic group be contained within one ward or one area of the hospital so that the nursing staff may be trained in the careful observation of patient's responses to diagnostic and therapeutic procedures and also in running drug profiles and watching patients during drug withdrawal." During September 1974, Annis (2) and I had occasion to develop an inpatient teaching program for nurses working in the pain control unit (PCU) of a general hospital. This program has been modified and refined since that time to include what we consider to be the key material necessary for the smooth functioning of the PCU nursing staff.

Only with a proper educational background can the nurse achieve the necessary skills to help the patient in pain, utilizing the latest accepted approaches. Classic nurses' training encompasses very little information about the pain patient; this is strange, since the nurse expends a great part of her working time handling such patients. Encyclopedias and textbooks of nursing deal with pain only by describing neurosurgical procedures and methods for caring for the postneurosurgical patient. Drug descriptions deal with narcotics only. Simple placebo therapy, for example, is not even mentioned (i.e., Lippincott's excellent *Encyclopedia for Nurses*). Since the nurse spends far more time daily with the PCU inpatient than the physician, the doctor relies heavily on her skills. In fact, without trained nurse specialists the inpatient pain control program is doomed to failure from the start. In our unit we rely heavily on the psychological staff for the teaching and training programs. However, all specialists, including the physiotherapists, rehabilitation and recreational therapists, and even the electrical engineers, help carry on the education program.

Our program, which follows, has been taught two nights weekly. This was necessary by virtue of the special circumstances connected with our general hospital, but it could effectively be taught in a continuous weekly program encompassing a period of two weeks.

1. Operant conditioning; behavior modification (role playing of real life situations)	30 hr
2. Psychodynamics	20 hr

3. The pain questionnaires; history forms; psychological testing instruments (i.e., M.M.P.I., T.A.T., Edwards Vocational Aptitude, etc.), and other paper work; nurses note taking and report forms — 4 hr
4. Needle therapies: Osteopuncture®; acupuncture; trigger zone therapy; nerve blocks, etc. — 8 hr
5. The transcutaneous neurostimulator: types, construction, methods of application, simple repair techniques — 4 hr
6. Abbreviated neuroanatomy; the central nervous system; the autonomic nervous system — 2 hr
7. Simplified neurophysiology; theories of pain and pain control — 4 hr
8. Multidisciplinary conference; approaches — 8 hr
9. Biofeedback training and relaxation therapy — 20 hr
10. Observation techniques of patient behavior (occult and overt) — 10 hr
11. Placebo therapy: its purpose, methods of handling patients requests for medication, etc. — 2 hr
12. Pain medications and other pharmacological data — 2 hr

The place of the PCU nurse should become as well established within the next decade, we feel, as the intensive care unit (ICU) and coronary care unit (CCU) nurse has become during the last decade. We also found that our intensive teaching program has created an unexpected outflow regarding the morale and enthusiasm of the nurses. Consequently, an *esprit de corps* has developed, which is transmitted to the patient who, in the final analysis, is the one whom we all hope to benefit the most.

REFERENCES

1. Bonica, J. J. (1974): In: *Recent Advances on Pain, Pathophysiology and Clinical Aspects*, edited by J. J. Bonica, P. Procacci, and C. Pagni. Charles C Thomas, Springfield, Illinois.
2. Annis, A. P. (1967): *J. Consult. Psychol.*, 14:9–17.

Advances in Pain Research and Therapy, Vol. 1,
edited by J. J. Bonica and D. Albe-Fessard.
Raven Press, New York © 1976.

Measurement of Pain: Problems and Issues

C. Richard Chapman

Departments of Anesthesiology, Psychiatry and Behavioral Sciences, and Psychology, University of Washington School of Medicine, Seattle, Washington 98195

"When you cannot measure it, when you cannot express it in numbers—you have scarcely, in your thoughts, advanced to the stage of Science, whatever the matter may be."—Lord Kelvin

The intimate linkage of pain with human suffering has caused scientists to regard this phenomenon with fascination, but few have attempted to approach pain with the scientific method. Many have asserted that science is concerned with systematic study of observable events; therefore, it cannot deal directly with pain, which is entirely private. Some theorists have argued strongly that pain can never be measured. Savage (12), for example, has stated, "Measurement, very generally, is the process of comparing an object within some dimension with standard objects within that dimension. In an attempt to measure pain, what would the standard objects be? Other pains or physical objects? If we employ pains, we are employing private objects which cannot be felt by any other person than the subject." Savage contends that pains, like visual afterimages, are essentially unmeasurable phenomena and that the arbitrary assignment of numbers to such occurrences does not constitute measurement.

The views of conservative measurement theorists, such as Savage, have done little to inhibit investigators who have sought measures of pain, and several procedures for indirect quantitation have been used extensively over several decades. Among these procedures are pain threshold, pain tolerance, and subjective rating scales. Unfortunately, retrospective study of experimental outcomes suggests that such methods have not performed as reliably as they should have. Broadly speaking, two problems have historically characterized pain research.

First, it has been difficult to reconcile clinical observations with the outcomes of laboratory studies in which investigators have attempted to measure pain phenomena. For example, pharmacological agents that have proven effective as analgesics in the clinic sometimes have no effect on pain threshold in the laboratory (1,2). The second difficulty is that laboratory studies are often inconsistent, so that observations obtained in one laboratory sometimes conflict with those reported by another laboratory where similar methodology is used (4,6,11). Such inconsistencies have raised doubts about the validity of some pain quantitation procedures and provided critics with a basis for arguing that algesiologists have failed in attempts to develop valid measurement techniques.

Now that worldwide interest in the scientific study of pain is gaining momentum rapidly, we must come to grips with the charges of our critics and form some perspective on our limitations. We must acknowledge that we have dealt with measurement issues pragmatically, and that time has revealed considerable inconsistency and relatively little progress in pain research. Furthermore, we must admit that there has been little evolutionary progress in pain measurement methodology over the last century, so that most of today's researchers are using outdated classic procedures, some of which are as much as a century old. This shortcoming appears conspicuous in light of the rapid and revolutionary changes in technology that have characterized the last century in science.

Those of us who have chosen to study pain phenomena must consider seriously the issues of measurement, for such considerations are absolutely fundamental, and the long-term success of our scientific ventures rests directly on how we choose to resolve these questions. The position taken by Savage (12) places us on the horns of two dilemmas. The first centers on the question of whether it is possible to measure pain at all, and the second is based on the assumption that measurement is possible. If pain is measurable, then are we to quantitate it objectively, subjectively, or are we to develop methods of objectively handling subjective experience?

In answer to the first question, we can say that pain is ultimately measurable. As the psychophysicist Stevens has pointed out (16), classic measurement principles are based on theory and not on some form of eternal truth. The theory was developed to meet the needs of science a century ago. Today science is quite different and we need to measure different things. This is a time to develop new measurement theory and new procedures. Stevens has argued that it is an error to bind ourselves to the limitations of classic concepts.

If pain is to be measured, how do we deal with the conflict of objective and subjective approaches? This question has no simple answer, and its resolution ultimately depends on the development of pain theory. However, examination of the concept of measurement and its implications for pain research helps shed some light on this issue.

THE MEASUREMENT CONCEPT

The following definition seems exceedingly simple, but close examination of it provides a basis for evaluating pain measurement methodology currently in use: measurement can be defined as the assignment of numbers to objects or events to represent quantities of attributes according to rules.

Although most theorists will accept this definition, some will contest it because it does not specify that the process of measurement requires operations; i.e., the employment of instruments or a set of special procedures that functions as a test instrument. In pain research, this means that subjective numerical estimations of pain states made by patients can be accepted as measures, even though the investigator did not undertake any special operations or use a test instrument to obtain the number. Without operations, some would argue, it is impossible to obtain empirically verifiable scores. That is, other investigators could not obtain the same numbers by replicating a set of procedures. The validity of subjective reports for pain research is thus a moot issue.

The following concepts in the definition of measurement merit special attention.

Rules and Operational Definition

The definition of measurement offered here implies that some operational definition of pain is necessary, since it refers to rules, and these depend on the operational definition of the investigator. The operational definition is used to link the mentalistic concept of pain to an observable event or physical object that can be measured. For example, if a cat has been subjected to electrical tooth pulp stimulation, downward movement of the jaw may be operationally defined as a pain response, and certain characteristics of this response can be measured; e.g., its speed or frequency. Thus the private event of pain may be operationally defined as a specific type of motor movement, and the parameters of such a behavioral act may be quantitated.

The validity of the operational definition of pain in any study can be judged on the basis of the theoretical assumptions adopted by the investigator.

Number Assignment

The rules of measurement are also concerned with the assignment of numerals to objects or events to create what is called a scale. The rules employed in the assignment of numbers in pain research determine the information content of the measurements obtained. For example, numbers may be assigned to acupuncture needles in order to indicate length, but they may also be assigned to patients to indicate diagnostic categories. In one instance precise differences among the numbers are meaningful and complicated arithmetical procedures can be carried out on them, but in the second instance numbers have no meaning beyond that of differentiating each type of patient from other types of patients. Table 1 lists several rules for the assignment of numbers during measurement, and it indicates the level of scaling produced, the relations that exist among the numbers, and operations permissible.

TABLE 1. *Rules for assigning numbers during pain measurement*

Rule	Scale	Relations among scores	Operations permissible
1. To equal objects or events, assign the same number	Nominal	Equivalence or non-equivalence	Classification
2. To the greater (smaller) object or event, assign the greater (smaller) number	Ordinal	Greater or lesser than	Data can be rank ordered
3. To objects or events separated by equal intervals, assign numbers separated by equal intervals	Interval	Known ratio of any 2 intervals	Arithmetical procedures
4. To objects or events that stand to one another in equal ratios, assign numbers that stand to one another in equal ratios	Ratio[a]	Known ratio of any 2 scale values	All of the preceding plus multiplication by a positive constant

[a] This is the only scale in which the number zero is assigned to indicate absolute absence of the property being measured.

The quality of measurement obviously ranges from simple classification to a high level of scaling. The level of scaling achieved is an important factor in the evaluation of pain measurement techniques.

Attributes

Regardless of the level of scaling attained, measurement necessarily concerns some particular feature of an object or event rather than the object or event itself; i.e., an attribute. For example, one does not measure a person; one can only measure the blood pressure, height, weight, or some other characteristic attributable to the individual by an observer. Attributes are conceptual dimensions along which events or objects can be compared or otherwise related.

Although this is a simple notion, it has important implications for pain research. In selecting an attribute to measure, the investigator is obligated, first, to select an attribute that does, in fact, exist and is relevant to pain. For example, an attempt to measure the amount of threat associated with a laboratory pain might be futile since most laboratory pain experiences are not threatening. A second obligation of the researcher is that he must carefully consider whether he is developing a measure that reflects several attributes or only one. A unidimensional measure determined by multiple attributes is likely to yield inconsistent experimental outcomes when it is compared across laboratories, and such measurements are characterized by low precision. The question of whether a given type of score mirrors several attributes or a single attribute is important and has rarely been considered by algesiologists.

TYPES OF PAIN MEASURES

The measurement concepts just discussed provide a basis for the evaluation of current methods of pain assessment. Quantitation procedures used in pain research may be divided into three classifications: measurement of events, measurement of objects, and subjective estimations. The three classifications will be discussed, beginning with the most concrete form of operational procedure and moving to the most abstract.

Measurement of Events

The events quantified in pain research are always behavioral (whether they are observed at the level of the receptor, the nervous system, or the organism as a whole), and generally such events consist of reflex or motor responses of animal or human subjects to noxious stimulation. Such attributes as speed or latency, intensity, and frequency are commonly assessed.

In human research, latency of response is often measured and interpreted as an index of pain tolerance. Thus the length of time that a subject will bear the pain of a tourniquet [Submaximum Effort Tourniquet Test (13)] or the immersion of a limb in very cold water [Cold Pressor Test (5)] before requesting termination of the stimulus is a latency measure. Similarly, quantitation of the number of seconds that a volunteer will tolerate a constant intensity of cutaneous radiant heat also constitutes a latency measure [D'Armour-Smith Procedure (3)].

Behavioral events are generally measured at interval or ratio levels of scaling so that they are robust measurement procedures. They are clearly operationalized and, therefore, characterized by empirical verifiability. Such indices are among the most reliable used in pain research since they tend to replicate well across experiments.

Validity poses a problem for users of event measures. A measure is valid to the extent that it quantifies that which it purports to quantify. In the study of animals or of humans who make no verbal responses, it is questionable if the behavior measured has occurred as a direct function of pain. For example, an investigator can stimulate the tooth pulp of a rabbit electrically and measure the intensity of a muscle twitch in the animal's neck in order to make inferences about pain. Eventually, it is observed that the muscle twitch response is a segmental reflex that remains when the animal undergoes light anesthesia. Since most current conceptions of pain hold that pain can occur only in a conscious organism, the investigator has developed an operational definition for pain which is inconsistent with accepted pain theory. Hence it can be argued that measurement of the muscle twitch is invalid as an index of pain. A unique problem associated with event measure is thus the difficulty of making inferences about pain on the basis of operational behavioral measurements.

In spite of such problems, a precedent for inference about abstract mental processes on the basis of behavioral measures may be found in psychological research. The study of animal and human learning processes offers a parallel, since learning is a conceptual abstraction that can never be studied directly. Learning is always inferred from the performance of subjects in laboratory tasks in accordance with carefully designed operational procedures. The example set by the prolific investigators in the learning field suggests that study of behavioral events in pain research is a promising area that merits increased attention as well as careful reflection.

Measurement of Objects

The objects studied in pain research are usually human or animal subjects, but they may be neurological structures, organs, or other living tissue. Each object is measured with regard to an abstract attribute ascribed to it by the investigator, and this can be assessed only indirectly. For example, a human subject may be measured with regard to an attribute termed "sensitivity to pain." Traditionally, the pain threshold has been adopted as an operational definition of sensitivity to pain.

Measurements of objects, as exemplified by pain threshold, are characterized by a high level of scaling; i.e., interval or ratio level, and they can be empirically verified. Curiously, pain threshold has a notoriously low reliability across laboratories (1), probably because of the assumptions made in the process of operationalization. To measure pain threshold, the investigator must deliver a series of stimulus intensities to the subject. He assumes that each stimulus generates a hypothetical sensation and that at some point increasing sensations become pain experiences. This point is assigned the number of the corresponding physical stimulus intensity as a measure. To make such a number assignment, the investigator must rely on the verbal report of the subject.

Although this procedure may seem straightforward, it is seriously complicated by its dependence on the verbal report of the subject. The investigator assumes that he is measuring a single attribute, sensitivity to pain, but in fact the threshold is also influenced by the subject's other attributes including cooperativeness, passive aggressiveness, anxiety, attention, expectancy, and suggestibility. Pain threshold is thus a measure reflecting many attributes rather than a single one, and its methodology requires extreme care. The relevancy of the threshold measure for concepts in pain theory has been declining in recent years as newer techniques have emerged.

The methodology of signal detection theory (sometimes called sensory decision theory) offers an alternative paradigm for arriving at measures of sensitivity to pain (17). Subjects are required to make rating scale responses to both noxious and innocuous stimuli over many trials. The frequencies with which the subject uses the various categories on the rating scale for each of the two stimuli are tabulated. A complex function which relates the rate of correct identifications of a noxious stimulus as painful to the rate of erroneous identifications of an innocuous stimulus as painful is then generated. The measure of sensitivity to pain so obtained reflects a singular attribute and is not influenced by other attributes that may cause the subject to make most of his responses at the high or low end of the rating scale. A second measure provided by this methodology reflects an attribute that might be termed "predisposition to report pain," or, more commonly, "response bias."

The operational procedures of signal detection theory are formal and complex. Measures of sensitivity to pain and measures of predisposition to report pain are scaled at interval levels. A shortcoming of signal detection procedures is that they are complex and time consuming, lacking the pragmatic appeal of threshold methodology. Some critics point out that detection theory methods are limited to rigorously controlled laboratory settings and question the relevance of this approach to real world pain phenomena.

Subjective Estimations

The use of numerical estimates of subjective pain states is perhaps the most frequently used method of pain assessment. For example, clinical pain may be evaluated by asking the subject to mark a 10-cm line labeled "no pain at all" at one end and "as bad as it could possibly be" at the other end (10). Typically, subjective estimates are assumed to reflect pain intensity, and the scores obtained are commonly treated as though they belong to an interval-level scale; i.e., they are averaged and tested statistically.

The obtaining of rating scale scores requires virtually no operations since the number is assigned by the subject rather than by the investigator. Since operations are nonexistent or trivial, some question if subjective estimates taken at face value qualify as measurements at all.

Critics (12) contend that measurement and estimation are two different processes. Asking an individual to estimate his body weight, blood pressure, or IQ is quite different from actually measuring these factors. Most investigators acknowledge that any estimate obtained is limited by the skills of the observer making the judgment, and it is distorted by a host of psychological and social factors in the test setting (14).

The arguments advanced by critics of subjective estimations are compelling. Their case is further strengthened by pointing out that subjective estimates do not qualify as interval-level scores. Hence they are by nature not suited for operations of addition, calculations of averages, or other procedures. The common practice of carrying out conventional statistical procedures on such numbers is highly questionable from the viewpoint of measurement theorists, although some attempts have been made to rationalize such undertakings (7,8).

Interestingly, some researchers have performed operations on subjective judgments to obtain measures. Sternbach et al. (15) have attempted to improve introspective estimation methods by having patients subjectively match the intensity of their chronic pain to the intensity of an experimental pain. Applying a tourniquet (which grows more noxious over time) to generate pain, Sternbach et al. asked patients to indicate when the clinical pain matched the tourniquet pain. The time from tourniquet application to the point of subjective equality was then accepted as an assessment of the clinical pain state. The ratio of clinical pain level to the total length of time that the patient could bear a tourniquet was then computed and multiplied by 100 to obtain a measure of pain severity. This procedure has a clear-cut set of operations and yields a score at a high level of scaling. Although the test may fail to measure a unitary attribute, it does illustrate an unprecedented approach to the assessment of clinical pain.

Stevens (16) has developed an unconventional procedure for measurement, termed power law scaling, which is also based on subjective reports. In Stevens' research, subjective magnitude estimations or other types of subjective judgments are obtained in response to the presentations of controlled intensities of stimulation, and a series of operations is performed on the estimations in order to arrive at a value. The measure obtained is an exponent that serves as a function relating stimulus intensity to intensity of sensation, according to the power law, $\psi = k\,\phi^n$, where ψ is the subjective intensity of sensation, ϕ is the stimulus intensity, k is a constant, and n is the power exponent. Since operations are carried out in order to arrive at a value for the exponent, measurement takes place. These methods have been applied to the study of pain only infrequently, but they indicate that it is possible to develop measurement procedures based on subjective estimations of sensory states.

Yet another promising approach to pain measurement based on subjective report is the multidimensional scaling procedure developed by Melzack and Torgerson (9). These investigators appropriately noted that clinical pain states are complex phenomena that cannot be adequately described by a single attribute. On the basis of language used by French-speaking and English-speaking Canadians to describe pain states, Melzack and Torgerson postulated that three attributes, evaluated simultaneously, could adequately describe a clinical pain problem. The following three dimensions were offered as a basis for measurement: sensory-discriminative, affective, and evaluative. Questionnaires given to patients served as test instruments that provided three-dimensional measures of pain states. Although this technique is young and likely to undergo further refinement, it offers great promise for the assessment of clinical pain.

CONCLUSION

Development of measurement methodologies is one of the unrecognized frontiers in pain research. An elusive mystery, pain is a private event that does not conveniently lend itself to study by means of conventional scientific methodology. Just as the clinician finds that his specialty has not prepared him adequately for dealing with intractable pain, the scientist finds that his discipline has difficulties in dealing effectively with pain as a focus for research.

Historically, we have been guilty of conceptually simplifying pain in order to measure it, like Procrustes, who amputated the feet of his guests in order to fit them into his bed. In recent years, however, creative investigators have demonstrated that unconventional approaches to measurement can open new avenues of scientific inquiry, and their example is laudable. It is a responsibility of each of us engaged in the study of pain to consider new approaches to measurement and to offer constructive, but rigorously critical, evaluations of procedures proposed by others. It is also our responsibility to generate interest among scholars whose skills or specialties differ from our own, and to actively encourage interdisciplinary research, for the complexity of pain merits a pooling of intellectual resources.

REFERENCES

1. Beecher, H. K. (1959): *Measurement of Subjective Responses: Quantitative Effects of Drugs.* Oxford University Press, New York.
2. Chapman, L. F., Dingman, H. F., and Ginzberg, S. P. (1965): *Brain,* 88:1011.
3. D'Armour, F. E., and Smith, D. L. (1941): *J. Pharmacol.,* 72:74–79.
4. Hardy, J. D., Wolff, H. G., and Goodell, H. (1952): *Pain Sensations and Reactions.* Williams & Wilkins, Baltimore.
5. Hilgard, E. R., Ruck, J. C., Lange, A. F., Lenox, J. R., Morgan, A. H., and Sachs, L. B. (1974): *Am. J. Psychol.,* 87(1–2):17–31.
6. Kutscher, A. H., and Kutscher, H. W. (1957): *Int. Rec. Med.,* 170:202–212, 228–230.
7. Labovitz, S. (1961): *Soc. Forces,* 46(2):151–170.
8. Labovitz, S. (1974): In: *Scaling: A Sourcebook for Behavioral Scientists,* edited by G. Maraned. Aldine Publishing Company, Chicago.
9. Melzack, R., and Torgerson, W. S. (1971): *Anesthesiology,* 34(1):50–59.
10. Pilowsky, I., and Kaufman, A. (1965): *Br. J. Psychiatry,* 111(481):1185–1187.
11. Procacci, P., Della Corte, M., Zoppi, M., Romano, S., Maresca, M., and Voegelin, M. R. (1974): In: *Recent Advances on Pain,* edited by J. J. Bonica, P. Procacci, and C. A. Pagni, pp. 105–147. Charles C Thomas, Publisher, Springfield, Illinois.
12. Savage, C. W. (1970): *The Measurement of Sensation: A Critique of Perceptual Psychophysics.* University of California Press, Berkley.
13. Smith, G. M., Lowenstein, E., Hubbard, J. H., and Beecher, H. K. (1968): *J. Pharmacol. Exp. Ther.,* 163(2):468–474.
14. Sternbach, R. A. (1974): *Pain Patients—Traits and Treatment.* Academic Press, New York.
15. Sternbach, R. A., Murphy, R. W., Timmermans, G., Greenhoot, J. H., and Akeson, W. H. (1974): In: *Advances in Neurology, Vol. 4: International Symposium on Pain,* edited by J. J. Bonica, pp. 281–288. Raven Press, New York.
16. Stevens, S. S. (1975): *Psychophysics.* John Wiley & Sons, New York.
17. Swets, J. A. (Ed.) (1964): *Signal Detection and Recognition by Human Observers.* John Wiley & Sons, New York.

Advances in Pain Research and Therapy, Vol. 1,
edited by J. J. Bonica and D. Albe-Fessard.
Raven Press, New York © 1976.

Signal Detection Theory Assessment of Pain Modulation: A Critique

Gary B. Rollman

Department of Psychology, University of Western Ontario, London, Ontario, Canada

When pain researchers attempt to modulate acute or chronic pain, they vary greatly in the methods they use to test the efficacy of their treatments. The persistent problem of pain measurement (1,11,20,25) centers on the difficulty in assessing the degree of discomfort felt by a patient and the need to disentangle sensory and emotional contributions to the pain response (18). Traditional pain and tolerance thresholds are not well suited for understanding the nature of pain modulation since they confound the sensory and motivational components.

A relatively new psychophysical methodology, signal detection theory or sensory decision theory (16), has held out the hope that some of these problems might be overcome. The theory presents a means by which one can independently measure the sensitivity and response bias of an observer, thus separating the sensory and cognitive factors underlying his performance.

Recognizing the desirability of independently assessing a subject's sensory experience and his proclivity for describing such an experience as painful, a number of pain researchers have adopted signal detection theory procedures in their investigations. This chapter summarizes and critically reviews this existing literature, suggesting that the use of the signal detection model is generally inappropriate and that the conclusions drawn by the authors may be unwarranted.

SIGNAL DETECTION THEORY

Clark (8) has provided an excellent account of the fundamental aspects of signal detection theory in the study of pain, and several other publications (e.g., 17,19,27) have demonstrated its wide applicability. The model assumes that the detection of a weak stimulus requires the observer to make a statistical decision. Since the stimulus, if it is there, is superimposed on a randomly varying background of internal "noise" arising from spontaneous neural discharges, each trial involves a decision as to whether the activity at that time is more likely to result from the signal added to the noise or from the internal noise alone. This decision is based on the magnitude of the sensory experience and the criterion adopted by the observer for making a positive decision.

In the simplest case, described in Fig. 1, the model assumes that both the noise and the signal plus noise distributions are normal or gaussian and of equal variance. When the signal is weak, the two distributions show considerable overlap. This is reduced as the signal strength increases, since the signal plus noise distribution then moves to the right. A parameter, d′, indicates the separation of the two hypothetical underlying curves and thus represents the observer's true sensitivity for detection of their difference.

An experiment involves a large number of noise or blank trials and a large number of trials presenting signal plus noise. Because of the overlap, the observer can never be certain whether or not a stimulus occurred. Therefore, he establishes a criterion for making an affirmative response, setting it to the right if he is conservative (thus minimizing "false alarms" at the cost of a reduced "hit" rate) and setting it to the left if he is more liberal (thus maximizing hits at the cost of increased false alarms). An independent parameter, described by various names, represents the observer's response bias or criterion. Changes in the subject's motivational state can shift the criterion and alter his hit rate (and thus his "threshold"), even though his sensitivity remains unaltered. However, d′ would remain constant.

The same arguments can be advanced to describe discrimination between two more intense stimuli, each of which is added to the internal noise. If stimuli are easily confused, the signal detection calculations (8) yield a low value of d′. Since pain studies require strong stimulus levels, investigators have typically examined discrimination after a variety of modulation procedures.

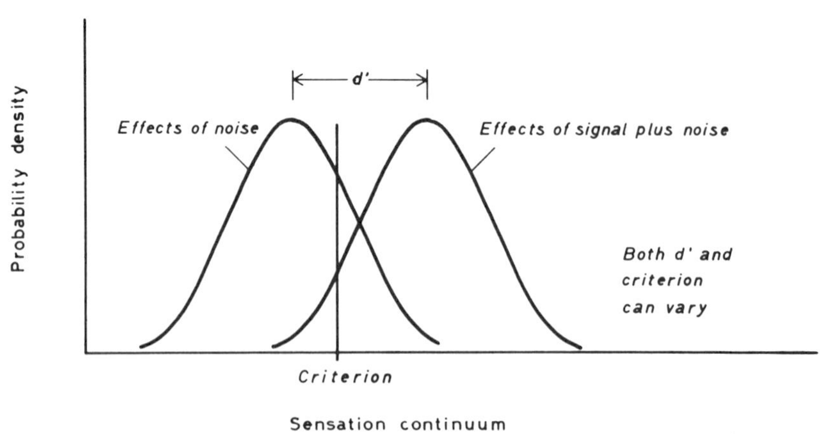

FIG. 1. Representation of the overlapping effects of noise and signal plus noise assumed by the signal detection theory model.

EXPERIMENTAL STUDIES

The typical pain experiment presented several intensities of a noxious stimulus, such as radiant heat or electric shock, which the observer was asked to rate on a scale ranging from "nothing" to "extremely painful." Rating scales have often been used in the signal detection framework since they are assumed to provide information based on a number of simultaneously held criteria rather than on a single one. Although Clark and Dillon (9) recommended that data from binary decisions (such as no-yes or low-high) rather than sensory intensity ratings be used to compute d′, all researchers have maintained the rating procedure.

Most of the studies have deviated from standard practice in a number of potentially important ways: subjects were asked to report the intensity of strong stimuli rather than confidence in their detection or discrimination ability; the scales often included as many as 13 categories; up to four different stimulus levels were intermixed with blank trials; and generally few trials per intensity were presented to each observer.

Clark (7) found that an orally administered placebo, described as a potent analgesic, increased the pain threshold but left the discriminability parameter unaltered. The effect of the placebo was to increase the criterion for issuing a report of pain. Clark and Mehl (12) concluded that older men and women show higher pain criteria than younger ones, and that older women also exhibit a reduction in sensitivity. Clark and Goodman (10) gave instructions to increase or decrease pain or tolerance thresholds, modifying behavior in the desired manner. Changes in the criterion, but not discriminability, caused them to conclude that suggestion (and, perhaps, hypnosis and counterirritation) forces subjects to alter the level of sensory activity required before they will verbally report pain, even though their sensations are unchanged.

Clark and Yang (13) applied signal detection theory to test the effects of a putative therapeutic agent, acupuncture, finding no significant differences in d′ between needled and control arms or between the periods before, during, or after the 15- to 20-min stimulation period. The criterion parameter was significantly higher in the experimental arm during acupuncture than in the control arm, leading to their conclusion that acupuncture altered the likelihood that subjects would admit to feeling pain, but did not change the pain experience.

Some Critical Remarks on Clark's Hypotheses

Clark proposed that sensory modulation alters the neural effects of a noxious stimulus, thus reducing the d′ in the same manner as if the physical intensity of that signal were weakened. Figure 2 demonstrates that this is not necessarily the case. If acupuncture truly functions as an analgesic by

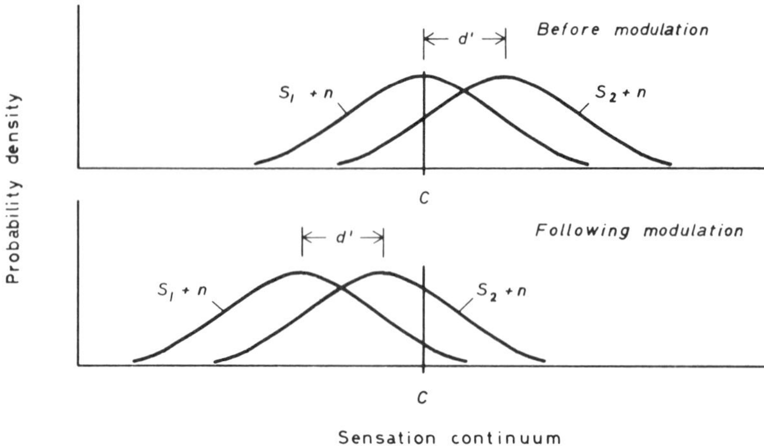

FIG. 2. Representation of the change produced by an analgesic modulation procedure. Sensory effects of noise plus both the weaker (S_1) and stronger (S_2) stimuli are reduced, but d′ remains constant.

modulating the neural response to potentially painful stimuli, the activity produced by both of the intense heat levels should be reduced. In that case, the distributions of both signal levels will be shifted to the left, but the discriminability index, d′, which represents the distance between them, could be unaffected. The sensory pain components of both stimuli could be greatly reduced, yet d′ would not change. The shift that would be observed is one in criterion level, but this would be illusory.

Clark's sensory magnitude criterion could be constant with respect to the level of activity required to elicit a report of pain, but one would mistakenly conclude from performing the signal detection calculations that it had shifted in a conservative direction. The basis for this problem is that no fixed distribution exists in pain modulation—both distributions are free to vary. As a result, acupuncture might act as a powerful analgesic, yet signal detection analysis would erroneously infer that only the subject's predilection for reporting pain had been affected. The same problem of interpretation exists for Clark's earlier studies as well. Suggestion (10) or placebo (7) or advancing age (12) could have affected a central biasing mechanism, inhibiting the response to all noxious stimuli, but the signal detection analysis would show that only the response bias had been affected.

Additional Studies

These difficulties plague other signal detection investigations of pain as well. Bloedel et al. (2) analyzed the modulating effects of peripheral nerve and spinal cord stimulation, reporting that dorsal column stimulation yielded both a lower d′ and a shift to a more conservative criterion, whereas transcutaneous stimulation primarily shifted the bias parameter. Again, it may be more appropriate to conclude that stimulation of the cord and nerve influenced the sensory impact of the thermal pulses and not, as they suggested, the criterion adopted for issuing pain reports.

Craig and Coren (14) exposed naive subjects to social models who simulated different levels of discomfort and pain susceptibility. Subjects used a 10-point scale to describe the effects of a random series of five levels of electric shock after being paired with a tolerant, intolerant, or control model. An index, related to d′, for the discriminability of adjacent pairs of stimuli was significantly increased for the subjects exposed to the intolerant model but was not altered for those in the tolerant modeling ground, even though both groups showed ratings that differed significantly from those of controls. They concluded that exposure to an intolerant model produced a change in the sensory experience of pain, whereas exposure to a tolerant one changed the response bias.

In addition to the difficulty of unambiguously interpreting a constant d′ in pain modulation experiments, Craig and Coren's study (14) presents another problem of data interpretation. It appears that they calculated d′ based on individual data points rather than on a receiver operating characteristic (ROC) curve fit to all the data. The sensitivity change occurred primarily at intermediate ratings. This point is too complex to receive much elaboration here, but it is important. For any pair of hit and false alarm rates, one can calculate d′ or look it up in published tables (e.g., 26). Such calculations and tables are based on a vital assumption: that the variance of the two underlying distributions is equal. Clark (7) showed that for thermal stimuli this may well be the case, but Rollman (22,23) found that it is not true for electrical or mechanical stimulation of the skin. When such signals are used the data must be plotted on ROC curves, and then special conventions (16) must be followed to determine d′ for distributions of unequal variance. Failure to do so can cause an experimenter to report a d′ shift when actually a criterion change occurred, or vice versa. As Theodor (28) has stated, "d′ is independent of response bias only when [the ratio of the variances of the underlying distributions] has been taken into account; . . . it is necessary to know [the ratio] in order to properly calculate d′."

Some of these same comments apply to the research of Chapman and his colleagues. Feather et al. (15), in a study similar to Clark's (7), found that d′ for discriminating two levels of radiant heat was uninfluenced by an oral placebo, although criterion was shifted in a more conservative direction. Again, a shift in sensory response to both the "warm" and the "painful" stimuli could have yielded this outcome. The same is true in a study by Chapman and Feather (4) on the analgesic effects of an oral tranquilizer, diazepam (10 mg). The drug significantly increased pain tolerance times to tourniquet-induced ischemia in comparison to both a matching placebo and

600 mg of aspirin. However, d′ for the discrimination of adjacent levels of radiant heat was not affected by the drug, nor was the criterion for pain response.

In a study cited earlier, Clark and Yang (13) concluded that, "the sole effect of acupuncture was to cause the subjects to raise their pain criterion in response to the expectation that acupuncture works." Chapman et al. (5) came to different conclusions in their study of the effects of bilateral needling of the hand on the discrimination of electrical stimuli at the dental pulp. The pain-attenuating effects of acupuncture were weak, but significant declines in d′ were observed. Since the criterion for describing their most intense stimulus as painful also increased, Chapman et al. (5) concluded that acupuncture's effects involve both sensory loss and alterations in response bias. They suggested a number of procedural differences that might result in their finding a sensitivity shift when Clark and Yang (13) failed to find one. However, they also determined d′ in a different manner from that used by Clark and Yang. Chapman et al. (5) used a technique presented by Richards and Thornton (21), which calculates a least squares fit to a straight-line ROC function on normal deviate coordinates. Even if Chapman et al. assumed unequal variances in their calculations, their values of d′ are subject to some error. A least squares procedure inaccurately assumes that the abscissa, the false alarm rate, is not free to vary. In addition, Richards and Thornton's (21) estimate of d′ for unequal variances calculates d′ at the point where the ROC curve intersects the 50% false alarm rate rather than where it intersects the negative diagonal (16).

OBJECTIONS TO THE RATIONALE OF SIGNAL DETECTION STUDIES OF PAIN MODULATION

Objections have been raised above to hypotheses about what should happen to the discriminability index if a modulation procedure were truly analgesic and to the methods sometimes used in making d′ calculations. These criticisms apply if it is valid to use the signal detection model to study pain. Is such validity apparent?

All of the cited studies do not, in fact, determine a bias-free estimate of how painful a stimulus seems to be and if the modulation procedure reduces that painfulness. Although this is what they purport to investigate, they ask merely if the strongest stimulus changes in discriminability from the next strongest. Is it critical that an analgesic, which drastically reduces the painfulness of a series of strong impulses, also reduces the ability to discriminate adjacent levels? If not, the premise of all of the studies is untenable.

One might suggest that d′ should be calculated between the potentially noxious levels and the zero intensity of the blank or noise stimulus. In fact, Chapman et al. (6) showed that 33% nitrous oxide reduced d′ for three levels of radiant heat when calculated against the zero intensity responses, but the gas "did *not* change sensitivity to the differences between adjacent nonzero stimulus pairs." Thus they concluded, "33 percent nitrous oxide did not interfere with the ability of the subjects to discriminate among nonzero stimuli, even though the gas did reduce absolute sensory sensitivity to each of the nonzero stimuli." This point has been overlooked in each of the later pain papers which refers to this experiment. There are good reasons for not examing d′ between a strong stimulus and a blank. But no good rationale has been advanced for studying d′ between adjacent nonzero intensities, as all other investigators have done.

It has been argued here that an analgesic need not reduce the discriminability of adjacent stimuli. It can also be argued that discriminability can be reduced in the absence of analgesic effects. Some intervention could render it more difficult to discriminate between two shocks or heat levels, thereby reducing the d′ between them, yet have little effect on the painfulness of the stimuli.

A procedure which claims that motivational changes have occurred when, in fact, they were sensory, which claims that sensory changes have occurred when, in fact, they were motivational, and which examines the discriminability of adjacent stimuli without measuring their noxiousness has no utility in the study of pain. Chapman's (3) statement that "the threshold has had its day in court, and it has proven to be largely unreliable" seems to be accurate. Signal detection theory, on the other hand, has permitted great conceptual and substantive advances in the study of human decision processes. But it has not yet proven that it can offer a bias-free estimate of the sensory and motivational changes produced by pain modulation. Until it does, pain researchers might be well advised to heed the caveat of Rosner and Goff (24), "Beware of psychophysicists bearing gifts."

ACKNOWLEDGMENTS

These investigations were supported by Grant AO-392 from the National Research Council of Canada and by a Leave Fellowship from the Canada Council. This chapter was prepared while the author was on leave at the Psychological Laboratories, University of Stockholm.

REFERENCES

1. Beecher, H. K. (1959): *Measurement of Subjective Responses: Quantitative Effects of drugs*. Oxford University Press, New York.
2. Bloedel, J. R., Erickson, D., and McCreery, D. B. (1974): *Abstracts of the Annual Meeting of the Neuroelectric Society,* 7:54.
3. Chapman, C. R. (1974): In: *Advances in Neurology, Vol. 4: International Symposium on Pain,* edited by J. J. Bonica, pp. 115–122. Raven Press, New York.
4. Chapman, C. R., and Feather, B. W. (1973): *Psychosom. Med.,* 35:330–340.
5. Chapman, C. R., Gehrig, J. D., and Wilson, M. E. (1975): *Anesthesiology,* 42:532–537.

6. Chapman, C. R., Murphy, J. M., and Butler, S. H. (1973): *Science,* 179:1246–1248.
7. Clark, W. C. (1969): *J. Abnorm. Psychol.,* 74:363–371.
8. Clark, W. C. (1974): *Anesthesiology,* 40:272–287.
9. Clark, W. C., and Dillon, D. J. (1973): *Percept. Psychophys.,* 13:491–493.
10. Clark, W. C., and Goodman, J. S. (1974): *J. Abnorm. Psychol.,* 83:364–372.
11. Clark, W. C., and Hunt, H. F. (1971): In: *Physiological Basis of Rehabilitation Medicine,* edited by J. A. Downey and R. C. Darling. W. B. Saunders Co., Philadelphia.
12. Clark, W. C., and Mehl, L. (1971): *J. Abnorm. Psychol.,* 78:202–212.
13. Clark, W. C., and Yang, J. C. (1974): *Science,* 184:1096–1098.
14. Craig, K. D., and Coren, S. (1975): *J. Psychosom. Res.,* 19:105–112.
15. Feather, B. W., Chapman, C. R., and Fisher, S. B. (1972): *Psychosom. Med.,* 34:290–294.
16. Green, D. M., and Swets, J. A. (1966): *Signal Detection Theory and Psychophysics.* John Wiley & Sons, New York.
17. Lusted, L. B. (1971): *Science,* 171:1217–1219.
18. Melzack, R., and Casey, K. L. (1968): In: *The Skin Senses,* edited by D. Kenshalo. Charles C Thomas, Publisher, Springfield, Illinois.
19. Pastore, R. E., and Scheirer, C. J. (1974): *Psychol. Bull.,* 81:945–958.
20. Procacci, P., Della Corte, M., Zoppi, M., Romano, S., Maresca, M., and Voegelin, M. R. (1974): In: *Recent Advances in Pain,* edited by J. J. Bonica, P. Procacci, and C. Pagni. Charles C Thomas, Publisher, Springfield, Illinois.
21. Richards, B. L., and Thornton, C. L. (1970): *Educ. Psychol. Meas.,* 30:855–859.
22. Rollman, G. B. (1969): *Percept. Psychophys.,* 5:377–380.
23. Rollman, G. B. (1974): *Percept. Psychophys.,* 16:291–294.
24. Rosner, B. S., and Goff, W. R. (1967): In: *Contributions to Sensory Physiology, Vol. 2.* Academic Press, New York.
25. Sternbach, R. A. (1974): *Pain Patients—Traits and Treatment.* Academic Press, New York.
26. Swets, J. A. (Ed.) (1964): *Signal Detection and Recognition by Human Observers.* John Wiley & Sons, New York.
27. Swets, J. A. (1973): *Science,* 182:993–1000.
28. Theodor, L. H. (1972): *Psychol. Bull.,* 78:260–261.

Advances in Pain Research and Therapy, Vol. 1,
edited by J. J. Bonica and D. Albe-Fessard.
Raven Press, New York © 1976.

Laboratory Pain Induction Methods for Human Analgesic Assays

B. Berthold Wolff, Thomas G. Kantor, and Patricia Cohen

Pain Research Group, New York University Medical Center, 550 First Avenue, New York, New York 10016

Laboratory pain induction methods for reliable and fast human analgesic screening have an important role in clinical pharmacology and pain research, and we have systematically studied such techniques. In view of Beecher's (1) well-known criticism of experimental pain, and some of our own earlier studies, based on both differential pain responses to various types of physical stimuli (3,7) and the apparent role of tissue depth and body locus (6), Wolff (5) outlined three major requirements for human analgesic assays with laboratory pain. These are: (a) measurement of suprathreshold pain, such as pain tolerance; (b) use of several pain induction methods involving different types of stimuli; and (c) stimulation of various body loci at different tissue depths in order to evaluate cutaneous, deep somatic, and visceral pain. Furthermore, the pain induction methods should obey the rules stated many years ago by Hardy et al. (2).

Originally, we studied three laboratory methods, involving radiant heat, cold pressor, and electrical stimulation. However, we found the radiant heat method to be equivocal for human analgesic assays, supporting Kutscher and Kutscher's (4) conclusions. In contrast, the cold pressor and electrical stimulation methods seemed promising and were used in the studies reported here. We have previously published details of these two methods (10). Briefly, the cold pressor method consists of placing the subject's hand in a lukewarm bath at 37°C for 2 min and then plunging it up to the wrist in an ice-water bath saturated with ice chips and approaching 0°C. The electrical stimulation method consists of placing the subject's second and fourth fingers in two 250-ml beakers filled with 10% saline serving as fluid electrodes and placed in series with a Grass stimulator, a specially built attenuator which controls the stimulus output and simultaneously drives a pointer around a dial graduated from 0 to 100, and a stimulus isolation unit. Trains of square pulses, continuously ascending or descending in current intensity, are administered. Both methods permit the measurement of three pain response parameters: (a) pain threshold, the point at which the subject first begins to feel pain (or at which the pain disappears during a descending trial); (b) pain tolerance, the point at which the subject no longer permits stimulation; and (c) pain sensitivity range (PSR), the difference between the tolerance and the pain threshold. In recent studies we have added another parameter, termed the drug request point, which lies between the pain threshold and pain tolerance and is the point at which the subject would take a mild pain-relieving drug were he to experience this pain intensity in "real" life.

In three previously published studies (8–10) we found that single doses of 10 mg morphine sulfate, 60 mg codeine sulfate, 1,000 mg aspirin, and placebo could be significantly differentiated. Pain tolerance appeared to be the most sensitive analgesic index.

The overall objectives of the four studies reported now were to: (a) test the ability of our pain-induction methods to yield significant dose discrimination, i.e., dose-response curves; and (b) evaluate various common mild and moderately potent oral analgesic agents as potential standard drugs for future assays.

METHOD

All four studies used paid, healthy adults. Drugs were always given orally with water under strict double-blind conditions using complete crossover designs. The cold pressor and electrical methods were always administered and the pain threshold, drug request point, pain tolerance, and PSR measured. Every experimental session consisted of no-drug base-line pain measurements, followed by drug ingestion, and then by rest and repeat post-drug pain measurements. The collected pain scores were transformed into ratio scores, being the ratio of the post-drug score over the base-line (no drug) score. These ratio scores were subjected to analyses of variance.

Study 1

Two doses, 100 and 200 mg, of a new Pfizer drug, CP-24,877 (2-amino-methylene-indan-l-one), were compared with doses of two controls, 65 mg *d*-propoxyphene (Darvon®) and placebo, in 24 subjects. In each of the four experimental sessions repeat pain measurements were made at 40, 80, and 120 min post-drug administration. The results indicated that: (a) dose/drug–response curves for pain tolerance and drug request point were significant ($p < 0.05$); (b) 65 mg propoxyphene was invariably the strongest analgesic and could always be differentiated from placebo; and (c) 200 mg CP-24,877 had significant ($p < 0.05$), but relatively mild, analgesic effects, peaking around 40 min. We found 100 mg CP-24,877 to be no better an analgesic than placebo.

Study 2

Three doses of aspirin—300, 600, and 1,200 mg—were compared to placebo. Examination of the data after 12 subjects had completed the study showed that although the lowest and highest doses of aspirin could be differentiated, the middle dose could not. Thus we did not obtain appropriate dose-response curves and decided to terminate the study.

Study 3

Two doses of a mild oral analgesic—aspirin (600 and 1,200 mg)—were compared with two doses of a moderately potent oral analgesic—codeine sulfate (60 and 120 mg)—and with placebo, using 30 healthy volunteers. The pain induction methods were repeated at 1 and 2 hr post-drug and, as usual, the scores were transformed into 60-min and 120-min post-drug over base-line ratios.

The cold pressor results (Table 1) indicated that: (a) significant dose/drug discrimination was obtained; (b) there was a very marked time effect because at 60 min all pain response parameters showed statistically high dose/drug discrimination (*p* ranging from 0.025 to 0.001), whereas at 120 min only pain tolerance and PSR yielded significant (*p* 0.05 and 0.025) dose/drug differences, suggesting analgesic peaking to be much closer to 60 than to 120 min post-drug; and (c) aspirin and codeine seemed to exert a differential analgesic effect on the cold pressor pain responses. Although codeine showed dose-response curves on each pain response parameter, pain tolerance was the most sensitive parameter. In contrast, for aspirin dose-response curves were obtained for both pain threshold and drug request point, but not for pain tolerance and PSR.

The electrical stimulation results differed somewhat from those for the cold pressor method. Table 2 shows that highly significant (*p* 0.005 and 0.001) dose/drug discriminations were obtained on all pain response parameters except PSR. There were no marked time differences between 60 and 120 min post-drug. Pain threshold and pain tolerance showed the greatest dose-responses for both aspirin and codeine. The control detection threshold, which is not a pain parameter, as expected showed no significant results.

TABLE 1. *Cold pressor method: F-values for one-way analyses of variance for drug effects for ratio scores*

		F	
Pain response parameter	df	60 min	120 min
Pain threshold	4;116	3.239[a]	0.879
Drug request point	4;116	6.787[b]	2.229
Pain tolerance	4;116	9.213[b]	2.858[c]
Pain sensitivity range	4;116	6.886[b]	3.359[a]

[a] $p < 0.025$.
[b] $p < 0.001$.
[c] $p < 0.05$.

TABLE 2. *Electrical stimulation method: F-values for one-way analyses of variance for drug effects for ratio scores*

		F	
Pain response parameter	df	60 min	120 min
Detection threshold	4;116	1.104	1.773
Pain threshold	4;116	5.331[a]	4.749[b]
Drug request point	4;116	4.657[b]	5.015[a]
Pain tolerance	4;116	5.521[a]	5.672[a]
Pain sensitivity range	4;116	2.369	2.770[c]

[a] $p < 0.001$.
[b] $p < 0.005$.
[c] $p < 0.05$.

Study 4

Two doses of *d*-propoxyphene—65 and 130 mg—were compared to placebo and 120 mg codeine in 24 subjects. A third laboratory pain-induction method—pressure algometer with stimulation of both ankles and thumb knuckles—was added to the cold pressor and electrical methods. Preliminary results indicated that: (a) pain tolerance yielded dose-response curves for propoxyphene with good discrimination from placebo on all three laboratory methods; (b) 120 mg codeine seemed more effective than 130 mg propoxyphene on both the cold pressor and pressure algometer methods but not on the electrical stimulation method; and (c) the pressure algometer appeared to be a less reliable method than the other two for analgesic assays.

CONCLUSIONS

On the basis of the results from these four studies, it has been concluded that:

1. The cold pressor and electrical stimulation methods yield significant dose-response curves for *d*-propoxyphene and codeine. However, it is more difficult to obtain significant dose responses for aspirin unless doses of 1,000 mg or above are used.
2. The pain tolerance seems to be the most sensitive pain response parameter for human analgesic assays, although some drugs may exert different effects on various pain response parameters.
3. The cold pressor and electrical stimulation methods appear to be more reliable for analgesic assays than the pressure algometer method.
4. Different pain-induction methods measure different components of the behavioral pain reaction and should thus be selected carefully for analgesic screening. Preferably, at least two different methods should be used in an assay.

5. Complete crossover designs are powerful statistical procedures for this type of human analgesic assay with experimentally induced pain and require relatively few subjects.

6. Laboratory pain-induction methods with healthy human volunteers appear to be promising for future fast and objective analgesic screening of new oral analgesic drugs.

ACKNOWLEDGMENTS

This work was supported in part by research grants GM-20228, National Institute of General Medical Sciences, Department of Health, Education and Welfare (USA), and DA4PG-017, Special Action Office for Drug Abuse Prevention, Executive Office of The President of The United States of America; a research contract from Pfizer, Inc.; and a research grant from Bristol-Myers Products, Inc.

REFERENCES

1. Beecher, H. K. (1959): *Measurement of Subjective Responses.* Oxford University Press, New York.
2. Hardy, J. D., Wolff, H. G., and Goodell, H. (1952): *Pain Sensations and Reactions.* Williams & Wilkins, Baltimore.
3. Jarvik, M. E., and Wolff, B. B. (1962): *J. Appl. Physiol.,* 17:841–843.
4. Kutscher, A. H., and Kutscher, H. W. (1957): *Int. Rec. Med.,* 170:202–222, 228–230.
5. Wolff, B. B. (1968): In: *Proceedings of the 3rd International Pharmacological Meeting, July 24–30, 1966, Vol. 9: Pharmacology of Pain,* edited by R. K. S. Lim. Pergamon Press, Oxford.
6. Wolff, B. B., and Jarvik, M. E. (1963): *Can. J. Psychol.,* 17:37–44.
7. Wolff, B. B., and Jarvik, M. E. (1964): *Am. J. Psychol.,* 77:589–599.
8. Wolff, B. B., Kantor, T. G., Jarvik, M. E., and Laska, E. (1966*a*): *Clin. Pharmacol. Ther.,* 7:224–238.
9. Wolff, B. B., Kantor, T. G., Jarvik, M. E., and Laska, E. (1966*b*): *Clin. Pharmacol. Ther.,* 7:323–331.
10. Wolff, B. B., Kantor, T. G., Jarvik, M. E., and Laska, E. (1969): *Clin. Pharmacol. Ther.,* 10:217–228.

Advances in Pain Research and Therapy, Vol. 1,
edited by J. J. Bonica and D. Albe-Fessard.
Raven Press, New York © 1976.

Multivariate Analysis of Pain Data

*Gary B. Cox and C. Richard Chapman

*Departments of Anesthesiology, *Psychiatry and Behavioral Sciences, and Psychology, University of Washington Medical School, University of Washington, Seattle, Washington 98195*

The human pain experience is a deceptively complex phenomenon. It is tempting to simplify one's thinking so that pain is construed as an evoked potential or a response to a questionnaire, but history has shown that such narrow perspectives give the investigator little that can contribute to the advance of pain theory or clinical pain control. Recent models for human pain stress the interaction of sensory experiences with emotions and drive states as well as socially determined value judgments (6). Study of the language used by patients to describe clinically significant pain problems similarly indicates that people suffering with pain conceive of it as a multifaceted combination of sensory, emotional, and evaluative or judgmental experiences (7).

What implication does the contemporary multifaceted conceptualization of pain have for the laboratory or clinical researcher? The basic issue becomes how the observed complexity can be adequately preserved and manipulated in the process of investigation so that studies of human pain do not caricature the phenomenon too severely. It is not enough to apply traditional measures and methods routinely to each new question for these have taught us little about pain in the past. Indeed, several factors are crucial for a truly informative experiment.

First, models of pain must attend to variables representing a broad range of conditions and events. Although pain involves changes in sensory states, it also involves changes in emotion, mood, and social behavior. Second, hypotheses must predict interrelations among two or more variables. That is, changes in mood and social behavior, as well as anxiety, may correlate with changes in pain, and the nature of these interactions is important. Third, experimental designs must be sophisticated, carefully thought out, and flexibly applied. Finally, data analyses appropriate to the design should be employed. This chapter addresses one aspect of the last consideration—the use of multivariate data analytic techniques.

Simple research designs and data analysis are always desirable. Unfortunately, simple procedures when appropriately applied usually imply phenomena that are well understood, well controlled, or both. The most pragmatic way to study complex and not well understood phenomena such as pain is to collect multiple measures of the important variables. If there is no single authoritative measure of pain, then an investigator may use several pain indices, and he may proceed similarly with variables relating to personality, interpersonal situations, physical pathology, and other factors. Complex data sets may also be useful when the researcher is satisfied that he has an adequate measure of some, say, personality variable, but he also wishes to relate pain simultaneously to social and physical variables. Either of these situations, and others as well, will lead to multivariate data sets; i.e., data sets containing multiple pain-related measures and/or multiple treatments and conditions. Many investigators would carry out a series of statistical tests on such data. However, the repeated application of simple univariate (i.e., single variable) tests (e.g., X^2, *t*-test) is completely inadequate for complex data analyses for two reasons.

First, several univariate tests performed on a single set of subjects can yield a significant result when none exists because inferential statistics are based on probabilities. If conventional significance levels are used, 5% of the time random variations in the data lead to falsely significant findings. Naturally, if two tests of significance are performed, the probability that one will be significant by chance is greater than 5%. As more tests are added, the probability that at least one of them will be significant by chance alone quickly becomes quite large.

Nor is it satisfactory to feel comfortable because several results out of a set of multiple tests are significant. Imagine that out of a large set of analyses four are significant, but that two of these results were found with two different measures of anxiety, and the other two with two different measures of pain. Presumably, there would be high correlations between the two variables in each pair, so that, given a significant result with one pain variable, the probability of the other also being significant is quite high. Additionally, in many situations anxiety and pain are correlated so that a significant effect on one implies significance with the other, so the four significant effects may be reduced to two, or perhaps to one. But how many meaningful effects are there, and how does one determine this? Single-variable techniques are simply not designed to provide an answer to this overall question, and for this reason they should not be used for multiple tests.

The second major reason for avoiding multiple univariate tests is that they can indicate marginal or even nonsignificant results when, in fact, the effects are highly significant. A data example is relevant here. Chapman and Cox (2) collected measures of pain, anxiety, and depression on each of 3 days (presurgically, first day after surgery, and third day after surgery) for three groups of surgical patients (renal transplant donors and recipients and patients undergoing general abdominal surgery). Table 1 presents the univariate analysis of variance results for the nine variables. Two of these results are significant and a third is borderline. However, overall probability for the multivariate analysis of variance (MANOVA) for the entire set of nine variables (i.e., three measures taken over 3 days) is much more highly significant than any of the individual tests. The apparent contradiction is because the multivariate procedure takes into consideration the relationships or interactions among the variables (this is accomplished by considering the correlations among the variables), and if these vary among groups, then significant results can be obtained even though the means for the separate variables do not differ among groups.

In the present example the three daily scores for each variable were transformed into trend scores over the 3 days (average score, linear trend—whether day three is higher or lower than the pre-test day, and curvilinear trend—how much of a peak there is on the middle day) and reanalyzed by MANOVA. The overall test of significance remains precisely the same as before because the total information in the data is exactly the same. However, although it is the same information, it has been rearranged and for that reason the pattern of individual variable results is altogether different. Table 2 shows that the curvilinear scores for pain and anxiety are highly significant, but nothing else is. Further analysis demonstrates that the overall significance for the nine variables is due solely to differences among the groups in the curvilinearity of their pain and anxiety scores over days, a finding that could never be detected given only the set of univariate results for the daily scores. In this case the use of multivariate procedures not only increased the investigators' power to evaluate hypotheses but also gave them new insight into the nature of the data set.

Although MANOVA (4) is a highly useful procedure, other types of multiple measure analyses are also available. For example, an investigator may focus his attention on the patterns underlying his large data set. Factor

TABLE 1. *Test of differences between groups on mean daily scores*

Test	F-ratio	Probability
Single-variable tests[a]		
Presurgical pain	3.579	0.034
Pain day 1	1.252	0.293
Pain day 3	3.545	0.035
Presurgical anxiety	3.113	0.051
Anxiety day 1	2.107	0.130
Anxiety day 3	2.289	0.110
Presurgical depression	2.294	0.109
Depression day 1	0.040	0.961
Depression day 3	1.715	0.188
Overall test[b]	2.175	0.007

[a] 2 and 64 df for all single-variable tests.
[b] 18 and 112 df for the overall test.

TABLE 2. *Results of multivariate analysis of variance on scores representing trends over days*

Test	F-ratio	Probability
Single-variable tests[a]		
Average pain	0.895	0.414
Pain–linear trend	2.342	0.104
Pain–quadratic trend	8.704	0.001
Average anxiety	0.442	0.657
Anxiety–linear trend	1.647	0.201
Anxiety–quadratic trend	9.914	0.001
Average depression	1.150	0.323
Depression–linear trend	1.770	0.179
Depression–quadratic trend	2.545	0.086
Overall test[b]	2.177	0.007

[a] 2 and 64 df for all single-variable tests.
[b] 18 and 112 df for the overall test.

analysis (8) and multidimensional scaling (9) are useful for this type of purpose. Additionally, an individual differences model of multidimensional scaling has recently become available, and it can be used for testing hypotheses about differences in structure (1). Or an investigator may be interested in either of two types of classification. First, data may be available for subjects known to belong to one of two or more groups (e.g., patients with pain and with physical pathology versus patients with pain but no apparent pathology), and one might wish to learn how to predict to which of the groups new patients will belong. Here one could employ discriminate function analysis (4) to learn how to use data to best assign new cases to known categories. Or one may have data for a large set of patients and suspect that there should be meaningful, but unknown, subsets of patients. For example, one might expect a large group of headache patients to fall into several distinct subgroups. In this case a clustering procedure would be appropriate (5). Other more specialized techniques exist but need not be mentioned here. Pain studies using one or another of these techniques are beginning to find their way into the literature (3,10,11), but certainly many other applications exist.

How does an investigator with a minimal background in statistical methodology go about developing multivariate research? The basic requirement is interdisciplinary collaboration. By collaborating with a biostatistician or a psychologist or other social scientist educated in statistical procedures, even the most clinically oriented researcher can employ multivariate techniques in the analysis of his data. In addition to active consultation, the researcher will require access to a suitable computer. In the United States most large academic installations provide Statistical Package for the Social Sciences (SPSS) or Biomedical Data (BMD) package programs, which are equipped to handle multivariate analyses.

The multivariate approach clearly is more complicated, more demanding, and more expensive than the traditional single-variable methodology. Is it worth the costs? The answer lies with the realization that the understanding and control of human pain is an exceedingly difficult challenge, and it will not yield to methods that are adequate for other seemingly similar areas of research. Traditional statistical methods and experimental designs that restrict testing to single variables are likely to lead to an unfortunate oversimplification of human pain. Although not a panacea, multivariate statistics may be of considerable value in clarifying and testing ideas about the cause and cure of pain problems.

REFERENCES

1. Carroll, J. D., and Chang, J. J. (1970): *Psychometrika,* 35:283–319.
2. Chapman, C. R., and Cox, G. B. (1976): *J. Psychosom. Res.* (*in press*).
3. Davidson, P. O., and Neufeld, W. J. (1974): *J. Psychosom. Res.,* 18:25–32.
4. Harris, R. J. (1975): *A Primer of Multivariate Statistics.* Academic Press, New York.
5. Hartigan, J. A. (1975): *Clustering Algorithms.* Wiley-Interscience, New York.
6. Melzack, R., and Casey, A. L. (1968): In: *The Skin Senses,* edited by D. Kenshalo. Charles C Thomas, Publisher, Springfield, Illinois.
7. Melzack, R., and Torgerson, W. S. (1971): *Anesthesiology,* 34:50–59.
8. Rummel, R. J. (1970): *Applied Factor Analysis.* Northwestern University Press, Evanston, Illinois.
9. Shepard, R. N., Romney, A. K., and Nerlove, S. B. (Eds.) (1972): *Multidimensional Scaling, Vol. I.* Seminar Press, New York.
10. Timmermans, G., and Sternbach, R. A. (1974): *Science,* 184:806–808.
11. Wolff, B. B. (1971): *J. Abnorm. Psychol.,* 78:292–298.

Advances in Pain Research and Therapy, Vol. 1,
edited by J. J. Bonica and D. Albe-Fessard.
Raven Press, New York © 1976.

Application of Laser to Psychophysiological Study of Pain in Man

Amiram Carmon, Joseph Mor, and Judith Goldberg

Departments of Behavioral Biology and Bio-Medical Engineering, Technion–Israel Institute of Technology, Technion City, Haifa, Israel

An important issue in pain research is the relation between a painful stimulus and a response indicating that the subject felt pain. Pain-inducing stimuli and painful sensations are difficult to define. The influence of subjective variables points out that pain is not only a sensory event but also a complex psychological process. In order to measure pain objectively, one must use stimuli that undoubtedly cause pain, and pain only, and record responses that unequivocally indicate that the subject had a painful experience (3). Since both problems are interdependent, they should be solved simultaneously. A possible solution is to find a stimulus that has physiologically been proven as painful and substitute verbal response with a physiological response, which is less prone to be influenced by personality, set, or cultural attitudes.

When pain is induced without other concomitant sensations, thermal nociceptors are most suitable as the target organs. They are activated only at noxious temperatures, i.e., in excess of 45°C, and they do not adapt easily (5). Noxious temperatures inhibit other thermal-sensitive fibers, and the message transmitted to the central nervous system is of pain and not of warmth. No parallel situation is found in mechanoreceptors (1). Thermal nociceptors can be activated and both thermal receptors and mechanoreceptors bypassed if heat is irradiated and not conducted from a mechanical contact and if high temperatures are reached quickly. Customary cutaneous heating by irradiation from incandescent sources (Hardy-Wolff-Goodell dolorimeter) is too slow and can result in stimulation of thermal receptors other than thermal nociceptors.

To overcome this technical difficulty, we have employed radiant heat by a new technique, an infrared laser beam. This technique permits heating to high temperatures within a few milliseconds, in contrast to the 250 to 300 msec required with the dolorimeter.

The problem of measuring pain objectively is even more complex. Among other psychophysiological measures, the electroencephalogram is widely used as a physiological indicator of both sensory percepts and cognitive and psychological states. Changes induced by peripheral stimulation are detected by averaging the EEG over many repetitions to single out an evoked response from the background noise. All EEG epochs sampled must be accurately time locked to the stimulus. Therefore, stimuli should be accurately timed and as brief as possible. The short burst of laser energy answers this timing requirement as well.

Details of the component parts, biophysics, and application of the laser to pain research have been published (4). This report briefly summarizes several psychologic and electrophysiologic investigations on pain and presents new data.

METHODS

The technique used (6) consisted of cutaneous stimulation by a brief exposure to the output of a CO_2 laser (8C Laser manufactured by The Israel Electro-Optical Industry). The laser output is a 20-mm diameter

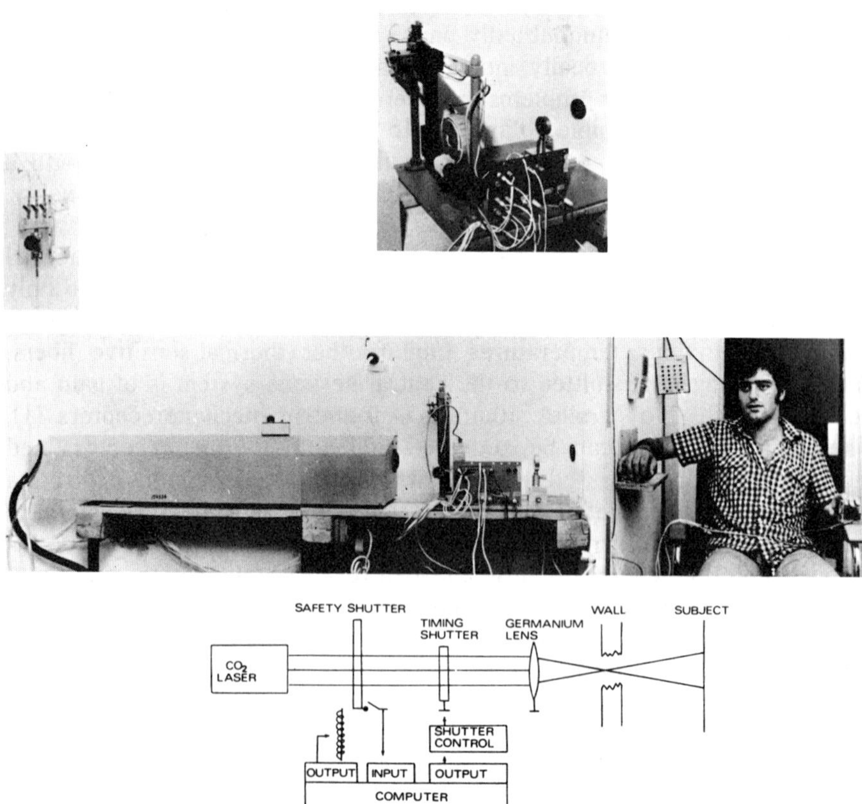

FIG. 1. Experimental set-up.

infrared beam (wavelength 10.6 μm) with 50 W maximum power. The diameter of the beam can be limited and the intensity increased by focusing it with a germanium lens. Electronic control of the output power is optional, but small increments of energy are best achieved by varying the duration of exposure and keeping output power at a fixed level.

To chop the output into a predetermined, discrete, brief stimulus, we used a system of two shutters: a solenoid-driven safety shutter of heavy-gauge blackened aluminum served as both gross control and heat sink, and a fast shutter was used for accurate timing. A PDP 11/45 computer controlled the activation of the heavy shutter at random intervals, received information that the shutter was open, and opened the fast shutter for a predetermined duration. The location and size of the stimulus were controlled by a germanium lens which follows the path of the beam (Fig. 1). The computer also received the EEG input from the subject for averaging and recording subjective responses. The subjects pressed one of a set of designated microswitches to indicate what they felt 2 sec after each stimulation. This delay was employed to avoid contamination of the sampled EEG by motor activity. All experiments were conducted in a temperature-controlled room. Outside noises were appropriately masked.

RESULTS

Psychophysical Pain Thresholds

Nine Ss (healthy paid volunteers) were tested by serial exploration. We measured for stimulations with both nonfocused (area 3.14 cm^2) and focused (area 0.28 cm^2) beams on the lateral side of the right forearm. Thresholds are best described by integrated energy, a term derived by multiplying stimulation power by exposure time:

$$2.39 \times \text{number of watts used} \times \text{duration in msec}$$
$$(1\ \text{W} = 1\ \text{J/sec or } 239\ \text{mCal}/1{,}000\ \text{msec}).$$

With the nonfocused beam, one could feel a nonnoxious sensation of warmth with a 180- to 240-mCal stimulus. A burning pain was felt when intensity was increased, and it was followed by a feeling of both burning and stabbing pain (380 mCal). With the concentrated beam the initial sensation was always a slight burning pain (110 to 130 mCal), followed by a moderate pinprick feeling (160 to 170 mCal), and then by a strong stabbing pain (210 to 230 mCal). Thresholds were stable even after more than 100 repetitions of the stimulus (intertrial interval was approximately 10 sec). Figure 2 depicts the time course of the stimulation.

Thresholds varied only slightly at different locations on the forearms. These changes were not systematically analyzed. No attempt was made to study other cutaneous locations.

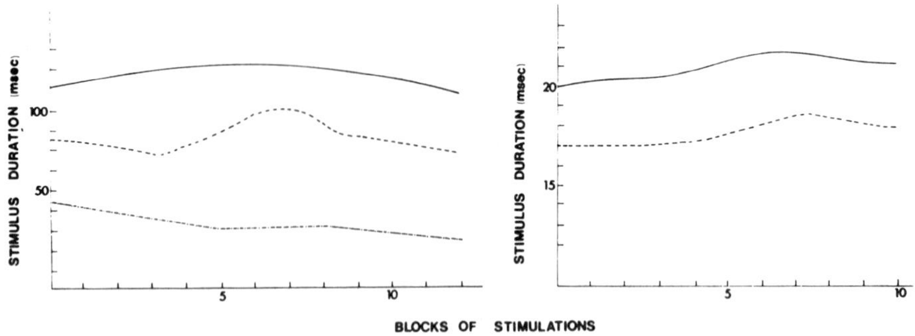

FIG. 2. Time course of sensory thresholds. Blocks refer to series of 6 to 10 repeated stimulations administered in ascending or descending order to measure thresholds. Subjective response: (–·–·), warmth; (––––), slight burn; (——), pain. **Left:** stimulus, 2.5 W/cm²; area, 3.14 cm². **Right:** stimulus, 15 W/cm²; area, 0.28 cm².

Electrophysiological Responses to Painful Stimuli

The EEG in 4 subjects was averaged in several sessions in order to disclose a cerebral evoked response. Initial results showed that a clear evoked response was obtained only to stimuli that caused pain and not to stimuli felt as warm. The most typical components were a negative wave with a peak latency at approximately 130 to 190 msec and a big positive wave with a peak latency at 240 to 360 msec. The two waves appeared in all subjects, were easily replicable, and were most prominent from the vertex. The peak-to-peak size of the negative-positive complex was 5 to 40 μV, and it showed an increase in amplitude concomitant with the increase in either stimulus intensity or subjective response (Fig. 3). The most prominent evoked responses were obtained with discrete stimuli (area 0.28 cm^2), and when the subjects felt pure pain without accompanying warmth.

COMMENT

The improvement in radiant heat stimulation obtained by applying the laser-emitted infrared beam resulted in several methodological gains. First, stimuli are discrete in both space and time. Second, there is little intersubject or intrasubject variability in the sensations produced. Technical difficulties such as habituation or sensitization are avoided. These characteristics enable the investigator to obtain for the first time what seems to be an objective indicator of pain—a cerebral evoked response that is correlated with the subjective feeling of pain. The significance of the electrophysiological signal obtained should be further investigated. However, its temporal and spatial attributes suggest that it probably signifies cerebral

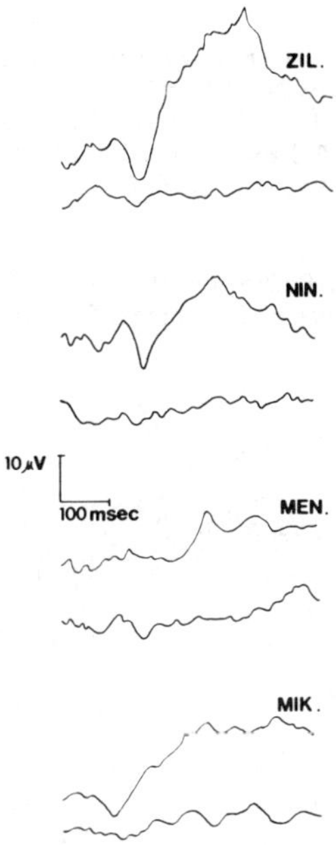

SUBJECTIVE RESPONSE	INTENSITY (mCal)	DURATION (msec)	AREA (cm^2)
PAIN	30	8	0.28
WARM	140	42	3.14
PAIN	30	8	0.28
WARM	150	40	3.14
PAIN	140	40	1.13
WARM	70	40	1.13
PAIN	380	45	3.14
WARM	170	45	3.14

FIG. 3. Examples of evoked responses to warm and painful stimuli. (Abbreviations on left refer to subjects.)

arousal (2) owing to pain. With further experimentation and technical refinements, it might be possible to substitute verbal responses with this signal and also to use it in studies of pain in animals.

SUMMARY

Brief stimulation by concentrated high-power infrared laser beam was used to induce warm sensations or pain. Preliminary results showed that magnitude of subjective response to pain was correlated with stimulus intensity. Habituation or sensitization to the painful stimuli was not observed. Thresholds were similar in all subjects investigated.

Cerebral evoked responses were also recorded with this stimulation. They were obtained when stimuli were painful but not when they were only warm. The significant components of the response were two late waves, in the form of a negative-positive complex, which were correlated with both stimulus intensity and the subjective feeling of pain.

ACKNOWLEDGMENT

This study was supported by a David Rose Grant.

REFERENCES

1. Burgess, P. R. (1974): In: *Advances in Neurology, Vol. 4: International Symposium on Pain,* edited by J. J. Bonica, pp. 11–18. Raven Press, New York.
2. Goff, W. R., Matsumiya, Y., Allison, T., and Goff, G. D. (1969): In: *Averaged Evoked Potentials: Methods, Results and Evaluations,* edited by E. Donchin and D. B. Lindsley. National Aeronautical and Space Administration, Washington, D.C.
3. McBurney, D. H. (1975): *Science,* 189:66.
4. Mor, J., and Carmon, A. (1975): *Pain,* 1:233.
5. Wall, P. D. (1974): In: *Recent Advances on Pain: Pathophysiology and Clinical Aspects,* edited by J. J. Bonica, P. Procacci, and C. Pagni. Charles C Thomas, Publisher, Springfield, Illinois.

Advances in Pain Research and Therapy, Vol. 1,
edited by J. J. Bonica and D. Albe-Fessard.
Raven Press, New York © 1976.

Peripheral and Spinal "Pain" Mechanisms and Their Modulation

A. Iggo

SRC Somatosensory Research Group, Department of Physiology, Faculty of Veterinary Medicine, University of Edinburgh, Edinburgh EH9 1QH, United Kingdom

Any account of the peripheral mechanisms of "pain" that draws on experimental work using animals has to be prefaced by the cautionary statement that pain is a conscious experience of humans and that we can only infer or deduce the possible mechanisms from animals studies. Nevertheless, many important advances in our knowledge of pain have been initiated in the laboratory and tested in the clinic. Equally important is the transfer of ideas in the other direction, from the clinic to the laboratory, and it is just this cross-fertilization that is one of the objectives of the International Association for the Study of Pain. In this chapter I shall outline the current state of knowledge of peripheral and spinal mechanisms.

PERIPHERAL MECHANISMS

During the last two decades a consensus has emerged from electrophysiological and morphological studies that the peripheral receptors are functionally organized to respond to specific stimuli and have a high degree of "selective sensitivity." The old ideas of specific nerve energies and the "adequate stimulus" have, in modified form, survived critical experimental evaluation, and the general conclusion is that three categories of cutaneous receptor exist: *mechanoreceptors, thermoreceptors,* and *nociceptors.* The evidence has been reviewed at recent symposia on "pain" (Recent Advances on Pain, Florence, 1972; Pain, Seattle, 1973; 24) and other review articles (25,29) are available for reference. It might be thought that a symposium on pain would be concerned principally if not exclusively with nociceptors. But as I will attempt to show, this is certainly not so—at least some of the mechanoreceptors may also play a part.

The following paragraphs summarize current knowledge of the receptor systems.

The mechanoreceptors in skin include a variety of organized, often encapsulated, structures that are extremely sensitive to small (< 10 μm or < 10 mg) displacements or forces applied to the skin surface. They are innervated by rapidly conducting myelinated axons ($>$4-μm diameter) with low thresholds for electrical stimulation. These mechanoreceptors are usually inactive in resting or undisturbed skin. Hairy skin in addition has sensitive mechanoreceptors with thin myelinated afferent fibers (1- to 3-μm diameter), some of which may be active in resting skin but only at low rates of discharge, as well as sensitive mechanoreceptors with nonmyelinated axons. All the mechanoreceptors can be stirred to vigorous activity by lightly brushing or pressing on the skin (e.g., drawing cotton wool over the surface).

The thermoreceptors (cold and warm receptors) are not excited by mechanical stimuli, may carry a resting discharge depending on skin temperature, and have small myelinated (1- to 3-μm diameter) or nonmyelinated afferent axons that are electrically less excitable than the large mechanoreceptor axons.

The nociceptors are much less excitable by mechanical or thermal stimuli than either of the above classes of receptors, but nociceptors are excited by more severe mechanical, thermal, and/or chemical irritants. There are at least two major subdivisions: *mechanical and thermal nociceptors.*

Mechanical nociceptors are excited by pinching, pricking, or scraping the skin, but not by severe heating or cooling of the skin. Some of the receptors have small to medium-sized axons (3 to 6 μm) and others are nonmyelinated ($<$ 1 μm), but none are as large as the largest mechanoreceptor axons. Consequently, the large axons from mechanoreceptors can be excited selectively by electrical pulses.

Thermal nociceptors (synonyms: heat receptors, polymodal nociceptors) are vigorously excited by high ($>$43°C) skin temperatures as well as by severe mechanical stimuli. They can be distinguished experimentally from warm receptors. In nonprimates the sensory axons are nearly all nonmyelinated, and therefore they are both slowly conducting and of low electrical excitability. In primates many of the axons are nonmyelinated, but some of them have small myelinated axons ($\simeq$ 1-μm diameter) in the proximal part of their paths. These, however, are of relatively low electrical excitability.

The deeper tissues of the body (muscles, joints, viscera) all contain nociceptors, most of which, like those from the skin, are supplied by thin myelinated or nonmyelinated axons of low electrical excitability. The relation between sizes of the sensory fibers (conduction velocity) and function of skin receptors is summarized in Fig. 1.

Modulation of the Peripheral Mechanisms

The peripheral mechanisms can be modified in their effectiveness at several sites and by various means. Beginning with the receptors them-

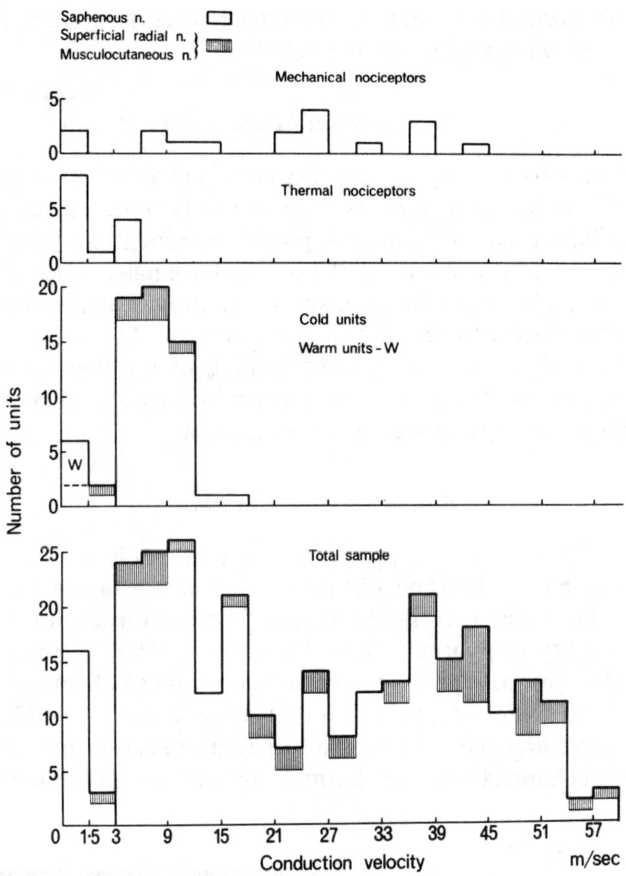

FIG. 1. Comparison of the conduction velocities of primate cutaneous sensory fibers to illustrate the slowness (and therefore small size) of the nociceptor and thermoreceptor afferent fibers. Balance of the axons in the bottom histogram are from sensitive mechanoreceptors (A. Iggo and H. Ogawa, *unpublished*).

selves, the possible sites of action include: (a) the transducer, which converts the natural stimulus to an electrical potential capable of generating impulses in the sensory fibers; (b) the axon terminal where the impulses start their journey to the central nervous system; and (c) the conducting axon, which stretches from the receptor to the central nervous system, traveling via the peripheral nerves, spinal nerves, and dorsal (posterior) roots and (for some visceral sensory axons) the ventral roots (12).

There are many possible causes of modulation – physiological, pharmacological, and pathological. Physiologically, there is the possibility of efferent control (as for the muscle spindles), but, except for some indication that the sympathetic system may have an effect, there is no firm evidence for such an action on normal nociceptors, and the nociceptors show no unusual sensitivity to norepinephrine or acetylcholine.

Physiological Modulation

Receptor sensitivity may be depressed or enhanced as a normal consequence of activity. If a noxious stimulation is repeated too frequently, it may be effective initially but less potent on repetition (23). This is because of changes in sensitivity of the active terminals, and if the stimulus is localized, a small change in its position to a previously unstimulated part of the receptive field can restore full effectiveness. In contrast, sensitivity may be enhanced, as follows radiant heating of the thermal nociceptors (4,23); consequently, there may be a period of greater excitation which, however, is followed by a depression of sensitivity.

Biochemical Modulation

The role in "pain" of polypeptides [such as bradykinin (BK)] of the amines (particularly 5-HT and histamine) and of prostaglandins (PG) continues to excite interest, from the point of both the receptor mechanisms and the possibility of pharmacological interference with painful conditions (Fig. 2). Although not highly specific in action, these chemicals can cause a discharge from some receptors with thin sensory fibers, in both skin (2,15) and muscle (16), and they are probably painful because they excite either or both the mechanical and the thermal nociceptors. There is no evidence

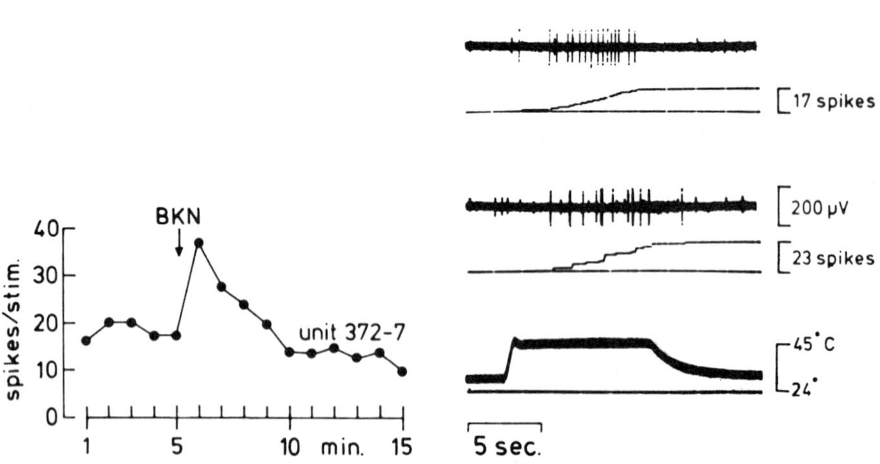

FIG. 2. Effect of intra-arterial bradykinin (Bk) in the response of a thermal nociceptor to radiant heat. **Left:** Sample responses of nociceptor. **Right:** Heat step. Total number of spikes in response (17, 23 spikes/stim in the illustrated responses) is plotted in graph at top, showing increment in response after Bk injection. (From ref. 2.)

that they act on an entirely different set of receptors. They may alter the sensitivity of the nociceptors (2)—modulation—so that natural stimuli are more effective and therefore more painful when the potentiating chemicals are present. In addition, the chemicals might interact and result in mutual enhancement or facilitation, even though the tachyphylaxis after, for example, BK does not alter sensitivity to 5-HT. Interactions are reported in human i.v. studies (35) where pretreatment with 5-HT enhances the subsequent response to injections of BK. Afferent nerve recording has also brought forward evidence that PGE_1, although not itself strongly excitatory (10), can potentiate the action of BK and 5-HT on sensory nerves (27).

These pharmacological studies may now provide an explanation for the analgesic effects of aspirin, which by interfering with the synthesis of prostaglandin may diminish the potency of chemalgogenic agents, such as 5-HT and BK (40), and also for the powerfully excitatory effect of intra-arterial BK on dorsal horn neurons (3).

Pathological Conditions

Pathological conditions can modify the peripheral pain mechanisms in many ways. Traumatic injury may lead to complete or partial denervation, which initially may cause anesthesia of the affected part. The processes of regeneration and their failure may lead to aberrations of the normal mechanisms and result in "painful" states arising during otherwise normal conditions. Examples are (a) *increased sensitivity of the regenerating nerve tip* where a mild physical stimulus may initiate a continued stream of sensory impulses (7); (b) *painful neuromas,* in which the nerve tip gives rise to a discharge of impulses that can be averted by pressure or even antidromic impulses (7,44); (c) *after distal transection of the peripheral nerve* (28), when impulses may even be initiated in dorsal root ganglion cells; and (d) *causalgia,* in which nerve injury leads to severe pain arising from completely untouched tissue—this may arise from a breakdown of the normal insulation between axons in the nerve trunk at the site of the injury and the initiation of impulses in sensory axons by motor impulses in sympathetic axons in the damaged tissue.

Peripheral deafferentation may lead to abnormal central states and thus cause pain. Because the general level of activity in the central pain pathways depends on the balance and kind of input in peripheral sensory nerves from the skin, muscles, joints, viscera, and other deep tissues, factors which cause absence of inputs in some pathways as a result of selective, partial, or complete deafferentation of a given part or tissue may give rise to pain or hallucinations of pain. This is an experimentally difficult area of investigation and exact knowledge is lacking.

Another condition of general interest is the inflammatory reaction that follows injury or infection. The "pain" arising in these conditions probably arises from the actions of chemalgogenic agents produced in or released from the inflamed tissues. I have already discussed the probable chemicals (5-HT, BK) which in very low concentrations can both cause "pain" and excite sensory nerve endings (2,15), although not in a specific way. The postulated action of aspirin-like drugs in blocking this kind of action (40) is an example of a second-order modulation of pain.

SPINAL MECHANISMS

A prudent scientist might be pardoned for eschewing any attempt to give a rational account of the spinal mechanisms involved in pain, in view of the flood of new papers on the physiology and pharmacology of the spinal cord. Some positive statements can, however, be made. First, the "pain" pathways lead through the dorsal horn of the spinal cord (or its equivalent in the brainstem). Second, the spinothalamic tract (the classic pain pathway) is well developed in primates, where it arises principally from cells in Rexed's laminae I, IV, and V (39), and less clearly present in cats (5), where it originates principally from laminae VII and VIII. Third, transmissibility of "painful" stimuli through the dorsal horn can be modified by segmental and descending mechanisms (19).

It is now possible to design experiments based on an exact knowledge of the functional characteristics of afferent nerves in cutaneous nerves—their diameters and electrical excitability and the characteristics of the peripheral receptors, as reviewed earlier in this chapter. To this extent, the experiments can be designed to answer specific questions in the hope that the central nervous system will yield less than ambiguous answers. On the other hand, experimental analysis still has to contend with the formidable problems presented by the central nervous system, often compounded by the technical difficulties of preparing and sustaining animal preparations in a satisfactory physiological state during the long periods required. The use of anesthetized animals is a continuing requirement for exact and quantitative analysis, but the possible interference caused by anesthetics (21) makes it necessary that the results and hypotheses be tested in unanesthetized animals. The pain-producing trials that may be demanded impose difficult moral problems on the investigators. Finally, there is the transfer of the new ideas for therapy to the clinic. I shall be concerned only with laboratory work in my account in the confident expectation that clinical aspects will be reviewed by other authors.

Dorsal Horn

The dorsal horn of the gray matter of the spinal cord receives input from cutaneous and visceral axons of all sizes and from some muscle afferents, as well as from descending tracts of supraspinal origin. The output from the dorsal horn enters long ascending pathways or short, more localized intersegmental connections. There is a degree of segregation of sensory fibers on entry to the cord, and the largest, coming from mechanoreceptors in the skin and muscles, send collaterals into the dorsal columns, where they ascend to dorsal column nuclei or to deeper parts of the spinal gray matter, in addition to any branches that may enter the dorsal horn from its medial border. The finer fibers, in contrast, send collaterals into the dorsal horn from its dorsal border (33). Since the nociceptors have thin sensory fibers, it would seem reasonable to look for their first actions in the dorsal horn; and since they do not have long collaterals traveling up the spinal cord or deep into the ventral horn, it seems equally sensible to expect to find the next stage in any "pain" pathway in the output of cells of the dorsal horn. This latter expectation is strengthened by the clinical evidence that "painful" states may be relieved, for example, by anterolateral cordotomy, which interrupts the spinothalamic tract fibers. These straightforward expectations are confounded by new knowledge that the responsiveness of dorsal horn cells is powerfully modified by descending control systems (14,43), which may selectively alter transmissibility through the dorsal horn (6).

The general picture that is emerging from contemporary work is that the dorsal horn contains a diversity of neurons organized into laminae and responding in several recognizable patterns to the inputs received from the periphery and from other, usually higher, levels of the nervous system. In my laboratory we have attempted to codify the lumbosacral dorsal horn cells according to their responses to an input from cutaneous and muscle receptors and have found four distinct classes (19,24).

Class 1 neurons are excited by afferent fibers from the cutaneous mechanoreceptors with large afferent fibers that can be excited vigorously by stroking or lightly pressing on the skin, but not by stimuli that excite only the thermal nociceptors. *Class 2 neurons* (Fig. 3) are also excited by the large mechanoreceptors but more powerfully by an input from the nociceptors (in spinal animals). (These cells probably correspond to the T cells described in the gate hypothesis.) *Class 3 neurons* (figure in Iggo et al., *this volume*) are not excited by the mechanoreceptors but are stirred to activity by an input from both thermal and mechanical nociceptors. *Class 4* or *"cold" neurons* are excited only by an input from thermoreceptors.

These four categories have their counterparts in the kinds of dorsal horn cells reported by most other laboratories (3,6,11,18,31,32,36,39,42), although they are not necessarily grouped in the same way and in several studies only the neurons projecting into tracts were investigated (6,39). The input connections to these various cells may be direct (i.e., monosynaptic) or indirect (polysynaptic), and any neuron may be reached both mono- and polysynaptically from the primary afferent fibers. The connections can be established with reasonable accuracy only in the physiological

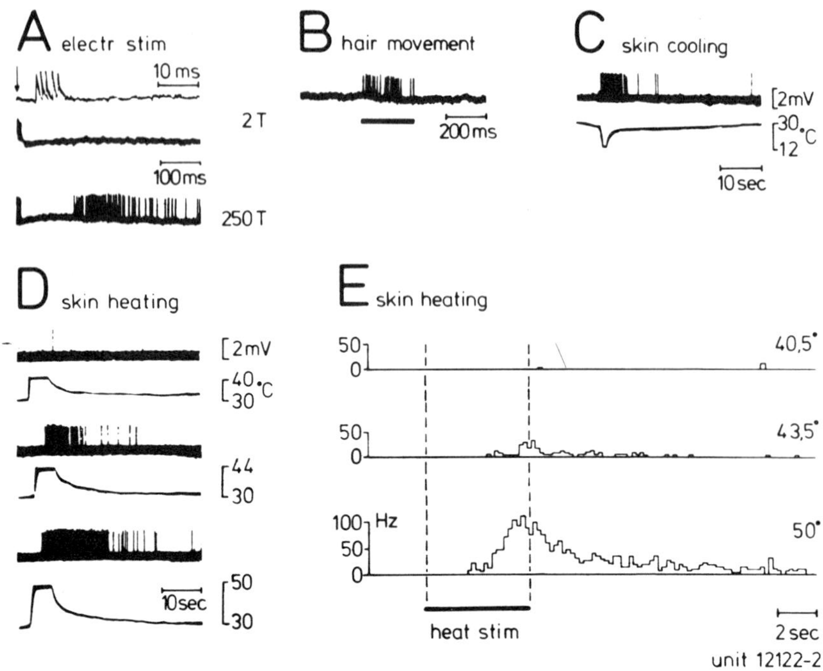

FIG. 3. Response of a class 2 neuron to various kinds of stimuli. **A:** Top 2 traces: electrical stimulation at 2 T (twice threshold of most excitable fibers) of both plantar nerves; bottom trace: electrical stimulation of plantar nerves at 250 T, which was above the threshold of C fibers. **B:** Hair movement (*bar*) on plantar surface of the foot. **C:** Skin cooling by ethylchloride evaporation; skin surface temperature recorded by a thermocouple is shown below. **D:** Heating the skin of the foot pad by radiation to 40°, 44°, and 50°C; skin surface temperatures measured with a thermocouple are shown below each record. **E:** Time course of discharge frequencies plotted as histograms during and after heating foot pad to various temperatures. Duration of heat stimulus indicated by bar below. Spinalized animal. Unit was 1,750 μm from cord dorsum and had polysynaptic connection to group 2 afferents. (From ref. 19.)

studies for the inputs from the fast axons from the mechanoreceptors. There is plenty of opportunity for the cells to be in complex neuronal interconnection, as would be expected from the morphological studies (33).

Of course, dorsal horn neurons can be inhibited as well as excited (22,32), although the synapses formed by primary afferent fibers are all excitatory. The inhibitory effects require the addition of at least one neuron to the chain, but once again there is no shortage of candidates among the small neurons of the dorsal horn.

Before considering these inhibitory actions, I will put the various classes of neurons into a spatial framework and also summarize our knowledge of the output from the dorsal horn into ascending pathways.

Laminar Organization

The dorsal horn of the lumbar spinal cord (Fig. 4) can be divided in several more or less clearly recognized layers, the laminae of Rexed (34). The great accuracy of locating recording sites has led to general use of cell marking at the time of recording using glass microelectrodes and electrophoretic deposition of dyes (e.g., pontamine sky blue) or electrolytic lesions. Reconstruction of electrode tracks from scalar coordinates is also used. The four classes of neurons I have described with positions of recording marked by pontamine sky blue are distributed in lamina I (all classes in monkey, classes 1, 2, and 3 in the cat). The substantia gelatinosa (laminae II and III) contains large numbers of small cells, most (or all) of which have eluded examination by electrophysiological methods; nevertheless, some unit recording of class 1, 2, and 3 cells has been reported. Lamina IV, which together with lamina V contains some of the largest cells in the dorsal horn, has most of the class 1 and 2 cells. Lamina V has cells with a mixed cuta-

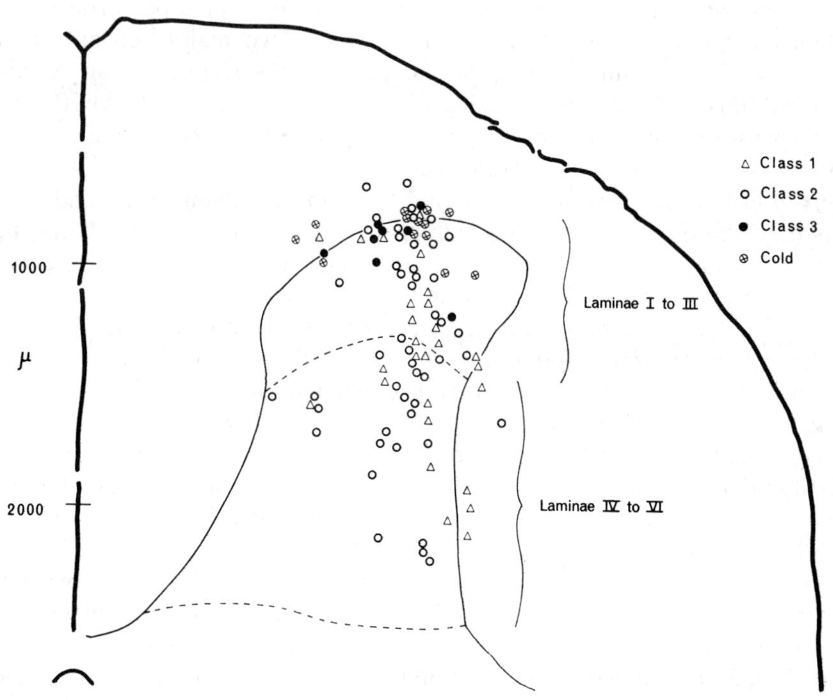

FIG. 4. Laminar organization of the spinal cord (based on Rexed's analysis) in the monkey with location of class 1–4 dorsal horn neurons. Nociceptor neurons (class 3) and cold-sensitive neurons are restricted to laminae I and II, whereas class 1 and 2 neurons, although also present there, are more widespread.

neous and muscle input and which show considerable convergence. A functional lamination is therefore present. The cells with an exclusively nociceptor input are most superficial, although not as a pure culture.

A dorsoventral stratification in the dorsal horn has been suggested with increasing convergence of the cutaneous fields at greater depths, together with an admixture of muscle afferent inputs particularly in lamina V and deeper. There is some indication of this in the relatively smaller sizes of the receptive fields in the more superficial laminae of the cord, but it is also evident, even in lamina I, that some cells are excited from the larger cutaneous afferents and others receive an excitatory input from the small myelinated and nonmyelinated muscle afferents.

Output from Dorsal Horn

The output from dorsal horn neurons has been studied mostly from the standpoint of long ascending pathways (6,37,39), by electrophysiological and neuroanatomical methods (often in combination), and most recently with horseradish peroxidase (38), which is proving to be a powerful tool in establishing neuronal tracts and connections. Two major sensory tracts arise in the dorsal horn—the spinothalamic and the spinocervical. A third possible sensory tract is the dorsal column postsynaptic system [DCPS (1)]. The spinothalamic tract has long been implicated in "pain," and current investigations (37,38) have established that the tract arises from two locations in primates, a few cells in lamina I and more in laminae IV and V. In cats the spinothalamic tract originates principally from more deeply located cells in laminae VII and VIII. The second major tract arising from the dorsal horn is the spinocervical, and its cells of origin are principally in lamina IV (6,37). Other outputs from the dorsal horn of interest from the point of "pain" are the short spinal interneurons, with axons in Lissauer's tract, running just ventral to the dorsal root entry and interconnecting with nine spinal segments (13) and with the cells of origin of the dorsal column postsynaptic units (1). There is no doubt of the importance of the former in modifying the activity of neurons in adjacent segments, but no detailed information is available on the properties of the individual units projecting into Lissauer's tract.

The functional attributes of various kinds of dorsal horn neurons projecting into the long sensory tracts (Fig. 4) have been established by electrophysiological studies (20,39,45). The class 1 cells (mechanoreceptor input) and class 2 cells (mechanoreceptor and nociceptor input) project into either the spinothalamic or the spinocervical tracts, whereas the class 3 (nociceptor driven) and cold cells project only in the spinothalamic (or crossed ventrolateral) tracts (20). These results can be interpreted as giving powerful support to the hypothesis that the class 3 cells, excited from the periphery only by nociceptors, may constitute an important pathway for the transmission of information interpreted as "painful." The role of the class 2 cells (driven by mechanoreceptors and nociceptors) remains equivocal. The DCPS tract has characteristics (1) that make likely the projection of some of the class 1 and 2 cells into it, especially the strong excitation of some of its component units by both light tactile and noxious stimuli.

Inhibitory Mechanisms of Dorsal Horn Neurons

The nervous system does not work by excitation alone, and in general there is always a balance of excitatory and inhibitory actions. In this respect the dorsal horn neurons are not exceptions. So far I have discussed excitatory inputs; the inhibitory actions on the dorsal horn neurons can be potent.

Supraspinal inhibition

Powerful tonic and selective inhibitory actions of supraspinal origin (14,37,43) in intact anesthetized animals can effectively shut down transmission from the nociceptors through the spinothalamic (20) and spinocervical (6,9) tracts, while leaving mechanoreceptor conduction relatively unimpaired or at most selectively modified. The effect of these tonic descending inhibitory actions is dramatic when tested by reversible block of the spinal cord. Class 2 cells may be strongly affected (Fig. 2); class 3 (nociceptor) cells may be inhibited to a lesser degree; and the class 1 (mechanoreceptor) cells are unaffected. Therefore, on balance in the intact animal, excitation from the peripheral nociceptors is most likely to enter the spinothalamic tract via the class 3 "nociceptor" neurons since the path through the class 2 cells is selectively closed.

Modulation of this pathway could be effected by altering the strength and distribution of the descending tonic inhibition, acting through interneurons in the dorsal horn. There may be several parallel sources of this kind of inhibitory action, e.g., the cerebral cortex (8) or the median raphe nuclei (30), and it is too soon to be able to give a concise or comprehensive story. In similar fashion, the pharmacological basis is under active investigation because of the potential clinical importance of the use of pharmacologically active agents in the treatment of pain.

Descending axons contain tryptamine, arising from neurons in the midline raphe nuclei of the brainstem end in the dorsal horn of the spinal cord. On depletion of their 5-HT, there is a reduction in the analgesic effect of morphine (41). Whether or not this is the same system as that which operates when morphine is injected into periaqueductal and periventricular sites (30) remains to be tested.

Segmental inhibition

A further important way in which inhibitory mechanisms can modulate possible "pain" pathways at the level of the dorsal horn is by a local or segmental selective suppression of the responses of class 2 and 3 dorsal horn neurons to nociceptive inputs (Fig. 2). These effects at the dorsal horn were established first for the class 2 cells in laminae IV and V (8,19,22,42). These are relatively large cells, and the preferential reduction in their responses to an excitatory input from nociceptors (or nonmyelinated fibers) was reported to the Seattle Congress (24). These class 2 cells are effectively suppressed by an input coming exclusively from the cutaneous mechanoreceptors, and the effect usually lasts only for the duration of the stimulation of the mechanoreceptors or their afferent fibers (19). The intriguing possibilities of these kinds of action have alerted investigators to their use in clinical situations and raised theoretical questions concerning the role of such class 2 dorsal horn neurons in "pain" and related conditions.

The possible segmental inhibition of the class 3 "nociceptive" neurons has been slower to be tested, but it is now established (26) that these cells can also have their excitability reduced by an input from the sensitive mechanoreceptors. This action, which is also limited to the duration of the afferent input, is not always expressed as potently on the class 3 as on the class 2 cells, but it may completely suppress the response of such a cell to a nociceptor input from cutaneous thermal nociceptors.

These descending and segmental inhibitory actions might be channeled through common interneuronal pathways in the dorsal horn, but this is not yet established. The tryptaminergic neurons of the brainstem (41) probably have an excitatory action on interneurons in the dorsal horn which, in their turn, may have inhibitory or excitatory effects. An interesting possibility is that such interneurons are also excited by afferent fiber collaterals, in which case a competitive or synergistic interaction between descending and segmental inhibitory inputs would be expected.

The mechanisms of the inhibitory actions in the dorsal horn are still under study, and it is not possible, for example, to say whether they are pre- or postsynaptic, or both. However, at least two synaptic mechanisms are involved in inhibition of afferent origin (17), one acting via a strychnine-sensitive transmitter site (glycine or its structural analogue as the transmitter) and the other, of longer latency, acting via a bicuculline-sensitive transmitter site (gamma-aminobutyric acid or its structural analogue as the transmitter). Here again is the possibility of selective pharmacological suppression or modulation of conduction through "pain" paths.

SUMMARY

In this general survey of the peripheral and spinal mechanisms of "pain," I have discussed only laboratory-based studies and tried to present a coherent account of current ideas. In such a synthesis it becomes necessary to take a stand on controversial issues, but in so doing I have attempted to adopt a position that can be justified by the facts available. In summary, my view of the facts is that there are selectively sensitive peripheral afferent fibers, some of which are well suited to function as detectors of "painful" stimuli. Their peripheral sensitivity can be enhanced or depressed, and their connections with the central nervous system are either interrupted or modified. The system of nociceptors parallels those of mechanoreceptors and thermoreceptors, which are normally called into full activity by non-damaging stimuli, but which also may be active during any natural stimulus that is sufficient to excite the nociceptors.

The central actions of inputs from all these peripheral receptors are played onto a diversity of dorsal horn cells, some of which are excited directly and others indirectly. There are at least four categories of dorsal horn cells, ranging from those unaffected by nociceptor input to those excited exclusively by such an input. The potency of excitatory actions on these cells is strongly affected by inhibitory mechanisms of both supraspinal and segmental origin, which can selectively depress the responses of some of these cells to noxious stimuli.

On the basis of the simplest hypothesis, it is possible to argue that there is a "pain pathway" through the dorsal horn, driven by an input in nociceptive afferent nerves, which is selective and exclusive. This "pain" channel can have its excitability modulated by both descending and segmental inhibitory systems acting via the dorsal horn to depress (and possibly enhance) conduction through it.

This "pain" channel is paralleled by other systems that are more open in that they can be excited by both sensitive mechanoreceptors and nociceptors, although normally a tonic descending mechanism effectively shuts off any input from the nociceptors. The role of this perhaps ancillary "pain" path remains enigmatic.

REFERENCES

1. Angaut-Petit, D. (1975): *Exp. Brain Res.,* 22:471.
2. Beck, P. W., and Handwerker, H. O. (1974): *Pfluegers Arch.,* 347:209.
3. Besson, J. M., Conseillor, C., Hamann, K.-F., and Maillard, M. C. (1972): *J. Physiol.,* 221:189.
4. Besson, P., and Perl, E. R. (1969): *J. Neurophysiol.,* 32:1025.
5. Boivie, J. (1971): *Exp. Brain Res.,* 12:331.
6. Brown, A. G. (1971): *J. Physiol.,* 219:103.
7. Brown, A. G., and Iggo, A. (1962): *J. Physiol.,* 165:28*P*.
8. Brown, A. G., and Short, A. D. (1974): *Brain Res.,* 74:338.
9. Brown, A. G., Hamann, W. C., and Martin, H. F., III (1974): *Adv. Neurol.,* 4:253.
10. Chahl, L., and Iggo, A. (1974): *Proc. Aust. Physiol. Pharmacol. Soc.*
11. Christensen, B. N., and Perl, E. R. (1970): *J. Neurophysiol.,* 33:293.
12. Clifton, G. L., Vance, W. H., Applebaum, M. L., Coggeshall, R. E., and Willis, W. D. (1974): *Brain Res.,* 82:163.
13. Denny-Brown, D., Kirk, E. J., and Yanagisawa, N. (1973): *J. Comp. Neurol.,* 151:175.
14. Fetz, E. E. (1968): *J. Neurophysiol.,* 31:69.
15. Fjällbrant, N., and Iggo, A. (1961): *J. Physiol.,* 156:578.
16. Fock, S., Franz, M., and Mense, S. (1973): *Pfluegers Arch.,* 339:R87.

17. Game, C. J. A., and Lodge, D. (1975): *Exp. Brain Res.*, 23:75.
18. Gregor, M., and Zimmermann, M. (1972): *J. Physiol.*, 221:555.
19. Handwerker, H. O., Iggo, A., and Zimmermann, M. (1975): *Pain,* 1:147.
20. Handwerker, H. O., Iggo, A., Ogawa, H., and Ramsey, R. L. (1975): *J. Physiol.*, 244:76*P*.
21. Heavner, J. E. (1975): *Pain,* 1:239.
22. Hongo, T., Jankowska, E., and Lundberg, A. (1968): *J. Physiol.,* 199:569.
23. Iggo, A. (1959): *Q. J. Exp. Physiol.,* 44:362.
24. Iggo, A. (1974*a*): *Adv. Neurol.,* 4:1.
25. Iggo, A. (1974*b*): In: *The Peripheral Nervous System,* edited by J. Hubbard, p. 347. Plenum Press, New York.
26. Iggo, A., Ogawa, H., and Cervero, F. (1976): *This volume.*
27. Juan, H., and Lembeck, F. (1974): *Arch. Exp. Pathol. Pharmacol.,* 283:151.
28. Kirk, E. J. (1974): *J. Comp. Neurol.,* 155:164.
29. Leek, B. F. (1972): In: *Handbook of Sensory Physiology, Vol. III/1. Enteroceptors,* edited by E. Neil, p. 113. Springer, Berlin.
30. Mayer, D. J., and Liebeskind, J. C. (1974): *Brain Res.,* 68:73.
31. Price, D. D., and Browe, A. C. (1973): *Brain Res.,* 64:425.
32. Price, D. D., Hull, C. D., and Buchwald, N. A. (1971): *Exp. Neurol.,* 33:291.
33. Réthelyi, M., and Szentágothai, J. (1972): *Handbook of Sensory Physiology, Vol. II,* p. 207.
34. Rexed, B. (1952): *J. Comp. Neurol.,* 96:415.
35. Sicuteri, F., Fanciullacci, M., Franchi, G., and del Bianco, (1965): *Life Sci.,* 4:309.
36. Tapper, D. N., Brown, P. B., and Moraff, H. (1973): *J. Neurophysiol.,* 36:817.
37. Taub, A. (1964): *Exp. Neurol.,* 10:357.
38. Trevino, D. L., and Carstens, E. (1975): *Anat. Rec.,* 181:494.
39. Trevino, D. L., Coulter, J. D., Maunz, R. A., and Willis, W. D. (1974): *Adv. Neurol.,* 4:167.
40. Vane, J. R. (1971): *Nature* [*New Biol.*], 231:232.
41. Vogt, M. (1974): *J. Physiol.,* 236:483.
42. Wagman, I. H., and Price, D. D. (1969): *J. Neurophysiol.,* 32:803.
43. Wall, P. D. (1967): *J. Physiol.,* 188:403.
44. Wall, P. D., and Gutnick, M. (1974): *Exp. Neurol.,* 43:580.
45. Willis, W. D., Trevino, D. L., Coulter, D. J., and Maunz, R. A. (1974): *J. Neurophysiol.,* 37:358.

Advances in Pain Research and Therapy, Vol. 1,
edited by J. J. Bonica and D. Albe-Fessard.
Raven Press, New York © 1976.

Use of Peripheral and Spinal Cord Stimulation in the Relief of Chronic Pain

Don M. Long

Department of Neurosurgery, The Johns Hopkins University School of Medicine, Baltimore, Maryland 21205

Electrical stimulation for pain relief is an ancient technique that was used even when electric fishes were the only available electrical generators. Electrical sources of many kinds were employed in the 18th and 19th centuries, and electrical stimulation continued to be used widely in medicine in the early portion of this century. The unlicensed availability of these machines and the often extravagant claims made for their efficacy no doubt contributed to a sudden decline in their use, so that for the past 30 years little has been written or said about the use of electricity in the treatment of chronic pain (33). Renewal of interest in the possibility of artificial stimulation of the nervous system for the relief of pain followed quickly on the publication of the gate theory by Melzack and Wall in 1965 (22). Their subsequent elaboration on the theories of pain increased interest in research in pain, and clinical trials based on the gate theory have led to a major effort to apply the principles of afferent stimulation for chronic pain in the past 10 years (1,23,24,26,43–45). These attempts have taken several forms. Electricity has generally been used because of its ease of application, portability, and safety. Electrical stimulators have been devised which may be applied to the skin or mucous membrane for excitation of peripheral receptors or peripheral nerves. Implantable stimulators have been devised for peripheral nerves, the posterior and anterior surfaces of the spinal cord, and the brain (9,10). The purpose of this chapter is to detail the experience to date with stimulations of the peripheral nervous system and the spinal cord for the relief of chronic pain.

TECHNIQUES

Transcutaneous Electrical Stimulation

Portable and stationary electrical stimulators which deliver a variety of electrical impulses to the skin have been available throughout this century. However, for the most part the electrical signal delivered was not a clearly defined wave form, and the engineering of these devices was certainly inadequate. The first satisfactory external electrical stimulators were designed in 1969 and became available for use in 1970. Since that time, several families of satisfactory models have been developed by different manufacturers and have been subjected to extensive clinical trials (18,34). These data are now becoming available for critical review.

The use of these stimulators has been empiric. In general, all investigators have simply applied them first in and around the areas where pain is perceived, and secondly over major nerve trunks destined for these areas (25). Clinical success has been said to occur when the use of such an external electrical stimulator is the only treatment for pain that the patient requires. The results obtained by a number of investigators have been remarkably constant (Table 1). Ebersold et al. (8) reported on 230 patients with pain of diverse chronic origin. Of these patients, 60% reported a significant effect on the pain, and in 43% stimulation alone was adequate treatment. Davis and Lentini (7) reported on 31 patients suffering from chronic spinal injury, and in 41% treatment with transcutaneous stimulation was adequate. Cauthern and Renner (6) treated 113 patients, and in 32% external electrical stimulation was satisfactory. In 100 patients Picaza and associates (32) had a 50% success rate. Long (18,19) found 33% of 400 patients adequately treated by external electrical stimulation, and 67% of the patients reported a significant effect on the pain. Loeser and co-workers (16) reported on 198 patients; 68% experienced an effect on the pain, but long-term relief was satisfactory in only 12.5%.

In the literature 972 cases have been described and are available for critical analysis (Table 2); 35% of these patients were satisfactorily treated by the use of external electrical stimulation alone. In 1973 a letter survey was conducted concerning the use of external electrical stimulation in four of the major pain treatment programs in the United States. This letter survey was answered by data on over 3,000 patients; 33% of these patients were said to have achieved satisfactory pain treatment by the use of external electrical stimulation alone. The number who achieved a beneficial effect

TABLE 1. *Reported results of transcutaneous stimulation in chronic pain*

Author	Number	Results
Ebersold	230	60% effect on pain; 43% satisfactory
Davis	31	41% satisfactory
Cauthern	111	32% satisfactory
Picaza	100	5% satisfactory
Long	400	67% effect on pain; 33% satisfactory
Loeser	198	68% effect on pain; 12.5% satisfactory

TABLE 2. *Summary of reported results of transcutaneous stimulation in chronic pain*

Patients (no.)	Results
972 (in print)	35% satisfactory
3,000 (personal review)	33% satisfactory

on the pain was approximately double this figure. Recently Nathan and Wall (29) have demonstrated the effectiveness of cutaneous stimulation in the relief of pain of postherpetic neuralgia.

Complications of this treatment form have been rare. The most common has been skin irritation by the electrode or tape required for the application of stimulating electrodes. The large number of patients who report a beneficial effect and the fact that Long has demonstrated the effectiveness of these devices in the relief of pain for over 1 year make it unlikely that this is a placebo effect. The efficacy of externally applied electrical stimulation for the treatment of chronic pain appears to be well demonstrated (14).

Temporary and Permanent Stimulation of Peripheral Nerves

One of the earliest implications of the principles of the gate theory for the relief of pain came with the development of implantable stimulating devices for chronic stimulation of peripheral nerves (43,44). Sweet (40), Shealy (34), and Long (17) all presented early data concerning the efficacy of this method. In addition to the development of implantable devices for the stimulation of peripheral nerves, the temporary stimulation of peripheral nerves for diagnostic purposes has now become a well-developed and well-accepted technique. It appears that these procedures are effective for pain of chronic nerve injury origin and probably constitute the method of choice for the treatment of the majority of these injuries. Their role in the treatment of pain which is not of nerve injury origin is much less secure (3).

Temporary Stimulation

Peripheral nerves may be stimulated for diagnostic purposes in a manner which is similar to nerve blockade of any type (5). Needles are selected which allow the passage of thin insulated electrodes to the general vicinity of the nerve after placement of the larger needle. These techniques are all carried out under local anesthesia, and no attempt is made to enter the nerve with either the needle or the electrode. After the needle is placed in the general vicinity of the nerve, the nerve is located by means of electrical stimulation. When adequate stimulation achieves motor or sensory phenomena in the distribution of the appropriate nerve, the stimulation is continued for 10 to 45 min. The usual parameters of stimulation are 0 to 10 V, 0 to 0.5 msec, and 0 to 60 Hz. Stimulations carried out for this period of time may produce objective hypalgesia but have had no permanent side effects. Pain relief during a period of such stimulation has a good predictive value for the use of an implantable stimulating device on the same nerve for pain treatment.

Implantable peripheral nerve stimulators are available from two firms. The stimulators are essentially cuff electrodes placed circumferentially around the nerve and then attached to a subcutaneous radio receiver implanted in some convenient location. Picaza et al. (32) and Long (17) have recently reported their experiences with these techniques. Picaza and associates (31) initially reported results in 100 patients with stimulation of peripheral nerves transcutaneously: pain was relieved in 50%, 23 implants were taken, and 20 patients attained 50% to 100% relief of pain. The same authors (32) later reported results of 50 implants with 34 patients achieving good-to-excellent pain relief.

The results of our peripheral nerve implants (38 cases) are found in Table 3. Pain relief was complete in 17 patients and partial in 7 others. However, it is readily appreciated that the majority of the failures occurred in sciatic nerve implants put in place for pain which involved both the leg and the low back, resulting from multiple spinal surgeries. The leg pain was predictively relieved, but the failure of these patients to achieve low back pain relief has placed them in the failure category. Restriction of the use of peripheral nerve stimulators for pain of nerve injury origin greatly improves these statistics.

Complications with this technique have been few. If carried out in an excessive manner, temporary stimulation may lead to muscular contraction that can be quite painful. No injuries to peripheral nerves have been reported to date. Complications of implantable devices are few. Nerves have been injured during manipulation for implantation of the device, and infection is an ever-present hazard with the implantation of foreign bodies. The most

TABLE 3. *Results of implanted peripheral nerve stimulators*

Site	Number	Pain relief: Complete	Partial	None
Brachial plexus	10	8	1	1
Ulnar	7	7	0	0
Median	2	1	0	1
Peroneal	1	1	0	0
Occipital	1	0	0	1
Sciatic	17	0	6	11
Total	38	17	7	14

serious complication has been the advent of late neurological disease deficit with apparent scarring around these nerves. This complication has not occurred in the author's series, but must be carefully considered as these patients are followed.

Spinal Cord Stimulation

The first electrical stimulators employed for clinical relief of pain were implantable stimulators designed to stimulate the large-diameter afferent fibers of the posterior columns (37,40). After the initial clinical trials by Shealy et al. (24) and by Sweet and his associates (41), a number of investigators (4,12,20,27,36) evaluated dorsal column stimulation as a treatment for chronic pain. The experiences of all of these individuals have now been synthesized into a relatively standard technique for patient selection, implantation of electrode system, and evaluation of success or failure of pain relief (21). Most investigators now choose patients by using some form of positive response to electrical stimulation as a predictor of success. A positive response to external electrical stimulation is considered the minimum to allow the implantation of a dorsal column stimulator.

Most investigators stimulate the spinal cord in some manner before implanting an electrical stimulator. The most common stimulation technique has been the placement of an electrode in the epidural space over the posterior columns of the spinal cord and activating it temporarily over a 2- to 3-day period. Another technique has been the stimulation of the anterior-posterior surface of the spinal cord by means of a free-floating subarachnoid electrode placed percutaneously usually at the C_2 level or in the lumbar region with subsequent manipulation of the electrode to its desired position under fluoroscopy (12). A third technique has been the actual intraparenchymal stimulation of the dorsal columns by fine electrodes that pierce the spinal cord (11). When this form of stimulation is clearly demonstrated to be of value, a permanent spinal cord stimulator can be implanted.

The placement of the stimulating systems has been varied. They have been placed at spinal levels from the lumbar thoracic junction to the high cervical region. The electrodes have been placed in the subdural-subarachnoid space, subdural-extra-arachnoid space, within the dura, and in the epidural space. Electrode types have been equally varied. However, none of these variables appear to have significantly influenced success, and the reported results are quite similar from investigator to investigator (42).

Sheldon and associates (38) have reported on 27 patients, 59% of whom had excellent-to-good results. Long and Erikson (20) treated 69 patients with excellent results in 17%. Patients achieving less than 100% relief of pain were considered failures. Shealy (35) has listed 80 patients with 15% excellent results and 31% fair-to-good results. Nashold (27,28) reported on 30 patients with excellent results or complete relief of pain in 23%. Of 130

TABLE 4. *Reported results of dorsal column stimulation*

Author	No. of patients[a]	Results (%)
Sheldon	27	59, good to excellent
Long	69	17, excellent
Shealy	80	15, excellent; 31, fair
Nashold	30	23, excellent
Nielson	130	25, excellent; 24, good
Pineda	76	21, excellent; 23, satisfactory
Burton	79	11, excellent; 48, satisfactory

[a] Total, 491 patients.

patients treated by Adams and Hosobuchi, Nielson (30) reported that 25% achieved total pain relief and 24% good pain relief. Burton (4) treated 75 patients with 11% excellent and 48% satisfactory pain relief (Table 4). Thus in 489 patients, implantation of dorsal column stimulators in 18% resulted in excellent relief of pain and in 37% satisfactory relief of pain for an overall success rate of 56%. Moreover, there has been a continual decline in the efficacy of dorsal column stimulation as a treatment modality. Initial studies suggested that over 80% of patients leave in the first 6 months and that there is then a steady decline in efficacy so that at 2 years or more only 18% remain completely free of pain (41) (Table 5).

The complications of dorsal column stimulation are those expected from a major procedure requiring thoracic laminectomy. Paraplegia has been reported. Cerebrospinal fluid fistula appears to be the most common complication, and infection occurs more frequently than one would expect without foreign body implantation. Late failures of stimulating devices are common. The most common functional complication appears to be the early or late failure of stimulation in a painful part. It appears that many patients achieve partial pain relief but are left incapacitated by an unrelieved portion of pain (41).

TABLE 5. *Summary of patients treated with dorsal column stimulation as reported in literature*[a]

Pain relief	Percent
Excellent	18
Satisfactory	37
	55

[a] 489 patients.

New Techniques of Spinal Cord Stimulation

Stimulation of the anterior and posterior surface of the spinal cord has been suggested on both an experimental and a clinical basis (15). There is not enough data yet to analyze the success of any of the techniques of anterior spinal cord stimulation. Preliminary studies suggest that it may be a satisfactory method of pain control, and this technique awaits further investigation.

Attempts to modify dorsal column stimulation to allow the percutaneous placement of epidural wire electrodes are currently underway. Only a small number of patients have been so treated, but initial studies suggest that the results will be at least as good as those obtained after operative dorsal column stimulation, and in fact they may be better. The lack of a need for a major operative procedure, the low complication rate, and the possibility of a two-stage procedure with temporary stimulation of the electrodes followed by internalization of the stimulating system if pain relief is satisfactory make this an alternative technique. Review of preliminary studies suggests that it will be effective. However, long-term studies are not available, and it is entirely possible that movement of electrodes and escalation of thresholds secondary to scarring around the epidurally implanted electrodes may limit the usefulness of this technique. Insufficient data are currently available to be certain about its efficacy.

DISCUSSION

The current status of electrical stimulation of the peripheral nervous system and spinal cord for the control of pain can be briefly summarized as follows. Externally applied electrical stimulation appears to be a feasible way of treating many pains of benign origin. Approximately one-third of patients with intractable pain of benign origin referred to chronic pain treatment centers respond to this method of pain therapy. Less serious pain responds predictably better, although insufficient studies have been carried out to delineate completely the use of the device in such problems as acute cervical and lumbar syndromes, acute visceral pains, pain of severe sprain or fracture, and similar problems. Available studies suggest that external electrical stimulation will be of great value in the treatment of postoperative pain, and this area requires further exploration (13).

Peripheral nerve stimulation is an excellent technique for the relief of pain of nerve injury origin. Patients who are relieved by temporary stimulations will be predictably relieved by implantable stimulating devices. These techniques are of less value in pain which is not confined to the distribution of a single nerve injury and must be applied with great care. However, the use of a peripheral nerve stimulator appears to constitute the method of choice for the treatment of pain of nerve injury origin.

Dorsal column stimulation has now been studied enough to allow several generalizations. The technique is promising but will provide complete pain relief in less than 20% of patients with severe chronic benign pain. A significant additional percentage will be improved by the use of the device, but the definition of improvement and the proof of betterment are difficult. The complication rate of this procedure is reasonably high. It appears that dorsal column stimulation should be practiced only by a few individuals skilled in its use and skilled in patient selection with all of the facilities of a chronic pain treatment program at their disposal.

Obviously, the simple relief of pain is not satisfactory therapy for many patients with chronic pain (39). The concept of a comprehensive pain treatment program is apparent, and treatment of the psychosocial ills of many of these patients is mandatory if satisfactory rehabilitation is to be achieved. Simple relief of pain is not adequate to achieve rehabilitation in many instances, and the complete facilities of a chronic pain treatment program are usually required to treat such patients satisfactorily (2). The availability of these kinds of facilities will remarkably reduce the number of patients considered to be candidates for any kind of intervention, and it has been our experience that no more than 10% of such patients admitted to our chronic pain treatment program will be considered as candidates for a major interventional procedure at the present time.

External electrical stimulation appears to be the most effective means of treating pain. Although it can be used advantageously in any comprehensive pain treatment program, it appears to be most effective for patients less seriously incapacitated than the average patient reaching a pain treatment program. Its use in the relief of acute pain must be explored further, but the initial data appear promising. Peripheral nerve stimulation is the method of choice for relief of pain of nerve injury origin. The combination of these simple techniques with a comprehensive pain treatment program has almost eliminated the use of operative dorsal column stimulation in our hands. However, the advent of the anterior cord stimulation and the possibility of using percutaneously implanted electrical stimulators may certainly change this picture if the initial success rates of these techniques can be maintained. The relief of pain by afferent stimulation appears now to be established. It is to be hoped that continued improvement in engineering design, application of these principles, and patient selection will improve the results currently obtained.

REFERENCES

1. Bloedel, J. R. (1974): *Clin. Neurosurg.*, 21:194–228.
2. Blumer, D. (1975): *Psychiatric Considerations in Pain in The Spine, Vol. 2,* edited by R. Rothman and F. Simeone. W. B. Saunders Co., Philadelphia.
3. Burton, C. (1973): Paper presented at the Annual Houston Neurological Symposium, Houston, Texas.

4. Burton, C. (1975): *Surg. Neurol.,* 4:171–180.
5. Campbell, J. N., and Taub, A. (1973): *Arch. Neurol.,* 28:347–350.
6. Cauthern, J. C., and Renner, E. (1975): *Surg. Neurol.,* 4:102–105.
7. Davis, R., and Lentini, R. (1975): *Surg. Neurol.,* 4:100–102.
8. Ebersold, M. J., Laws, E., Stonnington, H., and Stillwel, G. (1975): *Surg. Neurol.,* 4:96–100.
9. Hosobuchi, Y., Adams, J. E., and Rutkin, B. (1973): *Arch. Neurol.,* 29:158–161.
10. Hosobuchi, Y., Adams, J., and Rutkin, B. (1975): *Surg. Neurol.,* 4:91–93.
11. Hosobuchi, Y., Adams, J. E., and Weinstein, P. R. (1972): *J. Neurosurg.,* 37:242–245.
12. Hoppenstein, R. (1974): *Surg. Neurol.,* 4:187–195.
13. Hymes, A. C., Raab, D. E., Yonehiro, E. G., Nelson, G. D., and Printy, A. L. (1974): *Advances in Neurology, Vol. 4: International Symposium on Pain,* edited by J. J. Bonica, pp. 761–767. Raven Press, New York.
14. Indeck, W., and Printy, A. (1975): *Minn. Med.,* 58:305–309.
15. Larson, S., Sances, A., Cusick, J., Meyer, G., and Swiontek, T. (1975): *Surg. Neurol.,* 4:180–187.
16. Loeser, J., Black, R., and Christman, A. (1975): *J. Neurosurg.,* 42:308–314.
17. Long, D. M. (1973): *J. Neurosurg.,* 39:718–722.
18. Long, D. M. (1974): *Minn. Med.,* 57:195–198.
19. Long, D. M., and Carolan, M. T. (1974): *Advances in Neurology, Vol. 4: International Symposium on Pain,* edited by J. J. Bonica, pp. 755–759. Raven Press, New York.
20. Long, D. M., and Erickson, D. (1975): *Surg. Neurol.,* 4:134–142.
21. Long, D. M., and Hagfors, N. (1975): *Pain,* 1:109–123.
22. Melzack, R., and Wall, P. D. (1965): *Science,* 150:971–979.
23. Melzack, R., and Wall, P. (1970): *Int. Anesthesiol. Clin.,* 8:3–34.
24. Mortimer, J. T., Shealy, C. N., and Wheeler, C. (1970): *J. Neurosurg.,* 32:553–559.
25. Mountcastle, V. B., and Powell, T. P. S. (1959): *Johns Hopkins Med. J.,* 105:201–232.
26. Nashold, B. S. (1974): *Clin. Neurosurg.,* 21:311–322.
27. Nashold, B. S. (1975): *Surg. Neurol.,* 4:146–148.
28. Nashold, B. S., and Friedman, H. (1972): *J. Neurosurg.,* 36:590–597.
29. Nathan, P., and Wall, P. (1974): *Br. Med. J.,* 3:645–647.
30. Nielson, K. D., Adams, J. E., and Hosobuchi, Y. (1975): *J. Neurosurg.,* 42:301–307.
31. Picaza, J., Cannon, B., Hunter, S., Boyd, A., Guma, J., and Maurer, D. (1975*a*): *Surg. Neurol.,* 4:105–115.
32. Picaza, J., Cannon, B., Hunter, S., Boyd, A., Guma, J., and Maurer, D. (1975*b*): *Surg. Neurol.,* 4:115–127.
33. Ray, C. D., and Maurer, D. (1975): *Surg. Neurol.,* 4:82–91.
34. Shealy, C. N. (1974): *Clin. Neurosurg.,* 21:269–277.
35. Shealy, C. N. (1975): *Surg. Neurol.,* 4:142–146.
36. Shealy, C. N., and Mortimer, J. T. (1971): In: *Neuroelectric Research, Electroneuroprosthesis, Electroanesthesia and Nonconvulsive Electrotherapy,* edited by D. N. Reynolds and A. E. Sjoberg, pp. 146–150. Charles C Thomas, Publisher, Springfield, Illinois.
37. Shealy, C. N., Mortimer, J. T., and Hagfors, N. R. (1970): *J. Neurosurg.,* 32:560–564.
38. Sheldon, C. H., Paul, F., Jacques, D., and Pudenz, R. (1975): *Surg. Neurol.,* 4:127–133.
39. Sternbach, R. A. (1974): *Clin. Neurosurg.,* 21:323–333.
40. Sweet, W. H. (1968): *Trans. Stud. Coll. Physicians, Phila.,* 35:171–184.
41. Sweet, W. H., and Wepsic, J. G. (1968): *Trans. Am. Neurol. Assoc.,* 93:103–105.
42. Sweet, W. H., and Wepsic, J. G. (1974): *Clin. Neurosurg.,* 21:278–310.
43. Wall, P., and Gutnick, M. (1974): *Exp. Neurol.,* 43:580–593.
44. Wall, P., and Gutnick, M. (1974): *Nature,* 248:740–743.
45. Wall, P., and Sweet, W. (1967): *Science,* 155:103–104.

Advances in Pain Research and Therapy, Vol. 1,
edited by J. J. Bonica and D. Albe-Fessard.
Raven Press, New York © 1976.

Inhibition of Primate Spinothalamic Tract Neurons by Electrical Stimulation of Dorsal Column or Peripheral Nerve

R. D. Foreman, J. E. Beall, A. E. Applebaum, J. D. Coulter, and W. D. Willis

Marine Biomedical Institute and Departments of Physiology and Biophysics, Anatomy, and Psychiatry, University of Texas Medical Branch, Galveston, Texas 77550

Stimulation of the dorsal columns has been shown to control chronic pain in humans (11,13,15). The explanation for the effect is controversial. The procedure was based on the gate theory of pain introduced by Melzack and Wall (10). However, the details of this theory have been challenged on experimental grounds by a number of investigators (1,5,8,19). Furthermore, it has been suggested that the level of the interactions between dorsal column volleys and pain transmission may be at higher levels of the nervous system, rather than in the spinal cord (12). However, there have been reports of inhibition of transmission to spinal interneurons after dorsal column stimulation in cats (6,7). The present investigation demonstrates that dorsal column stimulation interferes with the activation of spinothalamic tract cells in the monkey spinal cord. The inhibition is similar to that produced by stimulation of large afferents in peripheral nerves. However, spinothalamic tract cells which can be activated by hair movement or other tactile stimuli are initially excited by dorsal column stimulation, and then they are inhibited.

METHODS

Recordings were made from the cell bodies of spinothalamic tract neurons in the dorsal horn of the lumbosacral enlargement or from the axons in the ventrolateral white matter at an upper lumbar level in the spinal cords of anesthetized monkeys (*Macaca mulatta* or *M. irus*). The neurons were identified by antidromic activation following stimulation within the caudal diencephalon (17). Natural mechanical stimuli were used to locate the receptive fields and to classify the responses (20). The classes of cells were hair movement, low threshold, and high threshold; these were distinguished on the basis of the weakest mechanical stimuli needed to excite them. Electrical stimuli applied to the appropriate peripheral nerves (left in continuity with the skin) excited the spinothalamic tract neurons (4). The discharges evoked by such stimuli served as a test of the effects of conditioning volleys in another peripheral nerve or in the dorsal column. Single stimuli were applied to either the peripheral nerve or the dorsal column, and the intervals between the conditioning and test stimuli were altered over the range of 5 to 150 msec. Lesions were placed in the dorsal column or in the lateral funiculus between the stimulating and recording electrodes to determine whether the effects were produced by a loop through the brain or by a volley descending directly in the dorsal column. The extent of the lesions was determined histologically. Intracellular records were made from some spinothalamic tract neurons using glass microelectrodes. Tests for changes in the excitability of primary afferents of the sural nerve were made using the technique of Wall (18).

RESULTS

Effects of Peripheral Nerve and Dorsal Column Volleys

The effects of stimulation of a peripheral nerve or of the dorsal column on the discharges of a spinothalamic tract neuron are shown by the curves in Fig. 1. The inhibition produced by a volley in either the plantar nerve or the dorsal column (stimulation was at T_5) lasted approximately 150 msec. This time course of inhibition was typical for all classes of spinothalamic tract neurons.

Dorsal column volleys typically did not excite high-threshold spinothalamic tract neurons, but they did cause a burst discharge of hair-activated

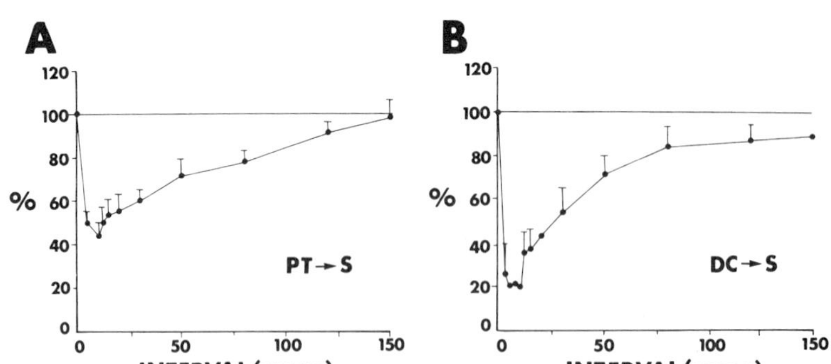

FIG. 1. Time course of depression of spinothalamic tract cell activity by volleys in peripheral nerve or in dorsal column. Neuron studied was excited by sural nerve stimulation. A conditioning stimulus applied to the plantar nerve (PT → S) did not cause a discharge of the cell, but instead produced the inhibition whose time course is shown in **A.** Comparable inhibition was produced by a dorsal column volley (DC → S), as shown in **B.** Points represent means of 10 values, and bars are SDs of the mean.

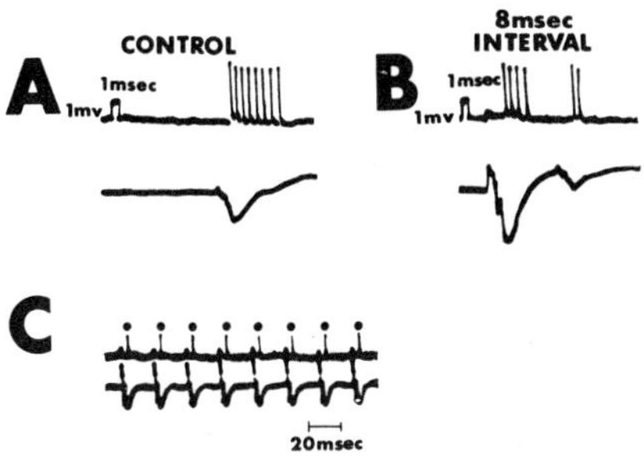

FIG. 2. Excitation of hair-activated spinothalamic tract cells by volleys in the dorsal columns. **A:** Discharge of a hair-activated spinothalamic tract axon after stimulation of common peroneal nerve. A conditioning volley in the dorsal column also excited the cell, **B,** but inhibited response to peripheral nerve stimulus. Conditioning-test interval was 8 msec, and some inhibition was still seen at intervals of at least 150 msec. **C:** Response of another hair-activated spinothalamic tract axon to repetitive dorsal column stimulation at a rate of 50 Hz. The neuron discharged after each stimulus, as shown by the dot over each response.

and low-threshold spinothalamic tract cells. An instance of this is shown in Fig. 2. The discharge in Fig. 2A was produced by stimulation of the common peroneal nerve in a spinothalamic axon which was also activated by hair movement over the dorsum of the foot. A volley in the dorsal column produced by stimulation at T_7 excited the cell, as shown in Fig. 2B. However, the dorsal column volley also depressed the discharge evoked by peripheral nerve stimulation. Another hair-activated spinothalamic axon was caused to discharge in a one-for-one fashion by a repetitive stimulus at 50 Hz applied to the dorsal column, as shown in Fig. 2C.

Pathway for Dorsal Column Inhibition

The pathway responsible for the effects of dorsal column stimulation was shown to include the collaterals of dorsal column fibers themselves. Figure 3A and B shows the inhibition of activity in a high-threshold spinothalamic tract neuron. When a lesion was placed in the dorsal column between the stimulating electrode and the recording site (Fig. 3D), the effects of dorsal column stimulation were eliminated, as shown in Fig. 3C (*open circles* versus *crosses*). The electrode continued to evoke a potential in the thalamus, indicating that it still was able to activate ascending pathways. Moving the electrode caudal to the lesion restored the effectiveness of the dorsal column stimulus in producing inhibition (Fig. 3C, *filled circles*). A lesion in the lateral funiculus did not change the inhibitory action, indicating that the effect did not depend on lateral pathways near the dorsal column, such as the corticospinal tract (2,3).

Mechanics of Inhibition

The volley descending in the dorsal column collides with incoming activity over certain kinds of afferent fibers. The fibers affected are more likely

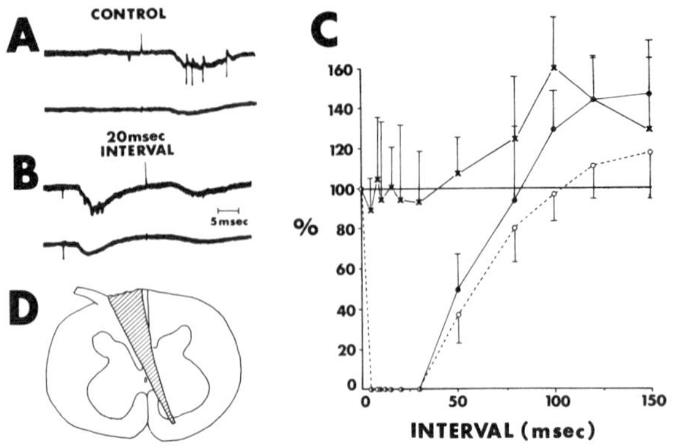

FIG. 3. Effect of dorsal column lesion on inhibition of spinothalamic tract neuron. **A:** Discharge of a high-threshold spinothalamic tract cell in response to electrical stimulation of skin within the receptive field. **B:** Discharge is inhibited when a stimulus is applied to the dorsal column at C_{7-8} 20 msec earlier than cutaneous stimulus. **C:** Full time course of inhibition is shown by curve through open circles. Dorsal column was then sectioned between the stimulating and recording electrodes. Inhibition was eliminated, as shown by curve through crosses in **C.** Inhibition was restored by moving the stimulating electrode caudal to the lesion, as shown by curve through filled circles in **C. D:** Maximum extent of the lesion. Points in **C** are means of 10 trials, and bars represent SDs of the mean.

to be involved in exciting the hair-activated and low-threshold classes of spinothalamic tract cells than the high-threshold ones. The intervals over which collision can be expected depend on the conduction distance from the dorsal column stimulus site to the periphery, but we estimate that these will not be much greater than 17 msec for the slowest A-β fibers under the conditions of our experiments. However, a much longer interval is expected in humans because of the greater distance involved. In addition to collision, the descending dorsal column volley undoubtedly produces synaptic effects in the dorsal horn at the lumbosacral enlargement. We have recorded inhibitory postsynaptic potentials intracellularly from spinothalamic tract neurons in response to dorsal column stimulation, and dorsal column volleys were shown to produce primary afferent depolarization at least of large cutaneous afferent fibers. Thus both postsynaptic and perhaps presynaptic inhibition may occur at the level of the cells of origin of the spinothalamic tract. In addition, there may be interactions at an interneuronal level.

DISCUSSION

The activity of spinothalamic tract cells was inhibited by volleys in large afferent fibers of peripheral nerve or of the dorsal column. The inhibition produced by a single conditioning volley lasted approximately 150 msec. It seems reasonable to suppose that the inhibitory effects account at least in part for the beneficial therapeutic effect of dorsal column stimulation for the relief of pain. The inhibitory action seems to be mediated by collaterals of dorsal column fibers that are invaded by the volley descending from the point of stimulation of the dorsal column at a midthoracic or cervical level. The mechanism of inhibition is probably complex, involving postsynaptic inhibition, perhaps presynaptic inhibition, and possibly actions at an interneuronal level. In addition, at least for spinothalamic tract neurons excited by afferents which also send collaterals rostrally in the dorsal column, the descending volley collides with the incoming activity in such fibers and so interferes with the activation of these types of spinothalamic tract cells. Our experiments do not exclude additional effects of dorsal column volleys at higher levels of the nervous system. Such actions appear to be likely, since dorsal column stimulation can produce pain relief which outlasts the period of stimulation of the dorsal columns by hours (11,13,16). This prolonged action is more likely to be accounted for on the basis of brain mechanisms than of spinal cord mechanisms.

The observation that hair-activated and low-threshold spinothalamic tract neurons are excited by dorsal column stimulation suggests that such cells are unlikely to be involved in pain transmission. An opposite conclusion was reached by Price's group on the basis of the thresholds and refractory periods of the axons responsible for the pain evoked by stimulation of the ventrolateral white matter of the cords of humans and monkeys (9,14). However, dorsal column stimulation is not painful using rates of 50 Hz or more, which do produce pain when applied to the ventrolateral white matter. Yet spinothalamic tract cells responding to a wide range of tactile and more intense stimuli can be activated in a one-for-one fashion by dorsal column stimuli at 50 Hz. It is possible, however, that an ascending volley in the dorsal column or other pathways interferes with pain transmission at higher levels.

SUMMARY

It is concluded that dorsal column stimulation, as well as peripheral nerve stimulation, can inhibit spinothalamic tract neurons in the monkey. This suggests that the therapeutic effects of dorsal column stimulation in humans can be attributed at least in part to a spinal cord action. The role of spinothalamic tract neurons activated by tactile as well as by more intense stimuli in pain transmission is questioned, since such neurons are excited by dorsal column stimulation, which in itself is not painful.

ACKNOWLEDGMENTS

The work was supported by a research grant from the National Institutes of Health, U.S. Public Health Service (NS 09743), by training grants from the NIH (NS 05743; GM 00459), and by a grant from the Moody Foundation of Galveston.

The authors wish to thank Gail Silver for her expert technical assistance.

REFERENCES

1. Burke, R. E., Rudomin, P., Vyklický, L., and Zajac, F. E. (1971): *J. Physiol.,* 213:185–214.
2. Coulter, J. D., Foreman, R. D., Beall, J. E., and Willis, W. D. (1975): Proc. 1st World Congr., Int. Assoc. for the Study of Pain, Florence.
3. Coulter, J. D., Maunz, R. A., and Willis, W. D. (1974): *Brain Res.,* 65:351–356.
4. Foreman, R. D., Applebaum, A. E., Beall, J. E., Trevino, D. L., and Willis, W. D. (1975): *J. Neurophysiol.,* 38:132–145.
5. Franz, D. N., and Iggo, A. (1968): *Science,* 162:1140–1142.
6. Handwerker, H. O., Iggo, A., and Zimmermann, M. (1975): *Pain,* 1:147–165.
7. Hillman, P., and Wall, P. D. (1969): *Exp. Brain Res.,* 9:284–306.
8. Jänig, W., and Zimmermann, M. (1971): *J. Physiol.,* 214:29–50.
9. Mayer, D. J., Price, D. D., and Becker, D. P. (1975): *Pain,* 1:51–58.
10. Melzack, R., and Wall, P. D. (1965): *Science,* 150:971–979.
11. Nashold, B. S., and Friedman, H. (1972): *J. Neurosurg.,* 36:590–597.
12. Nashold, B. S., Somjen, G., and Friedman, H. (1972): *Exp. Neurol.,* 36:273–287.
13. Nielson, K. D., Adams, J. E., and Hosobuchi, Y. (1975): *J. Neurosurg.,* 42:301–307.
14. Price, D. D., and Mayer, D. J. (1975): *Pain,* 1:59–72.
15. Shealy, C. N., Mortimer, J. T., and Hagfors, N. R. (1970): *J. Neurosurg.,* 32:560–564.
16. Sweet, W. H., and Wepsic, J. G. (1974): *Clin. Neurosurg.,* 21:278–310.
17. Trevino, D. L., Coulter, J. D., and Willis, W. D. (1973): *J. Neurophysiol.,* 36:750–761.
18. Wall, P. D. (1958): *J. Physiol.,* 142:1–21.
19. Whitehorn, D., and Burgess, P. R. (1973): *J. Neurophysiol.,* 36:226–237.
20. Willis, W. D., Trevino, D. L., Coulter, J. D., and Maunz, R. A. (1974): *J. Neurophysiol.,* 37:358–372.

Advances in Pain Research and Therapy, Vol. 1,
edited by J. J. Bonica and D. Albe-Fessard.
Raven Press, New York © 1976.

Anodal Blocking of Aδ Tooth Pulp Afferents

L. Vyklický, O. Keller, and *P. Jastreboff

*Institute of Physiology, Czechoslovak Academy of Sciences, Budějovická 1083, 142 20 Prague 4, Czechoslovakia; and *Nencki Institute of Experimental Biology, 3 Pasteur Street, Warsaw 22, Poland*

Differential blocking of fast-conducting afferent fibers by anodal current has been successfully employed in modern neurophysiology for studying the physiological role of slow-conducting afferent systems (5,7). Attention has also been aroused concerning the possibility of using anodal current to produce peripheral anesthesia, especially in controlling dental pain (6). It was recently shown in two laboratories independently that at least the reflex action and the field potentials elicited by tooth pulp stimulation can be blocked by direct current (4,2).

Our experiments were designed to follow the time course of the effects of anodal current on the field potentials in the brainstem and on the reflex activity evoked by electrical stimulation of the tooth pulp primary afferents.

METHODS

Experiments were performed on cats anesthetized with pentobarbital sodium (50 mg i.p.). Upper canine tooth pulp nerve was prepared for stimulation by drilling two small holes in the dentin. Stainless steel wire electrodes insulated except for 1 mm from their tip were inserted into the cavities with a small amount of amalgam and firmly pressed. The whole tooth was covered with dental cement to prevent displacement of electrodes or short-circuiting by saliva. Field potentials evoked by tooth pulp nerve stimulation were recorded from the rostral subdivision of the nucleus of the spinal trigeminal tract (NTSnV) approximately 6 mm rostral to the obex, 4 mm laterally from the midline at a depth of 4 to 5 mm, with 4 M NaCl microelectrodes (1,3). This group of 5 animals was immobilized with gallamine triethiodide and ventilated artificially with air, the end-tidal CO_2 levels being maintained at 3.6% to 4.6%. Another group of 4 animals was anesthetized but not immobilized, and the EMG activity was recorded with a coaxial needle electrode from the digastric muscle (4).

Anodal current from a constant current source was supplied to one of the electrodes inserted in the dentin of a canine tooth while the cathode was connected to the ear bars of the stereotaxic instrument or to a silver hook inserted in the neck muscles.

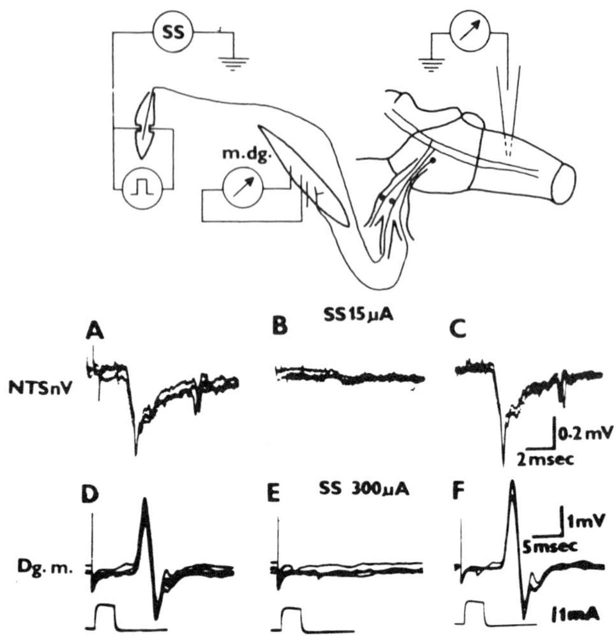

FIG. 1. Blocking effect of direct current (DC) on tooth pulp afferents; experimental arrangement. Field potentials **(A)** in rostral subdivision of the spinal trigeminal tract (NTSnV) and EMG activity **(D)** in digastric muscle (Dg.m.) evoked by single pulses to upper canine tooth pulp disappear when anodal current is applied between one of the stimulating electrodes and the indifferent electrode inserted in the neck muscle. In **A–C** the tooth pulp nerve was stimulated by rectangular pulses of 0.1 mA and of 0.1 msec duration, and in **D–E** intensity of stimuli was 1.3 mA and duration 0.1 msec. **C, F:** Recovery 30 sec after DC supply was discontinued. Stimulating pulses in **D–F** were monitored and recorded at a faster speed than the EMG activity. SS, DC intensity.

To exclude any interference between the stimulating and blocking electrodes, we applied the direct current (DC) in 2 additional cats through an electrode inserted into a separate cavity in the dentin that was drilled approximately 2 mm proximal from one of those in which stimulating electrodes were inserted. The results did not differ from those of the experiments in which DC was applied between one of the stimulating electrodes and the indifferent electrode. The anodal current and the stimulating current pulses were both monitored and measured.

Experimental arrangement is shown diagrammatically in Fig. 1. Current pulses of 0.1-msec duration applied to the tooth pulp nerve evoked full-size field potentials in the rostral subdivision of the NTSnV at the intensity of 0.1 to 1 mA, and jaw opening reflex was evoked at 0.5 to 2 mA.

RESULTS

The range of DC needed for blocking the impulse conduction of the tooth pulp afferents that are responsible for the reflex action varied between 6 and 300 μA. Recordings in Fig. 1 demonstrate that the anodal current of 15 μA was nearly sufficient to block the field potentials (Fig. 1B), whereas in another experiment 300 μA was needed for blocking the EMG activity accompanying the jaw-opening reflex (Fig. 1E).

It was found as a rule that the higher the intensity for stimulation, the higher was the DC needed for blocking. This finding can easily be understood because of higher sensitivity of the lower threshold nerve fibers to the blocking effect of DC (5,7). We, however, do not have an unequivocal explanation for the wide range of intensity of the DC needed for blocking the impulse conduction in the tooth pulp nerve in individual cats. The effectiveness of anodal current in blocking the tooth pulp afferents is presumably greatly influenced by its distribution in the pulp and the dentin, and therefore the values of DC do not indicate its actual density near the nerve fibers.

The blocking effect of the DC did not occur as an immediate event, but it developed over a period of time. This is demonstrated in Fig. 2 which shows depression of the field potentials elicited by stimuli of 1-mA and 0.1-ms duration after anodal current of 80 μA had been applied. In the lower part of Fig. 2 the amplitudes of the field potentials were plotted as percentages at various intervals after the DC had been applied. It can be seen that the time needed for a 50% blocking was 16 sec, and for a blocking greater than 80% the DC had to be applied for approximately 30 sec.

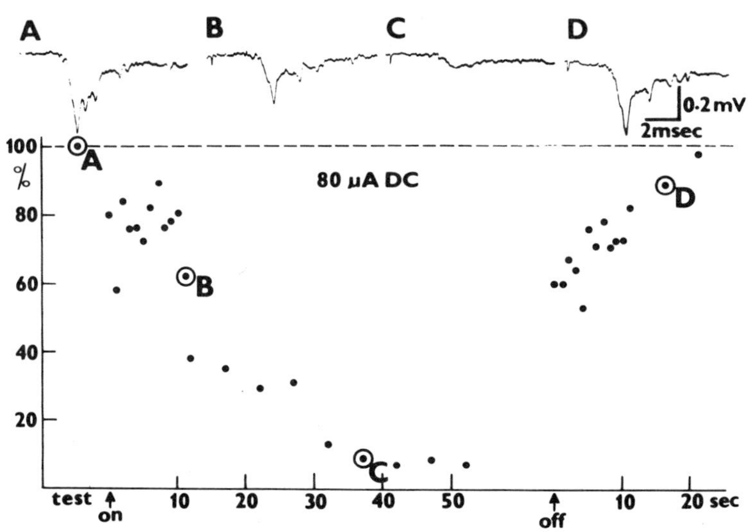

FIG. 2. Time course of the blocking effects of anodal current on tooth pulp afferents. **A–D:** Field potentials from rostral subdivision of the spinal trigeminal tract nucleus. In **B** and **C** the direct current (DC; 80 μA) was applied between one of the electrodes inserted in the dentin of an upper canine tooth and the indifferent electrode inserted in the neck muscle. Diagram shows time course of the blocking effects of DC. Amplitudes of the field potentials were plotted at various intervals after DC was switched on. Letters attached to some of the measurements correspond to the records **A–D.**

When the DC was discontinued, the recovery became rather fast. A 50% recovery of the amplitude of the field potentials was reached immediately, and recovery was complete after 20 sec. The time course of DC blocking action in other experiments varied only slightly. In the same animal the blockade could be repeated several times without significant changes in the time course of its development and recovery.

CONCLUSIONS

Assuming that the same afferent system participating in evoking the field potentials in NTSnV and the reflex activity in jaw-opening muscles is responsible for the activation of central pathways engaged in pain mechanisms, the application of anodal block appears a promising way to control the pain arising from the activity in tooth pulp afferents. The blockade does not, however, develop immediately after application of DC, and at least several seconds is needed for the effect. This may be one of the reasons why dental analgesia provided by DC was reported to be effective only in some and not in all patients.

REFERENCES

1. Davies, W. I. R., Scott, D., Jr., Vesterstrøm, K., and Vyklický, L. (1971): *J. Physiol. (Lond.)*, 218:515–532.
2. Fields, W. R., Tacke, R. B., and Savara, B. S. (1975): *Exp. Neurol.*, 47:229–239.
3. Greenwood, F. (1973): *Arch. Oral Biol.*, 18:771–785.
4. Keller, O., Vyklický, L., and Syková, E. (1972): *Brain Res.*, 37:330–332.
5. Mendell, L. M., and Wall, P. D. (1964): *J. Physiol. (Lond.)*, 172:274–294.
6. Newman, P. P. (1973): *Nature (Lond.)*, 243:474–475.
7. Zimmermann, M. (1968): *Pfluegers Arch.*, 301:329–333.

Advances in Pain Research and Therapy, Vol. 1,
edited by J. J. Bonica and D. Albe-Fessard.
Raven Press, New York © 1976.

Influence of Transcutaneous Neural Stimulation on the Pain Threshold of Human Teeth

J. M. Mumford

School of Dental Surgery, University of Liverpool, Liverpool L69 3BX, England

One feature of the gate control theory of pain (5) is that it has encouraged a fresh examination of pain problems together with experiments to test it and to make use of its concepts for therapeutic purposes. One form of therapy, transcutaneous neural stimulation, is the subject of this chapter.

A transcutaneous stimulator is a battery-powered electrical device that produces electrical impulses, the amplitude, duration, and frequency of which can be adjusted by the patient. A barrage of neural impulses are sent along the large nerve fibers to the central nervous system where they close the "gate," thus reducing or preventing the onward transmission of impulses from small fibers. Stimulation is applied by electrodes, which are normally moistened sponge pads, and one of these is placed over the painful area. The patient adjusts the electrical parameters to produce the maximum pain relief.

The equipment has been evaluated (1,14) and the peripheral mechanisms considered (16). The method has been used to treat acute pain, bringing relief in approximately 80% of cases (2,12–14). A similar success rate with either complete or partial relief of chronic pain has been reported (3,4, 12–14). A cautionary note has been raised (15), and technical manuals suggest special care with patients who have heart disease or cardiac pacemakers. Irritation of the skin and the possible harmful effects of muscle twitching especially in the face and around the eyes are also mentioned.

There is no doubt that the device is effective to some extent in some cases, and further investigation is desirable. This chapter describes the influence that such stimulation has on pain perception thresholds and pain tolerance levels of human subjects as determined by electrical stimulation of their teeth, a method described in earlier papers (6,9–11).

METHODS

The subjects were 8 dental students, 4 men and 4 women, aged 22 to 24 years. Measurements were made on their upper anterior teeth which were either intact or had small fillings well away from the electrode area.

The dental stimulator was a mains-powered, high-impedance, constant current generator. The square wave impulses were of 10-msec duration with a frequency of 50 Hz. The rate of rise of current, starting from 0, was electronically controlled at 2 μA per second.

The upper anterior teeth were isolated by folded dental napkins and dried, but not desiccated, by a stream of compressed air. The stimulating electrode (cathodal) had a contact area of 9.5 mm^2, and this was placed on the tooth's labial surface well clear of the gingival margin to reduce the possibility of surface conduction. The indifferent electrode, held in the subject's hand, included a microswitch which he pressed to allow current to flow. As soon as he felt a sensation in the tooth he released the microswitch and the meter reading was noted, this being the pain perception threshold value. (It was the mean current which in this case happened to be half the impulse peak, the mark-space ratio being 1:1). The same procedure was repeated for all six upper anterior teeth.

To determine the pain tolerance level, we repeated the procedure but the subject allowed the current to increase until it became so unpleasant that he did not wish to tolerate it any longer. He released the microswitch and the meter reading was noted to obtain the pain tolerance level.

The transcutaneous neural stimulator (STIMTECH EPC Personal) was powered by three 1.5-V batteries and generated square wave impulses of 50- to 300-μsec duration with a frequency of 10 to 100 Hz, each of the three scales being graduated from 0 to 10. Stimulation was applied via two circular sponge electrodes that had been moistened with water. One was applied to the infraorbital area, and the left side was used in each case to determine if any effect was greater on the ipsilateral side since this seemed a reasonable possibility. The subject adjusted the voltage control to produce a facial sensation. After about a minute this sensation diminished, so the voltage (and therefore current amplitude) was increased until the sensation in the subject's face was such that he thought it might have reduced pain had this been present. He then adjusted the pulse width and frequency to obtain the "best" sensation. For the 8 subjects the voltage control setting ranged from 1 to 5, the pulse width from 1 to 8, and the frequency from 1 to 7. While stimulation was continued, the pain perception threshold and pain tolerance were measured for all teeth as before.

After approximately 10 min, transcutaneous stimulation was stopped and the two pain levels were again determined.

During the experiments on pain tolerance some subjects reported that after stimulation of the first tooth they knew what to expect and could allow the current to rise during further stimulation of subsequent teeth. This meant that the first tooth might yield a falsely lower tolerance level than subsequent teeth; for this reason half the experiments were started with the left canine and half with the right canine.

Between each main group of readings (before, during, and after transcutaneous stimulation), the subject used a mouthwash to prevent the enamel from drying out for this would have allowed the electrical impedance to be raised unnecessarily (7).

The subject's lower eyelid frequently twitched, and this was avoided or reduced by moving the infraorbital electrode and by adjusting the current parameters. The subject's upper lip sometimes twitched.

RESULTS

The results are given in Tables 1 and 2. Subjects reported that during measurements on pain tolerance the sensation tended to become severe and then fade slightly before rising again, as though in waves. Twitching of the muscles of the lower eyelid was not completely controlled in some cases, but in no case did it continue after the experiments.

One subject reported that he became used to the burning sensation of transcutaneous stimulation but did not like the return to normal sensation. Another complained that his face became stiff, numb, and uncomfortable. Sensations in the tooth at the pain perception threshold were described as hot, cold, tingling, creeping, sharp, pressure, warm, and one subject was not sure. At the pain tolerance level the sensation was described as pain (mentioned four times), tingling, burning, cold, and sharper (than the pain perception sensation).

Transcutaneous stimulation was described as electrical, burning, throbbing, pulsating, and pleasantly tingling.

TABLE 1. *Effect of transcutaneous neural stimulation*[a]

	Pain perception threshold	Pain tolerance level
Before	6.6 (SD 2.7)	20.1 (SD 9.2)
During	7.6 (SD 3.4)	22.2 (SD 10.7)
After	8.6 (SD 4.4)	19.8 (SD 7.9) 20.4 (adjusted value)

[a] Readings in microamps.

TABLE 2. *Comparison of right and left sides*[a]

	Pain perception threshold		Pain tolerance level	
	Right	Left	Right	Left
Before	6.9	6.4	20.2	19.9
During	7.5	7.6	20.4	22.8
After	8.9	8.1	21.4	18.5

[a] Readings in microamps.

DISCUSSION

The pain perception threshold was raised during transcutaneous neural stimulation and was found to be even higher afterward, but the standard deviation was considerable (Table 1). Further analysis gave the following figures. There was no significant difference between the values before and during stimulation ($p > 0.05$) or between the values during and after stimulation. However, comparison of the results before and after stimulation revealed a significant difference ($p < 0.01$).

Separation of the results showed them to be approximately the same for right and left sides (Table 2). In other words, transcutaneous neural stimulation seemed to have no more effect on the ipsilateral side than on the contralateral side. This presumably means that the effect of transcutaneous stimulation is not confined to the first synapse but affects higher levels.

At the pain tolerance level the true peak value was not obtained in some cases because the high electrical impedance of dental enamel limited the current that could be passed. There were 6 such cases before, 4 during, and 13 after stimulation. Making an estimated allowance for this yields the adjusted value indicated in Table 1.

Since pain tolerance is associated with a wave-like rising and falling sensation, the author prefers to call it the pain tolerance level rather than the pain tolerance threshold, which suggests a discrete step. This value is also known as the severe pain threshold, and the same semantic objection is made. For the same reason, the pain tolerance level is less reliable as a particular value and this may partly account for the result of transcutaneous stimulation; statistical analysis revealed no significant difference between the mean values before, during, and after stimulation.

However, the pain tolerance level could be of value as indicating the range from pain perception to pain tolerance. The pain ranges were: 13.5 μA before, 14.6 μA during, and 10.7 μA after transcutaneous stimulation. Similarly, it is possible to derive the ratio of the pain tolerance level divided by the pain perception threshold; the author calls this the pain tolerance ratio. This was found to be 3.0 before, 2.9 during, and 2.3 after transcutaneous stimulation. Both the pain range and the pain tolerance ratio decreased, but this was mainly a secondary result of the rise in pain perception threshold. The base value for the pain tolerance ratio was similar to that obtained in earlier investigations (10,11).

The sensations that subjects reported at the pain perception threshold are similar to those reported in earlier investigations of the author. It may seem paradoxical that pain was not reported by any subject at the pain perception threshold, but they were asked to report the first sensation. This is acceptable since it is generally agreed that pain is the only sensation occurring in human teeth, although the author has frequently expressed reservations to this general view, based partly on results such as this. The subject is discussed elsewhere (8).

SUMMARY

The pain perception thresholds and pain tolerance levels of human subjects were determined by electrical stimulation of their teeth. This was repeated while transcutaneous neural stimulation was being applied to their faces and again after transcutaneous stimulation was terminated. The mean pain perception threshold afterward was significantly higher than before, whereas the mean pain tolerance level was not significantly different.

REFERENCES

1. Burton, C., and Maurer, D. D. (1974): *IEEE Trans. Biomed. Eng.*, 21:81–88.
2. Hymes, A. C., Raab, D. E., Yonehiro, E. G., Nelson, G. D., and Printy, A. L. (1974): In: *Advances in Neurology, Vol. 4: International Symposium on Pain,* edited by J. J. Bonica, pp. 761–767. Raven Press, New York.
3. Long, D. M. (1974): *Minn. Med.*, 57:195–198.
4. Long, D. M., and Carolan, M. T. (1974): In: *Advances in Neurology, Vol. 4: International Symposium on Pain,* edited by J. J. Bonica, pp. 755–759. Raven Press, New York.
5. Melzack, R., and Wall, P. D. (1965): *Science,* 150:971–979.
6. Mumford, J. M. (1965): *Arch. Oral Biol.,* 10:957–968.
7. Mumford, J. M. (1966): *Br. Dent. J.,* 121:178–179.
8. Mumford, J. M. (1976): *Toothache and Orofacial Pain.* Churchill Livingstone, Edinburgh (*in press*).
9. Mumford, J. M., and Newton, A. V. (1974): *Arch. Oral Biol.,* 19:145–149.
10. Mumford, J. M., Newton, A. V., and Ley, P. (1973): *Br. J. Psychol.,* 64:105–107.
11. Newton, A. V., and Mumford, J. M. (1972): *J. Dent. Res.,* 51:940–942.
12. Shealy, C. N. (1974*a*): *Med. Prog. Technol.,* 2:71–80.
13. Shealy, C. N. (1974*b*): In: *Advances in Neurology, Vol. 4: International Symposium on Pain,* edited by J. J. Bonica, pp. 775–782. Raven Press, New York.
14. Shealy, C. N., and Maurer, D. (1974): *Surg. Neurol.,* 2:45–47.
15. Sweet, W. H., and Wepsic, J. G. (1974): In: *Advances in Neurology, Vol. 4: International Symposium on Pain,* edited by J. J. Bonica, pp. 737–747. Raven Press, New York.
16. Taub, A., and Campbell, J. N. (1974): In: *Advances in Neurology, Vol. 4: International Symposium on Pain,* edited by J. J. Bonica, pp. 727–732. Raven Press, New York.

Advances in Pain Research and Therapy, Vol. 1,
edited by J. J. Bonica and D. Albe-Fessard.
Raven Press, New York © 1976.

Somatosensory Changes During Transcutaneous Electrical Analgesia

Ronald J. Ignelzi, Richard A. Sternbach, and Maureen Callaghan

Pain Unit, Veterans Administration Hospital, San Diego, California 92161

There have been few studies which examined the mechanism of electrical analgesia, and these have produced conflicting conclusions. Satran and Goldstein (2) observed a complete suppression of the somatosensory cortical evoked potential, which they interpreted as a "correlate" of the spinal gating mechanism. However, Taub and Campbell (3) and Campbell and Taub (1) reported that neurostimulation suppressed only the A-delta component of the averaged compound action potential recorded from the median nerve at the wrist, and they proposed that pain relief occurs because of peripheral blockade of smaller myelinated fibers, rather than because of a central inhibition. Torebjörk and Hallin (4) obtained similar results and concluded that peripheral inhibition or "fatigue" of smaller myelinated (A-delta) fibers was at least a part of the pain relieving mechanism, although central inhibition could not be ruled out.

As a test of the conflicting hypotheses (spinal gating versus peripheral inhibition), we decided to perform sensory testing during electrical analgesia. We hypothesized that if peripheral blockade of A-delta and C fibers occurred, we should see an alteration in pain and temperature sensitivity. On the other hand, if spinal gating occurred because of large-fiber stimulation, we should see an effect on all modalities.

METHODS

Two similar experiments were conducted. In the first, 18 patients with degenerative spine disease or peripheral nerve injury, producing pain in one limb primarily, and who obtained good to excellent pain relief with their stimulators (manufactured by Medical Devices, Inc.) were given a careful sensory examination of their painful limb without electrical stimulation, then with electrical analgesia using parameters of amperage and frequency which were customary for them. As a control, the contralateral (nonpainful) limb was then similarly tested, first without and then with stimulation. The second, similar study was conducted on 6 normal volunteers, testing one arm only and using similar stimulation parameters as those used by the patients. This study was designed as a control for a bias in the judgments of a chronic patient population.

Testing was conducted for sensitivity to pinprick, temperature, light touch, position sense, vibration, two-point discrimination, and pain threshold and pain tolerance to electric shock. Stimuli were not quantified but were the usual stimuli used in clinical neurological examination. Thus "pinprick" refers to touching with the sharp or dull end of a pin, in random order, five times each; responses were scored as the number of correct judgments, number of errors, and number of "cannot say" responses. Similarly, "temperature" refers to touching with a warm (90°F) and a cool (70°F) test tube, and the number of correct, incorrect, and uncertain responses were recorded. "Vibration" refers to a vibrating or nonvibrating tuning fork pitched at 256 Hz. "Position" sense refers to raising or lowering the digits, and "light touch" refers to brushing with a wisp of cotton. "Two-point discrimination" was measured in millimeter distances, and "pain" was recorded in voltages for lower pain threshold, mid-range ("mild") pain, and upper or maximum pain tolerance.

RESULTS

Data were analyzed in terms of frequency of occurrence of correct, incorrect, and uncertain responses (range: 0 to 5); the minimum discriminable distance between points (millimeters); and voltages at which pain threshold, mild pain, and pain tolerance were reported. Means and standard errors were calculated, and paired *t*-tests were performed on all data from all subjects for painful and unaffected limbs in the unstimulated and stimulated conditions.

Significant results are as follows: Without electrical stimulation, patients' painful limbs were less sensitive than their unaffected limbs (Table 1). Fewer correct responses were made to the sharp stimulus in pinprick ($t=2.15$; $p<0.05$) and also to the dull stimulus ($t=2.68$; $p<0.025$). There was poorer discrimination between two points on the painful limb than on the nonpainful limb ($t=2.44$; $p<0.05$). Temperature sensation was impaired: with the warm stimulus there were fewer correct responses ($t=2.43$; $p<0.05$) and more incorrect responses ($t=2.65$; $p<0.025$) for the painful as compared with the normal limb. With the cool stimulus there were fewer correct responses ($t=3.01$; $p<0.01$) and more uncertain responses ($t=3.56$; $p<0.01$) for the painful limb as compared with the unaffected limb. Light touch was also poorer in the painful limbs, with both fewer correct responses ($t=2.29$; $p<0.05$) and more incorrect responses than in the unaffected limbs. Position sense was also poorer in the painful limb, with fewer correct responses in the upward ($t=2.75$; $p<0.025$) and downward positions ($t=2.41$; $p<0.05$). There was no difference between the limbs in only two senses: vibration and electrical stimulation.

TABLE 1. *Sensitivity of painful vs nonpainful limbs in 18 chronic pain patients without electrical analgesia*

Modality	Difference	Significance
Pinprick: sharp	Painful limb less sensitive	0.05
dull	Painful limb less sensitive	0.025
Two-points	Painful limb less sensitive	0.05
Temperature: warm	Painful limb fewer correct responses	0.05
warm	Painful limb more incorrect responses	0.025
cool	Painful limb fewer correct responses	0.01
cool	Painful limb more uncertain responses	0.01
Light touch	Painful limb less sensitive	0.05
Position sense: up	Painful limb fewer correct responses	0.025
down	Painful limb fewer correct responses	0.05
Vibration	No difference	n.s.
Electrical	No difference	n.s.

During electrical analgesia patients showed improved sensitivity in their painful limbs as compared to the condition without stimulation (Table 2). There was a significant increase in the number of correct responses to the sharp pinprick ($t=2.41$; $p<0.05$) and to the dull stimulus ($t=2.68$; $p<0.025$). There was a nonsignificant tendency to improved two-point discrimination ($t=1.91$; $p<0.10$). There was an increase in the frequency of correct responses to the warm stimulus ($t=2.61$; $p<0.025$) and a decrease in the number of uncertain responses to the cool stimulus ($t=2.12$; $p<0.05$). Threshold to electric shock (pain threshold) was lowered ($t=2.60$;

TABLE 2. *Changes in sensitivity in painful limbs in 18 chronic pain patients with transcutaneous electrical analgesia*

Sensitivity indicator	Change with stimulation	Significance
Pinprick: sharp	Increase in correct responses	0.05
dull	Increase in correct responses	0.025
Two-points	Increase in correct responses	n.s. ($p<0.10$)
Temperature: warm	Increase in correct responses	0.025
cool	Decrease in uncertain responses	0.05
Electric shock: threshold	Lowered pain threshold	0.025
mild pain	No difference	n.s.
tolerance	No difference	n.s.
Light touch	No difference	n.s.
Position sense	No difference	n.s.
Vibration	No difference	n.s.
Skin temperature	Lowered	0.05

TABLE 3. *Changes in sensitivity in nonpainful limbs in 18 chronic pain patients with transcutaneous electrical stimulation*

Sensitivity indicator	Change with stimulation	Significance
Temperature: cool	Fewer correct responses	0.05
	More incorrect responses	0.05
All others	No differences	n.s.
Skin temperature	Lowered	0.005

$p < 0.025$), but mild pain and pain tolerance were not significantly altered. There were no significant changes in light touch, position sense, or vibration.

In the normal contralateral limb, comparable electrical stimulation resulted in some slightly impaired sensation compared to the condition without stimulation (Table 3). There were fewer correct responses to the cool stimulus ($t = 2.41$; $p < 0.05$) and more incorrect responses to the cool stimulus ($t = 2.36$; $p < 0.05$). These were the only significant changes, however.

In the study with 6 normal volunteers, the only significant change in sensitivity with stimulation was in two-point discrimination: this sense showed an improvement with stimulation ($t = 2.94$; $p < 0.05$).

An incidental finding of some surprise was made on 15 patients whose skin temperature was measured before and after stimulation. Stimulation significantly reduced skin temperature on both the affected and the unaffected limbs by about 2°F. In the painful limb this was significant at $p < 0.05$ ($t = 2.20$). In the normal side the difference was even more significant ($t = 3.90$; $p < 0.005$).

DISCUSSION

These results partly support both hypotheses tested. The fact that the painful limb is less sensitive than the normal limb in several modalities lends support to the concept of a central "gating" mechanism, in which small-fiber activity "holds the gate in a relatively open position" (5).

Second, the finding that at clinically effective parameters of stimulation electrical analgesia improves sensitivity in the painful limb supports the concept of the analgesic mechanism occurring by peripheral inhibition or blockade of the small fibers (whether by depolarization or by hyperpolarization). This is further supported by the failure to alter sensitivity in the normal limb except to impair cool temperature sensitivity. This also suggests that only some of the small fibers are "fatigued" by clinically effective stimulation, preventing the summation which results in pain but preserving the ability of other small fibers to transmit some temperature information.

The finding that skin temperature was lowered by electrical stimulation suggests that there was an enhancement of peripheral sympathetic activity. In some patients (not included in this study), electrical stimulation to relieve the pain associated with causalgia produces a peripheral warming. Thus electrical stimulation at higher voltages than used by the patients in this study can produce a peripheral blockade of sympathetic fibers, and at still higher voltages stimulation may involve the larger fibers. This may account for some of the differences between our results and those reported by others using normal subjects (1–4).

SUMMARY

Eighteen patients with pain primarily in one limb who obtained good to excellent pain relief with transcutaneous electrical neurostimulation were studied for sensory changes in the painful limb and in the normal contralateral limb before and during stimulation. Six normal volunteers were also studied before and during stimulation of one arm. The modalities tested were vibration, two-point discrimination, light touch, pinprick, position sense, temperature, and electric shock. It was found that without electrical stimulation, the painful limb was less sensitive than the contralateral limb. Electrical analgesia improved the sensitivity of the painful limb but had almost no effect on the normal limb except to impair temperature sensitivity in part. It was also found that skin temperature decreased significantly in both normal and painful limbs with stimulation. These findings support the concept of a spinal gating mechanism in clinical pain states, and they also support the hypothesis that clinical electrical analgesia occurs by means of peripheral blockade of some, but not all, small-fiber activity.

ACKNOWLEDGMENT

This work was supported by the Veterans Administration Hospital, San Diego, California.

REFERENCES

1. Campbell, J. N., and Taub, A. (1973): *Arch. Neurol.,* 28:347–350.
2. Satran, R., and Goldstein, M. N. (1973): *Science,* 180:1201–1202.
3. Taub, A., and Campbell, J. N. (1974): In: *Advances in Neurology, Vol. 4: International Symposium on Pain,* edited by J. J. Bonica, pp. 727–732. Raven Press, New York.
4. Torebjörk, H. E., and Hallin, R. G. (1974): In: *Advances in Neurology, Vol. 4: International Symposium on Pain,* edited by J. J. Bonica, pp. 733–736. Raven Press, New York.
5. Melzack, R., and Wall, P. D. (1965): *Science,* 150:971–979.

Advances in Pain Research and Therapy, Vol. 1,
edited by J. J. Bonica and D. Albe-Fessard.
Raven Press, New York © 1976.

Modulation of First and Second Pain by Peripheral Stimulation and by Psychological Set

Donald D. Price

Neurobiology and Anesthesiology Branch, National Institute of Dental Research, National Institutes of Health, Bethesda, Maryland 20014

Under certain circumstances a sudden application of a noxious stimulus to the distal portion of a limb results in the experience of an initial well-localized "stinging" or "pricking" pain followed by a less well-localized second burning or throbbing pain 1.0 to 1.5 sec later. If only a single stimulus is given, first pain is more intense than second pain and to some extent masks the latter. Second pain summates in intensity and duration with repeated stimuli and often has an unpleasant lingering quality. Reaction time measurements made before and during selective blockage of first pain by pressure applied to a nerve have confirmed that first and second pains are related to impulse conduction in A-delta and C fibers, respectively (2,6,9). Therefore, first and second pain can be related to separate afferent fiber groups and to different perceptual characteristics which they evoke.

Prolonged temporal summation and the capacity to outlast the stimulus duration are characteristics shared by experimentally induced second pain and by some pathological pain states such as postherpetic neuralgia and causalgia (1,4,6). These characteristics lead one to wonder to what extent these summation phenomena are attributable to exacerbations of existing physiological mechanisms. Recent studies and observations in our laboratory have shown that the second pain evoked by an abrupt noxious stimulus not only long outlasts the duration of the stimulus and summates at low stimulation frequencies, but it is susceptible to inhibition (6). Therefore, the phenomenon of second pain may serve as a useful guide to understanding physiological summation mechanisms that, under pathological conditions, become exaggerated. With these considerations in mind, it would be appropriate to review the results of our studies of first and second pain in relationship to physiological mechanisms of primary and secondary nociceptive neurons.

EFFECTS OF REPEATED STIMULI

In experiments now in progress (8), we have used constant wave form noxious heat pulses as a source of physiological stimuli that reliably produce

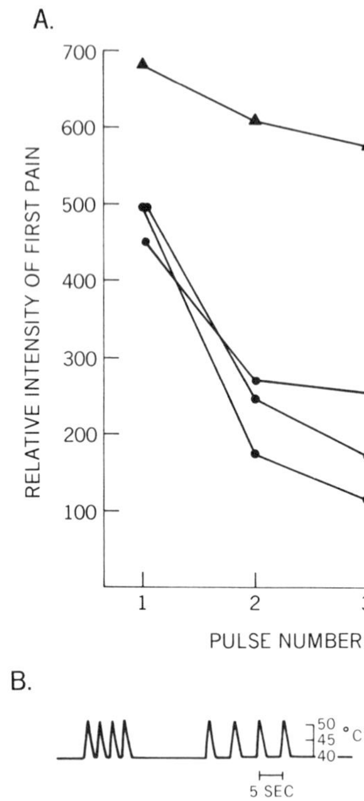

FIG. 1. First pain suppression. **A:** Magnitude estimations of first pain in response to trains of 4 consecutive heat pulses. Each train had an interpulse interval (IPI) fixed at 4, 40, or 80 sec. Subjects were instructed to squeeze a handgrip dynamometer in response to each first pain. These responses then were converted to magnitude estimations by having subjects estimate various handgrip forces. First pain decreased markedly with the IPIs used in this experiment. However, if the probe location changed between pulses, this decrement did not occur. Each point is the mean of 3 subjects (5 trials/IPI/subject). **B:** Standard heat pulses that produce first and second pain. Each pulse is constant in wave form and peak temperature (51.5°C). *Left,* pulses are repeated at 2.5-sec intervals; *right,* 5.0-sec intervals.

first and second pain (Fig. 1B). A train of four heat pulses generated by a contact thermode (1-cm diameter) is delivered to the back of the hand. During the heat pulse, the temperature at the thermode-skin interface is within the noxious range (45° to 51°C) for 0.7 sec. The interpulse interval (IPI) as well as all parameters of the heat pulses are programmed via a computer. The major dependent variables, perceived intensities of either first or second pain, are measured by magnitude estimation (cross-modality matching using a hand dynamometer). The distinction between first and second pain is made in all subjects by measuring their reaction times to the two pains. Changes in reaction times also serve to indicate selective blockage of A fibers by pressure applied to the ulnar nerve.

As illustrated in Fig. 1A, the perceived intensity of first pain decreases markedly with each successive heat pulse when the IPI is 40 sec or less. Several observations indicate that this progressive decrease is most likely owing to suppression of A-delta heat nociceptors. This suppression does not occur if the location of the probe changes between each successive pulse in the train. Such suppression also does not occur when electrical shocks are used. Finally, we have directly observed suppression of A-delta heat nociceptors by heat pulses similar to those used in our psychophysical experiments (*unpublished observations*).

In contrast to that of first pain, the perceived intensity of second pain does not decrease with successive heat pulses whose IPIs are 5 and 10 sec. Instead, the perceived intensity of second pain increases with each successive pulse at IPIs of 3 sec and 2.5 sec (Fig. 2). Several observations support the hypothesis that summation of second pain is most likely the result of central summation mechanisms activated by impulses in C fibers. This summation also can be obtained after blockage of first pain by pressure to the ulnar nerve (determined by a 1-sec increase in reaction time) and even when the location of the thermode changes between each heat pulse (Fig. 2). During blockage of first pain, second pain is consistently and reliably larger than in the unblocked condition ($p < 0.001$). An increase in perceived in-

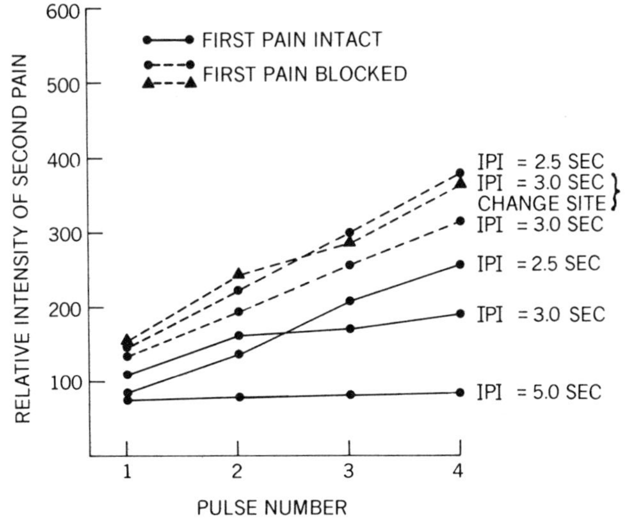

FIG. 2. Second pain summation. Magnitude estimations of second pain in response to trains of 4 heat pulses whose interpulse interval (IPI) was fixed at 5.0, 3.0, or 2.5 sec (*right*). Broken lines, condition wherein first pain is selectively blocked by pressure applied for 30 to 40 min to the ulnar nerve. Solid lines, condition wherein first pain is intact. Summation occurs with IPI of 3.0 and 2.5 sec before and during blockage of first pain and when probe location is changed between each pulse (*broken line* and *triangles*). Each point is the mean of 3 subjects (5 trials/IPI/subject).

tensity of second pain also occurs when constant current (9 mA) electrical shocks are delivered to the hand at frequencies greater than one every 3 sec. That summation of second pain is not due to sensitization of C-fiber polymodal nociceptors is further supported by our observations that responses of C-fiber polymodal afferents are partially suppressed by repeated noxious heat pulses (*unpublished observations*).

Central facilitatory mechanisms that could account for summation of second pain have been demonstrated in the spinal cord dorsal horn of spinalized cats and intact monkeys (3,7,10). In these preparations, long-latency discharges evoked in dorsal horn cells by electrical stimulation of C fibers increase in frequency and duration with each successive shock to C fibers, but only if the frequency of stimulation is greater than one every 3 sec. This long-term summation may have special relevance to Noordenbos' observations of the spatial and temporal summation characteristics of postherpetic pain (4). He found that multiple pinpricks applied at a frequency of about one every 3 sec resulted, after several applications, in an outbreak of unpleasant pain that spread over large areas and then wore off slowly once the pinpricks were terminated.

SUSCEPTIBILITY TO INHIBITION

We have found that second pain evoked by an intense electrical shock can be completely or nearly completely suppressed by mildly painful clamping of skin areas adjacent to the stimulus site or of skin areas of the contralateral limb (6). In contrast, first pain is much less affected by these same stimulation procedures. The greater susceptibility of second pain to peripherally induced inhibition may be related simply to the fact that with a single stimulus, second pain is less intense than first pain. In this regard, it is interesting that prolonged discharges evoked in dorsal horn neurons by C-fiber stimulation can be nearly completely inhibited by pinching skin areas that are outside and often contralateral to the excitatory receptive fields (5). Brief-latency discharges evoked in these same neurons by supramaximal A-fiber stimulation are less affected.

Psychological set also has different effects on the perception of first and second pain. We have assessed the effects of three different psychological sets on perception of first and second pain evoked by a single electrial shock (1). These sets include Past ("Place yourself in a previous experience that was free of any significant emotional tone"), Present ("Feel your foot that will be shocked"), and Future ("Think that you are about to be shocked"). When a single shock is given, second pain is never perceived in Past (0/10 Ss) and Future (0/10 Ss) sets but is always perceived by the same subjects in the Present set (10/10 Ss). First pain is perceived in all sets.

CONCLUSIONS

All of these results point to distinct functional differences between first and second pain. First pain gives information about the location, duration, and intensity of a noxious stimulus. If noxious heat pulses are repetitively applied to the same skin location, first pain decreases in intensity probably as a result of suppression of A-delta heat nociceptors. In contrast, second pain gives less information about the location and duration of the stimulus. It summates with low stimulus frequencies (one every 3 sec) as a result of activation of central facilitatory mechanisms that most likely occur in the spinal cord dorsal horn. Unlike first pain, second pain can be completely or nearly completely suppressed by psychological set and by central inhibitory mechanisms initiated by peripheral skin stimulation. Therefore, experimentally induced second pain may serve as a useful model in studying mechanisms that underly summation and inhibition of pathological pain and chronic pain.

REFERENCES

1. Barrell, J. J., and Price, D. D. (1975): *Percept. Psychophys.,* 17:163–166.
2. Lewis, T., and Pochin, E. E. (1938): *Clin. Sci.,* 3:67–76.
3. Mendell, L. M. (1966): *Exp. Neurol.,* 16:316–322.
4. Noordenbos, W. (1959): *"Pain,"* Elsevier, Amsterdam.
5. Price, D. D. (1969): Doctoral dissertation, University of California at Davis.
6. Price, D. D. (1972): *Exp. Neurol.,* 37:371–387.
7. Price, D. D., and Wagman, I. H. (1970): *Exp. Neurol.,* 29:383–399.
8. Price, D. D., Hu, J. W., Dubner, R., and Gracely, R. (1976): *Soc. Neurosci.,* 1:235.
9. Sinclair, D. C., and Stokes, B. A. R. (1969): *Brain,* 87:609–618.
10. Wagman, I. H., and Price, D. D. (1969): *J. Neurophysiol.,* 32:803–817.

Advances in Pain Research and Therapy, Vol. 1,
edited by J. J. Bonica and D. Albe-Fessard.
Raven Press, New York © 1976.

Analysis of the Action of Implanted Stimulating Devices Using Signal Detection Theory

James R. Bloedel, Douglas B. McCreery, and Donald L. Erickson

Departments of Neurosurgery and Physiology, University of Minnesota Medical School, Minneapolis, Minnesota 55455

The evaluation of the effectiveness of various methods for producing analgesia has been the subject of many studies pertaining to the psychophysics of pain perception. With the advent of the use of signal detection theory for this purpose, it has become possible to analyze a subject's responses to noxious stimuli over a range of stimulus intensities in terms of two parameters, bias and discrimination. In studies of known analgesic agents, all were shown to produce changes in discriminability (1,5, and W. C. Clark and L. Mehl, *unpublished observations*), whereas suggestion was shown to produce changes only in bias (2,3). On the basis of these results, investigators have made inferences concerning the nature of the perceptual and reporting processes involved in nociception (3). The process was considered to consist of two components, one pertaining to the sensitivity of the peripheral and central somatosensory systems (discriminability or sensitivity), and the other reflecting principally the subject's attitude and previous experience (bias). This model, together with the experimental results alluded to above, have served as the basis for arguing that a "true" analgesic effect (a state in which the patient actually feels less pain) must be accompanied by a change in discriminability. For this reason, the results showing that acupuncture produced only a change in bias were interpreted as implying that acupuncture produced no actual analgesia but only a change in the subject's criteria or response bias for describing a given stimulus as noxious (4).

The studies reported here were performed to determine the effect of electrical stimulation on experimentally induced pain using signal detection theory and, in addition, to evaluate the interpretation of changes in bias and discriminability which may accompany an analgesic effect.

METHODS

For this purpose, a device, described in detail elsewhere (6), was designed for applying temperature pulses of three amplitudes (2.5°, 3°, and 3.5°C) to the skin in a quantifiable, reproducible manner with an accuracy of

±0.2°C. The skin of the subject was preheated by the device to a base-line temperature of 34°C. Temperature pulses of three different intensities were applied in random order in sets of 24 consecutive trials applied 1.5 to 2 min apart in each of two sessions. After each trial, the thermode was placed on the next dot in a six-dot array placed either on the anterior surface of the thigh above the knee in patients with stimulating devices located on the cord, or on the skin in the distribution of the sciatic nerve in those with sciatic nerve implants. Each subject was given a neutral set of instructions regarding the purpose of the experiment and was instructed to describe each presentation of the thermal stimulus with one of the following categories: faintly warm (FW), warm (W), hot (H), faintly painful (FP), painful (P), and very painful (VP). Further details of the experimental paradigm can be found in a previous publication (6).

The results were plotted as receiver-operator characteristics (ROCs). The data presented in this chapter are from a preliminary study of a comparison of the effects of internally implanted and externally applied stimulating devices and their effect on the perception of noxious thermal stimuli. The conclusions drawn from these data are based on inspection of these changes in the ROCs from trials with the stimulating device on and with the device off. A more detailed study regarding the effect of external electrical stimulation has now been completed using a large enough number of subjects so that the data could be thoroughly examined using an analysis of variance technique (7). The conclusions from these studies have completely substantiated inferences based on inspection of the receiver-operator curves.

RESULTS

The results from three groups of patients in which implantable stimulating devices were evaluated are shown in Fig. 1. In all groups, electrical stimuli were applied in alternating blocks of six trials, with a 5-min interval between blocks. Patients with both dorsal column stimulators (Fig. 1, A and B) and sciatic nerve implants (C and D) showed a significant decrease of discriminability over a part of the temperature range during electrical stimulation as indicated by the shift of the ROC toward the main diagonal.

In the case of the dorsal column stimulator patients, the change in discriminability was evident in the lower part of the temperature range (T_1, T_2; Fig. 1A), whereas in the patients with the sciatic nerve implants, the discrimination change was most evident in the upper part of the temperature range (T_1, T_3; Fig. 1D). This finding indicates that the activation of these stimulating devices probably produced a change in the perception of these experimentally induced thermal stimuli. However, it is not possible to say whether the basis of the perceptual change is psychological or physiological (if indeed the distinction has any meaning from a physiological perspective). In addition, a marked change in bias was particularly evident in A, B, and D

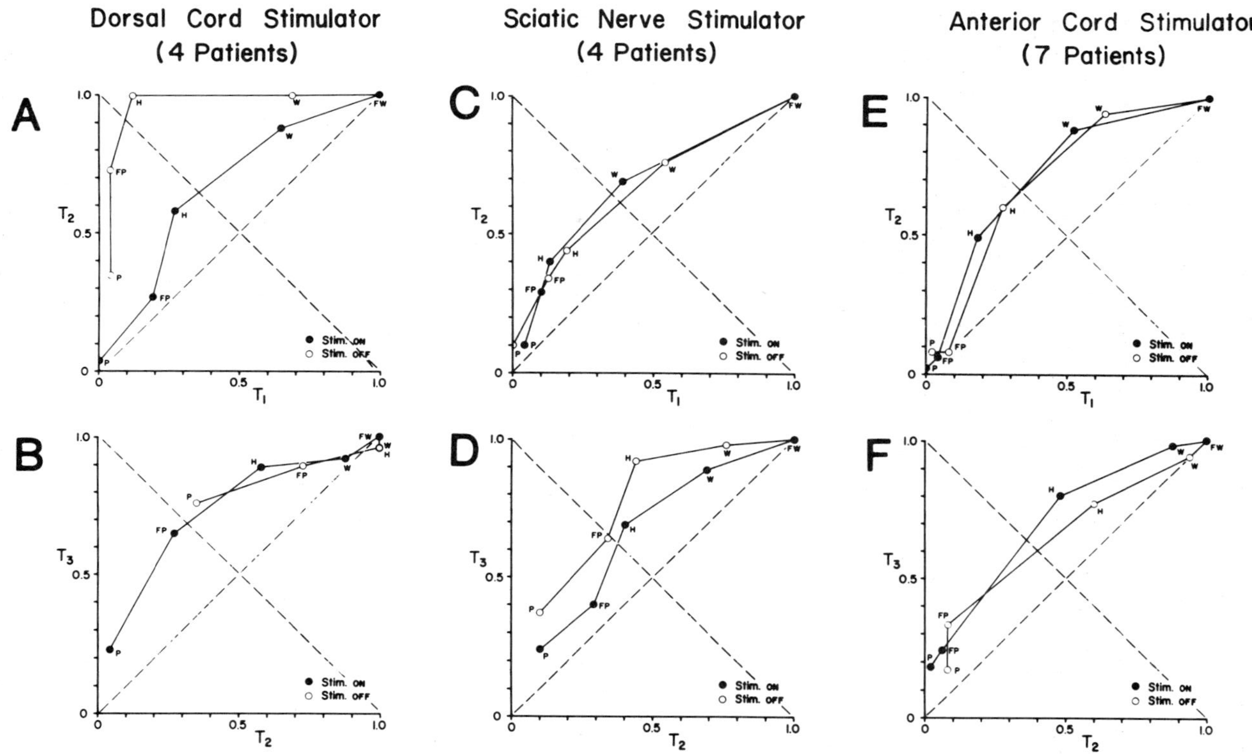

FIG. 1. Composite ROCs from a study involving patients with dorsal cord **(A,B)**, sciatic nerve **(C,D)**, and anterior cord **(E,F)** stimuating electrodes. Ordinate and abscissa of each point are the proportion of trials in which patients described thermal pulses of the intensity indicated beside the axes using the indicated category or a higher category. ROCs from stimulator-on and stimulator-off trials are shown together for comparison. Zero-discrimination and zero-bias loci are indicated by the principal and negative diagonals, respectively. Temperature pulse intensities were: T_1, 2.5°C; T_2, 3 °C; T_3, 3.5°C; all superimposed on a cutaneous base-line temperature of 34°C.

by the shift in the point on the ROC away from the negative diagonal for a specific response category. This finding shows that, when activated, certain types of implanted devices reduced the patient's tendency to describe the thermal stimulus as painful.

In contrast to the patients with implanted dorsal column stimulators and sciatic nerve stimulators, those in which a stimulating electrode was implanted on the anterior surface of the spinal cord showed no decrease in discriminability over any part of the temperature range with only a change in bias in some response categories (Fig. 1, E and F). As a group, these patients were either quite stoic or quite insensitive to the thermal stimuli as compared to the posterior column patients, as evidenced by the displacement of the "faintly painful" and "painful" points far down the ROC. Of the 7 patients in this group, 2 were tested and were considered on follow-up examination to be complete failures. An evaluation of their responses indicates little change between the trials in which the stimulator was off and those in which it was on. Therefore, the change in bias occurring in this group is principally due to changes in those patients in which the device was somewhat clinically effective.

DISCUSSION

According to the analysis of acupuncture analgesia by Clark and Yang (4), the results from the group of patients with anterior cord stimulators would be considered to indicate that no analgesic effect was produced with electrical stimulation applied to that region of the spinal cord. However, in a recent study of the effect of externally applied stimulation in our laboratory (7), it was shown that a statistically significant change in discriminability can be produced by suggestion implicit in neutral instructions. In addition, by comparing results in subjects in which the stimulator was not turned on with those from subjects in which it was activated, it was shown that the electrical stimulus can produce an increase in bias which cannot be totally ascribed to premonitions the subjects had concerning the likely effect of electrical stimulation. Consequently, bias changes cannot be totally ascribed to changes in patients' criteria for reporting pain because of suggestion. Furthermore, the results also show that such bias changes can occur without accompanying changes in discriminability between nonzero intensities of the thermal stimulus. It is therefore probable that both external stimulators and the three types of implantable stimulators considered above can produce "true analgesia."

In showing the analgesic effect of nitrous oxide, Chapman et al. (1) observed little change in discriminability when the responses to nonzero adjacent pairs of stimuli were examined. Clark and Yang (4) in analyzing changes in discriminability produced by acupuncture, which they feld did not produce actual analgesia, also used the responses to nonzero adjacent stimuli. Given this similarity, the lack of significant change in this parameter cannot be cited to show the absence of an analgesic effect on the basis of a comparison of their findings with those of Chapman et al. (1). Therefore, in addition to showing a definitive effect of electrical stimulation on experimentally induced noxious stimuli, the results of this study together with a study of the effect of external stimulation just completed in our laboratory (7) imply that the argument that a "true" analgesic should produce a decrease in discrimination must be reevaluated.

ACKNOWLEDGMENTS

This work was supported by a grant from Medtronic, Inc., Minneapolis, Minnesota, and by National Institutes of Health Grant NS09447–05.

REFERENCES

1. Chapman, C., Murphy, T., and Butler, S. (1972): *Science,* 179:1246–1248.
2. Clark, W. C. (1969): *J. Abnorm. Psychol.,* 74:363–371.
3. Clark, W. C. (1974): *Anesthesiology,* 40:272–287.
4. Clark, W. C., and Yang, J. C. (1974): *Science,* 184:1096–1098.
5. Dillon, D. J. (1973): *Proc. Am. Psychol. Assoc.,* 7:872.
6. McCreery, D., and Bloedel, J. R. (1975): *J. Assoc. Adv. Med. Instrum.* (*in press*).
7. McCreery, D., and Bloedel, J. R. (1975): *Submitted for publication.*

Advances in Pain Research and Therapy, Vol. 1,
edited by J. J. Bonica and D. Albe-Fessard.
Raven Press, New York © 1976.

Stimulation of the Vaginal Cervix Is More Effective Than Morphine in Suppressing a Nociceptive Response in Rats

*Barry R. Komisaruk, Vincent Ciofalo, and Miklos B. Latranyi

*Schering Corporation, Bloomfield, New Jersey 07003; and *Institute of Animal Behavior, Rutgers University, Newark, N.J. 07102*

In previous studies we demonstrated that vaginal stimulation in rats (pushing against the vaginal cervix with a plunger from a 1-cc syringe) abolished or markedly attenuated responses to noxious stimulation. Vaginal stimulation suppressed leg withdrawal in response to pinching the foot, and it also blocked facial twitches in response to pinching the ear, eyeblink in response to touching the cornea (9), vocalization squeaks in response to shocking the tail, and sensory thalamic responses to pinching but not to touching the skin (8,10). The present study was undertaken to compare the effectiveness of analgesic dosages of morphine sulfate with vaginal stimulation in a standard nociceptive test situation.

METHODS

The response measured was the latency for the rat to start to withdraw a hind foot from a pneumatic vise which gradually compressed the foot at a precisely controlled linearly increasing pressure (20 mm Hg/sec) according to the method of Randall and Selitto (12). One jaw of the vise was a rounded metal peg, the other was a flat metal disc. They were positioned lightly in contact with the dorsal and ventral surface of the foot, and then the pneumatic drive was activated simultaneously with a high-speed timer. As soon as the rat started to withdraw its foot, the vise was stopped and the latency recorded. If the rat did not withdraw its foot the vise was released at 15 sec, the maximum test duration.

Forty adult intact female Charles River C-D rats (190 to 240 g) were divided into four groups. All rats were pretested to determine the latency to withdraw the left and right foot from the vise. Each rat then received a subcutaneous injection of 0.1 ml of a 20% brewer's yeast suspension in water in the plantar region of the left foot (this produced a local inflammatory reaction, making the foot extremely sensitive to touch). One hour after the yeast injection, we measured the latency for each rat to withdraw its right and sensitized left foot from the vise. One group (m) then received a low dose of morphine sulfate 0.5 mg/kg i.p. (injection volume: 10 ml/kg); a second group (M) received a high dose of morphine sulfate 2.0 mg/kg i.p. (injection volume: 10 ml/kg); and a third group (s) received 10 ml/kg of physiological saline i.p.

Thirty minutes after administering this treatment, we again tested the withdrawal latency for the left and right foot in each rat. The fourth group received vaginal-cervical stimulation on this test. Vaginal stimulation was applied while the rat's foot was being positioned in the vise. Each rat received approximately 10 sec of vaginal stimulation before the vise pressure started to increase, and the vaginal stimulation was maintained until the rat moved its foot or the maximum test duration occurred. A force of 800 g was applied to the vaginal cervix using a tuberculin syringe modified as follows. The portion of the plunger that is normally pushed with the thumb was cut off with a sanding disc and the cut end was rounded and polished. Two springs (from retractable ball-point pens) were inserted into the syringe barrel and the syringe plunger was then inserted into the barrel. The polished end of the plunger was inserted into the vagina, and force was exerted against the cervix by pushing on the syringe barrel. The force thus exerted is proportional to the distance the springs are compressed. The amount of the compression required for a force of 800 g was previously determined by pressing the plunger against the platform of an animal scale and marking the corresponding position of the inner end of the plunger on the external markings of the syringe barrel. This force was maintained for the duration of the test. Thirty minutes after the test with morphine or vaginal stimulation, the rats were retested to determine if the effects of the treatment persisted.

RESULTS

As seen in Fig. 1, the base-line latencies to withdraw left and right foot ($pretest_1$) were essentially the same in all groups [range of all group means: 7.93 ± 0.42 (SE) to 8.62 ± 0.26 sec]. One hour after the yeast was injected into the left foot ($pretest_2$), the response latencies in that foot were markedly and uniformly reduced to a mean of under 2 sec (range: 1.37 ± 0.07 to 1.49 ± 0.13 sec), whereas the response latencies in the noninflamed control foot were similar to their previous levels (range: 7.35 ± 0.17 to 7.98 ± 0.23).

In the analgesia test ($test_1$), the withdrawal latency for the inflamed foot was significantly greater in each of the morphine groups (low dose, m: 5.39 ± 0.92; high dose, M: 13.02 ± 0.64) than in the saline controls (1.19 ± 0.04; $p < 0.001$). The Duncan multiple range test (5) was used for this and the following statistical analyses. The withdrawal latency for the noninflamed foot was higher than that of the comparable saline controls (7.70 ± 0.38) in the high-dose morphine group (10.74 ± 0.96; $p < 0.001$) but not in the low-dose morphine group ($p > 0.05$). Vaginal stimulation increased

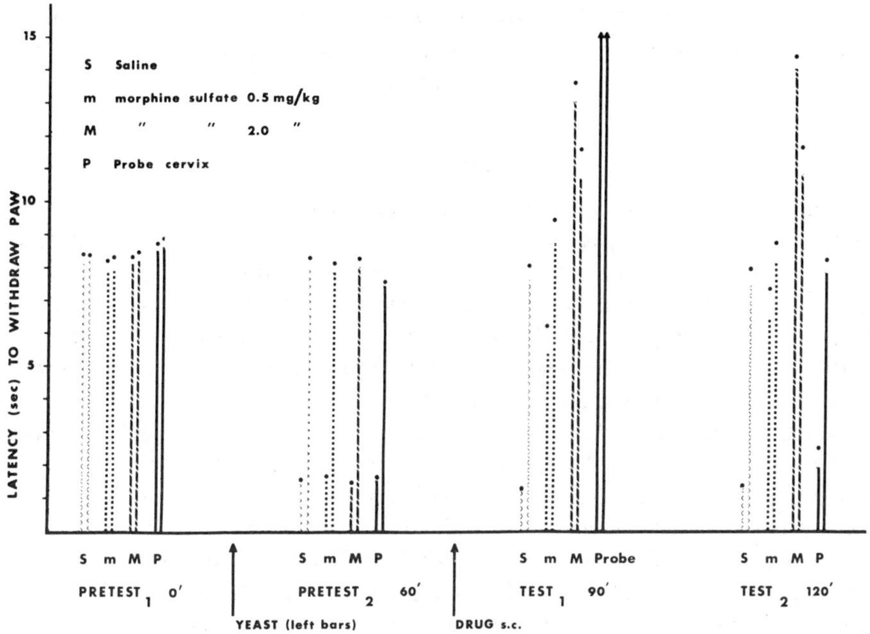

FIG. 1. Comparison of the effects of morphine sulfate and vaginal stimulation on the latency of foot withdrawal to a constantly increasing compressive force (represented as group mean ±SEM, in seconds) in 4 groups of 10 rats each. Left and right bars in each group represent withdrawal latencies for left and right foot, respectively. Pretest$_1$, time 0: withdrawal latencies when all rats were untreated. Pretest$_2$: withdrawal latencies measured 60 min after the left hind foot of each rat was injected with a yeast solution producing inflammation and sensitization. Test$_1$: withdrawal latencies measured 30 min after a subcutaneous (s.c.) injection of a low or high dose of morphine sulfate or saline or during vaginal stimulation. Test$_2$: withdrawal latencies measured 30 min later, when vaginal stimulation was not being applied.

the withdrawal latencies of inflamed or noninflamed paws to more than 15 sec, the predetermined cutoff point, in every single case. Vaginal stimulation was thus more effective than low-dose morphine in increasing the withdrawal latency of the inflamed or the noninflamed foot ($p < 0.001$). Vaginal stimulation was also more effective than the high-dose morphine ($p < 0.05$) in increasing the withdrawal latency of the noninflamed foot.

In the vaginal stimulation groups, no rat made any attempt to withdraw either foot before 15 sec. In a few cases we continued increasing the pressure in the sensitized foot for 20 to 25 sec, and even then there were no attempts to withdraw the foot.

When the rats were retested 30 min later (test$_2$), the foot withdrawal latencies for the saline and morphine groups were similar to those on the previous test (saline: sensitized 1.28 ± 0.04, nonsensitized 7.48 ± 0.43; m: sensitized 6.42 ± 0.96, nonsensitized 8.09 ± 0.58; M: sensitized 14.04 ±

0.37, nonsensitized 10.77 ± 0.84). Since the cervical probe was not applied on $test_2$, the latencies in this group returned to levels similar to those on pre-$test_2$ (sensitized 1.92 ± 0.56; nonsensitized 7.84 ± 0.37).

DISCUSSION

Our results demonstrate that in rats, probing against the vaginal cervix with a force of 800 g is more effective than 2 mg/kg morphine sulfate in blocking the foot withdrawal response to noxious stimulation. Other studies have shown that in this type of test, potent narcotic analgesics elevate the withdrawal latency of both the sensitized and nonsensitized paws, whereas anti-inflammatory analgesics and nonnarcotic analgesics such as aspirin raise the threshold of the inflamed paw only (14).

Since we are measuring a motor response, the present experiment does not reveal if the rats' perception of the noxious properties of the stimulus applied to the foot is altered by morphine and/or vaginal stimulation. There is no question that the cervical probing suppresses locomotor activity, for a rat can be slid stiff-legged across a table surface by simply probing against its vaginal cervix while applying no other restraints (7). On the other hand, thalamic neuronal responses to pinching but not to tactile stimulation are strongly suppressed by cervical probing, demonstrating that cervical probing can also block sensory responses to noxious stimulation (8,10). Furthermore, although vocalization in response to presumably noxious tail shock is abolished by cervical probing, vocalization in response to presumably non-noxious sudden lifting is not suppressed by cervical probing (8,10). Thus cervical probing blocks the vocalization response to noxious stimulation but does not block the ability of rats to vocalize. Thus we cannot yet conclude whether there are common aspects to the mechanism by which morphine and vaginal stimulation suppress responses to noxious stimulation.

One similarity is suggested in the condition of "Straub tail," in mice induced by high dosages of morphine, in which the tail, hind legs, and body become extended, the perineum protrudes, and the vertebral column shows lordosis (3,13). Activation of an extensor pattern is a characteristic effect of stimulation of vaginal cervix in rats (8); vaginal stimulation in addition to blocking responses to noxious stimulation also simultaneously strongly facilitates the lordosis response (elevation of head and rump and extension of tail and legs) to palpation of the flanks and perineum (7,8). Procedures that induce immobilization (tying a "tournique" around the Achilles tendon or a "twitch" around the nose in horses) are used during potentially painful veterinary procedures (6).

Morphine is also effective in increasing the latency for rats to flick the tail away from a hot light source (1,2). We have observed that cervical probing can block this tail-flick response in unanesthetized rats to the extent that the tail actually began to char (after 1 min) and yet the rats did not flick the tail or vocalize (11).

A force of as little as 100 g produces a significant increase in the shock intensity required to induce vocalization, and the effect of cervical probing on this threshold increases steadily as the force is increased to 800 g (4). The effectiveness of the cervical probing decreases after approximately 1 min of continuous stimulation, for the immobilizing effect wanes and the rat starts to turn and bite (11). Perhaps intermittent stimulation would prolong the effectiveness.

The question of whether there is a relationship between immobilization and blockage of pain perception is intriguing and requires further study.

ACKNOWLEDGMENTS

This article is contribution No. 225 of the Institute of Animal Behavior. We gratefully acknowledge the suggestions and encouragement of Dr. Philip N. Brody.

These studies were supported in part by Research Grant NIMH MH 13279 and Research Scientist Development Award Type II S-K02-MH 14711 (BRK) and by funds from the Alfred P. Sloan Foundation.

REFERENCES

1. Akil, H., Mayer, D. J., and Liebeskind, J. C. (1972): *C. R. Acad. Sci.* [D] (*Paris*), 274: 3603–3605.
2. Bass, W. B., and Vander Brook, J. J. (1952): *J. Am. Pharm. Assoc.*, 41:569–570.
3. Bilbey, D. L., Salem, H., and Grossman, M. H. (1960): *Br. J. Pharmacol.*, 15:540–543.
4. Crowley, W. R., Jacobs, R., Volpe, J., Rodriguez-Sierra, J. F., and Komisaruk, B. R. (1976): *Physiol. Behav.*, 16:483–488.
5. Edwards, A. L. (1968): In: *Experimental Design in Psychological Research, 3rd ed.*, pp. 130–134. Holt, Rinehart and Winston, New York.
6. Kaada, B. (1974): *Tidsskr. nor. Laegeforen.*, 94:422–431.
7. Komisaruk, B. R. (1971): In: *Steroid Hormones and Brain Function*, edited by C. H. Sawyer and R. A. Gorski, pp. 127–141. University of California Press, Berkeley.
8. Komisaruk, B. R. (1974): In: *Reproductive Behavior*, edited by W. Montagna and W. A. Sadler, pp. 97–129. Plenum Publishing Co., New York.
9. Komisaruk, B. R., and Larsson, K. (1971): *Brain Res.*, 35:231–235.
10. Komisaruk, B. R., and Wallman, J. (1973): *Soc, Neurosci.* (*Abs.*), 3rd Annual Meeting, 315.
11. Komisaruk, B. R., Rodriguez-Sierra, J., and Crowley, W.: *Unpublished observations.*
12. Randall, L. O., and Selitto, J. J. (1957): *Arch. Int. Pharmacodyn. Ther.*, 111:409–419.
13. Straub, W. (1911): *Dtsch. Med. Wochenschr.*, 1426.
14. Taber, R. I. (1974): *Adv. Biochem. Psychopharmacol.*, 8:191–211.

Advances in Pain Research and Therapy, Vol. 1,
edited by J. J. Bonica and D. Albe-Fessard.
Raven Press, New York © 1976.

Pain Modulation by Central Nervous System Stimulation

John C. Liebeskind

Department of Psychology, University of California, Los Angeles, California 90024

In recent years it has become quite clear that central stimulation not only can elicit pain but also can inhibit its elicitation by noxious peripheral stimuli. This chapter reviews some of the most recent evidence concerning central mechanisms of antinociception, focusing attention on a medial brainstem system with the specific and apparently endogenous property of pain inhibition.

BEHAVIORAL MANIFESTATIONS

Stimulation-produced analgesia (SPA) elicited from sites throughout the medial brainstem manifests itself in a number of characteristic ways [for a more detailed description, the reader is referred to the original papers by Reynolds (55) and by Mayer et al. (40); see also ref. 32].

Certainly the most salient feature of SPA is its potency. In the rat, it has been found equi-analgesic to morphine in doses ranging from 10 to 50 mg/kg, depending on the analgesia test (38). An effect of comparable magnitude has been reported in the cat (2,16,31,46–49) and monkey (18), and Richardson and Akil (57) obtained a dramatic degree of pain relief with medial brain stem stimulation in chronic pain patients. SPA may be reliably observed across a wide variety of pain tests including those utilizing pinprick (5), noxious heat (1,38,54,56,60) or cold (40), strong pinch (18,38,46,48,55,56), electric shocks applied to peripheral nerve (16,29), to the teguments (40,45), or to the tooth pulp (48,49), and the injection of chemical irritants into cutaneous (43) or visceral tissue (17). Particularly noteworthy is the fact that SPA from the medial brainstem may totally abolish even spinally mediated nociceptive reflexes (38,40), responses generally considered resistant to all but narcotic analgesic drugs (19). Evidence that an effect of this magnitude, reliability, and generality across measures can be obtained from stimulation elsewhere in the nervous system is so far lacking (see ref. 38).

In the rat, analgesia may outlast the period of brain stimulation by many minutes or even several hours (38,40). In the cat and monkey, on the other hand, analgesia has so far not been found to outlast brain stimulation by more than a minute or two (18,46,48,49). Fortunately, pain relief in man may endure for several hours after termination of a few minutes of central stimulation (57). Also in the rat, analgesia is sometimes seen to occur only within a restricted peripheral field such as the tail or the contralateral hindquarters (5,38,40); but again, this feature of SPA is less apparent in other species (46,48).

Brain stimulation resulting in analgesia may itself be rewarding, aversive, or neutral depending on the precise location of the stimulating electrode within the medial brainstem (32,38). Even from loci where both self-stimulation and SPA can be obtained, these two phenomena can be dissociated pharmacologically by administration of drugs that affect these behaviors in an opposite fashion (1,33,69). SPA may but need not be associated with various motor manifestations (40). In the best examples of the phenomenon in rat, cat, and monkey, it cannot be easily discerned when the stimulating current is being delivered. Cortical spiking has been seen to accompany SPA from a number of sites in the rat (56). However, it has also been reported that the elicitation of electrographic or motor seizures is negatively correlated with the occurrence of SPA in this species (38,56).

Finally, this powerful pain inhibition can take place with little apparent loss of acuity in other sense modalities (40). In fact, in the rat, complete analgesia is sometimes associated with hyperresponsiveness to light touch (40). Moreover, in the cat, SPA has been shown to block selectively the jaw opening (nociceptive) reflex to dental pulp stimulation without affecting a similar jaw-opening response evoked by innocuous tooth tap (49).

ANATOMICAL CONSIDERATIONS

SPA manifested as described above has been most frequently observed with stimulation of the caudal mesencephalic periaqueductal gray matter (PGM) (16,29,38,40,43,46,49,55,60). In the cat, stimulation of midbrain sites other than those in the immediate vicinity of the dorsal raphe nucleus in ventrocaudal PGM causes prominent aversive reactions, precluding adequate testing (16,31,46). In the rat, unlike the cat, where analgesia significantly outlasts the stimulation period, aversive reactions during central stimulation do not interfere with later analgesia testing. In part for this reason, we (38,56) and others (5) have obtained SPA in the rat from sites in dorsal and rostral PGM as well as from still more rostral regions of the caudal diencephalon where aversive reactions are common. Rhodes (56) has recently completed a comprehensive mapping in the rat of SPA sites rostral to the well-studied caudal PGM. Employing tail flick, hot plate, and pinch tests, she found the most potent and reliable effects within a more or less continuous medial system extending from the rostral PGM and pretectal region into the paraventricular nucleus of thalamus and the posterior hypothalamic area. The dorsomedial nucleus of thalamus and more lateral regions were notably lacking in effective SPA sites. Most successful placements in this study fell within the distribution of the periventricular system described by Krieg (27) and others. It is now known that monoamine-containing neurons [catecholaminergic (34) as well as tryptaminergic (13,15)] comprise important ascending portions of this system. The possible functional significance of this fact will be discussed below.

Two other loci caudal to PGM have been relatively well explored for possible sites of SPA. In a pilot investigation in the rat, J. M. Liebman (*personal communication*) found no evidence of analgesia to pinch from 15 stimulation sites within or close to the locus coeruleus, from which originates the dorsal noradrenergic bundle (63). On the other hand, several investigators have recently reported prominent SPA in the cat (48) and rat (44,54) from still more caudal sites near the nucleus raphe magnus. This region is known to contain the serotonin cell bodies whose axons descend in the dorsolateral funiculus and terminate in the dorsal horn of the spinal cord (14). Interestingly, Basbaum et al. (6) report that lesions of the dorsolateral funiculus block SPA from PGM stimulation in the rat, suggesting the possible involvement of these serotonin paths in SPA.

ELECTROPHYSIOLOGICAL OBSERVATIONS

SPA has been associated with marked alterations in spontaneous and pain-evoked electrical activity at several different levels of the neuraxis. In the dorsal horn of the cat, the responses of lamina V–type cells to even intensely noxious peripheral stimuli may be completely inhibited by PGM stimulation (31,46). Much recent evidence implicates these cells in central mechanisms of nociception (e.g., 8,9,66), and it is known that their activity (spontaneous and pain-evoked) is tonically modulated by supraspinal controls of brainstem origin (9,10,21,61,66). By contrast, lamina IV–type cells have no evident involvement in pain mechanisms, and their activity is unaffected by PGM stimulation (31,46). Similarly, morphine exerts a lamina-specific suppressive effect on the dorsal horn, it too affecting lamina V– but not lamina IV–type cells (26). Once again, the possible involvement in SPA of serotonin pathways is suggested by the finding that LSD, an anti-serotonin drug, blocks inhibition on lamina V–type cells stemming from PGM stimulation only when the stimulating electrode is near the serotonin cells of the dorsal raphe nucleus (20).

Indicating that the suppressive effects of SPA are related to sensory phenomena and not simply to spinal reflex mechanisms, several recent studies show SPA-induced inhibitory effects on pain-evoked electrical activity in supraspinal structures implicated in nociception. Casey et al. (11) report that PGM stimulation in the rat can block the response to noxious stimuli of neurons in the gigantocellular nucleus of the medial medulla. Akil and Richardson (2) show that PGM stimulation and morphine have comparable inhibitory effects in medial thalamic pain-evoked responses in the cat. Similarly, in experiments still in progress, we (44,45) are finding that analgesic doses of morphine and analgesic PGM stimulation in the fully awake, chronically implanted rat block pain-evoked multiple-unit and slow-wave responses in medial and ventrobasal thalamus as well as in the PGM. Responses to innocuous stimuli in these areas are generally not inhibited and are in some cases actually enhanced at the same time that pain responses are diminished. Stimulation outside PGM which fails to induce analgesia also fails to affect these electrical responses. In a pilot investigation, both SPA and morphine have been found to augment markedly the spontaneous multiple-unit activity in the serotonin-rich dorsal and median raphe nuclei, and especially in the nucleus raphe magnus (44).

RELATION TO MORPHINE'S MODE OF ACTION

The observations and insights deriving from the study of SPA appear to have both influenced and been influenced by a coincident series of dramatic developments in our understanding of the site and mechanism of morphine's analgesic action. Confirming and extending the original observations of Tsou and Jang (62), a number of studies have recently shown that the brain regions most sensitive to intracerebral microinjections of morphine are the same periaqueductal and periventricular structures found most clearly to support SPA (24,51,58,64,68). For example, Sharpe et al. (58) found that injections of 3 μg of morphine into the dorsal raphe nucleus caused analgesia of more rapid onset, greater magnitude, and longer duration than equivalent doses administered elsewhere in the midbrain, including the aqueduct. Similarly, in a study of morphine's ability to block "wet shake" behavior in rats, Wei et al. (68) found that injections of as little as 0.04 μg into the PGM were effective, whereas considerably higher doses were required in the numerous other areas tested.

Other evidence suggestive of morphine's site of action in the brain comes from the discovery of opiate receptor sites in the CNS (35,52). These sites are found to be unevenly distributed in the brain, with the PGM being one region showing a relatively high concentration (28). In other exciting work, Hughes (22) isolated an endogenous substance from brain tissue with specific morphine-like action in a bioassay. This action is blocked by the pure morphine antagonist, naloxone. Preliminary evidence indicates that the endogenous morphine-like substance has a distribution in the brain roughly similar to that of opiate receptor sites (22,50).

SPA and morphine analgesia share a number of properties in addition to possible site of action in the brain. For example, there is considerable evidence suggesting that they share an at least partly common set of pharmacological susceptibilities and hence, perhaps, a common underlying neurochemistry. Morphine analgesia and SPA both depend on the integrity of cerebral monoamine systems (1,67). Akil and Liebeskind showed that SPA from PGM stimulation in the rat is greatly reduced by either a dopamine receptor blocker (pimozide) or a serotonin synthesis inhibitor (PCPA) but is enhanced by a dopamine receptor stimulator (apomorphine) or the monoamine precursors, L-DOPA and 5-HTP. On the other hand, depletion of norepinephrine (disulfiram) led to an increase in SPA, and when a combination of drugs (AMPT + L-DOPA) was given such that norepinephrine levels were low and dopamine levels high, SPA was particularly potent. On the basis of these and other results, it was concluded that dopamine and serotonin facilitate SPA, whereas norepinephrine inhibits it (1). From a number of recent studies, a similar conclusion can be reached regarding the relation of the monoamines to morphine analgesia [see discussion in Akil and Liebeskind (1)].

The importance of serotonin and dopamine in SPA and morphine analgesia may relate to the presence of these neurotransmitters in those portions of the ascending periventricular system where SPA and opiate receptor sites have been found. Alternatively, excellent SPA has also been reported from the bulbar raphe system (44,48,54), whose serotonin-containing axons descend into the cord (14). These findings accrue significance in the light of recent work by Vogt (65) and by Proudfit and Anderson (53) showing a significant reduction in morphine analgesia after pharmacological interference with or electrolytic destruction of this bulbar raphe system. Their work suggests that the descending serotonin system is involved in morphine analgesia, just as the work of Basbaum et al. (6) implicates this path in SPA. Again, preliminary results from our laboratory indicate that both morphine and SPA augment multiple-unit activity in the bulbar raphe (44). Finally, Repkin et al. (54) report that morphine administration augments the presumed presynaptic inhibition of sensory input in primary afferent fibers in the cord and show that this effect can be blocked by the serotonin antagonist cinanserin. In sum, although these results are somewhat preliminary and have not yet been subjected to the test of time, they nonetheless clearly point to an important role for the descending serotonin system in centrifugal mechanisms of pain control.

Still another line of evidence linking the mechanism of SPA to that of morphine analgesia derives from the demonstration that naloxone, a specific morphine antagonist, reliably diminishes the potency of SPA in the rat (3,4) and cat (2,47). We have hypothesized (1) that SPA, like morphine analgesia, is mediated by activity at opiate receptor sites in the brain. We suggested that SPA may, via release or some other process, make the endogenous, morphine-like substance available for binding at these receptor sites, where naloxone can antagonize its action as it antagonizes the action of morphine. In a related study, Jacob et al. (23) report finding for the first time that small doses of naloxone can facilitate nociceptive reactions of rats and mice in the hot plate test. These authors similarly suggest that their results might favor the existence of an endogenous, morphine-like substance that serves tonically to inhibit nociceptive reactions. Naloxone, then, might facilitate responding by blocking this tonic inhibition.

Finally, Mayer and Hayes (37) have recently shown in the rat that tolerance develops with repeated exposure to SPA, then dissipates slowly over several weeks of nonexposure. Moreover, if animals are first made tolerant to morphine, then cross-tolerance to SPA can be seen. This effect also dissipates over several weeks after discontinuation of morphine administration. From this evidence it may be concluded once again that SPA and morphine analgesia share, at least in part, a common neural substrate. The property of tolerance development would, as Mayer and Hayes (37) suggest [see also Jacquet and Lajtha (24)], appear to reside within the neural substrate, manifesting itself after appropriate activation of the substrate by either electrical or chemical stimulation.

SUMMARY AND CONCLUSIONS

The findings reviewed above suggest, as we have previously concluded (1,32,38,40), that a neural substrate exists within the medial brainstem which serves normally to inhibit pain. This substrate may be activated by electrical stimulation and by morphine. It may be suggested that morphine acts directly at opiate receptor sites, whereas electrical stimulation may, at least in part, act on these sites indirectly via release of the endogenous, morphine-like substance. One important consequence of adequate activation of this pain-inhibitory substrate is the inhibition of transmission through spinal interneurons involved in the afferent conduction of the pain message. The exact site and nature of this inhibition in the cord are still unknown, but solid evidence is accumulating that the bulbospinal serotonin system is an important mediator of this effect. The possible importance in SPA of ascending serotonin and dopamine pathways must also be considered. In fact, it may be assumed that a number of sites, paths, and mechanisms of action other than those proposed here are involved in antinociception. In any case, there is no reason to believe that this process is either simply or narrowly represented in the nervous system.

The existence of a neural substrate with endogenous antinociceptive function implies the existence of physiological systems with normal access to this substrate. Unfortunately, there is not yet available a great deal of evidence relevant to this point. Melzack (42) and Kaada (25) have each suggested as one possible explanation of acupuncture analgesia that this form of peripheral stimulation has access to the medial brainstem. Lending a measure of support to this view, Mayer and co-workers (36,39) have presented evidence that naloxone antagonizes acupuncture analgesia in man.

There is also evidence that pain itself has ready and powerful access to the medial brainstem. Many studies implicate this brain region in the reception of pain-related information on the basis of its anatomical input from the anterolateral cord (e.g., 41) and its electrophysiological responsiveness to noxious stimuli (e.g., 7,12,30,45). More recently, Sherman and Gebhart (59) provided evidence for pain-induced biochemical alterations in this system. They report that pain significantly lowers glutamate levels in PGM of the rat, whereas morphine not only reverses this effect but also increases glutamate levels above normal.

It seems inevitable that a system subserving antinociception would be informed of the occurrence of pain. Yet this should not imply that nociceptive input to the medial brainstem is always capable of activating its pain-inhibitory function. For example, neural or humoral events associated with states of fear or anxiety might also normally have access to this system and serve to shut it down, thereby exacerbating or prolonging the experience of pain. It may well be, therefore, that the medial brainstem, having as it seems to a certain tonic level of activity, can be used to either reduce or augment the perception of pain.

ACKNOWLEDGMENT

The research conducted in my laboratory was supported by U.S. Public Health Service Grant NS 07628.

REFERENCES

1. Akil, H., and Liebeskind, J. C. (1975): *Brain Res.*, 94:279–296.
2. Akil, H., and Richardson, D. E. (1974): *Soc. Neurosci., 4th annual meeting.*
3. Akil, H., Mayer, D. J., and Liebeskind, J. C. (1972): *C. R. Acad. Sci.* [*D*] (*Paris*), 274: 3603–3605.
4. Akil, H., Mayer, D. J., and Liebeskind, J. C. (1976): *Science*, 191:961–962.
5. Balagura, S., and Ralph, T. (1973): *Brain Res.*, 60:369–379.
6. Basbaum, A. I., Marley, N., and O'Keefe, J.: *This volume.*
7. Becker, D. P., Gluck, H., Nulsen, F. E., and Jane, J. A. (1969): *J. Neurosurg.*, 30:1–13.
8. Besson, J.-M., Conseiller, C., Hamann, K. F., and Maillard, M. C. (1972): *J. Physiol.* (*Lond.*), 221:189–205.
9. Besson, J.-M., Guilbaud, G., and Le Bars, D. (1975): *J. Physiol.* (*Lond.*), 248:725–741.
10. Brown, A. G. (1971): *J. Physiol.* (*Lond.*), 219:103–125.
11. Casey, K. L., Keene, J. J., and Morrow, T. (1974): In: *Advances in Neurology, Vol. 4: International Symposium on Pain,* edited by J. J. Bonica, pp. 197–205. Raven Press, New York.
12. Chang, H. (1973): *Scientia Sinica,* 16:25–60.
13. Conrad, L. C. A., Leonard, C. M., and Pfaff, D. W. (1974): *J. Comp. Neurol.*, 156:179–206.
14. Dahlström, A., and Fuxe, K. (1965): *Acta. Physiol. Scand.* [*Suppl.*], 247, 64:5–36.
15. Fuxe, K. (1965): *Acta Physiol. Scand.* [*Suppl.*], 247:64.
16. Gebhart, G. F., and Toleikis, J. R. (1975): *Fed. Proc.*, 34:439.
17. Giesler, G. J., Jr., and Liebeskind, J. C. (1976): *Pain,* 2:43–48.
18. Goodman, S. J., and Holcombe, V.: *This volume.*
19. Grumbach, L. (1966): In: *Pain,* edited by R. S. Knighton and P. R. Dumke, pp. 163–182. Little, Brown and Co., Boston.
20. Guilbaud, G., Besson, J.-M., Oliveras, J.-L., and Liebeskind, J. C. (1973): *Brain Res.*, 61:417–422.

21. Handwerker, H. O., Iggo, A., and Zimmermann, M. (1975): *Pain,* 1:147–165.
22. Hughes, J. (1975): *Brain Res.,* 88:295–308.
23. Jacob, J. J., Tremblay, E. C., and Colombel, M.-C. (1974): *Psychopharmacologia,* 37:217–223.
24. Jacquet, Y. F., and Lajtha, A. (1974): *Science,* 185:1055–1057.
25. Kaada, B. (1974): *Tidsskr. Nor. Laegeforen,* 94:422–431.
26. Kitahata, L. M., Kosaka, Y., Taub, A., Bonikos, K., and Hoffert, M. (1974): *Anesthesiology,* 41:39–48.
27. Krieg, W. J. S. (1932): *J. Comp. Neurol.,* 55:19–89.
28. Kuhar, M. J., Pert, C. B., and Snyder, S. H. (1973): *Nature (Lond.),* 245:447–450.
29. Lewis, V. A., and Gebhart, G. F. (1975): *Fed. Proc.,* 34:757.
30. Liebeskind, J. C., and Mayer, D. J. (1971): *Brain Res.,* 27:133–151.
31. Liebeskind, J. C., Guilbaud, G., Besson, J.-M., and Oliveras, J.-L. (1973): *Brain Res.,* 50:441–446.
32. Liebeskind, J. C., Mayer, D. J., and Akil, H. (1974): In: *Advances in Neurology, Vol. 4: International Symposium on Pain,* edited by J. J. Bonica, pp. 261–268. Raven Press, New York.
33. Liebman, J. M., and Butcher, L. L. (1973): *Naunyn Schmiedebergs Arch. Pharmacol.,* 277:305–318.
34. Lindvall, O., Björklund, A., Nobin, A., and Stenevi, U. (1974): *J. Comp. Neurol.,* 154: 317–348.
35. Lowney, L. I., Schulz, K., Lowery, P. J., and Goldstein, A. (1974): *Science,* 183:740–753.
36. Mayer, D. J. (1975): *Neurosci. Res. Program Bull.,* 13:94.
37. Mayer, D. J., and Hayes, R. L. (1975): *Science,* 188:941–943.
38. Mayer, D. J., and Liebeskind, J. C. (1974): *Brain Res.,* 68:73–93.
39. Mayer, D. J., Price, D. D., Rafii, A., and Barber, J.: *This volume.*
40. Mayer, D. J., Wolfle, T. L., Akil, H., Carder, B., and Liebeskind, J. C. (1971): *Science,* 174:1351–1354.
41. Mehler, W. R. (1966): In: *Pain,* edited by R. S. Knighton and P. R. Dumke, pp. 11–32. Little, Brown and Co., Boston.
42. Melzack, R. (1973): *The Puzzle of Pain.* Basic Books, New York.
43. Melzack, R., and Melinkoff, D. F. (1974): *Exp. Neurol.,* 43:369–374.
44. Oleson, T. D., and Liebeskind, J. C. (1975): *Physiologist,* 18:338.
45. Oleson, T. D., and Liebeskind, J. C.: *This volume.*
46. Oliveras, J.-L., Besson, J.-M., Guilbaud, G., and Liebeskind, J. C. (1974): *Exp. Brain Res.,* 20:32–44.
47. Oliveras, J.-L., Guilbaud, G., and Besson, J.-M. (1975): *J. Physiol. (Paris),* 71:164.
48. Oliveras, J.-L., Redjemi, F., Guilbaud, G., and Besson, J.-M. (1975): *Pain,* 1:139–145.
49. Oliveras, J.-L., Woda, A., Guilbaud, G., and Besson, J.-M. (1974): *Brain Res.,* 72:328–331.
50. Pasternak, G. W., Goodman, R., and Snyder, S. H. (1975): *Life Sci.,* 16:1765–1769.
51. Pert, A., and Yaksh, T. (1974): *Brain Res.,* 80:135–140.
52. Pert, C. B., and Snyder, S. H. (1973): *Science,* 179:1011–1014.
53. Proudfit, H. K., and Anderson, E. G. (1974): *Pharmacologist,* 16:203.
54. Repkin, A. H., Proudfit, H. K., and Anderson, E. G. (1974): *Pharmacologist,* 16:203.
55. Reynolds, D. V. (1969): *Science,* 164:444–445.
56. Rhodes, D. L. (1975): Ph.D. dissertation, U.C.L.A.
57. Richardson, D. E., and Akil, H. (1974): *Abstr. 7th Ann. Meeting Neuroelectric Soc.*
58. Sharpe, L. G., Garnett, J. E., and Cicero, T. J. (1974): *Behav. Biol.,* 11:303–313.
59. Sherman, A. D., and Gebhart, G. F. (1975): *Life Sci.,* 15:1781–1789.
60. Soper, W. Y. (1976): *J. Comp. Physiol. Psychol.,* 90:91–101.
61. Taub, A. (1964): *Exp. Neurol.,* 10:357–374.
62. Tsou, K., and Jang, C. S. (1964): *Scientia Sinica,* 13:1099–1109.
63. Ungerstedt, U. (1971): *Acta Physiol. Scand. [Suppl.],* 367:1–48.
64. Vigouret, J., Teschemacher, H., Albus, K., and Herz, A. (1973): *Neuropharmacology,* 12:111–121.
65. Vogt, M. (1974): *J. Physiol. (Lond.),* 236:483–498.

66. Wall, P. D. (1967): *J. Physiol. (Lond.)*, 188:403–423.
67. Way, E. L., and Shen, F. (1971): In: *Narcotic Drugs: Biochemical Pharmacology,* edited by D. H. Clouet, pp. 229–253. Plenum, New York.
68. Wei, E., Sigel, S., and Way, E. L. (1975): *J. Pharmacol. Exp. Ther.,* 193:56–63.
69. Yunger, L. M., Harvey, J. A., and Lorens, S. A. (1973): *Physiol. Behav.,* 10:909–913.

Advances in Pain Research and Therapy, Vol. 1,
edited by J. J. Bonica and D. Albe-Fessard.
Raven Press, New York © 1976.

Modulation of Nociceptive Responses in the Thalamic Posterior Group of Nuclei

Willie K. Dong and Irving H. Wagman

Department of Animal Physiology, University of California, Davis, California 95616

Anatomical and electrophysiological investigations, particularly on the cat, have accurately delimited the boundaries and subdivisions of the thalamic posterior group of nuclei (PO). Afferent input from cortex (7,11–14,22–24), inferior colliculus (13,14,17), and spinal cord (2–4,8,11,13,14) have been traced to PO. Of particular significance with regard to somesthesia is the termination of axons from the dorsal column nucleus, lateral cervical nucleus, and spinothalamic tract onto the medial division of the posterior group (POm) and onto the medial portion of the magnocellular medial geniculate (MGmc), which collectively are termed "somatic" PO (2–4,11,13,14). Although all three spinal projections transmit low-threshold signals thalamopetally, only the spinocervicothalamic and spinothalamic projections contain axons that also carry high-threshold signals originating from dorsal horn cells (5,28). A majority of somatic PO neurons as determined by Poggio and Mountcastle (20) were "nociceptive" since noxious mechanical stimulation to the entire or part of the receptive field was required to excite these thalamic cells. However, this important observation has remained essentially unconfirmed (1,6,18,19).

The aims of the present study were to systematically reexamine the somatic PO for these nociceptive neurons with similar experimental procedures used by Poggio and Mountcastle (20) and, more importantly, to examine the interactions between responses to noxious and nonnoxious peripheral stimulation.

METHODS

Forty-six cats were studied under thiopental sodium and gallamine triethiodide. Cervical laminectomy exposing C_1 to C_4 spinal segments and craniotomy were performed to permit stimulation of the dorsal column surface and recording from single thalamic units with tungsten microelectrodes, respectively. The right and left dorsal columns were isolated from each other and from the dorsolateral funiculi by surgical section and by acetate film to limit spread of stimulus current. The contralateral superficial radial nerve was prepared for stimulation and recording the compound action potential in the usual manner. Temperatures of the spinal cord, nerve, and body were maintained within physiological ranges. Water and electrolyte balance were maintained by infusion of dextrose in lactated Ringer's. Hairs and skin surfaces were stimulated adequately by uncalibrated mechanical devices and electrically by subcutaneous electrodes. Joints were rotated and deep structures such as the periosteum were kneaded by hand. A pair of forceps for applying pressure to a fold of skin or across skin and bone, and a probe with blunt and sharp tips for applying pressure to the skin surface were both equipped with wire-resistance strain gages in order to deliver calibrated stimuli. The frequency of unit activity in relation to either electric or mechanical stimuli was analyzed by the dot-raster technique and by a digital computer. Histological verification of recording sites was determined by identification of electrolytic lesions made by the recording electrode at the end of each experiment.

RESULTS

We studied 258 neurons with somatic receptive fields extracellularly in POm and MGmc. Of these cells, 30% were determined to be "nociceptive." All had a slow or even negligible adaptation when driven by steady and intense mechanical stimulation of the noxious receptive field (Figs. 1A and 2A). Many cells had large and often bilateral receptive fields. Based on other response characteristics, these cells were classified into two groups: (a) 16% responded exclusively to noxious mechanical stimuli, that is, they were driven by either intense pressure to the skin alone or periosteal kneading and strong pressures applied across skin and bone; (b) 14% were composed of cells that responded differentially to both noxious and innocuous mechanical stimuli over separate (continuous or discontinuous) or overlapping receptive fields. Our present report is restricted to this latter group of nociceptive neurons.

These cells generated a specific sequence of responses when activated by: (a) stimulation of the dorsal column(s), (b) stimulation within the innocuous receptive field by electric shock to the skin, (c) brief skin displacement, or (d) activation of $A\beta$ or $A\beta\gamma$ nerve fibers. The response pattern to a single stimulus consisted of an initial discharge burst of short latency and duration followed by an inhibitory period of 40- to 150-msec duration, and then return to the resting level of discharge. There were no further changes in this discharge pattern after applying high-intensity shocks to the dorsal column(s) or to the purely innocuous part of the receptive field even at strengths sufficient to evoke $A\beta\gamma\delta$ or $A+C$ discharge.

In contrast, a high-intensity skin shock within the noxious receptive field or stimulation of $A\beta\gamma\delta$ or $A+C$ fibers in a nerve volley evoked a complex, patterned, prolonged discharge which followed the initial inhibitory period and which decreased over 1 sec or more before returning to resting level.

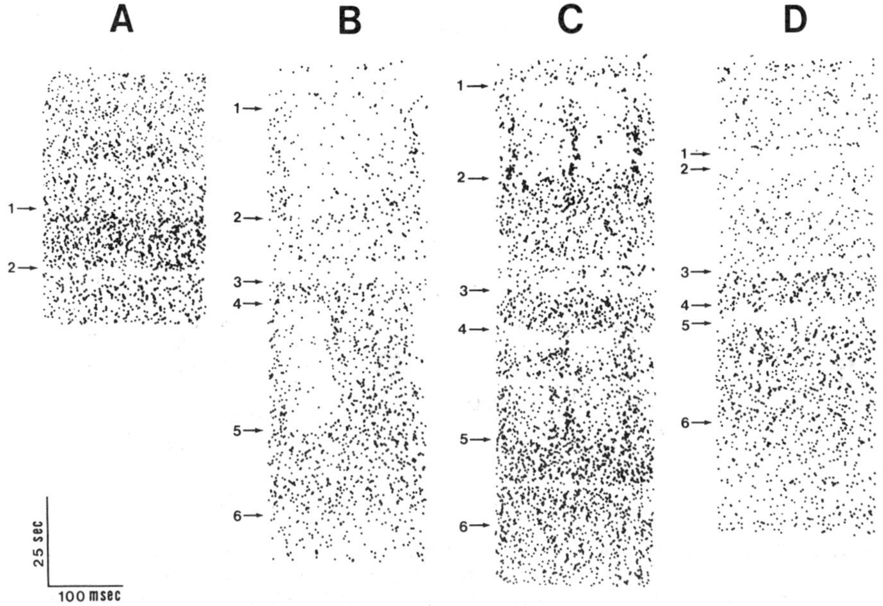

FIG. 1. Effects of dorsal column stimulation on resting and noxious evoked activity of a thalamic PO cell. Spike activity of a single unit is recorded as dots running left to right in 215-msec sweep lengths and displaced downward at the end of each sweep. Sweeps are tightly packed to illustrate lengthy records and thus are difficult to distinguish individually. Unit responds to both noxious deep periosteal kneading and nonnoxious tapping of skin along the entire contralateral and ipsilateral forelimbs. **A:** Resting discharge in upper- and lowermost series of records. Between arrows 1 and 2, a steady pinch (over 1 kg force) was applied with forceps across skin and bone of ipsilateral upper arm. **B, C, D:** Each column contains a similar sequence of events identically numbered. Top and bottom series of records show resting discharge. Between arrows 1 and 2, contralateral DC stimulated at 5/sec **(B)**, 10/sec **(C)**, and 50/sec **(D)**. Between arrows 2 and 3, resting discharge. At arrow 3, a steady pinch is applied to the ipsilateral upperarm. Between arrows 4 and 5, while pinch is maintained, DC is stimulated at 5/sec **(B)**, 10/sec **(C)**, and 50/sec **(D)**. At arrow 6, pinch is terminated.

Initial discharge bursts and reduction of resting or noxious evoked discharge due to DC shocks are seen in **B** and **C** during stimulation at 5/sec and 10/sec. The efficacy of DC stimulation at 5/sec and 10/sec in maintaining the inhibitory effects gradually diminishes with time. Resting discharge evidently increases after 10/sec shocks (**C**, record between arrows 2 and 3). Both initial bursts and resting or noxious evoked discharge are completely inhibited during DC stimulation at 50/sec **(D)**.

Somewhat similar response patterns evoked by activating low- and high-threshold peripheral inputs have been described in the spinal cord (15,16, 25,27).

Repetitive stimulation of the dorsal column(s) or of the innocuous receptive field has a marked inhibitory effect on both the spontaneous discharge and the discharge evoked by steady noxious mechanical stimulation and by excitation of $A\beta\gamma\delta$ or $A+C$ fibers. This inhibitory effect when evoked by

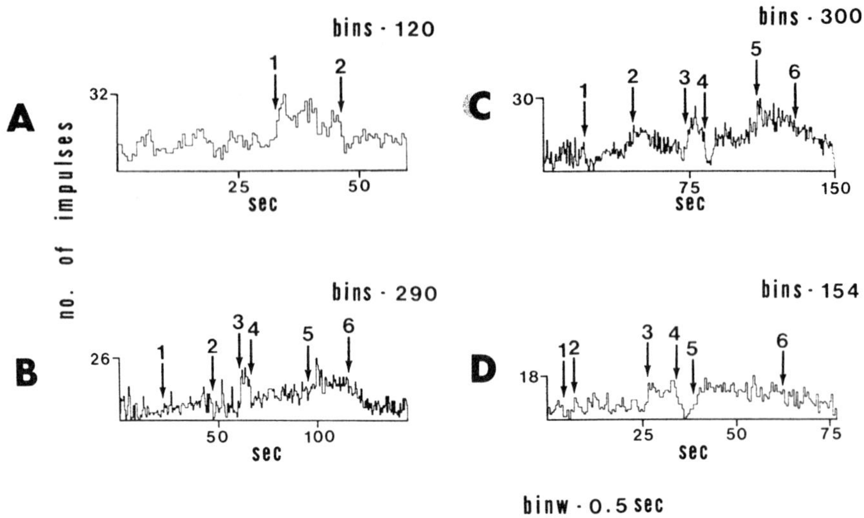

FIG. 2. Histograms representing results in Fig. 1. Seconds on abscissa are plotted in units of bin width (0.5 sec). Events in each histogram are numbered identically to those in Fig. 1. Although the discharge is reduced (Fig. 1 **B** and **C,** record between arrows 1 and 2) during DC stimulation at 5/sec and 10/sec, the total activity which includes the initial bursts is greater than activity at rest (Fig. 2 **B** and **C,** record between arrows 1 and 2). Noxious evoked activity is more effectively reduced by higher frequencies of DC stimulation. Compare Fig. 2 **B, C,** and **D,** records between arrows 3 and 6, and especially between arrows 4 and 5.

dorsal column stimulation at 5/sec and 10/sec is illustrated in the dot-raster records and histograms of Figs. 1 B and C and 2 B and C. The records clearly show the reduction of spontaneous activity (Fig. 1 B and C, records between arrows 1 and 2) and of noxious evoked discharges (Fig. 1 B and C and 2 B and C, records between arrows 4 and 5). In this example, however, note that the total activity resulting from dorsal column stimulation alone is above resting levels (Fig. 2 B and C, records between arrows 1 and 2) because the initial bursts occur at 200-msec and 100-msec intervals, respectively (Fig. 1 B and C, records between arrows 1 and 2). Stimulation at frequencies in which the interval between stimuli was equal to or less than the duration of the inhibitory period produced the most profound inhibitory effects on either spontaneous or noxious evoked activity. In many cells, the initial bursts to such stimulation were also completely inhibited. For example, when the dorsal column is stimulated at 50/sec, the initial bursts along with the spontaneous or noxious evoked discharges are almost completely inhibited (Figs. 1 D and 2 D).

Evidence from several experiments has shown that the low-threshold signals responsible for the inhibitory effects on these neurons may be transmitted both through a direct lemniscal pathway and through dorsal horn cells via extralemniscal projections to the somatic PO. When the dorsal columns are entirely lesioned within the C_2 and C_3 spinal segments, noxious evoked activity from the skin or by means of nerve stimulation can be inhibited by dorsal column stimulation either rostral or caudal to the lesion. However, less effective inhibition was observed with stimuli applied to the caudal site. Furthermore, the short latencies of the initial bursts elicited by stimulation of the dorsal column immediately rostral (2.0 to 2.5 msec) and caudal (5.0 to 5.5 msec) to the lesion indicate synaptically secure lemniscal and lemniscal-extralemniscal linked projections to PO. These short latencies indicate that much of the effect is due to thalamic projections only rather than to thalamocortical-thalamic projections.

COMMENT

Our results show that the somatic PO contains a relatively large number of neurons which respond to nociceptive skin stimulation. These results are in agreement more with those of Poggio and Mountcastle (20) than with those of others (1,6,18,19).

More significantly, we have shown that these neurons display an interaction between their noxious and nonnoxious elicited responses. This finding strongly suggests that the somatic PO is an important supraspinal site for modulation of nociceptive signals. The dorsal column–lemniscal input, in particular, exerts a powerful and direct inhibitory effect on somatic PO cells. A similar inhibitory action on nociceptive evoked responses of dorsal horn cells has been demonstrated by stimulation of either large primary afferents or dorsal columns (9,10,15). Thus it is possible that the reduction or elimination of noxious evoked responses in the somatic PO by stimulation of low-threshold primary afferents is a consequence of inhibitory mechanisms in both spinal cord and thalamus. These would include disfacilitation at the cord level, owing presumably to pre- and/or postsynaptic inhibition of nociceptive responses of dorsal horn cells (21,26), and activation of inhibitory mechanisms within somatic PO by low-threshold signals mediated directly by the dorsal column lemniscal projection and indirectly by dorsal horn cells via extralemniscal projections.

The inhibitory effects on the noxious evoked responses of somatic PO neurons by innocuous electrical or mechanical skin stimulation, and by stimulation of the dorsal column or low-threshold primary afferents may be one important inhibitory interactive process which underlies the suppression of chronic pain by employment of similar stimulating techniques clinically. The suppression of pain originating from large areas of the body by application of innocuous stimuli to the affected or unrelated parts, or by dorsal column and peripheral nerve stimulation, might be explained in part by wide somatic convergence and inhibitory mechanisms in the somatic region of the thalamic posterior group of nuclei.

ACKNOWLEDGMENTS

This work was supported in part by U.S. Public Health Service Grants NS07844 and RR00169 and by a grant from the California Medical Education and Research Foundation to Dr. H. S. Davis. W. K. Dong was a recipient of an A. P. Giannini Foundation Postdoctoral Fellowship.

REFERENCES

1. Berkley, K. J. (1973): *J. Neurophysiol.,* 36:940–952.
2. Boivie, J. (1970): *Brain Res.,* 19:333–360.
3. Boivie, J. (1971*a*): *Brain Res.,* 28:459–490.
4. Boivie, J. (1971*b*): *Exp. Brain Res.,* 12:331–353.
5. Brown, A. G. (1973): In: *Handbook of Sensory Physiology, Vol. 2: Somatosensory System,* edited by A. Iggo. Springer-Verlag, New York.
6. Curry, M. J. (1972*a*): *Brain Res.,* 44:439–462.
7. Curry, M. J. (1972*b*): *Brain Res.,* 44:463–481.
8. Curry, M. J., and Gordon, G. (1972): *Brain Res.,* 44:417–437.
9. Handwerker, H. O., Iggo, A., and Zimmermann, M. (1975): *Pain,* 1:147–163.
10. Hillman, P., and Wall, P. D. (1969): *Exp. Brain Res.,* 9:284–306.
11. Jones, E. G., and Burton, H. (1974): *J. Comp. Neurol.,* 154:395–432.
12. Jones, E. G., and Powell, T. P. S. (1968): *Brain Res.,* 10:369–391.
13. Jones, E. G., and Powell, T. P. S. (1971): *J. Comp. Neurol.,* 143:185–216.
14. Mehler, W. R. (1966): In: *Pain,* edited by R. S. Knighton and P. R. Dumke, pp. 11–32. Little, Brown and Co., Boston.
15. Mendell, L. M. (1966): *Exp. Neurol.,* 16:316–332.
16. Mendell, L. M., and Wall, P. D. (1965): *Nature,* 206:97–99.
17. Moore, R. Y., and Goldberg, J. M. (1963): *J. Comp. Neurol.,* 121:109–135.
18. Nyquist, J. K., and Greenhoot, J. H. (1974): *Exp. Neurol.,* 42:609–622.
19. Perl, E. R., and Whitlock, D. G. (1961): *Exp. Neurol.* 3:256–296.
20. Poggio, G. G., and Mountcastle, V. B. (1960): *Johns Hopkins Med. J.,* 106:266–316.
21. Price, D. D., Hull, C. D., and Buchwald, N. A. (1971): *Exp. Neurol.,* 33:291–309.
22. Rinvik, E. (1968*a*): *Exp. Brain Res.,* 5:153–172.
23. Rinvik, E. (1968*b*): *Brain Res.,* 8:237–254.
24. Rinvik, E. (1968*c*): *Brain Res.,* 10:79–119.
25. Wagman, I. H., and Price, D. D. (1969): *J. Neurophysiol.,* 32:803–817.
26. Wall, P. D. (1958): *J. Physiol.,* 142:1–21.
27. Wall, P. D., and Cronly-Dillon, J. R. (1960): *Arch. Neurol.,* 2:365–375.
28. Willis, W. D., Trevino, L., Coulter, J. D., and Maunz, R. A. (1974): *J. Neurophysiol.,* 37:358–372.

Advances in Pain Research and Therapy, Vol. 1,
edited by J. J. Bonica and D. Albe-Fessard.
Raven Press, New York © 1976.

Cerebral Modulation of Neuronal Excitability in the Cuneate Nucleus of the Macaque Monkey

*S. J. Jabbur, F. A. Harris, **M. A. Biedenbach, †R. W. Morse, and A. L. Towe

Department of Physiology and Biophysics, and Regional Primate Research Center, University of Washington School of Medicine, Seattle, Washington 98195

In the early 1960s, several studies showed that the excitability of neurons in the dorsal column nuclei of the domestic cat can be modified by direct stimulation of the anterior and posterior sigmoid gyri on either side of the brain (8,12,13,19). Nearly all neurons in these nuclei come under some form of cerebral influence—excitatory, facilitatory, or inhibitory. The excitatory and facilitatory influences come by way of the pyramidal tract (12,13), whereas the inhibitory influences apparently involve additional neurons in the medullary reticular formation (3,13,19). The effects on a particular neuron appear to be the same, whatever the effective cerebral site stimulated (*unpublished observations* by M. B. Bromberg compromise this statement). Neurons that are initially excited or facilitated by cerebral stimulation are concentrated deep and rostrally in the nuclei, are primarily touch sensitive, lack afferent inhibition (when tested with a conditioning stimulus outside the excitatory receptive field of the neuron), and infrequently respond antidromically to stimulation of the medial lemniscus (6,8). By contrast, neurons that are initially inhibited by cerebral stimulation are concentrated more superficially and in the middle third of the nuclei, are almost exclusively hair sensitive, show clear afferent inhibition (from a zone surrounding the excitatory receptive field), and frequently respond antidromically to stimulation of the medial lemniscus (6,8). A variety of other specific details are known from numerous other studies, but they are not of concern here.

In 1964 Andersen et al. (1) formalized the general scheme of organization of the dorsal column nuclei implied by these studies into a model wherein the primary afferent fiber terminals on cuneothalamic projection neurons receive a presynaptic depolarizing influence from cuneate interneurons, which themselves receive an excitatory influence from pyramidal

---

* Present address: Department of Physiology, School of Medicine, American University of Beirut, Lebanon.

** Present address: Department of Physiology, University of Texas Health Sciences Center, San Antonio, Texas 78284.

† Deceased.

tract neurons. Many of these interneurons were thought to receive convergent input from pyramidal tract and primary afferent fibers. In addition, some cuneate interneurons were thought to receive primary afferent fiber input only and to hyperpolarize the cuneothalamic projection neurons directly. This model made no statements about the magnitude of these effects. Recently, a somewhat more elaborate form of this general scheme, incorporating statements about magnitude, has been proposed by Blum, Bromberg, and Whitehorn (2). As all the foregoing studies, this last was based on observations from the domestic cat. The purpose of this chapter is to determine whether this general scheme of cuneate nucleus organization is tenable for members of the primate line.

METHODS

Rhesus monkeys (*Macaca mulatta*) were anesthetized with pentobarbital sodium, paralyzed with *d*-tubocurarine chloride and artificially ventilated on a positive-negative respiration pump. The dorsal column nuclei were exposed for recording, and pericentral cerebral cortex contralateral to the side of recording was exposed for stimulation. Bipolar stimulating electrodes were placed on the hand and foot foci of precentral and postcentral cortex, and a concentric electrode was placed caudally in nucleus ventralis of the thalamus. Additionally, bipolar needle electrodes were inserted into the tips of the digits of the forepaw ipsilateral to the side of recording; a bipolar needle electrode placed in the palm of the same paw served as a hunting stimulus source.

Recordings were made on a 0.5-mm grid, with a zero reference at the tip of the obex. Twenty electrode penetrations were made at each grid point (one penetration per site per animal), from 2 mm rostral to 4.5 mm caudal to the obex, and from 1.0 to 4.5 mm lateral to the obex, each penetration being carried to a depth of 3 mm below the dorsal surface. Recordings were made extracellularly through NaCl-filled glass micropipettes of 0.5- to 2.0-μm tip diameter. All data were photographically recorded and were also recorded on digital tape at 15-kHz sampling rate through a 25-nsec aperture with 6-bit amplitude accuracy, full scale. The data were analyzed automatically through a spike recognition program and checked for accuracy against the photographic records. In the sample of 2,038 cuneate neurons, many observations were made; only those pertinent to the issue of descending modulation of neuronal excitability are discussed here.

RESULTS

The most striking feature was that, unlike those in the cat, not all cuneate neurons in the monkey could be influenced by cerebral stimulation: in a sample of 1,431 adequately tested neurons, only 416 neurons showed a measurable cerebral influence. However, the magnitude of the effects on those neurons that could be influenced was considerably greater than that in the cat. Many of the cerebrally excited neurons readily responded to a single shock, and several could be shown unequivocally to be monosynaptically driven from the cortex. The second striking feature was that the cerebral effect was not always uniform on each neuron: some neurons showed mixed effects, according to the cerebral site stimulated. The distribution of these effects is shown in Fig. 1. Only 130 (31%) of the 416

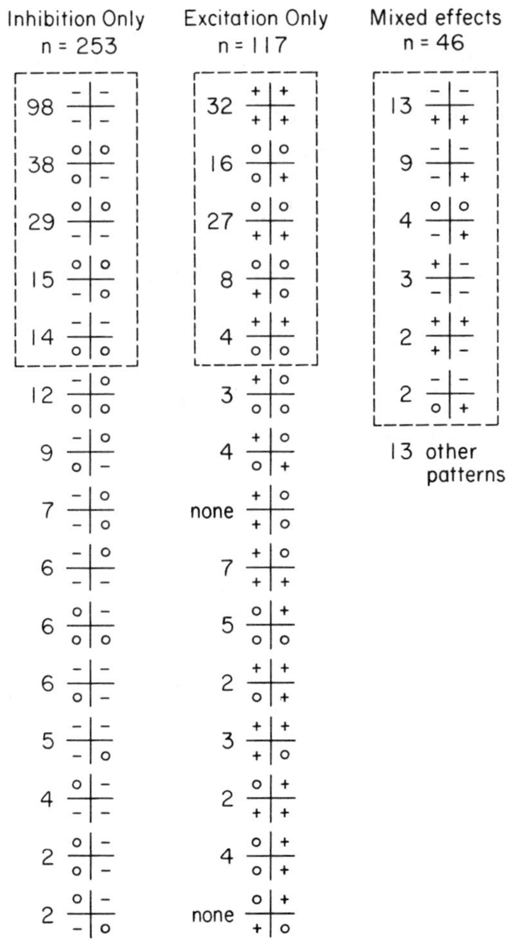

FIG. 1. Distribution of cerebral effects by major categories. Each block of four symbols shows one pattern of effects; number of neurons showing that pattern is at left of each block. Patterns: *upper left,* precentral foot focus; *lower left,* precentral hand focus; *upper right,* postcentral foot focus; *lower right,* postcentral hand focus. Symbols: −, inhibition; 0, no effect; +, excitation. Dashed fields include 75% of each sample.

affected neurons showed completely uniform effects, with 98 (24%) being inhibited and 32 (8%) being excited. Fully 46 (11%) of the neurons showed a mixture of excitatory and inhibitory effects, according to the cerebral site stimulated. These two features make the general scheme of organization proposed for the domestic cat inappropriate for the rhesus monkey.

A more detailed look at the distribution of cerebral effects is available in Fig. 2, where the relative proportions of neurons affected from each site are shown by categories of effects. The top left box, inhibition-only, shows the relative proportions for the sample of 253 cerebrally inhibited neurons. It is evident that inhibition comes with approximately equal probability from each of the four cerebral sites tested. On the other hand, if the neuron shows mixed effects, it is less likely to receive an inhibitory influence from the post-central hand region than from other regions of the cerebral cortex. When the inhibition-only and inhibition-mixed are added to yield inhibition-total, the distribution of effects is practically uniform from the four cerebral sites. The distribution of excitation is different, being less likely to result from stimulation of the pericentral foot foci than from the hand foci, and being most prominent from the postcentral hand focus.

Among the 1,431 neurons adequately tested for cerebral influence, 1,145 were also adequately tested for antidromic response to stimulation in nucleus ventralis posterolateralis of the thalamus. Only 204 (18%) of these were classed as cuneothalamic projection neurons. As shown in Fig. 3A, cuneothalamic projection neurons had a 0.5 probability of being influenced by cerebral stimulation, whereas the putative interneurons had only a 0.3 probability of being influenced. Further, Fig. 3B shows that there was no

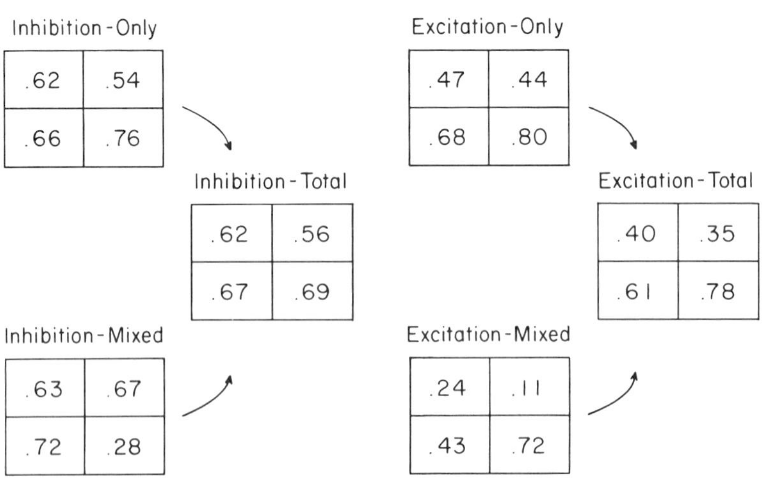

FIG. 2. Proportions of neurons in each major category showing effects, from each cerebral site. Same patterns as in Fig. 1. Middle pattern in each triad shows proportions after summing paired categories.

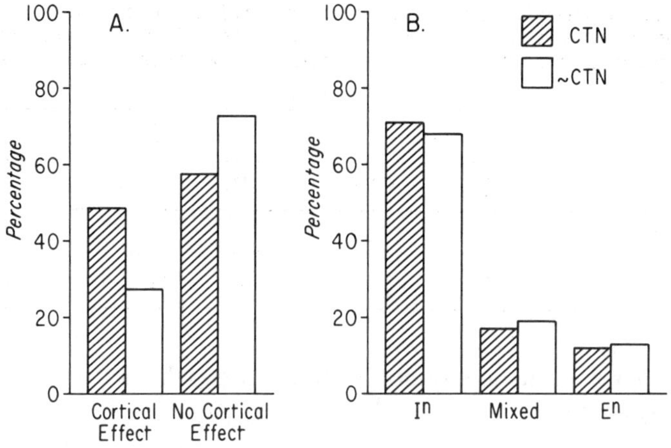

FIG. 3. Parcellation of cerebral effects on cuneothalamic projection neurons (CTN) and putative interneurons (~ CTN). **A:** Presence or absence of cerebral effects. **B:** Presence of cerebral effects, by major categories.

difference between cuneothalamic projection neurons and the putative interneurons in the types of cerebral effects to which they were subjected. This observation is incompatible with the general scheme of organization of the dorsal column nuclei proposed on the basis of observations from the domestic cat (1,2).

When partitioned into sets according to the number of digits to which each neuron was responsive—a crude measure of the size of each neuron's excitatory receptive field—the cuneothalamic projection neurons were found to distribute in nearly the same way as the putative interneurons. They showed only a slight relative increase over the putative interneurons in the single-digit category. This situation differs sharply from that described for the cat (1,7,8). Nor was a clear difference present according to the natural stimulus sensitivities of the neurons, as found in the cat (8).

Finally, in sharp contrast with the scheme for the cat, the shortest latency and strongest cerebral excitatory influences were found on cuneothalamic projection neurons, and many of these relationships could be shown to be monosynaptic (10). Table 1 shows that cuneothalamic projection neurons not only responded to cutaneous stimulation slightly earlier than the putative interneurons, but that they also responded earlier to cerebral stimulation. This latter observation may be confounded by the way in which latency was measured. Most putative interneurons required a short train of cerebral shocks, the latency being measured from the start of the train. If they received a weak monosynaptic input and required temporal summation, then the latencies stated may be misleadingly long. Also, neurons receiving an excitatory influence from the cerebral cortex responded significantly later

TABLE 1. *Mean first-spike response latencies of cuneothalamic projection neurons (CTN) and putative interneurons (~ CTN) to cutaneous cerebral and antidromic ($\bar{L}_{AD}$) stimulation, by major categories of effects.*

	Cutaneous $\bar{L}_1$		Cortex $\bar{L}_1$		$\bar{L}_{AD}$
Ctx effect	CTN	~ CTN	CTN	~ CTN	CTN
I^n	9.5	10.6	0	0	1.85
Mixed	9.6	12.9	7.0	11.9	1.61
E^n	12.1	13.5	4.3	12.2	2.22

than the other neurons to cutaneous stimulation, whether or not they were projection neurons.

DISCUSSION

The model of organization within the dorsal column nuclei of the cat is not descriptive of the cuneate nucleus of the monkey, nor is the pattern of descending cerebral influences consistent with that model. Only 29% of the neurons tested came under some form of cerebral influence. However, the effects were clearly stronger in the monkey (on those neurons that were affected) than in the cat. As in the cat, inhibition was more prevalent than excitation, but it involved cuneothalamic projection neurons and putative interneurons in equal proportions. Excitation was found on both types of neurons but was stronger on the cuneothalamic projection neurons. These observations cannot readily be brought into a simple model of organization within the dorsal column nuclei, and they show clearly the hazards in extrapolating across major phylogenetic lines, such as from carnivores to primates. Our present view suggests that fewer subcortical cells come under direct cerebral influence in primates than in carnivores, but that what cerebral influences exist are more potent in primates than in carnivores.

Control of Pain

The dorsal column–medial lemniscus system is not involved in the production of pain. On the other hand, information carried by that system modifies the sensation of pain. The gate control theory (14) proposes that large cutaneous afferent fibers "close the gate" to a hypothetical pain system. The theory provided a basis for development of a dorsal column stimulator; however, the theory is not validated by the observation that dorsal column stimulation relieves pain in certain selected patients (18). Orthodromic activity in addition to, or rather than, antidromic activity evoked by dorsal column stimulation may modulate the sensation of pain. Although Melzack and Wall (14) argued against the idea that pain is a primary sensation evoked via its own exclusive neural pathways, their "pattern" theory contains residual implications of specificity similar to those associated with the protopathic and epicritic systems envisioned by Head and Holmes (11). An alternative explanation for the success (albeit limited) of dorsal column stimulation is raised by clinical reports to the effect that "good pain relief occurs only in areas where a buzzing or tingling sensation is felt, radiating downwards throughout the body below the dorsal column electrode" (15). A "masking" sensation may be involved.

Such an idea is consistent with the modern pain specificity notion elaborated by Poggio and Mountcastle (17) and with the older notion of Head and Holmes (11). Emphasis is placed on the balance of impulse traffic in the dorsal column and anterolateral column systems rather than on inhibition of transmission in one system by activity in the other. Such "perceptual rivalry" might depend on the details of input processing at all levels of both systems rather than on a limited interaction between the two systems at the spinal level. If so, then detailed knowledge of information processing at all levels of both systems is required. Melzack and Wall (14) recognized such a possibility in connection with their putative "activity system for pain."

The foregoing ideas concerned with interactions along ascending systems are sufficient only for a system that acts as a passive receiver. A number of central processes—recognized in such concepts as set, expectation, attention, memory, and emotion—clearly modify sensation and perception. This modification was long thought to occur in the cerebral cortex, the sensory information arriving unmodified from the sense organs [see Mountcastle (16) for a modern statement of this ancient idea]. However, the discovery of cerebral modulation of ascending systems cast the nature of this interaction in a different perspective. Perhaps the system modifies its own input at all levels of ascending input (4,5,9). If so, pain input, by whatever route, should be no exception. Knowledge of the nature of this interaction should be important in formulating strategies for the control of pain.

ACKNOWLEDGMENTS

This work was supported by U.S. Public Health Service research grants NS 396 and NS 5136 from the National Institute for Neurological and Communicative Disorders and Stroke.

REFERENCES

1. Andersen, P., Eccles, J. C., Schmidt, R. F., and Yokota, T. (1964): *J. Neurophysiol.*, 27:1080–1095.
2. Blum, P., Bromberg, M. B., and Whitehorn, D. (1975): *Exp. Neurol.*, 48:57–78.
3. Cesa-Bianchi, M. G., and Sotgiu, M. L. (1969): *Brain Res.*, 13:129–139.
4. Clare, M. H., Landau, W. M., and Bishop, G. H. (1964): *Exp. Neurol.*, 9:262–267.
5. Fetz, E. E. (1968): *J. Neurophysiol.*, 31:69–80.

6. Gordon, G., and Jukes, M. G. M. (1962): *Nature*, 196:1183–1185.
7. Gordon, G., and Jukes, M. G. M. (1964*a*): *J. Physiol.* (*Lond.*), 173:263–290.
8. Gordon, G., and Jukes, M. G. M. (1964*b*): *J. Physiol.* (*Lond.*), 173:291–319.
9. Hagbarth, K. E., and Kerr, D. B. I. (1954): *J. Neurophysiol.* 81:305–318.
10. Harris, F., Jabbur, S. J., Morse, R. W., and Towe, A. L. (1965): *Nature*, 208:1215–1216.
11. Head, H., and Holmes, G. (1911): *Brain*, 34:102–254.
12. Jabbur, S. J., and Towe, A. L. (1961): *J. Neurophysiol.*, 24:499–509.
13. Levitt, M., Carreras, M., Chambers, W. W., and Liu, C. N. (1964): *Arch. Ital. Biol.*, 102:197–229.
14. Melzack, R., and Wall, P. D. (1965): *Science*, 150:971–978.
15. Mortimer, J. T. (1968): *EDC Report* No. 4-68-21.
16. Mountcastle, V. B. (1975): *Johns Hopkins Med. J.*, 136:109–131.
17. Poggio, G. F., and Mountcastle, V. B. (1960): *Johns Hopkins Med. J.*, 106:266–316.
18. Shealy, C. N., Mortimer, J. T., and Reswick, J. B. (1967): *Anesth. Analg.* (*Cleve.*) 46:489–491.
19. Towe, A. L., and Jabbur, S. J. (1961): *J. Neurophysiol.*, 24:488–498.

Advances in Pain Research and Therapy, Vol. 1,
edited by J. J. Bonica and D. Albe-Fessard.
Raven Press, New York © 1976.

Mechanoreceptive and Nociceptive Thresholds During Dorsal Column Stimulation in Man

U. Lindblom and B. A. Meyerson

Department of Neurology, Huddinge Hospital, 141 86 Huddinge, and Department of Neurosurgery, Karolinska Sjukhuset, 104 01 Stockholm, Sweden

The recently developed technique of electrical stimulation of the dorsal columns of the spinal cord, percutaneously or with implanted electrodes (6,8), for the relief of pain offers a possibility to study the effect of such stimulation on sensory functions. The first aim of the present investigation was to study how dorsal column stimulation (DCS) interfered with tactile and vibratory sensations, which are thought to be primarily dependent on the dorsal column system. The second aim was to measure the effect of DCS on some nociceptive functions in patients with chronic pain, and the third to seek an objective criterion for the adequate selection of patients for electrode implantation when tested with percutaneous DCS. For some unknown reason, it does not seem possible to predict the therapeutic effect of DCS from clinical data or preoperative transcutaneous nerve stimulation (TNS).

METHODS

The sample consisted of 10 patients with various types of chronic pain. The most common diagnoses were low back pain and causalgic postoperative pain. DCS was performed via implanted electrodes or percutaneously with Medtronics equipment. The sensory functions were studied with quantitative methods described in more detail elsewhere (3,4). The vibratory sense was tested with a 100-Hz sinusoidal stimulus, which was applied with a standardized technique at selected points, most often in the tarsal and carpal regions. The tactile stimulus consisted of a half-cycle sinusoidal pulse delivered from a mechanical stimulator and applied to the fingers, toes, or soles of the feet. The perception thresholds for both vibration and touch were determined with the method of limits and expressed in micrometers. Mechanical pain was induced with a flat forceps by which a fold of the skin was pinched and the threshold was determined in grams per square millimeter. The heat pain threshold was measured with a Peltier element device (MARSTOCK®) (7) by which the warmth-cold difference limen also could be studied.

RESULTS

DCS at a strength that reduced or abolished spontaneous pain regularly evoked paresthesias, which first appeared in the pain area. It is not known if this was owing to facilitation accompanying the pain state or simply to successful positioning of the electrodes on the dorsal columns. With increasing strength of DCS, the paresthesias spread distally in the trunk and leg. In some but not all cases paresthesias could be evoked, with high stimulus strengths, contralaterally to the side of the pain.

DCS at strengths which produced paresthesias caused an increase of the vibratory and tactile thresholds below the level of electrode implantation in all cases in which DCS was effective for pain relief. The threshold increase could be recorded even outside the area of paresthesias, for instance, in the leg when paresthesias were only in the trunk. It occurred also contralaterally, although this was less marked, when paresthesias were confined to the pain side. Occasionally the thresholds were influenced by DCS that was liminal or just subliminal for production of paresthesias.

The increase of the mechanoreceptive thresholds outlasted the DCS but recovered within some minutes, whereas pain usually did not recur for 1 hr or more. The optimal frequency of DCS for pain relief generally caused the greatest threshold increase, but there was no direct relation between the frequency and the threshold increase as would be the case if it were due solely to blocking of the primary afferent fibers.

DCS also interfered with the sensation evoked by a suprathreshold vibratory or tactile stimulus. Depending on the strength of DCS, the sensation produced by a mechanical stimulus of 2 to 10 times the threshold value could be blocked for poststimulatory periods of 5 to 30 sec. The sensation disappeared and reappeared gradually as is illustrated schematically in Fig. 1. The tactile sensation evoked by a pulse of two times the threshold amplitude, which was applied to the great toe, was successively reduced during DCS. When the strength of the DCS was just supraliminal for eliciting paresthesias in the pain area, which in this case was in the lower thorax, the tactile sensation gradually faded and disappeared after 100 sec of DCS (*open circles* in Fig. 1). When higher intensities of DCS were used, the disappearance time of the tactile sensation was reduced to 45 and 25 sec, respectively (*filled circles* and *triangles* in Fig. 1). In each experiment DCS was stopped as soon as the sensation was reported to have disappeared. After 5 to 10 sec it reappeared, and during the next 45 to 60 sec it gradually recovered to the original intensity.

The time course of the changes of both threshold and suprathreshold sensations during DCS and the fact that these changes could be recorded outside the area of paresthesias indicate that DCS exerts its influence on the mechanoreceptive functions by producing a central inhibitory state;

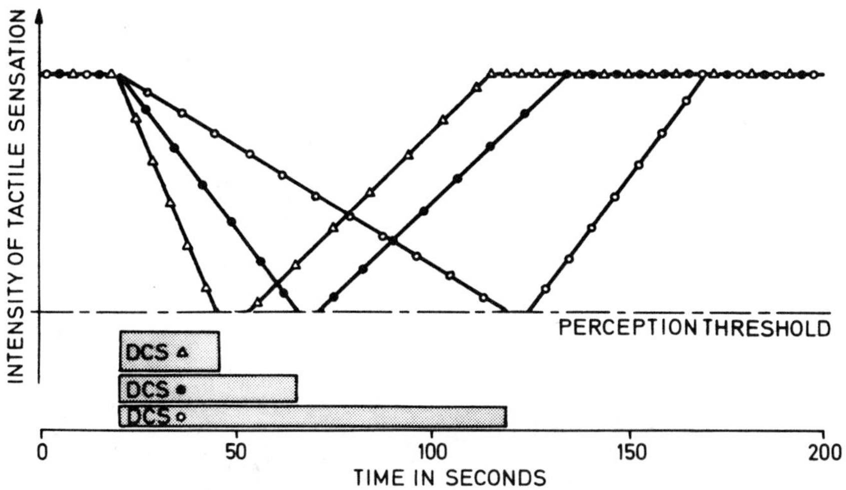

FIG. 1. Schematic illustration of effect of DCS on perception of a tactile stimulus applied to the volar surface of the great toe. Stimulus consisted of short mechanical pulses of 2 times threshold strength (450 μm), which were delivered at a rate of 3 Hz. DCS of 3 different strengths (and durations) was used: liminal for paresthesias in the pain area in the lower thorax region (○); slightly stronger with paresthesias also in the leg (●); and still stronger with paresthesias extending into the foot (△) but not into the toe where the tactile stimulus was applied.

DCS does not act simply by antidromic discharges or local blocking of the primary afferents.

In contrast to its effects on mechanoreceptive functions, DCS did not influence the normal pain threshold even though spontaneous pain was blocked. This was valid for pain evoked by both mechanical and heat stimulation and for different skin regions above and below the level of electrode implantation.

Some of the patients displayed causalgic-type hyperesthesia within the pain area. The nociceptive thresholds within these skin areas were abnormally low. Thus the mechanical pain threshold could amount to only 20% of the value obtained in the homologous, contralateral normal skin area. During DCS the lowered pain threshold increased toward normal values simultaneously with the gradual suppression of spontaneous pain. The higher threshold was sustained during the poststimulatory pain-free period which sometimes lasted for several hours. The heat pain threshold and the warmth-cold difference limen displayed similar changes as illustrated in Fig. 2. The difference in temperature when the patient felt the testing probe to be warm and cold, respectively, was considerably smaller, approximately 1°C (*upper left* in Fig. 2A), in the causalgic pain area compared to that in the homologous, contralateral unaffected skin area (*upper*

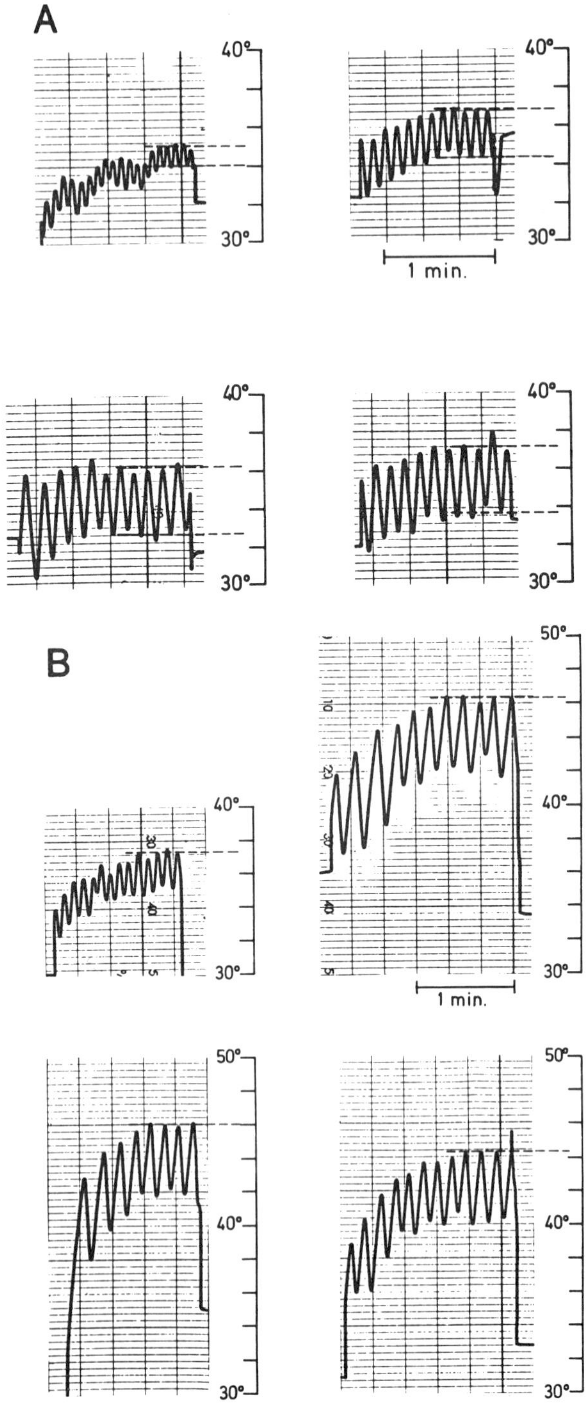
A
40°
30°
1 min.
B
50°
40°
30°
1 min.

right). During DCS the temperature difference limen gradually increased toward a normal value (*bottom records* in Fig. 2A). This change occurred simultaneously with the suppression of pain, although with a slightly different time course. Thus in the case illustrated in Fig. 2, the pain was abolished after 5 min. whereas the normalization of the temperature difference limen required another 15 min of DCS. In Fig. 2B are shown the changes in heat pain threshold caused by DCS. An abnormally low threshold was recorded in the pain area. After DCS, this threshold had increased to a level corresponding to that of the control side (lower records in Fig. 2B). The normalization of the pain threshold followed that of the temperature difference limen and persisted throughout the poststimulatory pain-free period.

COMMENTS

In a previous study (4,5) it was shown that the vibratory and tactile perception thresholds were increased during and after DCS. In the present chapter it has been demonstrated that also suprathreshold functions may be similarly influenced. For several reasons it is probable that these effects are due not to blocking of the primary afferents but to central inhibitory mechanisms.

The effects of DCS on the mechanoreceptive functions appeared in parallel with the suppression of pain but with a shorter time course. The two phenomena could be caused by related mechanisms. It may be significant that, among the examined patients, DCS had no effect on the pain in only 1 patient, and this was the only patient in whom the mechanoreceptive functions were uninfluenced.

In contrast to what has been found with TNS (1,2), DCS did not cause hypalgesia as tested by mechanical or heat pain stimulation of threshold strength. The nociceptive thresholds were changed only within hyperesthetic pain areas with disturbed nociception. These changes occurred simultaneously with the suppression of the spontaneous pain, and they are a further indication that DCS acts selectively on pathologic pain mechanisms and not on acute physiologic pain.

←

FIG. 2. Records obtained during thermostimulation of skin with Marstock® device to illustrate effect of DCS on warmth and cold sensations and on heat pain threshold in a patient with chronic postoperative abdominal pain and hyperpathia. Thermode was applied to pain area on the right side and to the homologous area on the left side, which served as control. **A:** *Right,* pain side; *left,* control. Warmth-cold difference limen (*dashed lines*) before (*top records*) and after (*bottom records*) 20 min of DCS of optimal intensity for pain relief. **B:** *Right,* pain side; *left,* control. Heat pain threshold (*dashed line*) before (*top records*) and after (*bottom records*) DCS as in **A.**

ACKNOWLEDGMENTS

The study was supported by grants from Karolinska Institutet and from the Swedish Medical Research Council (B75–14X–4256–02 and B75–14X–4505–02).

REFERENCES

1. Campbell, J. N., and Taub, A. (1973): *Arch. Neurol.*, 28:347–350.
2. Fields, H. L., Adams, J. E., and Hosobuchi, Y. (1974): In: *Advances in Neurology, Vol. 4: International Symposium on Pain,* edited by J. J. Bonica, pp. 749-754. Raven Press, New York.
3. Lindblom, U. (1974): *Brain Res.,* 82:205–210.
4. Lindbolm, U., and Meyerson, B. A. (1976*a*): *Pain,* 1:257–270.
5. Lindbolm, U., and Meyerson, B. A. (1976*b*): In: *Progress in Brain Research, Vol. 43: Somatosensory and Visceral Receptor Mechanisms,* edited by A. Iggo and O. B. Ilyinsky, pp. 237–241. Elsevier, Amsterdam.
6. Nashold, B. S., Jr., and Friedman, H. (1972): *J. Neurosurg.*, 36:590–597.
7. Schmidt, W. G., Lindbolm, U., and Fruhstorfer, H. (1976): *Pfluegers Arch.* (*in press*).
8. Shealy, C. N., Mortimer, J. T., and Hagfors, N. R. (1970): *J. Neurosurg.,* 32:560–564.

Advances in Pain Research and Therapy, Vol. 1,
edited by J. J. Bonica and D. Albe-Fessard.
Raven Press, New York © 1976.

Modulation of Experimentally Produced Pain in Man by Electrical Stimulation of Some Cortical, Thalamic, and Basal Ganglia Structures

Jan Gybels, Johan Van Hees, and Franco Peluso

Department of Neurology and Neurosurgery, K.U.L.,
Kapucijnenvoer 35, B-3000 Leuven, Belgium

In recent years, an important body of experimental evidence has been obtained in rat, cat, and monkey which strongly suggests that electrical stimulation of certain brain structures produces analgesia (6). However, in human, almost no such data are available except for a few clinical reports (5).

In this chapter, we describe results we have gathered in man on this problem during the last 10 years. A preliminary report has been published previously (1).

METHODS

To test the modulating effects of brain stimulation on pain sensation, we use a strategy in which the subject has to make comparisons of the subjective intensity of two equally noxious electrical skin stimuli St_1 and St_2, a brain structure being stimulated during the second noxious stimulus. Three categories of judgment are permitted: the sensation (S_2) provoked by the second stimulus is equal to ($S_2 = S_1$) or greater ($S_2 > S_1$) or smaller ($S_2 < S_1$) than the sensation (S_1) provoked by the first stimulus. This strategy is designed to avoid the use of a verbal response as an objective response without testing its reliability. The structures of the brain stimulated are determined by the use of scatterograms constructed from computer data [for stimulation details, see Gybels et al. (1), and for details of plotting stimulated brain structures, see Gybels et al. (2)].

RESULTS

In Fig. 1 are summarized the results obtained from 26 cooperative patients who underwent stereotactic surgery for a variety of diseases. The table in this figure shows that for the brain structures we could explore, hypalgesia could be obtained only from stimulation of the contralateral primary thalamic somatosensory relay nuclei ventralis posterolateral

Structure	Number of cases	Number of stim. (100 csec, 1 msec, 10 sec; 0.5 - 2 mA)	$S_2 < S_1$	$S_2 = S_1$	$S_2 > S_1$
Frontal cortex (area 9 ?)	9	160	24	102	34
Parietal cortex (area 19 ? - 39 ?)	12	119	39	50	30
Nucleus caudatus and Fundus striati	4	31	1	28	2
V.P.L. and Vcpc	17, 2] 19	290, 16] 306	141, 12] 153	112, 2] 114	37, 2] 39
C.M. - Pf.	3	23	2	19	2
V.L.	10	79	20	52	7

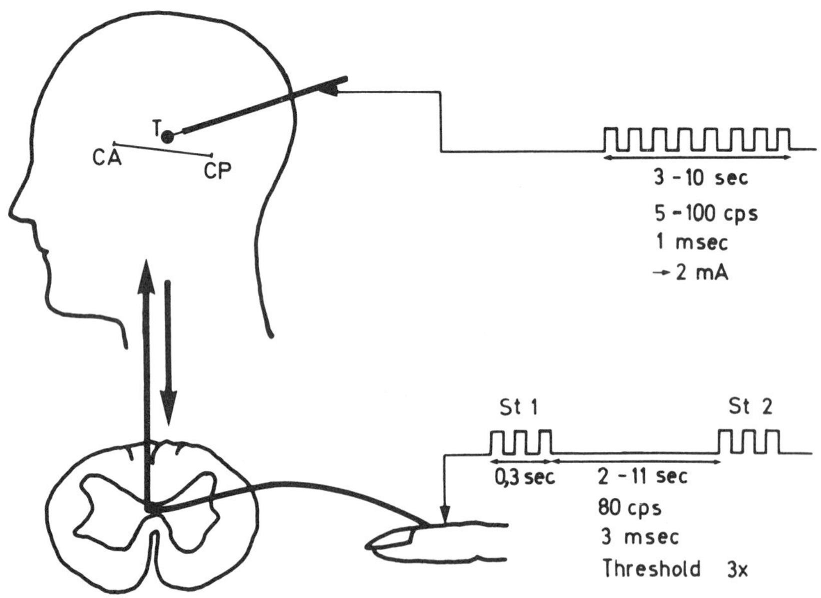

FIG. 1. Schematic representation of experimental arrangement for testing modulation of experimentally evoked pain by brain stimulation. Table shows results of stimulation.

(VPL), ventralis corporis (Vcpc), and possibly adjacent areas. The diminution or even disappearance of the pain sensation evoked by electrical stimulation of the skin was observed only when this noxious stimulus was around threshold, whereas for noxious skin stimulation at approximately three times threshold, no modulation of pain sensation was present. Together with the decrease of the experimental pain sensation by stimulation of VPL-Vcpc, the patients usually reported paresthesias, and sometimes movement was observed in the limb contralateral to the stimulated thalamus.

Stimulation of finger		Sensation	Result
weak	0.2 mA	touch	masking effect
threshold for	0.5 mA	pinprick	masking effect
2 to 3 × threshold	1.5 mA	disagreeable pinprick	no effect
20 to 30 × threshold on ischemic finger	10 mA	very disagreeable, burning	no effect

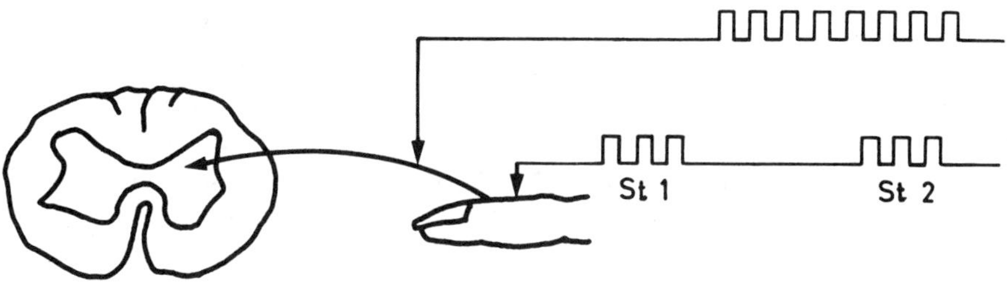

FIG. 2. Schematic representation of experimental arrangement for testing modulation of experimentally evoked pain by peripheral nerve stimulation. Table shows summary of results.

These results are comparable to those we obtained in a second type of experiment. Using the same experimental strategy, we stimulated the peripheral nerve innervating the area of skin on which the noxious electrical stimulus was applied. Results of these experiments are summarized in the table of Fig. 2.

DISCUSSION

In order to interpret the results presented in this chapter, one has to consider such factors as the use of electricity as a noxious stimulus, the estimation of the reliability of a verbal response, and the significance of experimental pain as a model for clinical pain. We refer the reader to the vast literature bearing on these problems.

Of considerable interest in the context of control of pain by brain stimulation is our finding that a decrease of peripherally evoked pain sensation was observed only when the specific somatosensory relay nuclei in the thalamus were stimulated. The central stimulus evoked paresthesias where the noxious stimulus was applied, and the noxious stimulus was not stronger than approximately three times threshold. This last value is far from the maximal pain and can be estimated at approximately 3 dols (J. Gybels, *in preparation*) on the pain scale as constructed by Hardy et al. (3). This makes one wonder, in view of reported clinical results (4), if the difference in terms of nervous activity between bearable and unbearable pain may be small indeed. In order to increase the significance of our findings, we should be able to extend our observations to those brain structures which when stimulated in animal experiments strongly suggest a powerful analgesic action. Up till now, we thought such stimulation was unacceptable for ethical considerations.

SUMMARY

We have tested in man the influence of electrical stimulation of the brain on an experimentally evoked pain sensation. The results showed that: (a) in the absence of paresthesias—as was the case when the frontal and parietal cortex, and nuclei centrum medianum, posterior, ventrolateralis, and caudatus were stimulated—no modulation of pain sensation was observed; (b) when the subject experienced paresthesias, as was the case with nuclei VPL-ventralis posterior mediale, Vcpc stimulation, there was a masking effect for pain sensation near the threshold. With more intense pain-provoking stimuli, no such effect was seen.

ACKNOWLEDGMENTS

We are grateful to Mrs. Feytons-Heeren and Mr. P. De Sutter for their skillful technical assistance. The investigation was supported by the F.G.W.O. (Grants 1212 and 20492) of Belgium.

REFERENCES

1. Gybels, J., Carton, H., Cosyns, P., and Peluso, F. (1972): In: *Pain: Basic Principles—Pharmacology—Therapy,* edited by R. Janzen, W. D. Keidel, A. Herz, and C. Steichele, pp. 128–131. Georg Thieme, Stuttgart.
2. Gybels, J., Kempen, D., Peluso, F., and Vanbael, M. (1974): *Confin. Neurol.,* 36:302–309.
3. Hardy, J. D., Wolff, H. G., and Goodell, H. (1948): *J. Clin. Invest.,* 27:380–386.
4. Hosobuchi, Y., Adams, J. E., and Fields, H. L. (1974): In: *Advances in Neurology, Vol. 4: International Symposium on Pain,* edited by J. J. Bonica, pp. 783–787. Raven Press, New York.
5. Long, D. M., and Hagfors, N. (1975): *Pain,* 1:109–123.
6. Oliveras, J. L., Redjemi, F., Guilbaud, G., and Besson, J. M. (1975): *Pain,* 1:139–145.

Advances in Pain Research and Therapy, Vol. 1,
edited by J. J. B·nica and D. Albe-Fessard.
Raven Press, New York © 1976.

Pain Patient Selection for Implantable Stimulating Devices

Donald L. Erickson, Margaret A. Michaelson,
and Atashi Acharya

*Department of Neurosurgery, University of Minnesota,
Minneapolis, Minnesota 55455*

Electrical stimulation of the nervous system for the relief of pain remains an investigative tool. None of the presently available implantable systems are so uniformly effective that success can be readily predicted in the treatment of a pain problem. Much of the initial enthusiasm has waned as the high percentage of early successes has often turned into a high percentage of late failures. Problems remain in both instrumentation and selection of appropriate patients. During the past 2 years, we have attempted to develop a set of criteria and a plan of preimplantation treatment that would allow us to select patients who are more likely to have effective pain relief with an implantable device. This plan was based on the assumption that the available implantable systems did physiologically affect the perception of pain. As will be evident from the results, this assumption may have been inaccurate, and in spite of attempting to resolve nonphysiologic social and emotional problems preoperatively, we have not been able to select accurately for success. We have, however, been able to evaluate more effectively the various implantable devices. This chapter presents what we believe to be a reasonable approach to the selection and evaluation of patients for implantation of stimulating systems.

METHODS

Criteria

It is well accepted that chronic pain patients have a multifaceted problem, including physical, social, and psychological aspects. The following criteria were established in an attempt to exclude possible secondary gains in the social and psychological realm related to surgical implantation.

1. The patient must have a clinically acceptable physiologic cause for his pain, for which there is no standard medical or surgical treatment.
2. The patient can have no major psychopathology, as assessed by clinical observation and psychological testing.
3. The patient must have a reasonably stable social setting. This is

divided into three areas: domestic, future plans, and financial stability. We prefer that the patient has a stable marriage, but certainly do not exclude other stable domestic settings. The patient must have rational future goals that are attainable regardless of the failure or success of the implant. Lastly, by financial stability, we mean that the implantation of the device will not document his disability or in any other way relate to a secondary financial gain. We accept the possibility that the improvement achieved with a successful system might allow him to become more employable, and in that way enhance his future earnings.

4. All patients must be completely off narcotics, barbiturates, and other similar analgesic medications.

5. The patient must have successful pain relief with a percutaneous trial of stimulation (2).

One might assume that if all the above criteria are met, the patient is functional and in need of no further treatment. Often this is true, but it is also observed that many patients remain entirely functional in spite of chronic pain problems. Those patients have what we would like to call a "pure pain" problem. One can have some degree of confidence that if such a patient reports pain control, the implanted system is indeed affecting pain on a physiological level, rather than indirectly through a host of social and psychological mechanisms. Most patients need a period of preimplantation treatment to attain the above criteria.

Behavioral Modification Pretreatment

The patients are admitted for a 2-week period of behavioral modification. Implantation is not generally discussed with them, and they are presented with the idea that behavioral modification will be the definitive treatment for them. If they successfully complete the behavioral modification program with drug detoxification and significant activity improvement, they will then be considered as candidates for implantation of a stimulating system. As one might expect, our experience has been that after the period of behavioral modification, most patients do not need or do not wish any further surgical intervention. Out of approximately 100 patients so treated in the past 18 months, only 10 have ultimately undergone some type of implantation. An additional 25 met the criteria for implantation initially or achieved them without a formal period of behavioral modification. We occasionally did an implant out of desperation in a patient who did not meet the criteria, but we were uniformly disappointed with the result.

RESULTS

The question of how to evaluate the success or failure of an implanted system has yet to be fully answered. Apparent success in a patient who has emotional disturbance, social dislocation, or drug addiction cannot

TABLE 1. *Results with various stimulating devices*

Type of stimulation	Cases	Success No.	Success %
Dorsal spinal cord	11	1	9
Peripheral nerve	16	8	50
Anterior spinal cord	8	4	50

necessarily be attributed to any physiologic effect of the device. A decrease in narcotic intake and increase in activity are often cited as criteria of success, but as has been established by behavioral modification studies, these may be the mechanisms of pain reduction rather than the result (3). It has been our experience that detoxification from narcotic drugs has rarely produced an increase in pain, and almost invariably produced a decrease in pain. Similarly, if a patient is extremely inactive because of a pain problem, he will experience much greater pain than when he is under a rational exercise program. We have also seen numerous patients who have claimed pain relief with an implantation but continue to be inactive and take narcotics at the same level as preoperatively. How, then, can one determine in a patient who has an apparently successful result with implantation whether the implanted device or the whole mileau of medical treatment has benefited him?

Our pretreatment program and criteria list is our attempt to eliminate all the extraneous factors that may confuse the evaluation of a patient's response to an implanted system. If indeed the patient is physically functional, drug-free, and has no apparent secondary gains from the implantation, one can then put more credence in his statement of the pain-relieving effect of the device. This coupled with objective improvement in activity are the measures of success in our clinic. It is our opinion that until such rigid demands are placed on the patients before implantation, we will continue to have the confusing contradictions regarding the results of the various implantable systems (1,5,6).

Using this plan of selection, we have evaluated results in dorsal cord stimulation, peripheral nerve stimulation, and anterior spinal cord stimulation (Table 1).

One must take into consideration that with this preimplantation treatment program, even if the device was a failure, the patient was prepared to function at a satisfactory level in spite of that failure. We therefore attempt to avoid the confusion that was present in some previous reports where the device was listed as a success but the patient was listed as a failure.

DISCUSSION

As one can see from the above results, our experience with dorsal column stimulation in this highly selected group is dismal. None of these patients have reported excellent pain relief or shown any objective signs in their life style which would indicate a bonified success, even though nearly all of them had a technically successful implant based on production of paresthesias covering their entire pain area. This might suggest that when one has eliminated the secondary gains, dorsal cord stimulation is less effective.

Our single, most frustrating problem in peripheral nerve stimulation has been the increasing sensory threshold, which makes continued use of the device impossible because of motor stimulation. In the 8 failures, only 2 were able to produce paresthesias at a submotor threshold. The patients with successful implants have continued to do well for a period of 12 to 18 months.

Our work with anterior spinal stimulation is of a preliminary nature but appears to offer some future promise (4). Because stimulation is at a subclinical threshold, the patient can function without continuous paresthesias. It is also possible to test the devices double-blind in a further effort to assess their physiologic function. Three of the four failures did not have a physiologically functioning system based on the inability to record evoked cortical potentials at a submotor threshold. Many technical problems have yet to be resolved in this form of stimulation.

CONCLUSIONS

Even with rigid criteria we have been unable to select successes uniformly, at least in part because none of the available systems are sufficiently predictable in their function on the nervous system. Nevertheless, we believe we can at least select patients who will report a meaningful result of the success or failure of a stimulating device. A further advantage of this preimplantation treatment and selection is that the patient is prepared to contend with his problem, even in the face of a surgical failure.

REFERENCES

1. Burton, C. (1975): *Surg. Neurol.*, 4:171–179.
2. Erickson, D. L. (1976): *J. Neurosurg. (in press).*
3. Fordyce, W. E., Fowler, R. S., Lehmann, J. F., DeLateur, B. J., Sand, P. L., and Treschmann, R. B. (1973): *Arch. Phys. Med. Rehabil.*, 54:399–408.
4. Larson, S., Sances, A., Jr., Cusick, J. F., Meyer, G. A., Swiontek, T. (1975): *Surg. Neurol.*, 4:180–186.
5. Long, D. M., and Erickson, D. E. (1975): *Surg. Neurol.*, 4:134–141.
6. Nashold, B. S., Jr. (1975): *Surg. Neurol.*, 4:146–147.

Advances in Pain Research and Therapy, Vol. 1,
edited by J. J. Bonica and D. Albe-Fessard.
Raven Press, New York © 1976.

Contribution of Thalamic Stimulation to the Physiopathology of Pain

G. J. Mazars, L. Merienne, and C. Cioloca

Saint Anne's Hospital, 75674 Paris, Cedex 14, France

An extensive study of electrical stimulation of the sensory pathways and relays, usually during surgical procedures for the relief of pain, suggested the use of electrical stimulation of the nucleus ventralis posterolateralis (VPL) for the relief of some types of intractable pain (6).

METHODS

Between 1962 and 1972, 17 patients had thalamic electrodes implanted and connected for several weeks to an externally placed stimulator. Since 1972, 28 patients have received an implanted stimulator with an electronic switch turned on by means of a magnet. Bipolar electrodes were stereotactically implanted in the portion of the VPL corresponding somatotopically to the site of pain (2,3–5).

The best parameters of stimulation are: 10/sec impulses of 2 msec, 1 V. Stimulation for 1 to 3 min produces a light feeling of "buzzing" or throbbing, which is never painful and is referred to the area of pain. In well-selected patients, pain "vanishes" after 1 to 3 min, even if no sensation is felt during stimulation. The relief of pain lasts for several hours or days, and a few daily stimulations are enough to prevent recurrence of the pain or to stop it when it recurs.

RESULTS

This procedure fails to relieve pain in: (a) true *tic douloureux* and thalamic syndromes with an actual lesion of the posterior thalamus, (b) nerve root compression, (c) pain due to cancer.

On the contrary, stimulation of the VPL resulted in complete control of pain in: (a) traumatic avulsion of the brachial plexus; (b) postradiotherapeutic lesions of the brachial plexus; (c) medullary and pontine cerebrovascular lesions; (d) postherpetic lesions; (e) analgesia dolorosa following alcohol block or Kirschner's operation; (f) some atypical trigeminal neuralgias including Benisti's syndrome (orbital pain following enucleation of the eyeball); (g) phantom limb pain; (h) caustic lesions and traumatic scars of large nerve trunks; and (i) paraplegias with diffuse spontaneous pain in both legs.

The specificity of action of stimulation of the VPL is consistent with the opinion that pain depends on two main physiological schemes: an excess of noxious stimuli and a lack of proprioceptive information due to interruption of discriminative sensory fibers or to a lesion of integration centers.

Additional evidence for this twofold mechanism is to be found in the following case histories demonstrating that in patients otherwise well relieved of their chronic pain by VPL stimulation, pain arising from peripheral lesions may need quite a different management.

Case Histories

Case 1 (Rich., 82 years). Traumatic avulsion of the brachial plexus; loss of discriminative sensibilities over the whole arm and shoulder; hyperpathia and causalgic pain. Thalamic stimulation controls the causalgia and hyperpathia for 2 to 24 hr, but mobilization of the shoulder remains painful because of periarthritis which requires periarticular injections of lidocaine.

Case 2 (Bis., 56 years). Post-traumatic amputation of the left arm with continuous and paroxysmal pain referred to the missing arm and a part of the stump. A dorsal column stimulator implanted in another hospital produced no improvement. Electrostimulation of the skin as well as of the median and ulnar nerves proved useless. Thalamic stimulation "rubs off" the pain for 2 to 6 hr, and the phantom is reduced in size and its shape modified. Although diffuse pain in the stump is well controlled, shoulder periarthritis is responsible for pain on mobilization of the joint and requires procaine and corticoid injections. Pressure on the scar produces some sharp "electric" pain even during thalamic stimulation, whereas procaine block of the median nerve is active for several hours.

Case 3 (Hui., 32 years). Amputation of the right leg after a dislocation of the knee. Diffuse excruciating pain is referred to the stump and the phantom limb. Rhizotomies of L_3-L_4-L_5, dorsal column stimulation, and resection of a supposed neuroma were ineffective. Electrical stimulation of the VPL leaves the patient pain free for several hours, although pressure at the extremity of the stump still produces unpleasant "electrical discharges" interfering with the use of a prosthesis.

Case 4 (Cas., 51 years). Breast cancer. Halstedt's operation and cobalt therapy resulted in massive sensory and motor impairment of the brachial plexus and severe trophedema improved by omentopexy. Anesthesia dolorosa extended over the arm and axilla. Neurolysis of the brachial plexus as well as procaine blocks of the plexus had no effect on pain. Electrostimulation of the VPL for 3 min left the patient pain free for several hours. A felon developed some time later on the left thumb, producing some sharp pain "about" the hand and persisting despite stimulation until the pus had been drained. In addition, the patient noted that periarthritis remained painful, although stimulation relieved pain in the arm.

DISCUSSION

How electrical stimulation of the VPL works is still an unsolved problem. It might be considered to act as a substitute for absent proprioceptive stimuli when pain is related to a lack of proprioceptive information owing to interruption of the large A fibers. Similarly, it acts when a lesion in some relay nucleus is responsible for a mechanism of deafferentation. The lack of action of dorsal column stimulation, which has been proven in some of our cases, shows that the control of pain is not the consequence of downward stimuli reaching a spinal "gate control system" via the dorsal columns.

The above-mentioned facts do not fit with Melzack's gate theory and tend to prove that the main level of integration of pain as such is in the posterior thalamus instead of the cord. It is our opinion that the electrodes placed by Adams et al. (1) in cases of chronic pain are in the VPL and not in the internal capsule as described by the authors. Thus their results fit fairly well with our own experience.

Stimulation of the VPL cannot be related to stimulation of the inferior and dorsal central nuclei of the raphe since the serotoninergic mechanism involved is mostly active on nociception (7). As a matter of fact, pain is relieved by thalamic stimulation, an anatomical background of sensory deafferentation is present, whereas pain related to some abnormal, excessive, or simply high level of nociception remains unmodified by thalamic stimulation. The two types of pain can exist simultaneously over the same area.

Operations combining interruption of the spinothalamic tract and stimulation of the VPL have already proved to be of some value in cancer pain and are to be extended to some other conditions.

ACKNOWLEDGMENTS

This work has been supported by the Fonds de recherches scientifiques, C.R.H.M. Hôpital St. Anne (Mr. O. Rouquet, Directeur), with the assistance of Biomedix Cy, who built the stimulators to our specifications.

REFERENCES

1. Adams, J. E., Hosobuchi, Y., and Fields, H. L. (1974): *J. Neurosurg.*, 41:740–744.
2. Mazars, G. (1975): *Surg. Neurol.*, 4:93–95.
3. Mazars, G., Merienne, L., and Cioloca, C. (1973): *Rev. Neurol.*, 128:273–279.
4. Mazars, G., Merienne, L., and Cioloca, C. (1974): *Neurochirurgie*, 20, 2:117–124.
5. Mazars, G., Merienne, L., and Cioloca, C. (1976): *Societe Medicale des Hopitaux de Paris (in press)*.
6. Mazars, G., Rogé, R., and Mazars, Y. (1960): *Rev. Neurol.*, 79:213–215.
7. Oliveras, J. L., Redjemi, F., Guilbaud, G., and Besson, J.-M. (1975): *Pain*, 1:139–145.

Advances in Pain Research and Therapy, Vol. 1,
edited by J. J. Bonica and D. Albe-Fessard.
Raven Press, New York © 1976.

Modification of Midbrain and Thalamic Evoked Responses by Analgesic Brain Stimulation in the Rat

Terrence D. Oleson and John C. Liebeskind

Department of Psychology, University of California, Los Angeles, California 90024

Previous reports (9,10) have shown that electrical stimulation of the midbrain central gray abolishes behavioral responses to painful stimuli without producing a generalized deficit in sensory, emotional, or motor responses. Brain stimulation–produced analgesia appears to reduce sensory responses to nociceptive stimuli selectively. Liebeskind et al. (8) and Oliveras et al. (13) have provided evidence that this inhibition may occur at the lowest central level of the somatic sensory pathway. They found that single units of the lamina V–type of the spinal cord exhibited reduced responsiveness to noxious but not to innocuous stimuli after stimulation of central gray. In contrast, units of the lamina IV–type, which principally respond to localized, innocuous stimuli, are not affected by midbrain stimulation.

The purpose of the present study was to extend this investigation of the neurophysiological effects of brain stimulation–produced analgesia to higher levels of the central nervous system. Different areas of the brain known to be activated by nociceptive stimuli were examined before and after central gray stimulation. Single units primarily responsive to nociceptive input have been observed in a number of brain regions including the ventrobasal thalamus (3,14), the medial thalamus (4,12), the central gray (1), and the bulbar reticular formation (2,5) of lightly anesthetized animals. Casey et al. (6) showed that the nociceptive responses of bulboreticular units are inhibited by central gray stimulation. In the present work, therefore, we studied the ventrobasal and medial thalamus and the central gray. As there is no *a priori* reason to suspect that pain perception is better reflected by the firing rates of individual neurons than by cell clusters or slow wave activity, we recorded both evoked potentials and multiple-unit responses. This technique allowed us to record neural and behavioral responses simultaneously in awake, only partially restrained rats. Since the perception of pain in animals can be assessed only by examination of the animal's behavior, alterations in neural activity owing to brain stimulation can be most appropriately related to behavioral analgesia when the two are simultaneously monitored.

METHODS

Bipolar stimulating electrodes were chronically implanted in the midbrain central gray, and concentric, bipolar recording electrodes (tip made from 100-μm formvar-coated, stainless steel wire) were placed in the contralateral central gray, the medial thalamus, and the ventrobasal thalamus of 30 albino rats. Testing began 2 weeks after surgery. Animals were restrained on a raised platform, and skin potential disc electrodes were attached to the left hindpaw and the base of the tail for differential recording. Shock needle electrodes were inserted into the right hindpaw, and heart rate and EMG needle electrodes were placed across the chest and neck, respectively. Leg flexion was quantified by fastening a string to the right hindpaw which led to a lever attached to a light (Fig. 1). The light then shone on a photocell potentiometer, and as the position of the lever varied when the animal lifted his paw, there was a corresponding alteration of the voltage applied across the potentiometer.

To minimize movement artifact contamination of the neural recordings, we passed the electrode wires through field effect transistor (FET) circuitry (15) mounted on the animal's head (Fig. 1) and then through low-noise Microdot cable before amplification. Simultaneous recording of multiple-unit and slow wave activity from the same electrode was achieved by differential filtering (18). Evoked potentials were obtained from the output of a low-pass filter, and multiple-unit responses were first high-pass filtered, then sent through a Schmitt trigger and integrated. EEG recordings were made from cortical screws. Behavioral responses and integrated multiple-unit activity were written on a polygraph, and evoked potentials and inte-

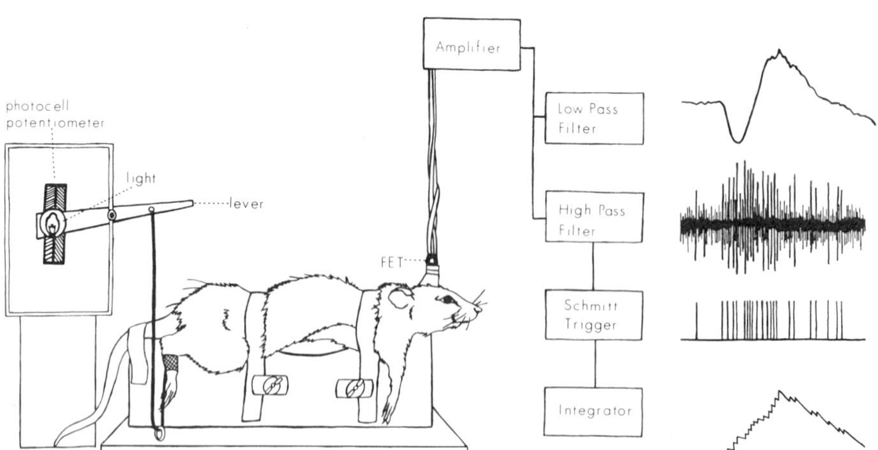

FIG. 1. Apparatus for restraining rat, measuring leg flexion, and selectively filtering evoked potential and multiple-unit responses.

grated multiple-unit responses were averaged by a Hewlett-Packard signal analyzer. Brain stimulation parameters from a constant current BERL stimulator were set at 50-Hz, 100-μsec pulses presented in 100-msec bursts at a rate of 3/sec, 1 to 10 mA.

RESULTS

Noxious pinprick, pinch, and shock elicited vigorous lifting of the leg, with the strongest flexion responses occurring after pinch. These specific limb reflexes were accompanied by vocalizations, large skin-potential responses (SPR), and strong neck electromyogram responses indicative of general body struggling. Initially, application of innocuous touch and air puff stimuli also elicited moderate leg flexion, SPR, and EMG responses, but these responses were smaller in amplitude and habituated within a few trials. Electrical stimulation in the vicinity of the midbrain central gray greatly reduced leg flexion responses to noxious stimuli in 24 of the 30 rats. Diminished leg flexion was accompanied by smaller SPR, little or no neck EMG response, and a total absence of vocalization. Thus the flexion response of the specific limb which was stimulated and the withdrawal reaction of the body as a whole, including autonomic as well as skeletal components, were reduced by central gray stimulation. Analgesic brain stimulation produced little or no alteration in tonic heart rate or cortical EEG.

In the ventrobasal thalamus (VB), medial thalamus (MT), and central gray (CG), the relative degree of neural responsiveness to the different somatic stimuli paralleled the findings for the initial behavioral responses. Multiple-unit responses to touch and air puff were of small amplitude and short duration, in contrast to the prolonged bursts of multiple-unit firing after pinprick, pinch, and shock. In those animals whose behavioral responses were attenuated by brain stimulation, there was generally a concomitant reduction in evoked potentials (EP) and multiple-unit responses (MUR) to noxious stimulation. These nociceptively elicited neural responses returned to prestimulation levels within 10 to 30 min, by which time the leg flexion responses were often only partially recovered.

Examination of the effectiveness of central gray stimulation in lowering the magnitude of evoked neural activity failed to reveal any substantial differences between the three brain areas. The base-to-peak amplitudes of the evoked potentials were attenuated by more than 40% in VB, MT, and CG (Fig. 2). In many instances, the reductions were as large as 70%. The one exception to this general observation was that short latency (< 15 msec) peaks in CG and VB were rarely attenuated by central gray stimulation, and in most cases these early peaks were actually enhanced by as much as 20% to 40%.

Reduced EP amplitude to noxious stimuli after brain stimulation was

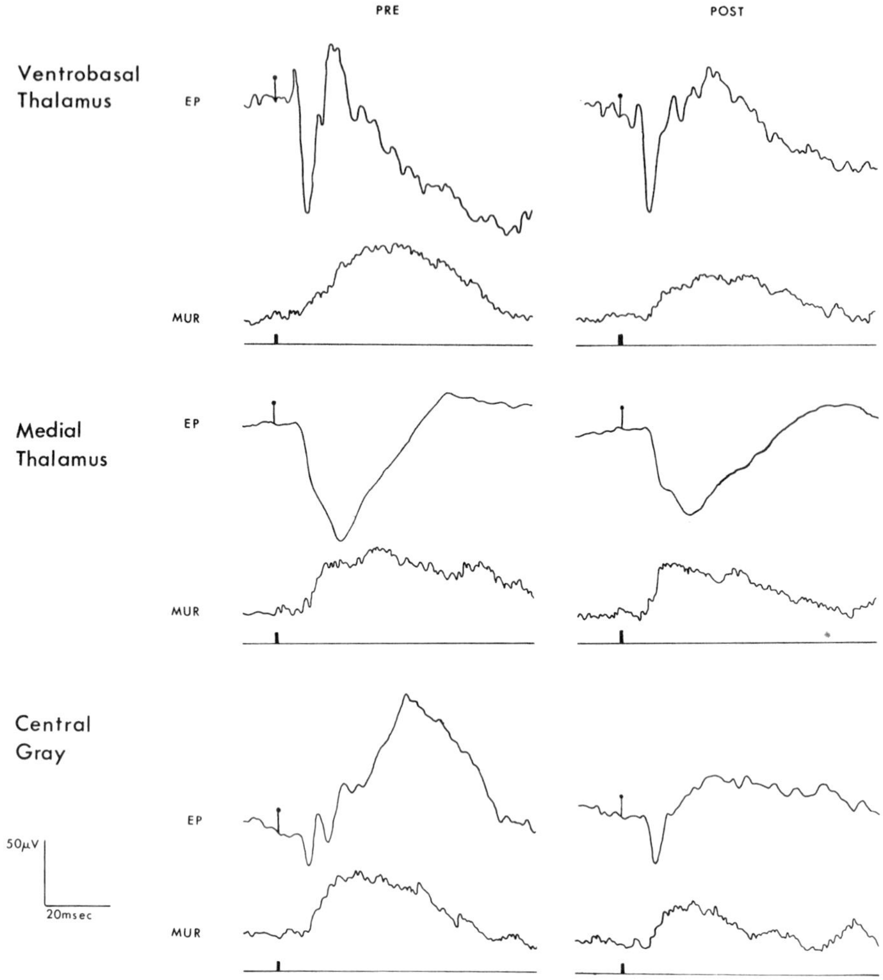

FIG. 2. Evoked potential and integrated multiple-unit responses to shock before and after brain stimulation.

accompanied by diminished MUR. For the great majority of placements, the amplitudes of the integrated MUR exhibited decreases of 50% or more, and the durations of the multiple-unit afterdischarges were considerably attenuated. These reductions in neural responses to nociceptive stimulation occurred against a background of prolonged increases in the spontaneous multiple-unit firing rate, particularly in central gray itself. At the same time, there was little or no attenuation of neural responses to innocuous air puff or touch (Fig. 3). In fact, there were frequently increases as large as 20% to 40%. In those placements outside CG, where brain stimulation failed to modify leg flexion responses, there was also little

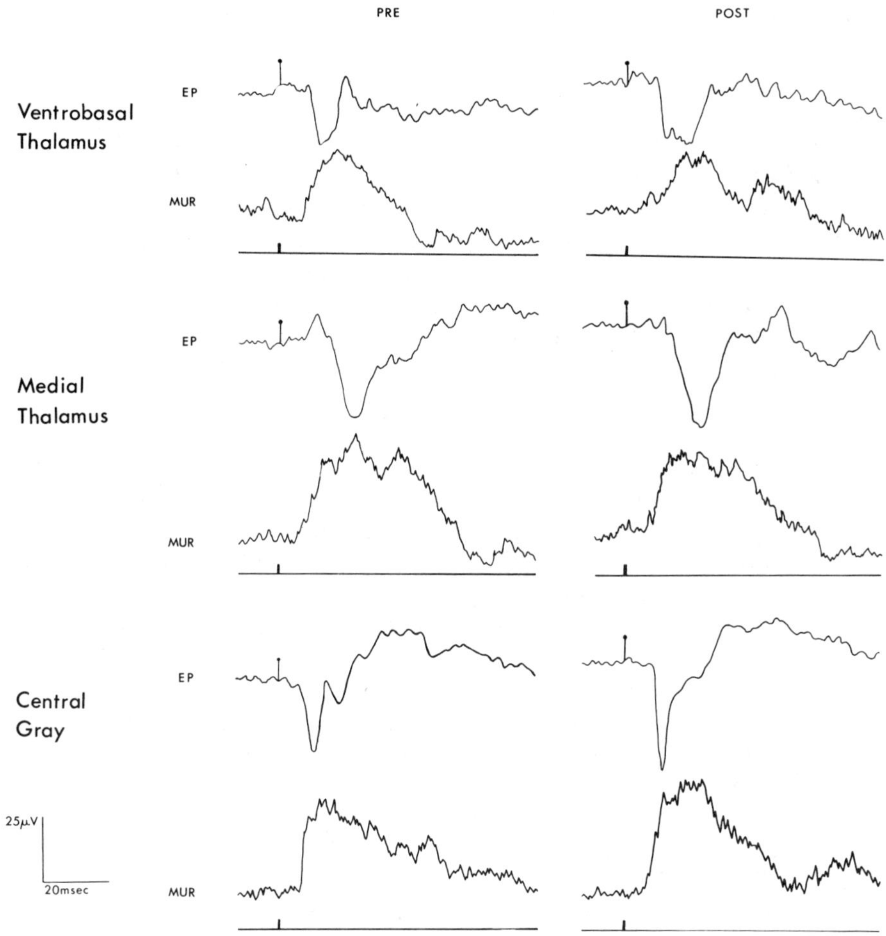

FIG. 3. Evoked potential and integrated multiple-unit responses to air puff before and after brain stimulation.

alteration of the neural response. The evoked potential amplitudes and the size of the integrated multiple-unit responses to both noxious and innocuous stimuli typically remained within 15% of control levels in these behaviorally nonanalgesic rats.

One week after testing with brain stimulation, animals were administered intraperitoneally an initial dose of 10 mg/kg morphine sulfate, then subsequently an additional dose of 20 mg/kg. Behavioral responses to noxious stimuli were only slightly diminished by 10 mg/kg of morphine but were almost totally abolished by the higher dose. Responses to pinch were the most resistant to modification by this drug. After morphine administration, most animals exhibited markedly lower evoked neural activity along with decreased behavioral responding to noxious input. The 20-mg/kg dose lowered evoked potentials by as much as 40%, yet, like brain stimulation, it often resulted in an enhancement of short latency components in CG and VB. After morphine administration, spontaneous multiple-unit activity was elevated; multiple-unit responses to pinprick, pinch, and shock were diminished; and responses to touch and air puff remained unchanged in the majority of animals. All behavioral and neural effects produced by morphine were reversed by naloxone. However, naloxone by itself did not alter the evoked neural responses nor did it antagonize either behavioral analgesia produced by brain stimulation or the concomitant reduction of evoked potentials and multiple-unit responses to noxious stimuli.

DISCUSSION

This study reconfirms earlier reports (9,10) that electrical stimulation of the midbrain central gray diminishes leg flexion responses to noxious stimulation, and it extends these findings to show that all components of the behavioral reaction to pain (including specific and general body movements, skeletal and autonomic responses) are reduced. The neural basis for this behavioral analgesia has previously been related to reduced unit responses in the spinal cord (9,13) and the lower brainstem (6). We found that neural responses in more rostral areas of the brain that normally are activated by nociceptive input are also attenuated by central gray stimulation. Both evoked potentials and multiple-unit responses in the ventrobasal thalamus, the medial thalamus, and the central gray were diminished, indicating that electrical stimulation of central gray modifies the slow wave field potential response as well as the evoked activity of local clusters of neurons. The specificity of this effect to pain modulation was underscored by the finding that neural responses to innocuous stimuli were not reduced and in fact could be enhanced. Moreover, when brain stimulation failed to attenuate behavioral reflexes, there was no consistent alteration of neural responses.

Previous discussions of brain stimulation–produced analgesia have suggested that this effect is not due to a functional lesion of a particular part of the pain pathway, but rather is due to the activation of a pain inhibitory system. That nociceptively elicited responses in thalamic projections of the somatosensory pathway were reduced to the same degree as those in central gray demonstrates indeed that the inhibitory effect is not simply limited to the disruption of neural activity around the stimulating electrode. The increase in spontaneous multiple-unit firing after brain stimulation, which was particularly evident in central gray, might reflect the active nature of the inhibitory process. Furthermore, enhancement of the earliest components of the central gray evoked potential, which was observed for both shock and air puff stimuli, might indicate a role for fast-conducting tactile elements of the somatic response in suppressing central responses to pain in a manner similar to the gating mechanism proposed by Melzack and Wall (11).

It has been suggested that brain stimulation–produced analgesia may act in a manner similar to morphine (e.g., 7). In this work, the effects of central gray stimulation were comparable to a dose of 20 mg/kg morphine. A lower dose of 10 mg/kg was not sufficient to reduce either leg flexion or neural responses to shock or pinch to the degree that was observed for brain stimulation. Morphine-induced reduction of thalamic and central gray evoked potentials to shock has been noted previously (16,17). Our further observation that there is a decline in multiple-unit responses, yet a slight rise in multiple-unit background firing rate, supports the hypothesis that morphine analgesia is owing to a tonically active inhibitory mechanism rather than to a simple blockade of central somatosensory transmission. Such an active inhibitory process was just suggested as the basis for brain stimulation–produced analgesia. That the two mechanisms are not totally comparable, however, is suggested by the finding that naloxone completely reversed the effect of morphine analgesia but had little or no effect on the analgesia produced by brain stimulation in this study. Since other researchers (cf., 7) have found that naloxone can modify brain stimulation–produced analgesia, further research is needed to clarify the circumstances under which naloxone exerts this effect. Experiments demonstrating that morphine is particularly effective when injected directly into the central gray (cf., 7) reinforce the conclusion from brain stimulation studies that the midbrain central gray not only responds to pain but also can serve to inhibit it.

ACKNOWLEDGMENTS

This work was supported by U.S. Public Health Service Grant NS 07628 and National Institute of Mental Health Grant MHTP MH 06415–18.

REFERENCES

1. Becker, D. P., Gluck, H., Nulsen, F. E., and Jane, J. A. (1969): *J. Neurosurg.*, 30:1–13.
2. Benjamin, R. M. (1970): *Brain Res.*, 24:525–529.
3. Berkeley, K. J. (1973): *J. Neurophysiol.*, 36:940–952.
4. Casey, K. L. (1966): *J. Neurophysiol.*, 29:727-750.
5. Casey, K. L. (1971): *Science*, 173:77-80.
6. Casey, K. L., Keene, J. J., and Morrow, T. (1974): In: *Advances in Neurology, Vol. 4: International Symposium on Pain*, edited by J. J. Bonica, pp. 197–205. Raven Press, New York.
7. Liebeskind, J. C. *This volume.*
8. Liebeskind, J. C., Guilbaud, G., Besson, J.-M., and Oliveras, J.-L. (1973): *Brain Res.*, 50:441–446.
9. Liebeskind, J. C., Mayer, D. J., and Akil, H. (1974): In: *Advances in Neurology, Vol. 4: International Symposium on Pain*, edited by J. J. Bonica, pp. 261–268. Raven Press, New York.

10. Mayer, D. J., Wolfle, T. L., Akil, H., Carder, B., and Liebeskind, J. C. (1971): *Science,* 174:1351–1354.
11. Melzack, R., and Wall, P. D. (1965): *Science,* 150:971–979.
12. Nyquist, J. K., and Greenhoot, J. H. (1974): *Exp. Neurol.,* 42:609–622.
13. Oliveras, J.-L., Besson, J.-M., Guilbaud, G., and Liebeskind, J. C. (1974): *Exp. Brain Res.,* 20:32–44.
14. Perl, E. R., and Whitlock, D. G. (1961): *Exp. Neurol.,* 3:256–276.
15. Rosetto, M. A., and Vandercar, D. H. (1972): *Physiol. Behav.,* 9:105–106.
16. Sinitsin, L. N. (1964): *Int. J. Neuropharmacol.,* 3:321–326.
17. Straw, R. N., and Mitchell, C. L. (1964): *J. Pharmacol. Exp. Ther.,* 146:7–15.
18. Verzeano, M., Dill, R. C., Vallecalle, E., Groves, P., and Thomas, J. (1968): *Experientia,* 24:696–698.

Advances in Pain Research and Therapy, Vol. 1,
edited by J. J. Bonica and D. Albe-Fessard.
Raven Press, New York © 1976.

Selective and Prolonged Analgesia in Monkey Resulting from Brain Stimulation

Stanley J. Goodman and Virginia Holcombe

Harbor General Hospital, and University of California Medical Center, Los Angeles, California 90024

There have been a number of reports demonstrating that electrical stimulation of the brainstem can produce analgesia or alteration of neurophysiological mechanisms apparently subserving nociceptive transmission (2,3,5–9). These studies have been done mainly in rats or cats and for the most part have not clearly identified the relationship between stimulation-produced analgesia and other stimulation-produced effects resulting from excitation of neighboring neural structures. In fact, many studies are based on analgesia testing done immediately after the application of brief stimulation specifically to minimize the chance of a false-positive judgment wherein nonresponse to painful stimulation is due to motor interference rather than to induced analgesia.

The motivation for this study was to extend earlier findings to a primate model as a strategy for research that might aid the development of better clinical methods for treating pain. The specific goals of this study were to define the nonanalgesic as well as the analgesic effects of stimulation, to determine the duration of analgesia during continuous stimulation, and to attempt to improve the stimulation-produced analgesia by pharmacologic means.

METHODS

Seven adult rhesus monkeys (*Macaca mulatta*) weighing between 4 and 6 kg were used. Under ketamine anesthesia, 40 electrodes were stereotaxically aimed at mesencephalic and diencephalic sites. Teflon®-insulated stainless steel wires 0.5 mm in diameter with 0.5 mm length bared were either arranged side by side (1 to 2 mm separation) or vertically spaced (3 to 5 mm tip separation). The electrode wires were attached to a miniature plug secured to the calvaria. The animals were housed in individual cages and were transferred to a primate chair for approximately 1 week per month for testing.

We used as our pain test animal responsiveness to an "alligator clip" applied to toes or tail. Clips were selected that were judged to be unequivocally painful by laboratory personnel when applied to fingertips: the pain was generally reported as sharp and localized over the first few minutes, thereafter causing a more diffuse throbbing pain. If the clip was applied for longer than 5 min, mild ecchymoses occasionally occurred. Therefore, the clip was never applied for longer than 1 min to the monkey, and care was taken to avoid any soft tissue injury as a direct result of pain testing. The monkey normally responded to the clip with a variety of dependable behavioral responses. Generally there was some restlessness and vocalization as the foot or tail was held. The response to tail clipping was most often prompt, forceful curling of the tail followed by tail wagging; in addition, the animal often shifted sitting positions and attempted to either reach the tail or bring the tail up alongside the trunk. The response to toe clipping was most often toe fanning, foot wiggling, tucking the leg under the buttocks, and variable attempts to remove the clip. Brain stimulation was judged to be causing analgesia only when there was no detectable behavioral response to the application of the clip for 30 sec, at which time the clip was removed.

Three monkeys received incremental oral L-DOPA over a 15-day interval based on other investigations demonstrating that brain stimulation analgesia can be enchanced by drugs potentiating dopamine systems (1).

Brain stimulation was applied using a constant current stimulator delivering symmetrical biphasic pulses at 150 cps with a pulse width of 0.5 msec and a delay of 0.5 msec between each component of the biphasic pulse. The animals were repeatedly studied over a 6- to 10-month interval. The animals were sacrificed under deep anesthesia and perfused with formalin. The brains were thinly sliced, stained for cells and myelin, and inspected for electrode tip localization.

RESULTS

Brain stimulation at 29 of the 40 sites caused reproducible and unambiguous analgesia. The current required to produce analgesia varied among brain sites from 0.25 mA to 6.0 mA and was a stable requirement over months of testing. Generally, when analgesia occurred with stimulation it was found equally bilaterally and in the tail—occasionally the foot ipsilateral to the side of stimulation had a higher threshold for stimulation than the contralateral foot. During short periods of stimulations (seconds to minutes) the analgesia ended abruptly with the termination of stimulation.

At all 29 sites from which analgesia could be produced, prominent nonanalgesic effects occurred such as hyperventilation, pupillary changes (miosis or mydriasis), conjugate eye deviation, head turning, and body rotation. The intensity of these nonanalgesic effects was directly related to the intensity of stimulation and inversely related to the duration of stimulation. For example, stimulation at a particular site caused only a tendency for left lateral gaze with the animal being able to gaze right to novel stimuli.

At higher intensity stimulation, the involuntary lateral gaze became constant, and the degree of lateral gaze became more extreme with increasing stimulus strength. However, the degree of lateral gaze deviation associated with a particular level of stimulation gradually decreased over several minutes of continuous stimulation, reaching some stable low point. If the stimulus-produced nonanalgesic effect was initially mild (e.g., just a tendency to lateral gaze), then after a few minutes of continued stimulation the nonanalgesic effect might have completely disappeared. This decremental manifestation of nonanalgesic effects over time pertained to every nonanalgesic phenomenon observed. We graded each nonanalgesic effect from a first to a maximum third degree and soon realized that most first- and second-degree effects faded during continued brain stimulation.

It proved useful to describe these complex induced analgesic and nonanalgesic effects in terms of a therapeutic index (TI):

$$\frac{\text{mA required for nonanalgesic phenomena}}{\text{mA required for analgesia}} = \text{TI}$$

The numerator consisted of values required to produce third-degree nonanalgesic effects after 2 min of continuous brain stimulation since lesser degrees of nonanalgesic effects were apt to disappear over time. At 15 electrode sites, analgesia occurred at lower currents than that needed to produce third-degree nonanalgesic effects, and the TI was therefore greater than 1. At nine sites analgesic and nonanalgesic effects occurred at the same stimulation intensity, so the TI was 1. At five sites prominent nonanalgesic effects appeared at lower stimulation intensities than did analgesia, and the TI was less than 1. At 11 remaining sites no analgesia was observed at stimulus intensities up to 10 mA, and we rated the TI as 0. Among the 29 sites yielding analgesic effects, the TI varied from 12.0 to 0.5 (Table 1).

In general, the most favorable stimulation sites ($T1 > 1$) were in the periaqueductal gray and the periventricular zone around the third ventricle (Fig. 1). Surprisingly, we were able to localize only 36 of the 40 electrode tips by directly viewing the tissue defect and surrounding gliosis associated with the tip. Anatomical reconstruction of the path of the remaining four electrodes indicated that those tips were in the third ventricle (2) or in the quadrigeminal cistern (2). One ventricular and one cisternal electrode yielded impressive analgesia with $T1 > 1$; the remaining two electrodes provided analgesia but with $T1 < 1$. Brainstem stimulation caused analgesic and nonanalgesic effects at stimulation currents below 1 mA, whereas diencephalic stimulation was usually at levels above 2 mA. However, the full range of TIs (from 0 to >1) was observed both within the brainstem and within the diencephalon (Table 1) and was observed with relatively low and high levels of stimulation intensity (Fig. 2).

During continued brain stimulation, analgesia was often maintained for 30 min or longer. We tested the animal for analgesia every 15 min and ob-

TABLE 1. *Degree of selectivity in brain stimulation analgesia: the therapeutic index*

Site	Therapeutic index	Current needed for: Analgesia (mA)	Current needed for: Nonanalgesia (mA)	Main nonanalgesic effect*
Reticular nucleus	12	0.25	3.0	R
? Third ventricle	5	2.0	10.0	T
Medialis dorsalis	5	2.0	10.0	H
Periaqueductal gray	4.3	0.4–0.5	2.0	H
Periaqueductal gray	4.0	0.5	2.0	T
Periventricular zone	3.0	1.0	3.0	H, LG
Anterior medial nucleus	2.5	1.5	3.75	R
Periaqueductal gray	2.0	1.0	2.0	R, LG
Periaqueductal gray	1.6	0.5	0.8	T
Reticular nucleus	1.6	0.25	0.4	LG
Parafascicularis nucleus	1.6	1.6	2.5	T
?Quadrigeminal cistern	1.4	3.5	4.90	LG
Pretectal area	1.3	0.4–0.5	0.6	LG
Periaqueductal gray	1.3	1.5	1.95	H
Medialis dorsalis	1.2	1.0	1.2	R
Tegmentum	1.0	0.4	0.4	H
Superior colliculus	1.0	1.0	1.0	LG
Superior colliculus	1.0	2.5	2.5	H, LG
Medialis dorsalis	1.0	0.7	0.7	R
Periaqueductal gray	1.0	0.7	0.7	LG
Superior colliculus	1.0	3.0	3.0	T
Lateralis dorsalis	1.0	0.4	0.4	H
Reticularis (thalamus)	1.0	3.0	3.0	R
Caudate nucleus	1.0	0.8	0.8	LG
Red nucleus	0.9	0.5	0.45	LG
Medialis dorsalis	0.8	4.0	3.0	LG
Tegmentum	0.6	0.7	0.4	LG
?Third ventricle	0.6	6.0	5.0	LG
?Quadrigeminal cistern	0.5	0.4	0.2	LG
Superior colliculus	0	>10.0	0.25	LG
Inferior colliculus	0	>10.0	0.35	LG
Superior colliculus	0	>10.0	0.35	LG
Medialis dorsalis	0	>10.0	0.6	LG
Caudate nucleus	0	>10.0	2.8	R
Nucleus ventralis posterolateralis	0	>10.0	2.8	H, LG
Lateralis dorsalis	0	>10.0	3.0	T, LG
Superior colliculus	0	>10.0	3.0	LG
Tegmentum	0	>10.0	5.0	T
Pretectal area	0	>10.0	4.5	LG
Medialis dorsalis	0	>10.0	6.0	H

* H, head turning; R, trunk rotation; LG, lateral gaze deviation; T, tremor.

served that analgesia persisted at times for several hours (Fig. 3). Since the nonanalgesic effects of stimulation always decreased over time, prolonged stimulation often revealed analgesia at its "purest": after 10 min or more of stimulation, the animal often appeared to be completely normal except that it did not respond to pain. The animal accepted food, ate, retreated from

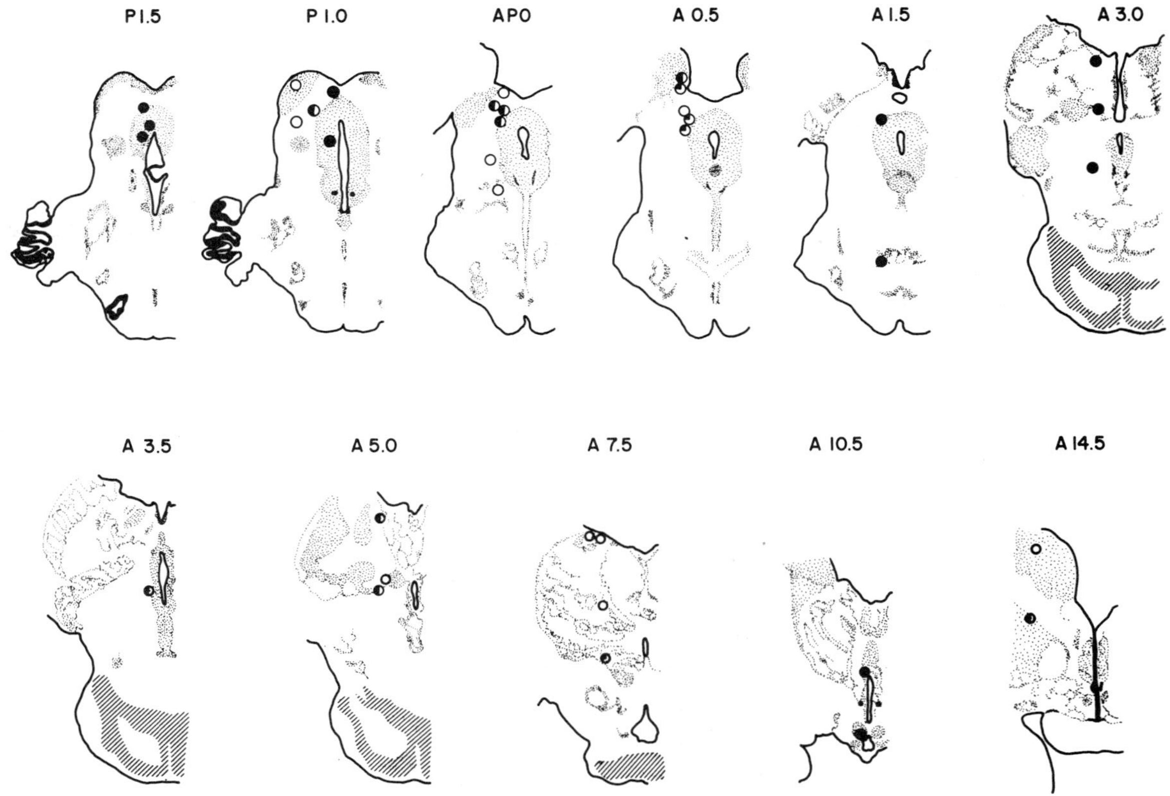

FIG. 1. Localization of 36 electrode tips. Tip sites displayed in terms of standard coronal planes from a stereotaxic atlas (11). Filled *circles,* electrode sites producing analgesia with TI > 1; *half-filled circles,* TI = 1; *quarter-filled circles,* TI < 1; *open circles,* sites producing no analgesia with stimulation intensities up to 10 mA.

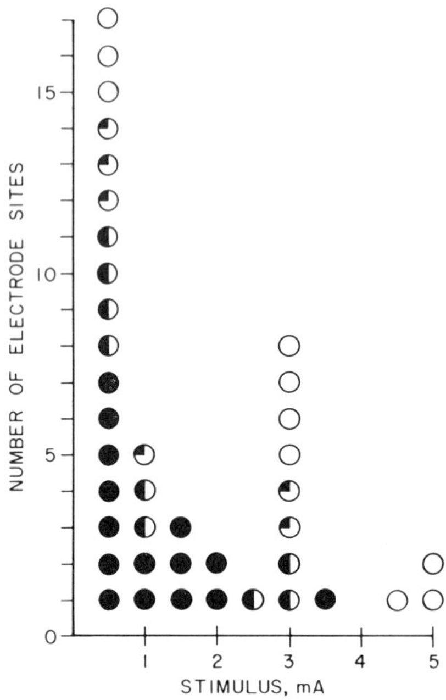

FIG. 2. Stimulus intensities at each electrode site required to produce the first prominent analgesic or nonanalgesic effect. Results represented by degree of darkening in circles, as in Fig. 1. The full range of TI (0 to >1) occurred both at sites requiring low-intensity stimulation below 1 mA and at sites requiring over 2 mA stimulation intensity.

human contact, and was normally oriented to novel stimuli. We could detect at times only two other stimulation-related phenomena: a stimulated animal made far fewer teeth-baring aggressive gestures to strangers than did a nonstimulated animal, and at times the former group of animals seemed to react excessively to light touch on the back or abdomen (hyperpathia?).

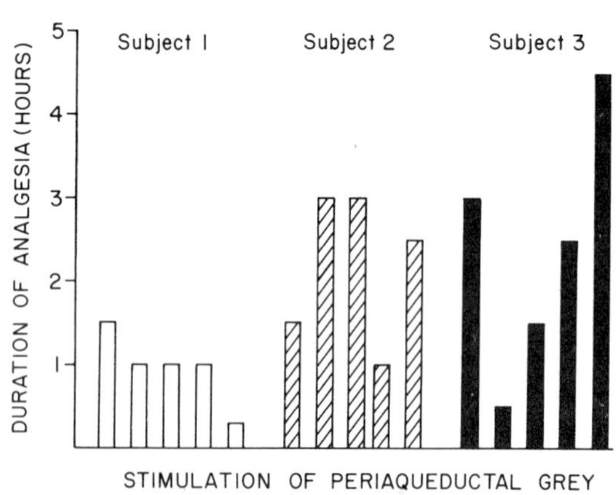

FIG. 3. Duration of analgesia during prolonged, continuous brain stimulation at 3 separate sites in 3 different subjects. Subjects tested for analgesia every 15 min after start of stimulation.

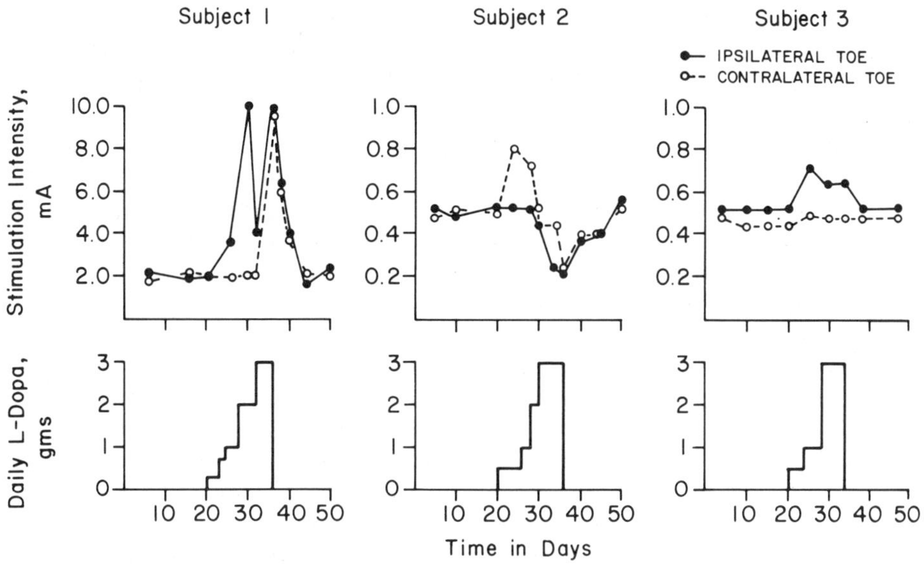

FIG. 4. Stimulation of periaqueductal gray. Effect of L-DOPA on analgesia threshold, 3 separate sites in 3 different subjects. Note that requirements for analgesia ipsilaterally and contralaterally became temporarily uncoupled. Subject 1 had an elevated analgesia threshold, subject 2 had an elevated and then reduced threshold, and subject 3 had just an ipsilaterally elevated threshold. Not shown: subjects 2 and 3 had a lowered TI during L-DOPA administration.

We attempted to enhance the therapeutic effectiveness of the stimulation-induced analgesia by administering L-DOPA. Seven sites in 3 animals were studied. We asked if the therapeutic index might be favorably increased, if the duration of maintained analgesia might be prolonged, or if the stimulus threshold to induce analgesia might be lowered with or without altering the TI. L-DOPA was administered in increasing doses over 15 days. We saw a variety of effects including uncoupling ipsilateral from contralateral analgesia, biphasic threshold changes that were first elevated and then reduced, and monophasic reduction of analgesic thresholds (Fig. 4). However, we observed no favorable gain in the TI (some temporary declines in TI) and no favorable prolongation of the analgesic effect.

DISCUSSION

In this study we assume that there is some commonality among the systems subserving acute pain and those subserving chronic intractable pain in man. This is supported by the observation that thalamic stimulation in man done for chronic pain does elevate pain threshold for a short period of time after stimulation; however, the alleviation of the chronic pain may far outlast the initial clinically demonstrable hypalgesia (10). In addition, dorsal column stimulation may elevate a clinical radiant heat dolorimeter pain threshold, although the intensity of spinal stimulation needed to elevate the pain threshold may well exceed that which the patient selects to treat the chronic pain (4).

These fragmentary observations support the idea that there are features common to both acute and chronic pain and that significant modulation of acute pain may well modulate chronic pain. However, no satisfactory chronic pain model has been developed for use in experimental animals, and the number of anatomic and physiological questions that can be asked and answered in patients is of necessity quite restricted. Thus this study was an attempt to develop a more "clinically" oriented set of observations, so we emphasize the ratio between stimulation-induced nonanalgesic and analgesic effects. The resulting therapeutic index used in this study was composed of observations made on breathing, eye movements, pupillary size, and movement of the head and neck. We observed that rather selective analgesia with a favorable TI could be produced by focal brain stimulation. However, further studies must define as part of an extended definition of the TI whether or not performance capabilities or cognitive function is disturbed by the apparent "best" analgesic stimulation.

In addition, strategies for prolonging analgesia must be developed based, e.g., on sequential stimulation of different analgesic sites or intermittent stimulation of a single site, thereby perhaps avoiding "depletion" of the desired effect. It is still not clear whether there are dependable excellent anatomical targets that will allow a higher yield of selective analgesia after electrode implantation. Is our current yield low because the anatomical target is so small, or is the yield low because the anatomical target is not both necessary and sufficient to subserve analgesia? Many questions remain which should serve as a stimulus for further clinically oriented laboratory research.

REFERENCES

1. Akil, H., and Liebeskind, J. (1975): *Brain Res.* 94:279–296.
2. Balagura, S., and Ralph, T. (1973): *Brain Res.,* 60:369–379.
3. Gebhart, G., and Toleikis, J. (1975): *Fed. Proc.,* 34:439.
4. Goodman, S. J. (1975): Presented at annual meeting, *Am. Assoc. of Neurologic. Surgeons.*
5. Lewis, V., and Gebhart, G. (1975): *Fed. Proc.,* 34:757.
6. Mayer, D., and Liebeskind, J. (1974): *Brain Res.,* 68:73–93.
7. Mayer, D., Wolfle, T., Akil, H., Carder, B., and Liebeskind, J. (1971): *Science,* 174:1351–1354.
8. Oliveras, J., Besson, J., Gilbaud, G., and Liebeskind, J. (1974): *Exp. Brain Res.,* 20:32–44.
9. Reynolds, D. (1969): *Science,* 164:444–445.
10. Richardson, D., and Akil, H. (1974): *Abstr. 7th Ann. Meeting Neuroelectric. Soc.*
11. Snider, R. S., and Lee, J. C. (1961): *A Stereotaxic Atlas of the Monkey Brain.* University of Chicago Press, Chicago.

Advances in Pain Research and Therapy, Vol. 1,
edited by J. J. Bonica and D. Albe-Fessard.
Raven Press, New York © 1976.

Analgesia Produced by Mesencephalic Stimulation: Effect on Bulboreticular Neurons

*Thomas J. Morrow and †Kenneth L. Casey

Departments of Physiology† and Neurology†, University of Michigan, Ann Arbor, Michigan 48104*

The medial medullary reticular formation in the region of nucleus gigantocellularis (NGC) appears to play an important role in mammalian pain mechanisms. There is anatomical (14) and physiological (1,5) evidence that the NGC receives input from somatically activated fibers ascending in the anterolateral quadrant of the spinal cord. A significant fraction of NGC cells are excited primarily or exclusively by electrical stimulation of Aδ peripheral nerve fibers, noxious somatic stimuli (1,5–7,11), and splanchnic nerve stimulation (18). The discharge of some NGC neurons has shown significant correlation with escape elicited by cutaneous nerve (3). Electrical stimulation of NGC has consistently elicited escape behavior in rat (10) and cat (2), and lesions in NGC or in the medial thalamus receiving NGC projections have elevated escape threshold or latency (8,9) in the cat.

Recent studies indicate that both narcotic analgesics and intracerebral electrical stimuli may activate a descending midbrain pathway which modulates the activity of ascending systems subserving pain. Electrical stimulation in the periaqueductal gray (PAG), particularly near the dorsal raphe nucleus, produces in rat and cat a marked analgesia which, in rat, outlasts the period of stimulation without any apparent loss of motor responsiveness to other stimulus modalities (12,13,16,19). Similarly, direct microinjections of morphine into the brain produce analgesia most effectively when delivered in the region of the PAG of rat (20) and monkey (17). Pharmacological experiments have emphasized the similarity of analgesia produced by MES (PAG) electrical stimulation and narcotic analgesics (12).

If the excitation of NGC neurons is an essential part of central pain mechanisms, those cells receiving somatic, and especially noxious, input should be depressed by analgesic stimuli. The experiments described here demonstrate the effect of analgesic electrical MES stimulation on somatically evoked NGC unit activity in the rat.

In preliminary experiments using lightly anesthetized rats, recordings from the medial medullary reticular formation showed that MES (PAG) stimulation inhibited 55% of all units driven by tail shock at 10- to 15-msec latencies. Excitability data revealed an immediate complete depression followed by gradual recovery to approximately 80% of control levels 400 msec after MES stimulation. Of the units excited primarily by noxious mechanical or thermal stimuli, 40% showed MES-induced depression, whereas none of the units responding only to tap or touch were affected.

These findings suggested a specific effect of MES (PAG) stimulation on NGC neurons, but their significance could be determined only by further experiments in the awake rat.

METHODS

Thirty-nine rats were implanted with bipolar MES stimulating electrodes (AP −0.6, ML 0.0, H −2.0). A screw-driven microelectrode drive chamber (T. J. Morrow, *unpublished observations*) was cemented over a skull opening for repeated penetrations into NGC (11 to 12 mm post-bregma, 0.2 to 1.0 mm lateral to and 8.5 to 9.5 mm below skull surface). After recovery (1 to 2 weeks), tail-flick latency was determined by at least 8 trials (repeated before each recording session) by placing the tail over a timed, thermally calibrated light source terminated by tail flick. The range of control tail flick latencies in all rats was 3.5 to 5 sec; at 4 sec, the temperature at the tail surface was estimated to be 45°C. MES stimulation (10 sec, 60-Hz train of 50 μsec, 1- to 4-mA pulses) was considered analgesic if tail flick latency increased to 8 sec, the maximum stimulus duration allowed (tail temperature estimated at 59°C). Ineffective MES stimulus loci were either clearly aversive or produced no shift in response latency at the parameters tested.

During NGC unit recording, tail shocks and thermal stimuli were routinely used to activate unit discharge. Manual mechanical stimulation was limited to face and tail. Unit activity was integrated for monitoring of spontaneous discharge rate and temporal correlation with thermal stimulus duration. Poststimulus histograms were generated to determine responsiveness to tail shock. During and after MES stimulation, the rat was observed for behavioral responses to auditory, visual, and olfactory stimuli. Tests of unit responses to somatic stimuli were usually applied at 1-min intervals throughout the post-MES stimulation analgesic period. Electrode placements were verified histologically.

RESULTS

Figure 1 shows that MES stimulation sites eliciting analgesia were located within the PAG. Ineffective loci were nearly always outside the PAG or within the cerebral aqueduct. Analgesia always persisted for 30 sec to 4 min after 10 sec of MES (PAG) stimulation. During analgesia, rats exhibited spontaneous movements and showed startle responses to loud sounds and visual threat.

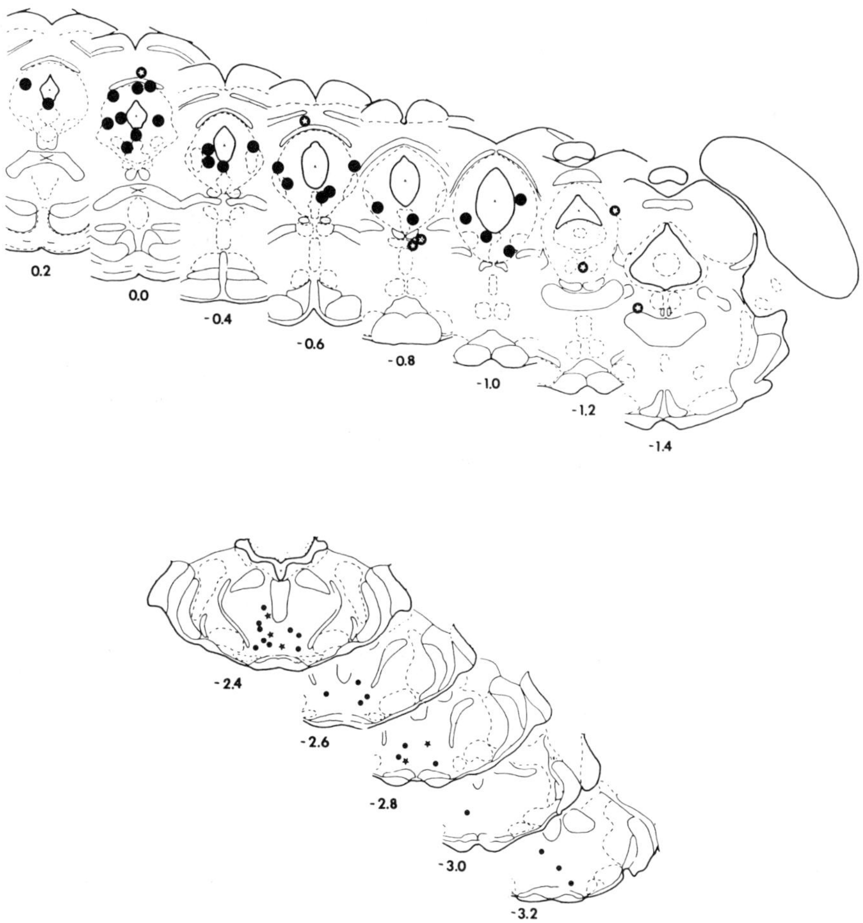

FIG. 1. Top: Location of tips of stimulating electrodes in awake rats. *Stars,* no analgesia; *filled circles,* analgesia elicited using stimulus parameters given in text. **Bottom:** Location of electrolytic lesions made along microelectrode tracks in awake rats. *Stars,* location along tracks in rats without analgesia; *filled circles,* rats with analgesia. (Drawings from Pellegrino, L. J., and Cushman, A. J., Appleton-Century-Crofts, New York).

The locations of marking lesions made along microelectrode tracks are shown in Fig. 1. Of the 193 units recorded, 167 (87%) were excited by some form of somatic stimulation including tail shock (151 units). Of those excited, 92 (55%) responded either exclusively (30 units) or with greatest discharge frequency (62 units) to strong thermal or mechanical stimuli eliciting escape responses and vocalization. Innocuous mechanical stimuli were exclusively effective in discharging 56 cells; 26 others were not responsive to any stimuli tested.

Units responding primarily to noxious thermal tail stimulation (56 units) invariably started to respond 150 to 450 msec before the tail flick response (Fig. 2). Peak discharge occurred near the time of tail flick; increased unit activity persisted for 1 to several seconds thereafter. Unit discharge was never associated with passive or spontaneous tail movements, but the latter were infrequent and never duplicated the abrupt movement of tail flick.

Nonanalgesic MES stimulation had no effect on the somatic excitation of 38 cells or on the spontaneous activity of 2 unresponsive units. Analgesic MES stimulation, however, markedly depressed the spontaneous and/or evoked activity of 100 (65%) of 153 NGC cells tested ($x^2 = 51.67$; $p < 0.001$). All but 1 of the units so affected were excited by somatic stimuli; unaffected units were more evenly distributed between the somatically responsive (30 units) and unresponsive (24 units) categories, suggesting that analgesic MES stimulation preferentially affects somatically activated cells ($x^2 = 43.93$; $p < 0.001$).

As shown in Fig. 3, the analgesic depression reduces NGC field potential

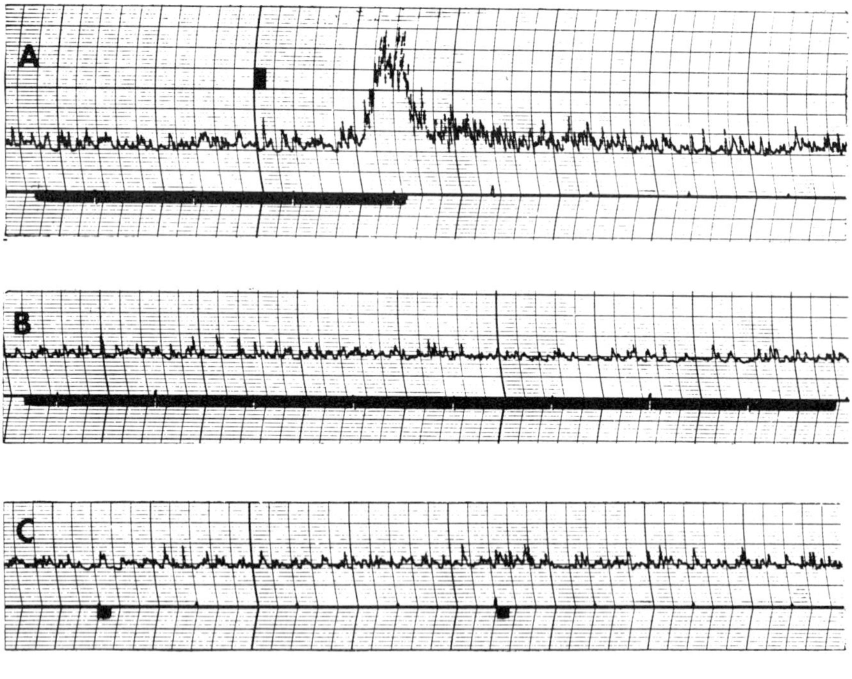

FIG. 2. Depression of NGC unit response to thermal stimulation by analgesic stimulation in awake rat. *Upper traces,* discharge frequency of single unit; *lower traces,* timing pulses (1/sec) and stimulus marker. **A:** Before analgesic stimulation. Unit begins response 3.4 sec after onset of thermal stimulation; tail flick terminates stimulus 325 msec later. Note prolonged poststimulus activity. (Vertical calibration, 20 spikes/sec.) **B:** During analgesia, 1 min after analgesic stimulation. No unit or behavioral responses during thermal stimulation for 8 sec. **C:** Before analgesia. No response to passive tail movements given at marks.

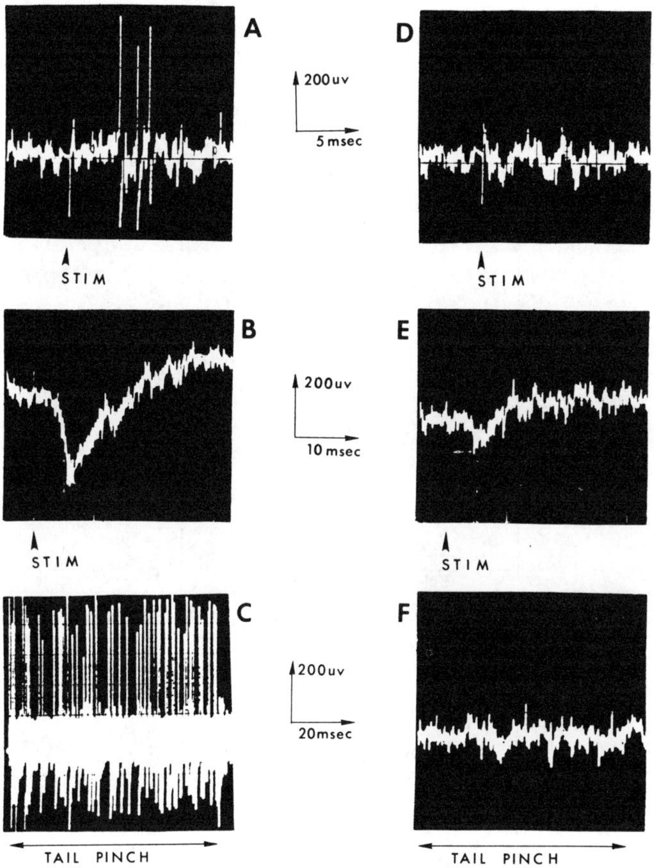

FIG. 3. Depression of NGC response by analgesic stimulation in awake rat. **A–C:** Before analgesia. NGC unit **(A)** and field potential **(B)** responses to tail shock; same unit responding during strong tail pinch **(C). D–F:** Same responses during analgesia 1 min after analgesic stimulation.

amplitude and eliminates the unit responses to tail shock and continuous strong tail pinch. Figure 2 shows a unit's integrated response to thermal tail stimulation before and after analgesic MES stimulation. In all instances of response depression, unit responsiveness recovered only when analgesia disappeared over the ensuing 30-sec to 5-min period.

The modality of the unit responses depressed by MES stimulation is shown in Table 1. The uniquely effective analgesic MES (PAG) stimulation clearly depressed the responsiveness of all types of units tested, including those responding exclusively to innocuous mechanical stimuli. The distribution of response depression, however, shows a significant modality pref-

TABLE 1. *Driven units: chronic preparations*

Type of stimulus	Analgesic animals: Responsive units No.	Analgesic animals: Responsive units %	Analgesic animals: Units inhibited by MES stimulation No.	Analgesic animals: Units inhibited by MES stimulation %	Nonanalgesic animals: Responsive units No.	Nonanalgesic animals: Responsive units %	Nonanalgesic animals: No. of units inhibited by MES stimulation
Tail shock	115	89	99	86	36	95	0
Multimodal (noxious and non-noxious)	45	35	39	87	17	47	0
Non-noxious only	27	21	13	48	3	8	0
Noxious only	48	37	42	88	8	22	0

Percentages shown in columns 1 and 3 are calculated from the total number of responsive units in analgesic and nonanalgesic rats, respectively. Percentages in column 2 are calculated from the number of units in each row of column 1.

erence ($x^2 = 6.11$; $p < 0.01$) for cells responsive to primarily or exclusively noxious stimulation.

DISCUSSION

The results show that analgesia produced by MES (PAG) stimulation is accompanied by a marked reduction in NGC unit responses to somatic stimuli. The significance of this finding depends, in part, on the behavioral specificity of MES-induced analgesia. It is possible that other sensory and motor functions, although less obviously affected, are modified during MES analgesia. NGC response depression could therefore reflect effects unrelated to analgesia, as is possibly suggested by the depression of units responding only to innócuous stimuli. Although this possibility is less likely in light of the significant depression preference for units responding to noxious input, the problem cannot be resolved without additional information about NGC and MES analgesia, some of which has been presented earlier in this chapter.

The results are nonetheless consonant with the hypothesis that NGC cells are an integral part of central pain mechanisms. In anesthetized and awake rats, a significant proportion of neurons responded primarily or exclusively to noxious somatic stimuli, confirming previous observations (10). The depressed excitability of NGC cells appeared related to the behavioral state of analgesia since it was present only during analgesia and was not elicited by nonanalgesic MES stimuli. Finally, analgesic MES stimulation preferentially affected somatically activated cells rather than generally depressing the spontaneous activity of both responsive and unresponsive units.

The mechanism by which MES (PAG) stimulation depresses NGC responses cannot be specified. MES (PAG)-induced depression of spinal cord dorsal horn responses is suggested by the findings of Oliveras et al. (16) in the cat. The excitability cycles obtained in our experiments, however, are more consistent with a supraspinal interaction since the early onset of NGC depression allows little time for bulbospinal conduction delay. Moreover, in rat and cat, there is no evidence for direct spinal projections from the mesencephalic reticular formation (15) or adjacent dorsal raphe nuclei (4). There is, however, anatomical evidence for a direct projection of dorsal raphe neurons to medullary NGC at the level of facial nucleus in rat (4). This direct descending connection could provide an anatomical basis for our findings since there is evidence that dorsal raphe neurons mediate MES analgesia (13,16).

Our observations cannot resolve the question of whether NGC has primarily a motor or sensory function. The buildup of unit activity preceding tail flick could be related to the recruitment of spinal motoneurons, the modulation of spinal sensory input, or the activation of suprabulbar mechanisms mediating sensory or motivational mechanisms. The functions they mediate, however, are probably related specifically to aversive behavior in response to noxious somatic stimuli.

ACKNOWLEDGMENTS

This research was supported by grants GM353, NS12581, and NS12015 from the National Institutes of Health, Department of Health, Education and Welfare.

REFERENCES

1. Casey, K. L. (1969): *Exp. Neurol.*, 25:35–56.
2. Casey, K. L. (1971*a*): *Int. J. Neurosci.*, 2:29–34.
3. Casey, K. L. (1971*b*): *Science*, 173:77–80.
4. Conrad, L. C., Leonard, C. M., and Pfaff, D. W. (1974): *J. Comp. Neurol.*, 156:179–205.
5. Fields, H. L., Wagner, G. M., and Anderson, S. D. (1975): *Exp. Neurol.*, 47:118–134.
6. Goldman, P. L., Collins, W. F., Taub, A., and Fitzmartin, J. (1972): *Exp. Neurol.*, 37:597–606.
7. Guilbaud, G., Besson, J. M., Oliveras, J. L., and Wyon-Maillard, M. C. (1973): *Brain Res.*, 63:131–140.
8. Halpern, B. P., and Halverson, J. D. (1974): *Behav. Biol.*, 11:215–229.
9. Kaelber, W. W., Mitchell, C. L., Yarmat, A. J., Afifi, A. K., and Lorens, S. A. (1975): *Exp. Neurol.*, 46:282–290.
10. Keene, J. J., and Casey, K. L. (1970): *Exp. Neurol.*, 28:155–166.
11. LeBlanc, H. J., and Gatipon, G. B. (1974): *Exp. Neurol.*, 42:264–273.
12. Mayer, D. J., and Hayes, R. L. (1975): *Science*, 188:941–943.
13. Mayer, D. J., Colfle, T. L., Akil, H., Carder, B., and Liebeskind, J. C. (1971): *Science*, 174:1351–1354.
14. Mehler, W. R., Feferman, M. E., and Nauta, W. J. H. (1960): *Brain*, 83:718–750.
15. Nyberg-Hansen, R. (1965): *J. Comp. Neurol.*, 124:74–100.
16. Oliveras, J. L., Besson, J. M., Guilbaud, G., and Liebeskind, J. C. (1974): *Exp. Brain Res.*, 20:32–44.
17. Pert, A., and Yaksh, T. (1974): *Brain Res.*, 80:135–140.
18. Preobrazhenskii, N. N., and Limanskii, Y. P. (1969): *Neirofiziologiia*, 1:177–185.
19. Reynolds, D. V. (1969): *Science*, 164:444–445.
20. Sharpe, L. G., Garnett, J. E., and Cicero, T. J. (1974): *Behav. Biol.*, 11:303–313.

Advances in Pain Research and Therapy, Vol. 1,
edited by J. J. Bonica and D. Albe-Fessard.
Raven Press, New York © 1976.

Spinal Cord Pathways Involved in the Production of Analgesia by Brain Stimulation

A. I. Basbaum, N. Marley, and J. O'Keefe

Department of Neurology and Physiology, University of California, San Francisco, California 94143; and Department of Anatomy, University College London, Gower Street, London WC1, England

INTRODUCTION

Over the past few years there have been several demonstrations of analgesia produced by electrical brain stimulation (EBS) (2,7–9). Only recently has attention been focused on the mechanisms by which EBS exerts its effect. Electrophysiological studies demonstrated that electrical stimulation in the region of the periaqueductal gray (PAG) of the cat, which is known to produce analgesia in freely moving animals, also inhibits the discharge of laminae I and V cells of the spinal cord (8). Furthermore, electrical stimulation not only produces analgesia but also blocks the flexor-withdrawal reflexes, indicating that descending inhibitory mechanisms are probably involved (7).

To test this hypothesis, we studied the effects of various spinal cord lesions on the analgesic properties of brain stimulation in the rat. We used the rat for two important reasons. First, most subtotal spinal cord lesions in the rat do not alter the animal's responsiveness to a noxious stimulus, so that analgesia is not induced by the lesion itself (3). Second, the location of the corticospinal tract (CST) in the ventral part of the dorsal funiculus allows selective destruction of descending tracts and possible delineation of the relevant systems mediating the descending inhibition. We also tested for the presence of self-stimulation, a measure of the rewarding properties of the brain stimulation, to determine if reward plays a role in the production of the analgesia.

METHODS

Female albino rats were used in this study. All surgical procedures were performed under a halothane, nitrous oxide, oxygen anesthetic mixture. Two bipolar electrodes (250-μm diameter insect pins insulated except for 500 μm at conical tip) were implanted bilaterally in each rat, using stereotaxic coordinates from the atlas of Konig and Klipell (6). Stimulation parameters were 100-ms trains of 50-Hz sin waves presented at three trains per second. Current intensities for the production of both analgesia and self-stimulatory behavior ranged from 20 to 1,000 μA.

To test for the presence of analgesia during EBS, we applied a small alligator clip to each of the four limbs. Each limb was tested separately before, during, and after stimulation. Analgesia was indicated by complete absence of the following signs: vocalization, localization of and attempts to remove the alligator clip, or attempts to escape from the test box. Flexion of the limb was also abolished during stimulation.

In 8 rats with complete analgesia of the four limbs, various spinal cord lesions were subsequently induced. Initially the lesions were placed at T_3, ipsilateral to the effective stimulating electrode. Five of these rats underwent a lesion of the dorsal part of the lateral funiculus (DLF); three of the dorsal columns. When the initial lesion had no effect, a second lesion was made at T_8. In all cases, at least 1 week intervened between surgery and retesting.

In addition to the tests of analgesia, all animals were tested for the presence of self-stimulation by allowing the rats to press a lever to self-administer the stimulation. No quantitative estimates of stimulation rates were made.

RESULTS

In agreement with previous authors, we found analgesia from sites within and adjacent to the dorsal raphe nucleus of the midbrain. Figure 1 illustrates the sites which supported analgesia and several representative negative sites. In general, analgesia covered the whole body; however, if one side was dominant, it was usually ipsilateral to the effective stimulating electrode. The analgesia was apparent within seconds of the onset of the stimulation and outlasted the stimulation for periods of a few seconds up to several minutes. All sites which supported analgesia also supported self-stimulatory behavior.

As expected, self-stimulatory behavior was never disrupted by spinal cord surgery; however, marked and consistent changes in the levels of analgesia produced by EBS were observed. Figure 2 is a reconstruction of all the spinal lesions. A unilateral lesion of the DLF ipsilateral to the analgesia-producing electrode completely abolished the analgesia of the hindlimb on the same side. There was a suggestion of hyperresponsiveness to placement of the clip and possible hyperesthesia to light touch. The level of analgesia was reduced on the contralateral limb. Absolutely no change in the analgesia of the forelimbs was observed.

In contrast, a unilateral (rat P-20 and P-23) or bilateral (rat P-19) lesion of the dorsal funiculus, which in all instances severed the ventrally located CST, had no effect on the EBS-induced analgesia. Not only does this rule out the CST as a mediator of the descending inhibition, but these data serve

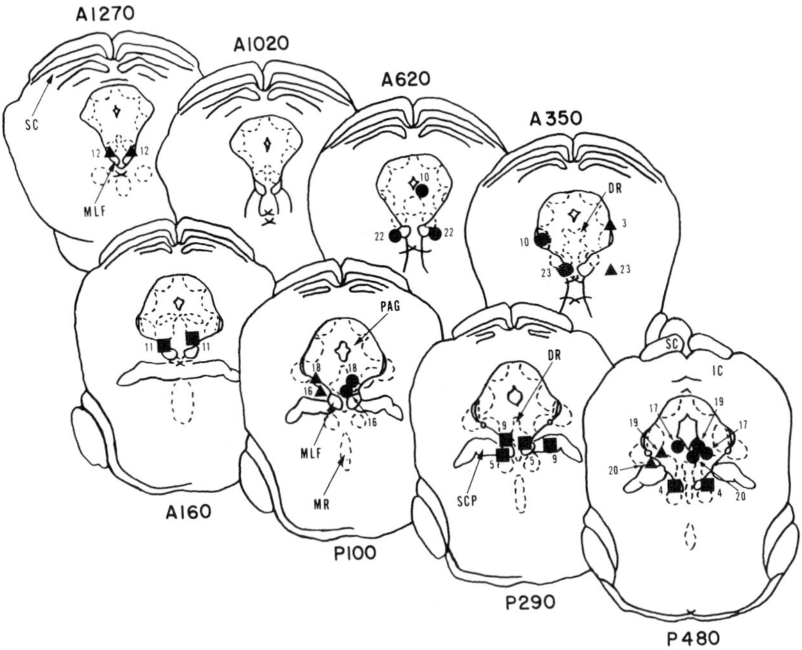

FIG. 1. Representative sections through the midbrain of the rat, taken from the atlas of Konig and Klippel (6), indicating electrode tip positions. *Squares,* analgesia-producing electrode, with less than whole-body analgesia—no spinal lesions performed; *circles,* electrode sites in rats in which subsequent spinal lesions were performed; *triangles,* some sites from which no analgesia was produced. Not all negative sites are indicated. SC, superior colliculus; MLF, medial longitudinal fasciculus; DR, dorsal raphe; MR, median raphe; PAG, periaqueductal gray; SCP, superior cerebellar peduncle; IC, inferior colliculus. Numbers refer to particular rat.

as controls for the effects of postsurgical trauma on the analgesic properties of EBS.

In the 3 rats with dorsal column lesions, a second lesion was induced ipsilateral to the first lesion and five segments caudal (T_8). In 1 rat, P-23, a subsequent lesion of the DLF abolished the analgesia, confirming the results of the previous five DLF lesions. In the remaining 2 rats, neither a Lissauer tractotomy (P-20) nor a lesion of the ventral part of the lateral funiculus (P-19) had any effect on the analgesia.

With continued testing, however, it was apparent that the effect of DLF section in disrupting the analgesia was transitory. In 3 rats—P-10, P-16, and P-17—the analgesia partially returned within 2 months. In 1 rat, P-18, there was complete return of the analgesia in both hindlimbs. To determine if crossing fibers mediated the recovery of analgesia, two subsequent operations were performed. Neither a lesion of the DLF at C_1 nor a lesion of the

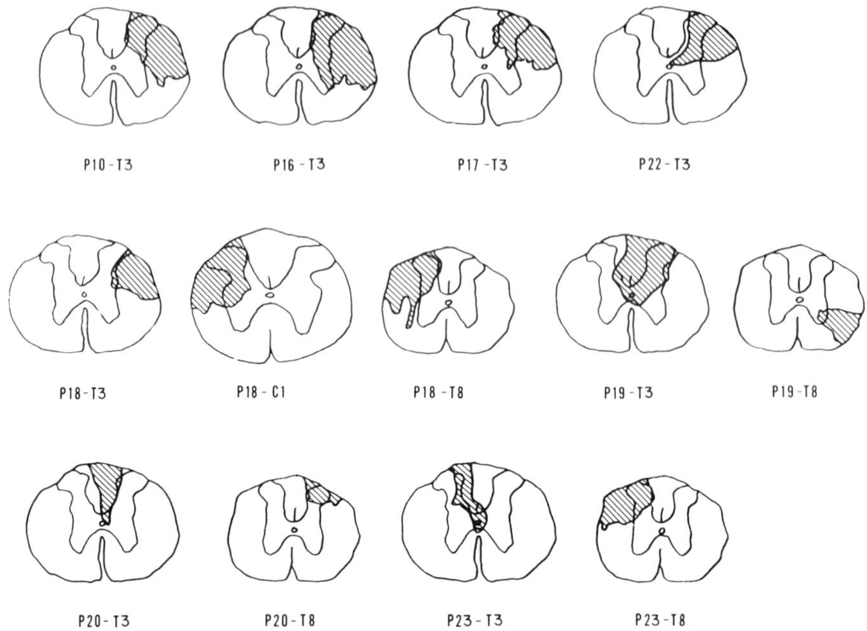

FIG. 2. Schematic reconstruction of spinal cord lesions. Hatched regions indicate extent of the lesion which was reconstructed from 50-μm serial sections alternately stained with cresyl fast violet and solochrome cyanide. The level of the lesion is indicated.

DLF at T_8 had an effect on the analgesia. No attempts were made to cut fibers of the ventral funiculus.

DISCUSSION

We conclude, therefore, that the dorsal part of the lateral funiculus ipsilateral to the analgesia-producing electrode plays a special role in the control of input by stimulation in the region of the periaqueductal gray of the midbrain. We can rule out the corticospinal tract as the critical descending system since a lesion of the dorsal columns had no effect on the analgesia. The question, of course, is what systems within the DLF mediate the descending inhibition which one presumes underlies the analgesia? Since no direct connections between the dorsal raphe and the spinal cord have been demonstrated (4), the cells of origin of the critical descending fibers in the DLF must be found elsewhere.

There have been several pharmacological studies demonstrating a relationship between aminergic systems and the control of pain by brain stimulation. For example, *p*-chlorophenylalanine, a serotonin synthesis inhibitor, antagonizes the analgesic properties of EBS (1). Furthermore, it has been demonstrated that a large number of the descending aminergic fibers of the caudal medulla course through the DLF to terminate in the dorsal horn (5). Taken together with the recent description of profound analgesia from sites in the serotonin-rich region of the caudal medulla (9), these data suggest that the mechanism of analgesia production from PAG stimulation is via synaptic linkage with the caudal medulla, and thence via aminergic fibers of the DLF which inhibit the discharge of dorsal horn cells that respond to noxious stimulation.

The return of analgesia after DLF section indicates, however, that other spinal systems must be involved. We have not ruled out a role for the ventral funiculus because of difficulty with surgical procedures. In addition, complex multisynaptic linkages between the midbrain, caudal medulla, and spinal cord may underlie the descending inhibition.

These results also substantiate the independence of the self-stimulatory and analgesic properties of EBS. Since the analgesia was abolished in the hindlimbs and maintained in the forelimbs, despite the continued presence of self-stimulation, it is clear that the rewarding properties of EBS do not underlie the observed analgesia.

ACKNOWLEDGMENTS

We would like to thank Prof. P. D. Wall for his continuing help and also Ms. Lynn Albertiri for histological assistance.

This work was supported by grants from the MRC and SRC (England) and from the Foundations' Fund for Research in Psychiatry.

REFERENCES

1. Akil, J., and Mayer, K. J. (1972): *Brain Res.*, 44:692–697.
2. Balagura, S., and Ralph, T. (1973): *Brain Res.*, 60:369–379.
3. Basbaum, A. I. (1973): *Exp. Neurol.*, 40:699–716.
4. Conrad, L. C., Leonard, C. M., and Pfaff, D. W. (1974): *J. Comp. Neurol.*, 156:179–206.
5. Dahlstrom, A., and Fuxe, K. (1965): *Acta Physiol. Scand.* [*Suppl. 64*], 247:5–36.
6. Konig, J. F. R., and Klipell, R. A. (1963): *The Rat Brain. A Stereotaxic Atlas of the Forebrain and Lower Parts of the Brain Stem.* Williams & Wilkins Co., Baltimore.
7. Mayer, D. J., Wolfe, T. L., Akil, H., Carder, B., and Liebeskind, J. C. (1971): *Science*, 174:1351–1354.
8. Oliveras, J. L., Besson, J. M., Guilbaud, G., and Liebeskind, J. C. (1974): *Exp. Brain Res.*, 20:32–44.
9. Oliveras, J. L., Redjemi, F., Guilbaud, G., and Besson, J. M. (1975): *Pain*, 1:134–145.

Advances in Pain Research and Therapy, Vol. 1,
edited by J. J. Bonica and D. Albe-Fessard.
Raven Press, New York © 1976.

Significance of the Membrane-Stabilizing Effect of Nonnarcotic Analgesics

R. Ziel and P. Krupp

Research Department, Pharmaceuticals Division, CIBA-GEIGY Limited, Basel, Switzerland

The group of drugs known as nonnarcotic analgesics includes a variety of substances with different chemical structures. In addition to their analgesic effects, they display antipyretic and anti-inflammatory properties. On the basis of findings reported by Lim (8), it is presumed that the analgesic action of these preparations may be mediated by a peripheral mechanism. The demonstration that the inhibition of prostaglandin synthesis is an essential feature of the activity of these compounds (12) gives grounds for assuming that their analgesic effect may also be attributable to this property (3). The degree to which they interfere with the biosynthesis of prostaglandins is, however, not as clearly correlated with their analgesic activity as with their antipyretic and anti-inflammatory effects (13). Various observations suggest that there may be other mechanisms that could account for the analgesic action of these drugs. For example, it has been reported that they exert a stabilizing effect on excitable membranes (2), which, according to Barker and Levitan (1), is associated with reduced conductance for potassium and chloride.

This chapter is concerned with experiments undertaken in an attempt to determine which of these various mechanisms is chiefly responsible for the analgesic effect of this class of compounds.

MATERIALS AND METHODS

Demonstration of Analgesic Activity

The analgesic efficacy of the compounds was assessed by reference to their influence on the writhing syndrome in the rat (R. Ziel, *unpublished observations*). This nociceptive reaction was induced in female rats weighing between 90 and 110 g by the intraperitoneal injection of 0.2 ml of a 3% solution of acetic acid. The resultant writhing movements were then assessed during an observation period of 20 min. The test compounds were administered orally in three different doses given to the animal 60 min before the intraperitoneal injection of the irritant. Their analgesic potency was estimated by interpolation of the dose required to reduce the number of writhing movements by 50%.

Influence of Prostaglandin Synthesis In Vitro

By analogy with the method described by Takeguchi et al. (10), the lyophilized microsomal fraction of bovine seminal vesicle or cerebral cortex was used as enzyme and ^{14}C-labeled arachidonic acid as substrate. The reaction mixture was incubated at 37°C in the presence of the cofactors 1-epinephrine and glutathione. The amount of PGE_2 formed was determined radiometrically after chromatographic separation of the extracted lipid fraction. The test compounds were added to the incubation mixture in at least three different concentrations.

Effect on the Excitability of Isolated Nerve

This experiment was carried out with the desheathed sciatic nerve of the frog (*Rana temporaria*) at room temperature. To determine its excitability, we introduced the nerve into a double chamber. One end was immersed in Ringer's solution and subjected to a bipolar maximal stimulus via platinum electrodes; the other end, attached to the recording electrodes, was immersed in paraffin oil. The action potentials were amplified and registered photographically. The test compounds were added to the Ringer's solution in various concentrations. Their activity was estimated by reference to the concentration required to diminish the amplitude of the action potential by 50% after incubation of the nerve for 10 min.

RESULTS AND CONCLUSIONS

The results obtained are listed in Table 1. All the nonnarcotic analgesics tested were active in the experimental models employed, although differences in their potency were noted depending on the particular system. They all exerted a dose-related inhibitory effect on the writhing reaction. The repeatedly demonstrated differences in their activity in this respect were also evident in our experiments in the rat.

The effect of the compounds on the biotransformation of arachidonic acid to PGE_2 was also dependent on the concentrations applied. In this *in vitro* assay also (Table 1) there were distinct differences in the potency of the compounds, consistent with the data reported in the literature (4,7,11). Approximately the same effects were observed, regardless of whether the microsomal fraction of the cerebral cortex or of the seminal vesicle was used as enzyme.

Similar results were obtained with regard to the inhibition of the excitability of the isolated nerve preparation. Nonnarcotic analgesics caused

TABLE 1. *Analgesic activity, inhibition of PGE synthesis, membrane-stabilizing effect, and partition coefficients of nonnarcotic analgesics*

Preparation	Analgesic activity[a] ID_{50} mg/kg p.o.	Inhibition of PG synthetase[b] ID_{50} μM	Membrane-stabilizing effect[c] ID_{50} mM	Partition coefficient[d] log P
Acetylsalicylic acid (Aspirin)	65	780	>100	−2.75
Aminopyrine (Pyramidon®)	30	1,300	38	0.88
Diclofenac sodium (Voltaren®)	2.5	0.3	1.5	1.13
Indomethacin (Indocid®)	2	0.4	10	1.0
Mefenamic acid (Ponstan®)	40	1.1	2	2.05
Oxyphenbutazone (Tanderil®)	60	120	>100	−0.06
Phenylbutazone (Butazolidin®)	35	100	40	0.7

[a] Writhing test, rat.
[b] Microsomal fraction of bovine cortex.
[c] Isolated nerve; concentration reducing action potential by 50% in 10 min.
[d] *n*-Octanol/water at pH 7.4.

TABLE 2. *Correlations between the activities of the compounds studied in various test systems*

Test system	Test system	Correlation coefficient	Significance
Analgesic activity[a]	Inhibition of PG synthetase[b]	0.306	>0.05
Analgesic activity[a]	Membrane-stabilizing effect[c]	0.842	<0.05
Membrane-stabilizing effect	Partition coefficient[d]	−0.820	<0.05
Inhibition of PG synthetase	Partition coefficient[d]	−0.406	>0.05

[a] Writhing test, rat.
[b] Microsomal fraction of bovine cortex.
[c] Isolated nerve, concentration reducing action potential by 50% in 10 min.
[d] *n*-Octanol/water at pH 7.4.

decrease in the amplitude of the action potential; both the degree and the rate of this response are dose dependent.

Table 2 shows that there is a clear correlation between the partition coefficients of the compounds in an octanol/water system and their membrane-stabilizing effect *in vitro*. Barker and Levitan (1) have also described a correlation of this nature in nonnarcotic analgesics. It is presumably attributable to interaction of the lipophil moiety of the molecule with the lipids of the membrane, leading to reorganization of the lipid layer of the biomembrane as a result of expansion (5,6,9). By contrast, the capacity of the compounds to interfere with the PG synthetase system is unrelated to their affinity for lipids, possibly because inhibition of this enzyme system is associated with a high degree of structural specificity (P. Krupp, *unpublished observations*).

Finally, there is no significant correlation between the inhibitory action of the nonnarcotic analgesics on PGE synthesis *in vitro* and their analgesic efficacy. There is, however, a significant relation between the concentrations at which they exert a stabilizing effect on nerve membrane and their analgesic action. This finding appears to indicate that the influence of these agents on membranes in general may have an important bearing on their analgesic potency. It would seem, therefore, that in the event of damage to the tissue, nonnarcotic analgesics may decrease the amounts of PGE precursors released from membrane-bound phospholipids by their membrane-stabilizing effect. The diminished amounts of PGEs formed during painful inflammatory reactions may thus not be entirely attributable to the inhibition of the PG synthetase system by these substances. It is, however, also conceivable that the membrane-stabilizing effect of this class of drugs leads to a reduction of the excitability of the pain receptors which are sensitized by PGE to other pain-inducing mediators of inflammation.

REFERENCES

1. Barker, J. L., and Levitan, H. (1974): In: *Advances in Neurology, Vol. 4: International Symposium on Pain,* edited by J. J. Bonica, pp. 503–512. Raven Press, New York.

2. Baust, W., Fischer, T., and Schaefer, H. (1957): *Arzneim. Forsch.,* 7:547–550.
3. Ferreira, S. H. (1972): *Nature* [*New Biol.*], 240:200–203.
4. Ferreira, S. H., Moncada, S., and Vane, J. R. (1971): *Nature* [*New Biol.*], 231:237–239.
5. Hansch, C., and Dunn, N. J. (1972): *J. Pharm. Sci.,* 61:1–19.
6. Jain, M. K., Wu, N. Y. M., and Wray, L. V. (1975): *Nature,* 255:494–495.
7. Ku, E. C., Wasvary, J. S., Court, R. H., and Wasvary, J. M. (1974): *Fed. Proc.* (Abs.) 33:590.
8. Lim, R. K. S. (1966): In: *Pharmacology of Pain,* edited by R. K. S. Lim, p. 169. Pergamon Press, Oxford.
9. Seeman, P. (1972): *Pharmacol. Rev.,* 24:583–655.
10. Takeguchi, C., Kohno, E., and Sih, C. J. (1971): *Biochemistry,* 10(12):2362–2376.
11. Tomlinson, R. V., Ringold, H. J., Qureshi, M. C., and Forchielli, E. (1972): *Biochem. Biophys. Res. Commun.,* 46(2):552–559.
12. Vane, J. R. (1971): *Nature* [*New Biol.*], 231:232–235.
13. Ziel, R., and Krupp, P. (1975): *Int. J. Clin. Pharmacol.,* 12:186–191.

Advances in Pain Research and Therapy, Vol. 1,
edited by J. J. Bonica and D. Albe-Fessard.

Modulation of Neuronal Activity in the Spinal Cord with Ketamine and Barbiturates

Guenter Corssen, Wilfred Nix, Clifford Holcomb, and Wilhelm Erdmann

Department of Anesthesiology, University of Alabama School of Medicine, Birmingham, Alabama 35233

After studying the effects of ketamine on single-unit activity on various dorsal horn Rexed laminae, Kitahata et al. (4) reported a marked suppressive effect on the spontaneous and evoked activities of laminae I and V, although the activities of laminae IV and VI were not significantly affected. Earlier reports of Conseiller's group (2) had also suggested a selective action of ketamine by documenting that it did not affect the response to innocuous tactile stimuli. In contrast, Strittmatter and Somjen (5) reported that barbiturates produced a uniform suppression of sustained potentials in the spinal cord without any evidence of selectivity among sensory tracts. Furthermore, barbiturates suppress synaptic transmission to the motor cells of the ventral horns more intensely than to the sensory relay cells of the fourth, fifth, and sixth layers of the dorsal horn. An explanation offered for the overall suppression afforded by barbiturates has been to attribute these effects to diminished level of neuronal activity. This, however, cannot explain the selectivity of action observed with ketamine.

The study reported in this chapter was designed to explore why a nonbarbiturate such as the phencyclidine derivative ketamine is selective in its pharmacologic action, whereas barbiturates such as thiopental lack this selectivity but exert an overall depressant effect on neuronal tissue function. A correlation of tissue Po_2, tissue perfusion, and neuronal activity as influenced by ketamine and thiopental could be expected to give some clue in answering this question. The experiments were performed in albino rats (Wistar).

METHODS

Rats were anesthetized with diethyl ether, relaxed with pancuronium bromide, tracheostomized, and artificially ventilated with N_2O/O_2 (2.1:7.9) using a 680 Rodent Ventilator connected to an endotracheal tube which was placed in the rat's trachea. Thirty minutes after the administration of diethyl ether was discontinued, the spinal cord was exposed through a

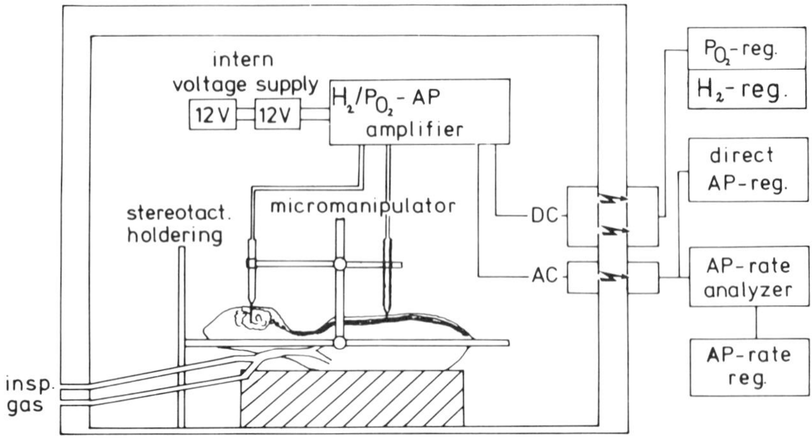

FIG. 1. Schematic diagram of the experimental setup. The rat is fixed in a stereotaxic hold inside a highly shielded chamber to avoid noise disturbance. Microelectrodes are driven into tissue (brain, spinal cord) by means of a micromanipulator. Information is led to a H_2/Po_2/AP amplifier which is driven by a 12-V battery. When feedback noise has to be abolished, output signals can be led to the recording equipment by light-emitting diodes which transmit information through the space between 2 shielding layers to light-receiving phototransistors.

laminectomy at the level of $T_{10\text{-}12}$ (Fig. 1). Microelectrodes were then inserted with a micromanipulator, and simultaneous recordings were obtained of action potentials, tissue Po_2, and tissue perfusion as previously described by Erdmann and Kunke (3). Both thiopental and ketamine were given via an intra-arterial catheter (brachial artery). Thiopental was given

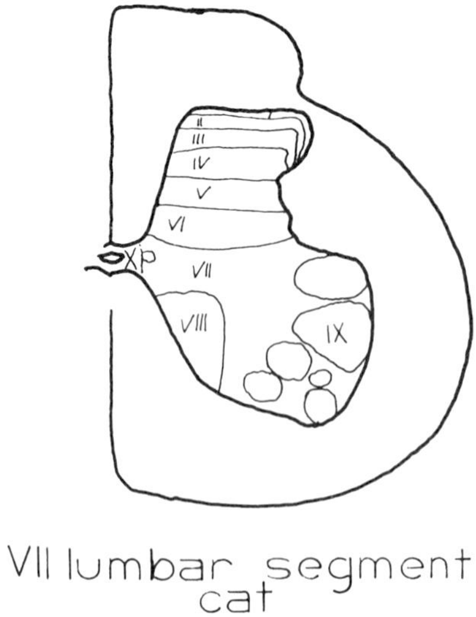

FIG. 2. Morphological structure (Rexed laminae) of gray matter of the spinal cord.

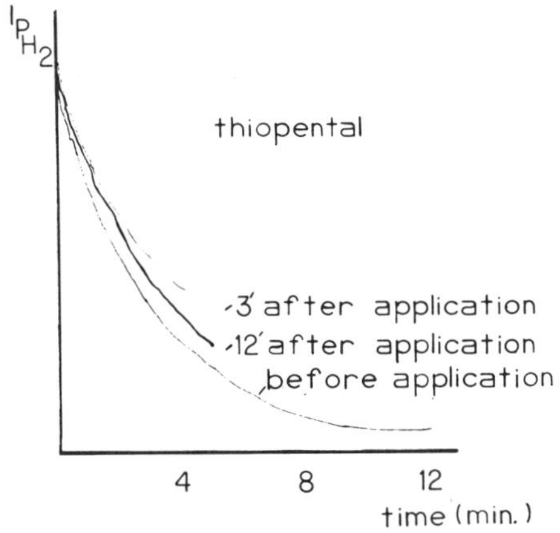

FIG. 3. H_2 clearance curves before and 3 and 12 min after thiopental application. The time course is decisively reduced (reduction of capillary perfusion) by thiopental.

in doses of 4 to 5 mg/kg and ketamine in doses of 2 to 3 mg/kg. The experiments were performed in a shielded cage in order to avoid noise interference. The electrodes were driven forward into the different laminae of the spinal cord (Fig. 2) 0.7 mm lateral to the dorsal spinal artery passing through a thin layer of white matter and entering the gray matter at lamina 1. The electrodes were left in this position while the above-mentioned recordings were continuously monitored.

RESULTS

Thiopental caused a significant decrease in tissue perfusion, thereby reducing oxygen supply to the spinal cord. In the gray matter of the dorsal horn with a rich capillary network, it could be shown that thiopental caused a 10% to 30% decrease (Fig. 3) in tissue perfusion. This phenomenon lasted from 12 to 20 min, at which time there was a gradual return to normal perfusion values. During hypoperfusion, there was a concomitant decrease in tissue Po_2 values from a normal of 10 to 20 mm Hg to 6 to 15 mm Hg (Fig. 4). A general suppression of action potentials throughout the dorsal horn laminae was also noticed during hypoperfusion and hypoxia. Although there was slightly less suppression of the potentials in the deeper tracts (laminae IV, V, and VI) as compared to the superficial tracts, this seemed to be anatomically rather than physiologically correlated. In the motor tracts of the ventral horn where tissue perfusion and tissue Po_2 are known to be much lower than in the dorsal horn, thiopental caused an even steeper decline in perfusion rate and therefore a more pronounced fall in tissue Po_2 to near 0 mm Hg combined with a marked suppression of action potentials.

Ketamine, on the other hand, showed no decrease in tissue perfusion or oxygenation (Fig. 5). In fact, in some instances a slight increase in perfusion

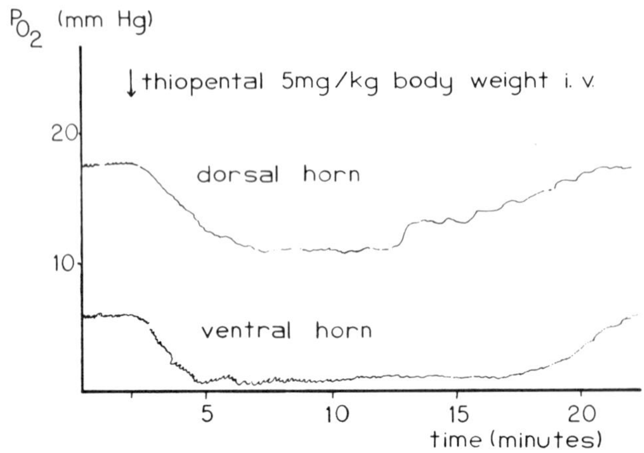

FIG. 4. Tissue Po_2 in dorsal and ventral horns of the spinal cord after thiopental application. A decisive drop in tissue Po_2 with differences in degree of hypoxia for the different regions is seen.

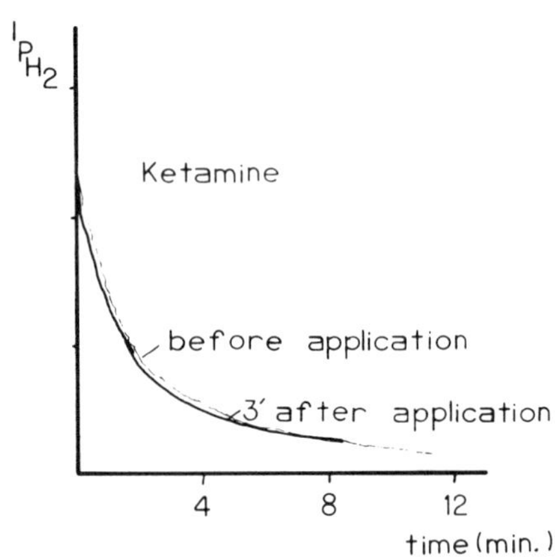

FIG. 5. H_2 clearance curves before and 3 min after i.v. application of ketamine. Change of the time course of the clearance curve is minimal, indicating that no decisive change of tissue perfusion occurs.

levels was observed. This may suggest increased usage of O_2 since no associated rise in tissue Po_2 was noted. These changes seemed to be random, however, and not specific to any particular lamina.

DISCUSSION

For the brain, it is well established that barbiturates cause a significant reduction in cerebral blood flow, while the oxygen consumption rate is decreased (1). For the microarea of the cerebral cortex, it has been documented that these changes are associated with marked reduction in tissue Po_2 (3). The results of the study presented here suggest that the thiopental-induced decrease of spinal cord capillary perfusion exceeds the decrease in tissue metabolism and oxygen consumption to such a degree that severe tissue hypoxia results. This observation seems to justify the assumption that the decrease in capillary perfusion may not be the mere result of autoregulation in response to reduced tissue metabolism, but that barbiturates may have some direct effect on the regulation of perfusion in the tissue. It also appears that the reduction of neuronal activity caused by barbiturates is mediated, at least in part, by the reduction of perfusion and tissue Po_2 levels.

Although ketamine is known to not interfere with the capillary perfusion/oxygen consumption ratio in the brain, the drug changes the rhythm of capillary perfusion as reported by Erdmann and Kunke (3). No changes of capillary perfusion in the spinal cord were observed. Alterations in rhythmic capillary flow patterns characteristic for the brain cortex are not found in the spinal cord. Therefore, it may be concluded that the neuronal suppression observed with barbiturates is probably owing to drug-induced tissue hypoxia, whereas ketamine's selective action in relation to nociceptive impulse conduction is likely to be due to a direct action on synaptic and neuronal units.

REFERENCES

1. Betz, E. (1972): In: *International Encyclopedia of Pharmacology and Therapeutics*, edited by A. Carpi, pp. 149–180. Pergamon Press, Oxford.
2. Conseiller, C., Benoist, J. M., Hamann, J. F., McMaillard, K., and Besson, J. (1972): *Eur. J. Pharmacol.*, 18:346–352.
3. Erdmann, W., and Kunke, S. (1973): In: *Oxygen Transport to Tissue*, edited by H. I. Bicher and D. F. Bruley, pp. 261–269. Plenum Publishing Co., New York.
4. Kitahata, L. M., Taub, A., and Kosaka, Y. (1973): *Anesthesiology*, 38:4–11.
5. Strittmatter, W. J., and Somjen, G. G. (1973): *Brain Res.*, 55:333–342.

Advances in Pain Research and Therapy, Vol. 1,
edited by J. J. Bonica and D. Albe-Fessard.
Raven Press, New York © 1976.

Observations on the Relationships Between Plasma Concentration and Analgesic Activity of a Soluble Acetylsalicylic Acid Derivative After Intravenous Administration in Man

V. Ventafridda and G. Martino

Pain Therapy Department, National Tumor Institute, Milan, Italy

The numerous studies concerning the kinetics and the metabolism of aspirin demonstrated that this drug is rapidly hydrolyzed to salicylic acid (2,9–13). In man, it has been observed that oral and intravenous administration of aspirin gives a contemporaneous increase in the plasma levels of acetylsalicylic acid (ASA) and of salicylic acid (SA). Rowland et al. (12) demonstrated that a peak plasma level of ASA is attained in 20 min and falls off in 1 hr, whereas the plasma level of SA reaches a plateau after 20 min and persists for several hours. Lester et al. (7) noted that ASA produces analgesia which is significantly superior to that produced by SA and that the period of analgesia corresponds to the period during which ASA is present in plasma. The advantage of aspirin over sodium salicylate has also been noted by several clinicians (3,5,6), and there is pharmacological evidence of the same superiority in animals (4).

Recently Barker and Levitan (1) have used an experimental nociceptor model consisting of isolated neurons from marine mollusk (*Navanax inermis*). They found that decreases in pH caused a decrease in membrane potential and conductance and thus served to decrease neuronal excitability. They also found that salicylate antagonized these effects by increasing membrane potential and conductance. For salicylate and a number of other compounds, they found a good correlation between reported analgesic activity in the vertebrate and activity in the system. In contrast, they found ASA (aspirin) to have a poor correlation between analgesic efficacy and activity in the model. They explained this discrepancy by citing the fact that aspirin is largely hydrolyzed to salicylate before reaching its site of action. The obvious conclusion was that it is probable that salicylate and not aspirin is the active agent producing the analgesic effect.

The discrepancy of the results cited above, together with our desire to elucidate a correlation between plasma levels of ASA and SA and analgesic efficacy in man, prompted us to undertake the present study. The aims of the study were to correlate analgesic activity of a soluble ASA derivative, lysine acetylsalicylate (Flectadol®), with measurements of plasma levels of ASA and its primary metabolite, SA.

METHODS

The trial was carried out in a group of 10 inpatients homogeneous in sex, age, and weight, and with similar pain owing to malignant tumors. Lysine acetylsalicylate was given in two regimens: intravenous injection of 1.8 g lysine acetylsalicylate in 6 patients; and intravenous injection of 1.8 g plus intravenous infusion of 4.5 g lysine acetylsalicylate in 4 patients (in all, lysine acetylsalicylate 6.3 g equivalent to ASA 3.5 g).

Plasma levels of ASA and SA were determined in all the patients 15, 30, 45, 60, 90, 120, 150, and 180 min after drug administration. All patients were asked before administration of drug and at specific time intervals afterward to grade the intensity and the relief of their pain according to the following scales:

Pain intensity		*Pain relief*	
Very severe pain	= 4	Complete relief	= 3
Severe pain	= 3	Moderate relief	= 2
Moderate pain	= 2	Slight relief	= 1
Slight pain	= 1	No relief	= 0
No pain	= 0		

The pretreatment intensity of pain was scored as 3.

Direct determinations have been made using gas chromatography employing the method of Rowland and Riegelman (10) partially modified by Lodi and Marozzi (8). A 5-ml sample of whole blood was placed immediately into a centrifuge tube containing heparin solution and potassium fluoride solution, the tube being kept in an ice bath. The blood was centrifuged and the plasma pipetted and stored at −30°C until required for analysis. (It is important to inhibit the enzymatic hydrolysis after withdrawal of blood samples because the hydrolysis of ASA in whole blood at 37°C is rapid with a half-life of approximately 30 min.)

Subsequently, 2 ml of plasma was pipetted into a centrifuge tube containing 0.5 ml potassium bisulfate solution, extracted with 6 ml of 20% ether and then centrifuged. The centrifuge tube was cooled at −10°C until aqueous phase froze. The ether extract was then injected into a conical gas chromatography tube and evaporated. The test tube was again cooled at −10°C. The concentrate was reextracted with 50 μl ether. The test tube was again cooled at −10°C for approximately 10 min and then shaken.

For gas chromatographic analysis, operating conditions were as follows: 1 μl of No-bis-(trimethylsilyl) acetamide (BSA) was accurately pipetted in a 10-μl Hamilton syringe; exactly 1 μl of ether-extracted solution was injected for analysis into the chromatograph. Thus the difficult silylation step described by Rowland and Riegelman (10) and recently by Thomas et al. (14) was avoided. A Fractovap model GI gas chromatograph with flame ionization detector fed with hydrogen (0.7 atm) and air (1 atm) and equipped with a column 2 meters long, filled with QF 1% on Gas-Chrom P conditioned at 145°C was used. Evaporator temperature was 180°C.

The retention times of SA and ASA were 138 and 312 sec, respectively, under the conditions described. Since SA concentrations generally are much larger than ASA concentrations, reduction of the attenuation switch (approximately 240 sec after introduction) would be necessary. Because the plasma levels of ASA fall rapidly, rise of the attenuation switch (up to 10 × 32) is necessary. "Zero time" analysis was performed first using a lower attenuation, generally 10 × 256 for SA and 10 × 32 for ASA. Measurements of peak heights of SA and ASA from samples corrected for the respective blank samples were compared with the standard values regarding dilution and initial plasma volume.

RESULTS

The results are summarized in Tables 1 and 2, and mean values are shown in Figs. 1 and 2 describing the plasma concentration times for ASA and SA after the administration of lysine acetylsalicylate and the contemporaneous scores for pain intensity and pain relief attained. The intravenous injection of lysine acetylsalicylate 1.8 g (corresponding to ASA 1 g) was followed immediately by high plasma levels of ASA and SA in the 6 treated patients (Fig. 1). The level of ASA fell rapidly, whereas that of SA remained high even after 3 hr. In parallel fashion, the lowest pain intensity and the peak pain relief were achieved about 60 min after administration, when ASA was found in extremely low concentrations. Pain intensity and pain relief scores remained constant and clearly correlated with plasma level of SA for 90 min. Thereafter, slight pain recurred and pain relief decreased slightly, both reaching maximum changes at 180 min in correlation with the lowest plasma levels of SA.

In the 4 patients given intravenous injection of lysine acetylsalicylate 1.8 g and an intravenous infusion of 4.5 g of the same drug (Fig. 2), the plasma levels of ASA fell to minimum after 1 hr, remained at the same level for 30 min, and reached a peak at 150 min, after which the levels declined. Contemporaneously, the plasma level of ASA rose to a first peak at 60 min, remained at that level for the ensuing 90 min, and rose further at 180 min. The plasma levels of ASA were always higher in these cases than in the previous 6 cases and for all observations. Even in these 4 cases the lowest pain intensity and the peak pain relief were achieved at 60 min. However, unlike the previous 6 cases, in these 4 cases no variation in pain intensity and pain relief was found. That is, both were unchanged in relation to the optimum levels reached during observation.

TABLE 1. *Personal data and pain intensity and pain relief scores after administration of lysine acetylsalicylate*

Case	Age	Weight (kg)	Diagnosis	Pain intensity 0′	15′	30′	45′	60′	90′	120′	150′	180′	Pain relief 0′	15′	30′	45′	60′	90′	120′	150′	180′	Side effects
1	52	63	Penis cancer	3	0	0	0	0	0	1	–	1	0	3	3	3	3	3	2	–	2	None
2	55	64	Histiocytic lymphoma	3	0	0	0	0	1	1	–	2	0	3	3	3	3	2	2	–	1	None
3	55	67	Lung cancer with bone metastases	3	4	3	2	2	1	1	–	1	0	0	0	0	1	2	2	–	2	None
4	54	64	Left laterocervical unidentified mass	3	4	2	1	0	1	1	–	2	0	0	1	2	3	2	2	–	1	None
5	56	63	Mammary carcinoma with bone metastases	3	3	2	1	1	1	1	–	1	0	0	1	2	2	2	2	–	2	None
6	54	64	Lung cancer with pelvis metastases	4	4	4	3	2	2	2	–	–	0	0	0	1	2	2	–	–	–	None
1	53	63	Lung cancer	4	4	3	3	2	2	2	2	2	0	0	1	1	2	2	2	2	2	None
2	55	65	Bone metastases in mammary carcinoma	3	2	1	0	0	0	0	0	0	0	1	2	3	3	3	3	3	3	None
3	54	64	Endometrial adenoma	3	1	1	0	0	0	0	0	0	0	2	2	3	3	3	3	3	3	None
4	56	66	Right lung cancer	4	3	1	1	0	0	0	0	0	0	1	2	2	3	3	3	3	3	None

Intravenous injection of 1.8 g (cases 1–6) and i.v. injection of 1.8 g + i.v. infusion of 4.5 g (cases 1–4).

TABLE 2. *Plasma levels of ASA and SA after administration of lysine acetylsalicylate*

	Plasma levels of ASA γ/ml								Plasma levels of SA γ/ml							
Case	15′	30′	45′	60′	90′	120′	150′	180′	15′	30′	45′	60′	90′	120′	150′	180′
1	25.80	1.55	1.00	0.80	nd	nd	—	nd	53.00	38.10	43.20	35.60	29.15	21.60	—	22.30
2	26.65	3.35	2.10	1.00	nd	nd	—	nd	58.50	69.20	62.10	56.80	59.10	60.80	—	36.80
3	nd	8.00	4.00	2.20	nd	nd	—	nd	50.00	37.50	53.10	52.80	46.10	47.50	—	34.70
4	61.00	18.30	13.40	6.10	nd	nd	—	—	126.00	125.00	130.60	104.30	64.70	66.50	—	—
5	25.65	6.05	1.50	nd	nd	nd	—	nd	59.45	47.35	40.50	37.35	39.50	29.80	—	32.80
6	4.30	4.70	4.20	2.30	1.20	1.10	—	—	7.50	29.60	42.50	35.00	27.80	41.60	—	—
Mean	28.68	6.99	4.37	2.48					59.08	57.79	62.00	53.64	44.39	44.63		31.65
SE	9.11	2.44	1.88	0.95					15.55	14.55	14.12	10.82	6.23	7.09		3.22
1	39.00	25.00	21.00	19.00	19.00	28.00	4.00	4.00	44.00	53.00	60.00	71.00	85.00	81.00	81.00	100.00
2	17.40	29.40	14.40	16.40	10.40	5.40	55.40	32.40	42.00	49.00	50.00	57.00	56.00	50.00	72.00	109.00
3	31.00	17.00	23.00	11.00	10.00	13.00	23.00	18.00	40.00	117.00	124.00	237.50	165.00	180.00	223.00	280.00
4	23.00	25.00	14.00	11.00	17.00	24.00	15.00	10.00	42.00	48.00	36.00	41.00	61.00	76.00	49.00	117.00
Mean	27.60	24.10	18.10	14.35	14.10	17.60	24.35	16.10	42.00	66.75	67.50	101.63	91.75	96.75	106.25	151.50
SE	4.71	2.58	2.29	2.01	2.29	5.16	11.06	6.14	0.82	16.78	19.47	45.7	25.22	28.57	39.50	42.97

Intravenous injection of 1.8 g (cases 1–6) and i.v. injection of 1.8 g + i.v. infusion of 4.5 g (cases 1–4) nd, not determined.

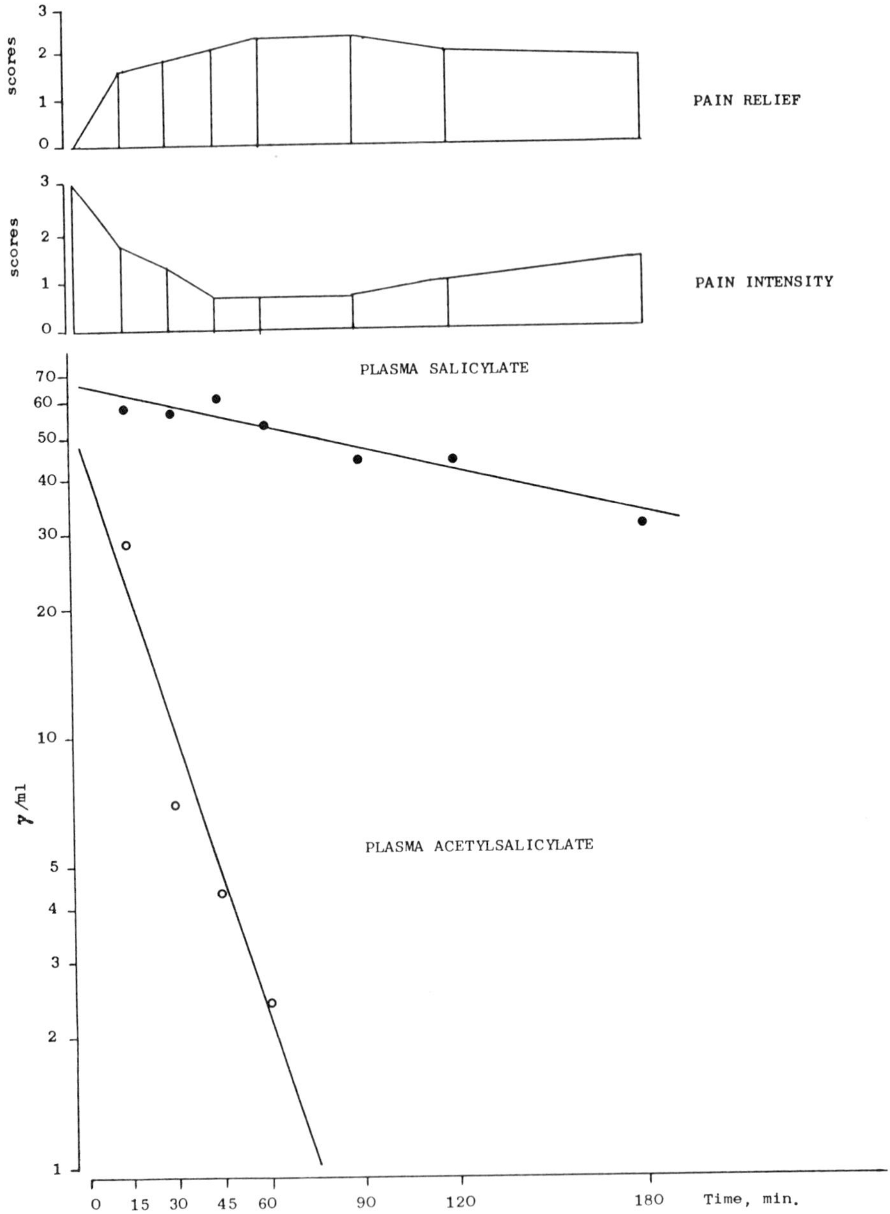

FIG. 1. Mean values of pain relief and pain intensity correlated with the mean plasma levels of ASA and SA after i.v. injection of 1.8 g lysine acetylsalicylate in 6 subjects.

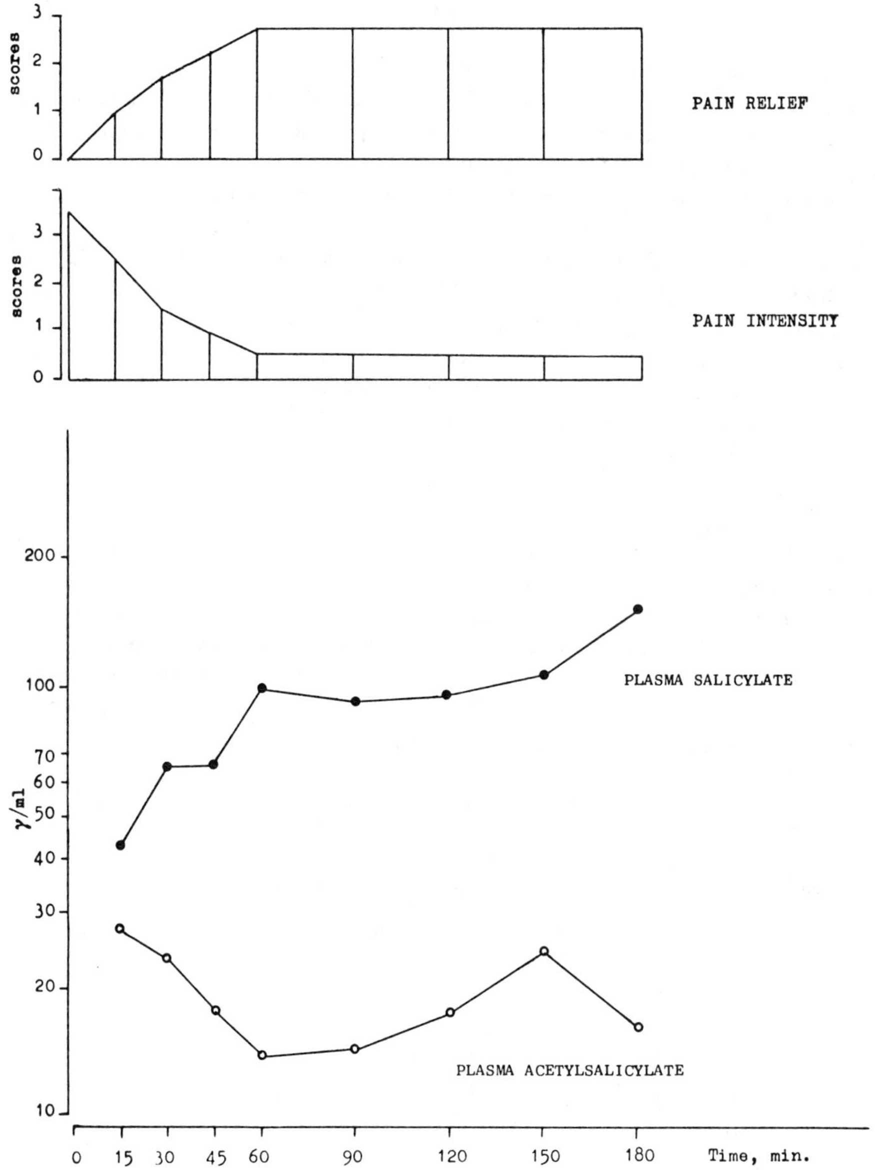

FIG. 2. Mean values of pain relief and pain intensity correlated with the mean plasma levels of ASA and SA after i.v. injection of 1.8 g + i.v. infusion of 4.5 g lysine acetylsalicylate in 4 subjects.

DISCUSSION

The results obtained are related to results previously reported in the literature regarding pharmacokinetics of ASA. Promptly after intravenous injection of ASA, the plasma acetylsalicylate reached a high level but was rapidly metabolized to SA. Consequently, the plasma level of SA promptly rises and remains high long after the plasma concentration of ASA has reached zero.

The analgesic effect is achieved during high plasma levels of SA when the hydrolysis of ASA has already occurred. Therefore, it appears that the analgesic effect of aspirin can be correlated not with its plasma levels but with the high plasma levels of SA, which are an index of good analgesia. The intravenous injection followed by intravenous infusion appears to be more manageable and efficacious in the relief of cancer pain.

SUMMARY

The discordant conclusions of the numerous studies regarding the pharmacokinetics of ASA prompted us to use a soluble ASA derivative, lysine acetylsalicylate, to correlate analgesic activity with measurements of plasma levels of ASA. The results we obtained after evaluating the relationship between the plasma levels of ASA and SA and the intensity of analgesic effect have demonstrated that analgesia occurs with high levels of SA and persists when ASA is already hydrolyzed.

REFERENCES

1. Barker, J. L., and Levitan, H. (1974): In: *Advances in Neurology, Vol. 4: International Symposium on Pain,* edited by J. J. Bonica, pp. 503–512. Raven Press, New York.
2. Davison, C. (1971): *Ann. N.Y. Acad. Sci.,* 179:249.
3. Duthie, J. J. R. (1963): In: *Salicylates. An International Symposium,* edited by A. S. J. Dixon, B. K. Martin, M. J. H. Smith, and P. H. N. Wood, p. 64. Little, Brown and Co., Boston.
4. Guzman, F., Braun, C., Lim, R. K. S., Potter, G. D., and Rodgers, D. W. (1964): *Arch. Intern. Pharmacodyn. Ther.,* 149:571.
5. Houde, R. W. (1958): *Personal communication.*
6. Lasagna, L. (1961): *Am. J. Med. Sci.,* 242:620.
7. Lester, D., Lolli, G., and Greenberg, L. A. (1946): *J. Pharmacol.,* 87:329.
8. Lodi, F., and Marozzi, E. *Unpublished investigation.*
9. Mandel, H. G., Cambosos, N. M., and Smith, P. K. (1954): *J. Pharmacol.,* 112:495.
10. Rowland, M., and Riegelman, S. (1967): *J. Pharm. Sci.,* 56:717.
11. Rowland, M., and Riegelman, S. (1968): *J. Pharm. Sci.,* 57:1313.
12. Rowland, M., Riegelman, S., Harris, P. A., and Sholkoff, S. D. (1972): *J. Pharm. Sci.,* 61:379.
13. Rowland, M., Riegelman, S., Harris, P. A., Sholkoff, S. D., and Eyring, E. J. (1967): *Nature,* 215:413.
14. Thomas, B. H., Solomonraj, G., and Coldwell, B. B. (1973): *J. Pharm. Pharmacol.,* 25:201.

Advances in Pain Research and Therapy, Vol. 1,
edited by J. J. Bonica and D. Albe-Fessard.
Raven Press, New York © 1976.

Nefopam Hydrochloride (Acupan®), A New Analgesic

Osvaldo N. Ré

Riker Laboratories, 19901 Nordhoff Street, Northridge, California 91324

Nefopam[1] is a new drug synthesized by Klohs et al. (7) at Riker Laboratories, Northridge, California. After extensive laboratory studies, it was introduced into clinical investigations in 1966. Early clinical studies revealed that the drug had mild antidepressant activity, and subsequently it was shown to have some analgesic efficacy. This report summarizes the results of the important studies carried out to date and the various aspects of nefopam.

NEUROPHYSIOLOGICAL PROFILE

Neurophysiological experiments in man by Gassel have revealed that nefopam enhanced the excitability of the motoneurons. These effects were opposite to the actions of other drugs (sedatives, tranquilizers) tested in this experimental model. The results provided substance to the following conclusions: nefopam was not a muscle relaxant and it did not behave as a sedative or a tranquilizer; indeed, it proved to be a fusimotor driver.

Concomitantly with the reflex studies described above, subjects participating in these trials were observed clinically and tests of intellectual performance were conducted as well. The overall characterization of this evaluation can be summarized as follows: subjects generally displayed a state of mental alertness, relaxation without drowsiness, no increase in motor activity, and no reduction of intellectual performance. Again, these effects were grossly different from those seen with sedatives and tranquilizers in subjects with a variety of musculoskeletal disorders.

SAFETY FACTORS

The safety of nefopam has been documented in a great number of studies involving more than 1,500 patients and/or normal subjects. Of special interest are two studies in which nefopam was administered in normal volunteers at a dose of 180 mg daily for 12 weeks with excellent overall

[1] Code name: R-738 (previously fenazoxine hydrochloride); chemical name: 3,4,5,6-tetrahydro-5-methyl-1-phenyl-1H2,5 benzoxazocine. Nefopam is an investigational drug in most countries. It is, however, commercially available in Mexico.

safety. The study by Klotz (8) failed to reveal a potential for abuse associated with the use of nefopam. In this regard nefopam shares some pharmacological actions with orphenadrine and diphenhydramine, and neither of the latter drugs has a history of abuse over many years of clinical use. Although no case of overdose has been reported to this date, clinical observation indicates that the symptoms of overdosage with nefopam may very well be indistinguishable from those of overdosage with atropine or orphenadrine, which, in turn, are indistinguishable from each other. If so, the treatment of overdose should be symptomatic/supportive, and one can anticipate that physostigmine may be of use in selected cases.

A blood loss study with ^{51}C technique (1) demonstrated a statistically significant ($p < 0.01$) increase in gastrointestinal bleeding after aspirin administration, whereas nefopam was not associated with such an increase.

METABOLISM

Metabolic studies have been carried out in man, monkey, dog, rabbit, and rat. The drug is rapidly absorbed and excreted. Approximately 85% is excreted within 24 hr of its administration, 90% of it being eliminated with the urine. Biotransformation is extensive and seven metabolites have been recovered.

In man, peak plasma levels occurred between 90 and 120 min, the half-life being approximately 4 hr. A dose of 20 mg of nefopam given parenterally is approximately bioequivalent to one of 60 mg administered orally.

MECHANISM OF ANALGESIC ACTION

Experiments conducted by Besson (3) revealed that nefopam did not alter the spontaneous or evoked activity of the lamina V cells of the dorsal horn of the cat, a phenomenon which was contrary to the depression of activity induced by anesthetics, morphinics, diazepam, and sedatives. The mechanism of action of nefopam remains, therefore, obscure.

CNS PROFILE

In addition to the already described effects of nefopam on the motoneuron pool (5), Basset et al. (2) have reported on the potentiation by nefopam of responses to norepinephrine and sympathetic nerve stimulation. Inhibition of the uptake of catecholamines, thus increasing their availability, is an action which nefopam shares with the tricyclic drugs and which may be related to its antidepressant effects.

Both pharmacological data and clinical observations clearly indicate that the CNS effects of nefopam are not amphetamine-like but rather are atropine-like.

ANALGESIC STUDIES

The studies on the analgesic efficacy of the drug which have been published or have been accepted for publication have included evaluation of analgesic efficacy of nefopam after parenteral or oral administration.

Parenteral Administration Studies

Gassel et al. (6) carried out a clinical trial on 20 patients with musculoskeletal pain. The experimental design was double-blind crossover by which each patient received on subsequent days a single i.m. dose of pethidine 50 mg, nefopam 20 mg, and placebo. The degree of pain relief was evaluated every 10 min for the first hour and again at 4 hr after drug administration. The Friedman two-way analysis of variance revealed that the relief of pain with nefopam was better than with placebo ($p < 0.01$), and that likewise pethidine was more effective than placebo ($p < 0.05$). There were no differences between the two active drugs. All drugs were tolerated well.

Sunshine (9) studied 74 patients with postsurgical pain. The experimental design was double-blind noncrossover by which patients received single i.m. doses of nefopam 10 or 20 mg or morphine 6 or 12 mg. Drug effects were measured in terms of sum of the pain intensity differences (SPID) and total pain relief. The relative potency, on a milligram basis, of nefopam to morphine was estimated to be 2 to 1 (or 20 mg of nefopam approximately equivalent to 12 mg of morphine). All patients tolerated both drugs well.

Oral Administration Studies

Gassel et al. (6) carried out a second clinical trial involving 80 patients with musculoskeletal pain given nefopam intramuscularly. The experimental design was double-blind noncrossover by which patients received either nefopam, 60 mg t.i.d., or matching placebo tablets for 3 days. The degree of pain relief was evaluated every 10 to 20 min during the hour after the first dose of day 1 (early pain relief). Drug effects were also evaluated over the 3-day period, but excluding the first hour of day 1 (late pain relief or continued pain relief). The Mann-Whitney U-Test revealed that nefopam was better than placebo at the 0.01 level of significance for early pain relief and at 0.02 for continued pain relief. Both regimens were tolerated well.

Workmon and Winter (11) have reported on 137 patients with musculoskeletal pain. The experimental design was double-blind noncrossover by which patients received single oral doses of nefopam 30 or 60 mg, aspirin 300 or 600 mg, or matching placebo tablets. Drug effects were measured in terms of SPID and total pain relief. Both active drugs were better than placebo without, however, reaching statistical significance. Nevertheless, positive slopes for both active drugs permitted us to estimate the relative potency of nefopam to aspirin to be 1 to 8.4. Nefopam also demonstrated a faster onset of action than aspirin. All patients tolerated the drugs well.

Cohen (4) studied 60 patients with musculoskeletal pain. The experimental design was double-blind noncrossover by which patients received nefopam 60 mg t.i.d. or aspirin 600 mg t.i.d. for 3 days. Both drugs afforded the same degree of relief over the 3-day period. Nefopam, however, demonstrated a superiority over aspirin in the onset of pain relief ($p=0.05$). All patients tolerated the drugs well.

Tobin and Gold (10) studied 24 patients with musculoskeletal pain. The experimental design was double-blind noncrossover by which patients received single i.v. doses of nefopam 10 mg, normal saline (12 patients), single oral doses of nefopam 60 mg, or matching placebo tablets (12 patients). The administration of both i.v. and oral nefopam was followed by greater analgesia than with placebo ($p < 0.01$). All patients tolerated the drugs well.

SUMMARY

Nefopam is a safe, effective analgesic that covers the entire range intensity depending on its dosage and route of administration. To this date, no evidence of abuse potential has emerged from clinical use. Nefopam is not a muscle relaxant, sedative, or tranquilizer. Psyche effects can be characterized by: a state of mild stimulation and mental alertness without increase in motor activity, relaxation without drowsiness, and no reduction of intellectual performance.

The CNS profile of nefopam includes: enhancement of the excitability of the motoneuron pool (human studies); inhibition of the uptake of catecholamines (animal studies); weak, atropine-like action (human studies); and no effects on the lamina V cells of the dorsal horn (animal experiments).

Nefopam has been shown not to induce gastrointestinal bleeding in man. The picture of overdose with Nefopam can be reasonably expected to be related to the atropine-like effects of the drug. The tablet form is absorbed quickly with a half-life of approximately 4 hr. A dose of 20 mg parenterally is approximately bioequivalent to 60 mg orally. Nefopam 20 mg parenterally appears to be approximately as potent as morphine 12 mg and meperidine 50 mg. Nefopam 60 mg orally appears to be approximately as potent as aspirin 600 mg with, however, a faster onset of action.

REFERENCES

1. Baltes, B. J., and Diamond, S. (1972): Riker files.
2. Bassett, J. R., Cairncross, K. D., Hacket, N. B., and Story, M. (1969): *Br. J. Pharmacol.*, 37:69–78.
3. Besson, J. M. (1974): Riker files.

4. Cohen, A. (1974): *Curr. Ther. Res.,* 16:184–193.
5. Gassel, M. M. (1973): *Electromyogr. Clin. Neurophysiol.,* 3:342–359.
6. Gassel, M. M., Diamantopoulos, E., Petropoulos, V., Hughes, A. C. R., Fernandez Ballesteros, M. L., and Ré, O. N. (1976): *J. Clin. Pharmacol.,* 16:34–42.
7. Klohs, M. W., Draper, M. D., Petracek, F. J., Ginzel, K. H., and Ré, O. N. (1972): *Arzneim. Forsch.,* 22:132–133.
8. Klotz, A. L. (1974): *Curr. Ther. Res.,* 16:602–608.
9. Sunshine, A. (1975): *Clin. Pharmacol. Ther.,* 17:245.
10. Tobin, W. E., and Gold, R. H. (1972): *J. Clin. Pharmacol.,* 12:230–238.
11. Workmon, F. C., and Winter, L., Jr. (1974): *Curr. Ther. Res.,* 16:609–616.

Advances in Pain Research and Therapy, Vol. 1,
edited by J. J. Bonica and D. Albe-Fessard.
Raven Press, New York © 1976.

Nefopam Hydrochloride (Acupan®) and Morphine Sulfate Comparisons in Man

*Abraham Sunshine and **Eugene Laska

**Arthur C. Logan Memorial Hospital, and New York University Medical Center, New York, New York 10016; and **Rockland State Hospital, Orangeburg, New York*

A new analgesic is under phase 3 investigation for a variety of painful clinical and experimental conditions. The drug, nefopam hydrochloride, is chemically distinct (Fig. 1) and pharmacologically unrelated to any presently known analgesic agent (4). It has no appreciable adverse gastric irritation effects (B. J. Baltes and S. Diamond, *unpublished observations*) and has demonstrated long-term safety over a period of 90 days in healthy volunteers, with no evidence of habituation or abuse (5).

Initial recognition of nefopam HCl as an analgesic was made by Gassel (3), who found it to have an electrophysiologic profile similar to that of pethidine. The relationship was borne out both in novel experimental pain investigations and in subsequent clinical tests in patients with orthopedic, fracture, or postsurgical pain conditions. Clinical trials by Tobin and Gold (8), Cohen (1), and Workmon and Winter (9), and unpublished data by Forrest and co-workers and by Gassel et al. confirm the analgesic effects of nefopam HCl. This chapter reports on a study designed to estimate the relative potency of nefopam HCl to morphine sulfate in the treatment of clinical pain.

METHODS AND MATERIALS

Adult male and female inpatients from the medical and surgical services at Arthur C. Logan Memorial Hospital participated in this study. A total of 74 such patients successfully completed all follow-up pain evaluations, being treated for fracture or somatic pain of moderate to severe intensity that required parenteral medication. They ranged in age from 20 to 76 years (Table 1) and had received no analgesics or tranquilizers for at least 4 hr before the administration of the test medications. All patients were fully informed regarding the nature and intent of this study and gave written consent indicating their willingness to participate.

The method of study has been described in detail elsewhere (7). Briefly, in design, it was double-blind single administration in which patients were

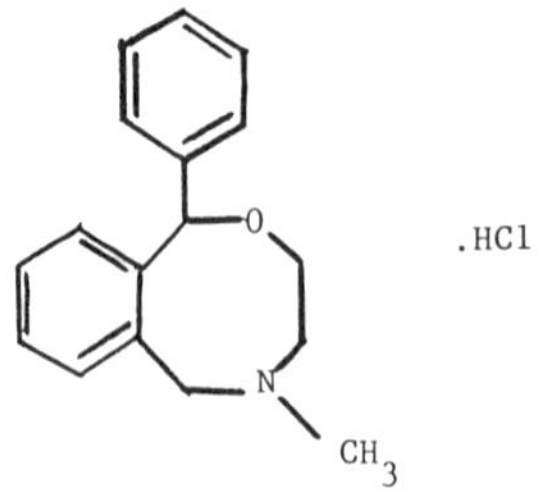

FIG. 1. Nefopam hydrochloride. Chemically, it is 5-methyl-1-phenyl-3,4,5,6-tetrahydro-1H-2,5-benzoxazocine hydrochloride.

randomly assigned to one of four treatment groups (Table 1). Weights of nefopam base in the 10- and 20-mg regimens were 8.74 and 17.48 mg, respectively; in the 6- and 12-mg morphine regimens, 4.51 and 9.02 mg, respectively. All dosages were given by the intramuscular route, and drugs were supplied in identical-appearing ampules, individually packaged and numbered for each patient. Randomization was such that in each group of 4 patients all four treatments were administered.

Successful entrants were questioned by the nurse-observer concerning the initial intensity of their pain (i.e., moderate to severe). Thereafter, two subjective measures of pain, intensity and relief, were used. The intensity scale had four graduations: 0 = no pain; 1 = slight pain; 2 = moderate pain; 3 = severe pain.

Relief was rated on a binary scale, wherein 0 was less than 50% and 1 was 50% or more. After base-line determination of pain intensity, patients were interviewed by the nurse-observer at 30 min and then hourly thereafter until the 6th hr after base line to ascertain both pain intensity and pain relief. If a patient asked for additional analgesics before 3 hr had passed after

TABLE 1. *Patient statistics*

	Nefopam HCl		Morphine sulfate	
Characteristic	10 mg	20 mg	6 mg	12 mg
Mean age (yr)	50 (20–67)	46 (20–71)	39 (23–76)	45 (20–73)
Mean weight (lb)	152 (98–200)	152 (100–200)	155 (128–185)	158 (96–265)
Mean height (in)	67 (60–74)	66 (61–71)	68 (63–74)	62 (59–78)
Sex				
Male	15	15	14	15
Female	3	5	3	2
Race				
White	5	5	4	5
Black	13	15	13	12
Initial pain intensities				
Severe	16	20	17	16
Moderate	2	0	0	1

taking the test drug, he was given conventional analgesics and removed from the study. However, after the arbitrary 3-hr mark, insufficiently controlled pain was also treated with conventional analgesics, but the patient's pain relief and intensity scores at the time of remedication were used for the remaining hours.

Pain intensity difference (PID) was calculated for each observation by subtracting the pain intensity at that moment from the premedication intensity. The weighted sum of the pain intensity differences (SPID) is obtained by multiplying each PID by the fraction of an hour since the previous observation and adding the result across all observations for each patient. Pain relief scores were similarly weighted and totaled for all seven post-medication observations to provide another estimate of analgesia (Total[1]) and yield a percent index of patients who had 50% or more relief.

Data thus obtained were recorded on the Cooperative Analgesic Card (2). In addition, pain site and type were recorded, as well as time of meals in relation to analgesic administration, patient demographic information, and any information on adverse reactions or side effects.

Data from these cards were analyzed by the bioassay method described in Laska et al. (6) with separate calculations for each variable listed below:

Pain 0: Initial pain score (which must be either 2 or 3) at time of drug administration.

Pain i: Pain intensity score at ith observation period (i – 1, 2, 3, 4, 5, 6, 7).

PID i: Pain 0 minus Pain i pain intensity differences.

SPID: Sum of the pain intensity differences (see above) across time, which is derived by subtracting the pain score at each observation from the initial pain level. These individual PID scores, weighted by the length of time since the preceding observation, are then added together, giving the SPID.

Relief i: Percentage of patients with 50% relief at the ith observation period.

Total: Percentage of patients with 50% relief or better (those with a relief score of 1) at each time point. These hourly percentages, weighted by the length of time since the preceding observation, are then added together, giving the Total.

The analyses include a calculation of the means, estimates of the slopes and intercepts of the dose-response curves, estimate of the relative potency with confidence curves, and analysis of variance including tests for linearity, parallelism, and pairwise *t*-tests.

RESULTS

Mean initial pain intensity scores varied for the four treatment groups between 2.9 and 3.0 (Table 2), but these differences were not statistically significant and thereby attest to the adequacy of randomization. No patients

---

[1] Total pain relief score.

TABLE 2. *Pain intensities (mean values and SEs)*

Observation periods	Nefopam HCl 10 mg	(SE)	Nefopam HCl 20 mg	(SE)	Morphine sulfate 6 mg	(SE)	Morphine sulfate 12 mg	(SE)
Base line	2.9	(0.07)	3.0	(0.0)	2.9	(0.6)	3.0	(0.0)
30 min	1.5	(0.17)	1.5	(0.17)	1.6	(0.16)	1.4	(0.16)
1 hr	1.4	(0.15)	1.2	(0.15)	1.3	(0.14)	1.3	(0.11)
2 hr	1.5	(0.16)	1.4	(0.18)	1.5	(0.15)	1.3	(0.13)
3 hr	1.7	(0.15)	1.4	(0.19)	1.6	(0.16)	1.4	(0.16)
4 hr	1.8	(0.20)	1.5	(0.20)	2.0	(0.19)	1.6	(0.19)
5 hr	2.4	(0.18)	1.7	(0.22)	2.1	(0.18)	1.8	(0.24)
6 hr	2.4	(0.17)	1.8	(0.22)	2.2	(0.17)	1.9	(0.22)

were dropped from the study because of side effects. Pain intensity scores presented in this table show greater mean analgesia with high doses of both nefopam HCl and morphine. These time-effect curves at the high and low doses were similar for nefopam HCl and morphine. The mean peak effect of nefopam HCl 20 mg and morphine 12 mg occurred at 1 hr. In concert, PID curves (Table 3, Fig. 2) were similar to pain intensity scores. Again, there was a definite tendency for the low- and high-dose curves of both drugs to remain juxtaposed over time.

In contrast to the above, relief scores showed higher initial values for morphine 12 mg versus nefopam HCl 20 mg (Table 4); however, these curves crossed between 4 and 5 hr. These differences were not significant, and the curves after 1 hr were essentially similar to those for both pain intensity and PID.

SPID values revealed a significant dose response for nefopam HCl (means: 6.1 and 8.7) and for morphine (means: 6.6 and 8.6), with the higher doses of each drug inducing greater analgesia (Table 5). This was significant at the 95% level. An estimate of relative potency of nefopam HCl versus morphine was 0.56, supported by a 95% confidence level of 0.23 to 1.13 (Fig. 3). The combined analysis of variance revealed a significant regres-

TABLE 3. *Pain intensity differences (means and SEs)*

Observation periods	Nefopam HCl 10 mg	(SE)	Nefopam HCl 20 mg	(SE)	Morphine sulfate 6 mg	(SE)	Morphine sulfate 12 mg	(SE)
30 min	1.4	(0.15)	1.5	(0.17)	1.3	(0.16)	1.6	(0.16)
1 hr	1.5	(0.14)	1.8	(0.15)	1.6	(0.14)	1.7	(0.11)
2 hr	1.4	(0.15)	1.6	(0.18)	1.4	(0.14)	1.7	(0.13)
3 hr	1.2	(0.13)	1.5	(0.19)	1.3	(0.16)	1.6	(0.16)
4 hr	1.0	(0.19)	1.5	(0.21)	0.9	(0.18)	1.4	(0.19)
5 hr	0.5	(0.16)	1.2	(0.22)	0.8	(0.17)	1.2	(0.24)
6 hr	0.5	(0.14)	1.1	(0.23)	0.7	(0.18)	1.1	(0.22)

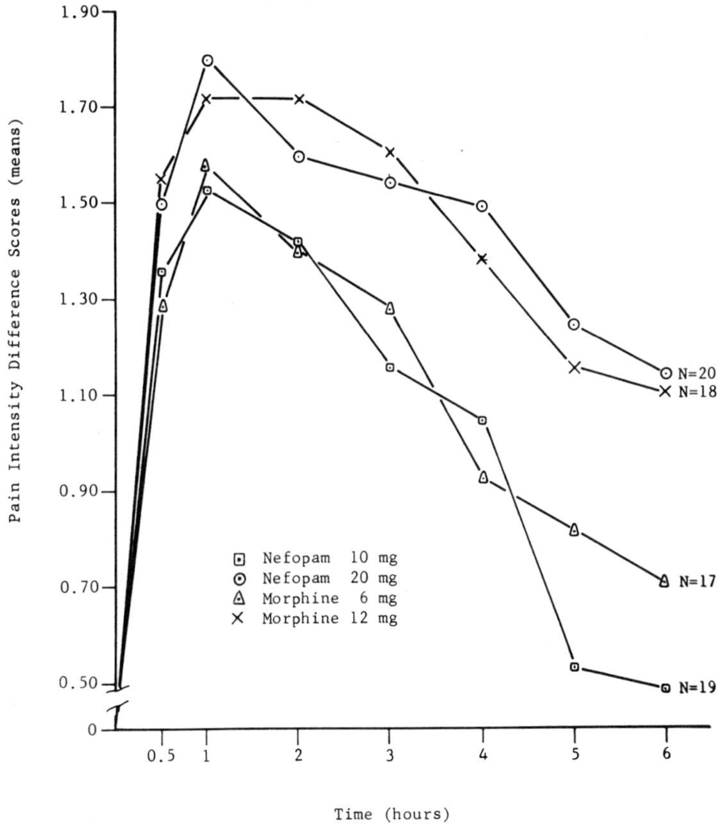

FIG. 2. Mean pain intensity difference scores in patients treated with nefopam HCl and morphine sulfate (each at 2 dose levels). Scores are calculated by subtracting the mean pain intensity score for each observation point from the pain intensity at the 0 hour. N = number of patients.

TABLE 4. *Pain relief*[a] *(means and SEs)*

Observation periods	Nefopam HCl				Morphine sulfate			
	10 mg	(SE)	20 mg	(SE)	6 mg	(SE)	12 mg	(SE)
30 min	0.68	(0.11)	0.70	(0.10)	0.59	(0.12)	0.72	(0.11)
1 hr	0.74	(0.10)	0.80	(0.09)	0.65	(0.12)	0.94	(0.05)
2 hr	0.74	(0.10)	0.75	(0.10)	0.65	(0.12)	0.89	(0.07)
3 hr	0.63	(0.11)	0.70	(0.10)	0.65	(0.12)	0.78	(0.10)
4 hr	0.53	(0.11)	0.70	(0.10)	0.53	(0.12)	0.72	(0.10)
5 hr	0.32	(0.11)	0.65	(0.11)	0.41	(0.12)	0.56	(0.12)
6 hr	0.32	(0.11)	0.55	(0.11)	0.35	(0.12)	0.50	(0.12)

[a] Rated per observation: 0 = less than 50% relief; 1 = 50% relief or more.

TABLE 5. *SPID (means and SEs)*

	Nefopam HCl				Morphine sulfate			
Variable	10 mg	(SE)	20 mg	(SE)	6 mg	(SE)	12 mg	(SE)
SPID	6.1	(0.54)	8.7	(1.0)	6.6	(0.80)	8.6	(0.90)

x^2, 7.874; $p < 0.05$ (cl = 0.23–1.13); df, 3.

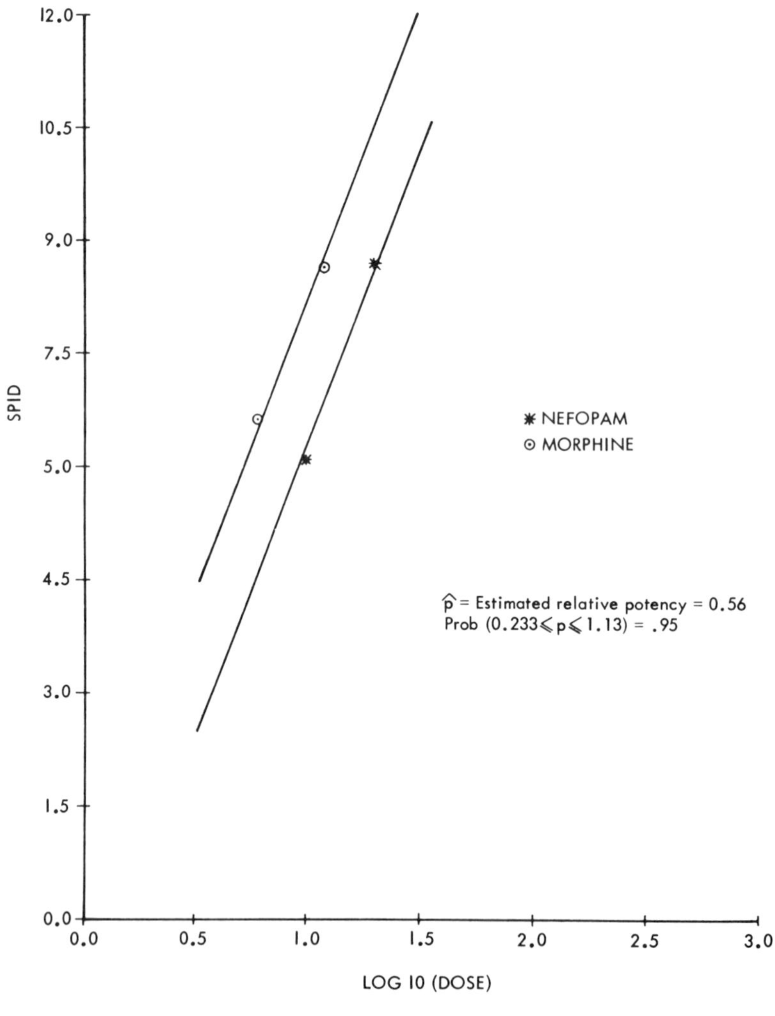

FIG. 3. Parallel line regression curves (potency 0.56) for SPID based on mg of drug base.

TABLE 6. *Total pain relief in all periods of observation (means and SEs)*

Variable	Nefopam HCl				Morphine sulfate			
	10 mg	(SE)	20 mg	(SE)	6 mg	(SE)	12 mg	(SE)
Total	3.2	(0.48)	4.1	(0.52)	3.2	(0.53)	4.3	(0.45)

x^2, 7.306; $p < 0.10$ (cl = 0.11–1.8); df, 3.

TABLE 7. *Summary of bioassay results in patients treated with nefopam hydrochloride or morphine sulfate*

Variable		Slope of standard[a]	Slope of test[b]	Potency[c]	Confidence levels[d]	
					Lower	Upper
Base-line		0.196	0.350	−0.479	−0.023	1.281
Pain[e]	30 min	−0.673	−0.087	0.726	0.262	40.454
Pain	1 hr	−0.250	−0.559	0.719	0.194	*
Pain	2 hr	−0.836	−0.245	0.513	0.002	1.764
Pain	3 hr	−0.858	−0.953	0.496	0.010	1.356
Pain	4 hr	−1.292	−1.136	0.774†	0.326	64.580
Pain	5 hr	−0.944	−2.054	0.533‡	0.026	1.811
Pain	6 hr	−1.151	−1.897	0.540‡	0.081	1.538
Relief[f]	30 min	0.445	0.052	0.844	0.396	210.129
Relief	1 hr	0.988	0.210	0.531	0.052	1.568
Relief	2 hr	0.803	0.044	0.512	0.001	1.844
Relief	3 hr	0.434	0.227	0.429	0.000	0.942
Relief	4 hr	0.641	0.577	0.571	0.077	2.361
Relief	5 hr	0.478	1.110	0.603‡	0.084	4.624
Relief	6 hr	0.489	0.778	0.617	0.173	2.706
PID[g]	30 min	0.869	0.437	0.617	0.168	2.805
PID	1 hr	0.445	0.909	0.620	0.191	2.497
PID	2 hr	1.031	0.595	0.507	0.000	1.948
PID	3 hr	1.053	1.303	0.496‡	0.004	1.426
PID	4 hr	1.487	1.486	0.713‡	0.295	6.241
PID	5 hr	1.140	2.404	0.527‡	0.188	1.028
PID	6 hr	1.346	2.247	0.533††	0.001	2.654
SPID[h]		6.715	8.707	0.560††	0.000	9.036
Total[i]		3.561	2.867	0.568†	0.115	1.822

[a] Slope of standard is the slope of the dose-response curve obtained with morphine sulfate.

[b] Slope of test is the slope of the dose-response curve with nefopam hydrochloride.

[c] Potency is an expression of the amount of nefopam hydrochloride necessary to give an analgesic effect equal to that of morphine sulfate.

[d] Confidence intervals were at ≥ 90% where indicated.

[e] Pain represents the pain intensity score for each observation period.

[f] Relief is the percent of patients with ≥ 50% relief at each observation.

[g] PID represents the difference of the pain intensity of each observation subtracted from base-line pain.

[h] SPID is the summation of all pain intensity difference scores.

[i] Total is the summation of all the relief scores.

* = > 999.999.

† Significant at 90% level.

‡ Significant at 95% level.

‡‡ Significant at 99% level.

sion and no significant deviation from parallelism. There was no significant difference between preparations averaged across both doses.

Total pain relief values also showed a significant dose response for nefopam HCl (means: 3.2 and 4.1) and morphine (means: 3.2 and 4.3) on analysis (Table 6). Based on this variable, relative potency of nefopam HCl to morphine was 0.57, with a 90% confidence interval of 0.11 to 1.8. The combined analysis of variance revealed a significant regression and no significant deviation from parallelism. There was no significant difference between preparations averaged across both doses. Thus the data on relative potency for SPID and total pain relief indicate approximate equipotency between 0.56 and 0.57 mg morphine and 1 mg nefopam HCl. A summary of these bioassay results is presented in Table 7.

Adverse Effects

There were no adverse effects observed or volunteered with nefopam HCl. One patient who received morphine 12 mg complained of dizziness, sweating, and nausea.

DISCUSSION

This study demonstrated that nefopam HCl has a time-effect curve similar to that of morphine, and that it is 0.57 times as effective as an analgesic. The incidence of adverse reactions in this small sample size did not differ between the two drugs. Previous work by others suggests that nefopam HCl has no abuse or habituation potential. Its animal pharmacological profile characterizes it as distinct from morphine in that it is not a respiratory depressant; if this distinction is confirmed in man, nefopam HCl will prove to be a significant advance in the management of pain.

SUMMARY

A new analgesic, nefopam hydrochloride, has a unique heterocyclic structure and is chemically distinct and pharmacologically unrelated to any presently known analgesic agent. We compared morphine sulfate and nefopam HCl in 74 patients who required parenteral analgesia for moderate-to-severe postoperative and somatic pain, using a single administration, two-dose level, double-blind design. A significant dose-response curve was obtained with nefopam HCl and with morphine. Analysis of variance revealed a significant regression and no significant deviation from parallelism. The time-effect curves for the two drugs were similar. The estimated relative potency of nefopam HCl to morphine indicates that 20 mg of nefopam HCl is the approximate equal of 12 mg of morphine. There were no adverse effects with nefopam HCl and one adverse effect with morphine.

REFERENCES

1. Cohen, A. (1974): *Curr. Ther. Res.,* 16:184–193.
2. Forrest, W. H., Belleville, J. W., Seed, J. C., Houde, R., Wallenstein, S. L., and Sunshine, A. (1963): *Serv. Center Bull.,* 2:1–10.
3. Gassel, M. M. (1973): *Electromyogr. Clin. Neurophysiol.,* 3:342–359.
4. Klohs, M. W., et al. (1972): *Arzneim. Forsch.,* 22:132–133.
5. Klotz, A. L. (1974): *Curr. Ther. Res.,* 16:602–608.
6. Laska, E., Gormley, M., Sunshine, A., Belleville, J. W., Kantor, T. G., Forrest, W. H., Siegel, C., and Meisner, M. (1967): *Clin. Pharmacol. Ther.,* 8:658–669.
7. Sunshine, A., Laska, E., Slafta, J., and Fleischman, E. (1971): *Toxicol. Appl. Pharmacol.,* 12:512–518.
8. Tobin, W. E., and Gold, R. H. (1972): *J. Clin. Pharmacol.,* 12:230–238.
9. Workmon, F. C., and Winter, L. (1974): *Curr. Ther. Res.* 16:609–616.

Advances in Pain Research and Therapy, Vol. 1,
edited by J. J. Bonica and D. Albe-Fessard.
Raven Press, New York © 1976.

Comparison of the Analgesic Effects of Morphine, Hydroxyzine, and Their Combination in Patients with Postoperative Pain

William T. Beaver and Grace Feise

Departments of Pharmacology and Anesthesiology, Schools of Medicine and Dentistry, Georgetown University, Washington, D.C. 20007

A great variety of major and minor tranquilizers and sedative-hypnotics have, at one time or another, been claimed to enhance or potentiate the effect of analgesics. The vast majority of these claims have been based on anecdotal evidence or uncontrolled clinical trials. However, when subsequent well-controlled analgesic studies have been performed, the sedative or tranquilizer in question has usually been found neither to have analgesic activity of its own nor to enhance the analgesic activity of concomitantly administered narcotics.

Hydroxyzine (Vistaril®, Atarax®), a minor tranquilizer with associated antihistaminic, antispasmodic, and antiemetic activity, is one of the many drugs claimed to potentiate potent analgesics. Initially, these claims were based on anecdotal evidence and results of uncontrolled trials. Recently, however, more sophisticated studies by Momose (2–6) in Japan and A. Sunshine (*personal communication*) in the United States have also indicated that hydroxyzine may have an analgesic-enhancing effect. The present study was undertaken to determine if hydroxyzine has analgesic activity of its own, if it enhances the analgesic effect of concomitantly administered narcotics, and if its antianxiety effect can be quantitated and is beneficial in patients with postoperative pain.

METHODS

Subjects for this study were postoperative patients from the general surgical and gynecologic services at Georgetown University Hospital in Washington, D.C. Patients likely to experience moderate-to-severe postoperative pain and for whom there was no contraindication to the administration of 8 mg of morphine in combination with 100 mg of hydroxyzine were interviewed the evening before surgery by the nurse-observer. At that time she explained the details of the study and solicited the participation of those patients who were cooperative and who appeared likely to communicate meaningful information about their pain.

The method of quantitating analgesia was a modification of that developed by Houde, Wallenstein, and Rogers (1). Test medications were administered on the first postoperative day by one nurse-observer only when patients complained of moderate or severe pain and only if at least 3 hr had elapsed since the last analgesic medication. Neither the patient nor the observer was aware of the identity of the medications, which were physically indistinguishable and identified only by an individual numerical code (the double-blind technique). Observations were made hourly for 6 hr after administration of the test medication or until the pain returned to the premedication level and another analgesic was required. Awakening the patient if necessary, the observer asked him to classify the intensity of his pain as none, slight, moderate, or severe, and to classify his estimate of relief from the medication as none, slight, moderate, good, or complete. In addition, a nine-item tension/anxiety questionnaire was completed at the time of drug administration and at 2-hr intervals thereafter. The observer also recorded apparent or volunteered side effects, but leading questions were avoided.

The study was of a 2×2 factorial design comparing placebo, 8 mg of intramuscular morphine sulfate, 100 mg of intramuscular hydroxyzine hydrochloride, and the combination of morphine 8 mg plus hydroxyzine 100 mg. The study was done on a single-treatment-only basis and was stratified for moderate and severe initial pain intensity. Twenty-four patients received each of the four treatments.

RESULTS

None of the 96 patients entering the study dropped out. Figure 1 depicts the time-effect curves for the four treatments using the change in pain intensity (pain intensity difference) parameter. The time-effect curves and statistical analyses based on pain relief estimates were similar. The placebo is obviously the least effective treatment. Morphine 8 mg appears, as would be expected, clearly superior to placebo, and this impression is confirmed by an analysis of variance using the appropriate orthogonal comparisons for a factorial study, which demonstrates a morphine effect significant to at least the 0.01 level.

The most surprising and intriguing result of this study is the clear-cut potent analgesic activity demonstrated by hydroxyzine. The time-effect curves of morphine and hydroxyzine are different in shape, with the analgesic effect of hydroxyzine peaking somewhat earlier than that of morphine. Although hydroxyzine appears somewhat less effective than morphine at the doses used, there is no statistically significant difference between the analgesic effect of hydroxyzine and that of morphine. An analysis of variance reveals a hydroxyzine effect significant at the 0.01 level. The top curve represents the effect of the combination of morphine 8 mg and hydroxyzine 100 mg. The analysis of variance shows a lack of a significant value for interaction between the two treatments, a finding which implies that the effects of hydroxyzine and morphine are additive.

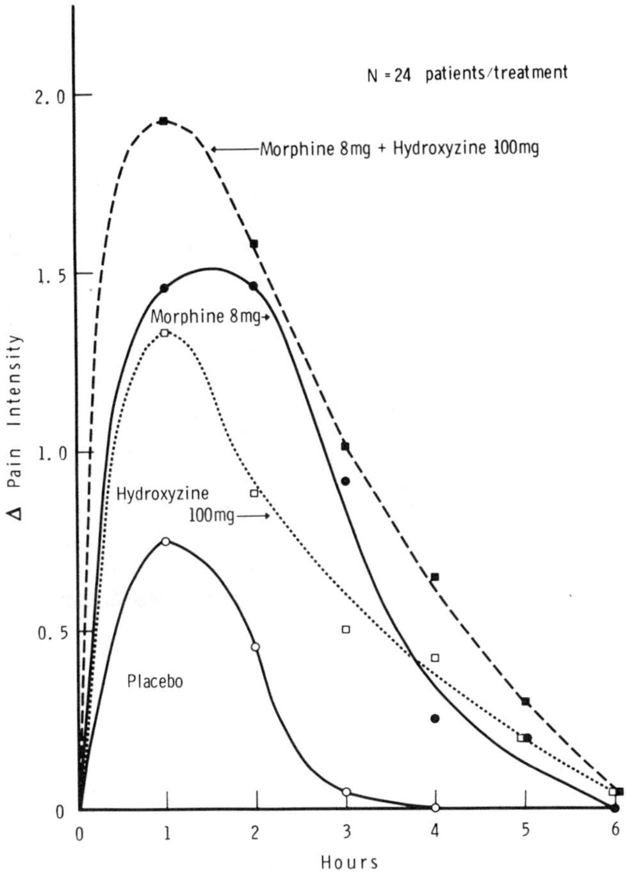

FIG. 1. Time-effect curves for placebo, morphine 8 mg i.m., hydroxyzine 100 mg i.m., and the combination of morphine 8 mg + hydroxyzine 100 mg i.m. using the change in pain intensity (pain intensity difference) parameter. Data from patients with moderate and severe initial pain are pooled.

Figure 2 depicts the time-effect curves for the four treatments when the results are plotted separately for those patients who initially had moderate pain and those patients who initially had severe pain. Statistical analysis reveals a significant superiority of both morphine and hydroxyzine to placebo in both groups of patients. However, although the effect of the combination is almost exactly additive in patients with severe initial pain, the effect of the combination appears no greater than that of morphine or hydroxyzine alone in patients with moderate initial pain. Since only 9 patients per treatment started with moderate initial pain, the significance of this apparent difference in response based on initial pain intensity is uncertain.

The mean tension/anxiety score for each treatment at the 2-hr observation point, adjusted for each patient's base-line tension/anxiety level,

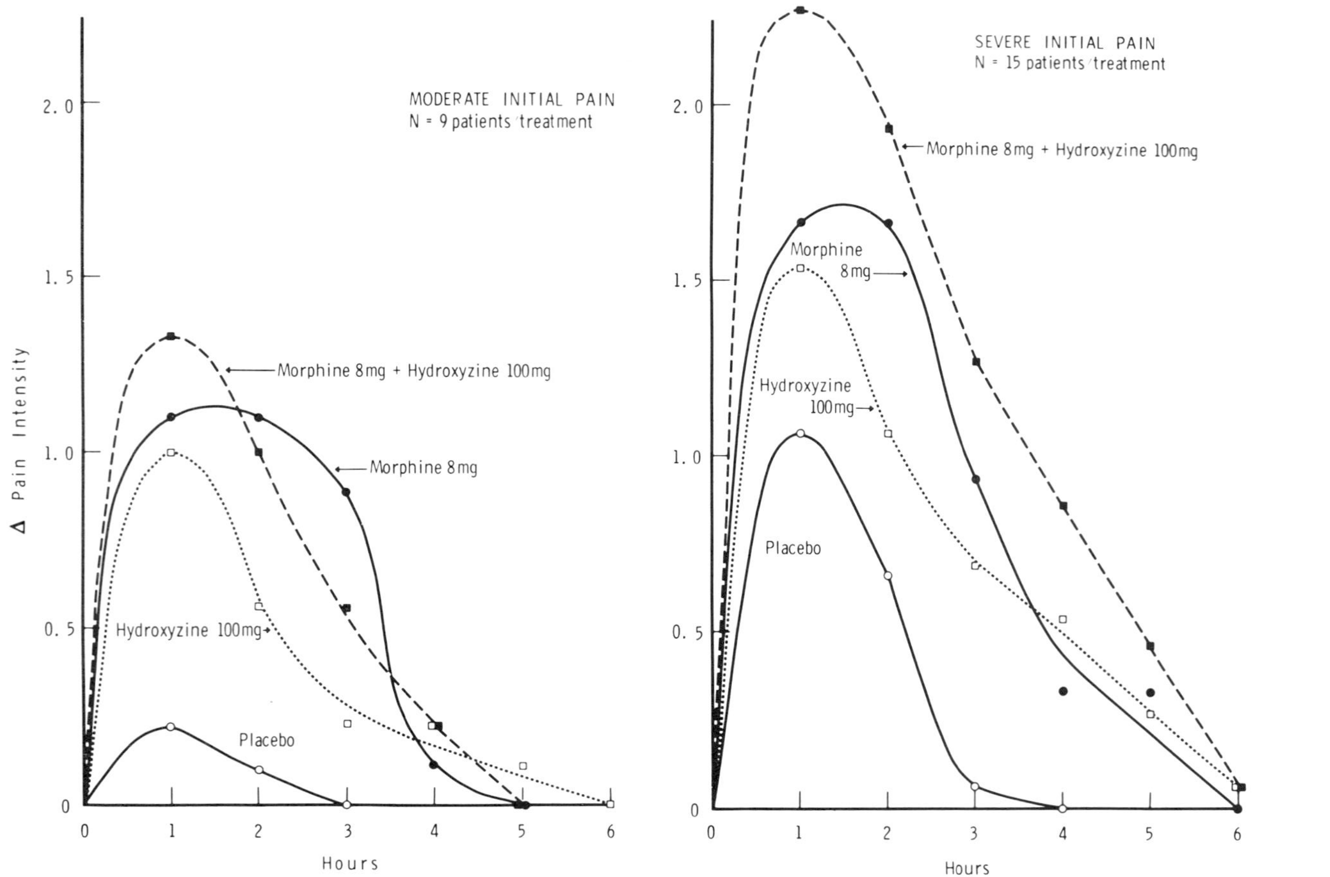

FIG. 2. Time-effect curves for placebo, morphine 8 mg i.m., hydroxyzine 100 mg i.m., and the combination of morphine 8 mg + hydroxyzine 100 mg i.m. using the change in pain intensity (pain intensity difference) parameter. Data from patients with moderate initial pain and severe initial pain are plotted separately.

closely paralleled the analgesic responses for both the total sample and the subpopulations of patients with moderate and severe initial pain considered separately. The most substantial differences between treatments are again apparent in the severe initial pain group. The combination was significantly more effective than any of the other treatments in the relief of tension/anxiety, whereas placebo was the least effective treatment. Morphine was also significantly more effective than placebo, but not significantly superior to hydroxyzine alone, which, in turn, was not significantly superior to placebo. It is not clear from the data what part of the relief of tension/anxiety produced by the active treatments is because of a specific tranquilizing effect and what part reflects the analgesic effect of these drugs.

The incidence and type of side effects encountered in this study were what one would generally expect in a postoperative population administered potent analgesics. Sedative-type side effects occurred in 3 patients on placebo, 19 patients on morphine 8 mg, 15 patients on hydroxyzine 100 mg, and 25 patients on the combination. The severity of sedative side effects did not differ substantially among the active drug treatments. Side effects other than sedative-type side effects did not occur with sufficient frequency to allow any meaningful analysis.

DISCUSSION

This study unequivocally demonstrates analgesic activity for a 100-mg dose of intramuscular hydroxyzine in the general range of that produced by 8 mg of morphine. In addition, the analgesic activity of hydroxyzine appears additive with that of morphine when the two drugs are given together. This observation is consistent with the hypothesis that the two drugs are producing analgesia by different mechanisms.

Although hydroxyzine has been marketed for a variety of indications for more than a decade, we are unaware of any previous study which has unequivocally demonstrated potent analgesic activity for this compound. Indeed, this type of activity would not be predicted on the basis of the available animal data. Since the pharmacologic profile of hydroxyzine is quite different than that of existing potent analgesics, and since hydroxyzine does not seem to have any dependence-producing properties, further studies of this agent and its congeners as analgesics certainly seem indicated.

REFERENCES

1. Houde, R., Wallenstein, S. L., and Rogers, A. (1960): *Clin. Pharmacol. Ther.*, 1:163–174.
2. Momose, T. (1970): In: *Proceedings of the 3rd Asian and Australasian Congress of Anesthesiology (Canberra)*, pp. 532–537. Butterworths, Sydney.
3. Momose, T. (1970*a*): *Iryo* (*Japan*), 24:919–924.
4. Momose, T. (1970*b*): *Iryo* (*Japan*), 24:1031–1034.
5. Momose, T. (1971): *Iryo* (*Japan*), 25:33–39.
6. Momose, T. (1973): *Iryo* (*Japan*), 27:257–265.

Advances in Pain Research and Therapy, Vol. 1,
edited by J. J. Bonica and D. Albe-Fessard.

Metabolic Studies of Hydroxyzine and Meperidine in Human Subjects

John E. Stambaugh and Irving W. Wainer

Department of Pharmacology, Thomas Jefferson University, Philadelphia, Pennsylvania 19107

The combination of narcotic analgesics, especially meperidine, with hydroxyzine hydrochloride (Vistaril®) is used in the clinical management of pain and as a preanesthetic medication. The rationale for this use is an enhancement of the analgesic properties of meperidine without a comparable increase in respiratory depression (4). Although the tranquilizing effect of hydroxyzine may play a role in this usage (2), there is evidence that there exists an alternate mechanism for the enhancement of meperidine analgesia. The clinical use of this combination has increased, yet no pharmacological basis of this potentiation has been reported. As part of our continuing study of the pharmacokinetics and metabolism of narcotic analgesics administered alone and in combination with other agents, we have attempted to define the mechanism of interaction between hydroxyzine and meperidine. Since initial clinical studies in our laboratory suggested that hydroxyzine altered the metabolism of meperidine, the following study using healthy volunteers was undertaken.

METHODS

We studied 12 volunteers determined as healthy by a complete medical evaluation along with laboratory tests to rule out any underlying organic disease, especially metabolic, cardiovascular, hepatic, or renal disorders. No subject had taken any medication for at least 4 weeks before the study. Each subject was fasted for 12 hr. All subjects fell within 10% of ideal weight as determined from Metropolitan Life Insurance Tables.

The subjects in the study were randomly divided into four groups of 3 subjects each, and dosages were prescribed according to a Latin square design. Each subject received 28 mg/m^2 of meperidine—corresponding to approximately a 50-mg total dose of meperidine—as a single deep intramuscular injection followed immediately by either sterile water (group A), or by 25 mg (group B), 50 mg (group C), or 100 mg (group D) of hydroxyzine hydrochloride also administered as a single deep intramuscular injection. During the four-way crossover experiment, each subject received placebo and each of the doses of hydroxyzine hydrochloride. Venous blood samples were collected at 1/4, 1/2, 1, 2, 4, 6, 8, and 24 hr after dosing. A cumulative urinary output was collected at each sampling time, including 24- and 48-hr periods. Serum levels of meperidine and the cumulative excretion pattern of meperidine and normeperidine were followed by gas-liquid chromatography as previously described (6,7). The serum time-concentration curves and the biological half-lives of meperidine and the total urinary excretion of meperidine and normeperidine were determined in a manner previously described and statistically analyzed (6,7).

RESULTS

The mean serum level for all groups reached its maximum at 1 hr with complete plasma clearance at 24 hr as shown in Fig. 1. The peak serum concentration expressed in μg/ml for group A (50 mg meperidine + placebo) was 0.182 ($\pm$0.047); for group B (50 mg meperidine + 25 mg hydroxyzine) it was 0.201 ($\pm$0.041); for group C (50 mg meperidine + 50 mg hydroxyzine) it was 0.243 ($\pm$0.073); and for group D (50 mg meperidine + 100 mg hydroxyzine) the peak serum concentration was 0.168 ($\pm$0.048). The biological half-lives ($t^1/_2$) were 3.70, 4.20, 3.90, and 4.40 hr for each of the groups, respectively. These results are consistent with the values previously reported for meperidine metabolism in humans in which a biological half-life of 3.65 hr was found after a 50-mg intramuscular injection (6). The serum time-concentration curves are also consistent with those previously reported. The analysis of variance (ANOVAR) of the data demonstrated that at every sampling time during the test there was no significant difference in the meperidine serum levels produced by the concomitant administration of meperidine and placebo or meperidine and the 25-, 50-, and 100-mg doses of hydroxyzine.

Significant levels of meperidine were detected in the urine 1 hr after dosing as shown in Fig. 2. The mean 48-hr cumulative excretion of meperidine for group A was 2.24 mg, which corresponds to 4.5% of the administered dose. The cumulative excretion for group B was 2.21 mg, or 4.2% of the administered dose. Similarly, for group C the cumulative excretion of meperidine was 2.46 mg, or 4.9% of the dose; and for group D it was 2.39 mg, or 4.8% of the administered dose. These levels are consistent with those previously reported (1,7), and, using the ANOVAR method, no significant difference was detected among the four groups at any of the sampling times.

Significant amounts of normeperidine did not appear in the urine until after hour 8 of the study as shown in Fig. 3. The mean 48-hr cumulative excretion of normeperidine for group A was 2.43 mg, or 4.9% of the administered dose; for group B it was 2.77 mg, or 5.5%; for group C it was 2.87 mg, or 5.7%; and for group D the cumulative excretion was 2.73 mg, or 5.5% of the administered dose. These results are consistent with the

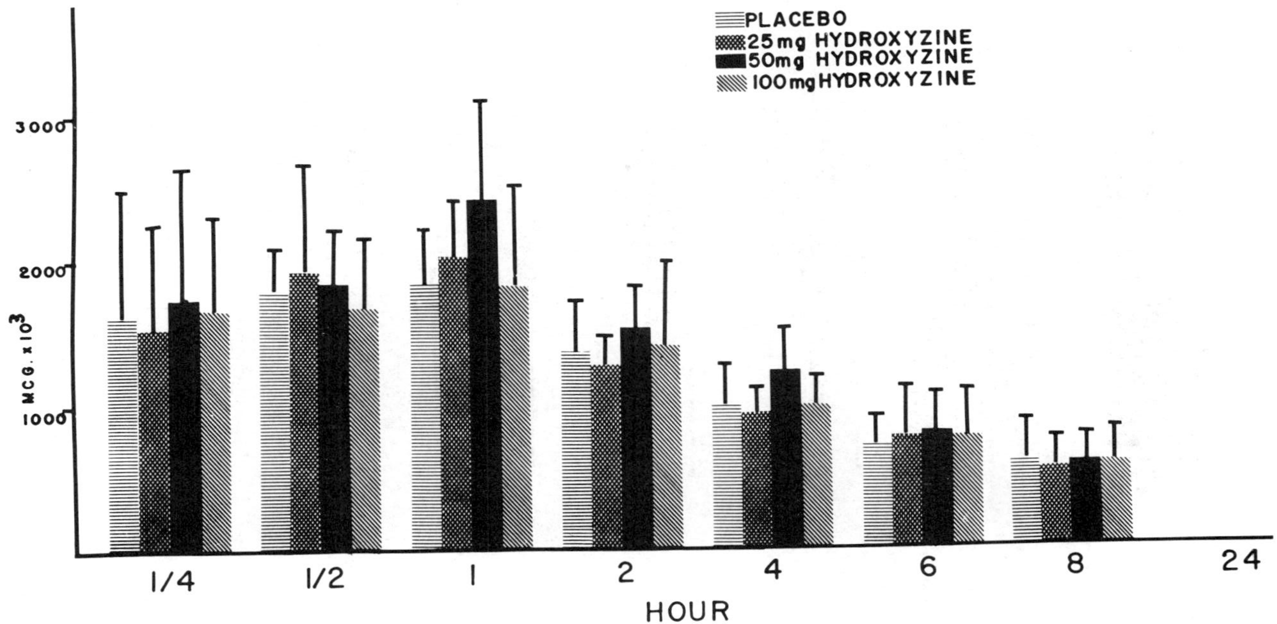

FIG. 1. Mean hourly serum levels of meperidine.

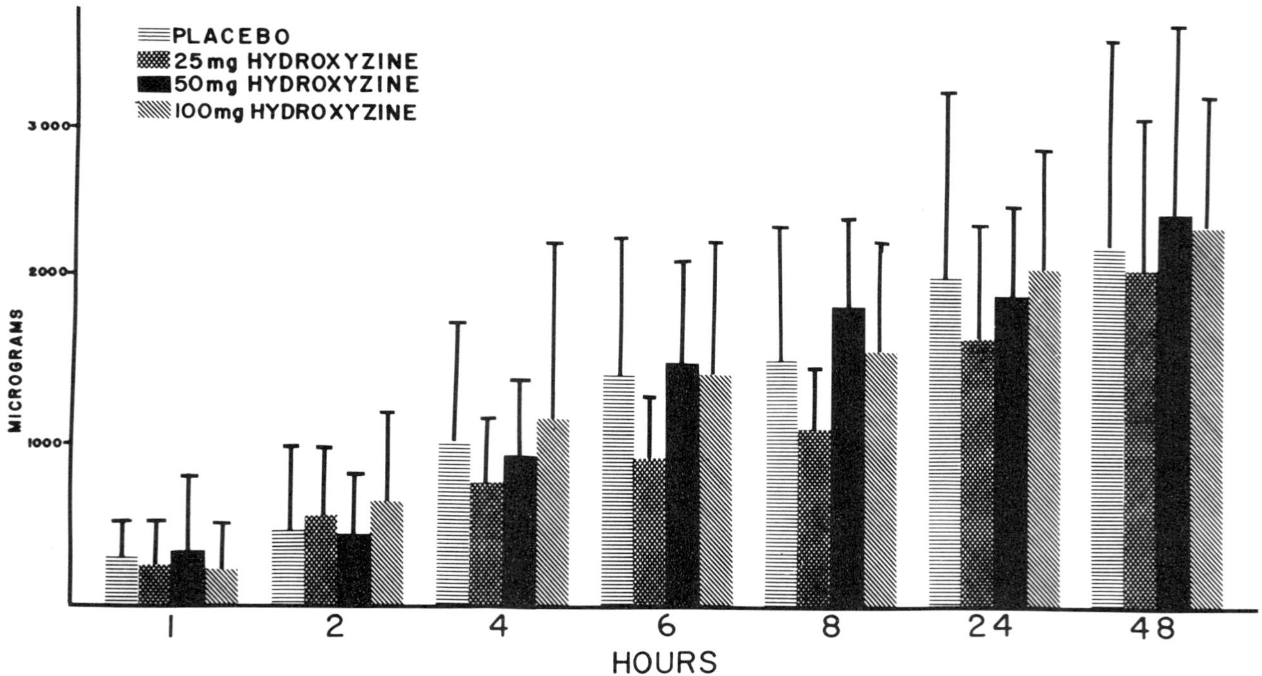

FIG. 2. Mean hourly cumulative excretion of meperidine.

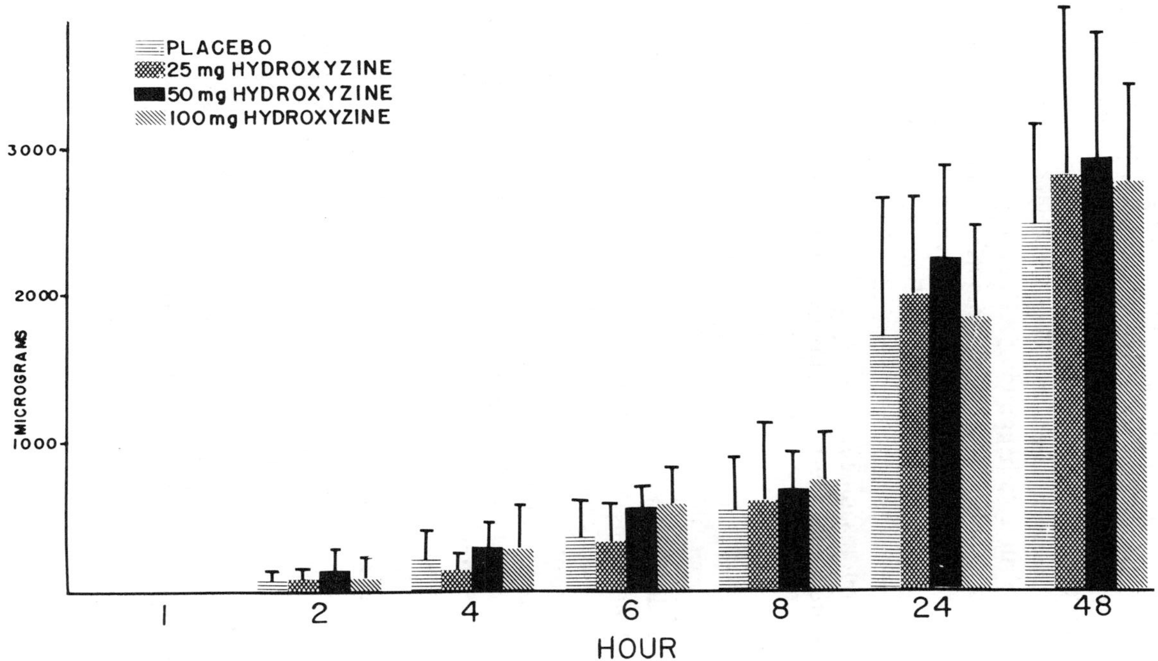

FIG. 3. Mean hourly cumulative excretion of normeperidine.

previously reported values of 5.0% and 6.2% (3,7). The ANOVAR of the data demonstrated that there were no significant differences among the four groups at any sampling time during the study.

The subjective symptoms reported in reply to the question, "How do you feel?" varied in each subject according to the level of the dose of hydroxyzine administered. Slight light-headedness, euphoria, and tiredness were reported by all subjects after receiving meperidine and placebo. At all dosage levels the subjects began to describe these symptoms within 20 min after dosing, and in most cases the symptoms lasted on the average of 1 hr. At the 50- to 100-mg dosage level of hydroxyzine, some subjects reported vertigo, nausea, dry mouth, and sweating. With the 100-mg dose of hydroxyzine, these symptoms lasted an average of 2.5 hr. The onset and severity of the latter symptoms appear to correlate directly to the dosage of hydroxyzine administered, and the symptoms were not observed with meperidine alone.

DISCUSSION

Since meperidine and normeperidine are central in the metabolic pathways, any alteration in the metabolism of the drug should be reflected by a change in the serum time-concentration curve, the biological half-life, or the urinary excretion pattern of meperidine or the normeperidine metabolite. On the basis of the above results, it appears that hydroxyzine does not alter the hepatic metabolism of meperidine, especially the rate of N-demethylation, as reflected in the cumulative excretion of meperidine and normeperidine. This study leads us to conclude that hydroxyzine hydrochloride does not alter either the pharmacokinetics or the metabolism of meperidine under our experimental conditions.

Thus any reported potentiation of the analgesic effect of meperidine by hydroxyzine hydrochloride appears not to be owing to an alteration in the pharmacology of meperidine. Lambertsen et al. (2) have suggested that the potentiation of meperidine by chlorpromazine is due to a direct summation of qualitatively dissimilar actions on the central nervous system. In addition, hydroxyzine has anticholinergic properties similar to those of chlorpromazine (5) and this latter property could increase the permeability of meperidine to the blood-brain barrier and account for the increased analgesia. However, distribution studies in our laboratory using male Wistar rats have shown that there is no alteration in the ratio between the serum concentration of meperidine and the concentration of the drug in the brain of the animal when meperidine is administered alone or in combination with hydroxyzine hydrochloride. We would therefore suggest that the observed clinical response to the hydroxyzine-meperidine combination is due not to a change in the pharmacology of meperidine but to an enhancement of analgesia, if indeed it does occur, arising from separate properties of the two drugs.

SUMMARY

The proposed potentiation of the analgesic effect of meperidine by hydroxyzine hydrochloride has been investigated. Twelve healthy subjects received 50 mg of meperidine hydrochloride and either placebo or 25, 50, or 100 mg of hydroxyzine hydrochloride on four separate occasions in a four-way crossover experiment. The serum time-concentration curves for meperidine and the urinary excretion patterns of meperidine and a major metabolite, normeperidine, were followed by gas-liquid chromatography. A statistical analysis of the data showed no significant differences in the serum time-concentration curves or the cumulative urinary excretion of meperidine and normeperidine resulting from the combinations of meperidine with placebo or hydroxyzine hydrochloride. It is concluded that hydroxyzine does not alter the pharmacokinetics or metabolism of meperidine, and it is suggested that if any analgesic enhancement does occur it involves a summation of effects in the central nervous system.

ACKNOWLEDGMENTS

This study was supported in part by a grant from Pfizer Laboratories, Inc.

The authors would like to thank Dr. H. Menduke for assistance in the statistical analysis of the experimental data and Dorothea Astl and Caprice Rogers for technical assistance.

REFERENCES

1. Burns, J. J., Berger, B. L., Lief, P. A., Wollack, A., Papper, E. M., and Brodie, B. B. (1953): *J. Pharmacol. Exp. Ther.,* 114:289–298.
2. Lambertsen, C. J., Wendel, H., and Logenhagen, J. B. (1961): *J. Pharmacol. Exp. Ther.,* 131:381–393.
3. Plotnikoff, N. P., Way, E. L., and Elliot, H. W. (1956): *J. Pharmacol. Exp. Ther.,* 117:414–419.
4. Reier, C. E., and Johnstone, R. E. (1970): *Anesth. Analg. (Cleve.),* 49:119–124.
5. Robins, G. S., and Zsigmond, E. K. (1972): *Anesth. Analg. (Paris),* 29:193–196.
6. Stambaugh, J. E., and Wainer, I. W. (1974): *J. Clin. Pharmacol.,* 14:552–559.
7. Stambaugh, J. E., and Wainer, I. W. (1975): *J. Clin. Pharmacol.,* 15:46–51.

Advances in Pain Research and Therapy, Vol. 1,
edited by J. J. Bonica and D. Albe-Fessard.
Raven Press, New York © 1976.

Studies of Tranquilizing Agents and Meperidine in Clinical Pain. Hydroxyzine and Meprobamate

Thomas G. Kantor and Frances P. Steinberg

New York University Medical Center, 550 First Avenue, New York, New York 10016

Anxiety on the part of the patient is very much related to his perioperative mental status when faced with either elective or nonelective surgery. The euphorigenic properties of most narcotic analgesics are considered to alleviate most of this problem. However, narcotics are not euphorigenic in many people and, in fact, dysphoria may often develop, which only adds to the anxiety. In addition to or separate from analgesic drugs (4), many different types of drugs have been used to allay anxiety. Not all perform a useful service for the patient.

We have previously noted that meprobamate in a 200-mg dose causes the perception of more pain by patients in the postoperative period than would be present without any analgesic; meprobamate is statistically worse than placebo in this regard (3). In our previous experiment, the anxiolytic properties of meprobamate were not explored.

In the present study, the anxiolytic antihistamine hydroxyzine is compared with meprobamate and with placebo for its effect on postoperative pain; in addition, their respective anxiolytic properties are examined.

Hydroxyzine is said to confer analgesia on its own when used in parenteral form and to augment the effect of meperidine when both are given parenterally in the postoperative period (5,6). A further portion of the presently reported study explores the possibility that oral hydroxyzine augments the analgesic effect of oral meperidine.

METHODS

Subjective response methodology as conceived by Beecher (1) and revised by Houde et al. (2) was used in this double-blind randomly assigned trial of 140 patients with postoperative pain at Bellevue Hospital in New York. Seven drug groups of 20 patients each were used in this study. The data records of 5 patients were dropped because of administrative reasons, such as double medication or patient dropout. Table 1 lists allocation of patients and drugs.

TABLE 1. *Allocation of patients and drugs*

Study group	No. of patients	Preparation given
1	19	Placebo
2	19	100 mg hydroxyzine
3	18	300 mg meprobamate
4	20	50 mg meperidine
5	19	100 mg meperidine
6	19	50 mg meperidine + 100 mg hydroxyzine
7	21	100 mg meperidine + 100 mg hydroxyzine

After signing appropriate consent forms, patients were medicated and then followed by nurse-observers at 30-min intervals for the first hour and then hourly for 6 hr. At each period of observation, they were queried as to their degree of pain on an ordinal scale ranging from 0 (meaning no pain) to 3 (meaning severe pain). No patient was selected for study who did not, at zero time, have either severe (3) or moderate (2) pain. At the same interval subsequent to dosing, patients were asked whether or not 50% or more of their starting pain was relieved. From these data, three derived scores can be obtained: (a) the total number of hours of 50% or better relief; (b) the individual pain intensity differences hour by hour subtracted from the starting pain; and (c) the sum of the pain intensity differences over the 6-hr period. Patients were also asked to report on a scale of 0 to 3 their degree of anxiety and degree of relaxation. In addition, the nurse-observer made an objective determination of anxiety independent from that of the patient.

RESULTS

There was no difference whatsoever in the objective or subjective reports of relaxation and/or anxiety as reported by the patient or as observed by the nurse-observers.

As to pain relief, neither hydroxyzine nor meprobamate was superior to placebo in respect to mean pain scores (Fig. 1), pain intensity difference (PID) scores (Fig. 2), or pain relief scores (Fig. 3). (Figures 1, 2, and 3 are all time-effect curves.) Meprobamate consistently gives less pain relief than the other two, but in no case are these statistically different from one another, possibly because of the relatively small number of patients on each data point.

When added to meperidine, hydroxyzine seems not to augment or diminish the analgesic effectiveness of the narcotic. Figure 4 shows the time-effect curves for mean pain scores, Fig. 5 shows the PID scores, and Fig. 6 shows

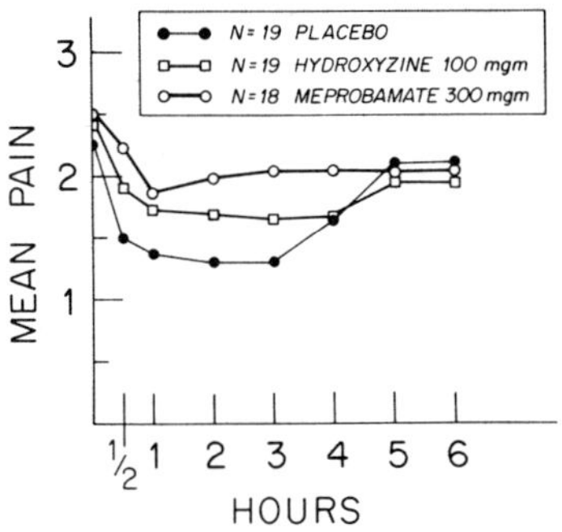

FIG. 1. Mean pain score on vertical axis: 3, severe; 2, moderate; 1, slight.

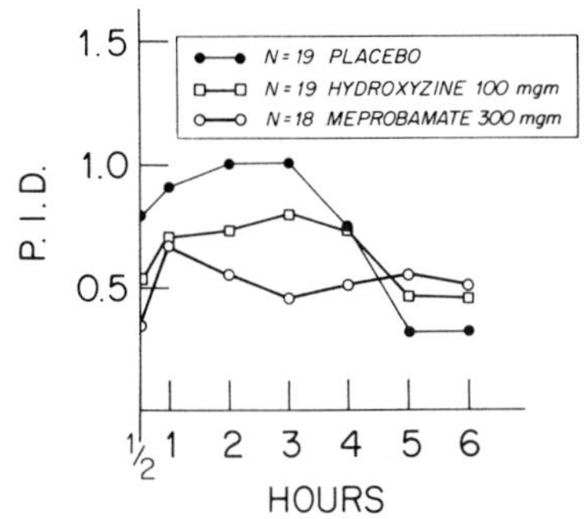

FIG. 2. Mean pain difference from starting pain on vertical axis.

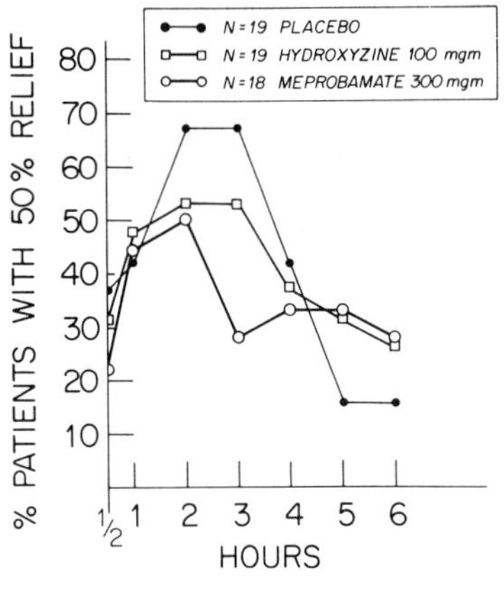

FIG. 3. Relief scores. Placebo curve is somewhat higher than that reported in many other studies.

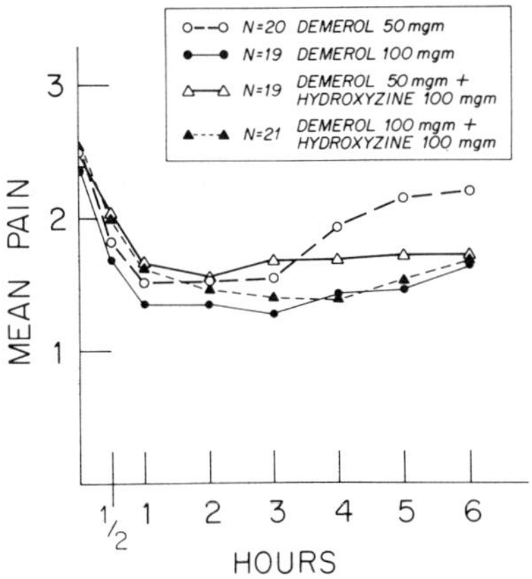

FIG. 4. Mean pain score on vertical axis: 3, severe; 2, moderate; 1, slight.

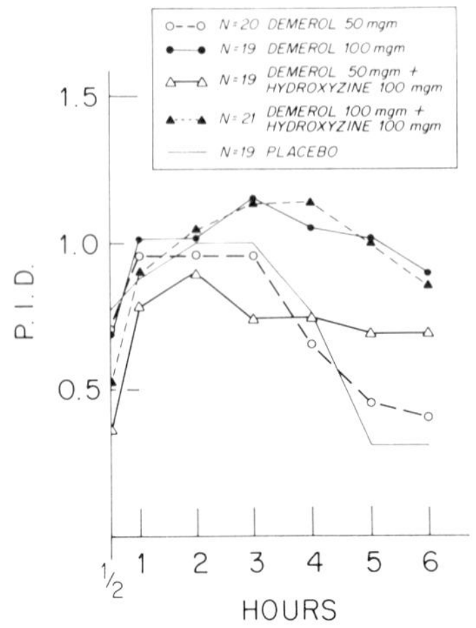

FIG. 5. Mean pain difference from starting pain on vertical axis.

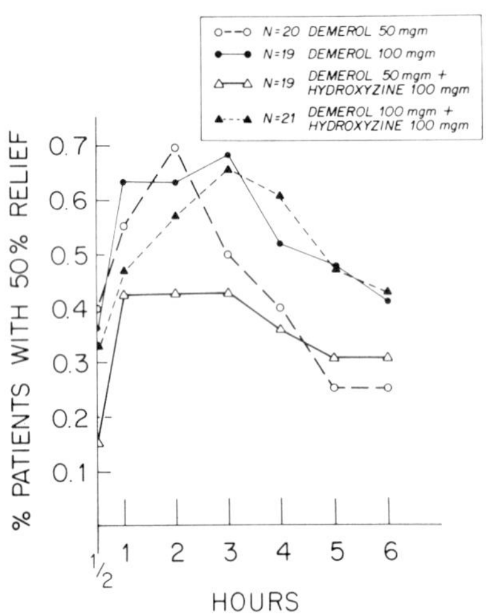

FIG. 6. Comparisons of pain relief scores.

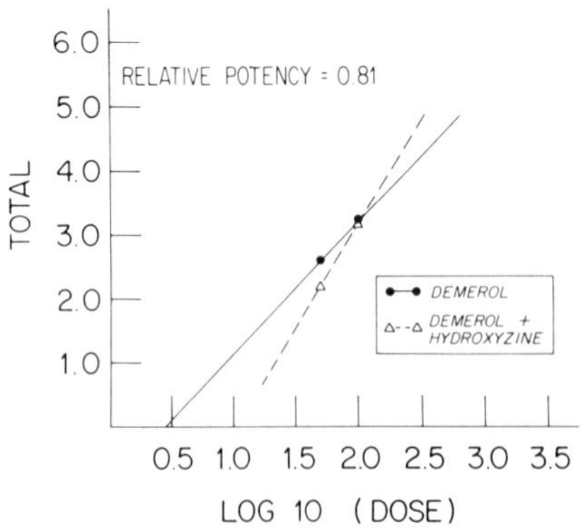

FIG. 7. Log dose–effect. Mean values for total hours of 50% relief on vertical axis.

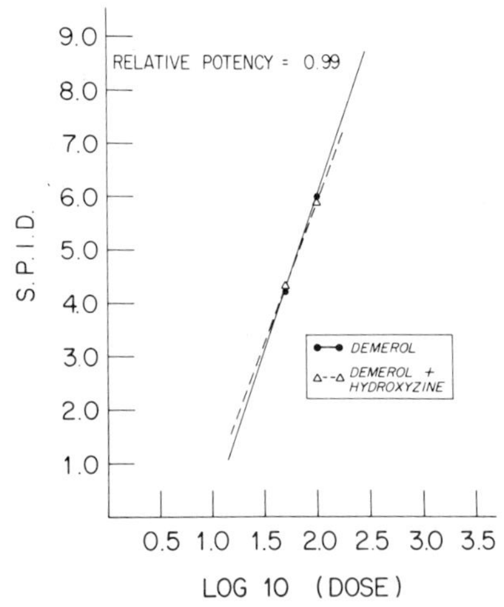

FIG. 8. Log dose—effect. Mean values for sum of pain intensity differences from starting pain on vertical axis.

the relief scores. In addition, log dose-effect curves are graphically depicted for the global parameters, total hours of 50% relief (Total), and sum of pain intensity differences (SPID) (Figs. 7 and 8). The relative potency for the parameter of Total gives a value of 0.81, and the relative potency when looked at for the more sensitive parameter, SPID, shows a value of 0.99. The confidence levels for these curves are 85% and 90%, respectively.

DISCUSSION

Although several studies suggest that hydroxyzine given parenterally has an analgesic effect and augments the effect of narcotics when given concurrently, this study shows oral hydroxyzine to be ineffective. Blood levels were not determined during this study, but it is known that hydroxyzine is metabolized in the liver and, to a great extent, excreted in the bile (7). The most obvious explanation for the disparity is that hydroxyzine is rapidly metabolized on its first pass through the liver. However, hydroxyzine when given orally is said to have sedative, anxiolytic, and antihistaminic properties. This further suggests the possibility that the parent drug alone has analgesic properties and that metabolites of the drug may give the other pharmacological effects. This discrepancy should be further explored by basic pharmacological studies in man.

ACKNOWLEDGMENTS

This work was supported in part by DA4PG-017, Special Action Office for Drug Abuse Prevention, Executive Office of the President of the United States of America, and by a research contract from Pfizer, Inc.

REFERENCES

1. Beecher, H. K. (1959): *Measurement of Subjective Response.* Oxford University Press, New York.
2. Houde, R., Wallenstein, S. L., and Rogers, A. (1960): *Clin. Pharmacol. Ther.,* 1:163–74.
3. Kantor, T. G., Laska, E., and Streem, A. (1973): *J. Clin. Pharmacol.,* 13:152–59.
4. Lear, E., et al. (1958): *J.A.M.A.,* 166:1438–44.
5. Mamose, T. (1971*a*): *Jpn. J. Anesthesiol.,* 20:908–9.
6. Mamose, T. (1971*b*): *Therapeutics,* 25:181–88.
7. Pong, S. F., and Huang, C. L. (1974): *J. Pharm. Sci.,* 63:1527–32.

Advances in Pain Research and Therapy, Vol. 1,
edited by J. J. Bonica and D. Albe-Fessard.
Raven Press, New York © 1976.

A Controlled Study on the Analgesic Activity of Indoprofen in Patients with Cancer Pain

G. Martino, V. Ventafridda, *J. Parini, and *A. Emanueli

*Pain Therapy Department, National Tumor Institute, and Medical Department, *Carlo Erba S.p.A., Milan, Italy*

The clinical investigation which we report in this chapter is part of the ongoing, long-term research being carried out in our department for the evaluation of new and old drugs in the treatment of cancer pain. As introduction, we emphasize that in any decision of what is the optimal method of relieving pain of patients with tumors, the stage of the disease is one of the most important factors to consider (7). The *first stage* is when patients have pain before or soon after surgical extirpation, radiation, and/or chemotherapy. This type of pain is not frequent and usually disappears after specific treatment. The *second stage* is when patients have widespread neoplastic disease but have a life expectancy of many months or years. In a high percentage of these patients pain may remain, disappear, or recur depending on the efficacy of the specific therapeutic regimen being applied. The *third stage* is when the patients have multiple parenchymal involvement and a life expectancy of not more than 3 months.

For patients who want to be managed with systemic analgesics, it is important to remember that aspirin and other nonnarcotic analgesics and the anti-inflammatory drugs such as phenylbutazone and indomethacin have a definite place in the management of cancer pain. These agents are especially useful in patients with mild-to-moderate pain owing to involvement of musculoskeletal structures and when an inflammatory reaction is present. On the other hand, there is a critical need for new potent nonnarcotic analgesics to control moderate-to-severe pain because the objective is to reduce or obviate the use of narcotic drugs.

In this chapter we report the results of clinical trials for the evaluation of the analgesic activity of a new nonnarcotic analgesic, indoprofen (2,3,6). This compound is a new phenylpropionic acid derivative with analgesic and anti-inflammatory properties (2). Pharmacological studies have clearly demonstrated its analgesic activity. In phenylquinone-induced writhing in the mouse, it has proven to be about 50 times as effective as acetylsalicylic acid (ASA) (2). Moreover, human studies have shown that indoprofen is rapidly and completely absorbed from the gastrointestinal tract (4). After oral administration peak plasma levels are reached between 30 min and 2 hr and are represented mainly by unchanged drug. Absorption may be considered complete since radioactivity recovered from feces after administration of ^{14}C-labeled compound is only approximately 4% of the dose as compared with 95% to 96% recovered from urine. The principal metabolite found in the urine is the glucuronide. After oral administration of indoprofen, its disappearance from the plasma follows at least a biexponential function and is almost complete in 24 to 48 hr. The plasma half-life of the slow disposition phase ranges between 2.2 and 5.4 hr.

METHODS

The aim of our trial was to evaluate the activity of indoprofen in relieving cancer pain and to ascertain how it compares in analgesic efficacy with two widely used compounds: ASA by mouth and pentazocine by intramuscular injection. The former was chosen because it represents the standard of reference for nonnarcotic analgesics with anti-inflammatory action, whereas the later was chosen because it is a widely used narcotic antagonist (5).

Three trials were carried out each involving 12 patients for a total of 36 patients. This group consists of 23 men and 13 women with a mean age of 55.4 ± 1.8 years (range 42 to 71); mean weight of 62.5 ± 2.0 kg (range 34 to 88); and mean height of 165.6 ± 1.1 cm (range 154 to 185). The patients were included in the study only if their pain before treatment was severe or very severe and presumably stable over periods of a few days. All subjects were in the second stage of the neoplastic disease. The number of patients with a specific type of neoplasm were as follows: lung cancer (8); cancer of the uterus (3); lymphoma and leukemia (3), bone metastases (4); cancer of the mouth, nose, and esophagus (4); breast cancer (5); cancer of the rectum (4); cancer of the testicle (2); and other tumors (3).

Each patient was treated three times with single doses of the drugs which were given in a randomized order. The three treatments were prepared in separate envelopes on which was indicated the order according to which they were to be given. The first treatment was given when the patient was admitted to the trial, and the pain intensity and relief were recorded over a period of 6 hr; when pain made another treatment necessary, the content of the second envelope was given to the patient, and so on. No other treatment that could interfere with the results of the trials was given. The investigation was carried out under double-blind conditions.

Two trials involved oral preparation given as capsules and were designed to compare: (a) a single dose of 200 mg of indoprofen, 600 mg of ASA, and a placebo; and (b) a single dose of 100 mg of indoprofen, 1,000 mg of ASA, and a placebo. The third trial was carried out to determine the analgesic activities of three dose levels – 15, 30, and 60 mg – of pentazocine. Analgesic effects of the drugs were assessed by the same physician throughout the trial. The interview method was similar to that used by Bellville et al. (1).

To assess the analgesic efficacy of the different preparations, we used the intensity of pain present before and after treatment. Pain intensity was graded according to the following rating scale: 0 = no pain, 1 = slight pain, 2 = moderate pain, 3 = severe pain, and 4 = very severe pain. Pain relief scores were also obtained, but by and large they did not supply additional information on the activity of the drugs. The differences in analgesic efficacy between preparations were calculated using analyses of variance.

RESULTS

The results of the first and second trials are depicted in Fig. 1. The graph on the left shows the modifications of pain intensity after oral administration of 200 mg of indoprofen, 600 mg of ASA, and placebo. It is clear that indoprofen is significantly more active than 600 mg of ASA. Comparison of indoprofen versus placebo is significant at the 5% level, whereas that of ASA versus placebo is not significant. With indoprofen the peak reduction of pain intensity as determined by averages was achieved after 3 hr when the mean score was slightly greater than 1. Specifically, from a pretreatment mean pain intensity score of 3.58 ± 0.14, indoprofen reduced the mean pain intensity to 1.50 ± 0.23 after 1 hr and to 1.08 ± 0.33 at 3 hr, and pain remained near this level for another hour before it started to rise again. In contrast, ASA reduced pain from 3.35 ± 0.15 to 2.5 at 1 hr and slightly lower at 3 hr. Although the placebo produced a similar reduction for the first 2 hr, subsequently the pain intensity returned to pretreatment level.

The graph on the right in Fig. 1 depicts the results of the second trial. The effects of both ASA at the dose level of 1 g and indoprofen at 100 mg were significantly different from those of placebo ($p < 0.05$). From a pretreatment mean score of 3.41 ± 0.14, an hour after 100 mg of indoprofen, the pain intensity was reduced to 1.66 ± 0.35. The values for 1,000 mg of ASA were 3.50 ± 0.15 and 1.75 ± 0.44, respectively. Thus indoprofen displayed the same analgesic effect as ASA with only one-tenth of the dose. By combination of estimates involving in the calculation two dose levels of indoprofen and ASA, we found the ratio of activity between these drugs to be 10.38. The peak reduction of pain intensity was obtained 1 hr after oral administration of indoprofen or ASA, and it was maintained under a mean score of 2 (moderate pain) for 4 hr. The percent reduction of the intensity of pain for both drugs was approximately 50% at the first hour. By combining the results of these two oral trials, we demonstrated a dose-related analgesic effect of indoprofen.

The dose-related analgesic effects of pentazocine are shown in Fig. 2. With the 60-mg dose of intramuscular pentazocine, the maximum reduction of the pain intensity was obtained after 60 min; from a basal mean score of 3.0, pain intensity was reduced to 1.67 ± 0.38 and remained well under 2 (moderate pain) for over 4 hr. The lowest average value was 43.4% under

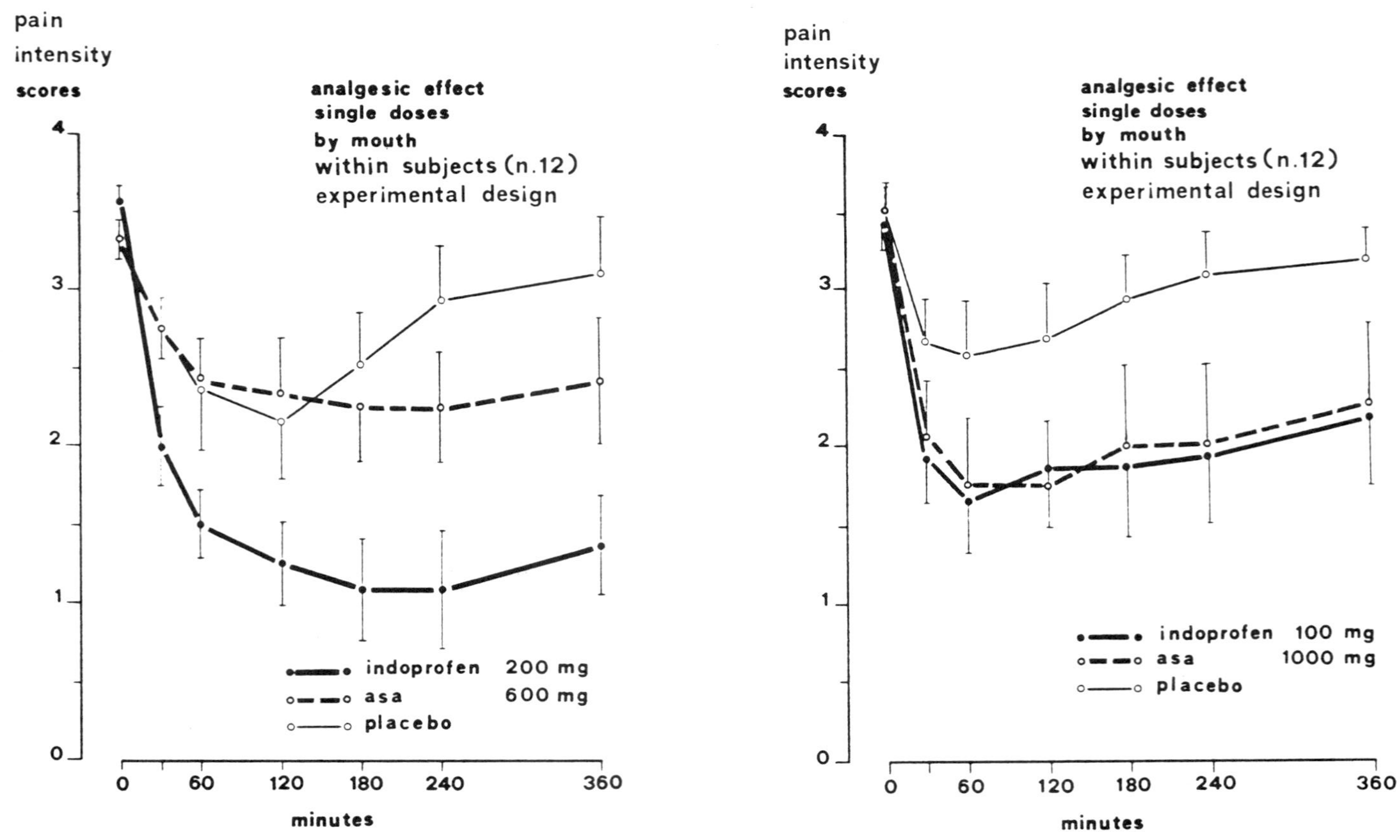

FIG. 1. Pain intensity scores of patients treated with single doses of placebo, ASA, and indoprofen by mouth. **Left:** Results of first clinical trial. **Right:** Second clinical trial. See text for details.

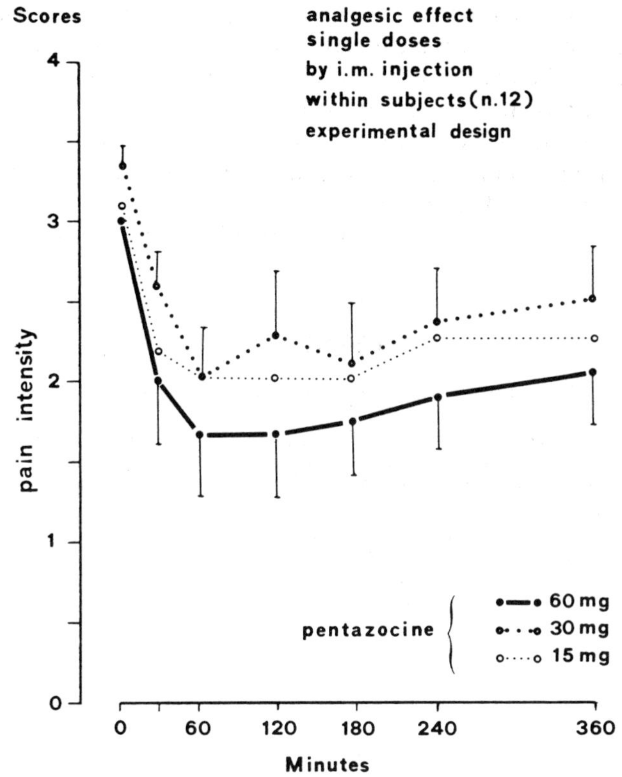

FIG. 2. Pain intensity scores of patients treated with pentazocine i.m.

the base value. Doses of 15 and 30 mg of pentazocine brought pain intensity down to a score of 2 at the most, but differences with the highest dose are not significant. The order of magnitude of the analgesic effect of intramuscular pentazocine as shown by our data is around that of 100 mg of indoprofen by mouth.

Side effects including gastric disturbances such as pyrosis and/or vomiting and sweating were seen with all drugs; there were four complaints with placebo, four with indoprofen, seven with ASA, and seven with pentazocine. Vertigo, drowsiness, and other psychic symptoms were experienced exclusively with pentazocine, which provoked 13 complaints.

CONCLUSIONS

The results of our trials have supplied information which substantiates the conclusion that indoprofen at a single oral dose of 100 or 200 mg is an effective analgesic for cancer pain. Moreover, the analgesic efficacy of 100 mg of indoprofen appears to be similar to that produced by 1,000 mg of ASA. Pentazocine given by intramuscular injection—which is considered preferable to oral administration—was comparable in activity to 100 mg of indoprofen. Surprisingly, the analgesic efficacy of the different doses of pentazocine did not vary much. This is probably due more to the experimental design and route of administration than to the number of patients involved. Among the three drugs considered in this chapter, pentazocine is the only one that may create significant clinical problems from its side effects (5).

REFERENCES

1. Bellville, J. W., Forrest, W. H., Jr., and Brown, B. W., Jr. (1968): *Clin. Pharmacol. Ther.*, 9:290–302.
2. Buttinoni, A., Cuttica, A., Franceschini, J., Mandelli, V., Orsini, G., Passerini, N., Turba, C., and Tommasini, R. (1973): *Arzneim. Forsch.*, 23:1100–1107.
3. Fuccella, L. M., Conti, F., Corvi, G., Mandelli, V., Randelli, M., and Stefanelli, G. (1975): *Clin. Pharmacol. Ther.*, 17:277–283
4. Fuccella, L. M., Goldaniga, G. C., Moro, E., Tamassia, V., Tosolini, G. P., and Valzelli, G. (1973): *Eur. J. Clin. Pharmacol.*, 6:256–260.
5. Miller, R. R. (1975): *J. Clin. Pharmacol.*, 15:198–205.
6. Ventafridda, V., Martino, G., Mandelli, V., and Emanueli, A. (1975): *Clin. Pharmacol. Ther.*, 17:284–289.
7. Ventafridda, V., Spreavice, R. (1974): *Int. J. Clin. Pharmacol.*, 9:174–179.

Advances in Pain Research and Therapy, Vol. 1,
edited by J. J. Bonica and D. Albe-Fessard.
Raven Press, New York © 1976.

Use of Psychotropic Drugs for the Treatment of Chronic Severe Pain

R. Kocher

Psychiatric and Neurological University Clinic, CH-4056 Basel, Switzerland

The introduction of psychotropic drugs, particularly thymoleptics and neuroleptics, has resulted in significant gains in the treatment of chronic severe pain due to a variety of conditions. The most important success has been achieved through a combination of drugs of both groups. Over a period of several years, the following drug combinations have been used (1,2):

Thymoleptics (first agent) and Neuroleptics (second agent):

Imipramine and levomepromazine
Chlorimipramine and levomepromazine
Trimipramine and levomepromazine
Imipramine and haloperidol
Chlorimipramine and haloperidol

This chapter reports the results we have obtained with these drug combinations and includes a discussion of the mode of action and the recommended dosage schedules.

CLINICAL MATERIAL

To date, 103 inpatients have been treated with one of these combinations for chronic severe pain caused by neurologic and rheumatic conditions. Most of these patients had to be hospitalized because the pain was resistant to therapy and the patients were in a bad condition. Some of them showed drug abuse or drug addiction.

The different clinical conditions managed with these drug combinations were: postherpetic neuralgia in 10 patients; lesions of the brachial and lumbosacral plexus in 26 patients; painful neuropathies and polyneuropathies in 10 patients; trigeminal neuralgia in 16 patients; degenerative diseases of the skeletal system in 21 patients; traumatic pain of the locomotor system in 5 patients; cancer in 5 patients; and other chronic pains of varied etiology in 10 patients.

In 12 patients the treatment had to be discontinued because of severe side effects consisting of somnolence or arterial hypotension (caused by levomepromazine in 10 patients) and urinary retention (caused by imipramine in 2 patients). Consequently, now we use haloperidol instead of levopromazine because it has the same and perhaps stronger neuroleptic effects and does not produce somnolence and arterial hypotension.

Of the remaining 91 patients, 9 had no significant improvement (pain remained the same and reduction of analgesics was impossible). These included 1 patient with painful mononeuritis complex, 1 patient with traumatic pain of the locomotor system, and 7 patients with degenerative diseases of the skeletal system, especially herniation of the intervertebral disc.

Among the 82 remaining patients, 60 experienced a fair-to-good result (less pain and reduction of analgesics) and 22 had very good results (complete relief of pain, termination of analgesic intake). Generally, fair-to-good results occurred in patients with painful neural and polyneuropathies, trigeminal neuralgia, degenerative diseases of the skeletal system (except in some patients with herniation of the intervertebral disc), traumatic pain of the locomotor system, and pain caused by cancer. Very good results were derived by patients with postherpetic neuralgia and by those with lesions of the brachial and lumbosacral plexus.

DISCUSSION

Advantages of Psychotropic Drugs

The advantages of using these combinations of psychotropic drugs include: (a) effectiveness in patients who have developed resistance to established treatment with analgesics; (b) absence of harmful side effects; (c) potentiation of analgesic effects; (d) reduction in the use of analgesics; and (e) prevention or reduction of the incidence of drug abuse and drug addiction. The last advantage is especially important because 20% of all medications prescribed are analgesics (3) and because drug abuse and drug addiction have markedly increased in recent years.

Mode of Action

How can we explain these good and encouraging results of combined treatment? The basis of the favorable outcomes exceeds probably that of either the purely thymoleptic or neuroleptic action of these psychotropic drugs. The psychotropic drugs have a variety of modes of action. When drugs are given in combinations, this action spectrum is certainly widened. Psychotropic drugs have been reported to have central and peripheral action.

Central Action

The central action of a therapy that combines psychotropic drugs consists essentially of alteration of pain perception and sensation. This leads to a "depersonalization of the pain," or to a certain "distance of the personality from the physical events" (4,5). Many patients made the statement: "I still have the pain, but it no longer hurts," or, "I still have the pain, but it is far away." In addition, thymoleptics and neuroleptics can interrupt or prevent the vicious cycle: pain → anxiety → depression → pain. In states of anxiety and depression, which often accompany chronic severe pain, combination therapy is more likely to interrupt or prevent this sometimes fatal vicious cycle than thymoleptics or neuroleptics applied alone.

Peripheral Action

A peripheral action possibly and even probably consists of involvement of the pain-producing substance, i.e., psychotropic drugs interfere in some way with the synthesis, metabolism, and/or elimination of pain-producing substances.

Dosage Schedule

A clear-cut dosage schedule has been established for inpatients and outpatients. A therapy based on these guidelines has been shown to be without relevant side effects. For outpatients the best combination consists of imipramine or chlorimipramine 25 mg by mouth three times daily, and haloperidol beginning with 0.5 mg two times daily and then carefully increasing the dosage to 1 mg two or three times daily.

For inpatients the best dosage schedule is as follows: chlorimipramine given via an intravenous infusion containing 25 to 50 mg of the drug in 250 ml of 5% glucose solution administered over the course of 2 to 3 hr daily. After 1 week this is changed to 25 mg given by mouth three times daily. At the same time, haloperidol is given in initial doses of 0.5 mg two times daily and then carefully increasing dosage to 1 mg two to three times daily.

If improvement occurs, this combination treatment should be continued for several weeks. In elderly persons the daily dosage of haloperidol should not exceed 1.5 mg daily. In the above-recommended dosage, haloperidol occasionally produces a Parkinson-like syndrome or acute dystonic reaction. In case of the former, an antiparkinsonian drug must be added; whereas in the latter case, haloperidol should be discontinued and one ampule of an anticholinergic drug promptly injected intravenously. To date we have treated 19 patients with this new combination. All showed an improvement except 1 patient suffering from a degenerative disease of the skeletal system and an underlying neurosis. Consequently, this new combined treatment of psychotropic drugs can be recommended for use in all patients with chronic severe pain. On the basis of past experience we predict that a definite improvement will occur in more than 80% of the patients thus treated.

REFERENCES

1. Kocher, R. (1968): *Praxis,* 57:1458–1464.
2. Kocher, R. (1967): *Praxis,* 63:1562–1567.
3. Lendle, L. (1966): *Med. Welt,* 21:1180–1189.
4. Linke, H. (1963): *Ther. Berichte,* 35:94–99.
5. Reisner, H. (1972): In: *Schmerz, Grundlagen-Pharmakologie-Therapie,* edited by W. Keidel, A. Herz, and C. Steichele, p. 186. Georg Thieme Verlag, Stuttgart.

Advances in Pain Research and Therapy, Vol. 1,
edited by J. J. Bonica and D. Albe-Fessard.
Raven Press, New York © 1976.

Postherpetic Neuralgia: Management with Antiepileptic and Tricyclic Drugs

V. S. Hatangdi, R. A. Boas, and E. G. Richards

Department of Anaesthetics and Pain Clinic, Auckland Hospital, Auckland, New Zealand

A wide spectrum of therapeutic measures has been tried for relief of the intractable pain of postherpetic neuralgia. These measures have ranged from drugs given empirically, like vitamin B_1, through the usual analgesics, to radical interruption of pain pathways.

Spontaneous neuronal hyperactivity with segmental pain has been described in the spinal cord of humans after traumatic paraplegia (7). Recently, similar experimental pain-like states with neuronal hyperactivity in the spinal trigeminal sensory nucleus have been demonstrated in cats (1).

Prompted by the findings in the above studies, we have employed a combination of antiepileptic and tricyclic antidepressant drugs in patients suffering from postherpetic neuralgia. This chapter describes our observations over a period of 3 years.

METHODS

Thirty-four patients suffering from pain of postherpetic neuralgia were seen at our Pain Clinic during the past 3 years. Duration of symptoms ranged from 3 months to 15 years, with over half of patients having had the disease for more than 10 years. Approximately 75% were over the age of 70, the oldest being 88 and the youngest 40. In 19 the thoracic segmental nerves were involved, 9 had lesions of lumbar nerves, 4 had cervical nerve involvement, and 2 had lesions of the ophthalmic division of the trigeminal nerve. A number of the patients were receiving various forms of analgesic and phenothiazine drugs with limited response.

Management

Patients were evaluated on the basis of the anatomical distribution of pain, its severity, and its duration. An inquiry was made into other systemic disorders and into all previous medication, with special reference to drugs likely to interfere with our drug treatment. Patients were then informed about the proposed therapy and possible side effects. Drug side effects are self-limiting and occur during the first 10 to 15 days of therapy.

Our current regime includes carbamazepine (Tegretol®) given to achieve specific measured blood levels, together with moderate doses of nortriptyline. This drug therapy may be combined with appropriate regional nerve blocks. Lidocaine, 1 to 1.5 mg/kg given intravenously during a paroxysmal attack, usually offered complete relief of lancinating pain within seconds of injection and provided an indication of the likely response to antiepileptic drugs by the oral route.

Drug Therapy

Therapy is begun with carbamazepine 600 to 800 mg/day (or diphenylhydantoin 300 to 400 mg/day in cases of intolerance to carbamazepine), together with 50 to 100 mg nortriptyline in divided doses, depending on the age and physical status of the patient. Those who live on their own are admitted to rest homes when necessary for nursing care during this period. At the end of 1 week, drug dosage is adjusted if required to achieve an acceptable degree of pain relief with minimal side effects and satisfactory carbamazepine level in the blood. The usual range of serum levels sought for carbamazepine is 8 to 12 μg/ml (10–40 μmole/1), and for diphenylhydantoin, 15 to 20 μg/ml (20–80 μmole/1).

When drug therapy was stopped because of side effects or other reasons, the paroxysms of acute pain quickly returned; when treatment was resumed, pain was relieved. A few patients have shown sustained remission when drugs have been discontinued after 3 to 6 months of treatment. In other patients therapy must be continued on a long-term basis.

Regional Nerve Blocks

Appropriate local anesthetic blocks were carried out once or twice a week in conjunction with drug therapy in 3 patients who were resistant to carbamazepine. The resulting block of all sensory input from the affected and adjoining dermatomes provided relief at the time and for increasing periods thereafter with subsequent blocks. Nerve blocks were also employed with success during a change to diphenylhydantoin in 5 patients who exhibited carbamazepine intolerance.

Patients were followed at the Pain Clinic for up to 4 weeks and in resistant cases for up to 3 months. Subsequent follow-up and supervision of drug therapy was carried out by the referring specialist or general practitioner, who was asked to arrange checks of serum levels of the antiepileptic drugs and of the white cell count every 3 months.

RESULTS

Improvements in sleep pattern and pain relief were noticed within 2 to 3 days of beginning drug therapy. Criteria for improvement were based on the patient's own assessment of the degree of pain relief, reduction of previous analgesic intake, improvement in sleep pattern, mental outlook, physical activity, and finally, our assessment of the reduced hyperesthesia in the involved area.

Of the 34 patients seen, 27 (79%) derived complete-to-good pain relief, while 3 of the remaining 7 had partial relief. Four others in the last group discontinued therapy because of drug intolerance. Thus of the 30 patients who continued medication without significant side effects, 27 (90%) had good-to-excellent pain relief (Fig. 1).

The lower range of serum levels (4 to 6 μg/ml) on a daily dose of 400 to 500 mg of carbamazepine was found to be effective in patients who had a short history of pain, usually of less than a year. Resistant cases or those with a pain history of over 10 years required higher doses (1,000 to 1,200 mg/day), which provided higher carbamazepine serum levels (8 to 10 μg/ml). However, 1 patient derived benefit only from a maximum dose of 1,600 mg daily, with a serum level of 15 μg/ml. Two patients on a long-term high-dose regime had recurrence of pain and were found to have very low serum levels. This is probably related to the enhanced metabolism of drugs as a result of enzyme induction. Based on the success achieved with psychotropic drugs (11), we have used fluphenazine (Anatensol®) in these 2 patients to further enhance relief.

Complications

Side effects, which were self-limiting, have been well documented (8) and occurred in over 60% of our patients during the first 2 weeks of therapy. In all, 22 patients had varying degrees of drowsiness; 18 of these also had dizziness, mild diplopia, tremors, and unsteadiness. Gastrointestinal symptoms of nausea, vomiting, anorexia, or a sense of fullness in the stomach

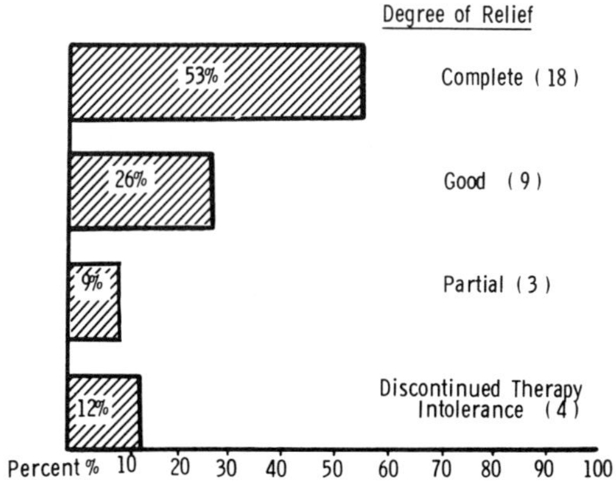

FIG. 1. Postherpetic neuralgia: Long-term results with antiepileptic and tricyclic drug therapy. Total no. of patients, 34.

were noted in 15 patients, the last two symptoms persisting for a few weeks even after the CNS effects had subsided. Most of those who had CNS side effects had serum carbamazepine levels of over 8 μg/ml. Other effects included postural hypotension in 6, dry mouth in 6, skin rash in 2, and urinary hesitancy/retention in 3 patients. Four patients discontinued therapy because of side effects and did not seek further treatment. Five others who showed intolerance to carbamazepine were treated satisfactorily with diphenylhydantoin. There has been no other morbidity of long-term drug therapy. Bone marrow depression or leukopenia was not noted in any of our patients.

DISCUSSION

The spontaneous paroxysmal quality of postherpetic pain and the provocation by minor stimulation within the involved area of deafferentation are suggestive of increased excitability leading to an inappropriately vigorous sensory response.

Intravenous lidocaine successfully relieved the paroxysmal pain in every patient for whom the agent was used, and this has provided a good correlation between the effect of lidocaine and anticipated improvement with carbamazepine. Lidocaine has been successfully employed to suppress ventricular arrhythmias—another form of spontaneous hyperactivity in conducting tissues. An extension of this concept prompted the use of lidocaine as a diagnostic aid and also provided intermittent short-term relief for acute exacerbations. It is of considerable interest that i.v. procaine at one time provided a useful form of therapy for postherpetic pain (3).

Earlier trials with antiepileptic agents in tic douloureux have demonstrated the usefulness of these agents in isolated cases of postherpetic neuralgia (4,12). More recently, tricyclic antidepressants have been successful alone (13) and in combination with other psychotropic drugs (10,11). The value of anticonvulsant drugs has been suggested recently in paroxysmal pain-like states (2) on the basis of electrophysiological evidence of epileptiform activity in deafferentated second-order neurons (1,2,7).

Nortriptyline and, more particularly, imipramine are closely related to carbamazepine. The improved response in our patients to a combination of the above two drugs may be owing to pharmacological potentiation or to a wider polysynaptic suppression. Imipramine is known to depress corticofugal inhibition of afferent activity in the spinal trigeminal nucleus of the cat and thus exert an anticonvulsant effect (6). Tricyclic drugs possibly interfere with synaptic mechanisms responsible for processing nociceptive impulses, so they may exert an analgesic effect in a restricted sense (5). Anticonvulsant agents, on the other hand, may increase the concentration of gamma-aminobutyric acid (GABA), which is possibly a transmitter for inhibitory synapses, thus resulting in cell membrane stability of hyperactive neurons (9).

Side effects of drug therapy have been observed in approximately 60% of our patients and cannot be avoided. Suppression of pain from postherpetic neuralgia using this regime is therefore achieved at the expense of CNS side effects, which are self-limiting and occur for 10 to 15 days during initiation of therapy. Patients should be warned of these side effects, and necessary home help or nursing care must be available in the first few days of therapy.

SUMMARY

Electrophysiological evidence of epileptiform activity in deafferentated second-order neurons has been demonstrated by other works, in both humans and cats. Based on the above hypothesis, we have employed carbamazepine to achieve specific measured blood levels, together with nortriptyline or imipramine in 34 patients with the intractable pain of postherpetic neuralgia. Intravenous lidocaine effectively suppressed the acute attacks of paroxysmal pain and provided a good indication of the anticipated improvement with antiepileptic drugs. Suppression of paroxysmal attacks may have to be brought about at the expense of the CNS side effects of the above drug combination. These effects are self-limiting and short lived (10 to 15 days) and occur during initiation of therapy. Follow-up to date (3 months to 3 years) indicates that 90% of patients who continued medications without significant side effects derived excellent-to-good pain relief.

REFERENCES

1. Anderson, L. S., Black, R. G., Abraham, J., and Ward, A. A. (1971): *J. Neurosurg.*, 35:444–452.
2. Black, R. G. (1974): *Advances in Neurology, Vol. 4: International Symposium on Pain*, edited by J. J. Bonica, pp. 651–658. Raven Press, New York.
3. Bonica, J. J. (1953): *The Management of Pain*, p. 866. Lea & Febiger, Philadelphia.
4. Braham, J., and Sara, A. (1960): *Lancet*, 2:892–893.
5. Deldeseo, D. J. (1967): *Dis. Nerv. Syst.*, 28:325–332.
6. Fromm, G. H., Amores, C. Y., and Thies, W. (1972): *Arch. Neurol.*, 27:198–204.
7. Loeser, J. D., Ward, A. A., and White, L. E. (1968): *J. Neurosurg.*, 29:48–50.
8. Mainardi, H. (1972): In: *Antiepileptic Drugs*, edited by D. M. Woodbury, J. K. Perry, and R. P. Schmidt. Raven Press, New York.
9. Mawdsley, C. (1972): *Scientific Foundation of Neurology*, edited by W. H. Critchley. Medical Books Ltd., London.
10. Merskey, H., and Hester, R. A. (1972): *Postgrad. Med. J.*, 48:594–598.
11. Taub, A. (1973): *J. Neurosurg.*, 39:235–239.
12. Vanderfield, G. (1964): *Med. J. Aust.*, 2:82–83.
13. Woodforde, J. M., Dwyer, B., McEwen, B. W., De Wilde, F. W., Bleasel, K., Connelly, T. J., Jr., and Ho, C. Y. (1965): *Med. J. Aust.*, 2:869–872.

Advances in Pain Research and Therapy, Vol. 1,
edited by J. J. Bonica and D. Albe-Fessard.
Raven Press, New York © 1976.

Periventricular Brainstem Structures as Sites of Acute and Chronic Opiate Action Related to Pain

A. Herz and E. Laschka

Department of Neuropharmacology, Max-Planck Institute of Psychiatry, 8 Munich 40, Kraepelinstrasse 2, Germany

Recently numerous investigators have studied the sites of action of morphine-like compounds in the central nervous system. There is now overwhelming evidence that brainstem structures lining the ventricular system (VS) are very important sites of opiate action. Data relevant to analgesia are given in this overview. In addition, recent studies that point to the brainstem as site of chronic opiate action and are also interesting in view of pain phenomena are discussed.

ANTINOCICEPTIVE EFFECTS IN RABBITS AND RATS

When our laboratory became interested in such localization problems about 7 years ago, a lot of data about morphine effects on sensory mechanisms were available; much of this work was done by recording EEG and evoked potentials (4). We started our work in freely moving rabbits and used the licking reaction, evoked by electrical stimulation of the tooth pulp, as a nociceptive test. (Terms such as pain and analgesia should be avoided in such types of experiments since little can be said about sensation.) Intraventricularly injected morphine was found to be 500 to 1,000 times more potent than that injected intravenously (6). This indicates that the sites of action are easily reached from the ventricular space and are probably located in periventricular structures. To define sites of action of morphine more precisely, we performed microinjections of morphine into various brain structures. These experiments, however, gave inconsistent results and it was difficult to exclude the uncontrolled spread of substance into the VS. A method was therefore developed permitting drug administration into restricted parts of the VS in freely moving animals (1). In principle, a eucerine plug into a certain part of the VS, for instance, into the aqueductus mesencephali, is applied; this plug restricts the spread of the drug injected into other parts of the VS. In our hands this method proved to be very useful for the study of localization aspects, especially when combined with autoradiographic control of the spread of the drug.

Depending on the site of injection and the location of the plug, big differences in the effect of morphine were observed. When the spread of the drug was restricted to the third and the lateral ventricles, the increase in stimulation threshold was small, even at morphine doses as high as 320 μg. The same was true when morphine was injected into the cisterna cerebellomedullaris (from where it reaches the outer surface of the brainstem) when a plug inserted into the fourth ventricle prevented the permeation of the drug into the VS. Strong effects were observed, however, when morphine (80 μg) was injected into the aqueduct in experiments with a plug in the third ventricle. This effect was also noted when in experiments with a plug in the aqueduct the drug was applied into the fourth ventricle. From these experiments it is concluded that the most sensitive sites for the inhibition of the licking reaction are located in the fossa rhomboidea; however, the caudal parts of the periaqueductal gray matter (PAG) must also be considered as sites of action; this is concluded from autoradiographs showing that the drug also reaches this region at least its caudal parts, in spite of the aqueductal plug (6,7).

In principle, very similar results were obtained in rats in which vocalization, elicited by electrical stimulation of the tail root, was used as a nociceptive test (E. Laschka and A. Herz, 1975, *unpublished observations*). A dose of 10 μg morphine injected into the lateral ventricle was almost ineffective when the spread of the drug into the caudal parts of the VS was blocked by a plug in the aqueduct. Moreover, the same dose induced a large increase in stimulation threshold when injected into the fourth ventricle with the plug located in the third ventricle. Only a weak effect was obtained when the location of the plug was in the aqueduct.

These results correlate rather well with those Jacquet and Lajtha (10,11) obtained in rats by the microinjection method; these authors stress the important role of the caudal parts of the PAG. In contrast, older results of Tsou and Jang (30) in rabbits and of Buxbaum et al. (3) in rats point to more rostrally located diencephalic structures. In view of our experiments one might argue that in addition to the periventricular brainstem, diencephalic structures not easily reached from the VS are also involved. However, this does not seem to be the case, at least in rabbits, where the action of systemically applied morphine could be fully reversed by the application of low doses of morphine antagonists restricted to the fourth ventricle (2).

EXPERIMENTS IN MONKEYS

Interesting results have been obtained recently by Pert and Yaksh (24) in rhesus monkeys using the pain titration technique in which the animal, by pressing a lever, can limit the intensity of noxious current delivered to the feet. Morphine was highly effective when applied by microinjection into periventricular sites extending from the lower portion of the third ventricle along the aqueduct into the fourth ventricle. Besides the periventricular/PAG, a second region of approximately the same extent but located about 5 mm more lateral showed less morphine sensitivity. At least the caudal parts of Pert's periventricular morphine-sensitive region correspond to the area that proved to be most sensitive in rabbits and rats. This is of interest in view of the different methods used. It indicates that regions sensitive to morphine in tests which use simple nociceptive reactions are also sensitive when using a test procedure in which pain sensation is tested. On the other hand, the morphine-sensitive areas cited in Pert's experiments extend to more rostrally located diencephalic structures, the hypothalamus and the medial thalamus. The complex test procedure used in the latter experiments makes the involvement of higher integrative centers understandable.

DESCENDING INHIBITIONS

Spinal cord transsection has long been known to reduce the sensitivity of polysynaptic (nociceptive) spinal reflexes to morphine. From experiments with transsection of the neuraxis at various levels in cats, Satoh and Takagi (27) concluded that morphine activates descending inhibitory mechanisms by an action on structures located in the lower brainstem. It has to be considered, however, that the reflex activity of the spinal cord itself is changed by spinalization (12). Therefore, experiments in intact rabbits, in which morphine was applied into separate parts of the VS, were performed (31). Injection of 20 μg morphine into the fourth ventricle blocked in the hind leg flexor reflex, whereas injection of much higher doses into the third ventricle, as well as into the cisterna cerebellomedullaris, was ineffective. Radioassay of ^{14}C-morphine showed only negligible amounts of morphine in the lumbar cord where the reflex is relayed. The inhibition of the reflex induced by systemically applied morphine could be reversed by intraventricular application of morphine antagonists. From these results it is concluded that a strong morphine-induced reflex inhibition originates from brainstem structures that are easily reached from the fossa rhomboidea. Autoradiography was used to identify these structures more exactly (28). The spread of morphine after intraventricular administration (which induces a strong antinociceptive effect) was compared with the spread of morphine after intracisternal injection (which is ineffective). The results of these experiments point to an area located in the superficial layers of the anterior parts of the fossa rhomboidea as site of origin of the descending inhibition. However, it cannot be definitely excluded that this critical area also extends somewhat more rostrally into the midbrain.

Some more recently obtained data point to a similar region as origin of inhibition of nociceptive spinal reflexes. In the experiments of Mayer and Murfin (20), morphine injection into the mesencephalic gray matter was most effective. Inhibition of discharge activity of lamina V dorsal horn cells was observed by Besson's group after electrical stimulation of the caudal part of the PAG near the dorsal raphe nucleus (23). Coagulation of the nucleus medianus raphe reduced the antinociceptive effect of morphine in the experiments of Samanin et al. (26).

The morphine-induced activation of descending inhibitory influences on the spinal cord is of interest in view of a possible more general mechanism of opiate action. Obviously, morphine is capable of inhibiting nociceptive reflexes from outside the reflex arc very effectively, and the morphine sensitivity of the links of the reflex arc itself is low. This may also hold for nociceptive reactions integrated in the brain where it is much more difficult to differentiate effects on the pathway from effects on structures modulating the reflex pathway.

CHRONIC OPIATE ACTION

Frequently repeated opiate intake induces tolerance and physical dependence, representing adaptive processes of the organism to exposure to the drug. When drug supply is interrupted or morphine antagonists are applied, physical dependence is unmasked by the appearance of a withdrawal syndrome. In general, the withdrawal signs represent the mirror image of the effects of acute morphine administration; for example, sedation is turned into excitation, respiratory depression into hyperpnea. One might also expect that the "nociceptive system" develops dependence and that this dependence is reflected by the withdrawal sign hyperalgesia. Recently Tilson et al. (29) showed in rats that the flinch-jump response to electrical stimulation of the feet is enhanced during morphine withdrawal.

To date little is known about the anatomical structure involved in the development of physical dependence and withdrawal. Our studies revealed the importance of brainstem structures in these processes in rabbits (8) and rats (15,16, see also 5). Intraventricular administration of morphine antagonists can precipitate a withdrawal syndrome similar to that induced by systemic antagonist administration. Administration of antagonists into the restricted anterior parts of the VS, consisting of the lateral ventricles and third ventricle, was rather ineffective in inducing abstinence signs, whereas administration of low doses of antagonist into the fourth ventricle precipitated an intense withdrawal symptomatology in both species. The sign "scream on touch," which was tested in the experiments with rats, could also be precipitated by lower doses of antagonists when injected into the fourth ventricle than when injected into the restricted anterior parts of the VS.

More quantitative results could be obtained when the flinch-jump response was evaluated in morphine-dependent rats and naloxone was applied either intraventricularly or into restricted parts of the VS (E. Laschka and A. Herz, 1975, *unpublished observations*). Intraventricular naloxone application induced a significant decrease in threshold for eliciting the flinch-jump response. A similar effect was obtained when naloxone was injected into the fourth ventricle, although the threshold remained unchanged when the same dose was injected into the lateral ventricle of animals with a plugged aqueduct. In experiments with some variation of the location of the plug, we got the impression that the effect was less pronounced when the aqueduct was scarcely involved. This is interesting in view of the withdrawal experiments mentioned above in which only the most caudal parts of the PAG proved to be important. The dose of naloxone used in these experiments was low (0.4 μg), and other withdrawal signs were only weakly precipitated by this dose. Thus, hyperreactivity to painful stimuli represents a sensitive withdrawal sign probably related to dependence development in periventricular brainstem structures involved in nociceptive mechanisms.

SUMMARY

Accumulating data point to periventricular structures in the upper brainstem as sites of the antinociceptive action of opiates. There is also some indication that a similar region is involved in withdrawal phenomena related to pain. Depending on the test and species, more rostrally located structures such as the medial thalamus, the hypothalamus, or the limbic system may also be involved in the antinociceptive opiate effect. As Nauta (22) has recently pointed out, the central gray represents a "nodal point" in conduction pathways that may constitute the lowest level at which pain is integrated. On the other hand, the sites where opiates exert their antinociceptive effect and the sites where pain is integrated are not necessarily identical. This has become especially clear for nociceptive spinal reflexes and may also be valid for the brain.

The significance of the periventricular upper brainstem structures for nociception and pain relief also becomes clear from the results obtained by electrical stimulation of brain areas. There are many parallel findings between stimulus-induced and morphine-induced antinociception, and even development of cross-tolerance between both phenomena has been shown (17,19,21).

Biochemical data also stress the important role of the upper brainstem as site of morphine analgesia. At least the dorsal nuclei of the raphe system, origin of ascending and descending serotonergic pathways, are located in the area which proved to be sensitive to morphine in the previous experiments. Many data show that serotonin is involved in pain mechanisms. Also, the locus ceruleus, origin of noradrenergic pathways, is located within this area. The role of this nucleus in pain mechanisms has been recently considered by Korf et al. (13).

Finally, investigations concerning the distribution of morphine receptors in various brain areas are of interest in this context. The brainstem, especially the PAG, of various species proved to be rich in opiate-binding sites (9,14), and a high stereospecific binding of levorphanol was found in the rhombencephalon (18). Recent results obtained by autoradiographic studies of opiates of high specific activity also revealed intense opiate binding in some areas of the medial brainstem (25). Although these data offer no proof of opiate action at these sites, they strongly support the data obtained by other methods.

REFERENCES

1. Albus, K. (1972): *Physiol. Behav.,* 8:569–571.
2. Albus, K., Schott, M., and Herz, A. (1970): *Eur. J. Pharmacol.,* 12:53–64.
3. Buxbaum, J. A., Yarbrough, G. G., and Carter, M. E. (1970): *Pharmacologist,* 12:211.
4. Domino, E. F. (1968): *Res. Publ. Assoc. Nerv. Ment. Dis.,* 46:117–149.
5. Herz, A. (1975): *Neurosci. Res. Program Bull.,* 13(1):92–94.
6. Herz, A., Albus, K., Metyš, I., Schubert, P., and Teschemacher, H. (1970): *Neuropharmacology,* 9:539–551.
7. Herz, A., and Teschemacher, H. (1971): *Adv. Drug Res.,* 6:79–119.
8. Herz, A., Teschemacher, H., Albus, K., and Zieglgänsberger, S. (1972): *Psychopharmacologia,* 26:219–235.
9. Hiller, J. M., Pearson, J., and Simon, E. J. (1973): *Res. Commun. Chem. Pathol. Pharmacol.,* 6:1052–1062.
10. Jacquet, Y. F., and Lajtha, A. (1974): *Science,* 185:1055–1057.
11. Jacquet, Y. F., and Lajtha, A. (1975): *Fed. Proc.,* 34:786.
12. Jurna, I., Grossmann, W., and Theres, C. (1973): *Neuropharmacology,* 12:983–993.
13. Korf, J., Bunney, B. S., and Aghajanian, G. K. (1974): *Eur. J. Pharmacol.,* 25:165–169.
14. Kuhar, M. J., Pert, C. B., and Snyder, S. H. (1973): *Nature,* 245:447–450.
15. Laschka, E., Herz, A., and Bläsig, J. (1976): *Psychopharmacologia (in press).*
16. Laschka, E., Teschemacher, H., Mehraein, P., and Herz, A. (1976): *Psychopharmacologia (in press).*
17. Liebeskind, J. C., Guilbaud, G., Besson, J.-M., and Oliveras, J.-L. (1973): *Brain Res.,* 50:441–446.
18. Lowney, L. I., Schulz, K., Lowery, P. J., and Goldstein, A. (1974): *Science,* 183:749–753.
19. Mayer, D. J., and Liebeskind, J. C. (1974): *Brain Res.,* 68:73–93.
20. Mayer, D. J., and Murfin, R. (1975): Satellite Symposium, Helsinki.
21. Mayer, D. J., Wolfle, T. L., Akil, H., Carder, B., and Liebeskind, J. C. (1971): *Science,* 174:1351–1354.
22. Nauta, W. J. H. (1975): *Neurosci. Res. Program Bull.,* 13(1):84–87.
23. Oliveras, J.-L., Besson, J.-M., Guilbaud, G., and Liebeskind, J. C. (1974): *Exp. Brain Res.,* 20:32–44.
24. Pert, A., and Yaksh, T. (1974): *Brain Res.,* 80:135–140.
25. Pert, C., Kuhar, M. J., and Snyder, S. H. (1975): *Life Sci.,* 16:1849–1854.
26. Samanin, R., Gomulka, W., and Valzelli, L. (1970): *Eur. J. Pharmacol.,* 10:339–343.
27. Satoh, M., and Takagi, H. (1971): *Eur. J. Pharmacol.,* 14:60–65.
28. Teschemacher, H., Schubert, P., and Herz, A. (1973): *Neuropharmacology,* 12:123–131.
29. Tilson, H. A., Rech, R. H., and Stolman, S. (1973): *Psychopharmacologia,* 28:287–300.
30. Tsou, K., and Jang, C. S. (1964): *Sci. Sinica,* 13:1099–1109.
31. Vigouret, J., Teschemacher, H., Albus, K., and Herz, A. (1973): *Neuropharmacology,* 12:111–121.

Advances in Pain Research and Therapy, Vol. 1,
edited by J. J. Bonica and D. Albe-Fessard.
Raven Press, New York © 1976.

Involvement of Central Transmitters in Narcotic Analgesia

G. Pepeu

Department of Pharmacology, University of Florence Medical School, Florence, Italy

We are all aware (13) that narcotic analgesics, besides their desirable analgesic action, exert a number of other central and peripheral actions such as respiratory depression, catalepsy, and reduction of intestinal motility. Furthermore, they induce tolerance and physical dependence. In exerting all these actions, narcotic analgesics either act on or indirectly involve the central and peripheral nervous systems. Both systems function through the synthesis, storage, release, and inactivation of various neurotransmitter substances responsible for the passage of the nervous impulse across the synaptic cleft. As an obvious consequence, whichever action of analgesic drugs we investigate, we can expect either direct or indirect changes in neurotransmitter function. It becomes difficult to ascertain which changes underlie the mechanism of action of narcotic analgesics, which are indirect effects, which changes are related to the antinociceptive properties, and which are side effects.

A large number of papers have dealt with the relationship between narcotic analgesics and neurotransmitters. The purpose of this chapter is to provide an overview of some of the most recent advances. Because of limitation of space, we shall call attention to only a few recent papers that shed some new light on the involvement of the neurotransmitters in the analgesic and addicting properties of these drugs. For a more comprehensive coverage of this field, we refer the reader to a number of recent books (8,27) and to our previous review (36).

GLUTAMATE

An example of how difficult it is to define the direct or indirect nature of the neurochemical effects of morphine is offered by the recent work of Sherman and Gebhart (44) showing that pain and morphine affect the level of glutamate in the central gray and the hypothalamus. Neurochemical analysis (26), uptake studies (30), and microiontophoretic applications on single neurons (11) suggest that glutamic acid is a possible transmitter in the sensory pathways. In mice a nociceptive stimulation (hot plate) brings about a decrease in the glutamate level in the central gray, a brain area involved in pain control mechanisms (29). Pretreatment with an antinociceptive dose of morphine not only antagonizes the pain-induced reduction of the central gray glutamate level, but it significantly raises glutamate above control values. The question arises as to whether the change in the glutamate level depends on the antinociceptive affect of morphine or is responsible for it. These findings are made even more intriguing by the observation that in the hypothalamus, a region not involved in the nociceptive system, morphine enhances the pain-induced decrease in glutamate possibly through a metabolic mechanism unrelated to antinociception.

DOPAMINE

That narcotic analgesics stimulate dopamine (DA) metabolism in the brain (9,17,41,46) is shown by the increase in the brain level of the DA metabolites 3,4-dihydroxyphenylacetic acid (DOPAC) and homovanillic acid (HVA) (1,16). Narcotic analgesics share this effect with other drugs such as neuroleptics (2). The stimulation of DA metabolism by neuroleptics has been interpreted as a consequence of the blockade of DA postsynaptic (3) and possibly presynaptic (38) receptors. Catalepsy, a symptom induced by neuroleptic drugs and to a lesser extent by narcotic analgesics, is considered to be caused by the blockade of DA receptors in the extrapyramidal and mesolimbic system (10). However, some recent evidence seems to prove that antinociception could also be related to a blocking effect of DA receptors by narcotic analgesics.

Van der Wende and Spoerlein (48) showed that in mice the dopaminergic agonists apomorphine and amantadine are antagonistic to morphine; conversely, dopaminergic antagonists such as spiroperidol, clothiapine, and perphenazine, but not adrenergic antagonists, potentiate morphine analgesia. The latter is by no means a new observation since the synergism between neuroleptic and narcotic analgesics is commonly exploited in clinical practice. Similar results have been presented by Eidelberg and Erspamer (15), who also found that haloperidol enhances morphine tolerance. Paalzow et al. (35) observed that pretreatment with L-DOPA antagonized pentazocine analgesia in the rat. It is also pertinent that pentazocine does not evoke catalepsy (1) while it increases DA turnover (46). Pretreatment with naloxone antagonizes the ability of morphine, pentazocine, and methadone to increase striatal DA turnover (46) but does not antagonize the increase in rat striatal HVA level induced by chlorpromazine (28).

NOREPINEPHRINE

Following the observation that the hypothalamic level of norepinephrine (NE) in the cat is decreased by acutely administered morphine (49) and that pretreatment with reserpine diminishes the antinociceptive effect of morphine in mice (43), a large number of investigations were devoted to the effect of narcotic analgesics on NE steady-state levels and turnover. The results are often conflicting, probably because of differences in the animal species used, in the doses of the different analgesics, and in the tests used for evaluating the antinociceptive activity. However, a possible role of NE in analgesia is supported by the recent work of Shiomi and Takagi (45). These authors reported that analgesic doses of morphine and pentazocine cause a dose-dependent increase in the concentration of normetanephrine, a NE metabolite, in the dorsal columns of the rat spinal cord. The effect was prevented by naloxone and by transsection of the spinal cord at C_1. The authors concluded that morphine and related analgesics enhance the activity of the bulbospinal inhibitory noradrenergic system, the terminals of which probably produce a postsynaptic inhibition of the dorsal horn neurons of the spinal cord (42). The dependency of the antinociceptive effects of morphine and other analgesic agents on spinal cord activity was also demonstrated after central monoamine depleting (21).

5-HYDROXYTRYPTAMINE

There is evidence to implicate the central 5-hydroxytryptamine (5-HT) pathways in the antinociceptive effect of morphine. The evidence is mainly based on experiments showing that a lowering of the level of brain 5-HT either by pharmacological procedures (18,20,47,50) or by selective lesions of 5-HT neurons in the brain (40) antagonized morphine analgesia. Conversely, the increase in brain 5-HT brings about a potentiation of morphine analgesia (31). Moreover, an increase in 5-HT turnover in morphine-treated animals was also reported (22,52,53). However, two recent studies demonstrate that morphine alone increases 5-HT turnover. Samanin et al. (39) showed that lesions of the midbrain raphe which produced a marked depletion of 5-HT in the forebrain antagonize the analgesic effect of morphine but not that of methadone, meperidine, codeine, or propoxyphene. Goodlet and Sugrue (19) showed that only morphine at a dose well in excess of that required for antinociception in rats significantly increases 5-HT turnover as demonstrated by a rise in brain 5-hydroxyindole acetic acid (5-HIAA); this rise is antagonized by naloxone. Pentazocine and methadone have no effect on 5-HIAA level; pethidine decreases it, but this effect is not antagonized by naloxone.

It appears from these experiments that 5-HT is not involved in the mechanism of action of the analgesic agents, with the notable exception of morphine, and that narcotic analgesics cannot be considered to act through identical neurochemical mechanisms.

Conflicting evidence makes it difficult to draw a definite conclusion about the role of 5-HT in both tolerance and physical dependence. According to

Way (51) and his group, the rate of brain 5-HT synthesis is increased in morphine-tolerant and -dependent mice, and a reduction in brain 5-HT synthesis, induced by pretreatment with *p*-chlorophenylalanine, is associated with a reduction in the development of tolerance to and physical dependence on morphine. On the other hand, a number of investigators have reported that tolerance and physical dependence can occur with no change in 5-HT turnover (7,32,53).

ACETYLCHOLINE

Narcotic drugs increase brain acetylcholine (ACh) levels and affect the release of ACh from different brain regions (see ref. in 36). Indirect (12) and direct (6) demonstrations have been given recently that narcotic analgesics can affect brain ACh turnover. However, species differences and differences among the brain regions make it difficult to interpret the result of the latter studies. Nevertheless, on the basis of all this evidence there is little doubt that narcotic analgesics affect the central cholinergic mechanisms. However, some of our recent results (33) cast some doubt on the relationship between morphine antinociception and brain ACh. In the frog no change in the antinociception threshold was found after morphine administration. Brain and spinal cord ACh levels were, however, increased by morphine when the doses of the drug did not cause remarkable behavioral excitation. Relevant to these results is the observation (4) that a marked decrease in ACh content induced by intraventricular administration of hemicholinium only slightly reduces the analgesic effect of morphine. Nevertheless, a close relationship seems to exist between the antinociceptive effect of cholinergic agents such as physostigmine and oxotremorine and changes in brain ACh levels (23,34).

Some evidence suggests that ACh may be involved in the development of the withdrawal syndrome. Domino and Wilson (12) observed that nalorphine and an abrupt (48 hr) withdrawal after chronic administration of morphine for 2 and 8 weeks significantly reduce the steady-state level of brain ACh. In agreement with these results, Jhamandas and Sutak (24) observed that the rate of spontaneous ACh release from the cerebral cortex is lower in morphine-dependent rats than in the control animals. Administration of naloxone and nalorphine to morphine-dependent rats was followed by a significant rise in the release of cortical ACh.

However, the severity of the morphine withdrawal syndrome precipitated by naloxone was not reduced by pretreatment with atropine or mecamylamine, with the exception of the autonomic signs (25); hemicholinium at a dose that markedly decreased brain ACh was also ineffective (4). According to Pinsky et al. (37), only the administration of choline reduces the severity of the withdrawal syndrome in rats. It should also be mentioned that if tolerance and physical dependence are induced by short-term morphine pellet administration, the naloxone-induced withdrawal syndrome is not associated with changes in the steady-state level of brain ACh (14).

CONCLUSION

The conclusion of this survey of recent literature on analgesic drugs and brain neurotransmitters is that all the neurotransmitters so far investigated —namely, ACh, DA, NE, 5-HT, and glutamic acid—are involved in the acute effects of these drugs and probably also in the antinociceptive effects. The discrepancies often found in the results from different laboratories are probably due to differences in the species, brain regions investigated, and methods used for evaluating the pharmacological effects of narcotic analgesics. The conclusion that narcotic agents act simultaneously on many neurotransmitter systems is also supported by the recent work of Bradley and Dray (5). These authors, using microiontophoretic application of morphine on single brainstem neurons in the cat, observed that morphine usually reduces and sometimes potentiates the excitation of neurons by ACh, NE, and 5-HT. As far as the development of tolerance, physical dependence, and the withdrawal syndrome is concerned, more experiments are necessary in order to evaluate fully the role of neurotransmitters.

REFERENCES

1. Ahtee, L., and Kääriänen, I. (1973): *Eur. J. Pharmacol.,* 22:206–208.
2. Andén, N. E., Butcher, S. G., Corrodi, H., Fuxe, K., and Ungersted, T. U. (1970): *Eur. J. Pharmacol.,* 11:303–314.
3. Andén, N. E., Corrodi, H., Fuxe, K., and Ungersted, T. U. (1971): *Eur. J. Pharmacol.,* 15:193–199.
4. Bhargava, N. L., Chan, S. L., and Way, L. (1974): *Eur. J. Pharmacol.,* 29:253–261.
5. Bradley, P. B., and Dray, A. (1974): *Br. J. Pharmacol.,* 50:47–55.
6. Cheney, D. L., Costa, E., Hanin, I., Racagni, G., and Trabucchi, M. (1975): In: *Cholinergic Mechanisms,* edited by P. G. Waser. Raven Press, New York.
7. Cheney, D. L., Goldstein, A., Algeri, S., and Costa, E. (1971): *Science,* 171:1169–1170.
8. Clouet, D. H. (1971): *Narcotic Drugs: Biochemical Pharmacology.* Plenum Press, New York.
9. Clouet, D. H., and Ratner, M. (1970): *Science,* 168:854–856.
10. Costall, B., and Naylor, R. Y. (1974): *Neuropharmacology,* 13:353–364.
11. Curtis, D. R., and Johnston, G. A. R. (1974): *Ergeb. Physiol.,* 66:97–188.
12. Domino, E. F., and Wilson, A. E. (1973*a*): *J. Pharmacol. Exp. Ther.,* 184:18–32.
13. Domino, E. F., and Wilson, A. E. (1973*b*): *Nature (Lond.),* 243:285–286.
14. Domino, E. F., and Wilson, A. E. (1975): *Psychopharmacology,* 41:19–22.
15. Eidelberg, E., and Erspamer, R. (1975): *J. Pharmacol. Exp. Ther.,* 192:50–57.
16. Fukui, K., and Takagi, H. (1972): *Br. J. Pharmacol.,* 44:45–51.
17. Gauchy, C., Azid, Y., Glowinski, J., and Cheramy, A. (1973): *Eur. J. Pharmacol.,* 22:311–319.
18. Genovese, F., Zonta, N., and Mantegazza, P. (1973): *Psychopharmacology,* 32:359–364.
19. Goodlet, I., and Sugrue, M. F. (1974): *Eur. J. Pharmacol.,* 29:241–248.
20. Gorlitz, B. D., and Frey, H. H. (1972): *Eur. J. Pharmacol.,* 20:171–180.
21. Grossman, W., Iurna, I., Nell, T., and Theres, C. (1973): *Eur. J. Pharmacol.,* 24:67–77.
22. Haubrich, D. R., and Blake, D. E. (1973): *Biochem. Pharmacol.,* 22:2753.
23. Howes, J. F., Harris, L. S., Dewey, W., and Voyda, C. A. (1969): *J. Pharmacol. Exp. Ther.,* 169:23–28.

24. Jhamandas, K., and Sutak, M. (1974): *Br. J. Pharmacol.,* 50:57–62.
25. Jhamandas, K., Sutak, M., and Bell, S. (1973): *Eur. J. Pharmacol.,* 24:296–305.
26. Johnson, J. L. (1972): *Brain Res.,* 37:1–19.
27. Kosterlitz, H. W., Collier, H. O. J., and Villareal, J. E. (1972): *Agonist and Antagonist Actions of Narcotic Analgesic Drugs.* Macmillan, London.
28. Kuschinsky, K., and Hornikievicz, O. (1972): *Eur. J. Pharmacol.,* 19:119–122.
29. Liebeskind, J. C., Guilbaud, G., Besson, J. M., and Oliveras, J. L. (1973): *Brain Res.,* 50:441–446.
30. Logan, W. J., and Snyder, S. H. (1971): *Nature* (*Lond.*), 234:296–299.
31. Major, C. T., and Pleuvry, B. J. (1971): *Br. J. Pharmacol.,* 42:512–521.
32. Marshall, I., and Grahame-Smith, D. G. (1970): *Nature* (*Lond.*), 228:1206–1208.
33. Nistri, A., Pepeu, G., Cammelli, E., Spina, L., and De Bellis, A. (1974): *Brain Res.,* 80:199–209.
34. Paalzow, G., and Paalzow, L. (1975): *Eur. J. Pharmacol.,* 31:261–272.
35. Paalzow, G., Paalzow, L., and Stalby, B. (1974): *Eur. J. Pharmacol.,* 27:78–88.
36. Pepeu, G., and Nistri, A. (1974): *Recent Advances on Pain,* edited by J. Bonica, P. Procacci, and C. Pagni. Charles C Thomas, Publisher, Springfield, Illinois.
37. Pinsky, C., Frederickson, R. C. A., and Vazquez, A. J. (1973): *Nature* (*Lond.*), 242:59–60.
38. Roth, R. H., Walters, J. R., and Morgenroth, V. H. (1974): In: *Advances in Biochemical Psychopharmacology, Vol. 12,* edited by E. Usdin. Raven Press, New York.
39. Samanin, R., Ghezzi, D., Mauron, C., and Valzelli, L. (1973): *Psychopharmacology,* 33:365–368.
40. Samanin, R., Gumulka, W., and Valzelli, L. (1970): *Eur. J. Pharmacol.,* 10:339–343.
41. Sasame, H. A., Perez-Cruet, J., Di Chiara, G., Tagliamonte, A., Tagliamonte, P., and Gessa, G. L. (1972): *J. Neurochem.,* 19:1953–1957.
42. Satoh, M., and Takagi, H. (1970): *Eur. J. Pharmacol.,* 14:150–154.
43. Schneider, J. A. (1954): *Proc. Soc. Exp. Biol. Med.,* 87:614–615.
44. Sherman, A. D., and Gebhart, G. F. (1975): *Life Sci.,* 15:352–357.
45. Shiomi, H., and Takagi, H. (1974): *Br. J. Pharmacol.,* 52:519–526.
46. Sugrue, M. F. (1974): *Br. J. Pharmacol.,* 52:159–165.
47. Tenen, S. S. (1968): *Psychopharmacology,* 12:278–285.
48. Van der Wende, C., and Spoerlein, M. T. (1973): *Res. Commun. Chem. Pathol. Pharmacol.,* 5:35–43.
49. Vogt, M. (1954): *J. Physiol.* (*Lond.*), 123:451–481.
50. Vogt, M. (1974): *J. Physiol.* (*Lond.*), 236:483–498.
51. Way, E. L. (1972): In: *Agonist and Antagonist Actions of Narcotic Analgesic Drugs,* edited by H. W. Kosterlitz, H. O. J. Collier, and J. E. Villareal. Macmillan, London.
52. Yarbrough, G. C., Buxbaum, D. M., and Sanders-Bush, E. (1971): *Life Sci.,* 10:977–983.
53. Yarbrough, G. C., Buxbaum, D. M., and Sanders-Bush, E. (1973): *J. Pharmacol. Exp. Ther.,* 185:328–335.

Advances in Pain Research and Therapy, Vol. 1,
edited by J. J. Bonica and D. Albe-Fessard.
Raven Press, New York © 1976.

Effects of Altering Brain Serotonin Activity on Human Chronic Pain

Richard A. Sternbach, David S. Janowsky, Leighton Y. Huey, and David S. Segal

Pain Unit, Veterans Administration Hospital, San Diego, California 92161; and Department of Psychiatry, University of California, San Diego, La Jolla, California 92037

Several lines of evidence from animal studies point to a serotonin-mediated pain inhibitory mechanism in the CNS. Inhibition of serotonin (5-HT) biosynthesis with para-chlorophenylalanine (pCPA) increases pain sensitivity, and intraperitoneal administration of 5-hydroxytryptophan (5-HTP), the immediate precursor of serotonin, restores both depleted serotonin levels and pain thresholds to normal (6,7,14). Lesions in the medial forebrain bundle similarly reduce serotonin levels and pain thresholds, and these effects are also countered by serotonin precursor administration (1,2,6,7). Cerebral ventricular injection of serotonin raises pain thresholds in rats and mice (3).

Morphine analgesia also seems dependent on a serotonin mechanism. Morphine induces a decrease in brain 5-HT (4,17). Morphine analgesia is antagonized by pCPA (4,14) and by reserpine (3,11), and this analgesia blockade is restored by administration of intracerebral serotonin and of 5-HT precursors. Conversely, intracerebral serotonin enhances morphine analgesia in rats (3,11).

Although such work in animals has been done with acute pain models, to our knowledge human chronic pain states have not been directly studied. In man, chronic pain is often associated with depression (12). We hypothesize that a common mechanism to account for increasing pain and depression with chronicity may lie in the depletion or decreased activity of brain 5-HT. To study this hypothesis we have begun to examine the effects of serotonin-altering agents on human chronic pain.

METHODS

Subjects

Patients who volunteered for the experiments were men, aged 22 to 60 years, hospitalized in the Pain Unit of the Veterans Administration Hospital, San Diego (5), for treatment of organic pain of long duration, usually musculoskeletal in origin (disc disease). All had demonstrable physical disease underlying their pain complaints. All were receiving various analgesics, usually nonnarcotic in nature, when they began the experiment, and most were also receiving electrical transcutaneous neurostimulation and flurazepam. For ethical and humane reasons, the treatment regimen existing at the start of a given study was continued unchanged throughout the phases of the experiment.

Pain Evaluations

Pain estimate. All subjects evaluated their average pain each day on a 100-point scale, with zero representing no pain and 100 representing pain excruciating enough to cause suicide.

Tourniquet test ratio. As described in detail elsewhere (13), the submaximum effort tourniquet technique has been adapted to measure the severity of clinical pain. The duration of arm ischemia required to match the patient's clinical pain level was noted and expressed as a percentage of the time required to reach the unbearable level. This test was performed triweekly.

Clinical pain level. The time, in seconds, required to match the severity of the clinical pain is the clinical pain level.

Maximum pain tolerance. The time, in seconds, required to reach the unbearable level of ischemic pain is the maximum pain tolerance.

Data were analyzed using each patient as his own control and applying one-tailed *t*-tests for paired results to each set of data.

Reserpine

Eleven patients received a dose of 0.5 to 1.5 mg reserpine administered on a single-blind basis at 9 A.M. and 9 P.M. daily on 2 or 3 consecutive days, followed and/or preceded by 3 or more days of matched placebos. Patients estimated their pain every 4 hr when awake, and the tourniquet test was given every other day.

Serotonin Precursors

Five patients received between 1.5 and 3.0 g/day of 5-HTP, in three divided doses daily, given in capsule form for 14 days, preceded or followed by 14 days of matched placebos. Three of these patients and two others received L-tryptophan (L-TP), gradually increased to maximum levels over a 4- to 6-day period to a maximum of between 7 and 10 g/day, given in grapefruit juice in three divided doses daily for 10 days, followed or preceded by grapefruit juice alone for 10 days. For both precursors, drugs were administered on a double-blind basis, the placebo–active drug sequence was counterbalanced, pyridoxine 100 mg was administered daily throughout the experimental active drug and placebo periods, and daily pain estimates and biweekly tourniquet tests were obtained.

Chlorimipramine

Nine patients received, on a double-blind basis using matched capsules, in counterbalanced order, either: (a) 14 days of chlorimipramine 150 mg p.o. hs, followed by 14 days of placebo p.o. hs, followed by 14 days of amitriptyline 150 mg p.o. hs; or: (b) 14 days of amitriptyline 150 mg p.o. hs, followed by 14 days of placebo p.o. hs, followed by 14 days of chlorimipramine 150 mg p.o. hs. Patients rated their pain daily and received triweekly tourniquet tests. Six were evaluated triweekly using Zung depression rating scales and were interviewed as to their symptoms and drug side effects. Amitriptyline was administered as an "active placebo" for chlorimipramine (Anafranil®). The latter is reported to have a selective effect of blocking the neuronal reuptake of 5-HT, thus increasing serotonin availability, while not increasing the availability of norepinephrine (8,9,15), as do other tricyclic antidepressants.

RESULTS

Reserpine

As shown in Table 1, there was a nonsignificant tendency for reserpine to increase pain. The tendency toward increased pain may be because of a decreased tolerance for pain, as reflected in the maximum pain tolerance component of the tourniquet test.

Serotonin Precursors

The sample groups of five L-TP and five 5-HTP trials were combined to give a serotonin precursor group of 7 subjects. The results, presented in

TABLE 1. *Effects of reserpine on pain in 11 chronic pain patients*

Pain indicator	Reserpine	Placebo[a]
Pain estimates (0–100%)	37 ± 5.5	34 ± 5.6
Tourniquet test ratio (0–100%)	51 ± 4.3	45 ± 7.2
Clinical pain level (sec)	138 ± 40	151 ± 49
Maximum pain tolerance (sec)	249 ± 68	299 ± 78

Data presented as averages ± SEM.

[a] All comparisons between active drug and placebo are not statistically significant.

TABLE 2. *Effects of serotonin precursors on pain in 7 chronic pain patients*

Pain indicators	5-HT precursors	Placebo[a]
Pain estimates (0–100%)	66 ± 4.2	68 ± 3.7
Tourniquet test ratio (0–100%)	60 ± 8.4	66 ± 7.4
Clinical pain level (sec)	238 ± 59	258 ± 54
Maximum pain tolerance (sec)	360 ± 83	397 ± 100

Data presented as averages ± SEM.
[a] All comparisons between active drug and placebo are not statistically significant.

Table 2, showed a nonsignificant tendency toward decreased levels of clinical pain, matched also by a trend toward decreased pain tolerance.

Chlorimipramine

Results for the last 3 days (pain estimates) and last two tourniquet tests for each drug and placebo phase are shown in Table 3. Chlorimipramine was found to be significantly more effective than placebo in decreasing patients' pain estimates; amitriptyline did not cause a significant decrease in pain when compared to placebo. Furthermore, with the tourniquet test, chlorimipramine was significantly more effective than placebo in increasing pain tolerance; amitriptyline was not.

In the 6 subjects tested, there were no significant differences in Zung depression ratings among the drugs (chlorimipramine, 50.3 ± 3.5; amitriptyline, 49.6 ± 4.3; placebo, 51.3 ± 4.3). Most patients said they preferred amitriptyline to chlorimipramine as an antidepressant, soporific, and anxiolytic agent.

DISCUSSION

These results are preliminary because, among other reasons, sample sizes are small and analgesics were continued throughout the studies, placing

TABLE 3. *Effects of chlorimipramine and amitriptyline on pain in 9 chronic pain patients*

Pain indicator	Chlorimipramine	Amitriptyline	Placebo[a]
Pain estimates (0–100%)	33 ± 4.7[b]	38 ± 7.1	40 ± 3.5
Tourniquet test ratio (0–100%)	42 ± 7.1	44 ± 5.7	47 ± 7.7
Clinical pain level (sec)	249 ± 82	215 ± 81	227 ± 55
Maximum pain tolerance (sec)	528 ± 137[c]	420 ± 124	438 ± 95

[a] Means ± SEs of last 3 days of each 2-week experimental phase.
[b] Paired $t = 2.198$; df = 8; $p < 0.05$ (1-tailed test) for chlorimipramine vs placebo.
[c] Paired $t = 3.098$; df = 8; $p < 0.025$ (1-tailed test) for chlorimipramine vs amitriptyline.

methodological limitations on the data. However, the results suggest that increased brain serotonin activity causes decreased pain, perhaps by increasing pain tolerance. We suspect that more significant results may have been obtained had we also administered an agent to block peripheral serotonin effects. Peripheral serotonin may increase pain, especially ischemic pain (10) as in the tourniquet test.

Amitriptyline did not significantly decrease pain, yet most patients subjectively preferred it to chlorimipramine as a mood elevator. Possibly this is because the effects of amitriptyline on norepinephrine reuptake enhance mood but allow norepinephrine to antagonize amitriptyline's analgesic serotoninergic effects (16).

SUMMARY

Pilot studies using reserpine, serotonin precursors, and chlorimipramine (a selective serotonin reuptake blocking agent) support the hypothesis that brain serotonin activity may be important in regulating the severity of human chronic pain. Increasing brain serotonin activity decreases pain levels and seems to do so by increasing pain tolerance. This finding supports conclusions from acute pain studies in animals and further suggests that decreases in central serotonin may account for increases in both depression and pain levels in human chronic pain.

ACKNOWLEDGMENT

This work was supported by Veterans Administration Research Grant MRIS-8131 to R. A. Sternbach.

REFERENCES

1. Akil, H. (1972): Doctoral dissertation, University of California, Los Angeles.
2. Akil, H., and Mayer, D. J. (1972): *Brain Res.,* 44:692–697.
3. Calcutt, C. R., Handley, S. L., Sparkes, C. G., and Spencer, P. S. J. (1973): In: *Agonist and Antagonist Actions of Narcotic Analgesic Drugs,* edited by H. W. Kosterlitz, H. O. J. Collier, and J. A. Villareal. University Park Press, Baltimore.
4. Fennessey, M. R., and Lee, J. R. (1970): *J. Pharm. Pharmacol.,* 22:930.
5. Greenhoot, J. H., and Sternbach, R. A. (1974): In: *Advances in Neurology, Vol. 4: International Symposium on Pain,* edited by J. J. Bonica, pp. 595–604. Raven Press, New York.
6. Harvey, J. A., and Lints, C. (1968): *Pharmacologist,* 10:211.
7. Harvey, J. A., and Lints, C. (1971): *J. Comp. Physiol. Psychol.,* 74:28.
8. Modigh, K. (1973): *J. Neural. Transm.,* 34:101–109.
9. Ross, S. B., Renyi, A. L., and Ogren, S. O. (1972): *Eur. J. Pharmacol.,* 17:107–112.
10. Sicuteri, F., Franchi, G., and Michelacci, S. (1974): In: *Advances in Neurology, Vol. 4: International Symposium on Pain,* edited by J. J. Bonica, pp. 39–44. Raven Press, New York.
11. Sparkes, C. G., and Spencer, P. S. J. (1971): *Br. J. Pharmacol.,* 42:230–241.

12. Sternbach, R. A. (1974): *Pain Patients: Traits and Treatment.* Academic Press, New York.
13. Sternbach, R. A., Murphy, R. W., Timmermans, G., Greenhoot, J. H., and Akeson, W. H. (1974): In: *Advances in Neurology, Vol. 4: International Symposium on Pain,* edited by J. J. Bonica, pp. 281–288. Raven Press, New York.
14. Tenen, S. S. (1968): *Psychopharmacologia,* 12:278–285.
15. Van Pragg, H. M., VandenBurg, W., Bos, E. R., and Dols, L. C. W. (1974): *Psychopharmacologia,* 38:267–269.
16. Verri, R., Graeff, F., and Corrado, A. (1968): *Int. J. Neuropharmacol.,* 7:283–292.
17. Way, E. L. (1972): *Fed. Proc.,* 31:113–120.

Advances in Pain Research and Therapy, Vol. 1,
edited by J. J. Bonica and D. Albe-Fessard.
Raven Press, New York © 1976.

Possible Involvement of Norepinephrine and 5-Hydroxytryptamine in the Antinociceptive Activity of Narcotic Analgesics

R. D. E. Sewell and P. S. J. Spencer

Applied Pharmacology Laboratories, Welsh School of Pharmacy, UWIST, Cardiff, CF1 3NU, United Kingdom

Although morphine and its derivatives have been used as analgesics for several hundred years, only recently has evidence emerged of the possible central mechanisms of action of the opiates. Considerable evidence now exists for a pharmacological interaction between the opiates and several putative central neurotransmitters. The evidence implicating individual agents has often been confusing or even contradictory, but a number of workers have successfully implicated acetylcholine, the catecholamines, and 5-hydroxytryptamine (see, for example, 3,4,8,17,18,21). Despite a general confusion about the roles of individual neurotransmitters, it is clear that changes in the metabolism of these biogenic substances are followed by changes in the antinociceptive activity of narcotic agonist and partial-agonist analgesics (5,9,10).

The present authors' interest in this problem began some years ago with the availability of methods for injecting materials directly into the brains of conscious mice (1) and rats (19). It seemed likely that the earlier, frequently contradictory results from studies with analgesics could be attributed to a number of factors, the most important being the inadequacy of many analgesiometric methods in laboratory animals, the effects of species differences, and the presence of interfering and often contrasting peripheral pharmacological effects from the various agents used to study the actions of analgesic substances. With the availability of the techniques for injecting materials directly into the brains of conscious animals, it was possible to study the pharmacological actions of agents whose distribution would now be restricted primarily to the central nervous system; there was also the advantage that some agents which would not normally gain ready access to the brain would now be helped to do so through the creation of a high concentration at the blood-brain barrier after intraventricular injection.

The present authors' earlier work with morphine and the biogenic amines was conveniently summarized in a paper presented in 1971 to the Aberdeen Symposium on "Agonist and Antagonist Actions of Narcotic Analgesics" (2). Since then, the work in these laboratories has been broadened to include a study of the interactions of a wide range of analgesics with biogenic substances, the work concentrating on the roles of norepinephrine (NE) and 5-hydroxytryptamine (serotonin; 5-HT). The original findings suggested that the actions of morphine were determined by the balance within the brain of the activities of two amines, NE and 5-HT, the latter amine being able to enhance markedly the actions of morphine. Recently, Samanin et al. (11), from their work with lesions in the midbrain raphe system, have claimed that the importance of brain 5-HT in the actions of morphine is not true for other narcotic agonist analgesics. We have more recently provided evidence to show that a wide range of analgesics do interact with both central NE and 5-HT (16). This chapter summarizes a number of more recent studies (13–15) supporting the general hypothesis that increases in available brain 5-HT enhance, while increases in available brain NE attenuate, the antinociceptive effects of both narcotic agonists and partial-agonist analgesics.

METHODS

Albino mice (ICI strain, weighing 18 to 22 g) and Wistar albino rats (200 to 300 g) were housed under constant conditions, and the laboratory temperature was maintained at approximately 22°C.

Tail Immersion Nociceptive Test in Mice

The technique has been described in full by Sewell and Spencer (16). Groups of 10 mice were restrained in individual plastic containers, and their individual nociceptive reaction times, in seconds, were determined when the tail was immersed in a water bath at 48°C. A rapid "flinch" in the whole body of the mouse, or, alternatively, a violent jerk of the animal's tail, characterized the nociceptive threshold. A 15-sec "cutoff" time was imposed on animals failing to show a response. The low temperature permitted repeated tests on each animal (16).

Tail Immersion Nociceptive Test in Rats

Groups of 5 rats were placed in individual restraining wire mesh containers, and their individual nociceptive reaction times, in seconds, were determined when the tail was immersed in a constant temperature water bath held at 55°C (6). The nociceptive endpoint was similar to that seen in mice, and a 15-sec cutoff was imposed. Repeated tests of nociceptive sensitivity were made on individual animals.

Evaluation of Antinociceptive Activity

Two types of assessment were made. In the first, dose-related effects of antinociceptive activity were measured over a full 100-min period. Nociceptive thresholds were determined at 20-min intervals, and the antinociceptive effect of each dose of agent was calculated by determining the area or "integral" of the graph of nociceptive response time (seconds) against duration of assessment period (100 min). The integral was then expressed as a percentage increase over the control value (integral in the absence of analgesic agent), and the dose-response lines illustrated in Fig. 1 were obtained in this way, plotting percentage effect against dose (see ref. 16).

Alternatively, in the second type of assessment, antinociceptive activity was expressed as a simple increase of nociceptive threshold (in seconds). For the amine interaction studies, this procedure was used at the time of peak effect for each individual analgesic drug (see Figs. 2 and 3). The values are expressed as group means (seconds ± SE), and the significance of difference between treatment groups is determined by Student's *t*-test.

Intracerebroventricular Injections

Intracerebroventricular (ICV) injections were made in conscious animals using techniques described by Brittain and Handley (1) and by Sparkes and

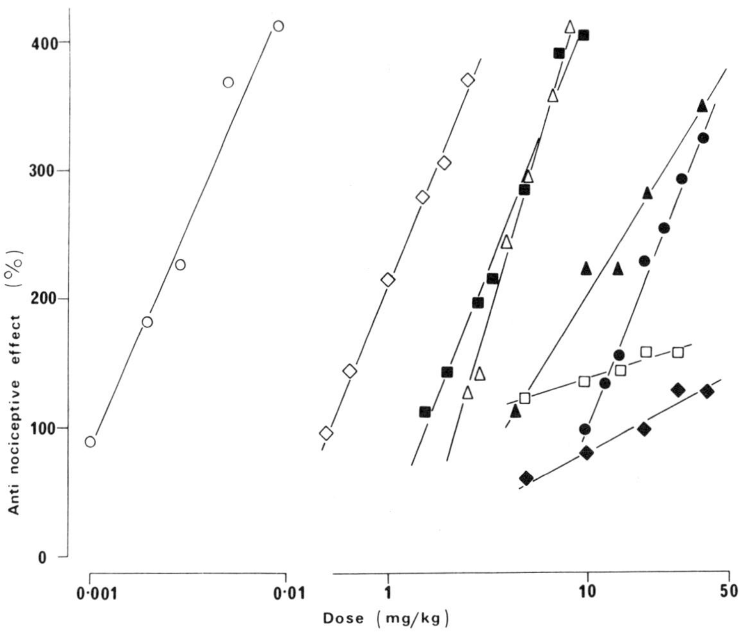

FIG. 1. Dose-response relationships in the mouse for representative centrally acting analgesics. For each dose of analgesic, nociceptive thresholds (sec) were determined at zero time and at 20-min intervals for a 100-min period. Antinociceptive effect was then assessed by calculating the area or "integral" of the graph between nociceptive threshold (sec) and duration of effect (100 min). Integral was then expressed as a percentage of the control (no drug) integral. Percentages are plotted as ordinates. Etorphine (○——○), diamorphine (◇——◇), morphine (■——■), AH 7921 (△——△), profadol (▲——▲), pethidine (●——●), pentazocine (◆——◆), and cyclazocine (□——□).

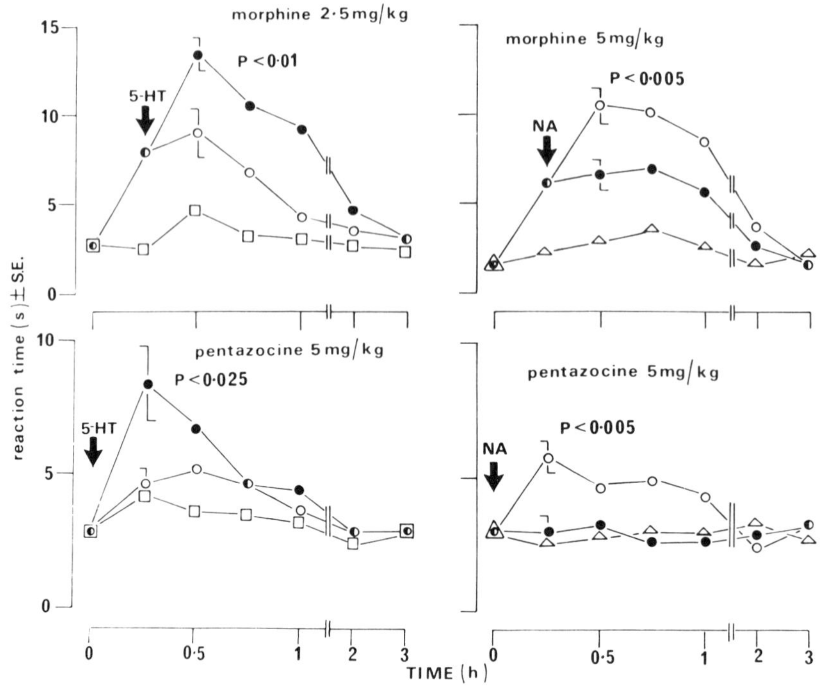

FIG. 2. Interaction in the mouse between morphine, pentazocine, and intracerebroventricularly injected 5-HT and NA. ICV injections of 5-HT (10 μg/mouse), NA (10 μg), or sterile saline (0.01 ml) were made 15 min (*arrow*) before the peak antinociceptive effect of morphine or pentazocine. Analgesic + ICV amine (●———●); analgesic + ICV saline (○———○); ICV 5-HT alone (□———□); ICV NA alone (△———△).

Spencer (19). A graduated Hamilton syringe was used in both mice and rats to introduce ICV volumes of 0.01 ml. ICV injections of 5-HT, NE, or vehicle were made using sterile apyrogenic 0.9% w/v NaCl solution. Doses in the text refer to the bases.

Subcutaneous Injection

The following drugs were used by subcutaneous injection: AH 7921 (3,4-dichloro-*N*-(1-dimethylamine)cyclohexylmethyl-benzamide), cyclizine, diamorphine hydrochloride (B.P.), etorphine hydrochloride, morphine hydrochloride (E.P.), pentazocine hydrochloride, pethidine hydrochloride, and profadol (m-(1-methyl-3-pyrrodinyl)phenol). We also used (+)-amphetamine sulfate (B.P.) and clonidine hydrochloride. All doses in the text refer to the salts.

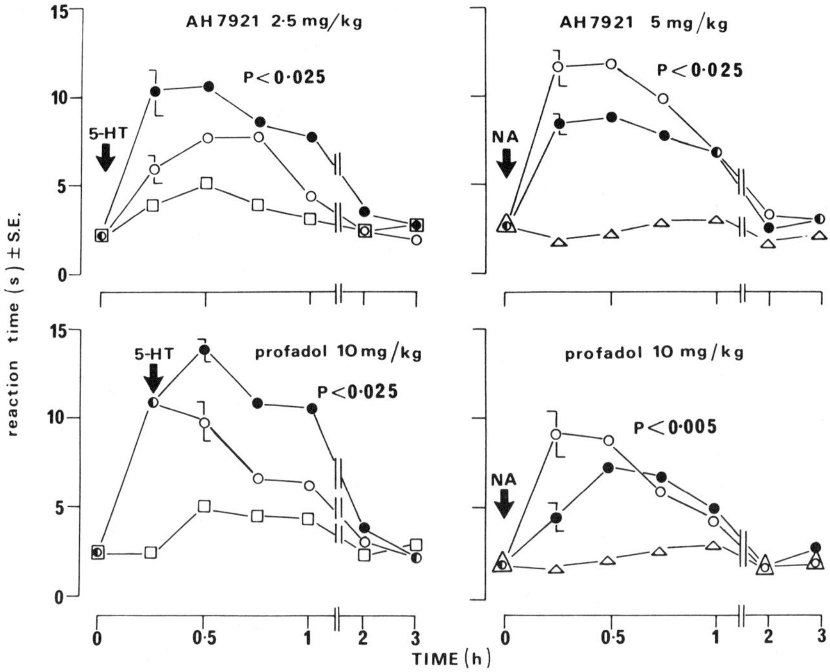

FIG. 3. Interaction in the mouse between AH 7921, profadol, and intracerebroventricularly injected 5-HT and NA. ICV injections of 5-HT (10 g/mouse), NA (10 g), or sterile saline (0.01 ml) were made 15 min (*arrow*) before the peak antinociceptive effect of AH 7921 or profadol. Analgesic + ICV amine (●———●); analgesic + ICV saline (○———○); ICV 5-HT alone (□———□); ICV NA alone (△———△).

RESULTS

Antinociceptive Activity of Various Centrally Acting Analgesics in the Tail Immersion Test

The early studies in these laboratories used the tail flick test in mice or a modified foot pressure test in rats (3), but in neither test do the partial-agonist analgesics possess a satisfactory dose-related, progressive antinociceptive effect. In contrast, marked antinociceptive activity is exhibited by a wide range of centrally acting analgesics, including the partial agonists, in the tail immersion tests in both mice and rats.

Figure 1 illustrates in mice the dose-response lines of representative narcotic agonist and partial-agonist analgesics. Although substantial dose-related activity was exhibited by the partial agonists pentazocine and cyclazocine, the differences in slopes illustrated in Fig. 1 are characteristic. Typically, steep slopes were obtained with naturally occurring (morphine), semisynthetic (diamorphine), and wholly synthetic opiates (etorphine), whereas similar steep slopes were obtained with nonopiates of known narcotic (pethidine) or suspected narcotic (profadol, AH 7921) properties. By contrast, the slopes of the partial agonists were much flatter and exhibited ceiling effects.

These studies were repeated in the rat, where qualitatively and quantitatively similar results were obtained. Dose-related antinociceptive activity was observed with both agonist and partial-agonist analgesics, and again typically steep slopes were obtained with the agonists, whereas flatter slopes with ceiling effects were obtained with partial agonists. Doses producing an antinociceptive effect of approximately 100% (100-min integral expressed as a percentage increase on the control integral) were: morphine 1.5 mg/kg, pethidine (9.0 mg/kg), pentazocine (10 mg/kg), and cyclazocine (15 mg/kg). These doses are substantially the same as those obtained in the mouse (see Fig. 1).

The antinociceptive effects of (+)-amphetamine and the centrally acting α-adrenoceptor agonist clonidine were also examined in mice and rats. As in other analgesiometric tests, both drugs exhibited substantial dose-related activity with dose-response line slopes intermediate in steepness between those of the narcotic agonists and partial agonists. Clonidine exhibited activity that was, weight-for-weight, five times more potent than that of morphine at an antinociceptive effect (100-min integral) of 100%, whereas at 250%, clonidine was only two and one-half times more potent because of its flatter dose-response line.

In subsequent studies reported below, we used submaximum doses of these agents, approximating to antinociceptive effects (100-min integrals) of between 150% and 250%.

Antinociceptive Activity of Analgesics After ICV Injections of 5-HT or NE

The abilities of intracerebroventricularly injected 5-HT to potentiate and of ICV NE to attenuate the antinociceptive activity of morphine are well documented (14,19). The present study describes interactions between ICV 5-HT and NE with a wider range of analgesics.

Figures 2 and 3 illustrate in mice the effects of ICV injections of 5-HT (10 μg per mouse) or NE (10 μg) on the antinociceptive effects of morphine (agonist), pentazocine (partial agonist), AH 7921, and profadol (the latter two drugs are nonopiates of suspected narcotic agonist activity). In every case, ICV 5-HT significantly potentiated ($p < 0.05$) whereas ICV NE attenuated ($p < 0.05$) the antinociceptive effects. Qualitatively identical effects were produced with the analgesics diamorphine, etorphine, pethidine, and cyclazocine.

When the studies were repeated in the rat, each of the same eight analgesics was affected by the ICV amines in a similar manner; 5-HT potentiated and NE attenuated antinociceptive effects.

In contrast, subcutaneous injections of 5-HT (300 μg per mouse or rat) and NE (300 μg) were without effect on antinociceptive activity.

Both (+)-amphetamine and clonidine were also examined for interactions, but qualitatively different effects were obtained. In the mouse, (+)-amphetamine was significantly potentiated by ICV NE ($p < 0.05$) but unaffected by ICV 5-HT. Clonidine's antinociceptive activity was unaffected by either amine. Similar results for both agents were obtained in the rat.

DISCUSSION

The present authors have already established that a substantial interaction exists between morphine and the biogenic amines 5-HT and NE when the latter are injected directly into the brain. The hypothesis has been advanced that the antinociceptive activity of morphine is determined by the balance within the brain of the activities or availabilities of 5-HT and NE; in particular, 5-HT enhances morphine's effects markedly (3). This view of a role for 5-HT is substantiated by many other reports (7,12,17,20). More recently, Samanin and his colleagues (12) failed to confirm this in analgesics other than morphine, and they advanced the possibility that morphine's reliance on brain 5-HT is atypical.

The tail immersion test of nociceptive sensitivity has the advantage that good dose-related antinociceptive activity is possessed by the partial agonists, and the interactions of submaximal doses of a wide range of analgesics with intracerebroventricularly injected amines have been studied in the present investigation. In both mice and rats, it has been found without exception that drugs with narcotic agonist activity (whether pure agonist or partial agonist) are potentiated by ICV 5-HT and attenuated by ICV NE, and these effects are central in origin. The study has included natural opiates (morphine), semisynthetic (diamorphine) and synthetic (etorphine) opiates, as well as nonopiate analgesics with known or suspected narcotic agonist properties (pethidine, AH 7921, and profadol). The partial agonists pentazocine and cyclazocine were also modified in an identical manner.

By contrast, (+)-amphetamine and clonidine interacted in a qualitatively different manner, yet both agents possessed good dose-related antinociceptive activity in this test in mice and rats, as well as in man.

It is concluded that the ability of ICV 5-HT to potentiate and of ICV NE to attenuate antinociceptive activity is a feature specific to analgesics with narcotic agonist or partial-agonist activity—and this holds true irrespective of the chemical structure of individual agents. It is further suggested that the nature of the interaction of an analgesic with intracerebroventricularly injected 5-HT or NE constitutes a simple acute test for the presence of narcotic agonist properties in new potential analgesics.

ACKNOWLEDGMENT

The authors are grateful to Messrs. Boehringer Sohn, Ingelheim, for their generous financial support of this work.

REFERENCES

1. Brittain, R. T., and Handley, S. L. (1967): *J. Physiol. (Lond.)*, 192:805–813.
2. Calcutt, C. R., Handley, S. L., Sparkes, C. G., and Spencer, P. S. J. (1972): In: *Agonist and Antagonist Actions of Narcotic Analgesics* edited by H. W. Kosterlitz, H. O. J. Collier, and J. A. Villareal, pp. 176–191. Macmillan, London.
3. Clouet, D. H. (Ed.) (1971): *Narcotic Drugs: Biochemical Pharmacology.* Plenum Press, New York and London.
4. Harris, L. S. (1970): *Fed. Proc.*, 29:28–32.
5. Harris, L. S., Dewey, W. L., Howes, J. F., Kennedy, J. L., and Pars, H. (1969): *J. Pharmacol. Exp. Ther.*, 169:17–22.
6. Janssen, P. A. J., Niemegeers, C. J. E., and Dony, J. G. H. (1963): *Arzneim. Forsch.*, 13:502–507.
7. Nicak, A. (1965): *Med. Exp.*, 13:43–48.
8. Radouco-Thomas, S., Singh, P., Garcin, F., and Radouco-Thomas, C. (1967): *Arch. Biol. Med. Exp. (Santiago)*, 4:42–62.
9. Saarnivaara, L. (1969*a*): *Med. Biol.*, 47:113–123.
10. Saarnivaara, L. (1969*b*): *Med. Biol.*, 47:180–190.
11. Samanin, R., Ghezzi, D., Mauron, C., and Valzelli, L. (1973): *Psychopharmacologia*, 33:365–368.
12. Samanin, R., Gumulka, W., and Valzelli, L. (1970): *Eur. J. Pharmacol.*, 10:339–343.
13. Sewell, R. D. E., and Spencer, P. S. J. (1974a): *J. Pharm. Pharmacol. Suppl.*, 26:92–93.
14. Sewell, R. D. E., and Spencer, P. S. J. (1974*b*): *Br. J. Pharmacol.*, 51:140–141P.
15. Sewell, R. D. E., and Spencer, P. S. J. (1975*a*): *Br. J. Pharmacol.*, 54:256–257P.
16. Sewell, R. D. E., and Spencer, P. S. J. (1975*b*): *Psychopharmacologia*, 42:67–71.
17. Sigg, E. B., Caprio, G., and Schneider, J. A. (1958): *Proc. Soc. Exp. Biol. Med.*, 97:97–100.
18. Slaughter, D. (1950): *Arch. Int. Pharmacodyn. Ther.*, 83:143–148.
19. Sparkes, C. G., and Spencer, P. S. J. (1971): *Br. J. Pharmacol.*, 42:230–241.
20. Tenen, S. S. (1968): *Psychopharmacologia*, 12:278–285.
21. Vogt, M. (1954): *J. Physiol. (Lond.)*, 123:451–481.

Advances in Pain Research and Therapy, Vol. 1,
edited by J. J. Bonica and D. Albe-Fessard.
Raven Press, New York © 1976.

Effects of Morphine and Meperidine in the Brainstem of the Cat

*J. L. Henry

Department of Research in Anaesthesia, McGill University, Montreal, Canada

Recently evidence has been presented which suggests that morphine may produce analgesia in the cat by an action on narcotic receptors in the spinal cord (2,5). Microiontophoretic application of morphine depressed the spontaneous activity and the responses to noxious cutaneous stimulation of spinal neurons classified as nociceptive but failed to alter the activity of those classified as nonnociceptive. Intravenous administration and iontophoretic application of naloxone, a specific narcotic antagonist, reversed the depression of nociceptive neurons by morphine.

Additional information has also been presented implicating other regions of the central nervous system as possible sites of action of narcotics. The most commonly suggested region is that of the periaqueductal gray (PAG) and the adjacent dorsal raphe nucleus (Rd), where microinjection of morphine may lead to analgesia in awake animals (6,10) and where electrical stimulation may produce an increase in the threshold of the behavioral response to noxious cutaneous stimulation (7,8).

In view of this information implicating the central gray as a possible site of action of narcotic analgesics, we attempted to determine if the narcotics morphine and meperidine have actions in the brainstem similar to those in the spinal cord. A preliminary report of some of this work has been presented (4).

METHODS

Adult cats were anesthetized with halothane in oxygen. For studies on the PAG and Rd, the animals were decerebrated at a just supracollicular level and the colliculi were exposed; for studies on the medial and lower brainstem, the animals were decerebrated at an intercollicular level and the floor of the fourth ventricle was exposed. After surgery anesthesia was discontinued. Exposed nervous tissue was covered with warm mineral oil to

* Present address: Laboratoire de Physiologie Nerveuse, Centre National de la Recherche Scientifique, Gif-sur-Yvette, France.

prevent drying. All animals breathed room air spontaneously. Core temperature was maintained at 38°C, and femoral arterial pressure was monitored continuously.

Seven-barrelled micropipettes with tips 4 to 6 μm were used for recording extracellular unit spikes and for iontophoresis. The central recording barrel contained 2.7 M NaCl. The contents of the remaining barrels included various permutations of morphine HCl (75 mM, pH 4.8), meperidine HCl (0.1 M, pH 5.2), naloxone HCl (25 mM, pH 6.2), sodium L-glutamate, acetylcholine chloride (ACh), norepinephrine bitartrate (NE), and 5-hydroxytryptamine bimaleinate (5-HT). One additional barrel contained NaCl of comparable pH to the narcotic solutions to be used as a control for artifacts arising from local changes in current and pH.

Selected sites of recording were identified by passing pontamine blue dye from one of the barrels and cutting paraffin sections. Nuclear structures were identified by counterstaining the tissue with cresyl violet.

RESULTS

Clear results were obtained from 76 of 150 units examined: 38 in the PAG and Rd, and 38 in the reticular formation. The effects observed during application of these drugs were of three types.

The first type of response, an increase in the rate of discharge, was observed at six sites in the reticular formation but was not observed in the PAG or the Rd. It was usually obtained with currents of 15 to 30 nA. The time course of this response was similar to the short-lasting excitation reported for morphine in the reticular formation in the rat (1).

The second type of response was a depression of discharge rate without a change in the amplitude of the spike. This response was observed at nine sites in the reticular formation but was not observed in the PAG or the Rd. It was usually obtained with currents of 15 to 30 nA. The time course of this response was similar to that reported for depression of nociceptive neurons in the spinal cord of the cat (2) and of reticular neurons in the rat (1).

The third type of response was a continual slow depression of both discharge rate and spike amplitude throughout the duration of the application, with full recovery usually taking 1 min or more. This response was observed at 12 sites in the reticular formation and at 26 sites in the PAG and the Rd. It was usually obtained with higher currents (40 to 100 nA). A typical response of this type is illustrated in the oscilloscope records of Fig. 1, taken from a unit in the dorsal raphe nucleus. Application of meperidine caused a slow reduction in spike amplitude with an accompanying reduction in discharge rate which is not easily seen in this record because of the high ongoing rate. Application of an equivalent control current failed to cause a change in discharge rate or spike amplitude. ACh caused a reduction in discharge rate without a change in spike amplitude. The change

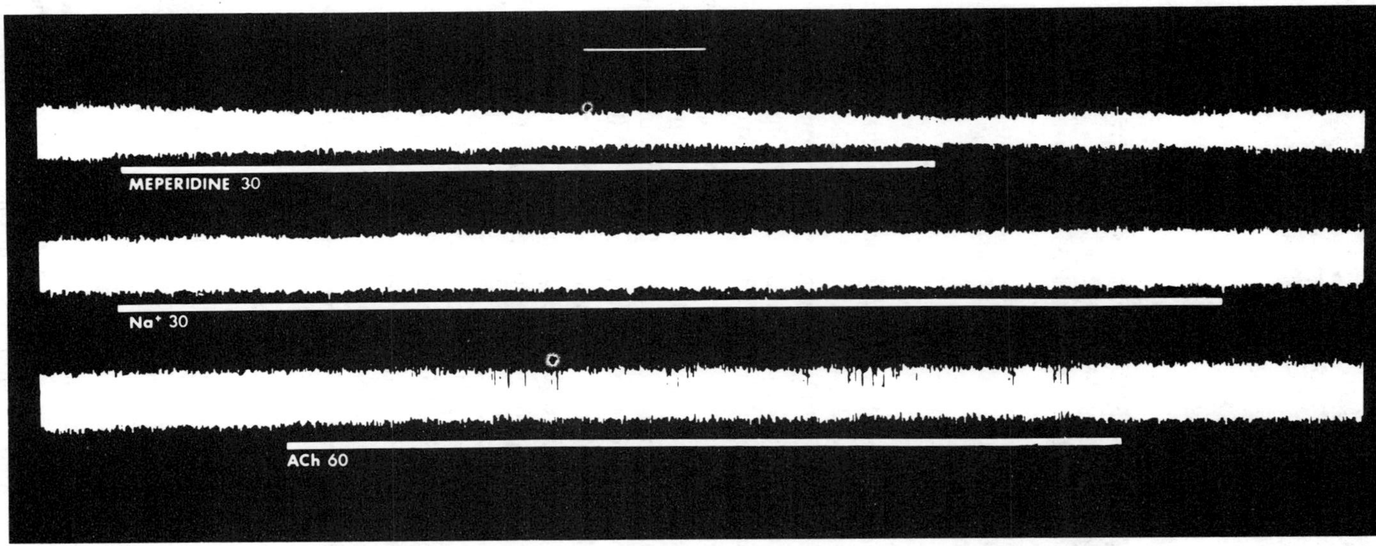

FIG. 1. Oscilloscope records of a unit in the dorsal raphe nucleus showing depression of spike amplitude by the iontophoretic application of meperidine. (Not obvious in these records is a similar depression of discharge rate.) Application of a control current through a barrel containing NaCl had no observable effect. Acetylcholine (ACh) caused a reduction in discharge rate without a change in spike amplitude. Iontophoretic currents are given in nA; time calibration above records is 5 sec.

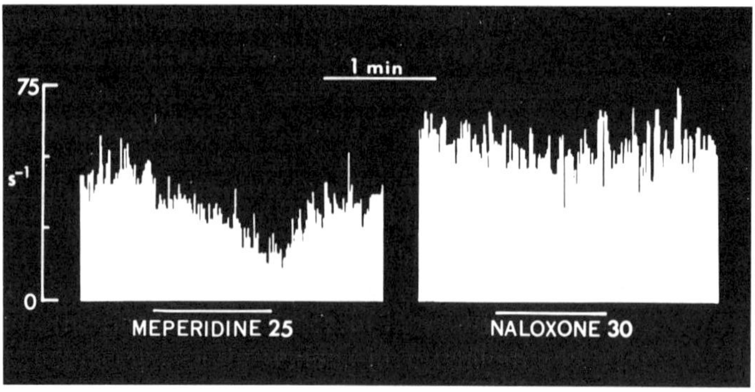

FIG. 2. Rate meter records of a unit in the PAG showing time course of the type 3 response (see text for definition) to meperidine application. Subsequent application of naloxone had no observable effect on this neuron.

in the rate of discharge of the type 3 response is better illustrated in the pen recorder tracings of Fig. 2, taken from a unit in the PAG. Meperidine caused a slow reduction in ongoing discharge, with a slow recovery, whereas naloxone failed to alter either discharge rate or spike amplitude.

Attempts were made to determine the effects of naloxone on the responses to iontophoretic application of morphine and meperidine. Applied by iontophoresis, naloxone failed to alter the type 3 responses of two neurons, one in the PAG and the other in the Rd. Intravenous administration of 0.4 mg/kg of naloxone, a dose greater than that of 0.05 to 0.25 mg/kg found sufficient to block narcotic depression of spinal nociceptive neurons (2), failed to alter the type 3 response of an additional unit in the PAG. In two cases the effects of iontophoretic application of naloxone were tested on type 2 responses from the reticular formation; in both cases it reduced the depression of discharge rate by 60 nA of meperidine.

Practically all units examined were excited by glutamate. Units excited by narcotic drugs were also excited by ACh and by 5-HT. NE had inconsistent effects on these units. Those that were depressed or failed to show a response to narcotics showed variable responses to ACh, NE, and 5-HT.

DISCUSSION

It has been found that iontophoretic application of the narcotic drugs morphine and meperidine elicits three types of responses from single units in the brainstem. One is excitation and is observed only from units in the reticular formation. Neurons excited by these drugs were also excited by ACh and by 5-HT. One possible explanation for this correlation is that the narcotic drugs may be producing this excitation by causing the release of endogenous ACh and/or 5-HT. Another possibility is that one mechanism of excitation is common to narcotics and to these putative transmitters. Present evidence is insufficient to allow precise conclusions, but the possibility that the excitatory actions of narcotics on these neurons are in some way linked to ACh and 5-HT is strengthened by the observations that narcotic activation of brainstem neurons in the rat is not antagonized by naloxone and that morphine enhances the excitatory response of these neurons to ACh (1).

A second response to narcotic drugs, a depression of discharge rate without a change in spike amplitude, was also observed only in the reticular formation. The variable responses of these neurons to ACh, NE, and 5-HT suggests that morphine and meperidine had an action independent of the actions of these putative transmitters. On the other hand, the reduction of this response by naloxone suggests that morphine and meperidine may have been causing depression by acting on a specific narcotic "receptor."

A third type of response, consisting of a depression of discharge rate together with a reduction of spike amplitude, was similar to that elicited by the local anesthetic procaine when applied to central neurons (3). This similarity, along with the observation that naloxone failed to alter this response, suggests that the narcotic drugs were interfering in a nonspecific way with spike-generating mechanisms and that a specific narcotic receptor was therefore not involved. This effect of narcotics, and the fact that it is observable at different levels of the central nervous system (see also ref. 2), suggests that this third type of effect may represent some more general action.

Thus the evidence of the present study suggests that the reticular formation contains two types of neurons that are sensitive to narcotic drugs: one type which is depressed by these drugs and is associated with a specific narcotic "receptor," and a second type which is excited by these drugs possibly by activation of mechanisms involving, or common to, some endogenous transmitters. The failure to observe either of these responses in the PAG or Rd, structures that have been implicated previously as possible sites of action of narcotic drugs (6,7), suggests that an involvement of narcotics with these structures may be indirect. Analgesia resulting from microinjection of narcotics into the PAG and Rd might then be accounted for by diffusion to nearby structures. This possibility of leakage to other structures is supported by evidence from studies on the distribution of radioactive narcotics injected into the ventricular system (9). It was concluded from these studies that the principal site of action of narcotics is in structures lying below the floor of the fourth ventricle, in an area corresponding to the region where the two genuine types of responses were observed in the present study.

ACKNOWLEDGMENTS

This project was assisted financially under the program of Research on Drug Abuse, Health and Welfare Canada, and by grants from the Medical Research Council of Canada.

The helpful advice of Dr. K. Krnjević throughout this project is gratefully acknowledged. The author is indebted to Mrs. Kiran Sudarshan for her careful preparation of histological material.

REFERENCES

1. Bramwell, G. J., and Bradley, P. B. (1974): *Brain Res.,* 73:167–170.
2. Calvillo, O., Henry, J. L., and Neuman, R. S. (1974): *Can. J. Physiol. Pharmacol.,* 52: 1207–1211.
3. Curtis, D. R., and Phillis, J. W. (1960): *J. Physiol.,* 153:17–34.
4. Henry, J. L. (1975): *Fed. Proc.,* 34:757.
5. Henry, J. L., and Neuman, R. S. (1974): *Proc. Can. Fed. Biol. Soc.,* 17:158.
6. Jacquet, Y. F., and Lajtha, A. (1973): *Science,* 182:490–492.
7. Mayer, D. J., Wolfle, T. L., Akil, H., Carder, B., and Liebeskind, J. C. (1971): *Science,* 174:1351–1354.
8. Reynolds, D. V. (1969): *Science,* 164:444–445.
9. Teschemacher, H., Schubert, P., and Herz, A. (1973): *Neuropharmacology,* 12:123–131.
10. Tsou, K., and Jang, C. S. (1964): *Scientia Sinica,* 8:1099–1109.

Advances in Pain Research and Therapy, Vol. 1,
edited by J. J. Bonica and D. Albe-Fessard.
Raven Press, New York ©1976.

Interaction of the Medial Thalamus and the Periaqueductal Gray in the Modulation of the Antinociceptive Actions of Morphine

T. L. Yaksh, J. C. Yeung, and T. A. Rudy

School of Pharmacy, University of Wisconsin, Madison, Wisconsin 53706

Both the central gray and the medial thalamus have been implicated by different laboratories in the mediation of the animal's response to aversive stimuli. In light of several experiments we report here, it is our working hypothesis that these two substrates represent a functionally interactive unit mediating the antinociceptive action of morphine.

Although it has been well documented that the periaqueductal gray is indeed sensitive to the direct application of morphine in a variety of species (2–4,8–10,12), we sought in the first series of experiments to establish its uniqueness in this regard. This was prompted because it has been shown that other brain regions including the caudate nucleus, the amygdala, and the medial thalamus also possess a significant capacity for stereospecific narcotic binding (7). The second series of studies was done to examine more closely the role of the medial thalamus.

FIRST SERIES

Methods

To carry out these investigations, we implanted 32 rats with arrays of two or three 24-gauge stainless steel cannulae and made microinjections of 0.5 μl into brainstem and forebrain sites ranging from 8 mm in front of to 3 mm behind the intra-aural line. Morphine was typically administered in doses of 5 μg with higher and lower doses being given in some instances to establish a dose-response relationship.

Sites were considered to be sensitive to morphine if: (a) a significant response was observed within 5 min of the injection of a mapping dose of 5 μg, (b) the effect was not obtained with sham injections, and (c) the effect was reversed by the systemic administration of naloxone (1 mg/kg). To ascertain the effect of the microinjection on reflexes, we systematically examined the withdrawal response to paw pinch and tail flick while its effect on the operant response to strong stimuli was determined by the 55°C hot plate and in some instances by the discrete trials shock titration procedure of Weiss and Laties (14).

Results and Discussion

In Fig. 1, we can see the effects on the hot plate and tail flick responses of a microinjection of morphine into an active site within the ventrolateral aspect of the periaqueductal gray. Within 5 min there was a significant elevation in the response latency of both measures. Moreover, as can be seen represented in the rat simicule, there was a rostrad ipsilateral depression in the rat's responsiveness to forceps pinch (*darkened region*). Although there is not space to discuss this interesting finding, we have observed both symmetrical and unilateral changes in responsiveness after such microinjections (15). Naloxone (1 mg/kg) given intraperitoneally (*second arrow*) completely reversed the elevated thresholds. The animal's response to pinch also returned to the preinjection state (not shown).

Figure 2 shows a series of rat brain sagittal sections ranging from 0 to 2.5 mm off midline in 0.5-mm increments. The open circles indicate sites where the microinjection of 5 μg of morphine produced no change in the analgesic thresholds. The black dots represent those sites where such a microinjection produced a significant elevation in the nociceptive threshold which was abolished by the administration of naloxone.

In this series of 268 sites, it is striking to observe the consistent localization of the distribution of the morphine-sensitive sites along the ventrolateral axis of the periaqueductal and periventricular gray (26 sites). This localization parallels the findings made by Pert and Yaksh in the primate brain (8,9). For the most part, after the microinjection these animals appeared no different from rats that had received an intraperitoneal dose of 20 to 30 mg/kg.

We have also observed the behavioral excitation or hyperreactivity previously reported by a number of laboratories (2,6,10) and more recently studied by Jacquet and Lajtha (3,4). In this response, after the microinjection of morphine the animals exhibit a markedly exaggerated response to auditory clicks and most especially to light touch such as obtained with a puff of air. In contrast, these animals are completely nonresponsive to otherwise aversive levels of stimulation, i.e., gradually applied pinch, heat to the feet or tail, and electric shock. This effect was most frequently observed after the microinjection of as little as 3 μg unilaterally into the caudal regions of the periaqueductal gray. Similar responses were elicited after more rostral injections, but correspondingly higher doses were required. In all cases, the effect could be reversed by the administration of naloxone. We stress that although not all rats displaying an elevated nociceptive threshold were hyperreactive, all hyperreactive animals observed were analgesic to otherwise aversive levels of stimulation.

In contrast to the central gray, other regions that also bind morphine stereospecifically were not shown to alter the animal's responsiveness to aversive stimuli, including the caudate nucleus, the amygdala, and in

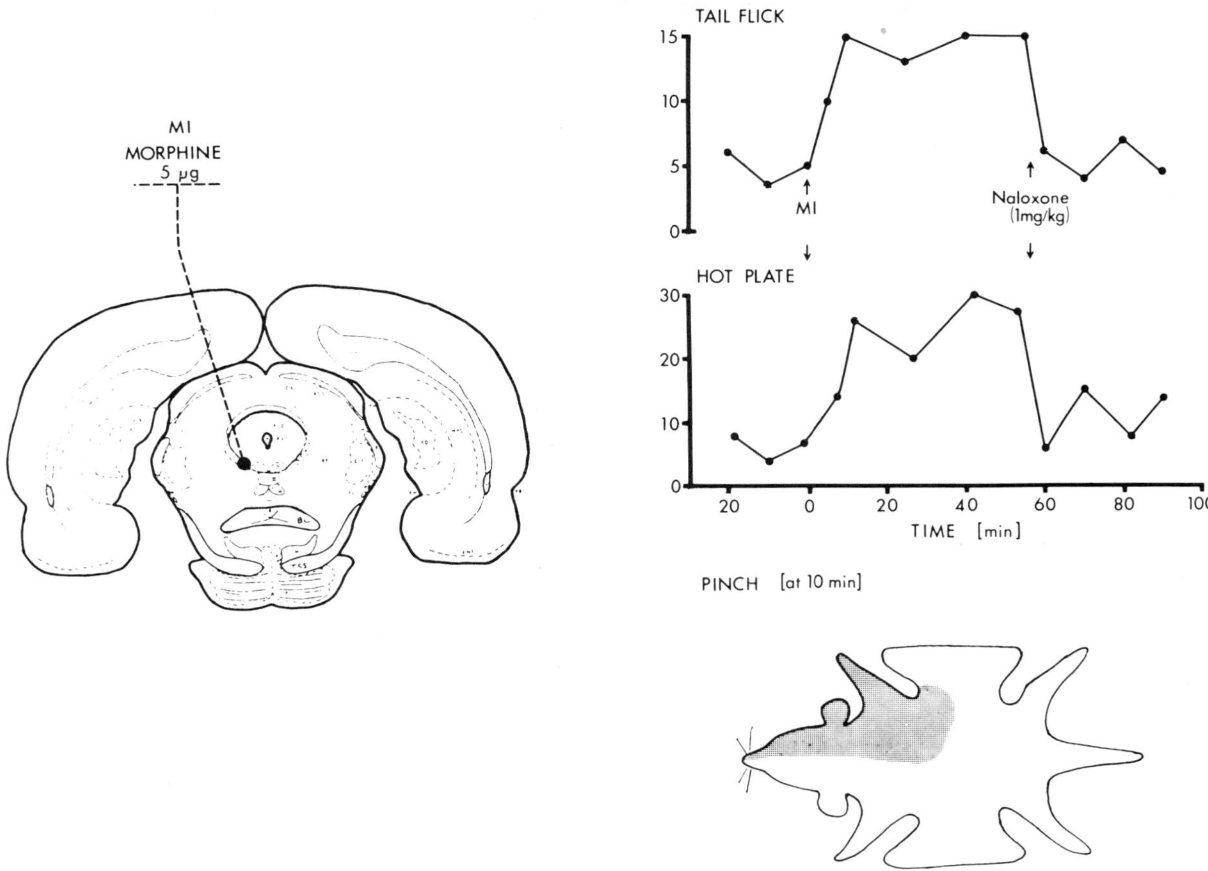

FIG. 1. Microinjection of morphine sulfate (5 μg) into rat brain site indicated by dot in the right ventrolateral quadrant of the periaqueductal gray. Responses of the animal after microinjection (MI) of morphine at the arrow on tail flick (*upper right*), hot plate (*middle right*), and forceps pinch (*lower right*) are shown. Shaded area is body region where forceps pinches did not elicit either squeaking or a withdrawal-biting response. At the second arrow, naloxone (1 mg/kg) was administered intraperitoneally.

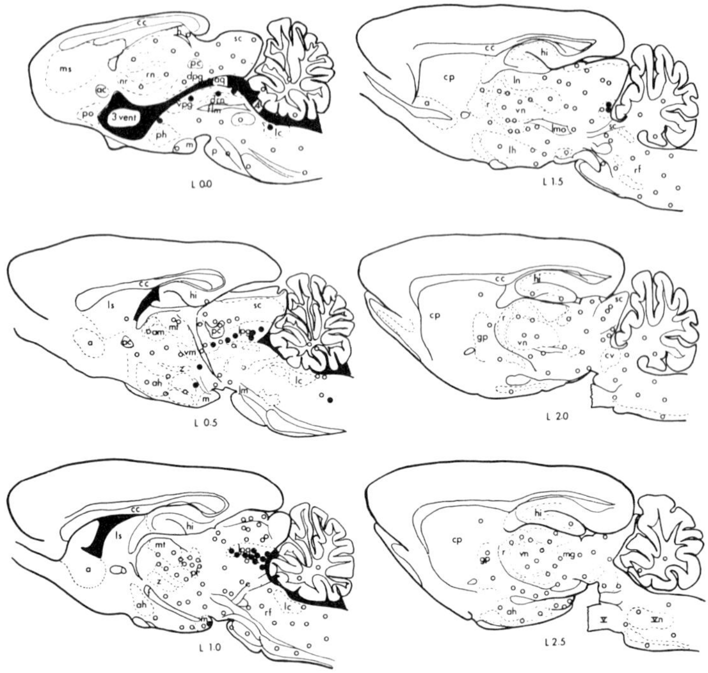

FIG. 2. Sagittal rat brain sections taken in planes 0 to 2.5 mm off midline in 0.5-mm steps. Open circles, sites where morphine microinjection (5 μg in 0.5 μl) did not elicit any change in the analgesic threshold as measured by hot plate and tail flick. Black dots, microinjection sites where similar injections produced an increased threshold. Abbreviations: a, nucleus accombens; ac, ant. commissure; ah, ant. hypothalamus; am, ant. medial nucleus of thalamus; aq, aqueduct; cc, corpus callosum; cp, caudate putamen; cv, caudal nucleus of lat. lemniscus; dpg, dorsal periaqueductal gray; drn, dorsal raphe nucleus; flm, med. longitudinal fasciculus; gp, globus pallidus; h, habenula; hi, hippocampus; lc, locus ceruleus; lh, lat. hypothalamus; lm, med. lemniscus; ln, lat. nuclei of the thalamus; lpg, lat. periaqueductal gray; ls, lat. septum; m, mammillary body; mg, med. geniculate; ms, med. septum; mt, med. thalamic nuclei; nr, nucleus reuniens; pc, posterior commissure; po, preoptic region; r, reticular nucleus of thalamus; rf, reticular formation; sc, superior colliculus; vn, ventral nuclei of thalamus; vpg, ventral periaqueductal gray; z, zona incerta; 3 vent, third ventricle; v, trigeminal nerve; Vn, trigeminal nucleus.

particular the medial thalamus. We were somewhat surprised to observe no behavioral effects in the medial thalamus because work by a number of investigators (11,13) has implicated this region in the development of narcotic tolerance. Similarly, we have observed that microinjections of morphine into this region can produce EEG synchronization in the rat, but of course no analgesia (J. C. Yeung and T. L. Yaksh, *unpublished observations*).

SECOND SERIES

Methods

We initiated a second set of experiments to examine more closely the possible role of the medial thalamus in the altered thresholds produced by morphine. In these experiments, electrolytic lesions were made in the medial thalamus by passing a 1-mA DC anodal current through a 28-gauge stainless steel needle, acutely inserted during pentobarbitol sodium (Nembutal®) anesthesia. The same analgesic measures as described in the previous experiments—shock titration, hot plate, and tail flick tests—were employed. After a 2-week recovery period, dose-response curves were obtained for intraperitoneally administered morphine sulfate over a range of 6 to 20 mg/kg in each of the sham and lesioned animals. Doses were administered 7 to 12 days apart in a counterbalanced fashion.

After the experimental series were completed, the rat was perfused and the brain cut on a freezing microtome at 40 μm. Cells and fibers were stained according to the method of Klüver and Barrera (5).

To determine the degree of relative damage, we drew the lesioned areas from sequential histological sections and the area of damage determined on each of the sequential plates by means of graphic planimetry. These procedures are described in more detail elsewhere (16).

Results and Discussion

From these experiments, we made three principal observations. First, the lesions alone had no detectable effect on the animal's nociceptive threshold as measured by the tail flick, hot plate, or shock titration tasks. Second, lesion size *per se* was not correlated with the animal's responsiveness to morphine. Third, lesions that specifically incorporated more than 40% of the medial thalamus produced a shift to the left in the morphine dose-response curves obtained on each of the three tasks. (In these experiments, we have defined the medial region as being composed primarily of the nucleus medialis dorsalis, the nucleus reuniens, the nucleus paraventricularis, the nucleus parafascicularis, and the habenula.)

For the shock titration and the hot plate tests, these shifts in the dose-response curves to the left were parallel, whereas there was a statistically significant increase in the slope of the dose-response curve for the lesioned group on the tail flick test. Figure 3 presents the ED_{50} for morphine for each of the three groups (greater than 40% lesion; less than 40% lesion and sham operates) on the three tasks (shock titration, hot plate, and tail flick). As can be seen in the group in which greater than 40% of the medial thalamus was destroyed, there is a statistically significant decrease in the amount

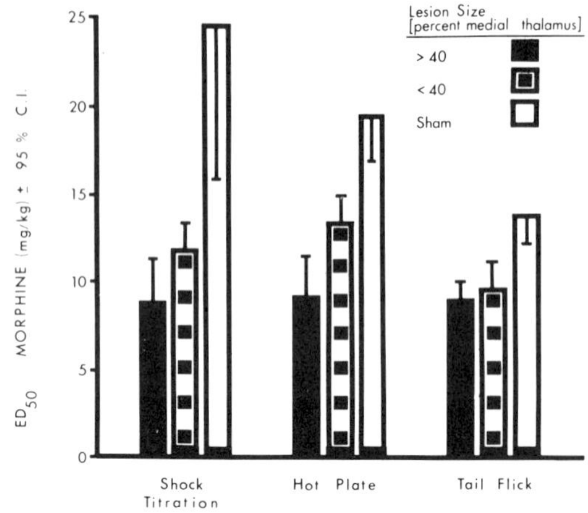

FIG. 3. Summary of mean $ED_{50} \pm 95\%$ confidence intervals (C.I.) of morphine for rats having greater than 40% of medial thalamus destroyed ($N = 8$), those with less than 40% of medial thalamus destroyed ($N = 12$), and sham operates ($N = 6$) on the shock titration, hot plate, and tail flick tests.

of morphine required to produce a given level of antinociception on all tasks. The fact that the animal remained able to perform the relatively complex operant shock titration task, as well as the fact that monotonic dose-response curves could be obtained, indicates that the lesion alone or the lesion in the presence of morphine did not simply block responding in the animal in an all-or-nothing fashion.

We also discount the possibility that the enhanced effect represents a possible opening of the blood-brain barrier by the lesion, thus facilitating the entry of morphine into brain. Lesion size alone had no correlation with the degree of potentiation. Moreover, the effect was not diminished as a function of time after the lesion. As the blood-brain barrier begins to recover its integrity after lesions, one would expect a diminution of the interactive effects as a function of time after lesion. This was not observed. Finally, in preliminary studies we have repeated these experiments by producing reversible lesions with the microinjection of a local anesthetic, dibucaine (10 μg) into this region of the medial thalamus. A similar potentiation of the action of systemic morphine was observed (T. L. Yaksh, J. C. Yeung, and T. A. Rudy, *in preparation*).

GENERAL DISCUSSION

The significance of the observation that morphine, acting only within the periaqueductal gray, can induce profound changes in the animal's response to otherwise aversive stimuli cannot be overestimated. It clearly represents a quantum difference in conceptualization from the hypothesis that narcotic action requires a diffuse effect on central nervous system activity. Although other structures may be sensitive to morphine, as indicated by their ability to bind narcotics, and may participate in some way in modulating an animal's response to different aspects of the environment, no other region can produce such an intense response after the local administration of morphine, which indicates the unique importance of this structure as a sufficient substrate through which narcotics can act to modulate the processing of ascending sensory information.

It is clear from the present experiments, however, that modulation of the animal's response to noxious stimuli can be affected at more than one level. Lesions of the medial thalamus alone had no effect on the analgesic threshold but in fact served to potentiate narcotic analgesia, which strongly suggests that certain structures may interact with the periaqueductal gray to antagonize the analgesic action of morphine. In view of the antinociceptive action of morphine in the periaqueductal gray, its lack of effect when injected into the medial thalamus, and a potentiation of the narcotic analgesia when the medial thalamus is destroyed, the medial thalamus appears to play a role functionally antagonistic to that of the periaqueductal gray. As this mesencephalic region has strong connections with the medial thalamus, it is possible that the periaqueductal gray in the presence of morphine may exert an excitatory influence on the medial thalamus.

Casey and Keene (1) have clearly shown that excitation of certain medial thalamic units is associated with aversive stimuli. Thus such an excitatory influence by morphine might serve paradoxically to antagonize the antinociceptive action of morphine subserved by other mechanisms within the central gray. In this regard we feel that it is significant that some microinjections of morphine into the periaqueductal gray can produce a hyperexcitability to light cutaneous and auditory stimuli which is concurrent with the increased thresholds observed on the several analgesia tasks.

Therefore, even these incomplete data clearly indicate that a portion of the neural substrate mediating the animal's response to aversive stimuli in the presence of a narcotic analgesic may reside in the functional and anatomical relationship that appears to exist between the medial thalamus and the periaqueductal gray.

ACKNOWLEDGMENT

We would like to thank Ms. Ping Huang and Ms. Diane Kietzke for their technical assistance in this work.

REFERENCES

1. Casey, K. L., and Keene, J. J. (1973): *Unit Analysis of the Effects of Motivating Stimuli in the Awake Animal,* pp. 113–129. Charles C Thomas, Publisher, Springfield, Illinois.

2. Herz, A., Albus, K., Metys, J., Schubert, P., and Teschemacher, H. (1970): *Neuropharmacology,* 9:539–551.
3. Jacquet, Y. F., and Lajtha, A. (1973): *Science,* 182:490–492.
4. Jacquet, Y. F., and Lajtha, A. (1974): *Science,* 185:1055–1057.
5. Klüver, H., and Barrera, E. (1953): *J. Neuropathol. Exp. Neurol.,* 12:400–403.
6. Lotti, V. J., Lomax, P., and George, R. (1953): *J. Neuropathol. Exp. Neurol.,* 12:400–403.
7. Pert, C. B., and Snyder, S. H. (1973): *Science,* 179:1011–1014.
8. Pert, A., and Yaksh, T. (1974): *Brain Res.,* 80:135–140.
9. Pert, A., and Yaksh, T. (1975): *Pharmacol. Biochem. Behav.,* 3:133–138.
10. Sharpe, L. G., Garnett, J., and Cicero, T. J. (1974): *Behav. Biol.,* 11:303–313.
11. Teitlebaum, H., Catraväs, G., and McFarland, W. (1974): *Science,* 185:447–451.
12. Tsou, K., and Jang, C. S. (1964): *Scientia Sinica,* 13:1099–1109.
13. Wei, E., Sigel, S., Loh, H. H., and Way, E. L.: *J. Pharmacol. Exp. Ther.,* 195:480–487.
14. Weiss, B., and Laties, V. (1958): *Science,* 128:1575–1576.
15. Yaksh, T. L., Yeung, J. C., and Rudy, T. A. (1976): *Brain Res.* (*In press.*)
16. Yeung, J. C., Yaksh, T. L., and Rudy, T. A. (1975): *Clin. Exp. Pharmacol. Physiol.,* 2:261–268.

Advances in Pain Research and Therapy, Vol. 1,
edited by J. J. Bonica and D. Albe-Fessard.
Raven Press, New York © 1976.

Effects of Morphine and Other Narcotics in the Spinal Cord of the Cat

O. Calvillo, J. L. Henry, and R. S. Neuman

Department of Research in Anaesthesia, McGill University, Montreal, Canada

Relatively little is known about the site of action of narcotics in the central nervous system. Various structures have been suggested: one such structure is the spinal cord. We have reported that morphine applied by microiontophoresis in the spinal cord of the cat depresses the discharge of neurons responding to noxious heat but has little effect on those that respond only to nonnoxious stimuli (3). This depressant effect was abolished by naloxone applied by microiontophoresis and administered intravenously. It was suggested that narcotics may produce analgesia by a direct depressant effect on spinal nociceptive pathways. To test this suggestion, we examined the effects of intravenous morphine on the withdrawal reflex of decerebrated spinalized cats and the effects of morphine, meperidine (Demerol®, pethidine), and fentanyl on functionally identified spinal neurons in chloralosed or decerebrated cats.

METHODS

The spinal cord was transected at T_{12}, and spinal segments L_6 through S_1 were exposed and covered with warm mineral oil. In order to avoid hypoventilation secondary to narcotic administration and to ensure that the single-unit responses to noxious stimuli were not secondary to reflex movements of the limb being stimulated, we paralyzed the animals with pancuronium bromide (Pavulon®, Organon®) or gallamine trethiodide (Flaxedil®, Poulenc®) and ventilated them mechanically. In experiments with nonparalyzed cats the withdrawal reflex elicited by the application of noxious heat was recorded with a force transducer attached to a foot. The threshold temperature for the withdrawal reflex was 45° to 50°C measured with a bead thermistor on the skin.

Single-unit neuronal activity was recorded extracellularly with glass micropipettes filled with a solution of 0.5 M sodium acetate and 2% pontamine blue. Neurons were identified by their responses to cutaneous stimulation of the following types: (a) strong pressure (600 g over an area of 5 mm^2) applied with a calibrated forceps; (b) noxious heat from a projector lamp (the threshold temperature for neuronal responses to noxious heat was similar to that for the withdrawal reflex); and (c) light mechanical stimulation applied with von Frey hairs and small jets of air. Noxious stimuli were defined according to the criteria of Burgess and Perl (2) and of Bessou and Perl (1).

Dorsal horn neurons were classified in three main groups: (a) neurons that respond only to noxious stimuli; (b) those that respond to noxious as well as to innocuous stimuli; and (c) those that respond only to innocuous stimuli. Selected sites where nociceptive neurons (groups 1 and 2) were recorded were marked by releasing pontamine blue iontophoretically from the microelectrode. They were found in the marginal layer of the dorsal horn, lamina 1 of Rexed, and in deeper layers, laminae IV to VI.

RESULTS

Morphine (1.1 to 2 mg/kg) caused a depression of the withdrawal reflex within 2 min of its intravenous administration; this depression was reversed by intravenous naloxone (0.1 to 0.3 mg/kg) within 6 min, causing an initial rebound overshoot of the response, which then returned to control magnitude in 5 to 10 min. Morphine (0.8 to 3 mg/kg), meperidine (10 to 25 mg/kg), and fentanyl (30 to 40 μg/kg) depressed the ongoing firing of nociceptive neurons and also their responses to applications of noxious heat to the plantar surface of the foot (Fig. 1). These depressions were consistently reversed by intravenous naloxone (0.1 to 0.3 mg/kg) within 2 to 6 min.

Because narcotics can have a nonspecific effect on spinal sensory pathways, they were also tested on responses generated by stimulating hair receptors with a jet of air. In the doses mentioned above, these drugs had no effect or a slight depressant effect on these responses (Fig. 2).

Selective blockade of nociceptive but not of nonnociceptive responses of these neurons with multiple inputs suggests that narcotics may have a presynaptic effect. According to unpublished observations (O. Calvillo, 1975), intravenous morphine (1.5 to 6 mg/kg) did not affect the responses evoked by noxious heat and recorded from the medial plantar nerve, suggesting that neither the skin receptors nor the peripheral nerves subserving them were important sites of action of the narcotics.

In further studies of possible presynaptic effects of narcotics, the excitability of primary afferent fibers of cutaneous nerves was tested in the dorsal horn using the technique described by Wall (6). Morphine, meperidine, and fentanyl produced an increase in excitability of A fibers, although the action on C fibers is as yet unknown. This effect was usually but not always reversed by naloxone.

DISCUSSION

Our results support the data reported by Krivoy and Huggins (5), who suggested that narcotics may depolarize the terminal region of primary

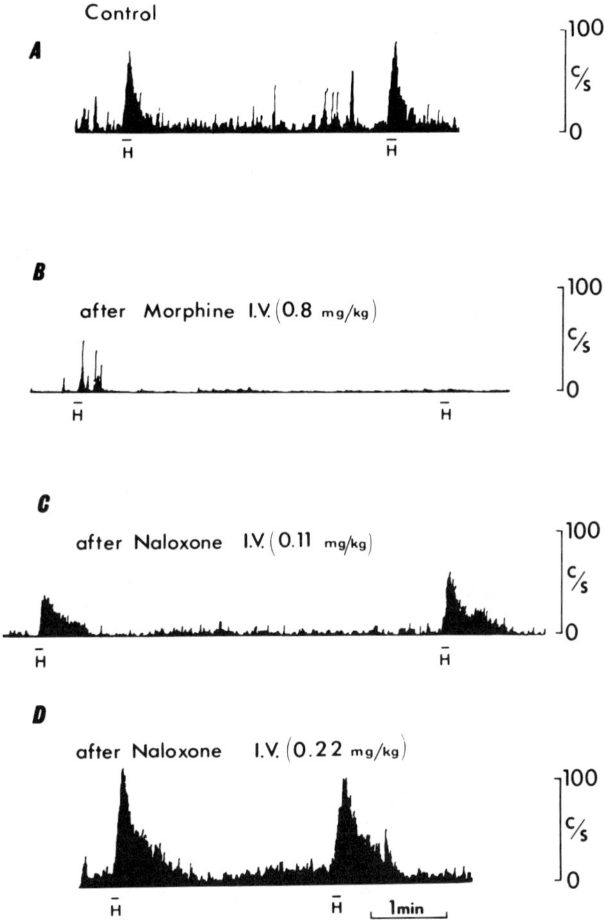

FIG. 1. Effects of i.v. morphine on firing rate, expressed in counts per second (C/S), of a nociceptive neuron in the dorsal horn responding to noxious heat (H; indicated by a short horizontal bar) applied to plantar surface of the hind foot. **A:** Control applications of heat; **C:** 60 min after record **B,** naloxone induces a partial reversal; **D:** complete reversal after a further dose of naloxone.

afferent fibers. Such a presynaptic action may contribute to their analgesic effect. Our results do not rule out the possibility that narcotics may have a postsynaptic effect as well. Reversal of the depressant effects of narcotics by naloxone indicates that they were acting on specific opiate receptors.

According to the suggestion of Herz and Teschemacher (4), narcotics may produce analgesia by activating a descending inhibitory system originating in the brainstem which inhibits transmission of nociceptive information at the spinal level. Since all animals in our study were spinalized, these experiments show that for narcotics to produce analgesia the brainstem need not be involved. Although our results thus suggest that narcotics

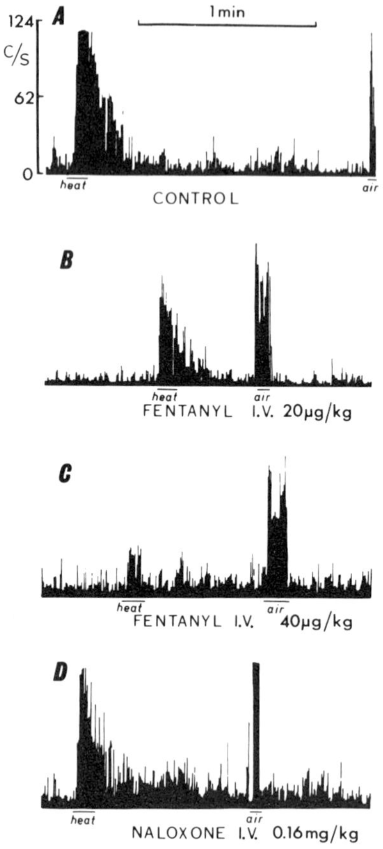

FIG. 2. Effects of i.v. fentanyl on firing rate (in counts per second) of a neuron responding to noxious heat and to a jet of air applied to receptive field on the hind foot. **A:** Control heat and air application. **B:** After fentanyl, note depression of heat response but not of air response. **D:** Reversal of the depressant effect of fentanyl by naloxone.

depress nociceptive transmission in the spinal cord, the possibility that narcotics may have an effect also in the brainstem cannot be eliminated.

ACKNOWLEDGMENT

This work was assisted financially under the program of Research on Drug Abuse, Health and Welfare Canada, and by the Medical Research Council of Canada.

REFERENCES

1. Bessou, P., and Perl, E. R. (1969): *J. Neurophysiol.*, 32:1025–1043.
2. Burgess, P. R., and Perl, E. R. (1967): *J. Physiol.*, 190:541–562.
3. Calvillo, O., Henry, J. L., and Neuman, R. S. (1974): *Can. J. Physiol. Pharmacol.*, 52:1207–1211.

4. Herz, A., and Teschemacher, J. (1971): In: *Advances in Drug Research, Vol. 6: Activities and Sites of Action of Morphine-like Analgesics,* edited by N. J. Harper and A. B. Simmonds. Academic Press, New York.
5. Krivoy, W., and Huggins, R. A. (1961): *J. Pharmacol. Exp. Ther.,* 134:210–213.
6. Wall, P. D. (1958): *J. Physiol.,* 142:1–21.

Advances in Pain Research and Therapy, Vol. 1,
edited by J. J. Bonica and D. Albe-Fessard.
Raven Press, New York © 1976.

Morphine Antagonists and Morphine-Induced Depression of Activity in Cat Ventrolateral Tract Axons

I. Jurna and W. Grossmann

Pharmakologisches Institut der Universität des Saarlandes, 665 Homburg/Saar, Federal Republic of Germany

Morphine antagonists such as levallorphan or naloxone are generally considered to have little or no agonist action. Because of a relatively high affinity for the morphine receptor at cell membranes, they displace the morphine molecule and thus antagonize the effect of morphine.

INTERNEURONAL ACTIVITY

In a previous investigation performed on spinal cats, it was found that morphine 2 mg/kg injected intravenously markedly reduced the number of impulses discharged by interneurons near motoneurons and activated by stimulation of dorsal roots with single pulses (Fig. 1). Levallorphan 0.2 mg/kg did not change the interneuron activity in the absence of morphine (Fig. 1 B). However, in contrast to what might have been expected from a displacement of morphine from its receptor sites, levallorphan not only antagonized the effect of a preceding injection of morphine but also increased the number of impulse discharges above the control level (Fig. 1).

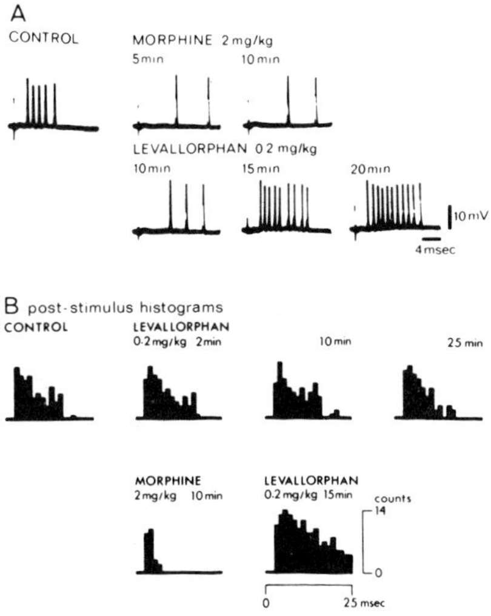

FIG. 1. Effect of morphine and levallorphan on the impulse discharge of 2 interneurons (**A** and **B**) to stimulation of dorsal roots with single pulses in cats spinalized at the lower thoracic level. **A:** Intracellular recording; stimulation of dorsal root L_7 (from ref. 5). **B:** Post-stimulus histograms of impulse discharges; 12 consecutive responses sampled in each recording; stimulation of dorsal root S_1 (I. Jurna and W. Grossmann, *unpublished result*).

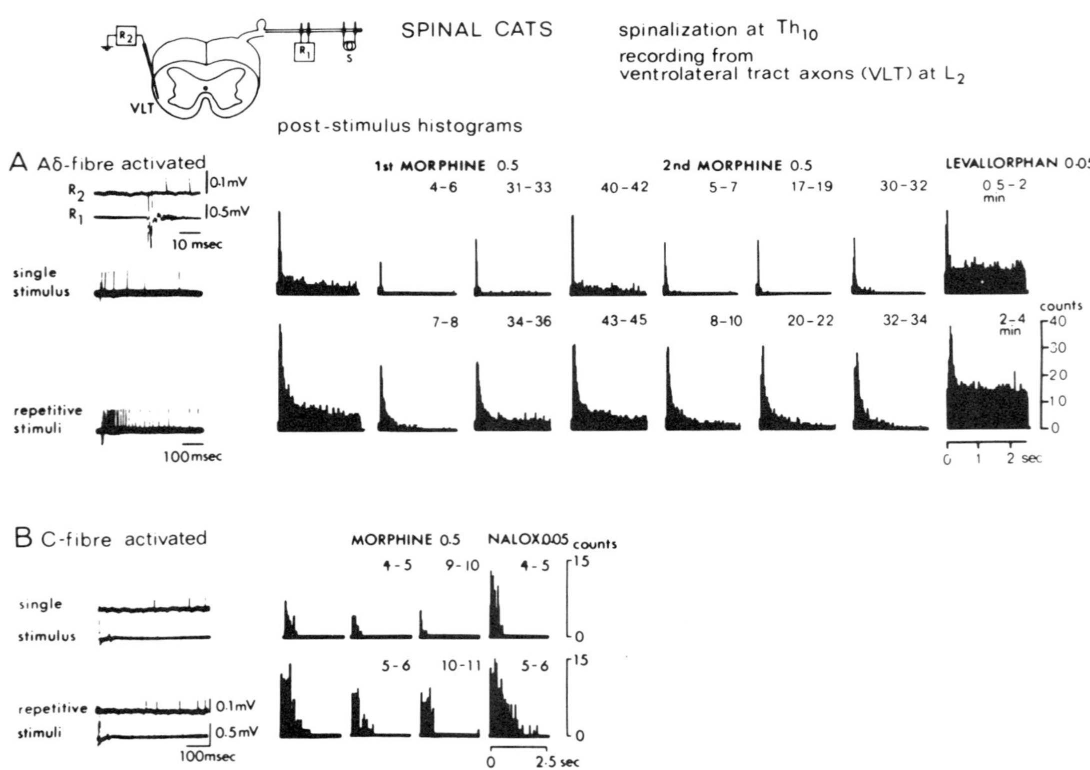

FIG. 2. Effect of morphine and naloxone on the impulse discharges evoked in VLT axons by stimulation of Aδ fibers **(A)** and C fibers **(B)** of the sural nerves in 2 cats spinalized at T_{10}. Recordings were made from the sural nerves stimulated (R_1) and from VLT axon (R_2) at L_2. Inset shows electrode arrangement. Recordings at left in **A** and **B** show impulse discharges of VTL axons (upper tracings, R_1) and compound action potentials of the sural nerve (lower tracings, R_1). Following recordings are poststimulus histograms of 12 consecutive responses each. Stimulation was performed with single pulses (single stimulus; repetition rate 0.25 Hz) or with trains of pulses (repetitive stimuli; stimulation frequency 300 Hz, 10-sec duration of train, repetition rate of train 0.25 Hz). Number at top of each histogram indicates the time after drug injection at which the recording was made.(**A,** from ref. 6.)

This result is in accord with the observation that morphine antagonists administered shortly after morphine may exert an excitatory effect on polysynaptic reflexes in chronic spinal dogs (6,4).

VENTROLATERAL TRACT AXONS

Methods and Results

Ventrolateral tract (VLT) axons in the cat spinal cord were found by Pomeranz (5) to be activated by noxious stimuli applied to the skin as well as by electrical stimulation of skin nerves.

Spinal Cats

In spinal cats, the activity evoked by electrical stimulation of Aδ and C fibers of the sural nerves with single pulses and trains of pulses was depressed by an intravenous injection of morphine in a dose as low as 0.5 mg/kg (Fig. 2). Naloxone 0.05 mg/kg reversed the depressant effect of morphine: the activity in the VLT axons was higher after morphine and naloxone than before morphine (Fig. 2). When given without morphine,

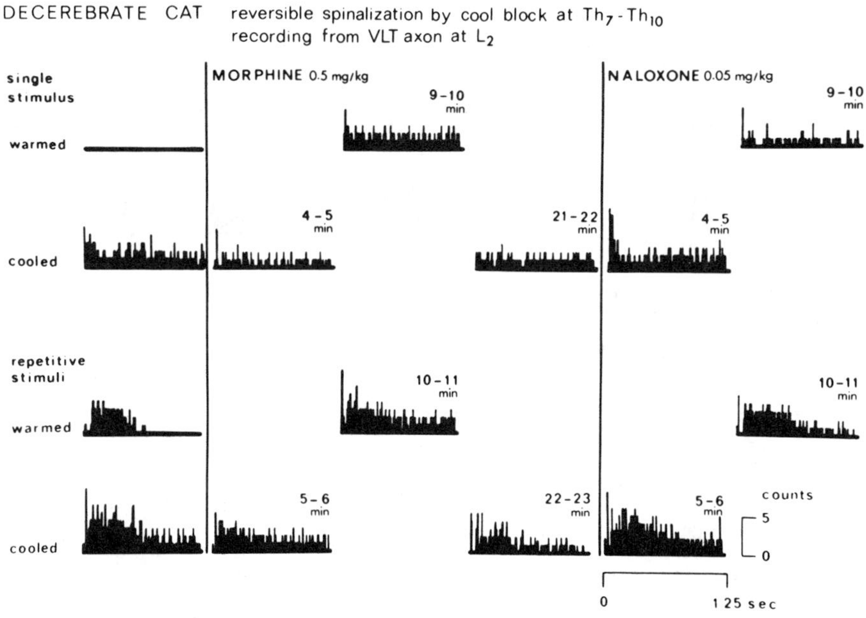

FIG. 3. Effect of morphine and naloxone on impulse discharges evoked in a VLT axon in an intercollicularly decerebrate cat without (warmed) and during (cooled) reversible spinalization. Activity in the VLT axon was evoked by ipsilateral stimulation of sural nerve with single pulses (single stimulus; top 2 rows of recordings) and with trains of pulses (repetitive stimuli; bottom 2 rows of recordings) and recorded at L_2. Each poststimulus histogram is the result of 12 consecutive responses.

the antagonist did not change the activity in the axons. Similar observations have been made by Le Bars et al. (3) when studying the effect of morphine on the activity of lamina V neurons in the cat spinal cord.

Decerebrate Cats

In intercollicularly decerebrate cats, reversible spinalization was produced by applying cool block to the spinal cord above the site of recording

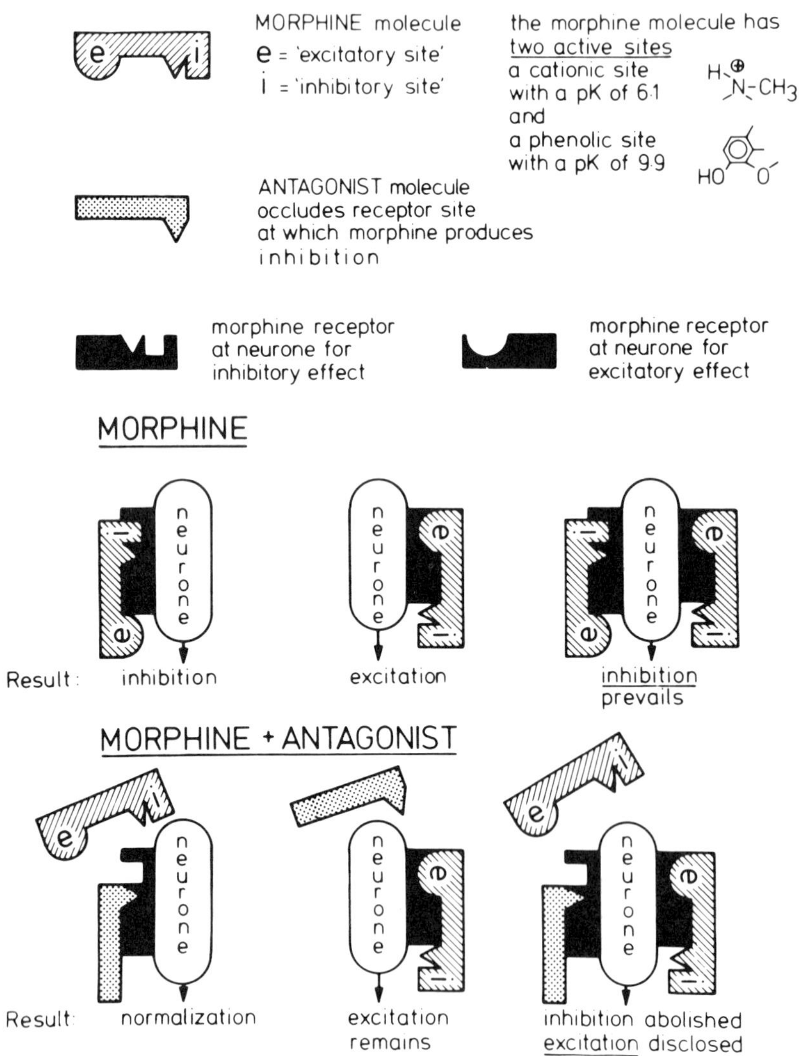

FIG. 4. Interaction between molecules of morphine and morphine antagonists at neuronal receptors and the effects resulting from it.

the activity from VLT axons. This resulted mostly in an increased impulse discharge to Aδ- or C-fiber stimulation (Fig. 3), probably because of disinhibition of impulse transmission to the VLT axons. Morphine 0.5 mg/kg depressed the activity in VLT axons during cool block, whereas in the preparation with an unimpaired descending impulse conduction, the activity in VLT axons could be enhanced even after morphine (Fig. 3). Naloxone 0.05 mg/kg reversed the depressant effect of morphine during cool block and diminished the "excitatory" effect of morphine in the nonspinal preparation (Fig. 3).

CONCLUSIONS

In spinal cats, morphine inhibited the activity of: (a) interneurons which, in all probability, are involved in flexor reflexes including nociceptive reflexes, and (b) VLT axons activated by Aδ- and C-fiber stimulation. The depressant effect is reversed by morphine antagonists. In addition to the depression exerted at the spinal level, morphine reduced the descending inhibition of the impulse transmission from Aδ and C fibers to VLT axons in intercollicularly decerebrate cats. Naloxone restored the descending inhibition. It is proposed that morphine acts on two types of receptors at the neuronal membrane (Fig. 4), one mediating inhibition of neuronal activity and the other mediating excitation. When both receptor types are present on one neuron, inhibition prevails. Morphine antagonists, by occluding the "inhibitory" receptor only, unmask the excitatory effect of morphine.

ACKNOWLEDGMENTS

This investigation was supported by the Sonderforschungsbereich 38 "Membranen" and the Stiftung Volkswagenwerk.

REFERENCES

1. Grossmann, W., and Jurna, I. (1974): *Eur. J. Pharmacol.,* 29:171–174.
2. Jurna, I., Grossmann, W., and Theres, C. (1973): *Neuropharmacology,* 12:983–993.
3. Le Bars, B., Ménétrey, D., Conseiller, C., and Besson, J. M. (1974): *J. Pharmacol.* (Paris), 5 (Suppl. 2):58.
4. Martin, W. R., and Eades, C. G. (1964): *J. Pharmacol. Exp. Ther.,* 146:385–394.
5. Pomeranz, B. (1973): *Brain Res.,* 50:447–451.
6. Wikler, A., and Carter, R. L. (1953): *J. Pharmacol. Exp. Ther.,* 109:92–104.

Advances in Pain Research and Therapy, Vol. 1,
edited by J. J. Bonica and D. Albe-Fessard.
Raven Press, New York © 1976.

Possible Physiological Significance of Enkephalin, an Endogenous Ligand of Opiate Receptors

Hans W. Kosterlitz and John Hughes

Unit for Research on Addictive Drugs, University of Aberdeen, Marischal College, Aberdeen, AB9 1AS, Scotland

The evidence for the presence of one or more endogenous ligands of the opiate receptors is now so convincing (2–5,10–15) that it will be useful to consider their possible physiological significance and the consequences of their interaction with exogenously administered narcotic analgesics. One of these ligands, enkephalin, has been isolated from the brain of several species in our laboratories (3,4) and obtained in sufficiently pure condition from pig brain to make possible an investigation of its structure. Results obtained so far indicate that we are dealing with a heptapeptide consisting of one tyrosine, one phenylalanine, one methionine, one unidentified, and three glycine amino acids (5 and J. Hughes and T. Smith, *unpublished observations*). Recently evidence has been accumulated indicating the presence of a second enkephalin-like compound (J. Hughes and T. Smith, *unpublished observations*). It differs from enkephalin 1 in several chromatographic systems.

SOME PHARMACOLOGICAL PROPERTIES OF ENKEPHALIN

Enkephalin has a rapid onset and offset of action in inhibiting morphine-sensitive transmission in the mouse vas deferens which has been used for the monitoring of the progress of purification of the brain extracts (5). Its onset of action is at least as fast as that of normorphine, which in this preparation is the most rapidly acting of all available narcotic analgesics. The rate of recovery from the action of enkephalin is considerably higher than that from normorphine, probably because of its rapid enzymatic degradation (4,8). There is no evidence of tachyphylaxis after repeated applications. These properties of enkephalin fullfil one of the essential conditions if a compound is to be considered as a neurotransmitter or neuromodulator.

Extensive pharmacological or neurophysiological investigations have so far been impossible in view of the availability of only small amounts of pure enkephalin which have been used for structural examination. Once the structure has been established, it is hoped that sufficient quantities of the synthetic material can be prepared.

An observation that was at first difficult to understand was that higher concentrations of naloxone ($K = 13$ nM) are required to antagonize the depressant action of enkephalin on the vas deferens than are needed to antagonize normorphine ($K = 2$ to 3 nM) (5). This finding acquired additional significance when it was shown that in the guinea pig ileum and mouse vas deferens similarly high concentrations of naloxone ($K = 9$ to 11 nM) are required to antagonize the agonist effects of certain benzomorphans, which are distinguished by high antinociceptive activity without substituting for morphine in the morphine-dependent monkey (6). These observations suggest that these benzomorphans and enkephalin may interact with an opiate receptor different from that with which morphine and other narcotic analgesics of high physical dependence activity interact.

Evidence that enkephalin may act as an inhibitor of certain neuronal mechanisms has been obtained in several ways. For instance, it has been shown (16) that release of acetylcholine evoked by electrical stimulation of the myenteric plexus of the guinea pig ileum is enhanced by the narcotic antagonist naloxone (Fig. 1). Moreover, this effect is stereospecific since only the (−)– isomer (GPA 1843) and not the (+)– isomer (GPA 1847), of another antagonist, β-5-phenyl-9-methyl-2-allyl-2′-hydroxy-6,7-benzomorphan, increases electrically evoked acetylcholine output. This finding suggests that the antagonists prevent the effect of enkephalin which is present in the guinea pig ileum in a concentration of approximately 0.8 μg equivalents of normorphine per gram of tissue (5). This concept that enkephalin or similar ligands control inhibitory influences is supported by the observations that naloxone increases the nociceptive responses of rats and mice to thermal stimuli (7) and inhibits the antinociceptive effect of electrical stimulation of the periaqueductal gray of the brainstem of rats (1).

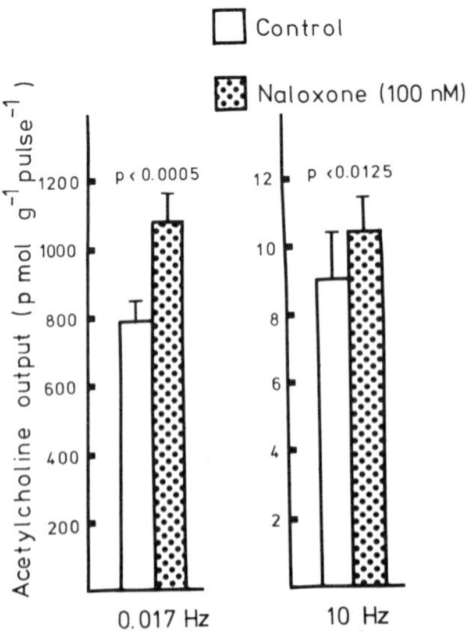

FIG. 1. Mean acetylcholine output from the myenteric plexus–longitudinal muscle preparation of the guinea pig ileum in the absence and presence of naloxone (100 nM). Stimulation (0.5 ms, supramaximal voltage) at 0.017 Hz ($N = 22$) or 10 Hz ($N = 7$). Output is given without subtraction of spontaneous output which is suppressed during stimulation. Increase was 277 ± 34 pmole g^{-1} pulse^{-1} ($p < 0.0005$) at 0.017 Hz and 1.55 ± 0.51 pmole g^{-1} pulse^{-1} ($p < 0.0125$) at 10 Hz. (Reproduced, with permission, from ref. 16.)

POSSIBLE ROLE OF ENKEPHALIN IN OPIATE TOLERANCE AND DEPENDENCE

If endogenous enkephalin has effects that are similar to those of exogenously applied opiates, then the possibility has to be considered that the somatic and autonomic hyperactivity observed after withdrawal of opiates from dependent animals may be due to an inactivation of the inhibitory mechanisms normally controlled by enkephalin. The interaction between endogenous enkephalin and exogenous opiates may be therefore of importance for the interpretation of tolerance and dependence associated with the chronic intake of opiates (8).

If opiates are administered with the intention of increasing the effects of the inhibitory mechanisms controlled by enkephalin, e.g., to produce analgesia, this control will eventually pass from endogenous enkephalin to the exogenous opiates. Since tachyphylaxis is an outstanding pharmacological characteristic of all opiates, a state of tolerance will arise in which increasing amount of opiate will be required to maintain the inhibitory mechanisms at a level of activity sufficient to prevent signs of withdrawal. This situation may be made more severe by a possible negative feedback from the constantly stimulated opiate receptors, resulting in a decreased rate of enkephalin synthesis. Thus the central nervous system will be wholly dependent on the concentration of exogenously supplied opiates for the maintenance of essential inhibitory mechanisms.

When the opiates are withdrawn suddenly, these inhibitory mechanisms will become inactive because any enkephalin that may be available will be unable to stimulate the opiate receptors until they have regained their sensitivity. It may be assumed that the loss of the inhibitory mechanisms normally controlled by enkephalin accounts for many, but not necessarily all, of the symptoms of the withdrawal syndrome. The duration of this syndrome depends on the rate at which the opiate receptors regain their sensitivity and on the restoration of normal enkephalin synthesis if this had been suppressed by a feedback mechanism.

The acuteness of the withdrawal syndrome caused by the administration of naloxone or other antagonists to dependent animals could be readily explained by the proposed hypothesis. The block of the opiate receptors by the antagonists also inactivates any action by enkephalin on these receptors and thus causes an even more severe inactivation of the inhibitory mechanisms than withdrawal of exogenous opiates.

An observation which at first sight does not seem to correlate well with this hypothesis is the relatively small effect caused by the injection of even large doses of naloxone in animals not dependent on opiates. Experiments have to be specially designed for the demonstration of such effects, which are much less dramatic than those observed in dependent animals. Evidence of a blocking effect by naloxone of the normal controlling action of enkephalin or similar ligands has already been mentioned—namely, increase in the nociceptive responses of rodents to thermal stimuli (7), inhibition of the antinociceptive effects of electrical stimulation of the periaqueductal gray of the brainstem (1), and increase in electrically evoked acetylcholine release from the myenteric plexus of the guinea pig ileum (16).

POSSIBLE MORPHOLOGICAL BASIS OF THE EFFECTS CAUSED BY ENKEPHALIN

In principle, there are three possibilities of control of an inhibitory mechanism by enkephalin (Fig. 2). The inhibition could be postsynaptic, presynaptic, or due to a modulatory effect on the nerve terminal in which both enkephalin and the compound responsible for interneuronal transmission are present. In the first two circumstances two neurons would be involved, whereas in the third circumstance enkephalin would be released from the nerve terminal on which it acts by inhibiting the release of the neurotransmitter.

On present evidence, it is difficult to distinguish between the three possibilities since no decisive electrophysiological evidence is available as far as the central nervous system is concerned. In the peripheral nervous system, the action of opiates can occur in the absence of ganglion cells, as, for instance, in the isolated nictitating membrane of the cat (8). In the myenteric plexus of the guinea pig ileum, intracellular recording has shown that morphine does not alter the membrane potential of ganglion cells and does not affect intraneuronal transmission (9). These observations make it unlikely that postsynaptic inhibition is the basis of the action of opiates, although findings obtained in the peripheral nervous system may not necessarily hold for the central nervous system. The most likely options may therefore be the two other models shown in Fig. 2, namely, presynaptic inhibition or inhibitory modulation.

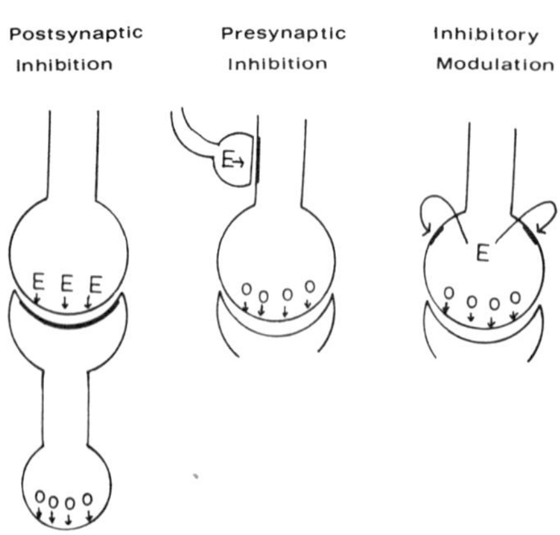

FIG. 2. Possible morphological basis for mechanism of action of enkephalin. (Reproduced, with permission, from ref. 8.)

ACKNOWLEDGMENTS

The experimental work on which this paper is based was supported by grants from the National Institute on Drug Abuse (DA 00662), the U.K. Medical Research Council, and the U.S. Committee on Problems of Drug Dependence, NRC-NAS.

REFERENCES

1. Akil, H., Mayer, D. J., and Liebeskind, J. C. (1972): *C.R. Acad. Sci.* [*D*] (*Paris*), 274: 3603–3605.
2. Cox, B. M., Opheim, K. E., Teschemacher, H., and Goldstein, A. (1975): *Life Sci.*, 16:1777–1782.
3. Hughes, J. (1975*a*): *Neurosci. Res. Program Bull.*, 13:55–58.
4. Hughes, J. (1975*b*): *Brain Res.*, 88:295–308.
5. Hughes, J., Smith, T., Morgan, B., and Fothergill, L. (1975): *Life Sci.*, 16:1753–1758.
6. Hutchinson, M., Kosterlitz, H. W., Leslie, F. M., Terenius, L., and Waterfield, A. A. (1976): *Br. J. Pharmacol.* (*in press*).
7. Jacob, J. J., Tremblay, E. C., and Colombel, M.-C. (1974): *Psychopharmacologia*, 37:217–223.
8. Kosterlitz, H. W., and Hughes, J. (1975): *Life Sci.*, 17:91–96.
9. North, R. A., and Henderson, G. (1976): *Life Sci.* (*in press*).
10. Pasternak, G. W., Goodman, R., and Snyder, S. H. (1975): *Life Sci.*, 16:1765–1769.
11. Terenius, L. (1975): *Neurosci. Res. Program Bull.*, 13:39–42.
12. Terenius, L., and Wahlström, A. (1974): *Acta Pharmacol. Toxicol.* [Suppl.] (*Kbh.*), 35 (I):55.
13. Terenius, L., and Wahlström, A. (1975*a*): *Acta Physiol. Scand.*, 94:74–81.
14. Terenius, L., and Wahlström, A. (1975*b*): *Life Sci.*, 16:1759–1764.
15. Teschemacher, H., Opheim, K. E., Cox, B. M., and Goldstein, A. (1975): *Life Sci.*, 16:1771–1776.
16. Waterfield, A. A., and Kosterlitz, H. W. (1975): *Life Sci.*, 16:1787–1792.

Advances in Pain Research and Therapy, Vol. 1,
edited by J. J. Bonica and D. Albe-Fessard.
Raven Press, New York © 1976.

Clinical Assessment of Narcotic Agonist-Antagonist Analgesics

R. W. Houde, S. L. Wallenstein, and A. Rogers

Sloan-Kettering Institute for Cancer Research, New York, New York 10021

From time immemorial, drugs have, in some form or another, been employed by man to modify pain and suffering. In more recent times, however, we have come to appreciate more fully the influence of a wide variety of physical and psychological factors that can alter perception of and reaction to pain and thus confound the assessment of any of our efforts to relieve pain. The issues are particularly complex when considering systemically acting drugs whose effects are greatly modified not only by interactions with other drugs but also by their own repeated administration, as is the case with our most effective analgesics, the narcotics.

The search for new potent analgesics lacking the tolerance- and physical dependence–producing properties of morphine and its surrogates led, almost three decades ago, to the rediscovery of the narcotic antagonist properties of certain *N*-substituted opiates (1,7) and, shortly thereafter, to the serendipitous discovery that some of these drugs were also in themselves potent analgesics (4). Although some measure of success has been attained in developing potent, nonaddictive analgesics, new problems of considerable practical and theoretical import have also come to light in the course of assaying this class of drugs.

Clinical investigation has played a vital role in directing attention to the narcotic agonist-antagonist, for not until nalorphine was evaluated in well-controlled studies in patients with pain were its analgesic properties even suspected. Indeed, the initial clinical trials were concerned merely with devising ways of combining nalorphine with morphine so as to prevent morphine's undesired side effects without interfering with its analgesic actions. Some early clinical reports suggested that this had been achieved, but our studies of nalorphine-morphine interaction led us to different conclusions (2).

In patients with chronic pain due to cancer, a biphasic dose-effect curve was obtained when increasing doses of nalorphine were administered with fixed doses of morphine. We interpreted this as showing progressive antagonism of the analgesic effects of morphine by nalorphine, followed by the emergence of an analgesic action of nalorphine itself. On the other hand, increasing the dose of nalorphine in the combination appeared only to increase the frequency and severity of adverse side effects, particularly of the psychotomimetic type. Because of these untoward effects, nalorphine never achieved any popularity as an analgesic itself, but it raised hope that other narcotic agonist-antagonist analgesics might be developed which would be free, or relatively free, of the capacity to produce undesired psychotomimetic effects.

Pentazocine, a benzomorphan analogue of nalorphine (Fig. 1), has thus far been the only one of the many agonist-antagonists developed which has been introduced into practice as an analgesic in the United States. Although this drug does not produce dependence of the morphine type, it is now well known that it is not devoid of abuse liability or of the potential for producing psychotomimetic effects. In our studies in cancer patients with chronic pain, we have found it to be only about one-sixth as potent as morphine in terms of its total analgesic effect and to have a relatively short duration of action. Compared to its agonist potency, pentazocine had been reported to be a weak antagonist, but we found that it would precipitate abstinence in patients who had been receiving large doses of narcotics.

On investigating the effects of the concomitant administration of pentazocine and morphine, we found that the results were strikingly influenced by the patients' prior narcotic experiences. In patients judged to be nontolerant, the effects of pentazocine and morphine were simply additive and narcotic-like, whereas in tolerant (and presumably physically dependent) patients, pentazocine progressively interfered with the analgesic action of

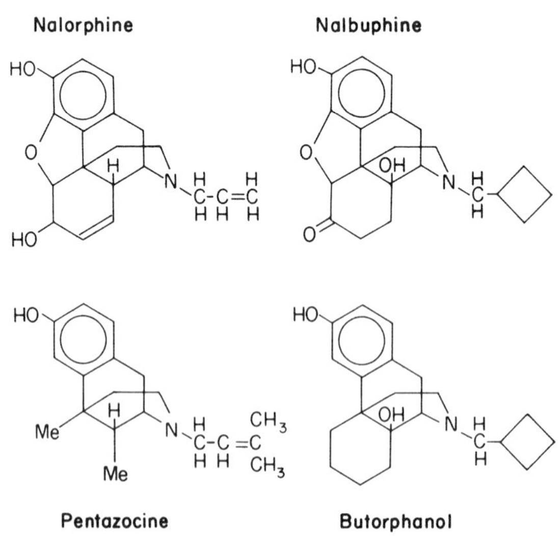

FIG. 1. Structural formulae of nalorphine (N-allyl-normorphine) and representatives of the benzomorphan (pentazocine), oxymorphone (butorphanol) series of narcotic agonist-antagonists.

morphine. The doses of pentazocine in this study ranged from 20 to 80 mg in the nontolerant patients and from 10 to 40 mg in the tolerant patients, administered either alone or with an 8-mg dose of morphine sulfate. Dose-related dysphoric and psychotomimetic effects were observed in both groups of patients, although in the tolerant patients concomitant signs of narcotic withdrawal were also observed. These results appear to support the "receptor dualism" hypothesis of Martin(5) and to suggest that narcotic tolerance is associated with some lessening of the affinity of morphine for its receptor relative to pentazocine. Of some interest, too, was that tolerance to narcotics did not appear to convey cross-tolerance to the psychotomimetic effects of pentazocine.

Most recently, we have been involved in the study of two new investigational drugs which, although more potent antagonists than pentazocine, were felt to be less likely to produce psychotomimetic reactions. Nalbuphine is an *N*-cyclobutylmethyl derivative of naloxone and butorphanol, an analogous morphinan (Fig. 1). The studies of these two drugs consisted of double-blind, twin-crossover relative analgesic potency assays in cancer patients with either postoperative or chronic pain. The drugs, however, were not compared to one another nor to a common standard drug.

NALBUPHINE STUDY

Methods

Nalbuphine had been reported to be equal to or slightly greater than morphine in analgesic potency (W. H. Forrest, *personal communication*) and about one-quarter as potent as nalorphine as an antagonist (3). The assay was originally designed as a series of sequentially related experiments comparing intramuscular doses of nalbuphine ranging from 2.5 to 20 mg with doses of pentazocine of 30 to 60 mg. As this progressed, it became apparent that a surprisingly large proportion of the patients were developing psychotomimetic reactions, so that the doses of both study drugs were halved and the subsequent range of doses was 1.25 to 10 mg of nalbuphine and 15 to 30 mg of pentazocine.

RESULTS

The results of the study to date indicate that nalbuphine is about four times as potent as pentazocine but that at equianalgesic doses, pentazocine has a higher peak effect and shorter duration of action. Both drugs produced similar dose-related morphine-like effects in patients with either postoperative or chronic pain, but distressing dysphoric reactions occurred with much greater frequency and severity with pentazocine than with nalbuphine in equianalgesic doses. Visual hallucinations and distortions of body image and personality were observed in 7 of 27 patients after pentazocine 60 mg and in 1 of 74 patients after nalbuphine 20 mg and in 2 of 42 patients after the 10-mg dose. Nalbuphine would thus appear to have a more favorable therapeutic ratio than pentazocine, even though it is a more potent antagonist.

BUTORPHANOL STUDY

Methods

Butorphanol had been previously reported to be approximately 10 times as potent as morphine as an analgesic and to have narcotic antagonist activity approximately equal to that of nalorphine. In our studies, which were similar in design to that of the nalbuphine-pentazocine assay mentioned above, intramuscular doses ranging from 0.5 to 4 mg of butorphanol were compared with 8- and 16-mg doses of morphine sulfate. As in the previously mentioned study, transient but disturbing psychotomimetic effects were observed in the course of this assay, and it was necessary to eliminate the 4-mg dose of butorphanol part way through the study.

Results

Analysis of the data in 114 patients who have complete crossover comparisons to date indicate that the time-effect curves are quite similar and that butorphanol in this study is approximately four times as potent as morphine sulfate. The undesired side effects after butorphanol included dose-related effects similar to those of morphine but also included dysphoric and psychotomimetic reactions similar to those observed with pentazocine and nalbuphine. These were observed in 6 of 18 patients after the 4-mg dose of butorphanol and in 6 of 33 patients after the 2-mg dose. Although all but a few of these were patients with postoperative pain, many had been receiving analgesics for pain before surgery, and there were significant differences in this respect between these patients and those participating in the nalbuphine-pentazocine assay. Consequently, direct comparison of the adverse effect potentials of nalbuphine and butorphanol from these studies is scientifically indefensible and could be misleading.

DISCUSSION

This report has been an attempt to show some of the complexities of evaluating the agonist-antagonist analgesics in the clinical setting. The interactions of nalorphine and pentazocine with the prototype narcotic, morphine, would seem to indicate that there is no simple way of expressing relative agonist-antagonist potency of these drugs in analgesic terms, for diametrically opposite results were obtained under different experimental conditions. We observed, for example, that combining graded doses of nalorphine with morphine produced a biphasic analgesic dose-effect curve in nontolerant patients, whereas similar experiments with pentazocine and morphine seemed to produce only additive narcotic effects. On the other hand, when the same experiment was carried out in narcotic-tolerant and physically dependent patients, only antagonistic effects were noted. Although some of the newer generation agonist-antagonists appear to come closer than pentazocine to the realization of the potent nonaddictive analgesic objective, neither nalbuphine nor butorphanol was found to be devoid of the potential for producing distressing dysphoric and psychotomimetic reactions so characteristic of this class of drugs. Tolerance to these effects has been observed to develop during repeated administration of those agonist-antagonists, but in our studies tolerance to narcotics did not seem to impart cross-tolerance to these adverse effects. These data are felt to support the concept of "receptor dualism" proposed by Martin (6) and to indicate further that narcotic tolerance is associated with a conformational change in the narcotic receptor.

ACKNOWLEDGMENTS

This work was supported by grants from the National Research Council—National Academy of Sciences Committee on Problems of Drug Dependence, U.S. Public Health Service Grant #CA 08748-09 from the National Cancer Institute, and Grant #DA4P016 from the National Institute of Drug Abuse.

REFERENCES

1. Eddy, N. B., and May, E. (1973): In: *Advances in Biochemical Psychopharmacology, Vol. 8: Narcotic Antagonists,* edited by M. C. Braude, L. S. Harris, E. L. May, and J. E. Villarreal. Raven Press, New York.
2. Houde, R. W., and Wallenstein, S. L. (1956): *Fed. Proc.,* 15:1434.
3. Jasinsky, D. R., and Mansky, P. A. (1972): *Clin. Pharmacol. Ther.,* 13:78–90.
4. Lasagna, L., and Beecher, H. K. (1954): *J. Pharmacol. Exp. Ther.,* 112:356–363.
5. Martin, W. R. (1967): *Pharmacol. Rev.,* 19:463–521.
6. Martin, W. R., Gorodetzky, C. W., and Thompson, W. O. (1973): In: *Agonist and Antagonist Actions of Narcotic Analgesic Drugs,* edited by H. W. Kosterlitz, H. O. J. Collier, and J. E. Villarreal. University Park Press, Baltimore.
7. Unna, K. (1943): *J. Pharmacol. Exp. Ther.,* 79:27–31.

Advances in Pain Research and Therapy, Vol. 1,
edited by J. J. Bonica and D. Albe-Fessard.
Raven Press, New York © 1976.

Long-Term Use of Diamorphine in Advanced Cancer

Robert G. Twycross and Shari J. Wald

Department of Clinical Studies, St. Christopher's Hospice, 51–53 Lawrie Park Road, London, SE26 6DZ England

Very little information is available concerning the long-term effects of narcotic analgesics when administered regularly to relieve persistent pain. This has resulted in predictions being made on the basis of animal and human volunteer studies. For example, in a review article on narcotic analgesics (4), comments about tolerance in patients were supported by references, on the one hand, to a short-term infusion study in pain-free dogs (5) and, on the other, to ex-addicts (3). However, in the studies using ex-addicts at the Addiction Research Center in Lexington, the emphasis has been on inducing tolerance and physical dependency as rapidly as possible by using maximum tolerated doses rather than administering the drugs in doses and at intervals comparable to a clinical regimen (2). Although such studies have been useful in predicting abuse liability, their relevance to clinical practice is questionable. The present study was undertaken to determine diamorphine (heroin) requirements when administered for extended periods of time to patients with advanced cancer.

METHODS

About 500 patients with malignant disease are admitted annually to St. Christopher's Hospice, and more than 80% of these receive diamorphine. The initial dose is increased until the patient is free of pain throughout the 4 hr between drug rounds. The aim is to titrate the level of analgesia against the patient's pain and to maintain continuous relief by giving the next dose before the effect of the previous one has fully worn off. With the aid of a night sedative, many patients do not require a 2 A.M. dose. A phenothiazine is usually administered concurrently, commonly prochlorperazine. Other drugs are prescribed when indicated clinically.

For this study patients who had received diamorphine regularly for at least 12 weeks were selected from approximately 3,000 patients with cancer admitted between July 1967 and June 1974. A total of 115 patients fitted this criterion, had a mean age of 61 years, and were divided into five groups according to survival after prescription of diamorphine (Table 1). Diamorphine was administered by mouth in an elixir containing a fixed 10-mg dose

TABLE 1. *Patients grouped according to survival*

Group	1	2	3	4	5	Total
Survival (weeks)	12–13	14–17	18–25	26–41	42+	12+
Female	13	16	17	13	14	73
Male	10	6	15	6	5	42
Total	23	22	32	19	19	115

of cocaine hydrochloride (1) or by injection using ampules of freeze-dried diamorphine hydrochloride. Starting doses ranged from 2.5 mg by mouth to 40 mg by injection every 4 hr and were similar in all five groups. About two-thirds of the patients were initially prescribed 2.5 mg or 5 mg of diamorphine hydrochloride every 4 hr. A starting dose in excess of 10 mg 4-hourly was confined almost exclusively to those patients who had previously been receiving morphine or diamorphine.

Dose-time charts were prepared. Visual analysis indicated that in many there was an initial phase when the dose ($r = -0.23$; $p < 0.05$) was increased several times followed by a prolonged phase when the dose was increased less often or not at all. The following definitions were applied: *Phase of initial pain control* (phase 1)—from the beginning of treatment until the beginning of the first "plateau" or "plateau-descent." A plateau was defined as any period of 2 weeks or more during which the dose of diamorphine was not increased, and a plateau-descent as any period of 2 weeks or more during which the dose of diamorphine was reduced. *Phase of continuing pain control* (phase 2)—from the beginning of the first plateau or plateau-descent until the last day of the last plateau or plateau-descent. *Phase of terminal pain control* (phase 3)—from the end of the last plateau or plateau-descent until death.

RESULTS

There was a negative correlation between age and starting dose significant at the 0.1 level ($r = -0.23$, $p < 0.05$). In all but 5 patients diamorphine was prescribed to control pain. In 3 patients it was prescribed primarily to control cough and in 2 for general distress. The latter received only a minimal dose until pain subsequently was relieved. There was no correlation between maximum dose received and survival ($r = -0.08$). Approximately two-thirds of the patients received diamorphine by mouth until death (44%) or until a few days beforehand (19%); 28% required parenteral treatment intermittently or for a more prolonged period; only 9% received diamorphine exclusively by injection. All received other drugs in addition to diamorphine (Table 2). Of these, 37 patients went home for varying lengths of time;

TABLE 2. *Common adjuvant medication*

Medication	Percentage of patients in each group receiving medication 1	2	3	4	5	Total (%)
Phenothiazine	100	100	100	100	100	100
Corticosteroid	70	55	69	47	89	66
Antidepressant	17	32	41	42	68	39
Anxiolytic	21	41	38	39	21	32
Second analgesic[a]	48	59	62	39	47	52

[a] Includes anti-inflammatory drugs, e.g., aspirin and phenylbutazone.

on average, they spent slightly more time at home than in the hospice. As expected, proportionately more in groups 4 and 5 were discharged (55%) than in group 3 (28%) and groups 1 and 2 (15%). Apart from a paraplegic, they were fully mobile, although some of the more elderly required a cane or other walking aid. More than 80% of the patients survived longer than expected.

Phase I was present on more than two-thirds of the dose-time charts. The mean length, including all 115 patients, was 8 days (SD $\pm$ 8) with an average rate of rise of 6 mg a day. No significant differences were noted between the groups or sexes in either the duration of the phase or the rate of rise of dose. Of those patients who did not have an initial phase, 4 had had no previous analgesics and 2 only paracetamol. These patients were satisfactorily controlled on the smallest dose prescribed, 2.5 mg by mouth every 4 hr. Eight others had already been stabilized on morphine or diamorphine before admission, and five had been receiving another potent oral analgesic. In 7 patients phase 1 lasted more than 3 weeks, and all but one of these completed the phase on above average doses (20 to 60 mg 4 hourly).

The one constant feature of all 115 dose-time charts was the phase of continuing pain control: every patient had at least one period of at least 2 weeks when the dose did not increase. In fact, on the average, patients had three periods of more than 6 weeks when the dose either remained the same or was reduced (Table 3). Phase 3 was recorded in 64 patients, and its mean length was 5 days (SD $\pm$ 7) with an average rate of rise of 18 mg/day. In 48 of these patients, dose was adjusted once or twice within 2 weeks of death. The median 4 hourly maximum dose for all patients was 30 mg by mouth; the median final dose was 20 mg. Case notes of 5 patients in group 5 are recorded (Table 4); dose-time charts are shown in Fig. 1.

TABLE 3. *Numerical analysis of phase 2*

Group	N	Percentage of treatment in phase 2	Direction of dose change: Up	Direction of dose change: Down	Direction of dose change: No overall change	No. of plateaus	No. of plateau-descents	Total	Average no. per patient	Average duration (days)	Ratio of plateau-descents to plateaus	Average rate of change (mg/day)
1	23	84	17	4	2	35	14	49	2	33	0.40	+0.46
2	22	89	19	2	1	36	17	53	2.5	30	0.47	+1.45
3	32	92	24	5	3	48	41	89	3	43	0.85	+1.02
4	19	94	11	6	2	31	25	56	3	66	0.81	+0.29
5	19	96	11	7	1	48	48	96	5	51	1.00	+0.02
Total	115		82	24	9	198	145	343	3	45	0.73	+0.64

TABLE 4. *Case histories*

Name	Sex	Age (years)	Primary site	Initial condition and treatment	Subsequent course
V.H.	F	62	Breast	Pain in left hip; nausea and vomiting. Able to walk with crutches. Dipipanone-cyclizine prescribed; replaced a week later by diamorphine, chlorpromazine, and prednisone because of severe back pain.	Became fully mobile. Several episodes of pain relating to fresh metastatic activity; diamorphine increased but subsequently reduced. Went home for more than 3 months. Eventually readmitted with pneumonia and died within hours.
V.E.	F	49	Ovary	Generally unwell and depressed. Abdomen swollen; intermittent epigastric and lumbar pain. Fully mobile. Improved by general supportive measures and amitriptyline. Diamorphine, chlorpromazine, and prednisone prescribed after 11 weeks for abdominal pain.	Condition flucutated over the next 9 months. Diamorphine then increased on account of discomfort and dyspnea associated with increasing abdominal distension due to ascites. Had several abdominal paracenteses. Troubled by obstructive vomiting; changed to phenazocine tablets as elixir seemed to exacerbate vomiting. Subsequently prescribed i.m. diamorphine when oral medication no longer feasible.
J.B.	M	66	Bronchus	Prescribed regular diamorphine and promazine after 4 weeks when less well, increasingly dyspneic, and anxious. Continued to receive digoxin, frusemide, and a bronchodilator.	Dose of diamorphine doubled after $2\frac{1}{2}$ weeks. Marked improvement in mood and ability after prescription of prednisone. After several months, diamorphine was tailed off. Maintained on promazine, prednisone, digoxin, and bronchodilator. After 8 months, transferred to another unit where he remained until his death.
A.B.	F	61	Breast	Dyspnea, chest pain, anorexia, vomiting; weak and depressed. On cortisone and amitriptyline; diamorphine and promazine added.	Remained weak and had episodes of recurrent depression. Able to walk short distances with help. Intermittent bone pain at varying sites. Later some doses given parenterally because of recurrent vomiting.
C.W.	F	32	Breast	Severe lumbar pain caused by metastasis in lumbar spine. Almost bedfast. Intermittent nausea; breathless on exertion. When admitted was on diamorphine and dipipanone-cyclizine q. 4 h. Parenteral diamorphine with oral chlorpromazine prescribed. Posthypophysectomy replacement therapy continued.	Fully mobile when discharged after 5 weeks. Readmitted several times because of back pain. Diamorphine replaced by phenylbutazone and propoxyphene-co after first nerve block. Second block not so successful; later represcribed diamorphine and chlorpromazine. Patient and family required continued support; benzodiazepines needed at times of additional stress. Trimipramine replaced by amitriptyline after 14 months. Patient still alive.

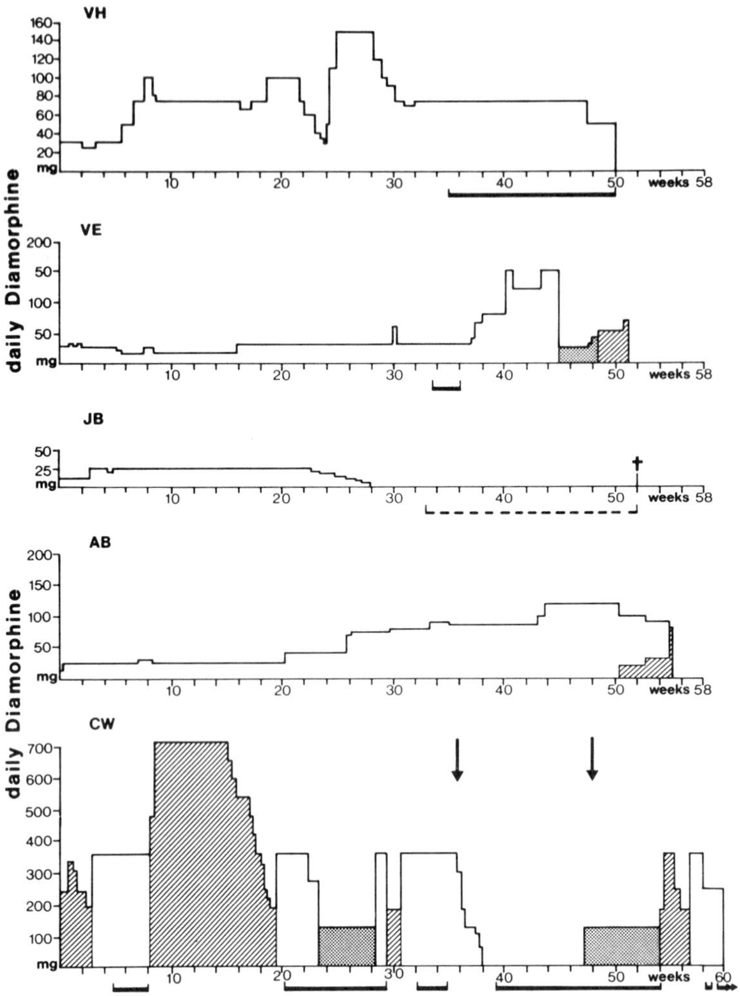

FIG. 1. Dose-time charts relating to case histories in Table 4. *Open squares,* diamorphine by mouth; *hatched areas,* diamorphine by injection; *dotted areas,* other narcotic analgesic (V.E., C.W.); *arrow,* phenol-in-glycerine nerve block; *horizontal bar,* time spent at home. V.H., V.E., and A.B. received diamorphine up to the time of death; C.W. is still alive.

DISCUSSION

In an earlier review of 500 consecutively admitted patients (7), it was concluded that the longer the duration of treatment, the slower the rate at which diamorphine requirements increased. The data in Table 3 further elucidate this point. Not only did the average number of plateaus and plateau-descents increase from group 1 to 5, but their average duration increased from approximately 4 to 8 weeks. (The apparent "fall-off" in group 5 is because 1 patient who is still alive after 5 years required diamorphine for only 16 weeks.) Further, there was a definite increase in the ratio of plateau-descents to plateaus as one moved from group 1 to group 5 ($p < 0.01$). This means that the longer a patient survived after the prescription of diamorphine, the greater the likelihood of a reduction in dose. Dose reductions were made on a trial and error basis in patients who had improved generally over a number of weeks and who had had no recent episodes of "breakthrough" pain. Reductions were also made after successful intrathecal nerve blocks in 5 patients and after treatment with a cytotoxic agent or radiation in a number of others. A total of 9 patients, all in group 5, stopped receiving diamorphine; 3 stopped taking diamorphine altogether; 4 patients stopped for more than 4 months; and 2 stopped for approximately 3 weeks.

Used as part of a pattern of total care, diamorphine—and presumably other narcotic analgesics—may be used for far longer periods without concern about addiction or tolerance (7). Pain unrelieved by other measures should be the main criterion for the prescription of a narcotic analgesic in advanced cancer. Optimal doses vary considerably; "maximum" or "recommended" doses, derived mainly from postoperative parenteral single-dose studies, are not applicable in advanced cancer. Furthermore, the top of the analgesic ladder is not reached simply by prescribing diamorphine because it may be given in a wide range of doses, e.g., 5 to 100 mg 4 hourly by mouth, after which injections can be used.

Because most patients have other symptoms, polypharmacy is generally necessary. For example, it is standard practice at the hospice to administer a phenothiazine concurrently with diamorphine. Half the patients die within 2 weeks of admission, and the incidence of nausea and vomiting appears to be higher in these patients than in patients with less far-advanced cancer. Moreover, diamorphine precipitates or exacerbates emesis in a number of patients. Many patients tend to be anxious or fearful on admission, and in these the routine use of a phenothiazine is doubly beneficial. Prochlorperazine 5 mg is commonly prescribed, but in patients with a marked emotional component to their pain this is often replaced by promazine, chlorpromazine, or, occasionally, methotrimeprazine. Promazine and chlorpromazine are also used to control confusion, delirium, and psychotic manifestations.

For approximately 16% of all patients admitted to the hospice, tricyclic antidepressants are prescribed, whereas in this review 39% received one. When this figure is broken down, it is apparent that there is a progressive increase from group 1 to 5 (Table 2): the proportion in group 5 was significantly greater than that in the other groups ($p < 0.01$). There was no history of previous depressive illness in the majority. It is, however, known that long-term treatment with a phenothiazine may cause depression (6). Even so, the patients were all receiving diamorphine and, if on oral medication, cocaine; two-thirds were also receiving a glucocorticosteroid. Unfortunately, there is no way of determining whether the onset of depression was precipitated by a protracted illness *per se*, was a side effect of treatment, or both.

Diamorphine clearly cannot be regarded as a panacea for terminal cancer. In the patients reviewed, it formed the common factor in a variety of individually determined drug regimens. Additional analgesic measures such as radiation, nerve blocks, or cytotoxic drugs were necessary in several instances, and anti-inflammatory agents were commonly used when pain was caused by a metastasis in bone. Diamorphine's main advantage over other potent analgesics appears to be its solubility; 100 mg of the hydrochloride dissolves in 0.2 ml. It is available in the United Kingdom in freeze-dried ampules, and if necessary a large amount can be injected in a small volume. No significant differences appear to exist between orally administered diamorphine hydrochloride and morphine sulfate when used as at St. Christopher's and when given in equianalgesic doses (9). A trial to evaluate the effect of the cocaine in the mixture has recently been completed and has demonstrated that patients are significantly more alert when receiving cocaine (R. G. Twycross, *in preparation*).

Work needs to be done comparing diamorphine with other potent analgesics such as methadone and levorphanol and comparing cocaine with other cerebral stimulants. Drowsiness is probably more related to the patients' general condition than to the effect of diamorphine or other narcotic analgesics *per se* (8). Further, the whole area of analgesic-tranquilizer combinations needs careful evaluation. Despite the gaps in our knowledge, the evidence suggests that diamorphine—and presumably other narcotic analgesics—are much safer in clinical practice than many doctors have hitherto believed.

SUMMARY

A total of 115 patients with advanced cancer received individually optimized doses of diamorphine hydrochloride regularly for 12 weeks or more to relieve pain or, occasionally, other symptoms. Patients were divided into five groups according to survival, and the initial, continuing, and terminal rates or rises in dose were determined. The initial and final phases were comparable in all five groups, but the rate of rise in the intermediate phase decreased serially from group 1 to group 5. Dose reductions were common, and the median final dose was less than the median maximum dose. There was no correlation between the maximum dose and survival. Only 9% received diamorphine exclusively by injection. Diamorphine was discontinued either permanently or for a prolonged period in 9 patients. One-third of the patients were able to go home for varying lengths of time.

The data support the hypothesis that, generally, increases in dose are necessitated by increased pain rather than by tolerance. The adjuvant use of phenothiazines and antidepressants is discussed. Diamorphine and possibly other narcotic analgesics appear to be safer in clinical practice than has been generally supposed. The need for further research is emphasized.

ACKNOWLEDGMENTS

We thank Dr. Cicely Saunders, Medical Director of St. Christopher's Hospice, for permission to study patients' case notes. The work was supported by grants from the Department of Health and Social Security and the Sir Halley Stewart Trust.

REFERENCES

1. *British Pharmaceutical Codex* (1973): Pharmaceutical Press, London.
2. Isbell, H. (1948): *Ann. N.Y. Acad. Sci., 51:108–122.*
3. Jasinski, D. R., Martin, W. R., and Hoeldtke, R. (1971): *Clin. Pharmacol. Ther.,* 12:613–649.
4. Martin, W. R. (1973): *Br. J. Hosp. Med.,* 10:175–178.
5. Martin, W. R., and Eades, C. G. (1961): *J. Pharmacol. Exp. Ther.,* 133:262–270.
6. Merskey, H. (1974): In: *Relief of Intractable Pain,* edited by M. Swerdlow. Excerpta Medica, Amsterdam.
7. Twycross, R. G. (1974): *Int. J. Clin. Pharmacol.,* 9:184–198.
8. Twycross, R. G. (1975): *J. Med. Ethics,* 1:10–17.
9. Twycross, R. G. (1976): *J. Int. Med. Res.,* 4 (Suppl. 2): 58–67.

Advances in Pain Research and Therapy, Vol. 1,
edited by J. J. Bonica and D. Albe-Fessard.
Raven Press, New York © 1976.

Local Anesthetics as Modulators of Neural Information

George A. Condouris

Department of Pharmacology, College of Medicine and Dentistry of New Jersey, New Jersey Medical School, 100 Bergen Street, Newark, New Jersey 07103

The study of the intimate mechanisms involved in processing neural information, including pain, requires an evaluation of each morphologic and functional component of afferent and efferent systems. Our interest in the modulation of neural information relates to the potential role of the axonal element in the mechanism of drug action on sensory systems. It is known that drugs like local anesthetics, besides causing a block of nerve conduction, can modify other functional properties of axonal membranes. We have reported, for example, that local anesthetics prolong the refractory period of the nerves to a degree that far exceeds any reported previously (1,2). In the rat peripheral nerve, lidocaine extends the refractory period approximately 40-fold; and in the amphibian nerve it extends the refractory period by more than 200-fold. This dramatic dampening of the membrane recovery process is most conspicuously manifested by the curtailment of high-frequency activity in the axon, that is, by Wedensky inhibition (3).

METHODS AND RESULTS

Figure 1 illustrates high-frequency failure in the isolated sciatic trunk of the frog which was treated with a low concentration of lidocaine (0.2 mM). Impulse trains were evoked by stimulating the trunk at various frequencies with a constant intratrain frequency. The top records show the response of the trunk before lidocaine; the bottom records show that this local anesthetic limits the upper frequencies that can be faithfully conducted. That is, this drug provokes a high-frequency failure. The patterns of failure depicted here reflect the loss of constituent fibers in the trunk; therefore, they provide a statistical description of the behavior of a population of fibers.

In similar types of experiments on single fibers, high-frequency failure is manifested in a significantly different way (Fig. 2). Procaine was applied to a single myelinated fiber from the frog. Before treatment this fiber could respond reasonably well to frequencies as high as 400 Hz, as is shown in the control column on the left. When affected by procaine, this fiber lost its

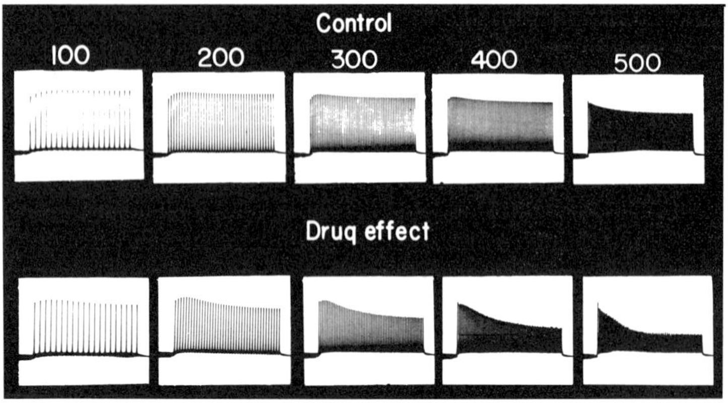

FIG. 1. Effect of lidocaine on high-frequency failure. Trains of compound action potentials from the isolated desheathed sciatic trunk of the bullfrog. Nerves were stimulated with square pulses at the tibial-peroneal bifurcation and the impulse conducted centrally through 5 mm of untreated axon, then through 15 mm of trunk treated with drug dissolved in Ringer's solution. Impulses emanating from the segment were recorded oscillographically 5 mm central to the treated margin. Temp. 22°C.

ability to conduct impulses consistently above 200 Hz. Thus at 200 Hz, after conducting nine impulses, the axon's membrane was "silent." At higher frequencies the number of conducted impulses was even less, and the period of silence correspondingly longer. Note, however, in the center panels for 200 Hz and 400 Hz that the membrane can recover after a period of silence, so that actually the axon passes not only shorter trains followed by a period of silence, but also trains in which interimpulse intervals are no longer uniform. The consequence of this pharmacologic effect is the transmission of distorted information.

To explore this phenomenon further, we reasoned that under natural conditions nerve fibers seldom transmit impulses in neat trains of constant frequency but, in fact, conduct impulses whose frequencies are modulated in complex ways.

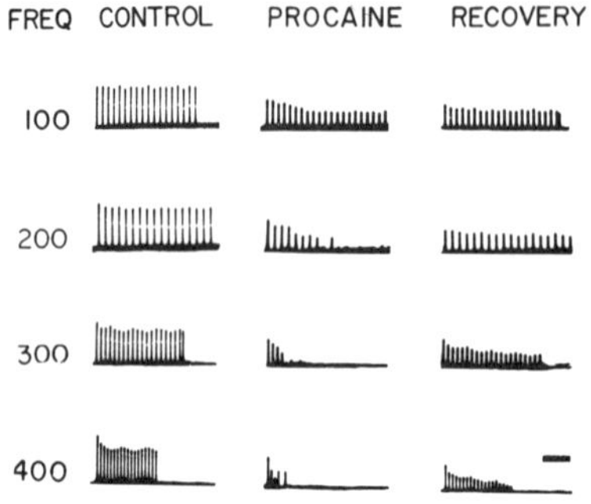

FIG. 2. Trains of impulses conducted through an 8-mm length of drug-treated single myelinated fiber from the bullfrog. General methods as in legend for Fig. 1. Temp. 23°C.

It was logical therefore to investigate high-frequency failure with axonal impulse patterns that were actually generated by a sensory end organ in a natural way. For this we observed in the anesthetized cat the response of single 1a afferent fibers receiving impulses from the spindle of the soleus muscle when the muscle was stretched through various lengths. With increasing stretch the overall frequencies of the afferents were, of course, increased. The patterns were passed through a window discriminator, and the pulse output of the discriminator was recorded on tape. These taped pulse patterns were used to drive an electronic stimulator that evoked activity in an isolated frog trunk *in vitro*. In this way we could study drug action in trunks repeatedly with standard "natural" patterns and could therefore follow the drug action without involving the sensory generator or the central synapses. The fiber groups examined were the $A_{\alpha\beta}$ groups, which correspond to the 1a afferents of the cat.

Some results from this approach are illustrated in Fig. 3, which shows the devastating distortion of the information by lidocaine. The upper row in each pair of records shows the "natural" pattern of the 1a's that was put into the trunk, and the lower row shows the pattern coming out of the segment of nerve treated with 0.75 mM lidocaine. This drug concentration caused virtually no change in the action potential derived from low-frequency stimulation. (See, for example, panel a, left side.) The beginning of high-frequency failure is seen in the middle of panel a where the compound potential undergoes significant decline. In this first sample of information from the spindle there is no total block of conduction, and the axons recover their conduction function when the interimpulse interval is suitably long.

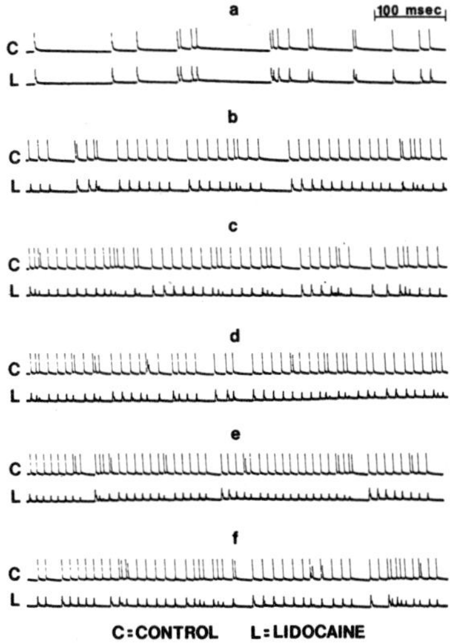

FIG. 3. Lidocaine distortion of spindle information. Compound potentials from isolated desheathed sciatic trunk of the bullfrog. (See Fig. 1 for general methods.) Patterns of activation of impulses were derived as explained in text. Top row of each pair of records shows nerve response before drug was applied; bottom row of each pair shows drug effects on same input patterns. Temp. 22°C.

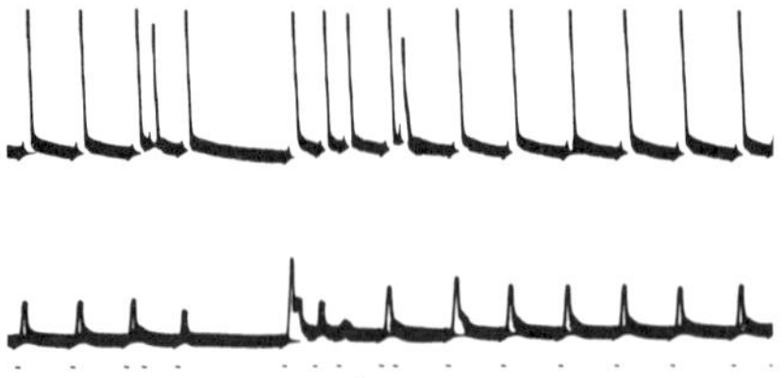

FIG. 4. Enlargement of part of the record in panel e of Fig. 3.

When the overall impulse frequency is increased and is maintained, a more drastic disturbance is visualized, as in panel b. Note that in this sample the spike amplitude remains low continuously, indicating a prolonged conduction block for some fibers. Also note an occasional total block, i.e., all the fibers fail to respond to the stimulus when the impulse frequency is on the high side, such as 400 Hz on the left and right. What is crucially important in these records is that there is no steady state of high-frequency failure. It is under constant change and depends on the intrinsic frequencies being conducted and on the duration of the barrages of higher frequencies.

Two portions of the records are shown in greater detail in Figs. 4 and 5. In Fig. 4 we see in the upper row that the fibers in the trunk respond well to the pattern presented to them. (The 1-msec dashes at the bottom of these records mark the applied stimulus.) Nearly all can follow even the highest intrinsic frequency, which is approximately 500 Hz. Lidocaine, however, has curtailed conduction in approximately 75% of the fibers, as is shown by the reduced amplitudes on the left. Moreover, lidocaine has totally abolished the ability of any fiber to respond to the 500-Hz frequency, as is shown by the absent impulse at the fourth mark. When the interstimulus interval is prolonged, fibers again can conduct, as is illustrated by the enlarged action potential. Still, these fibers succumb to persistent moderate frequencies and fail to respond to 500 Hz.

Finally, Fig. 5 shows an ultra-high-frequency input (approximately 800 Hz) in two bursts where fibers had difficulty even before drug was administered. Lidocaine converts a three-response pattern to a single response, thus not only lowering the average frequency but also changing the internal patterns.

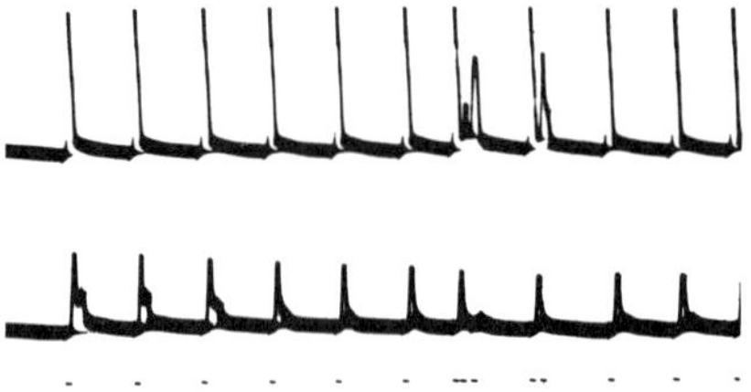

FIG. 5. Enlargement of part of the record in panel f of Fig. 3.

CONCLUSIONS

These experiments support the following concepts: Subblocking concentrations of local anesthetics can modify the information–carrying capacity of axons. The pharmacologic effect of the anesthetics on the membrane is to prolong the period of refractoriness, thereby limiting the high-frequency responsiveness of nerves. In addition to, and as a consequence of, limiting high-frequency activity, the drugs cause a drastic distortion in the impulse patterns transmitted by individual nerves. Finally, the alteration of patterns in individual axons leads to a disorganization of neural information that may depend on convergence of physiologically locked groups of fibers.

In terms of the modulation of the nervous system by drugs, this last effect of local anesthetics suggests that drugs can affect neural information transfer not only at the generation site and at the synaptic sites, but at the conducting element as well. The contribution of the axonal site to systemically administered drugs has not been evaluated. The experiments reported here indicate that the actions of local anesthetics on the axon are more profound when natural patterns of impulses are conducted than when the nerves are activated by artificial patterns of trains or by single impulses. It is conceivable, therefore, that subtle forms of high-frequency failure in axons may be detectable with systemically administered drugs and may indeed play some role in the pharmacologically induced modulation of neural information in the nervous system.

ACKNOWLEDGMENT

This work was supported in part by Grant No. 5R01 NS 06901 from the National Institutes of Health, Bethesda, Maryland.

REFERENCES

1. Condouris, G. A. (1966): *Pharmacologist,* 8:187.
2. Condouris, G. A. (1968): *Epilepsia,* 10:224–227.
3. Wedensky, N. E. (1903): *Pfluegers Arch.,* 100:1–144.

Advances in Pain Research and Therapy, Vol. 1,
edited by J. J. Bonica and D. Albe-Fessard.
Raven Press, New York © 1976.

Effect of Tetracaine and Epinephrine on Intrathecal Second Messengers—Cyclic AMP and Cyclic GMP

R. C. Balagot, M. Bilandzic, S. Kang, B. Kwan, V. Bandelin, and B. Ecanow

Chicago Medical School, Department of Anesthesiology, Veterans Administration Hospital, Downey, Illinois 60064

The currently accepted mechanism for local anesthetic action on nerves seems to be interference with propagation of the nerve action potential (NAP). The cationic local anesthetic amines (procaine, tetracaine) have an affinity for the phospholipids of biomembranes and displace Ca^{2+} bound to the negatively charged polar heads of the phospholipids (4,5,7,10). This physicochemical action occurs at the inner aspect of the cell membrane next to the cytoplasm and apparently affects phosphatidyl serine, which preponderantly binds the Ca^{2+} ion (9,11). This site also seems to be near the membrane sodium pore. All of the preceding phenomena are brought about by a membrane-expanding effect caused by the physical presence of the amine anesthetic in the membrane and its replacement of the cation Ca^{2+} as proposed by Seeman (14). If cationic anesthetics displace Ca^{2+} from the membrane and diminish monovalent cation flux, should not there be an increase in cerebrospinal fluid cation concentration after intrathecal injection of a local anesthetic?

In answer to the above query, we had reported (1) that injection of tetracaine (a cationic local anesthetic amine) intrathecally into human subjects provoked a highly significant decrease in CSF concentration of the cations Ca^{2+}, Na^{+}, Mg^{2+}, and K^{+} in the first 2 min postinjection, and the concentration remained significantly depressed at 5 min but was back to normal by 10 min. It did not matter whether the solution was hyperbaric or hypobaric in relation to CSF. This momentary decrease in CSF cationic concentration was contrary to expectation—we had expected an increase. One explanation was suggested by Mela (9) who showed that butacaine, chlorpromazine, and antihistamine drugs facilitated the uptake of Ca^{2+} by mitochondria. Mel'a explained this effect as because of the ability of the local anesthetic to diminish the buffering capacity of the inner mitochondrial membrane and facilitate its development of a high pH gradient. The high pH gradient she felt might also be true in nervous tissue, and it explains the anesthetizing action of tetracaine. Although cationic local anesthetics act faster in an alkaline than in a nonalkaline medium and, as Mela has shown in mitochondria, local anesthetics facilitate Ca^{2+} uptake and consequently a high pH gradient in mitochondria, such has not been demonstrated in nerve axons. Other mechanisms may be involved.

Rasmussen (12) has demonstrated increased permeability of plasma membrane to Ca^{2+} on stimulation of cyclic adenylase by a "first messenger" and subsequent release of cyclic AMP (cAMP), which in turn increases mitochondrial membrane permeability to Ca^{2+}. Flux of Ca^{2+} will be from extracellular fluid and mitochondria to cytoplasm. Goldberg (8) has shown that acetylcholine and other substances like oxytocin, calcitonin, insulin, polypeptide hormones, serotonin, histamine, epinephrine, and prostaglandin $F_{2\alpha}$ stimulated production of cyclic guanidine monophosphate (cGMP) intracellularly. Perpetuation of a high cGMP level was shown to be dependent on stimulation of cyclic guanylase by Ca^{2+} (13). Presumably, then, Rasmussen believed that in some cell systems an extracellular first messenger stimulated plasma membrane receptors that increased membrane permeability to Ca^{2+}, which in turn stimulated cyclic guanylase intracellularly to raise levels of cGMP.

Thus both cyclic nucleotides are intimately related to membrane Ca^{2+} flux. This chapter deals with an examination of such mechanisms.

METHODS

In one series of 12 patients undergoing different surgical operations, spinal anesthesia was induced with tetracaine (10 mg), glucose (10% – 1 ml), and epinephrine (0.5 mg) in 5 cases and without epinephrine in 7 cases. CSF samples (2 ml) were obtained before injection of the anesthetic and again 2 and 5 min after injection. To determine cation concentration (Ca^{2+}, Mg^{2+}, Na^{+}, and K^{+}), we used 1 ml of the CSF sample; the other milliliter was employed to determine cAMP levels by radioimmunoassay.

In a second series of 12 patients, 5 received tetracaine with glucose and epinephrine, and 7 without epinephrine. Simultaneous determination of cAMP and cGMP was done using radioimmunoassay on CSF samples obtained pre-drug and 2 and 5 min post-drug intrathecal injection.

RESULTS AND DISCUSSION

In the first series, mean value of cAMP in CSF for all 12 subjects before injection of tetracaine was 0.30 ± 0.05 (SE) pmoles/ml. There was no significant change at 2 and 5 min in cAMP with or without addition of epinephrine to the spinal anesthetic.

In the second series (Table 1), mean value in all 12 subjects was 0.39 ± 0.05 (SE) pmoles/ml. Again, there was no significant difference between

TABLE 1. *CSF cyclic nucleotide*[a] *changes caused by tetracaine and epinephrine*

Nucleotide	Control	2 Min	5 Min
cAMP	0.42±0.09	0.37±0.25	0.39±0.09
(with epinephrine)		0.43±0.23	0.45±0.23
cGMP	3.94±0.71	4.24±0.57[b]	4.57±0.98
(with epinephrine)		1.76±0.69[b]	2.20±1.04

[a] In pM/ml±SEM.
[b] $t=2.79$; $p=1.0\%$.

CSF cAMP values at 2 and 5 min as compared to control with or without epinephrine in the anesthetic solution.

Control value of cGMP was 3.07±0.64 (SE) pmoles/ml. There was no significant change in cGMP values at both 2 and 5 min post-drug injection without epinephrine as compared to control. However, CSF cGMP values obtained at 2 min showed a significantly lower value for patients receiving tetracaine with epinephrine as compared to the group that had no epinephrine—*t*-value was 2.79 and *p* was close to 1% (2,3).

The control values for CSF cAMP were much lower than those previously reported by Cramer et al. (6)—6 to 24 pmoles/ml. Our value ranged in 24 patients from 0.30 to 0.39 pmoles/ml. More studies will have to be done to obtain the correct range for normal values. Interestingly enough, cGMP, which is supposed to predominate intracellularly and in much smaller amounts than cAMP, had a greater value in CSF—10 times more. The significance of this finding eludes us at the moment.

The significant drop in CSF cGMP value at 2 min in patients who received epinephrine added to spinal anesthetic may be explained on the basis of epinephrine reciprocally inhibiting cGMP while stimulating cAMP production. However, cAMP in this instance did not increase materially, which nullifies this explanation partly.

This cGMP drop at 2 min also coincided with the most significant decrease of the cations Ca^{2+}, Mg^{2+}, Na^{+}, and K^{+} in spinal fluid. Assuming that Mela was correct in her findings that cationic local anesthetics facilitated entry of Ca^{2+} through membranes—mitochondrial or plasma—the migration of the divalent cation Ca^{2+} into the cytoplasm either failed to stimulate cyclic guanylase to facilitate production of cGMP or was overwhelmingly nullified by the inhibiting action of epinephrine.

SUMMARY

The average value for cAMP in human CSF was found to vary from 0.30±0.05 (SE) to 0.39±0.05 (SE) pmoles/ml. cGMP was found to be 3.07±0.64 (SE) pmoles/ml.

Epinephrine added to tetracaine when this drug was employed as a spinal anesthetic significantly decreased CSF cGMP levels. The mean value for cGMP was 4.24 ± 0.57 (SE) pmoles/ml in CSF without epinephrine as compared to 1.76 ± 0.69 (SE) pmoles/ml in CSF with epinephrine.

Epinephrine did not materially increase CSF cAMP.

ACKNOWLEDGMENT

We wish to thank Mrs. Margaret Gorman for doing the radioimmunoassay of the material.

REFERENCES

1. Balagot, R. C., Kosaphandhu, P., Kwan, B. K., Tumaneng, L. T., and Ecanow, B. (1974): Abst. Scientific Papers, ASA, October, pp. 327–328.
2. Batson, H. C. (1956): *An Introduction to Statistics in the Medical Sciences*, pp. 16–20. Burgess Publishing Co., Minneapolis.
3. Beyer, W. H. Ed. *Handbook of Tables for Probability and Statistics*, p. 226. The Chemical Rubber Co., Cleveland.
4. Blaustein, M. P., and Goldman, D. E. (1966[a]): *J. Am. Physiol.*, 49:1043–1063.
5. Blaustein, M. P., and Goldman, D. E. (1966[b]): Science, 153:429–432.
6. Cramer, H., Ng, L. K. Y., and Chase, T. N. (1973): *Arch. Neurol.*, 29:197–199.
7. Feinstein, M. B. (1964): *J. Gen. Physiol.*, 48:357–374.
8. Goldberg, N. D. (1975) In: *Cell Membranes, Cell Biology and Pathology*, edited by G. Weissman, pp. 185–201. H. P. Publishing Co., New York.
9. Mela, L. (1968): *Arch. Biochem. Biophys.*, 123:286–293.
10. Narahashi, T., Yamada, M., and Frazier, D. T. (1969): *Nature (Lond.)*, 223:748–749.
11. Ohki, S. (1970): *Biochem. Biophys. Acta*, 219:18–27.
12. Rasmussen, H. (1975) In: *Cell Membranes, Cell Biology and Pathology*, edited by G. Weissman, pp. 203–212. H. P. Publishing Co., New York.
13. Schultz, G., Hardman, J. G., and Schultz, K. (1973): *Proc. Natl. Acad. Sci. U.S.A.*, 70:3889.
14. Seeman, P. (1972): *Pharmacol. Rev.*, 24:583–655.

Advances in Pain Research and Therapy, Vol. 1,
edited by J. J. Bonica and D. Albe-Fessard.
Raven Press, New York © 1976.

Dissociation of Cold, Warm, and Hot Sensibility During Ulnar Nerve Block and Surface Anesthesia

*H. Nolte, H. Fruhstorfer, U. Pfaff, *H. Radtke, and M. Zenz

**Institute of Anaesthesiology, County and Municipal Hospitals, Minden, Germany; and Institute of Physiology, University of Marburg, Marburg/Lahn, Germany*

Receptors responding specifically to innocuous or noxious thermal stimulation are present in the skin of the primate. These receptors have slowly conducting axons belonging to the groups C or Aδ. Whereas the axons of warm receptor neurons seem to be mainly unmyelinated, a great proportion of cold receptors have thinly myelinated axons. Receptors responding to noxious heat have myelinated as well as unmyelinated axons (2,4).

So far, there is no direct evidence that cold, warm, and heat receptors elicit the sensations of cold, warm, and painful hot, respectively. One possible way to gain insight into this relation is to observe changes in sensation when the afferent conduction in one fiber group is blocked leaving the other one unaffected. In this study the loss of warm, cold, and pain sensibility was examined during differential chemical block of the ulnar nerve and related to the block of other sensory, motor, and vegetative functions dependent on certain nerve fibers. Additionally, in a further study, the changes in warm, cold, and hot sensibility were examined during surface anesthesia. In both studies simple reaction time (RT) served as an indicator of afferent conduction.

METHODS

In the first study the subject (S) was sitting in a chair with his hand resting comfortably on a specially designed stimulation and recording apparatus (3,9). He regularly received a cycle of four stimuli to which he had to respond in a typical way. The four stimuli were cold, pinprick, warm, and a sound, each preceded by a short tone pip. The cycle duration was 1 min. Cold and warm pulses of 10°C amplitude were presented to the glabrous skin of the right hypothenar region by a thermode kept at an adapting temperature of 30°C. The pinprick was delivered by a needle slowly driven against the hypothenar region with a linearly growing force reaching 150 g after approximately 4 sec. The S had to respond to the stimuli by pressing a key as soon as he perceived them, and the RT was measured. In the case of the pinprick, the S had additionally to report when, after the injection of the anesthetic, the pinprick felt no longer sharp but blunt. During the sound, the S had to abduct his right little finger with maximal force against a water-filled balloon, and the resulting pressure was recorded. At the same time the temperature difference between the skin of the right little finger and the index finger was measured in order to determine the degree of vasodilatation.

At the beginning of an experimental session, the S was trained in the procedure. Then the ulnar nerve was blocked by injecting 2 ml of an anesthetic just proximal to the right ulnar sulcus. Immediately after the injection, stimulation was begun.

Thirty-nine subjects received mepivacaine 1%, and the latency of the resulting nerve block was determined. In 11 Ss both ulnar nerves were blocked by etidocaine 1% and 0.5% and by bupivacaine 0.5% and 0.25% in two separate sessions. Here latency and duration of nerve block were determined.

In the second study surface anesthesia was performed in 12 Ss by applying tetracaine 2% to the inner surface of the upper lip. Thermal stimuli were presented to the anesthetized mucous membrane, and the Ss had to react as soon as they perceived the stimuli. The thermal pulses started from an adapting temperature of 30°C and had the following intensities: cold 20°C, warm 40°C, and hot 50°C. Again RTs were measured.

The experiment consisted of three parts: First, every 30 sec the S received a cold or warm pulse before and after application of tetracaine. After warm sensation had been blocked for 2 min, ethanol 40% was applied to the mucous membrane and the stimulation was continued. Second, the same stimulus cycle was presented before and after application of ethanol 40% alone. Third, warm and hot stimuli were presented before and after application of tetracaine.

The whole stimulation procedure as well as the processing of the recorded data were controlled by a PDP-12 computer.

RESULTS

Injection of mepivacaine into the ulnar nerve caused a dissociated loss of warm and cold sensibility in the hypothenar region: warm sensibility was lost significantly earlier than cold sensibility (Wilcoxon signed rank test, $p < 0.01$). The loss of warm sensibility was preceded by the block of vasomotor efferents; simultaneously with the warm sensibility block, pinprick sensation changed from sharp to blunt. When both warm and cold sensibility were completely blocked, touch was still perceived and the force of the affected muscle was reduced to approximately 60% of the original value (Table 1). The loss of a thermal quality was preceded by a significant increase in RT.

TABLE 1. *Latency of block of sensory afferents and vasomotor efferents*

Stimulus	Latency (min; mean ± SD)
Cold	16.35 ± 14.60
Warm	12.85 ± 11.60
Pain	12.81 ± 10.99
Vasomotor	8.08 ± 6.34

Vasomotor efferents were regarded to be blocked when skin temperature had exceeded 25% of its final peak amplitude. The change in pinprick sensation from sharp to blunt was taken as the beginning of analgesia. Ulnar block by mepivacaine 1%; 39 Ss.

Similar results were obtained when the nerve was blocked with etidocaine or bupivacaine (Fig. 1). Again warm sensibility was lost significantly earlier than cold sensibility ($p < 0.01$), and warm sensibility block lasted significantly longer than cold sensibility block ($p < 0.01$). On the whole, nerve functions were recovered in the reverse order from which they had been lost; only sympathetic efferents recovered earlier when the nerve was blocked by etidocaine. None of the Ss reported that a thermal sensation before being blocked had changed its quality in the sense that a cold stimulus

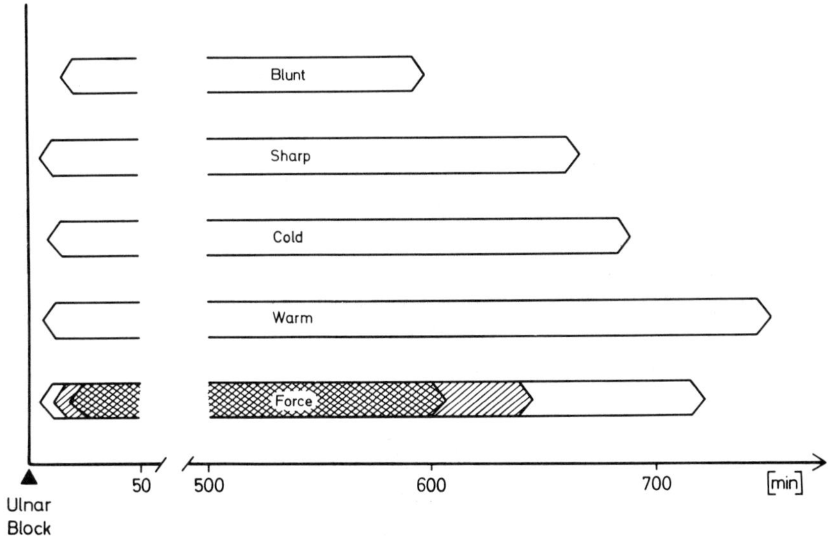

FIG. 1. Mean latency and duration of nerve block for the forces 75%, 50%, and 25% of the normal value. Data are combined from 44 ulnar blocks in 11 Ss by etidocaine and bupivacaine (both with epinephrine).

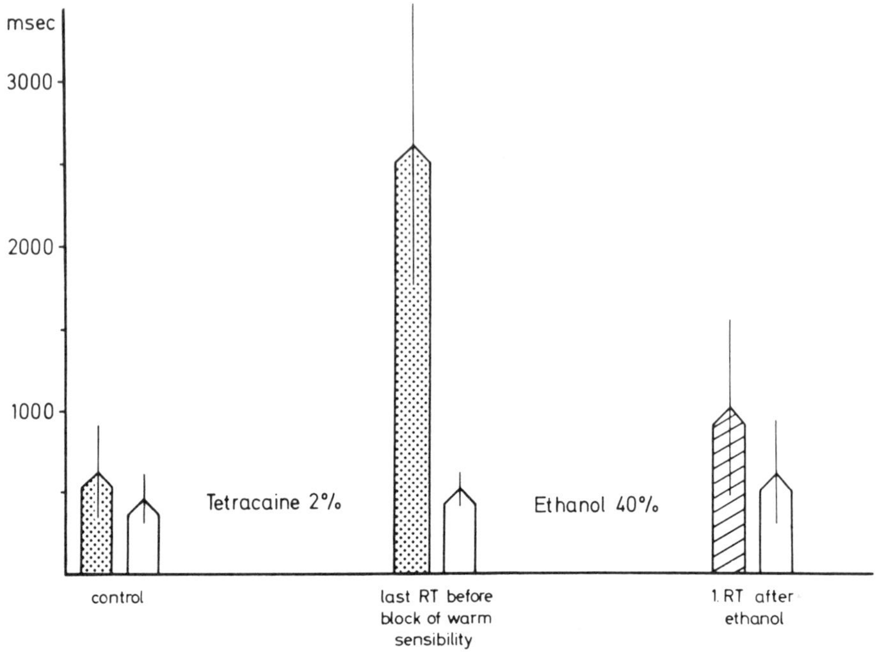

FIG. 2. Reaction times (mean ± SD) of 12 Ss to warm (*dotted*) and cold (*open*) stimuli after application of tetracaine 2% to inner surface of the upper lip. Ethanol 40% was applied 2 min after the loss of warm sensibility; warm stimuli were perceived again, but as stinging hot (*hatched*).

was perceived as warm, tactile, or painful. Similarly, there was no persisting thermal sensation when one thermal quality was blocked.

In surface anesthesia warm sensation was on the average blocked after 4.3 min without affecting cold or hot sensation; the RTs for cold and hot stimuli increased, however, significantly. If 2 min after warm sensibility had been lost ethanol was applied to the mucous membrane, the warm stimuli were perceived again, but now as stinging hot (Fig. 2). Application of ethanol alone without preceding tetracaine did not affect cold sensation but changed the sensation of the 40°C stimuli from warm to stinging hot; the RTs did not change significantly.

DISCUSSION

This study has confirmed that chemical nerve block causes a dissociated loss of nerve functions: after the block of sympathetic efferents warm sensibility is lost, followed significantly later by the loss of cold sensibility. At the time of warm sensibility block, a pinprick sensation changes from sharp to blunt and motor force is reduced to approximately half of its normal value. The increase in RTs before a sensory quality is lost indicates that spatial summation occurs in the afferent pathways and that the progressive loss of afferent fibers is compensated by temporal summation. When warm sensibility is blocked with cold sensibility still intact, no persisting cold sensation appears; this shows that thermal indifference is not achieved by simply combining the information from both warm and cold receptors. After the block of cold sensation, the thickly myelinated axons of cold-sensitive mechanoreceptors (1) are still conducting; as cold stimuli are not perceived at all at that moment, cold stimulation of these receptors probably does not lead to a conscious sensation. The finding that the sharp sensation of a pin-prick is blocked significantly shorter than warm sensation supports the assumption that sharp pain is at least partly mediated by thin myelinated fibers (2,7).

During surface anesthesia only warm sensation is blocked, whereas cold and hot stimuli are still perceived. This indicates that heat sensation is mediated by special receptors differing from warm receptors. When warm sensation is blocked, warm stimuli can be perceived again if ethanol is applied to the mucous membrane; but the same stimulus perceived as warm before is now perceived as stinging hot, similar to the 50°C stimulus in intensity and quality. If only ethanol is applied, warm stimuli are also perceived as stinging hot. This can be interpreted as indicating sensitization of these heat receptors by ethanol.

Heat receptors have been found with both myelinated and unmyelinated axons (2,5,6,10,11). Although sensitization of these heat receptors has been demonstrated only in polymodal nociceptors with C fibers (2,5,8,11), several facts indicate that heat receptors with Aδ fibers participate in heat sensation described here: heat sensation is not blocked like warm sensation by surface anesthesia; unlike warm sensation heat sensation begins instantly; RTs to heat stimuli are too short to be mediated by receptors with C fibers situated deeper than warm receptors.

These results support the hypothesis that in man cold, warm, and heat sensations are mediated by different receptor neurons that could correspond to the specific thermal receptors identified in the skin of primates.

REFERENCES

1. Brown, A. G., and Iggo, A. (1967): *J. Physiol.* (*Lond.*), 193:707–733.
2. Burgess, P. R., and Perl, E. R. (1973): In: *Handbook of Sensory Physiology, Vol. 2: Somatosensory System,* edited by A. Iggo. Springer, Heidelberg and New York.
3. Fruhstorfer, H., Zenz, M., Nolte, H., and Hensel, H. (1974): *Pfluegers Arch.,* 349:73–82.
4. Hensel, H. (1973): In: *Handbook of Sensory Physiology, Vol. 2: Somatosensory System,* edited by A. Iggo. Springer, Heidelberg and New York.
5. Iggo, A. (1974): In: *Advances in Neurology, Vol. 4: Pain,* edited by J. J. Bonica, pp. 1–10. Raven Press, New York.

6. Iggo, A., and Ogawa, H. (1971): *J. Physiol.* (*Lond.*), 216:77–78P.
7. Landau, W. M., and Bishop, G. H. (1958): *Science,* 128:712–714.
8. Perl, E. R., Kumazawa, T., Lynn, B., and Kenins, P. (1974): In: *Proceedings of the Academy of Sciences of the USSR, Symposium on "Tissue Reception."* Leningrad.
9. Radtke, H., Nolte, H., Fruhstorfer, H., and Zenz, M. (1975): *Acta Anaesthesiol. Scand.* [*Suppl.*], 60:17–20.
10. Sumino, R., Dubner, R., and Starkman, S. (1973): *Brain Res.,* 62:260–263.
11. Zimmermann, M., and Handwerker, H. O. (1974): In: *Advances in Neurology, Vol. 4: International Symposium on Pain,* edited by J. J. Bonica, pp. 29–34. Raven Press, New York.

Advances in Pain Research and Therapy, Vol. 1,
edited by J. J. Bonica and D. Albe-Fessard.
Raven Press, New York © 1976.

Accuracy of Needle Placement During Diagnostic and Therapeutic Nerve Blocks

Theresa Ferrer-Brechner and Verne L. Brechner

Department of Anesthesiology, University of California at Los Angeles, School of Medicine, Los Angeles, California 90024

In the management of acute or chronic pain, the use of nerve blocks can be a valuable diagnostic tool in determining the appropriateness of a surgical approach. The classic way of accomplishing this task is to rely on geometrical formulas based on anatomical landmarks for the proper placement of the needle. In certain nerve blocks, precise needle placement is mandatory, especially if the results are to be used as a prediction for the success of surgical ablation of specific nerves or nerve roots.

In recent years, aids in ensuring proper needle placement include use of roentgenograms. However, use of roentgenograms for guiding accurate needle placement during every diagnostic and therapeutic nerve block is practically impossible in a busy pain clinic. In the last year at UCLA Pain Management Clinic, we accomplished diagnostic and therapeutic nerve blocks with the classic method using anatomical landmarks. In a select group of patients, fluoroscopy and permanent films were taken to demonstrate needle placement. We gathered the following informative data.

METHOD

We studied 30 patients while they received either diagnostic or therapeutic nerve blocks. The blocks performed were stellate ganglion ($N=6$), lumbar somatic ($N=5$), paravertebral lumbar sympathetic ($N=5$), celiac ($N=8$), thoracic somatic ($N=2$), and sacral nerve root ($N=4$) blocks. The procedures were performed in the radiology area where fluoroscopy was available. After the patients were positioned correctly, the particular blocks were initially performed without the aid of fluoroscopy, adhering strictly to the anatomical landmarks recommended by a standard textbook on regional block (1). After the needle was apparently satisfactorily placed, fluoroscopy was performed to locate needle placement and permanent anteroposterior and lateral X-rays were taken. To verify the location of the needle tip, we injected 1.5 cc of meglumine diatrizoate (Renografin® 60) in 1.5 cc of 1% xylocaine. If the needle was inaccurately placed, it was repositioned under fluoroscopy and another X-ray was taken. Then the usual volume of local anesthetic to complete the block was injected and in some patients the local anesthetic was mixed with meglumine diatrizoate to demonstrate the extent of spread of the solution. The patients were then transported to outpatient surgery to recover.

RESULTS

Although the blocks were done with strict adherence to recommended anatomical landmarks, there was a high incidence of error as to exact location of the needle. The most consistently successful block was the stellate ganglion block, and the most consistent blocking error was the somatic block.

The results demonstrating the number of successes and failures with various nerve blocks studied are listed in Table 1.

Table 2 summarizes the common errors in needle placement (see below) that we had encountered.

Stellate Ganglion Block

During the performance of the stellate ganglion blocks, the tip of the needle, which was intended for the transverse process of the seventh cervical vertebra, consistently hit the body of the sixth or seventh cervical vertebra. If repositioning of the needle was attempted so that it could be near the transverse process, the patients experienced paresthesias. If injection was done at this point, unnecessary sensory and/or motor

TABLE 1. *Radiological studies of diagnostic and therapeutic nerve blocks*

Type of block	Total no.	Needle placement in error	Needle placement adequate
Stellate ganglion block	6	1	5
Lumbar somatic block	5	4	1
Celiac plexus block	8	2	6
Paravertebral lumbar sympathetic block	5	1	4
Sacral somatic block	4	3	1
Thoracic somatic block	2	1	1
Total	30	12 (40%)	18 (60%)

TABLE 2. *Radiological studies during nerve blocks: common errors*

Type of block	Error
Stellate ganglion block	Needle in body of C_6 or first rib instead of transverse process
Lumbar somatic block	Needle placement above or below intended interspace; injection of 2 cc spreads from 2–3 segments; needle too lateral and/or superficial
Celiac plexus block	Too superficial
Paravertebral sympathetic block	Too superficial; injection of 10 cc produces spread of 3 segments
Thoracic somatic block	Too lateral, usually on rib
Sacral somatic block	Too lateral and/or superficial; needle easily bent away from intended sacral foramina

block resulted with the sympathetic block, especially when higher concentrations of local anesthetics were used. Injection of 20 cc of local anesthetic with meglumine diatrizoate caused widespread diffusion of the solution anterior to transverse processes of C_6, C_7, and T_1 vertebrae.

Lumbar Somatic Block

Lumbar somatic block had a high incidence (4 out of 5) of error with needle placement. The most common and significant error was that the needle was placed at a different interspace than the one intended to be blocked. The needle could also be too lateral and/or superficial. During insertion of the needle, a patient complained of paresthesia of appropriate dermatome, but when fluoroscopy was performed the needle was found to be too lateral and superficial and was therefore grossly inaccurately placed for a somatic block. Another significant finding was that injection of 2 cc of solution had, surprisingly, a spread of two to three segments.

Celiac Plexus and Paravertebral Sympathetic Block

The most common error of these blocks was the superficial placement of the needle. This is understandable because of the depth involved for placement of the needle. Patients experienced paresthesias if the needle was more superficially located than intended because of proximity to somatic outflow. Injection of 10 cc of solution was demonstrated to spread three segments.

Sacral Somatic Block and Thoracic Somatic Block

With sacral somatic blocks, one common error was that the needle was too lateral and was easily bent away from the sacral foramina. With the thoracic somatic block, the needle tip rested on the rib instead of on the transverse process. With the high risk of pneumothorax, this procedure should be done always with the use of radiological guidance.

DISCUSSION

Our study shows that performance of nerve blocks with use of anatomical landmarks can have a 40% error in needle placement. Although this error should be compensated for by the use of large volumes of local anesthetics during therapeutic blocks and blocks used for surgical anesthesia, the precise location of needle during diagnostic nerve blocks is mandatory because only a small volume of local anesthetics can be used to limit the block and the spread of local anesthesia to specific nerves or ganglia.

The highest incidence of error during diagnostic blocks seems to be during performance of somatic nerve blocks. Injection of even as small as 2 cc of solution can cause a spread of three segments of spinal nerve roots. When a patient is a possible candidate for rhizotomy, somatic nerve blocks are used to predict the results and to offer the patient a temporary feeling as to how the areas blocked would feel after surgery. If the nerve block has been unknowingly performed in a level other than the one intended, and/or if the spread of local anesthesia involved more than the specific nerve roots intended, the patient may have an unnecessary rhizotomy in the incorrect levels and not obtain any pain relief. This could be one of the reasons for the 25% to 45% failure of pain relief as cited by White (2,3) after posterior rhizotomy. Therefore, in using somatic blocks to predict the success of rhizotomy, one has to be precise as to what level is being blocked and one must use a small volume of local anesthetic (as small as 0.5 to 1 cc) to limit the spread of the solution to other spinal nerve roots. We feel that roentgenograms are mandatory during performance of diagnostic somatic block.

In contrast, blocking autonomic plexuses such as stellate ganglion, celiac plexus, and lumbar sympathetic plexus requires larger volumes of local anesthetics. However, since these plexuses are deep in the body, the most common error is the superficial or posterior location of the needle. This tends to place the needle at the area of somatic outflow, and injection at this site can produce somatic block instead of pure sympathetic block, and therefore evaluation of response can be confusing.

In the management of the pain patient in whom various factors other than precisely performed nerve block can influence the results, we feel that accurately performed nerve blocks should be assured so that proper interpretation can be made.

SUMMARY

Thirty nerve blocks were performed adhering strictly to suggested anatomical landmarks. Fluoroscopy and anteroposterior and lateral X-rays were then taken after placement of needle. We found 40% error in needle placement. The highest incidence of error was with performance of somatic blocks, in which the needle was placed in improper interspace and the injection of a small amount of local anesthetic caused a block of three levels. It is therefore recommended that roentgenograms be done during performance of somatic block for it to be of use in predicting the outcome of surgical ablation.

REFERENCES

1. Moore, D. (1967): *Regional Block,* 4th Ed. Charles C Thomas, Publisher, Springfield, Illinois.
2. White, J. C. (1964): *Henry Ford Hospital International Symposium,* pp. 287–297. Little, Brown & Co., Boston.
3. White, J. C. (1973): In: *Neurologic Surgery, Vol. 3,* edited by J. Youmans, pp. 1702–1717. W. B. Saunders Co., Philadelphia.

Advances in Pain Research and Therapy, Vol. 1,
edited by J. J. Bonica and D. Albe-Fessard.
Raven Press, New York © 1976.

Lumbar Sympathectomy—a Percutaneous Chemical Technique

R. A. Boas,* V. S. Hatangdi, and E. G. Richards

Department of Anaesthetics and Pain Clinic, Auckland Hospital, Auckland, New Zealand

The value of lumbar sympathectomy is well recognized in the treatment of peripheral vascular disease or sympathetic overactivity of the lower limb. Surgical sympathectomy has long been the standard treatment, but it carries risks of intra- and postoperative complications. It also entails hospitalization for a week or more. Permanent chemical sympathectomy, on the other hand, can be done on an outpatient basis with less morbidity than and similar efficacy as surgical sympathectomy (2,5). This chapter describes a simplified, two-needle technique of lumbar sympathectomy using 7% phenol dissolved in radiopaque contrast medium—Conray 420 (70% sodium iothalamate in water).

METHODS

Forty-seven chemical sympathectomies were performed over a period of 3 years in 44 patients. Two patients had failed to benefit from previous surgical sympathectomy, and three others required bilateral blocks; a few were performed as urgent procedures within hours of the patients' referrals.

Peripheral vascular disease was the indication in 39 patients, and 5 were referred for relief of post-traumatic sympathetic dystrophy. The youngest patient was 18 years, the oldest 90 years, and more than 75% were over the age of 70 with associated cardiac and respiratory problems.

Patients were evaluated on the basis of history, the degree and site of pain, nutritional ischemia, ulceration, or gangrene. The referring vascular surgeons had previously undertaken arteriography when indicated. Diagnosis of sympathetic dystrophy was confirmed by the history of previous trauma or surgery and the presence of a cold, blue, perspiring foot with skin, hair, and nail changes.

Technique

Chemical sympathectomy is carried out as an outpatient procedure in the operating theater. The essential requirement is the availability of

* Preseat Address: Pain Clinic, University of Massachusetts Medical Center, Worcester, Massachusetts 01605.

televised X-ray screening with provision for two-plane visualization. Details of the procedure are explained to the patients in general terms, and a preliminary iodine patch test is carried out. The patient lies prone on an X-ray table over three pillows supporting his head, chest, and pelvis. An intravenous infusion is set up and the blood pressure is monitored. Cutaneous thermistor electrodes are strapped to each foot over the base of the great toe, little toe, and middorsum of both the affected foot and the other foot, which acts as a control. Base-line skin temperatures are recorded using a telethermometer, allowing approximately 30 min for the unexposed foot temperatures to stabilize at ambient temperature of 20°C.

After 5 mg of diazepam and local anesthetic skin infiltration, two 20-gauge BD sympathectomy needles 12.5 cm in length are inserted 6 to 8 cm lateral to the third and fourth lumbar vertebrae. Needles are directed to reach the ventrolateral aspect of the middle of the third and fourth lumbar vertebral bodies, their positions being checked with the image intensifier. In the AP projection the tip of the needles should lie 0.5 cm medial to the outer edge of the body, whereas in the lateral projection it lies at, or just short of, the anterior border of the vertebrae.

After negative aspiration tests, a small quantity (0.25 to 0.5 ml) of 7% phenol in Conray 420 is injected to confirm a localized spread of solution as seen on the screen. Should the radiopaque solution disperse rapidly along a blood or lymphatic vessel, as can happen even after negative aspiration, the position of the needle must be readjusted. Phenol in Conray is then injected slowly through each of the two needles, and the spread of solution is monitored on the X-ray screen. The quantity of phenol, determined by the actual spread of solution (Fig. 1), varies from 3 to 5 ml through each needle.

Injection should be painless and offer no resistance, indicating that the agent is in the correct tissue planes. Saline, 1 to 2 ml, is used to flush the needles as they are withdrawn and total screening time has been limited to an average of 3 min. Anteroposterior and lateral X-ray films are taken for future reference and records.

The patient is left in the prone position for up to 30 min and then transferred on a bed to the recovery ward and kept under observation for 1 hr.

Cutaneous temperatures are measured before the injection and at every 15 min over the next hour after sympathectomy.

Phenol in Conray Mixture

This is made by dissolving phenol crystals in Conray 420 (70% sodium iothalamate in water) to give 7% phenol in Conray, passed through a 1.2-μm millipore filter and stored in 10-ml ampules. Ultraviolet spectrometric analysis of the phenol-Conray mixture indicated that phenol in Conray exists as a physical mixture without free iodine and without chemical combination or degradation of the constituents.

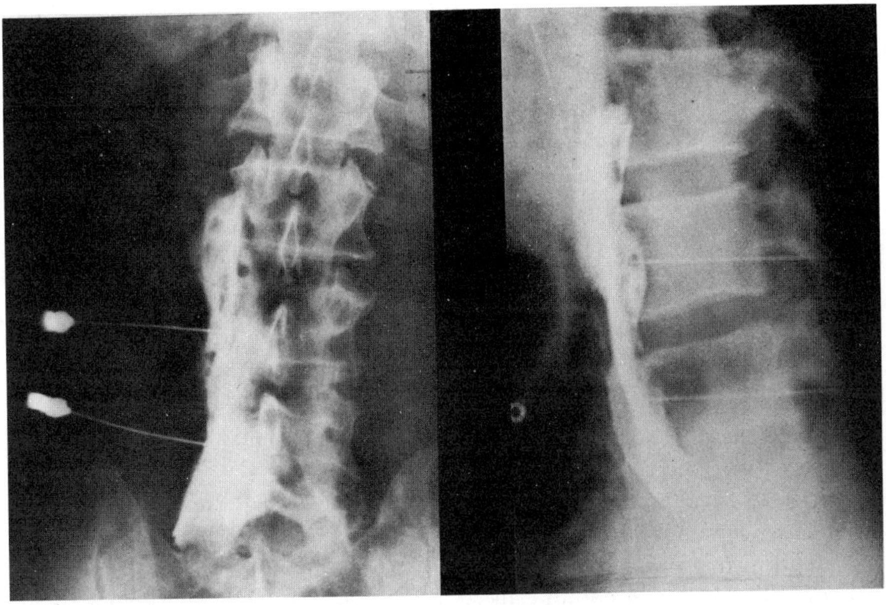

FIG. 1. Spread of phenol in Conray 420 in anterior and lateral projections.

RESULTS

Immediate

Effectiveness of sympathectomy was confirmed by improvement in circulation to the foot rendering it pink and warm with a rise in cutaneous temperature within 30 to 45 min and relief of rest pain in the majority. Rise in skin temperature after sympathectomy was in the range of 1° to 11°C with an average of 5°C. Maximum rise of the order of 9° to 11°C was noted in those patients with sympathetic dystrophy. No systemic reactions to phenol were encountered in our series.

Short-Term Follow-up

Patients were followed at our clinic for 1 month after sympathectomy. Subsequent follow-up was carried out by the referring specialist or general practitioner. In the follow-up period to date (of 3 months to 3 years), the only complication encountered as a result of sympathectomy was groin dysesthesia in the distribution of the genitofemoral nerve in 3 patients. The symptoms were transient, lasting from 2 to 5 weeks, and were of no great concern to the patient. This incidence of groin dysesthesia after surgical sympathectomy is as high as 35% (4), and as yet there is inadequate explanation for the mechanism of this condition. Somatic nerve involvement was excluded in these 3 cases on the basis of (a) absence of anesthesia in the distribution of the genitofemoral nerve, and (b) lack of radiological evidence of spread of phenol toward the intervertebral foramina or psoas sheath, through which the nerve courses.

Long-Term Follow-up

To date long-term follow-up indicates that sympathectomy appears to be permanent, as is shown by a pink foot with well-sustained skin temperatures in 81% of patients. Those who failed to derive benefit had extensive arterial disease with severe limitation of inflow through collateral vessels as the main cause. Failure can also be because of occurrence of shunting through an arteriovenous channel or precipitation of complete closure of already stenosed vessels (3).

Of the 35 patients who initially had rest pain, 71% obtained relief, which is an improvement over figures reported after surgical sympathectomies (3). Visual confirmation of predetermined spread of neurolytic agent permits an extended block of sympathetic fibers over three to four vertebral segments as well as catering for any aberrant sympathetic outflow. Healing of ischemic ulcers was noted in 8 (53%) of the 15 patients who had toe ulceration, and this figure compares favorably with results after surgical sympathectomy (1).

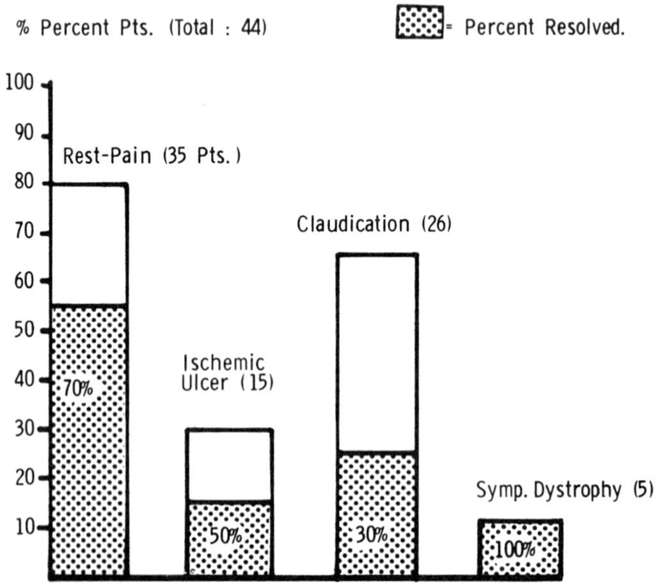

FIG. 2. Long-term follow-up results after lumbar chemical sympathectomy (1972 to 1975).

Claudication improved in 30% of the 26 patients who had this complaint. The incidence of improvement of claudication after sympathectomy varies from 13% to 75% (1,6). Reid et al. (5) found that improvement of claudication after chemical sympathectomy was 30% to 40% in patients with occlusion of the superficial femoral or femoropopliteal artery, although the incidence was only 11% in those with aortic-iliac occlusion. Sympathectomy was well sustained in all 5 patients with sympathetic dystrophy (Fig. 2).

In 2 patients sympathectomy helped in the demarcation of established gangrene of the toes, which were subsequently amputated. Following moderate improvement after sympathectomy, 2 patients were able to proceed to reconstructive surgery. Below knee amputation was carried out in only 4 patients followed in this series to date.

With this technique we have had none of the major complications encountered by other workers (5) employing percutaneous sympathectomy.

Up to the time of this writing, two deaths unrelated to sympathectomy have been recorded. One patient died of acute myocardial infarction 2 years later; the other died after 6 months from respiratory failure because of severe chronic obstructive pulmonary disease.

CONCLUSIONS

A two-needle technique of performing lumbar sympathetic block using 7% phenol in Conray 420 is described. Television X-ray screening is essential for the precision and success of the block.

The combination of phenol in Conray helps prevent inadvertent entry into vessels and, above all, confirms the desired anatomical spread of solution. Spectrometric analysis of this solution has confirmed the stability of this mixture. A wide and complete block achieved by this technique caters for aberrant sympathetic outflow.

The procedure entails minimal discomfort to the patient and is risk-free, requiring no hospitalization. It can be readily carried out at short notice in cases of rapidly progressing ischemia.

Results are comparable in both degree and duration of clinical response to those achieved by surgical sympathectomy. Based on the success of this technique, we recommend that this form of sympathectomy be used not only in poor risk patients but also as a standard procedure.

REFERENCES

1. Gillespie, J. A. (1960): *Br. Med. J.*, 2:1640–1642.
2. Lofstrom, B., and Zetterquist, S. (1967): *Acta Med. Scand.*, 182:23–39.
3. Myers, K. A., and Irvine, W. T. (1966): *Br. Med. J.*, 1:943–947.
4. Raskin, N. H., Levinstson, S. A., Hoffman, P. M., et al (1974): *Am. J. Surg.*, 128:75–78.
5. Reid, W., Watt, K. J., and Gray, T. G. (1970): *Br. J. Surg.*, 51:45–50.
6. Smithwick, R. H. (1957): *Surgery*, 42:567–578.

Advances in Pain Research and Therapy, Vol. 1,
edited by J. J. Bonica and D. Albe-Fessard.
Raven Press, New York © 1976.

Radiofrequency Denaturation in Occipital Pain: A New Approach in 114 Cases

Horst G. Blume

Clinical Associate Professor, Department of Neurosurgery, University of South Dakota, and Chief of Neurosurgery, St. Vincent Hospital, 809 Badgerow Building, Sioux City, Iowa 51101

Pain originating at the head-neck junction and radiating into the distribution of the major or minor occipital nerves can be generally referred to as occipital neuralgia and/or myalgia, regardless of actual C_2 nerve root involvement. One of the primary causes of occipital pain is trauma to the neck, especially when the head is abruptly rotated or hyperextended. However, any movement of the atlantoaxial joint can potentially irritate the C_2 nerve root with its sensory and sympathetic fibers or activate some myofascial trigger points. Many of the patients in this study suffered from so-called whiplash injury resulting from rear-end collisions or other automobile mishaps.

Treatment has typically involved a number of conservative approaches, such as neck stabilization with a cervical collar, traction, manipulation, occipital nerve blocks, steroids, hot and cold applications, ultrasound, electric current, and various medications. Avulsion of the greater occipital nerve has been performed successfully, but it usually results in recurrence of pain (4,6). Other surgical procedures, including division of the C_2 and C_3 posterior rootlets (1–4,7,8), have yielded more permanent results. However, more elaborate surgery such as cervical disc fusion may be required.

The present study uses a new approach that selectively denaturizes myofascial elements near the anatomical course of the main trunk of the major occipital nerve. The procedure involves percutaneous radiofrequency electrocoagulation, which I refer to as denaturation, in the region of the occipital nerve. The objective is to alleviate pain at the head-neck junction as well as any pain radiating into the region of the occipital nerve.

TECHNIQUE

The procedure may be performed in the outpatient department or in the doctor's office. A small area is shaved and "prepped" around the point of needle insertion which is 2 cm lateral to the midline and 3 cm below the occipital protuberance on the painful side. Interestingly enough, this is also the most tender spot at the head-neck junction. In the majority of cases the distance of entry was between 2 and 2.5 cm lateral to the midline (range 2 to 3.5 cm) and 3 cm below the occipital protuberance (range 2 to 3.5 cm). The actual lesion is approximately 2 cm below the occipital protuberance since the thermoelectrode is advanced cephalad at an angle of 45° to skin. (The probe tip itself is not really a "thermoelectrode" but merely radiates the radiofrequency energy, which in turn is converted to thermal energy through molecular friction resulting in protein coagulation.)

A local anesthetic such as 2% Xylocaine is injected into the skin of the scalp down to the periosteum. A special 14-gauge needle from the Radionics Spinal Facet Rhizotomy Kit is inserted at an angle of 45° to the skin pointing cephalad and nearly perpendicular to the occiput and advanced until the tip touches the occipital bone. The stylet is removed and replaced with the temperature-sensing radiofrequency thermoelectrode; the bare probe tip is inserted down to the periosteum. The guiding needle sleeve is withdrawn beyond the skin surface (Figs. 1 and 2).

The thermoelectrode and a wide-area skin surface-ground electrode are connected to the active and inactive inputs, respectively, of the radiofrequency lesion generator. The location of the thermoelectrode bare tip can be verified by applying a constant stimulation of 50 pulses per second

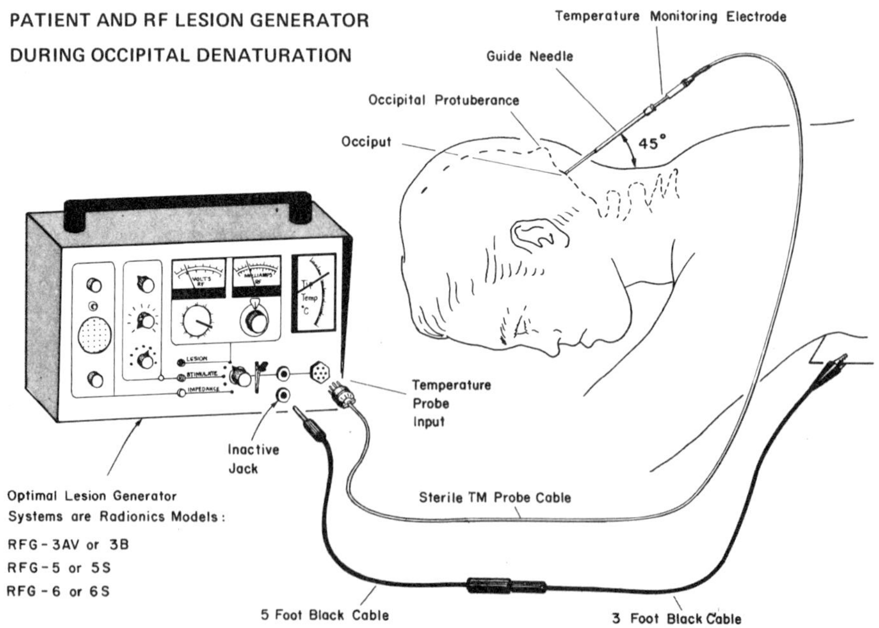

FIG. 1. Schematic drawing of the radiofrequency lesion generator with its connection to the thermoelectrode and ground. The temperature monitoring electrode is visualized with its tip in one location over the occipital bone.

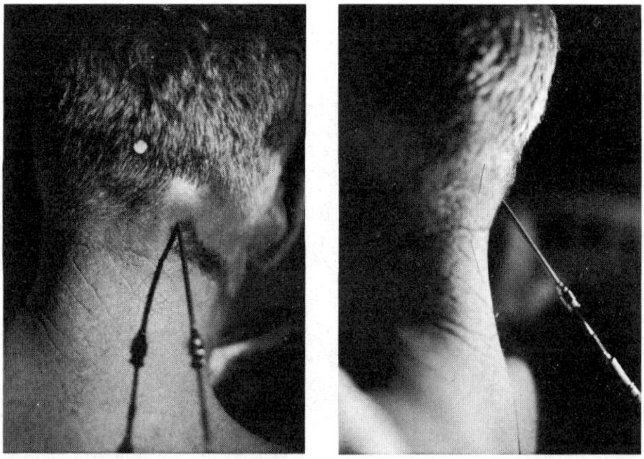

FIG. 2. Left: Temperature monitoring electrode in position with point of needle entry on skin surface 2 cm lateral to midline and 3 cm below occipital protuberance. **Right:** Lateral view to show direction of TM electrode; its angle with respect to the skin is about 45°.

and gradually increasing the output voltage up to 5 V. The patient experiences what is usually described as a tingling sensation at the head-neck junction. Confirmational electrical stimulation and X-ray films are not required in this technique (Fig. 3).

The heat denaturation is now done by raising the radiofrequency generator power until the electrode tip temperature reaches 85°C on the RFG panel meter, and this is held for 120 sec as read on the timer. The lesion around the uncoated tip will be a prolate spheroid with an axis of approximately 8 mm and a maximum diameter of 4 mm.

In the first 20 patients, only a single lesion was made on the affected side, whereas the remainder received a pair of lesions in each of three sections of the suboccipital region, as depicted in Fig. 4. The first lesion at 10 o'clock of each pair is closest to the superior neuchal line. The thermoelectrode with the guide needle is positioned by moving along the periosteum with the beveled edge down. After insertion, the guide needle is withdrawn and the first lesion is made at the point depicted by the dotted line in Fig. 4. Following the denaturation, the thermoelectrode is withdrawn 1 cm caudally and at all times is kept in contact with the periosteum for the second lesion indicated by the end of the solid line. The same techniques are followed for the other sections at 12 and 2 o'clock.

Patients with bilateral symptomatology and pain more prevalent on one side should have bilateral denaturations for a higher success rate.

After the probe is withdrawn, temporary compression is applied and ice packs are used to comfort the patient. In the occasional extremely sensitive patient, short anesthesia such as that induced by methohexital sodium (Brevital®) may prove helpful.

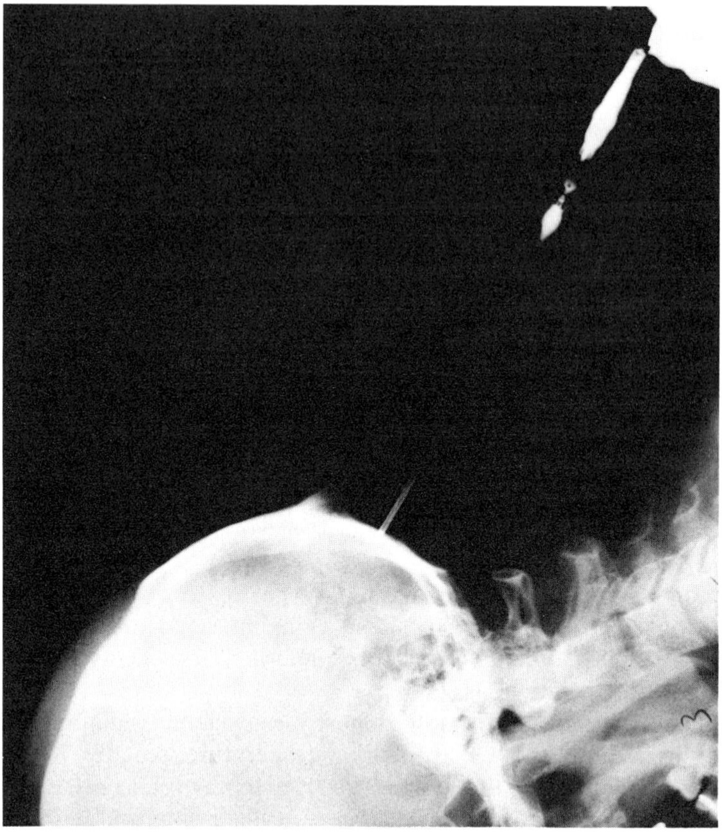

FIG. 3. Lateral X-ray film of occipital region visualizing entire thermoelectrode with its tip touching occipital bone 2 cm below the occipital protuberance where one of the denaturations takes place; X-ray confirmation is not essential.

RESULTS

The following criteria were established for evaluating the effectiveness of radiofrequency denaturation in relieving occipital pain: excellent—complete abolition of all pain originating at the head-neck junction and radiating into the distribution of the greater occipital nerve; good—relief of all pain except for transitory discomfort or mild occasional ache in the region of the greater occipital nerve; fair—significant (approximately 50%) reduction in frequency and intensity of pain; no result—pain remained unchanged. Included in the last group are patients whose pain recurred within 6 months.

The procedure has been applied to 114 consecutive cases with follow-up periods of 6 to 24 months.

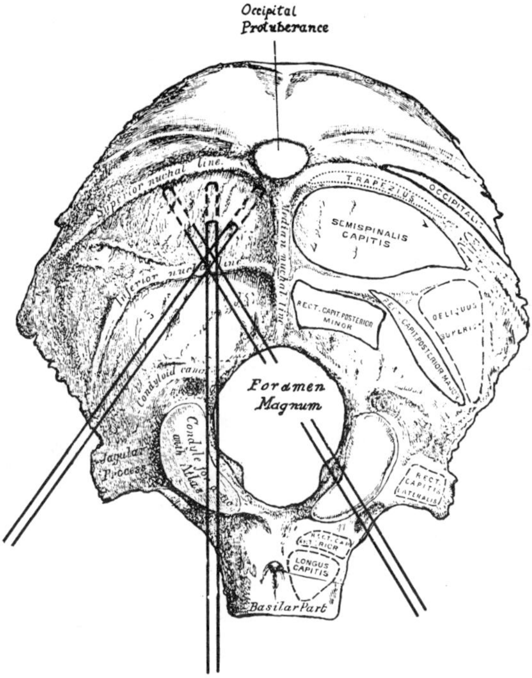

FIG. 4. Diagram of the positions of the thermoelectrode in three sections; the relationship to the occipital bone is shown on the left side and to muscles on the right side. Since additional lesions in each direction provide better results, the probe is usually first advanced to the side depicted by the dotted lines and following denaturation the probe is withdrawn to the location indicated by the solid line where a second lesion is made. In this typical case, the patient received denaturations at six points.

Table 1 summarizes the overall effectiveness of radiofrequency denaturation in relieving occipital pain. According to the established criteria, 78.1% of the patients exhibited good-to-excellent results, whereas 21.9% showed no results or only fair results.

TABLE 1. *Summary of results in 114 consecutive patients treated with denaturation in the greater occipital nerve territory*

Result	Number	Percent	
Excellent	84	73.7	78.1
Good	5	4.4	
Fair	5	4.4	21.9
None	20	17.5	

TABLE 2. *Results in patients with traumatic or nontraumatic origin of occipital pain*

	Traumatic			Nontraumatic	
Result	Number	Percent		Number	Percent
Excellent	55	72.0	78.6	29	76.3
Good	5	6.6		0	
Fair	4	5.3	21.3	1	23.7
None	12	16.0		8	
Total	76			38	

TABLE 3. *Overall results in patients with present or absent anatomical abnormalities*

	Abnormalities present			Abnormalities absent		
Result	Number	Percent		Number	Percent	
Excellent	56	68.3	74.4	29	90.7	
Good	5	6.1		0		
Fair	2	2.4	25.6	2	6.2	9.3
None	19	23.2		1	3.1	
Total	82			32		

Table 2 compares the effectiveness of treatment in patients whose occipital pain was either traumatic or nontraumatic in origin. The results in both groups conform closely with the overall percentages of good and excellent results.

Table 3 compares the results in patients with and without anatomical abnormalities. Patients without obvious abnormalities exhibited 90.7% excellent results, whereas those with confirmed abnormalities such as cervical spondylosis and disc disease showed 74.4% good-to-excellent results.

In 11 cases the initial denaturation was carried out bilaterally; results were excellent in 9 patients, all of whom had post-traumatic occipital pain. The 2 patients who experienced no results suffered pain of unknown origin.

The denaturation procedure was repeated in a total of 30 patients. Ten of these patients were re-treated on the same side with 50% good-to-excellent results. The other 20 patients in this group had their pain abolished previously on the prevalent side. After denaturation on the opposite side, 67% had excellent results and 33% showed no results.

DISCUSSION

The high success rate achieved with the denaturation procedure invites comments on the mechanisms that produce the analgesic effect. Several hypotheses can be proposed, but further research and more sophisticated diagnostic techniques are needed before these mechanisms can be explained conclusively.

Since the denaturations are near the occipital nerve and its branches, it would seem logical to consider the effect as arising from a modification of the function of the nerve fibers. The carefully temperature-controlled denaturation relieves occipital pain practically without any sensory deficit, and it is tempting to suggest that it selectively destroys pain-carrying fibers but leaves the sensory fibers relatively intact. Only 11% of the patients had transitory mild hypalgesia lasting for a few days up to a few weeks, and only 2% of the patients reported a permanent, mild sensory deficit.

If change in nerve function cannot account in part or entirely for the relief of pain by denaturation, then the existence of myofascial pain-triggering points should be considered. The occipital muscles and their envelopes and attachments can be the causative factor in the creation of pain. To answer the question of whether denaturation inactivates the pain-triggering points requires sophisticated diagnostic techniques and an extensive histopathological analysis.

Another possible explanation is that denaturation creates a focus of irritation, and this focus, even though in the scar phase, produces a relatively constant ascending input that may modify the pain impulses in some way. A similar mechanism is suggested by Melzack and Wall's (5) "gate control" theory of pain abatement, whereby external stimuli when applied to large fiber bundles interfere with small-fiber pain impulses at the first spinal synapse.

The relief of frontal headaches associated with occipital pain suggests another explanation. These headaches are probably caused by pain impulses rising from the mid-to-upper cervical region through short internuncial neurons into the trigeminal nucleus. Perhaps the denaturation process has interrupted the reflex arch.

A psychosomatic component in occipital pain cannot be ignored, and it has been considered in several patients. Nevertheless, excellent results were obtained and no recurrence of original pain or displacement of pain has been established.

The percentage of excellent results in the group without anatomical abnormalities exceeded the 30% effectiveness that could be accepted as a purely "placebo" effect. Prior to radiofrequency denaturation, 50% of all the patients underwent one or more occipital nerve blocks using a local anesthetic mixed with cortisone, and this resulted in only temporary relief of occipital pain.

The importance of precision temperature control should be emphasized since we are dealing with a selective denaturation of tissue. Following this guideline, the procedure has entailed minimal risk, low morbidity, and no complications.

REFERENCES

1. Buer, E. E. (1956): *Formen des Posttraumatischen Kopfschmerzen (der Neuralgische Schmerz)*, 111 p. Georg Thieme Verlag, Stuttgart.
2. Chambers, W. R. (1954): *J.A.M.A.*, 155:431–432.
3. Hunter, C. R., and Mayfield, F. H. (1949): *Am. J. Surg.*, 78:743–751.
4. Mayfield, F. H., and Hunter, C. R. (1952): Presented at meeting of American Academy of Neurological Surgery, October 1, New York.
5. Melzack, R., and Wall, P. D. (1965): *Science*, 150:971–979.
6. Roaf, J. (1948): *Am. J. Surg.*, 76:567–577.
7. Wanke, R., and Bues, E. (1953): *Chirurgie*, 24:306–311.
8. White, J. C., and Sweet, W. H. (1969): *Pain and the Neurosurgeon. A Forty Year Experience.* Charles C Thomas, Publisher, Springfield, Illinois.

Advances in Pain Research and Therapy, Vol. 1,
edited by J. J. Bonica and D. Albe-Fessard.
Raven Press, New York © 1976.

Clinical Evaluation of Subarachnoid Neurolytic Blocks in Intractable Cancer Pain

V. Ventafridda and G. Martino

National Tumor Institute, Via Venezian, 20100 Milan, Italy

The injection of neurolytic agents into the subarachnoid space is considered by many clinicians as one of the simplest and most effective methods of relieving intractable cancer pain (1,3,5–7). Nevertheless, certain factors make the procedure difficult and the results unpredictable. One of these is the presence of disease of the spinal column due to either the age of the patient or the disease process itself. Such a defect makes it difficult for the patient to assume the specific position needed for the injection and consequently prevents the neurolytic agent from affecting the posterior rootlets of the spinal segments involved in the pain. A second factor is the instability of the chemical agent in the cerebrospinal fluid. When the neurolytic agent is combined with a radiopaque medium, we note the diffusion of the substance from the target area with every movement of the thoracic and abdominal cage. A third consideration is that even if there is evidence of a chemical rhizotomy after the injection, it is not possible to know whether the neurolytic agent has caused a reversible or irreversible interruption of nociceptor fibers. Sometimes not only the posterior rootlets but also some of the anterior rootlets are affected, resulting in skeletal muscle weakness, visceral dysfunction, or both.

Another important consideration is that it is difficult to produce a selective damage of C and A-delta fibers because other fibers can be affected (9). Recent electromicroscopic studies on rootlet specimens after intrathecal injection showed different degrees of fragmentation of the myelin sheath and axon degeneration. In animal experiments it has been found that remyelinization of surviving axons occurs in a short time and thus increases the number of functioning fibers (2). For this reason the results are often reversible and of short duration.

Since this method is usually performed only on patients with inoperable or recurrent cancer, it is important to consider the specific mechanism by which the tumor involves nerve fibers directly or indirectly. Neoplastic invasion can be localized in highly pain-sensitive tissues like fascial periosteum, tumor cells can infiltrate nerve trunks, or the tumor can cause obstruction of a hollow viscus or a larger artery with consequent ischemic pain or a large vein with consequent edema and pain. An inflammatory process is often present in the superficial tissues of the tumor with a well-defined area of pain. The pain and related symptomatology can vary in intensity and location and can either be due to direct involvement of nerves by the lesion or be referred far from the neoplastic invasion. Obviously, it is essential to know accurately the mechanism of pain and the nociceptive pathways involved.

With this background, we present an analysis of results obtained with neurolytic blocks achieved with either alcohol or phenol in glycerine in a total of 227 patients treated at the National Cancer Institute of Milan, Italy. In this chapter we will not include data on the specific type of neurolytic agent used, but rather we want to focus on the anatomic area or structure involved by the neoplasm and its type as diagnosed by X-ray, scintigraphic, or lymphangiographic studies and considered to be the source of pain. The pain was well localized and monolateral in most patients, with the exception of some of those with terminal cancer.

RESULTS

The results for each patient were classified as: good when the block produced complete relief of pain for more than 6 days; and poor when the block produced partial or no pain relief. We have also analyzed the number of blocks performed for each type of pain syndrome, the mean duration of pain relief after a single injection in each patient who had a good result with each specific type of lesion, and the incidence of complications. Many patients underwent several injections in order to extend or enhance the degree of pain relief.

A total of 319 neurolytic blocks were performed. The patients have been segregated into three groups according to the spinal segments involved by the neurolytic block. In the first group we have included patients with pain localized in the cervical and upper thoracic region (C_7 to T_5); in the second group the pain involved the abdominal area or the posterior part of the trunk (T_5 to T_{12}); patients in the third group had pain mostly in the pelvis, sacrum, and lower limbs (L_1 to S_5).

Among the patients in the first group (Table 1) were those mostly affected by lung cancer (Pancoast's tumor) and breast cancer with neoplastic involvement of the thoracic wall and the brachial plexus monolaterally. Patients whose neoplastic invasion involved the thoracic wall including the skin obtained remarkably good relief of pain with neurolytic blocks. In contrast, the results were poor when the tumor involved the parenchymal tissue. Analgesia of the brachial plexus produced functional complications of the homolateral arm and a dysesthesia lasting a few weeks.

The pain in patients of the second group (Table 2) was caused primarily by neoplastic involvement of the viscera except that in some patients the pain was caused by tumor involvement of the abdominal wall. Apart from

TABLE 1. *Group 1—subarachnoid neurolytic blocks for pain in the cervical and thoracic area (C_7–T_5)*

Patients (no.)	No. of blocks	Area of tumor involvement	Good results No.	Good results % (of patients)	Mean duration of pain relief (days)	Complications
17	23	Chest wall	12	71	21	0
25	42	Lung and chest wall	11	44	12	2
11	13	Lung and pleura	1	9	10	1
27	39	Upper lung, brachial plexus	15	56	18	14
9	15	Vertebral	3	33	16	2
Total 89	132		42	47		19 = 21.34%

these latter patients, the results with neurolytic blocks for cancer pain of the viscera have been extremely poor. We encountered some complications in patients affected by radicular pain from vertebral disease that had also caused a slight muscular weakness in the lower limbs. Pathologic conditions in the spinal cord itself do not respond to pain relief and are vulnerable to complications.

Patients in the third group (Table 3) usually are in the last stages of the disease. In many of these patients there was neoplastic invasion of the viscera and surrounding soft tissues with lymph node involvement. In others, the neoplasm involved skeletal structures of the pelvis and lower limbs. Some of these patients had loss of sphincter function with bilateral pain syndrome in the sacral and lumbar areas. In these latter cases, neurolytic blocks produced more satisfactory results with a total regression of pain for

TABLE 2. *Group 2—subarachnoid neurolytic blocks for pain in abdominal and dorsal area (T_5–T_{12})*

Patients (no.)	No. of blocks	Area of tumor involvement	Good results No.	Good results % (of patients)	Mean duration of pain relief (days)	Complications
15	18	Splancnic (pancreas, liver, bowels)	3	20	8	1
9	14	Kidney, ureter	1	11	9	2
18	21	Abdominal and dorsal wall	15	83	27	5
11	15	Vertebral	5	45	18	7
Total 53	68		24	45		15 = 28.3%

TABLE 3. *Group 3—subarachnoid neurolytic blocks for pain in the pelvic, sacral, and lower limbs area (L_1–S_5)*

Patients (no.)	No. of blocks	Area of tumor involvement	Good results No. (of patients)	Good results %	Mean duration of pain relief (days)	Complications
14	21	Visceral + soft tissues	7	50	9	4
13	19	Visceral, soft tissues, + bone structure	6	46	14	6
10	12	Pelvic bone structure	7	70	12	7
21	37	Perineal	18	86	11	13
16	18	Sacral bilateral	15	94	21	16
11	12	Lower limbs	10	91	25	11
Total 85	119		63	74		57 = 67%

at least 3 weeks. The same can be said for pain localized to lower limbs; therefore, one can use a single large administration of the neurolytic drug, especially if there is no concern about ambulation. In contrast, the results have been poor in patients with predominant visceral pain.

It is also difficult to obtain prolonged relief of pain in the perineal area because of the high incidence of complications. Even with the most careful and accurate technique (8), S_2 and, more often, S_3 roots usually are not spared by the block. Therefore, the only way to minimize complications is to do a unilateral block. In the last group, complications were more frequent than in the other two groups. Most of the complications (Table 4) did not last more than 1 month. Sometimes bladder and rectal disturbances were the

TABLE 4. *Complications after 319 subarachnoid neurolytic blocks in 227 patients*

Duration	Muscle weakness No.	Muscle weakness %	Paresis No.	Paresis %	Bladder/rectal disturbances No.	Bladder/rectal disturbances %
Less than 1 week	17	7	3	1	6	3
Less than 1 month	11	5	16	7	13	6
Greater than 1 month	9	4	5	2	11	5

Results of neurolytic subarachnoid blocks in 227 patients

Pain relief	Mean time pain relief (days)	Complications
56.3%	15.4	40.1%

price that the patient had to pay in order to have pain relief. Muscle weakness and paresis were rapidly improved with rehabilitative therapy.

As noted in Table 4, the overall results among our group of patients were good in approximately 56%, with the mean duration of pain relief of 15.4 days. The incidence of complications in the entire group was approximately 40%. Our results are not as good as those reported by others (3,4) but, as previously mentioned, patients who derived only partial relief were not included in the "good" results.

CONCLUSIONS

Our experience suggests that neurolytic subarachnoid blocks must be restricted to those patients with advanced metastatic cancer with severe monolateral and well-circumscribed pain and in whom the neoplastic involvement is related to specific spinal segments. Notwithstanding the figures and complications, we believe that this technique properly executed (good positioning, right needle placement, and careful injection) still has a definite albeit limited place in cancer pain therapy. For patients who are still in good general condition and in whom the disease has not reached the terminal stage, neurosurgical interruption, like cordotomy and rhizotomy, may be a better form of therapy.

REFERENCES

1. Bonica, J. J. (1953): *The Management of Pain,* pp. 488–509. Lea & Febiger, Philadelphia.
2. Flanigan, S., and Boop, W. C. (1973): *Clin. Neurosurg.,* 21:229–238.
3. Hay, R. C., Yonezova, T., and Derrick, W. S. (1959): *J.A.M.A.,* 169:1315–1320.
4. Kuzucu, E. Y., Derrick, W. S., and Wilber, S. A. (1966): *J.A.M.A.,* 195:541.
5. Maher, R. M. (1955): *Lancet,* 1:18.
6. Maher, R. M. (1963): *Lancet,* 1:965.
7. Mark, V. H., White, J. C., Zervas, N. T., Ervin, F. R., and Richardson, E. P. (1962): *N. Engl. J. Med.,* 267:589.
8. Mehta, M. (Ed.) (1973): *Intractable Pain,* pp. 179–180. W. B. Saunders Co., Philadelphia.
9. Nathan, P. V. (1965): *J. Neurol. Sci.,* 2:7–29.

Advances in Pain Research and Therapy, Vol. 1,
edited by J. J. Bonica and D. Albe-Fessard.
Raven Press, New York © 1976.

Cardiorespiratory Effects of Treatment of Postcholecystectomy Pain by Pethidine or Intercostal Block

C. Devaux, D. Franckhauser, E. Dumeny, and P. Gauthier-Lafaye

Department of Anesthesiology, University of Strasbourg, France

DISCUSSION GÉNÉRALE

De l'étude la première série, nous pouvons tirer les conclusions suivantes:

Tout ce qui a été dit auparavant par Bromage, Whahba, Bonica, Holmdahl, Sjögren, Wright, se trouve confirmé sur le plan de la fonction respiratoire, spécialement au niveau de la fixation de l'oxygène (élévation de la PO_2 et de la saturation) en sont les reflets au niveau de la gazométrie sanguine.

Par contre, nous n'avons pas retrouvé d' étude comparative du transit intestinal post-opératoire, on ne peut donc que constater cette grande différence de résultats, en se rappelant que les effets sur le transit intestinal, de l'ouverture du péritoine sont majorés par l'action secondaire du morphinique.

Pour la seconde série de notre étude, la revue de la littérature ne nous a pas donné d'exemples de mesure du débit cardiaque au cours de la phase douloureuse post-opératoire. Cependant, on ne peut qu'être frappé par la similitude des courbes des quatre malades de chaque série. Les variations brutales de débit cardiaque au cours de l'analgésie réalisées par la Pethidine (−15 à 25% et + 60 à 80%) doivent conduire à penser que l'administration de ce produit, du fait de ses effets secondaires sur le plan cardio-circulatoire, reste à discuter surtout lors des 10 premières heures post-opératoires.

Les variations de ces mêmes débits cardiaques chez les malades analgésiés par bloc intercostal sont beaucoup moins amples (−0% et + 10 à 15%), et ne peuvent donc que majorer les effets de la dynamique ventilatoire, dans le cadre d'une meilleure saturation oxyhémoglobinée, d'où amélioration de l'oxygénation tissulaire.

Les variations comparatives des ΔPAP et ΔRPT reflètent ce qui se traduit au niveau des débits cardiaques couplées avec le pouls, l'accélération de celui-ci dénote la sommation des effets sympathomimétiques de la douleur et para-sympathomimétiques de la Pethidine en fonction de la dose administrée; cependant il reste que c'est le seul avec le Dextromoramide que l'on peut utiliser actuellement au cours de la phase post-opératoire immédiate sans support ventilatoire mécanique.

A l'opposé l'utilisation de morphine et en dehors du risque de toxicomanie non négligeable, de même que les autres analgésiques puissants type Fentanyl, Phénopéridine, Piritramide, ne peuvent être utilisés qu'avec l'assistance ventilatoire mécanique.

Cependant le relevé de nos mesures de débit cardiaque, ΔPAP-ΔRPT concorde avec le profil de l'activité de la Pethidine: Début d'action: 5 minutes; Activité maximale: 15 minutes; Durée d'activité maximale: 47 minutes, tel qu'il a été proposé par Viars et De Castro.

Quant à l'étude comparative de la gazométrie sanguine artérielle, celle-ci est le reflet et la conséquence sur le plan de l'hématose et de la circulation, de ce qui a été discuté auparavant.

Advances in Pain Research and Therapy, Vol. 1,
edited by J. J. Bonica and D. Albe-Fessard.
Raven Press, New York © 1976.

Nerve Blocks and Contingency Management in Chronic Pain States

*Steven F. Brena and **Irving P. Unikel

*Emory Pain Clinic, and Departments of *Anesthesiology and **Psychiatry, Emory University School of Medicine, Atlanta, Georgia 30322*

Results are presented of a treatment program employing operant conditioning procedures and sympathetic nerve blocks in an outpatient setting to increase the activities and range of behavior of selected patients with chronic pain. Furthermore, the utility of the Minnesota Multiphasic Personality Inventory (MMPI) in the selection of patients for such treatment was investigated.

First considering the psychodiagnostic question, we administered the MMPI to 77 patients with a variety of chronic pain states and to a control group of 51 medical patients with other diagnoses. All were patients who had been referred by a physician for psychological assessment. The two groups showed clearly elevated, distinct, and different MMPI profiles. The mean profile obtained for the chronic pain patients represents what has been called the "conversion valley" pattern (2). There are elevations of the Hypochondriasis (Hs) and Hysteria (Hy) scales, and both of these are greater than the Depression (D) scale.[1] The control medical patients display the mean profile: Hs > D > Hy.

Considering the distinction between the two profiles in the framework of learning theory, drawing on the earlier analysis by Meehl (ref. in 2), we feel that the behavior reflected in the profile of the chronic pain patients involves operants and is "purposive." Secondary gain predominates and an operant may be strengthened or its strength maintained by reward. On the other hand, the psychosomatic symptoms manifested by the medical controls are respondent and "non-purposive," and secondary gains do not contribute significantly to symptom maintenance. The latter is hypothesized to be a function of anxiety and associated physiological hyperreactivity. Therefore, the results of our psychological assessment suggested that the MMPI would be useful in predicting patients who would benefit from an operant conditioning program, and that chronic pain patients were included in this

[1] These results have since been reproduced and cross-validated on a different sample of patients.

category (whereas control medical patients should benefit most from different procedures emphasizing anxiety reduction).

The contingency management program that we designed for chronic pain patients employed principles of operant conditioning and extended the findings with inpatients of previous investigators—e.g., Fordyce et al. (1)—to an outpatient setting. Thus each patient's behavior occurred in its natural environment, allowing a wider range of activities and presumably increasing the potential for the maintenance and generalization of treatment effects. Subjects received medical treatment in the form of nerve blocks for symptomatic relief of painful sensation as reinforcement that was contingent on appropriate behavior. Specific behavioral requirements were determined for each patient involving programmed changes in the amount, intensity, and variability of selected activities. The patients were also required to remain free of habit-forming drugs.

Initial evaluation included a medical examination and psychological and behavioral assessments. Before the contingency management program, the use of habit-forming drugs was discontinued, using drug withdrawal methods when necessary. Only aspirin or similar drugs were allowed. Daily activity was recorded for a 1-week period to determine a base line.

Subsequently, changes in daily activities were prescribed as was appropriate in each case. Emphasis was placed on the necessity and desirability of performing various activities from the patient's point of view. Prescribed activities increased from "up-time," such as walking, through more strenuous tasks such as household chores, exercises, and active sports.

Nerve blocks were administered weekly when the patient achieved the prescribed criteria until six nerve blocks had been received. Sympathetic nerve blocks were performed by routine techniques currently described in textbooks, using 0.25% butylpipecoloxylidide hydrochloride (Marcaine®) with epinephrine. Daily recording of activities was maintained for 4 weeks after the termination of the treatment program. Patients were given follow-up evaluations at intervals of 4 weeks and 6 months after treatment (Fig. 1).

The results indicate that the amount of activity was increased during the contingency management program and was maintained up to 6 months by patients completing the program. These data represent a total of 54 patients completing the program. Four-week follow-up evaluations were completed on 35 of the 54 patients, and 6-month evaluations were completed on 6 of those 35 patients. Follow-up evaluations were pending for the remainder of the 54 patients.

Since all patients who complete the program increase in their activities by definition, a conservative estimate of the success rate for the program was computed by comparing the 54 patients who completed the program with the total of 83 patients who began the program (i.e., including all patients who dropped out or did not meet the requirements of the program). The success rate obtained was 65%.

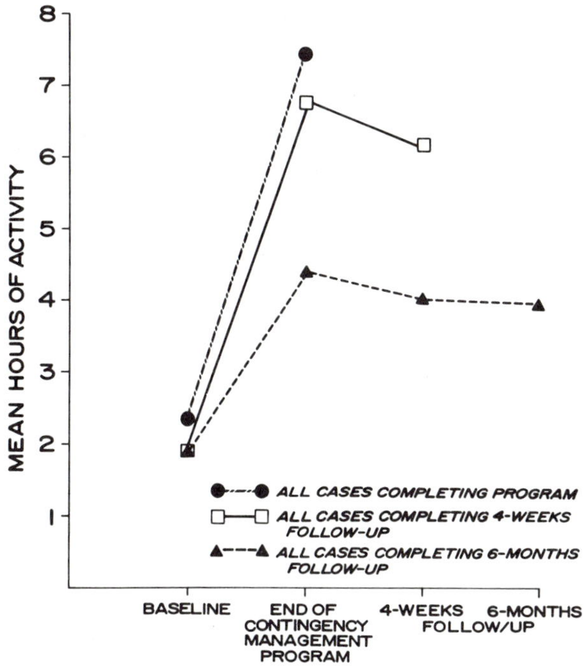

FIG. 1. Mean hours of activity at base line, end, and follow-up of contingency management program for chronic pain states.

It should also be noted that computing the results of the subgroup of 24 patients who completed the program in approximately the past 2 months and those of the 9 comparable dropped patients yielded a success rate of 74%. The data suggest an increase in program effectiveness over time, since newer patients included in the program achieved higher levels of activity as a result of the program. This improvement was presumably because of refinement of the procedures, although it must be further investigated and analyzed.

Although the results reported here focus on increases in the amount of activity, increases in the intensity and variability of activities were generally obtained and maintained. Patients who were formerly spending much of their time in bed or otherwise limiting their activities because of chronic pain learned to perform normal household chores, became involved in recreational activities, and even returned to their jobs in certain cases. This treatment program therefore appears to be effective overall. A study is underway to extend these findings and to determine the relative effectiveness—individually and in combination—of components of the program such as contingency management, nerve blocks, and placebo effects on activity and on a number of other dependent variables.

REFERENCES

1. Fordyce, W. E., Fowler, R. S., Lehmann, J. F., DeLateur, B. J., Sand, P. L. and Trieschmann, R. B. (1974): In: *Annual Review of Behavior Therapy Theory and Practice 1974,* edited by C. M. Franks and G. T. Wilson, pp. 691–712. Brunner/Mazel, New York.
2. Gilberstadt, H., and Duker, J. (1965): *A Handbook for Clinical and Actuarial MMPI Interpretation,* 134 pp. W. B. Saunders Co., Philadelphia.

Advances in Pain Research and Therapy, Vol. 1,
edited by J. J. Bonica and D. Albe-Fessard.
Raven Press, New York © 1976.

Psychiatric Aspects of the Control of Pain

H. Merskey

The National Hospitals for Nervous Diseases, Queen Square, London WC1N 3BG, England

There are many observations in literature generally which illuminate the problems that have been discussed. Of all those available the one I like best is from Montaigne (8), *"Nous sentons plus un coup de rasoir du chirurgien que dix coups d'epée en la chaleur du combat."* (We feel one nick from the surgeon's scalpel more than 10 blows of the sword in the heat of combat.) In that sentence we see the magnification of pain by anxiety and the dissipation of it by more extreme arousal.

The contribution by Sternbach makes it abundantly clear that psychological and other factors are of much importance in the production and relief of pain. It is not necessary for me to dwell on the point. My task is to review the psychiatric strategies available to relieve or control pain. I should also take into account the strategies we possess to relieve patients, which is of course not quite the same thing as relieving pain, since it sometimes happens that anxiety or depression or other mood changes may persist even after pain is relieved. However, that is not too frequent a problem, although the converse occurrence, the persistence of pain after the relief of an abnormal mood, is, I think, somewhat more common.

In talking about the psychiatric strategies, I should like to deal not so much with the fine details of psychiatric diagnosis and treatment, which always seem rather amorphous to the uninitiated, but with the leads psychiatry may be able to give a nonpsychiatrist.

REALITY OF PAIN

The first priority of the psychiatrist in the pain clinic is to establish for all patients, without exception, that their pain is treated as real. All too frequently patients are told that they are "imagining" their pain, when no physical cause can be found for it. It is actually rather hard to imagine a pain; it is even difficult, as Ernest Jones noticed (4), to recollect the experience of severe pain. If patients have pain for psychological reasons, and many do, this must usually occur because of the operation of mental mechanisms that produce it independently of the patient's conscious wishes. Such pain may depend on a mechanism of muscle tension and anxiety but may also arise as a conversion symptom or as a depressive or, very rarely, a schizophrenic hallucination (6). In all these cases the reality of the patient's experience must be honored; and it will still prove possible to discuss with him the emotional state that may be producing or exacerbating his pain.

It is easier to honor the patient's experience if we keep in mind that whatever the physical basis for a pain it can be known to an individual only through his consciousness. Thus pain is only and always a psychological experience. As such it can be discussed only in psychological terms.

I do not for one moment deny that we all want to know a lot more about the fascinating physical mechanisms that often correspond to these psychological experiences we call pain. But I want to insist that even if we do not find a physiological or pathological mechanism we should not deny the patient's pain. The patient's experience is the first and basic datum for all clinicians, and the psychiatrist in the pain clinic who discusses the symptoms seriously and carefully with the patient will almost always secure a positive and cooperative response, even from those patients who initially resent the referral. The physician, surgeon, or anesthetist, who normally takes this approach in any case, is in at least as strong a position and can use it to inquire into the patient's mood and personal life so as to discover if there is an important psychological factor promoting the pain.

RESENTMENT AND REST

Nevertheless, many patients with pain do express resentment. Thus in a controlled study (5), 30 out of 76 (39%) of psychiatric patients with pain expressed resentment, whereas only 5 out of 37 (14%) of a group without pain were resentful. Of the 30 in the larger group, 15 patients blamed their relations or other people in their environment for their circumstances and their pain. Three patients blamed doctors alone for the way they were and 12 patients blamed both doctors and others impartially. It seems that resentment is aroused in patients with pain fairly readily, and that it is easily attached to doctors and others, but that we are not quite the main object of this ill-feeling.

It is likely that a few patients with special dynamic problems are destined to focus their resentment specifically on doctors. Cramer et al. (1) showed in a penetrating study of some patients with the so-called Munchausen syndrome that physicians had been particularly important in the early lives of those individuals—and had occupied roles in which they were, at different times, and in the patient's view, both helpful and unhelpful. But such cases are rare, and the majority of patients with pain who turn against doctors probably do so because they are disappointed in their hopes of cure and dissatisfied with the attention the doctor gives them. Sometimes certainly this arises because, with patients we have failed to cure, we are disappointed and become brusque. Those of us who venture to give a great deal of time to treatment as well as to diagnosis inevitably like best those patients who are treated successfully.

Some psychiatric techniques that all physicians can practice are to avoid this sort of response, to be aware of one's own reactions, to be patient and detached, and to remain sympathetic. This approach is not a monopoly of psychiatrists, nor do psychiatrists always manage it as well as we should, but perhaps we have to use it more often than other specialists. Therefore I regard it as one of those psychiatric strategies that sometimes relieves the pain and more often relieves the patient.

Another aspect of resentment deserves brief mention but strong emphasis. In England since the work of John Hilton (3) in 1863 on rest and pain, we have been indoctrinated with the belief that pain produces rest and that the rest is beneficial to injured parts. I would not be in the least surprised to find that a similar doctrine holds sway throughout the world. Yet this reasonable and well-accepted point of view ignores an important biological phenomenon. Pain is an indication of damage to the body and of possible danger. There are times, for example, when pain is inflicted by an aggressor, when the response should be one of vigorous action. As with anxiety that action may be fight or flight. We should expect that patients with visceral pain or joint pain may not be ready to be active. Many patients with pain of nerve lesions, which is often referred to the skin—the barrier between the body and the outside world—may well show aggression. We know in fact that irritability is an important part of some pain syndromes. We all think it wise to avoid a bear with a sore head, an English expression I expect to find in many other languages. There is indeed some formal evidence from psychologists (12,13) that pain provokes aggression. We need hardly be surprised, and we ought to keep this in mind as part of our understanding of how to deal with patients with pain.

In one situation the sympathetic approach to pain may not be entirely justified: when patients are conscious that they can get some special advantage, particularly compensation, from their pain. In the case of back pain, compensation problems often occur and are compounded by the fact that rest tends to relieve the pain. Thus both physical and conscious psychological causes clearly combine to make patients reduce their activity and perhaps overemphasize their discomfort.

The unconscious psychological or intrapsychic advantage from pain can be tackled by interpretative psychotherapy. But a financial advantage from pain cannot be handled that way. Instead, two centers have reported the behavioral management of patients with chronic low back pain (2,10). Those who run behavioral management programs for the patients of this sort are fully aware that they are not transforming the subjective situation and that they leave themselves open to misunderstanding. Yet beneficial results in terms of a better life and more active mobilization of the patient undoubtedly can be obtained on occasion by deliberately ignoring his misery and encouraging him to do things about which he overtly used to complain. It is not a perfect solution.

Indeed, I do not think we have an adequate solution for the diagnostic and therapeutic problems and the personal relationships involved in dealing with patients who complain of low back pain without significant physical and psychological evidence in support of their complaint. This is especially so when low back pain serves to take patients away from some activity they dislike or promises some monetary reward. This is one of the unsolved problems of the pain clinic. It is hard to say to a patient whose pain is made worse by activity and who yet has little evidence to support either an organic or a psychiatric diagnosis, "You are making more of your pain than you should be doing." Nevertheless, some of Sternbach's matching techniques (10) for comparing the patient's spontaneous pain with induced pain allow us to recognize that the level of spontaneous pain about which the patient may complain may be trivial. In those cases it is possible to take a fairly firm line, but only after full examination and study.

GUIDANCE AND SUPPORT

I now come, albeit briefly, to the major phenomena with which the psychiatrist has to deal in his ordinary consultative work. These phenomena are not unique to patients with pain. They affect equally patients with anxiety, depression, and to some extent even those with schizophrenia and postoperative psychoses. All major depressing, stressful, alarming, or intractable life events may provoke emotional reactions in the individual. Every physician must tease out the strands of the provoking situation, straighten a tangled network of interactions, relieve tension on some of those strands, perhaps increase it on others so that an undue burden is taken off a patient, and generally act as a wise adviser. The physician probably has to go somewhat beyond the role of a simple adviser and do some things that involve interference in the patient's life and relationships with other people. It is, I think, hypocrisy to pretend that doctors do not intervene, at times actively, in the conduct of their patients' lives and do not give them much more positive advice than they are nominally supposed to do. Yet as a young psychiatrist I was taught, and indeed earlier in this chapter I suggested, that we should follow a more passive pattern and treat all patients with an attitude of neutral detached sympathy. For the beginner this is excellent advice. For the experienced doctor it is also excellent advice, but when the interventions are likely to be favorably received by all parties, the experienced doctor will take steps to encourage people to do things that strictly he should leave to the patient to decide. It is not a neutral act to tell a man to take his wife out more often or to change his job, but sometimes this may be necessary. Such advice must always be given tentatively, never vigorously or against significant resistance by the patient.

MEDICATION

Let me turn next to the use of drugs in psychiatry and in the control of pain. I cannot review this subject at length in this chapter, but two points can be made. First, as is well known, some antidepressant drugs are miraculous in their effect on patients with pain that seems to have an organic origin. One of my patients was recently relieved of gross postthoracotomy intercostal neuralgia by the simple application of a vibrator and cold spray followed by enough amitriptyline to enable him to sleep at night. After 18 months of helpless misery he is now actively looking for work. I do not know if this is because of the cure of a depression, which was certainly present, or cure of a pain that might have been causing the depression. This dilemma confronts us repeatedly. However, all doctors treating pain—not only psychiatrists—can benefit from becoming familiar with one or two antidepressant drugs and using them carefully in a dosage that is adjusted precisely for each individual.

In the case just cited, it is not clear whether the patient improved because of an antidepressant or an analgesic effect of the drug. We could, however, assume that it was an antidepressant effect. In other cases the psychiatric drugs that relieve pain are patently not those one would choose for either anxiety or depression. They are usually phenothiazines, which today are really indicated only for patients with schizophrenia—among the psychiatric syndromes—and certainly not for those with neurosis or depression, which they can make worse. Yet several phenothiazines, e.g., chlorpromazine, methotrimeprazine (9), pericyazine (7), and fluphenazine (11), have all been praised in the relief of pain. I label these drugs "psychiatric" because their main oral use is in psychiatric work, and they certainly are tranquilizers that act on higher functions of the central nervous system. But they probably also have an additional analgesic effect.

OTHER TECHNIQUES

Many other psychiatric techniques are available, including relaxation, suggestion, and deep psychotherapy for a few patients who have intractable human problems that seem to be causing their pain; electroshock therapy for those with severe depression; and biofeedback, particularly for patients with headache (where results seem fairly promising) and perhaps for those with other pain syndromes as well. Biofeedback is an important area in which systematic information is being offered us today, and about which we shall certainly want more in the next few years. At the moment it seems likely that it will find a useful place in the treatment of tension headache and migraine.

REFERENCES

1. Cramer, B., Gershberg, M., and Stern, M. (1971): *Arch. Gen. Psychiatry,* 24:573.
2. Fordyce, W. (1974): In: *Advances in Neurology, Vol. 4: International Symposium on Pain,* edited by J. J. Bonica, pp. 415–422. Raven Press, New York.
3. Hilton, J. (1950): In: *Rest and Pain,* edited by E. W. Watts and E. Philipp. G. Bell, London.
4. Jones, E. (1957): *Int. J. Psychoanal.,* 38:255.
5. Merskey, H. (1965): *J. Psychosom. Res.,* 9:299.
6. Merskey, H. (1968): *Postgrad. Med. J.,* 44:297.
7. Merskey, H., and Hester, R. N. (1972): *Postgrad. Med. J.,* 48:594.
8. Montaigne, M. E. de (1865): In: *Essais,* edited by J.-V. Le Clerc, pp. 374–375. Garnier Freres, Paris.
9. Sigwald, J., Hebert, H., and Quentin, A. (1957): *Sem. Hop. Paris,* 33:1137.
10. Sternbach, R. A. (1974): *Pain Patients: Traits and Treatment.* Academic Press, New York.
11. Taub, A., and Collins, W. F. (1974): In: *Advances in Neurology, Vol. 4: International Symposium on Pain,* edited by J. J. Bonica, pp. 309–315. Raven Press, New York.
12. Ulrich, R. E. (1966): *Am. Zoologist,* 6:643.
13. Ulrich, R. E., Hutchinson, P. R., and Azrin, N. H. (1965): *Psychol. Rec.,* 15:111.

Advances in Pain Research and Therapy, Vol. 1,
edited by J. J. Bonica and D. Albe-Fessard.
Raven Press, New York © 1976.

Mechanisms of Hypnotic Pain Control

Martin T. Orne

The Institute of Pennsylvania Hospital, and University of Pennsylvania, Philadelphia, Pennsylvania 19139

The dramatic pain suppressant effect of hypnoanesthesia has for a long time been a source of fascination and controversy. Surgical procedures ranging from appendectomies to thyroidectomies and from cesarean sections to open heart surgery have been carried out with hypnosis as the sole anesthetic, providing impressive and tangible evidence of the effectiveness that psychological factors can have in suppressing pain. Although it cannot be doubted that these procedures have been carried out with hypnosis, the interpretation of this fact remains a source of controversy.

In this chapter we shall seek to clarify questions about the reality of hypnoanesthesia, to juxtapose clinical evidence with laboratory data, and to address the apparent paradox that although over 90% of the population shows an increase of pain threshold with appropriate hypnotic suggestions, only a small percentage of unselected subjects can enter deep hypnosis. Finally, an effort will be made to suggest that two different kinds of psychological mechanisms are likely to be involved in the production of hypnotically induced analgesia.

REALITY OF HYPNOANESTHESIA

The induction of hypnosis is a remarkably simple procedure. The patient is instructed to focus his attention, to think about his eyes growing heavy, and to drift off as if to sleep. Typically the procedure takes only a few minutes. No drug is given and nothing dramatic is done to the patient. Nonetheless, moments later a suitable individual responds to suggestions that his body is becoming insensitive to pain, and as these suggestions are continued, it becomes possible to carry out surgical procedures.

This course of events is startling to the modern observer, not because surgery can be carried out on a relaxed and comfortable patient (a great many anesthetics allow this to occur) nor even because the patient is awake and comfortable (either local or regional anesthetics permit such a course of events) but rather because there is no obvious mechanism to account for the suppression of pain. The problem is further complicated by the absence of clear-cut physiological changes associated with entering hypnosis. Although suggestions of drowsiness may cause the patient to look like he is asleep, he continues to respond to the hypnotist's voice, shows no unique changes in the EEG, and is able to perform complex cognitive tasks without difficulty. Given appropriate suggestions, the patient may show every evidence of being wide awake, but nonetheless he will assert that he feels no discomfort even as major surgery is being carried out. The idea that a psychological process, occurring relatively quickly and easily in normal individuals and unaccompanied by unique physiological changes, can cause such profound alterations in an individual's response to obviously painful stimuli seems to fly against common sense expectations. It is hardly surprising that some observers are loath to accept the patient's assertion that he feels no pain under these circumstances.

Although the patient is for the most part relaxed during surgery, careful observation reveals that as the surgeon pulls on the peritoneum or manipulates some other organ richly endowed with pain receptors, changes in both heart rate and respiratory patterns can be seen to occur, at times associated with facial grimaces that might suggest pain. Not only is it possible to observe such changes in the naturalistic setting of the operating room, but in carefully controlled laboratory studies the subject who is in deep hypnosis and reports total insensibility to pain nevertheless shows the kinds of changes in heart rate and galvanic skin response (GSR) usually associated with pain stimuli (6).

These inconsistencies in the hypnotic response have long confused investigators and have raised serious questions in the minds of some observers about the reality of hypnotically induced anesthesia. Thus one way in which the phenomenon has been explained is to contend that the hypnotized patient is so eager to please the hypnotist or is so anxious to maintain the role of being a hypnotized subject or has some other personal—or even ulterior—motive that he is willing to bear the pain and make believe that he is comfortable. Much in the way the Greek stoics or the American Indians placed great emphasis on a brave man's ability to bear pain without outward signs of suffering, so, the argument goes, does the hypnotized subject strive to control both the external appearance of pain and his verbal reports. Only the physiological response and his occasional inability to suppress a facial grimace reveals his suffering.

The physiological data clearly indicate that pain perception must take place at least at the level of the thalamus, whereas other evidence to be discussed shows that pain perception also occurs at the cortical level.

Several investigators (1,3,4) have observed that when painful stimuli are applied to a hypnotically anesthetized limb a deeply hypnotized subject will assert verbally that he feels no pain, but at the same time he may indicate by means of automatic writing his appreciation of pain at another level. Automatic writing is a phenomenon relatively easily induced by giving a deeply hypnotized subject a pencil and the suggestion that the pencil will begin to write without his awareness of what is being written or, for that matter, that writing is occurring at all. Most interestingly, if the subject is asked to examine the material he has produced he will often disown it and insist that the ideas and sentiments expressed are not his own. Automatic writing is one of the procedures used by Morton Prince in his classic studies of coconsciousness, and there is a not inconsiderable body of poetry and mystical literature produced by means of automatic writing which, once learned, can also be carried out in the waking state. The best known example of such poetry is in the work of Gertrude Stein.

Recently Hilgard (2) has extended his systematic studies of hypnoanalgesia using a technique of automatic speaking. In addition to the usual kinds of verbal pain reports which are obtained while the subject is exposed to ischemic muscle pain, he instructs his deeply hypnotized subject that when he places his hand on the subject's right shoulder, that part of him which is not normally responsive but aware of all aspects of his experience will provide its own verbal pain report. When the subject is asserting that he feels no pain, Hilgard obtains pain ratings from what he terms the "hidden observer," which clearly indicates a considerable degree of pain at another level of awareness. Interestingly, however, these reports are given without the affect of suffering which would otherwise accompany them. Thus, although the deeply hypnotized subject reports experiencing no pain, the "hidden observer" typically reports awareness of some pain, but characteristically less than one would expect from the same subject exposed to the same stimulus in the waking state.

These data indicate that pain is perceived at a cortical level but not that the individual is merely suppressing his suffering. Thus patients who have had surgery under hypnoanesthesia continue to assert the effectiveness of the suggested pain relief long after surgery; even when pressed by skeptical friends, they continue to insist postoperatively that they did not in fact endure any suffering. These patients also require little if any postoperative analgesia, a behavior that is often markedly different from that which the same patients exhibited after prior surgery. When hypnoanalgesia is used in other contexts such as the treatment of intractable pain, as in terminal cancer, the need for narcotics is rapidly reduced and usually eliminated. In each of these instances one can still argue that the patient is somehow trying to please the hypnotist, but in many instances even such an implausible argument cannot be maintained. For example, one woman who had delivered a child with hypnoanesthesia moved to another city and went to great trouble to seek another obstetrician who used this technique. If she had really suffered discomfort and merely inhibited its expression during the original delivery, it is difficult to understand why she would choose to go through such a charade yet another time.

In a laboratory context analogous evidence can be cited. Typically, subjects participating in pain experiments will assert not only to the investigator himself but also to their friends away from the laboratory that they experienced no discomfort in the hypnoanalgesic condition. Not infrequently a subject who has taken part in such a study, when asked if he would be willing to participate in a similar experiment in the future, indicates that he is quite prepared to repeat the hypnoanalgesia segment but under no circumstances would he repeat the waking control part of the study, which involved his having to experience the same pain stimuli without hypnosis. Although it is difficult to prove that subjects are not willfully lying when they describe their experience during hypnoanalgesia, such an explanation is extremely implausible, and no proponents of such a view have been able to persuade volunteers to undergo major surgery without any form of anesthesia.

The absence of objective measures of pain needs to be recognized as a serious problem in all pain research, and indeed studies of hypnotically induced analgesia have been particularly sensitive to the problems of the validity of subjective reports—issues that need to be addressed in evaluating any reported analgesic effects. Certainly care must be taken to obtain subjects' reports in a context that is most likely to maximize honest reporting. Moreover, although it would be desirable to have an index of pain other than subjective reports, it should be kept in mind that these reports are the only meaningful way of indexing pain, which is after all a subjective experience—whether or not it is associated with concomitant physiological alterations. From our point of view, neither a physiological response nor a behavioral response can ever be more than an imperfect correlate of pain. The phenomenon itself resides in the patient's subjective experience of suffering, which may be more or less adequately reflected in a particular measure employed in a particular study.

In summing up the phenomenon of hypnotically induced analgesia, it seems clear that some deeply hypnotized subjects are able to tolerate surgical pain and analogous painful stimuli in the laboratory while asserting that they feel no discomfort. With appropriate techniques these subjects report an awareness of pain at another level without, however, evidence of suffering. The patient who asserts that he feels no pain seems to be truthful in asserting what he is actually experiencing, even though at some cortical level pain is perceived. However, the mechanisms by which hypnoanalgesic effects can be explained remain to be elucidated.

NATURE OF HYPNOTICALLY INDUCED ANALGESIA

It is well known that psychological factors affect pain perception. Consider, for example, the athlete who sustains a fracture but continues until the game is completed without even becoming aware of an injury that normally would cause exquisite pain; the dental patient who suffers intensely and on reaching the dental chair is no longer aware of his pain;

the patient who obtains profound relief from an injection of saline; and so on. There is a tendency to group all psychological mechanisms together, assuming somehow that they are similar or even the same. Particularly the placebo effect is generally conceived of as a form of suggestion closely related to hypnosis.

Because it is not possible to review here the voluminous literature on hypnotic analgesia, we will limit ourselves to research in our laboratory which addresses the particular relationship between hypnotic analgesia and the placebo effect (5). First, we sought to compare the effect of hypnotically induced analgesia with the effect of placebo. Second, we wished to study the effect of suggestions of analgesia on highly hypnotizable subjects as opposed to unhypnotizable subjects. An elaborate experimental design was developed to control for experimenter bias and similar problems in research by employing two groups of subjects, one that was highly hypnotizable and the other unable to respond to hypnosis. A hypnotic induction procedure is employed where there is no test of response to hypnotic suggestion that would result in a different response in these two groups of subjects. The two groups are treated in the identical manner by an investigator who is unaware of the subjects' past experience with hypnosis. These conditions make the procedure closely analogous to the double-blind technique used in psychopharmacology.

This approach takes advantage of the fact that the ability to enter hypnosis is a remarkably stable attribute of the individual. After three sessions the correlation between two succeeding standardized measures of hypnotizability is in excess of 0.9. It is therefore feasible to test subjects several times, selecting the two groups to be compared from the two ends of the distribution: those who are consistently highly responsive and those who are consistently unresponsive over repeated sessions. Since one group is essentially unresponsive to hypnotic suggestions, any effects observed in that group cannot be ascribed to hypnosis. At the same time, both groups will try to follow instructions to the best of their ability and be responsive to verbal and nonverbal cues indicating how they should behave. The one problem with this control group is that unhypnotizable subjects will have failed to respond in several experiences, and although it is possible to keep the hypnotist blind as to their status, they themselves will be aware that they are in essence unresponsive. Consequently, these subjects may well perceive the demands of the experimental situation quite differently. To solve this subtle but crucial problem in the design, we modified the procedure by including a special session designed to convince the unhypnotizable group that they could actually respond to hypnotic suggestions sufficiently well for the purposes of the study.

Another hypnotic session was arranged for the unhypnotizable subjects with a different hypnotist who employed a technique based exclusively on relaxation. Great care was taken not to test the ability of these subjects to respond to hypnotic suggestions and thereby avoid providing feedback that would indicate to them their continuing inability to respond. The subjects were treated as though they were responding extremely well to the particular procedure being employed. Even unhypnotizable individuals reach a state of profound relaxation under these circumstances. Once this had occurred, the hypnotist began to suggest analgesia of the right hand, again taking great care to induce the suggestion slowly and deliberately.

The analgesia suggestion was tested with electric shocks from an inductorium, and each subject was asked to compare the intensity of the shock in the analgesic hand with that in the normal hand. Although these subjects had been unhypnotizable, all of them experienced a considerable degree of analgesia because (unknown to them) the setting of the transformer was altered appropriately—they actually received less shock to the hand where analgesia had been suggested than to the normal hand. This manipulation was done carefully and within plausible limits. As a consequence, these subjects expressed considerable fascination and pleasure with the success of the analgesia suggestion. Careful postexperimental discussion supported the behavioral observations that these individuals were indeed persuaded about their ability to respond to analgesia suggestions. One subject who still doubted his responsiveness was excluded from participation.

This unusual manipulation resulted in a group of subjects who were essentially unresponsive to hypnosis as established by careful evaluation long before the experiment (and that persisted after the study), but who nonetheless believed themselves to be capable of responding to a particular form of hypnotic induction and to the suggestion of analgesia.

Subjects were then solicited for an experiment involving pain tolerance, and during a base-line session their tolerance for ischemic pain was established. The experimental population consisted of 12 highly hypnotizable and 12 unresponsive subjects. They were required to perform work that was quantified by the length of time pain was tolerated as well as by the amount of water they were able to pump while blood flow was occluded by means of a blood pressure cuff inflated to 200 mm Hg. Subjects were urged to pump as long as they could, and the initial pain threshold (when the sensation in the arm was first noticeably painful) and pain tolerance (when pain was so unbearable that they were unable to continue) were noted.

After the initial base-line session, all subjects returned and were tested by an experimenter who was not familiar with their previous hypnotic experiences in a session where a relaxation method of hypnotic induction was employed and analgesia was induced in one arm. The same technique of assessing pain threshold and tolerance that was used during the first session to test hypnotically induced analgesia was employed.

All subjects were asked to return for yet a third session. It was explained to them that during this session a drug would be used to help establish how effective hypnotic analgesia really was. It was pointed out that a powerful new analgesic drug was being employed that was known to suppress ischemic muscle pain. It was implied that the drug would work well and that this would allow us to see how closely hypnotic analgesia could approximate the drug effect. The experimenter himself believed he was administering dextropropoxyphene (Darvon®) and placebo in a double-blind manner. The pharmacy, however, had delivered two bottles, both of which were placebo: one had been labeled Darvon® and one placebo. The secretary then made up the usual envelopes from these bottles. Since no one in the laboratory other than myself was aware that there was no active drug, we created a firm belief in the experimenter that he was carrying out a drug study. However, all subjects received placebo, making the entire sample available for analysis.

Figure 1 summarizes our findings of the effect on pain threshold: the more sensitive, albeit less reliable, measure of analgesic response clearly

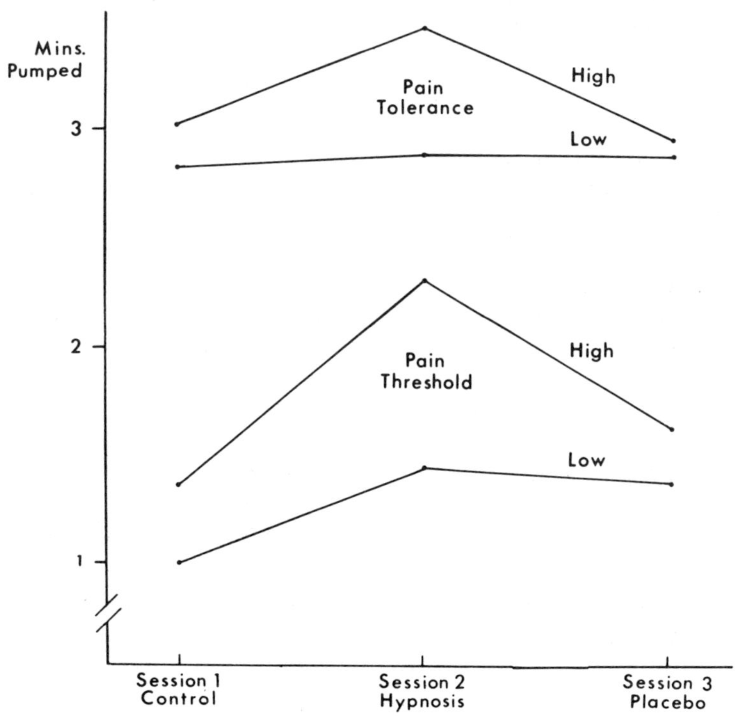

FIG. 1. Length of time pumped in relation to pain threshold and pain tolerance for Ss of high and low susceptibility to hypnosis during control, hypnotic analgesia, and placebo ischemic muscle pain performance.

shows that both groups responded to the hypnotic induction procedure. Although the pain threshold of the highly hypnotizable group is raised considerably more than that of the insusceptible group, the increment in pain threshold of the insusceptible group is nonetheless significant. In contrast, the change in pain threshold to placebo is identical in the groups. The pain tolerance findings show little change in the nonhypnotizable as opposed to a dramatic change in the hypnotizable group in response to posthypnotic suggestion.

The relationship between the response to hypnosis and the response to placebo is particularly interesting. Contrary to what is generally believed, there was no difference in the placebo response between the highly hypnotizable subjects and those who were insusceptible. On the other hand, the relationships between the placebo response and the effect of hypnotic analgesia were very different in these two groups. Thus in the unhypnotizable subjects the response to hypnotically induced analgesia correlated with the response to placebo 0.76, $p < 0.01$. In the highly hypnotizable group the correlation was totally insignificant, $r = 0.06$. These data strongly support our view that if the hypnotic procedure is expected to be effective by the subject it can exert a nonspecific placebo effect on his response to a painful stimulus. Note that the level of response to placebo in unhypnotizable subjects is, on the average, the same as that to hypnosis. The highly responsive subject, on the other hand, derives more benefit from hypnosis than he does from placebo. Moreover, the fact that the amount of relief yielded is uncorrelated with the amount of relief obtained with placebo in this group strongly suggests that two independent mechanisms are involved.

The placebo effect stems from the patient's belief in the drug's effectiveness, and it follows therefore that any other procedure that can evoke analogous patient expectancies will produce pain relief because of the same mechanism. In this sense it is appropriate to speak of a placebo effect of hypnosis that will occur in hypnotizable and unhypnotizable individuals alike, provided they both share the conviction that the procedure will be helpful. We were able to show that the nonspecific effect that is a function of the hypnotic procedure and independent of the patient's response to hypnosis results in a modest but nonetheless highly significant analgesic action. On the other hand, the specific effect of suggestions of hypnotic analgesia in the highly hypnotizable individual will result in a much more profound level of analgesia, which we expect will be additive with the nonspecific placebo component that can occur in all individuals.

CONCLUSIONS

What are the implications of these findings? As we pointed out earlier in this report, 90% of patients are helped by hypnotic analgesia in a dental context. However, this means that the patient becomes less anxious, allows the administration of local anesthetics, and is easier to manage. These important benefits do not require profound levels of analgesia but can be achieved by suggested relaxation and the associated analgesia owing to nonspecific placebo components inherent in the procedure. On the other hand, surgical anesthesia, in which the patient is exposed to profound pain stimuli, requires highly responsive hypnotic subjects since in these instances the control of pain involves a phenomenon best conceived of as a negative hallucination for pain. Much research on hypnosis has shown that any kind of negative hallucination, be it visual, auditory, or tactile, is difficult and requires considerable hypnotic skill on the part of the patient. This can be achieved only in a relatively small proportion of the population. Although motivational factors affect this proportion to some degree, 20% seems the likely upper limit.

These findings help explain the clinical observation that hypnosis is helpful in a high proportion of patients. Parenthetically it should be added that direct hypnotic suppression is rarely ever indicated in the treatment of functional pain. Enduring results with functional pain are achieved only when the contingencies associated with the symptom are fully understood and appropriately dealt with. On the other hand, hypnosis is ideally useful in helping to ameliorate transient pain induced by the physician or chronic pain of organic origin. Even the unhypnotizable subject will benefit from the hypnotic procedure because of its placebo component, and it may serve to renew hope, to reengage the patient in meaningful activities and thus decrease his somatic preoccupation, thereby greatly facilitating his functioning. Further, if the patient happens to belong to the approximately 20% of the population who have the skill of experiencing profound hypnotic phenomena, there is a good likelihood of almost complete relief owing to the specific effect of hypnotic suggestion on the hypnotizable individual. Since hypnosis in the treatment of organic pain is uniquely safe, non-habit forming, and easily applied, especially in conjunction with training in self-hypnosis, an appropriate therapeutic trial of this procedure is definitely indicated before considering the invasive or mutilating procedures that have been widely used in an effort to control pain.

ACKNOWLEDGMENTS

The substantive research on which this paper is based was supported in part by grant #MH 19156 from the National Institute of Mental Health and in part by the Institute for Experimental Psychiatry.

REFERENCES

1. Estabrooks, G. H. (1957): *Hypnotism,* Rev. ed., E. P. Dutton & Co., New York.
2. Hilgard, E. R. (1973): *Psychol. Rev.,* 80:396.

3. James, W. (1889): *Proc. Am. Soc. Psychical Res.,* 1:548.
4. Kaplan, E. A. (1960): *Arch. Gen. Psychiatry,* 2:567.
5. McGlashan, T. H., Evans, F. J., and Orne, M. T. (1969): *Psychosom. Med.,* 31:227.
6. Shor, R. E. (1962): In: *Hypnosis: Current Problems,* edited by G. H. Estabrooks, p. 54. Harper & Row, New York.

Advances in Pain Research and Therapy, Vol. 1,
edited by J. J. Bonica and D. Albe-Fessard.
Raven Press, New York © 1976.

Responses to Painful Stimuli During Animal Hypnosis

Giancarlo Carli, Francesca Farabollini, and Giuliano Fontani

Institute of Human Physiology, Strada del Laterino 8, 53100 Siena, Italy

The term "animal hypnosis" is commonly used to indicate several kinds of prolonged, reversible immobility responses that can be produced in animals by different types of sensory stimuli (13). The only immobility studied in great detail is that obtained by the mechanical method of inversion, which consists of holding the animal in reverse position and keeping it there until fully relaxed. Once immobility occurs, it persists without further restraint. Termination of this condition may occur either spontaneously or after different types of sudden stimuli (tactile, acoustic, or painful). This immobility response is not species specific: it is present in fish, reptiles, and birds, whereas in mammals it is easily obtained only in rabbits and guinea pigs (10,13,18,25).

CHARACTERISTICS OF ANIMAL HYPNOSIS IN THE RABBIT

The main characteristics of animal hypnosis elicited by inversion and restriction are briefly summarized below.

Electroencephalogram

During the induction procedure and at the onset of hypnosis, low-voltage fast activity in the EEG and pupillary dilatation are constantly recorded. As hypnosis continues, the EEG pattern tends to reflect high-voltage slow wave activity coupled with myosis. Occasionally, periods of low-voltage fast activity associated with mydriasis may occur spontaneously or after sudden sensory stimuli (2,17,26).

Motor System

During hypnosis there is hypotonia and depression of mono- and polysynaptic reflexes (2). This depression is constantly observed and lasts for the whole episode of hypnosis. The suppression of spinal reflexes is still present in hypothalamic and precollicular decerebrate rabbits. Moreover, the rigidity observed in the acute decerebellate hypothalamic rabbit ceases during hypnosis. However, when a postcollicular decerebration is performed, the manipulations leading to hypnosis in the intact rabbit have no effect, and the characteristic hypertonia of the low decerebrate rabbit is not affected (3).

Cutaneous Stimulation

The input from cutaneous afferents stimulated in supine position is not essential for hypnosis induction or maintenance since hypnosis can be elicited in rabbits having a complete denervation of the dorsal and dorsolateral skin area (6). The possible role of deep receptors (mainly muscle and joint afferents) stimulated in the inverted position has not been determined.

Blood Pressure and Heart Rate

During the manipulations involved in hypnosis induction, there is a long-lasting hypertension that persists during the initial seconds of the hypnotic episode (4). Later on, in the hypnotic state itself, blood pressure and heart rate resume the levels of the control periods, although—especially in hypnoses of longer duration—these levels may also decrease below control values (4,17).

Pavlovian and Avoidance Conditioning

Using pavlovian conditioning procedures, one can condition heart rate changes during hypnosis at the same rate as in the control state (9). In rabbits trained to avoid an electric shock (unconditioned stimulus, UCS) to the foot in response to a 4-sec sound (conditioned stimulus, CS), extinction in the control state proceeds much faster if extinction procedures are applied also in the hypnotic condition (5). If the performance of these animals is tested during hypnosis, only a few or no avoidance responses occur in the initial trials. Later on, after additional training during hypnosis, rabbits learn to interrupt CS and prevent UCS. Hypnosis termination always follows the performance of the avoidance task. When the animals are tested alternatively in control and in hypnotic conditions, the performance in the control trials is not affected by the presentation of the stimulus during hypnosis (5).

Duration

When hypnosis is produced at regular intervals, a reduction in duration is recorded (14,20). On the other hand, several fear-producing stimuli (10–12) such as electric shock, loud noise, suspension over a visual cliff, and confrontation with a simulated predator presented just before hypnosis induction result a significant increase in hypnotic duration. These results support the hypothesis which assumes that animal hypnosis is a consequence of fear stimuli (23).

FEAR HYPOTHESIS

Ratner (23) first elaborated the fear hypothesis in a model that could be experimentally tested. He assumes that "any stimulus, such as a natural predator, that functions as a threatening stimulus, elicits a sequence of responses as a function of the *distance between this stimulus and the animal*. . . . As the defensive distance between the threatening stimulus and the animal is reduced by movement of this stimulus, a sequence of responses occur. . . . First the animal is alert (freezes), then it moves away; as the distance reaches zero, it struggles or fights; and finally, as the defensive distance remains at zero, it becomes immobile and unresponsive (animal hypnosis)."

This elegant formulation stimulated a long series of experiments performed mainly by Gallup (10) and his collaborators. In short, it has been shown that any manipulation that presumably involves fear increases hypnosis duration (10). Ratner (23) also suggested "to bring the animal into the laboratory to determine the specific characteristics of a stimulus that elicits a response." Unfortunately, this important behavioral control has never been performed in Gallup's experiments (10), and the effects of the stimuli used were never recorded in the nonhypnotic condition. For instance, we don't know whether a chicken confronted with a sham predator at different distances would freeze or move away. Although there is no doubt that fear potentiates hypnosis duration and induction, manipulations are fear-producing procedures that precede hypnosis, and more precise behavioral and neurophysiological parameters should be adopted to define the fear response in the control state. Moreover, for hypnosis studies, the study of hypnotic duration should be associated with the recording of several physiological correlates (EEG, heart rate, spinal reflexes, etc.).

EFFECTS OF PAIN

It has been shown in this laboratory (6) that subcutaneous injection of formalin (38%) into the dorsal region of the rabbit foot elicits several adversive reactions (running and shifting movements, licking of the affected foot, etc.) that are associated with an EEG activity of low-voltage fast waves typical of intense emotional states. In the nonhypnotic condition these discomfort manifestations persist, with decreasing intensity, for approximately 1 hr. Hypnosis can be produced in this condition of continuous pain. Moreover, if hypnosis is elicited when the pain reactions are less intense, i.e., 15 min after formalin injection, it is characterized by a predominance of rhythms of high-voltage slow activity in the EEG (6). At the end of the hypnotic episode, in the control state, both the discomfort reactions and the activation rhythms in the EEG are again recorded.

A series of experiments is now in progress in this laboratory which is an attempt to elucidate the mechanisms involved in the suppression of the pain response during animal hypnosis. After a procedure of habituation (20), hypnosis duration was reduced below 45 sec within 2 to 3 weeks. In these subjects the main results obtained were the following: (a) increase in hypnotic duration was recorded when hypnosis was induced during a condition of continuous pain, i.e., 5 min after formalin injection; (b) naloxone (5 mg/kg, i.v.) injected 3 min after formalin abolished the potentiation of hypnotic duration elicited by the painful stimuli; (c) in absence of painful stimuli, morphine (1 mg/kg, i.v.) elicited an increase in hypnotic duration, and this potentiation was abolished by naloxone; (d) morphine (5 mg/kg, i.v.) did not prevent the initial pain manifestations after formalin injection. However, after 5 to 8 min, it elicited catalepsia and high-voltage slow waves in the EEG.

On the basis of these results, our working hypothesis assumes that a pain-suppressing mechanism is active during animal hypnosis.

ANALGESIA HYPOTHESIS

Mayer and Liebeskind (21) have recently suggested that analgesia from either central gray stimulation or morphine activates identical supraspinal mechanisms on the basis of several experimental results: both types of analgesia are reduced by depletion of serotonin by *p*-chlorophenylalanine (p-CPA) (1,19,27), both are antagonized by naloxone, and the sensory block is more likely occurring at spinal cord levels in consequence of supraspinal modulatory mechanisms (8,16,22,24). As for hypnosis, recent experiments (15) have shown that the potentiation of hypnotic duration by morphine (7) is abolished by p-CPA. The results mentioned in previous sections indicate that during animal hypnosis elicited in a condition of continuous nociceptive stimulation, the pain response is blocked by mechanisms that exhibit similar effects on morphine at both spinal cord (immobility, depression of polysynaptic reflexes) and cortical levels (high-voltage slow waves in the EEG). Moreover, both hypnosis and morphine are more effective on continuous, moderate pain, and the increase in hypnotic duration after both formalin and morphine is abolished by naloxone. We suggest the existence of an analgesic mechanism during hypnosis mainly in a condition of continuous nociceptive stimulation. The formulation of the analgesia hypothesis is justified by the confidence that this hypothesis can be experimentally tested by applying more direct approaches (evoked potentials, single-unit recordings, etc.). This hypothesis does not exclude the possibility that fear or other emotional components are associated with the painful stimuli, and it does not pretend to explain the general mechanisms responsible for animal hypnosis or its causation.

REFERENCES

1. Akil, H., and Mayer, D. J. (1972): *Brain Res.,* 44:692–697.
2. Carli, G. (1969): *Arch. Ital. Biol.,* 107:219–234.
3. Carli, G. (1971): *Arch. Ital. Biol.,* 109:15–26.
4. Carli, G. (1974): *Electroencephalogr. Clin. Neurophysiol.,* 37:231–237.
5. Carli, G., Coltelli, M., and Sabourin, M. (1974): *Brain Res.,* 66:365–366.
6. Carli, G., Lefebvre, L., Silvano, G., and Vierucci, S. (1974): *IRCS,* 2:1542.
7. Davis, W. M. (1963): *Arch. Int. Pharmacodyn. Ther.,* 142:349–360.
8. Dewey, W. L., Snyder, J. W., Harris, L. S., and Howes, J. F. (1969): *J. Pharm. Pharmacol.,* 21:548–550.
9. Draper, D. C., and Klemm, W. R. (1967): *Psychol. Rec.,* 17:13–21.
10. Gallup, G. G. (1974): *Psychol. Bull.,* 81:836–853.
11. Gallup, G. G., Nash, R. F., Donegan, N. H., and McClure, M. K. (1971): *Psychol. Rec.,* 21:513–519.
12. Gallup, G. G., Nash, R. F., Potter, R. J., and Donegan, N. H. (1970): *J. Comp. Physiol. Psychol.,* 73:442–445.
13. Gilman, T. T., and Marcuse, F. L. (1949): *Psychol. Bull.,* 46:151–165.
14. Gilman, T. T., Marcuse, F. L., and More, A. U. (1950): *J. Comp. Physiol. Psychol.,* 43:99–111.
15. Hicks, L. E., Maser, J. D., Gallup, G. G., and Edson, P. H. (1975): *Psychopharmacologia,* 42:51–56.
16. Irwin, S., Houde, R. W., Bennet, D. R., Hendershot, L. C., and Seevers, M. H. (1951): *J. Pharmacol. Exp. Ther.,* 101:132–143.
17. Klemm, W. R. (1966): *Electroencephalogr. Clin. Neurophysiol.,* 21:365–372.
18. Klemm, W. R. (1971): In: *Neurosciences Research, Vol. 4,* edited by S. Ehrenpreis and O. C. Solnitzky. Academic Press, New York.
19. Lee, J. R., and Fennessy, M. R. (1970): *Eur. J. Pharmacol.,* 12:65–70.
20. Lefebvre, L. (1974): M.A. dissertation, Université de Montréal.
21. Mayer, D. J., and Liebeskind, J. C. (1974): *Brain Res.,* 68:73–93.
22. Oliveras, J. L., Besson, J. M., Gilbaud, G., and Liebeskind, J. C. (1974): *Exp. Brain Res.,* 20:32–44.
23. Ratner, S. C. (1967): In: *Handbook of Clinical and Experimental Hypnosis,* edited by J. E. Gordon. The Macmillan Company, New York.
24. Sato, M., and Takagi, H. (1971): *Jpn. J. Pharmacol.,* 21:671–672.
25. Scotti de Carolis, A., Carruyo, L., and Longo, V. G. (1969): In: *The Present Status of Psychotropic Drugs,* edited by A. Cerletti and F. J. Boué. Excerpta Medica Foundation, Amsterdam.
26. Silva, E. E., Estable, C., and Segundo, J. P. (1959): *Arch. Ital. Biol.,* 97:167–177.
27. Tenen, S. S. (1968): *Psychopharmacologia,* 12:278–285.

Advances in Pain Research and Therapy, Vol. 1,
edited by J. J. Bonica and D. Albe-Fessard.
Raven Press, New York © 1976.

Neurophysiology and Acupuncture: A Review

Birger Kaada

Institute of Neurophysiology, University of Oslo, Oslo, Norway

EFFECTIVENESS AND TIME COURSE OF ACUPUNCTURE ANALGESIA

Before discussing the possible mechanisms of acupuncture analgesia, we should review a few facts concerning the degree and characteristics of the effect. There can be no doubt that acupuncture has a certain relieving effect on acute pain in surgery. This was the conclusion reached by the Norwegian medical delegation to The Peoples' Republic of China in October 1973 after having witnessed approximately 30 major operations (6). In view of previous information that had reached the Western world it was surprising, however, to learn the following.

First, acupuncture in surgery was nearly always given in combination with relatively large doses of hypnotic and analgesic drugs: 100 mg of phenobarbital the evening before the operation or 2 hr before and 1 mg/kg of pethidine i.m. or i.v. 30 min before the operation. The latter dose was repeated frequently during the operation. Finally, a supplement of local anesthesia with procaine was given to many patients.

Second, acupuncture in surgery was not used as frequently as one might be led to believe by the news media. The method was mostly used in the years after the Great Cultural Revolution. In 1967 to 1968 it was used in nearly 60% of all operations done in some hospitals. In 1972 this figure had dropped to 20% to 26%, in 1973 to 15% to 20%, and the last reports in 1974 (3,10,11) gave a percentage of only 5 to 6 at some of the largest hospitals which previously had been among the most enthusiastic proponents of acupuncture in surgery.

Third, the criteria for what the Chinese called the "success rate," which was around 85% to 90% for most types of operations, were different from those a Western anesthesiologist would require. Some patients experienced pain to a degree that would not be tolerated by patients in the Western world. Pain relief according to Western criteria was obtained in at most one-third of the patients operated on under acupuncture analgesia, i.e., in only a small percentage of the total number of operations, and this even in combination with drugs and after careful selection of the patients.

The degree and time course of acupuncture analgesia are shown in Fig. 1. The upper record, from a report by the Peking group (10), illustrates the

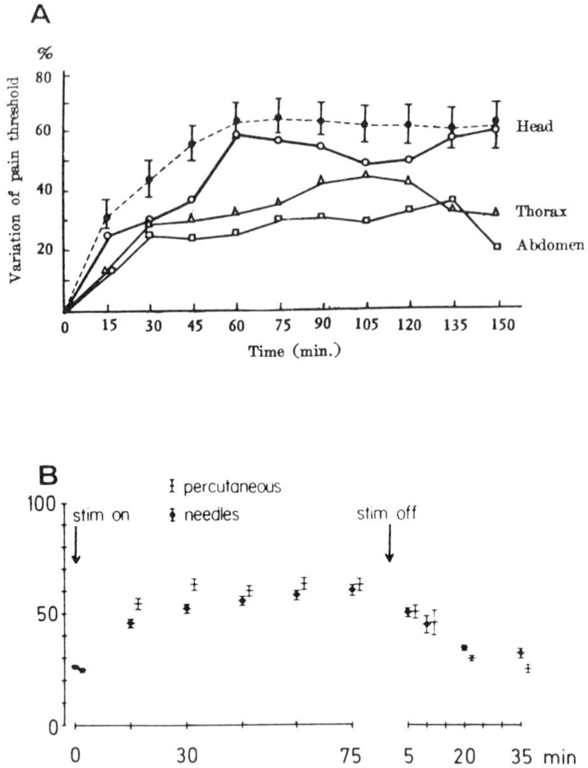

FIG. 1. A: Rise in pain threshold, as measured by a potassium ion algometer, in response to continuous needling of the *ho-ku* point (Li4) of the hand in normal volunteers studied by the Peking group (10). Dotted line represents the average pain threshold during intermittent needling. (From ref. 10.)

B: Similar experiment on students in Sweden. Increase in pain threshold, measured as the current needed to produce pain when applied to dental surface, and expressed as mean values and SEM. Conditioning electrical low-frequency stimulation of hands and cheeks via needles in 14 students and via surface electrodes (percutaneous) in 12 students. Ordinate, pain threshold in μA. Stimulation during time indicated between arrows. (From ref. 2.)

rise in pain threshold measured in the skin of the head, thorax, and abdomen over a period of 150 min in response to a continuous needling of the *ho-ku* point (between the first and second metacarpal bones on one hand) in normal volunteers. There is a gradual increase in pain threshold in the first 30 to 40 min affecting all points tested, although somewhat differently, indicating a relative specificity. This is also the typical time course of the analgesic effect seen in operations: on low-frequency stimulation (1 to 2/sec) the operation usually started after 20 to 30 min of continuous acupuncture, manually or electrically.

The lower record shows a similar experiment on Swedish volunteers (2). Again there is an increase in pain threshold, measured as the current needed to produce pain from the dental pulp (which contains pain fibers only) on low-frequency stimulation of peripheral nerves from the cheeks and hands. The effect may outlast the stimulation for a considerable period of time, even for some hours. One never obtains a painless condition by such a procedure, only an increase in pain threshold, as seen from both series of experiments. Similar results are reported by other investigators (C. R. Chapman et al. and D. J. Mayer et al., *this volume*).

The Chinese sometimes also used high-frequency stimulation (80 to 100/sec) in electroacupuncture, but they did not realize that one is then most likely dealing with a different mechanism with different clinical characteristics, as is demonstrated in this and in other chapters in this book (see below).

MECHANISM OF ACUPUNCTURE ANALGESIA

The theories that have been advanced to explain acupuncture analgesia belong to three categories: (a) the traditional Chinese meridian or channel theory; (b) theories based on neurophysiological data; and (c) theories claiming that pain is relieved by psychophysiological mechanisms.

Meridian Theory

There is no experimental support whatsoever for the first theory, the Chinese philosophical explanation of the life energy, *ch'i.* According to this concept, the *ch'i* flows through the body in a network of 12 main channels or meridians, and its excess or deficit produces pain and disease. This imbalance is corrected by inserting needles into various specific points along the course of the meridians near the surface of the body. These meridians are unrelated to the known nervous, circulatory, or lymphatic systems. However, when one compares the main acupuncture points with the branches of the cutaneous nerves (Fig. 2), the acupuncture points usually are near the nerve branches. The same holds true for all parts of the body and usually also for the deep muscular nerves. Also, in many instances the main acupuncture points are located within the dermatome of the diseased organ, corresponding to the well-known cutaneovisceral reflexes (Head's zones). It is known clinically and experimentally that stimulation of the skin may inhibit pain impulses from the visceral organ within such a segment (ref. in 5). In accordance with this fact, Chang Hsiang-tung, a Western-trained neurophysiologist from the Institute of Physiology in Shanghai, has recommended that the acupuncture needles be inserted into the same segmental areas as those involved in the surgery.

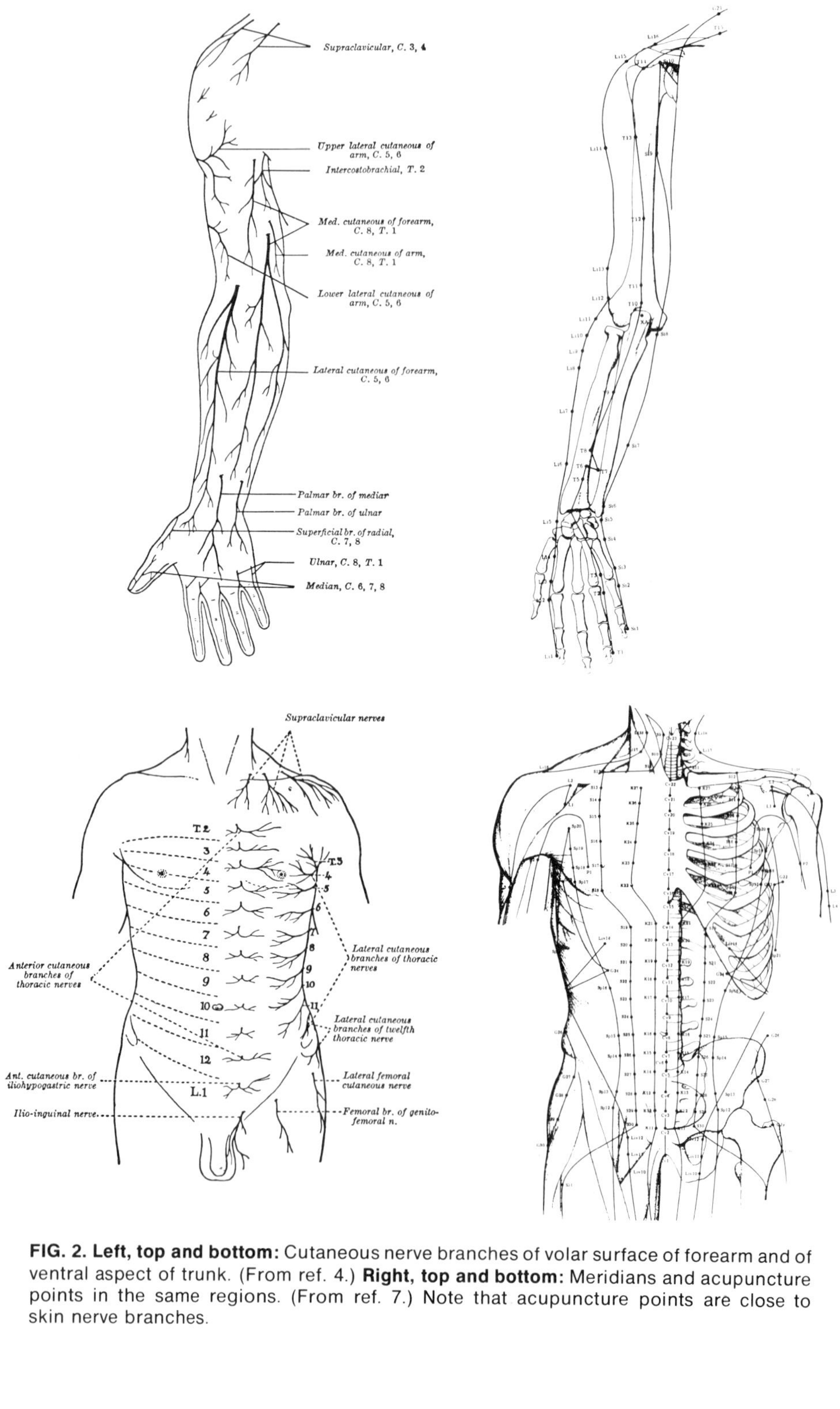

FIG. 2. Left, top and bottom: Cutaneous nerve branches of volar surface of forearm and of ventral aspect of trunk. (From ref. 4.) **Right, top and bottom:** Meridians and acupuncture points in the same regions. (From ref. 7.) Note that acupuncture points are close to skin nerve branches.

Neurophysiological Explanations

These observations strongly indicate the involvement of nervous mechanisms in acupuncture analgesia. There can be no doubt that the acupuncture effect, like the analgesic effect of transcutaneous peripheral nerve stimulation, is due to afferent nervous impulses. This is also evidenced by the fact that acupuncture analgesia fails to develop on the hypesthetic side in hemiplegic patients or during a procaine-induced conduction block of the nerves innervating the acupuncture site (ref. in 5).

Attempts have been made to identify receptors and types of afferent nerve fibers activated by acupuncture. The Shanghai group of physiologists concluded that maximal effects were obtained when group 2 afferent nerve fibers were activated, in particular those carrying impulses from deep pressure receptors and muscle stretch receptors (ref. in 5). This is in line with the clinical and experimental observations that analgesia requires a rather strong electroacupuncture or transcutaneous peripheral stimulation, preferably a stimulus which causes jerky movements of the muscles and one which is at a level just below that tolerated by the patient. The importance of high stimulus intensities is elaborated on by Andersson and Holmgren (*this volume*) and by Melzack and Jeans (*unpublished observations*). The beneficial effects of some physiotherapeutic procedures such as deep connective tissue massage appear to be based on the same principle as the acupuncture effect.

Turning to the spinal cord, interest in the neural mechanisms of pain perception and suppression has more recently been focused by the "gate control theory" advanced by Melzack and Wall in 1965 without any relation to acupuncture effects (9). In brief, impulses generated by noxious painful stimulation are carried to the spinal cord by small-sized C fibers and A-delta fibers. These are blocked at their synapses in the spinal cord by simultaneous stimulation of large-sized myelinated A fibers, thus preventing pain impulses from reaching higher levels of the central nervous system. The detailed mechanism behind this spinal inhibition is not known, but important data are presented by Iggo (*this volume*). This, however, does not invalidate the unquestionably empirical and experimental observation that pain impulses are inhibited at a spinal level. Most likely this is a pre- and postsynaptic inhibition elicited at a segmental level by activity in the primary afferents as suggested by Andersson and Holmgren (*this volume*). Further, this inhibition requires high-frequency conditioning stimulation; it appears almost immediately and it does not outlast stimulation for any considerable time. This inhibition is the basis for the treatment of patients with chronic pain by transcutaneous electrostimulation and dorsal column stimulation, as well as for the suppression of pain by vibration stimuli. Acupuncture also reduces "pain discharges" in cells of the medial thalamus and midbrain reticular formation (ref. in 5).

There must, however, also be another mechanism to account for the gradual increase in pain threshold in the course of 20 to 30 min. This effect is further characterized by its elicitation by low-frequency stimulation (1 to 2/sec), and it appears to be more widespread. This type of stimulation is usually employed in surgical acupuncture, and the response corresponds to the time course encountered in these patients.

In a pilot study we have tested the pain-relieving effect on various types of chronic pain using high- as well as low-frequency transcutaneous electrical stimulation. It appears that high-frequency stimulation causes an almost immediate and short-lasting effect that is strictly segmental, whereas low-frequency stimulation in the same patients has an effect that comes on gradually, may outlast stimulation for several hours, and is more widespread.

The slow time course of this effect suggests that a humoral chemical factor is possibly involved. Three independent studies in China have suggested that such an anti-pain factor may be produced in the brain on acupuncture (ref. in 5). Significant analgesia was obtained in 30 pairs of rabbits: cerebrospinal fluid was collected from an acupunctured group of 30 animals and injected into the ventricles of 30 normal rabbits. There was a significant rise in pain threshold in the latter, whereas a similar number of experiments without acupuncture failed to show this effect.

Similar results were obtained in crossed-circulation experiments in which 30 min of acupuncture in one rabbit caused a marked elevation in pain threshold in both animals. In control groups with no acupuncture, no change in pain threshold ensued. I have not yet seen the full report of these exciting experiments, and we will have to await the details before definite conclusions can be drawn. Similar crossed-circulation experiments have also been performed by Takeshige et al. (*this volume*) and with the same results.

The nature of this postulated humoral factor is not known. Nevertheless, it has been demonstrated (ref. in 5) that large doses of reserpine given to the animals 24 hr before acupuncture increase the analgesic effect. This might suggest that a monaminergic substance such as serotonin or norepinephrine might be liberated.

In the past few years a so-called serotonin system of neurons has been described descending mainly from the midline or raphe nuclei of the midbrain, and perhaps also from higher and lower levels of the periventricular gray substance, and exerting an ~~anti~~analgesic effect on stimulation (Fig. 3). I have previously postulated (5) that this system might be activated in acupuncture and responsible for the slowly increasing and prolonged pain-relieving effects in surgical acupuncture. Direct electrical stimulation of these nuclei or local microinjection of morphine into this region selectively blocks pain impulses in the dorsal horn of the spinal cord leaving other sensory modalities relatively unaffected. Such descending impulses also block the flexion reflex, which is always associated with pain elicited from

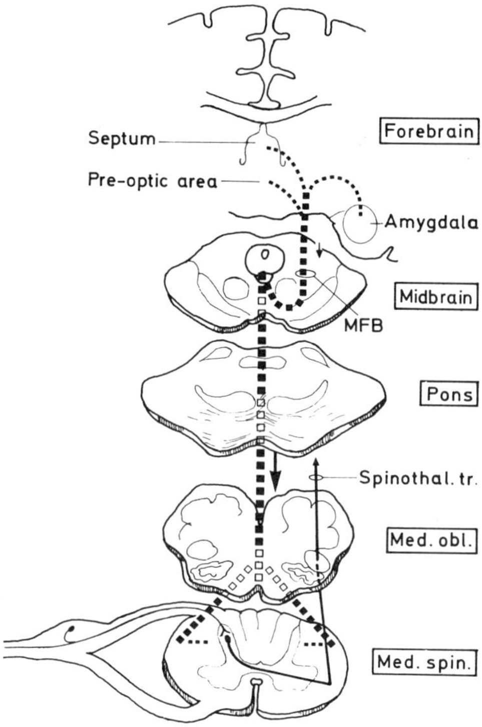

FIG. 3. Schematic diagram of a postulated midline (raphe) "serotonin system" in midbrain, lower brainstem, and periventricular gray of 3rd ventricle, exerting an analgesic or antinociceptive effect. Analgesia derives from activation of cells in the midline by electrical stimulation or microinjection of morphine. Descending impulses inhibit transmission of impulses evoked by painful stimulation and associated flexion reflex. (From ref. 5.)

the periphery. Lundberg and collaborators in Gothenburg (ref. in 5) have shown that reserpine, after injection of a monoamine oxidase inhibitor, also has this blocking effect in the acute spinal cat, most likely through liberation of serotonin from presynaptic terminals of descending monoaminergic tracts. Reserpine alone is effective in the decerebrate but not in the acute spinal cat, indicating an action on the brainstem "serotonin neurons." Perhaps low-frequency transcutaneous or acupuncture stimulation activates these cells in the brainstem by gradually liberating sufficiently large quantities of serotonin to stimulate the cells of the descending midline system. It is known that these midline cells may be activated directly through an ascending ventral cord path and through a dorsal column component. Two recent studies have actually demonstrated that direct stimulation of these brainstem nuclei requires an induction time of 15 to 20 min to produce analgesia (8), and also that acupuncture stimulation increases the serotonin content in the lower brainstem (1). The crucial experiment would be to eliminate the analgesic effects of acupuncture and transcutaneous peripheral nerve stimulation after selective destruction of the raphe nuclei.

Further support for this hypothesis is given by Mayer et al. (*this volume*), who have demonstrated that a specific narcotic antagonist, naloxone, may antagonize the analgesic effect of the pain inhibitory system of the brain as well as of manual acupuncture in man. Further, Takeshige and coworkers (*this volume*), using a serotonin synthesis inhibitor, blocked the analgesia induced by acupuncture with low-frequency stimulation.

The importance of the stimulus frequency in peripheral nerve stimulation on the degree and time course of the analgesic effect is also stressed in several recent studies (S. A. Andersson and E. Holmgren, E. A. M. Frost et al., and S. I. Heller and Y. Omara, *this volume*), and different mechanisms for acute and chronic pain are suggested.

I have also suggested (5) that the so-called animal hypnosis or still reaction, which occurs in a great variety of animals and is characterized by immobility and reduced responsiveness to external stimulation, is dependent on the midline serotonin system. Takeshige et al. (*this volume*) present some experimental evidence in support of this view.

Psychophysiological Mechanisms

Bearing in mind that psychological factors such as attention, anxiety, and past experience play a considerable role in pain perception and experience, it is of great interest that some raphe nuclei receive projections through the medial forebrain bundle (MFB) from limbic brain areas (Fig. 3), such as the amygdala, septum, anterior, cingulate, and orbital cortex of the frontal lobe. Ablation of these areas is known to reduce anxiety, and their stimulation also inhibits the flexion reflex associated with pain (ref. in 5). This might represent a neural substrate for the psychological and emotional factors involved in acupuncture.

Acupuncture analgesia has also been explained as owing to hypnosis, suggestion, or a placebo effect. These theories have found support in the fact that acupuncture does not work in all patients. However, all Chinese acupuncturists claim that these failures are because of anxiety rather than hypnosis. It is also well known from a number of studies that more anxious persons show greater pain responses than do more relaxed subjects (ref. in 5). Decreasing anxiety reduces such responses. The success of producing analgesia and pain relief by placebos, suggestion, and acupuncture is to a great extent a matter of reducing anxiety. The ability of Chinese physicians to minimize anxiety and tension through careful patient selection and drug administration most likely accounts for their greater success with acupuncture analgesia. In China confidence in the method is also created by cultural, educational, and ethnic factors that contribute to the effects obtained. Experimental evidence for the great influence of psychological factors on acupuncture analgesia is presented in several studies (e.g., C. R. Chapman et al. and C. M. Hossenlopp et al., *this volume*).

In conclusion, a combination of neurophysiological and psychophysiological mechanisms appears to be responsible for the analgesia obtained by acupuncture.

REFERENCES

1. Acupuncture Anaesthesia Research Group, Human Medical College, Changsha (1973): *Chin. Med. J.*, 8:105.
2. Andersson, S. A., Ericson, T., and Holmgren, E. (1973): *Brain Res.*, 63:393–396.
3. Bonica, J. J. (1974): *J.A.M.A.*, 229:1317–1325.
4. Davies, D. V., and Coupland, R. E. (Eds.) (1967): *Gray's Anatomy, 34th edition.* Longmans, Green & Co., Ltd., London.
5. Kaada, B. (1974): *Tidsskr. Nor. Laegeforen.*, 94:422–431.
6. Kaada, B., Hoel, E., Leseth, K., Nygaard-Østby, B., Setekleiv, J., and Stovner, J. (1974): *Tidsskr. Nor. Laegeforen.*, 94:417–442.
7. Mann, F. (1972): *Atlas of Acupuncture. Points and Meridians in Relation to Surface Anatomy.* W. Heinemann Medical Books Ltd., London.
8. Melzack, R., and Melnikoff, D. F. (1974): *Exp. Neurol.*, 43:369–374.
9. Melzack, R., and Wall, P. D. (1965): *Science*, 150:971–978.
10. Peking Acupuncture Anaesthesia Co-ordinating Group (1973): *Sci. Sinica*, 16:447–456.
11. Wall, P. (1974): *New Scientist*, 3:31–34.

Advances in Pain Research and Therapy, Vol. 1,
edited by J. J. Bonica and D. Albe-Fessard.
Raven Press, New York © 1976.

Acupuncture "Anesthesia": A Critical View

Arthur Taub

Section for the Study and Treatment of Pain, Department of Anesthesiology, Yale University School of Medicine, New Haven, Connecticut 06510

The most striking claims of success of acupuncture (3,14) in the relief of pain are in the area of surgical anesthesia (1,4,7,8,11,12). I propose to examine these claims. My comments are based on data obtained during a visit to China in May 1974 as a member of a group sponsored by the Committee on Scholarly Communication with the People's Republic of China. My opinions, of course, are my own and do not necessarily reflect those of other members of the group or of the Committee.

Since its development in about 1958, the procedure of acupuncture "anesthesia" has not been widely used in surgical procedures in China (4,7,8,11,12). Chinese anesthesiologists produce anesthesia probably 90% of the time with local, regional, or general anesthesia (4). General anesthesia is used relatively infrequently, since Chinese patients prefer being awake during surgery, sleep and coma being equated in popular thought with the departure of the soul from the body (6). Very little evidence is available to indicate that acupuncture is used in the relatively primitive interior of China as a surgical anesthetic, and it would appear that acupuncture anesthesia is used rarely in major Eastern Chinese surgical centers on an experimental basis and where trained anesthesiological backup is available (4). It is used in elective surgery only and never as an emergency procedure or on the battlefield. It is not used in old or "poor risk" patients. It is used in infants with "mummification." When used in juveniles, rarely, probably for splenectomy alone, it requires "basal narcosis." In veterinary surgery, it is considered highly experimental, is generally unsuccessful, and is not widely practiced.

Acupuncture anesthesia as practiced in China today is predicated on careful physical and psychological selection of patients. They must be in generally good health. They must be emotionally stable; that is, capable of lying motionless, awake, on an operating table for several hours. They essentially volunteer for the procedure, and compulsion, in the sense of physical or pharmacological coercion, is not used. Patients have heard of acupuncture anesthesia through Communist Party organs, from their friends, or from other patients in the hospital, and, of course, are familiar with acupuncture in medicine. School children are taught to accept needling as harmless, beneficial, and politically correct. In general, those patients selected have also been found to tolerate preliminary acupuncture testing, painful to Western observers (P. D. Wall, *personal communication*).

The few surgical procedures for which acupuncture anesthesia is suitable must be classic; that is, straightforward, with minimal exploration and with no complications expected. Otherwise, conventional regional or general anesthesia is used. The surgical approach and technique are fitted to the anesthesia, stimulation of nociceptors being avoided so far as is possible.

There is no uniformly accepted system in China for the use of acupuncture in surgical anesthesia. Such factors as number and position of needles, manual or electrical stimulation, and parameters of stimulation vary widely within and between hospitals. They are said to be experimental. In Peking we were told that one surgeon allows his patients to choose the site of needle placement. The number of needles used has decreased during the past few years to, in many cases, the absolute minimum: one.

When acupuncture is used today as an anesthetic, generally speaking, patients are premedicated with parenteral barbiturates (100 to 300 mg, up to 500 mg phenobarbital i.m.); narcotic analgesics (50 to 100 mg of meperidine i.v.), which may be repeated each 2 hr during surgery; and anticholinergic, sedating, and amnesic agents (0.3 mg scopolamine s.c.). Local anesthesia may be used for incision through and manipulation of fascia, pleura, and peritoneum, the viscera, and, on occasion, the skin. Local anesthesia is an integral part of the acupuncture anesthesia technique. Its use generally depends on whether a stimulus adequate to evoke a report of pain is planned to be delivered to the skin or viscera. On occasion, local anesthesia is also provided by direct electrical tetanic fatigue of peripheral nerves (1,5,13).

Acupuncture is most successful as an anesthetic in operations on insensitive viscera such as the thyroid and where reflex relaxation is not required. Operations on the abdominal viscera, however, done under acupuncture anesthesia are said to face three major unsolved problems at present: incomplete analgesia, incomplete muscular relaxation, and pain from visceral traction.

Acupuncture anesthesia produces neither anesthesia nor analgesia in the conventional sense (8). This may be seen by examining a classification system (Table 1) for the "effectiveness" of acupuncture anesthesia used in Shanghai (12). It includes four grades. There is no grade for complete analgesia. Grade I, or excellent anesthetic effect, allows for "slight pain" during the procedure, permits the use of intravenous meperidine at a rate of 1 to 1.5 mg/kg/2 hr, and allows the use of local anesthesia. Grade II, or good anesthetic effect, permits "occasional light groans for pain" during the procedure, as well as changes in blood pressure, pulse rate, and respiratory rate, permits the use of intravenous meperidine at a rate of 1 to 1.5

TABLE 1. *Results of acupuncture anesthesia in 10 kinds of operations*

Kind of operation	No. of cases	Grade I	Grade II	Grade III	Grade IV	Effective Rate (%)	Rate of grades I & II combined (%)	Rate of grades II, III, & IV combined (%)	Rate of grades III & IV combined (%)
Craniotomy	606	210	216	157	23	96.2	70.3	65	30
Operations for detachment of retina	1,374	443	569	98	264	80.7	73.6	68	26
Operations for thyroid	670	365	209	65	31	95.4	85.7	46	14
Total laryngectomy	121	65	36	11	9	92.6	83.5	46	17
Pulmonary resection	656	116	171	346	23	96.5	43.7	82	56
Mitral commissurotomy	100	33	41	21	5	95.0	74.0	67	26
Open heart surgery under extracorporeal cardiopulmonary circulation	72	9	47	7	9	87.5	77.8	88	22
Subtotal gastrectomy	763	129	343	261	30	96.1	61.9	83	38
Abdominal hysterectomy	590	203	236	67	84	87.4	79.9	66	26
Internal fixation of fracture with three-flanged nail	462	240	178	28	16	96.5	90.5	48	10
Total	5,414	1,813	2,046	1,061	494				

A table taken from a report by the Shanghai Acupuncture Anesthesia Coordinating Group, published in 1973, detailing statistics on the "effectiveness" of acupuncture anesthesia. The original table calculates statistics up to "Rate of grades I and II combined." The remainder of the table was calculated by the author.

mg/kg/2 hr, and allows the use of local anesthesia. Grade III, or moderate anesthetic effect, permits "obvious pain sensation" during the procedure, with "obvious changes in blood pressure, pulse rate and respiratory rate." Intravenous meperidine usage permitted is 1.5 to 2 mg/kg/2 hr, and a "moderate amount of local anesthesia" is used. With grade IV, or poor anesthetic effect, "marked pain" is experienced during the procedure; there are "obvious to marked changes in blood pressure, pulse rate and respiratory rate"; and it becomes "necessary to shift to drug anesthesia in order to accomplish the operation." In China, grades I, II, and III are considered "effective." In the West, of course, it is likely that only that portion of grade I in which pain is absent would be so considered.

It is instructive to examine statistics published by the Shanghai Acupuncture Anesthesia Coordinating Group in August 1973 (12) on results of the use of acupuncture anesthesia. As one example, we may select pulmonary resection. Out of 656 cases of pulmonary resection under acupuncture anesthesia reported on, 116 were said to have obtained a grade I anesthetic effect, 171 a grade II effect, 346 a grade III effect, and 23 a grade IV effect. The "effective rate" was reported as 96.5% including grades I, II, and III. Only 18% of the patients, however, experienced no pain or slight pain (grade I). The remaining 82% (grades II, III, and IV) experienced severe pain and physiological changes, and in 4% (grade IV) pain was severe enough to require a change to drug anesthesia during the operation. These statistics lead to the conclusion that acupuncture, with all its adjuncts as used in selected major surgery in China at present, may be associated with significant pain in as much as 82% of instances.

It is not at all clear what distinguishes the remaining 18%, those reporting either no pain or slight pain, from the others. From the available statistics, it is not possible to determine the proportion of patients, in fact, reporting no pain. From the description of the classifications used in the derivation of the statistics, it is not possible to distinguish those patients receiving no local analgesia from those patients receiving local analgesia; nor is it possible to determine the precise amount of premedication in each instance. These, of course, are the major physical factors, in addition to acupuncture, acting to produce analgesia, and they are the major ways in which modern acupuncture for surgery differs from any classic or modern (9) unsuccessful attempt. From the available evidence, it is not possible to determine further to what extent social class, level of education, previous experience, or Party membership relates to the report of slight pain or no pain. At maximum, 18% reporting no pain is a small percentage indeed. It is not predictable who will belong to this group. It appears surprising therefore that when it is known, or at least published, that more than 8 out of 10 patients undergoing pulmonary resection in this manner will suffer significant pain during an operation that patients volunteer for the procedure. Of course, it may be clear that physicians know these statistics, but it is not so clear that patients know them.

It is of interest to examine how the individual patient in China may be motivated to undergo surgery with acupuncture anesthesia. It is hardly necessary to tell anyone in China about acupuncture or to point out that acupuncture anesthesia is a unique product of the amalgamation of Chinese with Western medicine. Such specific medicopolitical indoctrination or harangue is unnecessary in China, a positive attitude toward acupuncture being present. On the other hand, the patient is encouraged to think of general anesthesia in terms only of the production of unconsciousness and a number of undesirable side effects. The possible benefits of general anesthesia in ensuring ventilation, muscular relaxation, and vagal blockade are not explained. The alternatives to general anesthesia, other than acupuncture anesthesia, particularly the relative innocuousness of complete regional or local anesthesia, are not presented. The patient is told that if pain reaches an intolerable level, either general or local anesthesia is available to control it. Thus the patient, socially motivated to do so and possessing only partial information imparted to him by his fellows and by his physicians, undertakes to submit to acupuncture anesthesia with the belief that he will benefit by reduced side effects, and that an adequate anesthetic backup is available. This overall indoctrination and selection process is similar to the procedure called natural childbirth in the West. Both procedures require special patient selection, social motivation, a conviction on the part of the patient that analgesic agents are deleterious, and a determination to withstand pain and discomfort and not to request analgesia. Both procedures are limited in their applicability to straightforward situations, permit the introduction of local anesthesia and narcotic analgesics, and provide a general or regional anesthetic backup. Acupuncture anesthesia may be usefully termed, by analogy, natural surgery.

After having said all this, we must admit that there is no question but that a small and, as yet, undetermined proportion of patients undergo major surgery while receiving acupuncture without local anesthesia and without intravenous narcotic analgesics. I probably saw such patients in China. They did not complain of pain. However, only if we assume that it is not possible at any time for selected patients to undergo selected major surgery without any anesthesia and not complain of pain can we conclude that the insertion and/or activation of acupuncture needles has an effect on the pain experience. But we cannot assume this. The same kind of anecdotal evidence regarding patients undergoing major surgery under acupuncture needle anesthesia alone without report of pain can be gathered about patients who have undergone major surgery for various reasons without any local or narcotic analgesic, or needle anesthesia, whatever and have denied pain. Also, tissue-destructive pubertal and other cultic rites in which pain is steadfastly denied (10) have been well described in the past. The uncontrolled observation of random patients undergoing major surgery associated with the manipulation of acupuncture needles, although interesting and heuristic, cannot indicate that these needles are in any substantive way related to the denial of pain.

There is an alternative to this latter assumption. We conventionally accept that the nonspecific, or "placebo," effect is associated with a denial of pain in approximately 33% of instances (2). This figure is an average only and was not obtained for pain during surgery. It is perfectly reasonable to suppose that placebo reactivity is variable and that a smaller proportion of patients undergoing major surgery would be "placebo reactors." Perhaps 18%, in China, is the correct figure for pulmonary resection. Although this may sound surprising at first, it was just as surprising originally to accept the notion that 33% of patients in pain from causes other than surgery could actually be relieved in the West by nonspecific means.

The most reasonable position to adopt at present, in my opinion, is that acupuncture may, perhaps, eventually be shown to relieve pain, probably poorly, but that evidence from acupuncture anesthesia as currently produced in China is no evidence for, and is some evidence against, this hope.

REFERENCES

1. Anonymous (1974): *The Principles and Practical Use of Acupuncture Anaesthesia.* Medicine and Health Publishing Co., Hong Kong.
2. Beecher, H. K. (1959): *Measurement of Subjective Responses. Quantification of Effects of Drugs.* Oxford University Press, New York.
3. Bonica, J. J. (1974*a*): *Anesthesiology,* 40:175–186.
4. Bonica, J. J. (1974*b*): *J.A.M.A.,* 229:1317–1325.
5. Campbell, J. N., and Taub, A. (1973): *Arch. Neurol.,* 28:347–350.
6. Croizier, R. C. (1968): *Traditional Medicine in Modern China. Science, Nationalism, and the Tensions of Cultural Change,* pp. 325. Harvard University Press, Cambridge.
7. Dimond, E. G. (1971): *J.A.M.A.,* 218:1558–1563.
8. Kaada, B., Hoel, E., Leseth, K., Nygaard-Østby, B., Setekleiv, J., and Stovner, J. (1974): *Tidsskr. Nor. Laegeforen.,* 94:417–442.
9. Mann, F. (1973): *Lancet,* (Sept. 8):563–564.
10. Melzack, R. (1973): *The Puzzle of Pain,* pp. 231. Basic Books, New York.
11. Quinn, J. R., Ed. (1973): In: *Medicine and Public Health in the People's Republic of China.* U.S. Department of Health, Education, and Welfare, P.H.S., N.I.H. Publication No. NIH 73-67, pp. 333.
12. Shanghai Acupuncture Anesthesia Coordinating Group (1975): *Acupuncture Anesthesia. An Anesthetic Method by Combination of Traditional Chinese and Western Medicine.* Shanghai Acupuncture Anesthesia Coordinating Group, Shanghai.
13. Taub, A., and Kane, A. (1975): *Pain,* 1:125–138.
14. Veith, I. (1972): *The Yellow Emperor's Classic of Internal Medicine* (translation). University of California Press, Berkeley.

Advances in Pain Research and Therapy, Vol. 1,
edited by J. J. Bonica and D. Albe-Fessard.
Raven Press, New York © 1976.

Comment on the Chapters of Taub and Kaada

Luciano Roccia

Department of Surgery, University of Torino, Torino, Italy

I think that, combined with modern medicine, acupuncture analgesia can be of great help not only in anesthesiology but especially in pain therapy. By the same token, I think that the so-called acupuncture anesthesia cannot have a place in our modern world where technology and pharmacology give us sophisticated equipment and drugs that have permitted raising the technique of anesthesia to an almost perfect level. We cannot suggest to our patients a form of analgesia that has a success rate of 80% to 90% in the best cases. However, to deny completely the analgesic and therapeutic value of acupuncture also means to ignore completely what acupuncture is. Unfortunately, we often tend to deny what our reason cannot explain, perhaps to hide our ignorance. On the other hand, to admit that acupuncture is the panacea for all pain means to be completely blind and false, and to be charlatans.

The experience of three trips to the Peoples' Republic of China, a stay of 1 month alone in hospitals in Peking and Shanghai, and wide personal experience in my own hospital prompt me to comment. My work in this field includes over 500 acupuncture analgesias for general surgery, gynecology, orthopedics, ophthalmology, ear, nose, and throat surgery, dentistry, and other procedures; 8 years of experimental and clinical research on acupuncture; and the direction of a pain clinic in which more than 100 patients are treated every day also with acupuncture. I congratulate Dr. Kaada on his objectivity, but I take great issue with the comments and evaluation made by Dr. Taub, who I believe must have been inaccurately informed in China and has transmitted inaccurate data to you.

I will emphasize some of Dr. Kaada's statements: first, the traditional theory of meridians is no longer followed by Chinese researchers and physicians, who are trying to explain the action of acupuncture on the basis of modern neurophysiology. Second, electrical stimulation is not absolutely necessary for surgical analgesia with acupuncture; simple manual manipulation of the needles is sufficient. With manual stimulation in our experience we have success not only in surgery but also in experimental research where we managed to cancel the nociceptive component of the trigeminal-facial reflex in the electromyogram in man. Third, the experiments of Prof. Chang of Shanghai on the medial thalamus have been repeated with the same results in France by Rabischong and Niboyet at the University of Montpellier. Moreover, we have repeated in Italy, with success, the experiments of crossed circulation, which strongly suggest the production of a humoral analgesic factor under acupuncture. Finally, the experience of over 500 acupuncture analgesias for surgery performed in Europe with success enables me to emphasize that it is not absolutely indispensable to be Chinese to undergo this technique.

To Dr. Taub I would like to emphasize that acupunctural analgesia with a history of only 15 years must be considered in an experimental stage, and therefore it inherently has many problems that must be solved. In any case, it is not absolutely true that acupuncture analgesia is characterized by failure. We can only say that there are failures in those patients in whom acupuncture analgesia is not indicated. During my trips to China I was not content to see only what the Chinese wanted to show me. After I returned home, I experimented with this technique and I now have extensive statistics of my own in this field. I would like to ask Dr. Taub if he did the same, since he did not refer to this in his chapter.

It is absolutely false that meperidine (pethidine) is used in doses of 200 to 500 mg. In most cases only 50 mg is given. Only in unsuccessful cases is the dosage increased before changing to general anesthesia. Many patients are operated on with acupuncture without any previous medication. The statistics presented by Dr. Taub are not valid outside the Chinese context, and his method of evaluating them cannot, from my point of view, be considered valid. Our criterion of success, considering the usual parameters such as blood pressure, pulse rate, and EEG, is based mostly on the patient's report. Most of them say they would undergo acupuncture analgesia again if necessary, and many of them have had surgery with general anesthesia previously.

Our experience shows that most of the Chinese data can be considered reliable when referred to cases in which acupuncture analgesia is indicated. This is the most important factor I would like to emphasize. People always consider acupuncture analgesia applicable to any case of surgery without considering the strict limits of this method. Yet our experience has shown us that acupuncture analgesia is not applicable to more than 15% to 20% of surgical patients. In these patients most of the Chinese data can be accepted.

Advances in Pain Research and Therapy, Vol. 1,
edited by J. J. Bonica and D. Albe-Fessard.
Raven Press, New York © 1976.

Acupuncture Analgesia: Evidence for Activation of a Pain Inhibitory System as a Mechanism of Action

David J. Mayer, Donald D. Price, Joseph Barber, and Amir Rafii

Medical College of Virginia, Richmond, Virginia 23298; and National Institute of Dental Research, Bethesda, Maryland 20014

Western attempts to understand and explain analgesic effects of acupuncture may be categorized in two theoretical approaches. The first uses knowledge of neurophysiological mechanisms, whereas the second presumes that psychological processes such as hypnosis, suggestion, or a placebo effect are involved (4). These two approaches need not be mutually exclusive since such "psychological" processes necessarily have a neural basis. The possible contribution of several of these factors in any clinical application of acupuncture analgesia makes any simple explanation of its mechanisms difficult.

Our investigations of experimentally induced acupuncture analgesia have tested the possibility that at least one of the mechanisms of acupuncture analgesia ultimately involves activation of the same descending pain inhibitory system that is activated by morphine and by electrical stimulation of periaqueductal and periventricular gray areas of the midbrain (1,6–8). Furthermore, we have tested the possibility that hypnosis involves activation of this same pain inhibitory system.

Our test was simply to determine whether acupuncture analgesia or hypnotic analgesia could be reversed with naloxone, a specific narcotic antagonist. The rationale for this test is based on observations that acupuncture analgesia, brain stimulation–produced analgesia, and morphine analgesia have some similar characteristics. All of these procedures take some time to reach maximal effectiveness as well as to disappear. Both morphine analgesia and stimulation-produced analgesia can be antagonized by naloxone (1,6). Thus an antagonism of acupuncture or hypnotic analgesic effects by naloxone would provide evidence that one or more of these phenomena involve activation of a pain inhibitory system.

METHOD

Five groups of human subjects were used. These included an acupuncture group ($N = 35$), a control group on which only repeated measures of pain threshold were performed ($N = 40$), a "placebo" control group ($N = 31$), a naloxone base-line group ($N = 30$), and a hypnosis group ($N = 14$). Experimental pain was evoked in all subjects by electrical stimulation of an upper or lower canine tooth with a commercially available tooth pulp vitality tester. Pain thresholds were measured by increasing the stimulation voltage in small increments until the subject reported the stimulus as definitely painful. A base-line pain threshold was established from the average of 3 to 4 measurements made at 5-min intervals. Pain threshold was also measured at 5-min intervals for 30 min during each of the above treatments. Subjects in the acupuncture group, the naloxone base-line group, and the hypnosis group were given either 0.8 mg naloxone hydrochloride (intravenously) or an equal volume of sterile saline 5 min after their 30-min treatment period. Approximately one-half of each group received naloxone. Drugs were administered in a double-blind procedure. Pain thresholds were measured 5, 10, and 15 min after injection. Treatment conditions (i.e., acupuncture, hypnosis) were maintained during these postinjection periods.

An acupuncture needle was inserted into each of the two *ho-ku* points and manual acupuncture was performed (4). Typically, this procedure produced irradiating and sometimes painful paresthesia, which disappeared as soon as manipulation of the needles was terminated. Thus, to eliminate effects of distraction, needle manipulation was performed for only 2 min out of the 5-min intervals between pain threshold measurements and never during the measurements themselves. The "placebo" group was instructed at the end of a 30-min nontreatment period that they were receiving a powerful analgesic drug. Instead, they were given an intravenous injection of saline. The naloxone base-line group received no analgesic treatment. At the end of a 30-min nontreatment period, one-half of this group received either naloxone or saline on a double-blind basis. This group was used to test effects of naloxone on base-line pain threshold. The hypnosis group received hypnotic instructions from one of us (J.B.), and each subject was given suggestions for: (a) subsequent analgesia to the stimulus, and (b) amnesia during the remainder of the experiment for these suggestions.

RESULTS

The results of the various treatments and the subsequent effects of naloxone and saline on treatment-induced increases in pain threshold are shown in Table 1. Acupuncture increased pain thresholds by 27% after 30 min of treatment. This increase, although not large, was reliably different than that of the repeated measures control group ($p = 0.0003$, t-test) and was also reliably different than the very small increase observed for the placebo group ($p < 0.01$, t-test). The largest increase, 85%, was observed for the hypnosis group, and all subjects in this group showed an analgesic effect. Interestingly, the placebo instruction combined with the saline injection did not reliably alter the pain threshold.

Of the 35 acupuncture subjects who had more than a 20% increase in pain

TABLE 1. *Treatment results*

Treatment	Change in pain threshold (% base line)	Pain threshold after naloxone (% base line)			Pain threshold after saline (% base line)		
		5 min.	10	15	5 min.	10	15
None ($N=40$)	7	—	—	—	—	—	—
Acupuncture ($N=35$[a])	27/35[a]	8	18	30	43	40	37
Placebo ($N=31$)	7	—	—	—	7	4	8
Hypnosis ($N=14$)	85	85	85	85	86	86	86

[a] Twenty of these subjects in whom a greater than 20% increase in pain threshold occurred were tested with saline or naloxone.

threshold, 20 were given naloxone (9 subjects) or saline (11 subjects). As indicated in Table 1, naloxone reduced pain thresholds to the level of the no treatment group and the placebo group. This reduction was highly reliable when measured at 5 min postinjection ($p < 0.003$, *t*-test, within subjects comparison) and was also reliable at 10 min postinjection ($p < 0.05$, *t*-test). In contrast, a slight increase in pain threshold occurred when saline was injected. Neither naloxone nor saline affected subjects in the naloxone baseline group and in the hypnosis group measured 5, 10, and 15 min postinjection. The result with hypnosis is consistent with that reported by Hilgard and Goldstein (2).

Another response difference distinguished the hypnosis and acupuncture groups. The analgesic effect often outlasted the acupuncture treatment by several minutes or even hours, whereas the analgesic effect of hypnosis could be terminated immediately by the hypnotist.

DISCUSSION

It is evident that under our conditions acupuncture produces a small but reliable increase in pain threshold and that this increase can be reversed with naloxone. It is unlikely that our acupuncture effects are related to any extent to placebo effects or to hypnosis. Placebo, unlike acupuncture, failed to alter pain thresholds. It is not unusual for placebo manipulations to be ineffective in modifying experimental pain (5). This negative result indicates that the increase in pain thresholds produced by acupuncture is unlikely to be a placebo effect. Unlike acupuncture, hypnotic analgesia was not antagonized by naloxone nor did it outlast the treatment period. Thus hypnosis is not likely to be a factor in our production of acupuncture analgesia.

These results support the hypothesis that acupuncture analgesia ultimately activates a pain inhibitory system that is also activated by narcotic analgesics and by electrical stimulation of the mesencephalic central gray area. The somewhat slow induction period and the long-lasting effects of acupuncture indicate a neurohumoral mechanism that is also consistent with the characteristics of the periaqueductal-periventricular analgesic system (6–9). Such an explanation is strongly supported by recent isolation from these structures of a substance with narcotic analgesic properties (3). Thus our data support the view that acupuncture ultimately causes the release of such a substance.

Our results also have bearing on the relative efficacies of acupuncture and hypnotic analgesia. Although the induction period for acupuncture analgesia is long and sometimes painful, we found that hypnosis was painless and anxiety reducing. More importantly, our acupuncture procedure, which employed needling of both *ho-ku* points, produced only small increases in pain threshold when compared to hypnosis. In addition, great variability was present in the analgesia produced by acupuncture, and no response to needling (i.e., paresthesia) was found to be a reliable predictor of the increase in pain threshold.

ACKNOWLEDGMENTS

This research was partly supported by Public Health Service Grant DA 00576 to D. J. Mayer. We thank Marjorie Robertson for technical assistance during these experiments.

REFERENCES

1. Akil, H., Mayer, D. J., and Liebeskind, J. C. (1972): *C. R. Acad. Sci.* [*D*] (*Paris*), 274:3603–3605.
2. Hilgard, R., and Goldstein, A. (1975): *Proc. Natl. Acad. Sci. U.S.A.*, 72:2041–2043.
3. Hughes, J. (1975): *Brain Res.*, 88:295–308.
4. Kaada, B. (1974): *Tidsskr. Nor. Laegeforen.*, 94:422–431.
5. Kuhn, R. A., and Bromiley, R. B. (1951): *J. Pharmacol. Exp. Ther.*, 101:47–55.
6. Liebeskind, J. C., Mayer, D. J., and Akil, H. (1974): In: *Advances in Neurology, Vol. 4: International Symposium on Pain,* edited by J. J. Bonica, pp. 261–268. Raven Press, New York.
7. Mayer, D. J., and Hayes, R. (1975): *Science,* 188:941–943.
8. Mayer, D. J., and Liebeskind, J. C. (1974): *Brain Res.*, 68:73–94.
9. Melzack, R., and Melinkoff, D. F. (1974): *Exp. Neurol.*, 43:369–374.

Advances in Pain Research and Therapy, Vol. 1,
edited by J. J. Bonica and D. Albe-Fessard.
Raven Press, New York © 1976.

Failure of Acupuncture to Produce Localized Changes in Subjective Cold Pain Ratings

*B. Lynn and E. R. Perl

Department of Physiology, University of North Carolina School of Medicine, Chapel Hill, North Carolina 27514

In a previous study (7,8) it was found that acupuncture produced only small, widely spread increases in pain threshold and decreases in pinprick discrimination. It seemed possible that our failure to find the spatial pattern of changes predicted by acupuncturists was because of using tests that involved only threshold levels of pain, and that tests involving stronger stimulation might reveal a different pattern of changes. The publication of a number of reports (2,4,10,11) which claimed that suprathreshold pain assessments were reduced by acupuncture of traditional points, but not by acupuncture at "placebo" points, further encouraged us to reexamine the efficiency of acupuncture using similar tests.

A method for producing graded cold pain at a variety of places on the body surface was therefore developed. The results obtained using it to study changes during acupuncture are reported herein.

METHODS

Stimuli were generated by placing the end of a cold metal cylinder (diameter 38 or 51 mm) firmly on the skin. Alcohol at temperatures of 0° to −3°C was continuously circulated through the cylinder. Subjects were asked to indicate when the resulting sensation (a) became painful, (b) reached a level that was half the maximum tolerable, and (c) became intolerable. From these responses, stimuli were assigned quantitative pain ratings. At any particular time, a stimulus was given a rating of 0.5 if the pain threshold had not been reached; a rating of 1.5 if threshold had been exceeded but the second criterion (half-way to intolerable) had not been reached; a rating of 2.5 if the second criterion had been passed but the stimulus was not yet intolerable; and a rating of 3.5 if the stimulus had already become intolerable. Thus a score of 1 on this scale represents threshold pain and a score of 3 represents the maximum tolerable pain.

*Present address: Department of Physiology, University College London, Gower Street, London, WC1E 6BT, England.

Two series of 12 subjects were tested. Those in series 1 were tested on the anterior surface of the neck, on the abdomen, and on the lateral surface of the upper thigh. Needles were inserted bilaterally in the lower leg [points *tsu-san-li* (stomach 36) and *san-yin-chiao* (spleen 6)], in the external ears (ear points "abdomen" and "stomach"), or at all four points. These points have been used for abdominal operations (1), and experienced, trained acupuncturists (Dr. W. Mao and Dr. T. C. Lee) predicted that they would produce maximum changes in pain reactions at the abdominal test area.

Subjects in series 2 were tested only on the neck and abdomen. Six of them received acupuncture at *ho-ku* (LI4) and *nei-kuan* (EH6) on the hands and forearms; the target area for these points was on the neck, and these points have been used for surgery there (1). The other 6 subjects in series 2 had needles inserted at points on the lower leg [*yang-ling-ch'uan* (spleen 9) and *san-yin-chiao*]. As before, these leg points were chosen to produce a maximum effect on the abdominal test area.

All subjects were paid male volunteers who gave their informed consent before the experiment started. Each took part in only one test session. A different paid volunteer-observer assisted with each experiment. Both subjects and observers were students or university staff; they knew that the experiments were concerned with analgesia but professed no knowledge of the expected relation between acupuncture points and affected region.

The acupuncture was carried out by an experienced acupuncturist. The experimenters played no part in carrying out the acupuncture, and the acupuncturist took no part in carrying out the sensory tests.

Acupuncture needles were inserted manually, and a suitable local reaction was elicited by hand twirling. When the needles were satisfactorily sited, electric pulses (from a Chinese type 6–26 stimulator) were passed between unilateral pairs of needles at a frequency of 3 to 7 Hz.

Each test session lasted approximately 2.5 hr. The first hour was spent in explaining the tests to the subject and observer and in practicing them. Next a series of control determinations of cold pain sensitivity was made. After this the acupuncture was started. Finally, a further series of sensory tests was carried out during the electroacupuncture. Testing was done in blocks, and within each block every area was tested once. The order in which areas were tested was switched and equated between blocks. Four blocks of tests were given both before and during acupuncture in series 1, whereas five blocks were given in series 2. Subjects were assigned to particular experimental plans at random.

RESULTS

Different subjects varied considerably in their reaction to the cold stimulus. Some subjects found that it rapidly produced an unpleasant radiating pain, although others experienced only mild pain. There were large differences, consistent from subject to subject, in the sensitivity of the three skin areas. The neck area was most sensitive and the leg area was least sensitive.

For all the areas examined, subjects usually found the cold pain stimulus less painful during acupuncture than before it. In order to compare results in different areas and in different subjects, we have calculated changes in ratings for durations of stimuli that produced the same average level of pain. Thus for insensitive areas, ratings for stimuli of relatively long duration have been calculated, whereas for a sensitive area a shorter stimulus duration has been used.

It is important to know if the average level of pain selected makes a difference to the results, and this can be assessed by comparing the changes at different average levels. Such comparisons have in fact not revealed any differences. An example is shown in Fig. 1A and B. The average decreases in pain ratings during acupuncture were very similar in this area regardless of whether an average level of 1.0 (threshold pain) or 2.0 (half-way to intolerable pain) was selected.

The average decrease in ratings during acupuncture was 0.46 units. This decrease is highly statistically significant ($p < 0.001$), and 5% confidence limits are 0.30 and 0.61 units (see Fig. 1C). All test areas showed a similar change during acupuncture.

The average changes at acupuncture "target" areas and at nontarget

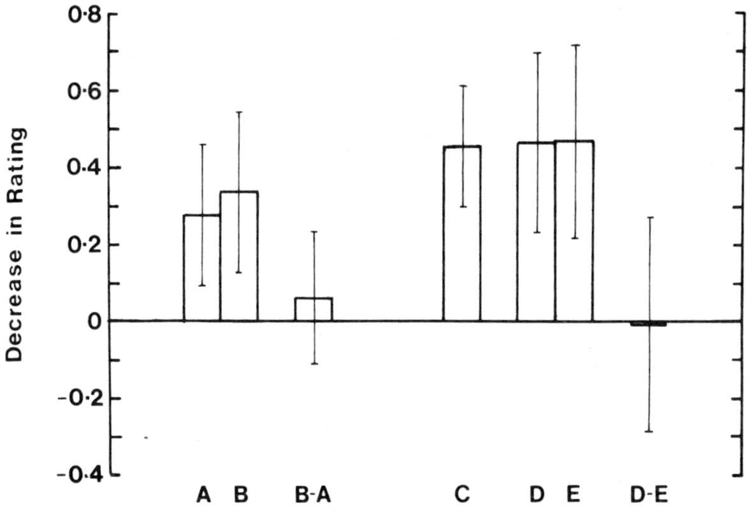

FIG. 1. Decrease in cold pain ratings during acupuncture. Mean ±5% confidence limits. **A,B:** Neck test area, 23 subjects; **A:** decrease when mean pain rating is 1; **B:** decrease for mean rating of 2; **B-A:** difference in decrease at mean ratings of 1 and 2; **C:** average for all test areas in 22 subjects; **D:** decrease at acupuncture "target" areas; **E:** decreases at nontarget control areas; **D-E:** difference between target and nontarget areas.

control areas are shown in Fig. 1D and E. The difference between these two is only 0.006 units (±0.28, 5% confidence limit). This difference is clearly not significant. This pattern of changes occurred with all the acupuncture points used; no points produced clear-cut differences in specific test areas.

DISCUSSION

These results indicate that acupuncture is as ineffective in reducing strong experimental pain as it had previously proved to be against threshold pain (7,8). The average changes were small and might well have been because of fatigue, the expectations of the subjects, and/or some other nonspecific factor. The crucial comparison between acupuncture target areas and other control areas produced a convincing negative result. There is only a 1 in 20 chance that a difference of 0.28 units or more (on a scale in which 2 units represents the tolerable range of pain sensations) was missed. It is conceivable that our acupuncture procedures were inadequate; however, they were consistent with modern Chinese practice (1) and with descriptions of traditional Chinese medicine. Finally, our results are similar to those of two Chinese groups who also failed to find any "specificity" of acupuncture points in relation to their classic target loci (5,9).

Other writers, however, have claimed that the meridian theory may be important because bigger changes in pain sensitivity were observed when "real" (classic) acupuncture points were used than when "new" or "placebo" acupuncture points were employed (2–4,10,11). Such studies, which involve comparisons with "placebo" points, suffer from two serious deficiencies. First, there is no satisfactory way to ensure that the intensity of needle stimulation is similar at different points. In fact, one report (10) stated that needle sensations were different at placebo acupuncture points, although other studies (2,3) did not find this. This is important since it has been reported that the sensory changes during transcutaneous electrical stimulation depend markedly on the strength of stimulation (6). The second, more serious problem is that the acupuncturist knows which are placebo points. This opens the door to all sorts of subtle influences. The small differences reported in these studies between the effects of acupuncture at different loci could well be due solely to such influences.

SUMMARY

Suprathreshold cold stimuli were rated slightly less painful on the average by 22 subjects during acupuncture than before it. Changes were similar on the neck, abdomen, and thigh, even though on the basis of traditional Chinese concepts one of these areas was always expected to be more affected than the others with the particular points used. This result confirms earlier findings using pain threshold measurements. We conclude that the classic meridan theories have little value when one is trying to select acupuncture points for anesthetizing a particular region of the body.

ACKNOWLEDGMENTS

This study was supported by U.S. Public Health Service Grant No. 21099. We wish to thank Prof. F. F. Kao (Department of Physiology, S.U.N.Y., Brooklyn, N.Y.) for advice and encouragement, Dr. W. Mao (Department of Anesthesiology, University of North Carolina School of Medicine, Chapel Hill, N.C.) for advice and for carrying out the acupuncture, and Dr. T. C. Lee (New York) for advice about the design of the experiments.

We would also like to acknowledge the assistance of the Clinical Research Unit at the North Carolina Memorial Hospital where this investigation was carried out; the Clinical Research Unit is supported by U.S. Public Health Service Research Grant No. RR-46 from the General Clinical Research Centers Branch of the Division of Research Resources.

REFERENCES

1. Acupuncture Editorial Group (1972): *Acupuncture Anesthesia.* People's Publishing Society, Shanghai. (Translation by J. E. Fogarty International Center, 1975. D.H.E.W. Publication No. (N.I.H.) 75–784.
2. Anderson, D. G., Jamieson, J. L., and Man, S. C. (1974): *Can. J. Psychol.,* 28:239–244.
3. Berlin, F. S., Bartlett, R. L., and Black, J. D. (1975): *Anesthesiology,* 42:527–531.
4. Chapman, C. R. (1975): Paper presented at Acupuncture Research Conference, N.I.H., Bethesda, Maryland, on March 14.
5. Chiang, C. Y., Chang, C. T., Chu, H. L., and Yang, L. F. (1973): *Scientia Sinica,* 16:210–217.
6. Holmgren, E. (1975): *Am. J. Chin. Med.,* 3:133–142.
7. Lynn, B., and Perl, E. R. (1975): *J. Physiol.,* 245:83–85P.
8. Lynn, B., and Perl, E. R. (1975): Paper presented at Acupuncture Research Conference, N.I.H., Bethesda, Maryland, on March 14.
9. Research Group of Acupuncture Anaesthesia (1973): *Chin. Med. J.,* 3:35.
10. Stacher, G., Wancura, I., Bauer, P., Lahoda, R., and Schulze, D. (1975): *Am. J. Chin. Med.,* 3:143–149.
11. Stern, J. (1975): Paper presented at Acupuncture Research Conference, N.I.H., Bethesda, Maryland, on March 14.

Advances in Pain Research and Therapy, Vol. 1,
edited by J. J. Bonica and D. Albe-Fessard.
Raven Press, New York © 1976.

Pain Threshold Effects of Peripheral Conditioning Stimulation

Sven A. Andersson and Eddy Holmgren

Department of Physiology, University of Göteborg, Fack, S-400 33 Göteborg 33, Sweden

A number of clinical studies have suggested that high-frequency electrical stimulation (50 to 200 Hz) of the dorsal columns or of peripheral nerves suppresses the perception of chronic pain (21,22,25,26,28). The hypalgesia is supposed to be due to a segmental inhibitory action of the transmission in the pain pathways by impulse activity in fibers mediating other somatic modalities (20). Low-frequency stimulation (1 to 3 Hz) has also been reported to relieve pain (12,16,27). In contrast to the almost immediate hypalgesia produced by high-frequency conditioning stimulation, low frequencies are reported to reduce the sensation of pain gradually and the poststimulation pain suppression is more long lasting. The reports are mainly based on the patients' subjective experience of changes in pain sensation, which is difficult to evaluate objectively. The aim of the present studies was to quantify experimentally the pain suppressive effect by measurements of the pain threshold in healthy subjects during conditioning stimulation at various frequencies and intensities applied segmentally and nonsegmentally with regard to the area of induced experimental pain.

MATERIALS AND METHODS

The investigation was performed on 34 subjects from the same class of dental students. The pain thresholds were established by applying electrical current from the cathodal side of a constant current stimulator, Bofors Pulp Tester (4,19), to the carefully cleaned and dried surface of intact teeth through a probe with a contact surface of 1 mm^2. The anodal side of the stimulator was connected to a handle with a switch used by the subjects to indicate the first sensation of pain. The current passing through the tooth at this moment was recorded. The current could be varied between 0 and 100 μA and consisted of 10-msec square wave pulses at a frequency of 5/sec.

On the test occasion the actual pain threshold of each tooth was based on several individual measurements. Usually three teeth in the upper and three in the lower jaw were used. Conditioning stimulation was given through sterilized needles or surface electrodes (area of contact 2 to 4 cm^2) applied bilaterally to the cheeks in the region of the exit of the infraorbital nerve and/or to the hands in the regions between the metacarpal bones I and II. Electrical conditioning stimulation at the frequencies of 2, 10, or 100 Hz was performed at these sites with pulses of short duration (less than 1 ms).

The intensity of the conditioning stimulation was usually increased gradually during the first 10 min of a session to a level which could be just tolerated by the individual subject and then only slightly adjusted. A strong beating sensation and forceful muscle contractions were elicited in arms and face. In the beginning of a test session the pain threshold of each tooth to be used was established two to three times at 15-min intervals. If reproducible threshold values were not obtained in a certain tooth, the results were discarded. During the conditioning stimulation which usually lasted 60 to 75 min the pain threshold was regularly measured at intervals of 15 min, and the pain threshold was followed for approximately 30 min during the postconditioning period.

In an initial survey the average pain threshold effects in each individual were correlated with certain personality factors such as the degrees of neuroticism and extraversion-introversion, established by the Eysenck Personality Inventory (3), and the hysterical-nonhysterical factors and the psychasthenic-sthenic character established by the MNT Scale (18).

RESULTS

Effects of Conditioning Stimulation at 2 Hz—General Characteristics

All subjects included in this study were tested according to a standard procedure. A reproducible and stable control level was established for each tooth in which the pain threshold should be followed during the session. The threshold was again established 15 to 20 min after the mere application of the needles or surface electrodes, and no change of the pain threshold was observed. The values of the control thresholds were distributed as shown in Fig. 1B. Fig. 1A illustrates the average change of the pain threshold during and after conditioning stimulation of hands and cheeks at 2 Hz expressed as multiples of the control values. The threshold increased gradually during the first period of conditioning and decreased slowly toward the control value in the poststimulation period.

In each individual the threshold increase was rather similar in all tested teeth in both the upper and lower jaw (2). The time course of the effect was similar whether the conditioning stimulation was given with needles or with surface electrodes and in all subjects except 3 who did not show any increase of the pain threshold. The interindividual variation of the threshold effects was considerable, however, as shown in Fig. 1B. Conditioning stimulation during 60 min increased the threshold from a mean value of

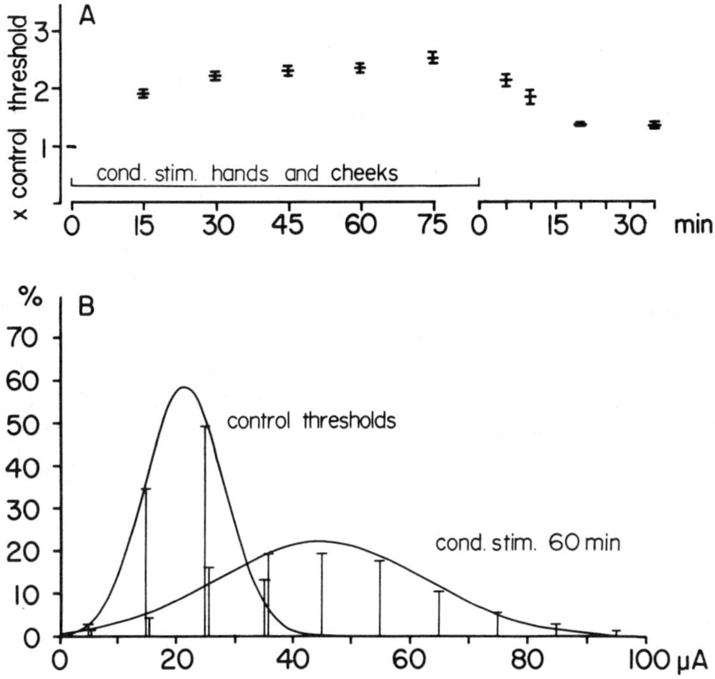

FIG. 1. A: Pain threshold increase of conditioning electrical stimulation at 2 Hz of hands and cheeks. Pain threshold measured as the minimum current which produced pain when applied to the dental surface. Calculated values, expressed as mean and SEM in this and following diagrams, are based on measurements from 6 teeth in each of 30 students and are given as multiples of control values. **B:** Histograms of distribution of the individual pain thresholds of tested incisors (teeth 1+, −1) in the control situation and after conditioning stimulation at 2 Hz during 60 min. Bell-shaped curves show the appearance of a normally distributed sample of data corresponding to the calculated mean values and SDs.

21.6 μA, SD 6.7 μA, to a mean of 45.2 μA, SD 17.7 μA. The bell-shaped curves included in Fig. 1B indicate how a normally distributed sample of data should appear in correspondence with the calculated mean values and standard deviations.

In order to elucidate the possible role of psychological suggestive mechanisms as a basis for the interindividual variation of the effects, we performed a correlation analysis, using Pitman's test (5), between the amplitude of pain threshold increase and various personality traits (see Methods). No significant correlation was found to any of the personality traits studied.

Effects of Segmental and Nonsegmental Conditioning Stimulation

To evaluate the relative contribution to the pain threshold increase from stimulation of hands and cheeks at 2 Hz, we stimulated each of these sites separately. Stimulation of only the cheeks gave an increase of the pain threshold which did not differ from that of the combined hand and cheek stimulation. Stimulation of the hands only was usually ineffective, and the pain thresholds of the teeth remained at the control levels throughout a test period of 60 to 75 min in spite of very high intensity of the conditioning stimulation. Only in 1 out of 9 tested subjects did the pain threshold increase, and in this case the effect was rather similar to that obtained by stimulation of the cheeks. A certain effect on the pain threshold of teeth by conditioning of the hands could, however, be revealed as illustrated in Fig. 2A, which is based on threshold measurements from a group of 4 subjects. In these subjects the pain threshold did not change during stimulation of hands only. When stimulation of the cheeks was added the threshold gradually increased to approximately 2.7 times the control value. After discontinuation of the conditioning of the cheeks, the threshold decreased first rapidly but leveled off at approximately 1.8 times the control value. When the conditioning via

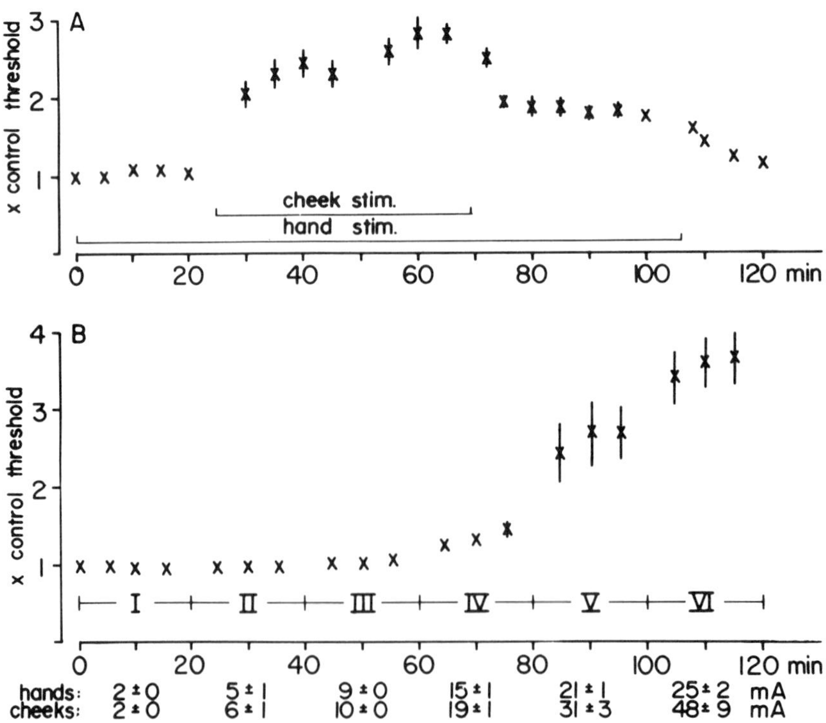

FIG. 2. Effects on the tooth pain threshold. **A:** Conditioning stimulation at 2 Hz of hands followed by a combined stimulation of hands and cheeks and then by stimulation of hands only. **B:** Conditioning stimulation at 2 Hz of hands and cheeks at 6 different intensity levels, I–VI. Results obtained from teeth in both jaws. Mean intensity of the conditioning current (±SEM) given at bottom.

the hands was also discontinued, the threshold returned gradually to the control level.

Effects of Graded Intensities of the Conditioning Stimulation

In a group of 4 subjects the pain threshold was established when the intensity of the conditioning stimulation of hands and cheeks at 2 Hz was increased in steps, each based on the subjective experience of the induced sensations and the distribution of the elicited muscle contractions (13). The strength of the conditioning current in milliamperes was also measured, and the values are given in Fig. 2B. At each level the intensity was kept constant for 20 min, and the thresholds of four teeth in the upper and lower jaw were determined three times. At the lowest intensities giving subliminal (I), just supraliminal sensation (II), and weak beating sensations with weak muscle contractions (III), the pain threshold did not change. At level IV, giving stronger beating sensations and distinct muscle contractions at all the stimulation sites, the threshold increased slightly. The intensity level V could be just tolerated for at least 60 min and elicited strong beating sensations and large muscle contractions in arms and face. This intensity corresponded to that used in other series of this study. The stimulation intensity was very strong at level VI and could be tolerated only with obvious difficulties for 20 min. At both levels V and VI the threshold increased significantly and similarly in the teeth of the upper and lower jaws.

Threshold Effects of Higher Conditioning Frequencies

The results of conditioning stimulation at similar intensities with 2 and 10 Hz, obtained in a group of 7 subjects, are compared in Fig. 3 together with a typical example of the threshold effects in tooth +3 in 1 subject conditioned with 100 Hz applied to the cheeks. Conditioning at 10 Hz increased the threshold more rapidly than at 2 Hz, but the threshold decreased during the ongoing stimulation and the poststimulation effect was rather small. Conditioning stimulation with 10 or 100 Hz of the hands only gave no effects on the pain threshold of teeth. A very high intensity conditioning at 100 Hz of the cheeks induced an instantaneous increase of the threshold mainly in the upper canine teeth. The threshold decreased rapidly, however, during the continuing conditioning. No threshold change appeared in the teeth of the lower jaw.

SUMMARY AND COMMENTS

The results indicate that somatic stimulation interferes with the perception of pain, an effect which during the actual experimental conditions did not seem to be related to any of the measured personality traits. The

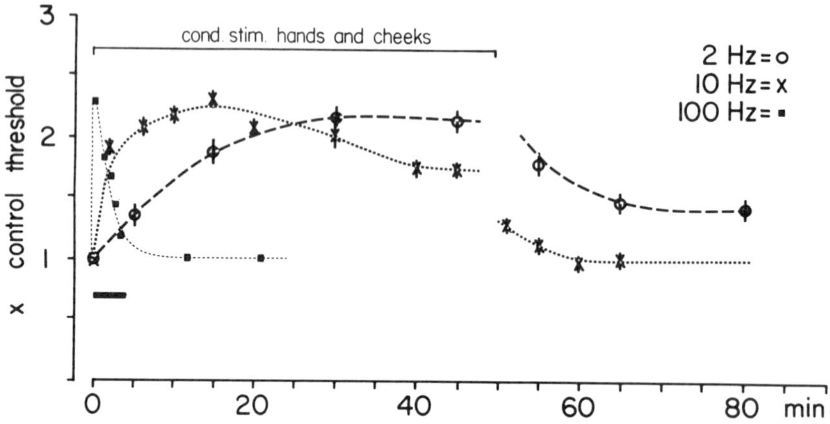

FIG. 3. Characteristic effects of different conditioning stimulation frequencies on pain threshold. Stimulations at 2 and 10 Hz were performed during 50 min, and threshold values represent measurements of 4 teeth in each of 7 subjects. Duration of stimulation at 100 Hz is indicated by the heavy bar below the curve, which is a typical example from 1 subject. Curves drawn tentatively.

pain threshold increase was most pronounced during conditioning at low frequencies. The notion that the threshold increase is because of basic physiological rather than psychological mechanisms is supported by observations in an ongoing study of chronic cats in which low-frequency conditioning stimulation of the infraorbital nerves increases the threshold of behavioral pain responses induced by electrical stimulation of the tooth pulp. The high intensity required to induce the change in the pain threshold at both low- and high-frequency conditioning stimulation suggests that the suppressive effects on the transmission in the pain pathways are owing to activity in high-threshold afferents, most likely including afferents from the muscles, rather than to activity in low-threshold afferents only, as previously suggested (20).

Apart from the frequency of the conditioning stimulation, the most pronounced threshold effects were obtained when conditioning and pain stimuli were applied in close proximity, indicating a topographical relationship between the pain afferents and afferents inhibiting the message in these afferents. The pronounced differences in the time course of the effects produced by low (2 Hz) and high (100 Hz) frequencies indicate that the interactive mechanisms are different. At high frequencies the effect is probably due to pre- and postsynaptic inhibitory interactions between the pain afferents and other high-threshold afferents at the input stage of the central nervous system and with characteristics similar to those revealed by studies on the control of the transmission from high-threshold afferents to flexor motoneurons (7,15,17,24,29). In the present study the experimental pain was evoked by stimulation of A-delta fibers (1,6), i.e., tooth pulp afferents. It may be that chronic pain is related to an abnormal C-fiber activation of pain pathways. The obvious discrepancy between the high intensities required to induce the observed transient change in pain threshold and the moderate intensities reported to suppress the perception of chronic pain could be related to a more efficient depression of the transmission from C fibers than from A-delta fibers.

The slow time course changes in pain threshold at low frequency of conditioning stimulation may reflect a resetting of more complex mechanisms involving the descending control systems known to exert a tonic inhibition on the transmission from mainly high-threshold afferents to ascending pathways (8–11,14,23). It is suggested that these systems give a negative feedback, mainly directed to the segments receiving an intense barrage of impulses from the sites of conditioning stimulation, but that transmission from pain afferents may also be influenced more generally as indicated by the presence of a certain nonsegmental effect on the pain threshold.

ACKNOWLEDGMENTS

This work was supported by the Swedish Medical Research Council (project no. 14X-55) and by Magnus Bergvalls Stiftelse.

REFERENCES

1. Anderson, K. V., and Pearl, G. (1974): *Exp. Neurol.,* 43:281–283.
2. Andersson, S. A., Ericson, T., Holmgren, E., and Lindqvist, G. (1973): *Brain Res.,* 63:393–396.
3. Bederoff-Petersson, A., Jägtoft, K., and Åström, J. (1971): *EPI Eysenck Personality Inventory, Ed. 2.* Skandinaviska Testförlaget, Stockholm.
4. Björn, H. (1946): *Swedish Dent. J.* [*Suppl.*], 39:1–101.
5. Bradley, J. V. (1968): *Distribution—Free Statistical Tests.* Prentice-Hall, Englewood Cliffs, New Jersey.
6. Brookhart, J. M., Livingston, W. K., and Haugen, F. P. (1953): *J. Neurophysiol.,* 16:634–642.
7. Eccles, J. C. (1964): *The Physiology of Synapses,* Springer-Verlag, Berlin, Heidelberg, New York.
8. Engberg, I., Lundberg, A., and Ryall, R. W. (1968*a*): *J. Physiol.,* 194:201–223.
9. Engberg, I., Lundberg, A., and Ryall, R. W. (1968*b*): *J. Physiol.,* 194:225–236.
10. Engberg, I., Lundberg, A., and Ryall, R. W. (1968*c*): *Acta Physiol. Scand.,* 72:115–122.
11. Engberg, I., Lundberg, A., and Ryall, R. W. (1968*d*): *Acta Physiol. Scand.,* 72:123–133.
12. Eye, Ear, Nose and Throat Hospital of Shanghai First Medical College, Shanghai (1973): *Chin. Med. J.,* 2:18 (Abstract in English).
13. Holmgren, E. (1975): *Am. J. Chin. Med.,* 3:133–142.
14. Holmqvist, B., Lundberg, A., and Oscarsson, O. (1960): *Arch. Ital. Biol.,* 98:60–80.
15. Hongo, T., Jankowska, E., and Lundberg, A. (1966): *Exp. Brain Res.,* 1:338–358.
16. Kaada, B., Hoel, E., Leseth, K., Nygaard-Østby, B., Setekleiv, J., and Stovner, J. (1974): *Tidsskr. Nor. Laegeforen.,* 94:417–442.
17. Lundberg, A. (1972): Symposial paper, *4th International Biophysics Congress,* Moscow.
18. Marke, S., and Nyman, E. (1958): *Manual Till MNT-Skalan.* Skandinaviska Testförlaget, Stockholm.
19. Matthews, B., and Searle, B. N. (1974): *Br. Dent. J.,* 137:307–312.
20. Melzack, R., and Wall, P. D. (1965): *Science,* 150:971–979.

21. Meyer, G. A., and Fields, H. L. (1972): *Brain,* 95:163–168.
22. Nashold, B. S., and Friedman, H. (1972): *J. Neurosurg.,* 36:590–597.
23. Oliveras, J. L., Besson, J. M., Guilbaud, G., and Liebeskind, J. C. (1974): *Exp. Brain Res.,* 20:32–44.
24. Schmidt, R. F. (1971): In: *Reviews of Physiology,* pp. 20–101. Springer-Verlag, Berlin, Heidelberg, New York.
25. Shealy, C. N., and Maurer, D. (1974): *Surg. Neurol.,* 2:45–47.
26. Shealy, C. N., Mortimer, J. T., and Hagfors, N. R. (1970): *J. Neurosurg.,* 32:560–564.
27. Thoma, H., Benzer, H., Mayrhofer, O., and Pauser, G. (1975): *Anaesthesist,* 24:32–38.
28. Wall, P. D., and Sweet, W. H. (1967): *Science,* 155:108–109.
29. Whitehorn, D., and Burgess, P. R. (1973): *J. Neurophysiol.,* 36:226–237.

Advances in Pain Research and Therapy, Vol. 1,
edited by J. J. Bonica and D. Albe-Fessard.
Raven Press, New York © 1976.

Changes in Thermal Discriminability and Pain Report Criterion after Acupunctural or Transcutaneous Electrical Stimulation

*W. Crawford Clark, **Wayne Hall, and †Joseph Yang

**N.Y. State Psychiatric Institute; Departments of *Psychiatry and †Anesthesiology, College of Physicians and Surgeons, Columbia University, New York, New York 10032; and **University of New South Wales, Australia*

According to Melzack and Wall's (7) gate control theory of pain perception, selective electrical stimulation of afferent large-diameter myelinated nerve fibers should produce peripheral analgesia. The effectiveness of percutaneous and transcutaneous electrical stimulation (TES) for the relief of pain has been demonstrated in clinical pain by Wall and Sweet (8) and in experimental thermal pain by Krasnegor et al. (6). The gate model has also been used to explain pain relief following acupuncture, although the neural basis is vague. In the present study, the effectiveness of TES was compared to that of acupuncture by obtaining response data under comparable physical (same thermal stimulus intensities) and methodological (analysis by signal detection theory) conditions.

The purpose of this study is not to demonstrate that TES and acupuncture raise the pain threshold, that is, decrease pain responses. Rather, it is to determine the source of this change. The recent advance in psychophysics known as signal detection theory makes it clear that the traditional "50% pain threshold" is an unresolvable mixture of sensory (physiological) and attitudinal (psychological) variables. Signal detection theory yields two measures of the subject's performance. The physiological parameter, d', provides a measure of discriminability which is independent of psychological (nonsensory) variables; d' is directly related to the amount of sensory information available. For example, Clark and Yang (4) have demonstrated that partial block of the median nerve with an infiltration of dilute mepivacaine decreases d'. The psychological parameter, L_x, locates the subject's response criterion, that is, his willingness or reluctance to report the presence of pain. For example, Clark (2,3) has demonstrated that the administration of a placebo described as a potent analgesic raises the pain report criterion L_x without influencing d'.

PROCEDURE

In both the acupuncture and TES studies, approximately 12 thermal stimuli were presented at each of six intensities (0, 120, 240, 305, 370, and

425 mcal · sec^{-1} · cm^{-2}) to six patches of India ink on either (a) the volar surface of each forearm (acupuncture) or (b) the palmar aspect of the thumb and lateral two fingers innervated by the median nerve in each hand (TES). Skin temperature was monitored every 15 min. The subjects were instructed to rate each presentation along a 12-category intensity scale with categories ranging from "nothing" through various degrees of heat and pain to "withdrawal."

The acupuncture procedure has been described by Clark and Yang (4) and by Clark et al. (5), the sites and duration of the stimulation being standard for surgery of the arm. For the TES procedure, electrode sites at the volar surface of the left wrist (cathode) and the left upper arm (anode) were prepared by wiping the skin with alcohol and vigorously rubbing with Offner electrode paste. The stimuli provided by a Grass stimulator and isolation unit were 0.1-msec monophasic square wave pulses at 100 Hz and 18 mA with an amplitude of 31 V (small, 0.8-cm^2 electrode).

The wrist electrode was moved and voltage increased until paresthesias and slight muscle twitching occurred in the region of the hand innervated by the median nerve. After the initial thermal test period (Pre), the median nerve was stimulated transcutaneously for 5 min before and for 12 to 15 min during the next thermal test period (During). The transcutaneous stimulation was then stopped and thermal testing continued for periods Post-1 and Post-2. The limb was partially enclosed in an electric blanket to maintain a constant temperature because preliminary observations revealed that the electrical stimulation decreased the temperature of the hand, presumably because vasomotor fibers were stimulated.

RESULTS

For d' the analysis of variance revealed no significant differences between the acupunctured and control arms, nor among the Pre, During, and Post-1 and -2 acupuncture periods (Table 1). None of the interactions were significant. d' varied with respect to stimulus intensity ($F=3.74$; df=4/40; $p<0.05$). [A t-test at 0 to 120 mcal · sec^{-1} · cm^{-2} suggests that d' decreased after acupuncture ($t=6.26$; df=11; $p<0.01$); however, in view of the absence of a significant main effect for Period, this result must be considered spurious.] Furthermore, there was no difference between the acupunctured and control arms either during or after acupuncture. A separate analysis of variance for the criterion for reporting "very faint pain" or pain of a higher intensity L_{VFP} revealed a tendency to raise report criteria during the test ($F=7.38$; df=2/20; $p<0.005$). In response to the 305 to 370 mcal · sec^{-1} · cm^{-2} stimuli, the subjects set a higher L_{VFP} criterion (fewer reports of pain) in the acupunctured arm during the acupuncture period than Pre or Post ($t=2.33$; df=11; $p<0.05$).

The results of TES of the median nerve appear in Table 2. Inspection of

TABLE 1. d′ *and* L_x *in control* (C) *and acupunctured* (A) *arms,* N=*12*

Time		Stimulus intensity (mcal · sec⁻¹ · cm⁻²) 0–120	120–240	240–305	305–370	370–425	Mean	L_{VFP} at 305–370
Pre	C	1.70	1.64	0.88	1.36	1.30	1.37	0.72
	A	1.90	1.04	1.03	1.44	1.37	1.36	0.99
During	C	1.86	1.12	1.16	1.39	1.49	1.40	0.61
	A	1.78	1.11	1.00	1.46	1.42	1.35	1.35
Post	C	1.44	1.29	1.00	1.41	1.73	1.37	1.49
	A	1.34	1.40	1.10	1.40	1.76	1.40	1.03

TABLE 2. d′ *and* L_x *in control* (C) *and electrically blocked* (E) *hands;* N=*6*

Time		Stimulus intensity (mcal · sec⁻¹ · cm⁻²) 0–120	120–240	240–305	305–370	370–425	Mean	L_{VFP} at 305–370
Pre	C	2.04	1.93	1.92	1.31	1.19	1.68	0.70
	E	2.09	1.56	1.17	1.89	1.18	1.58	0.63
During	C	2.50	1.67	1.12	1.49	0.77	1.51	0.63
	E	1.94	0.99	0.97	1.18	1.05	1.23	1.38
Post-1	C	2.23	1.33	1.57	1.79	0.63	1.51	0.78
	E	1.96	1.64	1.25	2.00	0.89	1.55	0.80
Post-2	C	2.04	1.62	1.53	1.96	0.99	1.63	0.69
	E	2.40	1.60	1.70	1.70	0.98	1.68	0.85

the data suggests that TES was effective in reducing d' at all thermal intensities but the highest. However, less than 30 min later (period Post-1) values of d' returned to their initial levels and remained there (period Post-2). The distraction and discomfort induced by TES did not affect values of d' obtained concurrently in the control arm (period During). In response to the 305 to 370 mcal · sec^{-1} · cm^{-2} stimuli, the subjects set a markedly higher L_{VFP} criterion (fewer pain reports) in the stimulated arm only during TES.

DISCUSSION

Both TES and acupuncture raised the pain report criterion, higher values of L_{VFP}. This decrease in the proportion of pain reports suggests that both treatments produced an analgesic effect. However, TES of the median nerve decreased discriminability, d', of thermal stimuli; in contrast, acupuncture failed to alter d'. A decrease in d' is known to occur after the administration of a recognized analgesic (4), presumably because neural transmission has been attenuated. Thus the results suggest that TES, but not acupuncture, suppresses experimental pain. The use of signal detection theory in this study ensures that this conclusion is not caused by a "placebo effect." The analgesia that followed TES was short in duration, an effect which according to Wall and Sweet (8) is to be expected with an intact nervous system.

Chapman and co-workers have used signal detection theory to examine dental analgesia. Contrary to the findings of the present study, they report that acupuncture and TES (C. R. Chapman, M. E. Wilson, and J. D. Gehrig, *personal communication*), as well as nitrous oxide (1), decreased d' and conclude that each of these procedures produces an analgesic effect. Is it possible to explain these discrepant results? Differences in the acupuncture procedure, psychophysical technique, or pain locus might account for the disagreement, but as Clark et al. (5) point out, this seems unlikely. Chapman et al. (*personal communication*) note that the "on-site" acupunctural stimulation of the hands may have made it difficult for the subject to attend to the weaker dental stimuli, and hence lowered d'. The finding that the "off-site" (placebo) acupuncture group showed no decrement in d' argues against this interpretation, but it remains, as Chapman et al. (*personal communication*) note, a possibility since *ten ch'i* should be absent in the "off-site" group. In the present study the effects of distraction or decreased vigilance were demonstrated to be absent since the d', based on simultaneous measurements of an untreated locus, was not decreased during either acupuncture or TES. Such a control should be used whenever possible.

Finally, the possibility must be entertained that the difference in conclusions lies in the statistical treatment of the results rather than in the data themselves. In their recent study Chapman et al. (*personal communication*) found significant decreases in d' at the lowest level of stimulus intensity. In the present study we, too, found a decrease in d' at the lowest intensity, which was significant according to a t-test. However, this finding had to be discounted in view of the lack of a statistically significant main effect in the analysis of variance. Regardless of how this result is viewed, it seems obvious that acupuncture exerts at best a very weak effect relative to analgesic drugs or TES.

ACKNOWLEDGMENTS

This work was supported in part by National Institutes of Health Grants NS09263 and FR 05650.

REFERENCES

1. Chapman, C. R., Gehrig, J. D., and Wilson, M. E. (1975): *Anesthesiology*, 42:532–537.
2. Clark, W. C. (1969): *J. Abnorm. Psychol.*, 74:363–371.

3. Clark, W. C. (1974): *Anesthesiology,* 40:272–287.
4. Clark, W. C., and Yang, J. C. (1974): *Science,* 184:1096–1098.
5. Clark, W. C., Yang, J. C., and Hall, W. (1975): *Science,* 189:65–68.
6. Krasnegor, N. A., Jennings, J. R., Orr, W. C., and Fields, H. L. (1972): *Psychon. Sci.,* 26:74–76.
7. Melzack, R., and Wall, P. D. (1965): *Science,* 150:971–979.
8. Wall, P. D., and Sweet, W. H. (1967): *Science,* 155:108–109.

Advances in Pain Research and Therapy, Vol. 1,
edited by J. J. Bonica and D. Albe-Fessard.
Raven Press, New York © 1976.

Signal Detection Evaluation of the Effects of Acupuncture on the Perception of Painful Dental Stimulation

*C. Richard Chapman, **Michael E. Wilson, and †John D. Gehrig

**Departments of Anesthesiology, Psychiatry and Behavioral Sciences, and Psychology; **Department of Anesthesiology; and †Department of Oral Surgery; University of Washington School of Medicine, Seattle, Washington 98195*

In recent years acupuncture analgesia has emerged as a major issue in pain research. Since Chinese physicians first demonstrated that patients can undergo major surgery with no significant analgesic treatment beyond acupunctural stimulation, two major issues have developed in the work of Western investigators. The first is the question of whether acupuncture stimulation brings about a sensory loss, and the second is that of determining the relative importance of psychological factors.

Acupuncture studies focusing on pain threshold have indicated that some perceptual changes can be detected in the laboratory. Chinese investigators (12) induced pain in human volunteers using potassium iontophoresis dolorimetry and recorded pain threshold over time in various parts of the body. Applying acupunctural stimulation, they observed a gradual increase in pain threshold over time, which seemed to reach stable state after 30 or 40 min. Other Chinese researchers (6,10) have found similar phenomena using cutaneous shocks to induce pain. Andersson and his collaborators in Sweden (1) studied changes in the dental pain threshold in response to acupunctural stimulation. Using electrical stimulation of the tooth pulp, they examined pain threshold over time in volunteers and reported a gradual increase in the limen with acupunctural stimulation of the hands and cheeks, which was similar in pattern to that reported by the Chinese. Unlike the Chinese, however, the Swedish investigators administered acupunctural stimulation to sites in the same neurological segment used for dolorimetric testing. Stimulation of the hands alone resulted in a trivial increase in dental pain threshold, whereas stimulation of the hands and cheeks together, or the cheeks alone, resulted in a substantial analgesic effect.

Using radiant heat dolorimetry, Berlin et al. (2) investigated the effects of acupuncture on the perception of cutaneous pain in the forearms of vol-

** Present address: Bristol Royal Infirmary, Bristol, England.

unteers. These investigators chose not to study pain threshold because it has been a highly controversial measure, and instead they measured the duration of time subjects would accept a continuous heat stimulus before terminating it because of pain. Response latencies to painful stimuli were increased significantly by acupunctural stimulation, whereas treatment of sites not considered acupuncture points had less effect on response times. Berlin and his associates (2) cautioned that acupuncture's effects, although significant, were quite small, and they noted that it was not possible to separate physiological changes from changes in attitude or emotional set which might affect response latency.

Although these results suggest that acupunctural analgesia merits further scientific investigation, they have not conclusively demonstrated that acupunctural stimulation changes sensory processes. As Berlin et al. (2) noted, psychological factors such as attitudes, beliefs, or expectations may determine performance in a laboratory task. Pain threshold may increase in response to reduction in sensory functioning, and it may also be elevated as a result of changes in psychological states.

SUMMARY OF METHODOLOGY

Recently, efforts have been made to evaluate acupunctural analgesia using the methodology of signal detection theory. These procedures permit the investigator to obtain separate and statistically independent measures of sensory sensitivity to painful stimulation and response bias (or willingness to report the stimulation as painful). The signal detection theory has been the subject of several textbooks, and Clark (7) wrote a definitive article describing its application to pain research.

Signal detection procedures require that the experimenter set up a task in which his subject makes judgments about two or more levels of stimulation, one of which may be zero. For example, one might use several levels of electrical current delivered to the tooth pulp and include a null stimulus among them. Each stimulus would be presented briefly for many trials, and the various stimuli would occur in pseudo-random order. It is essential in such a study that the task be difficult for the subject so that he always faces uncertainty about how to respond. This forces the subject to make errors as well as accurate judgments.

A unique characteristic of signal detection methodology is that it uses both the subject's errors and his correct responses. In such a task as the one just described, all of the information about the subject's behavior may be derived from two variables. The first of these is hit rate, or the percentage of trials on which a noxious stimulus is presented and is appropriately judged as painful. The second variable is false-affirmative rate, or the proportion of trials on which a nonnoxious stimulus is incorrectly identified as painful. The theory of signal detection is based on the assumption that a lawful relationship exists between the rate of correct responses and the rate of errors, and the two measures, sensitivity to pain and response bias, are derived from this relationship (13).

APPLICATION

We will describe briefly the results of two experiments in which we have applied the methodology of signal detection theory to the study of acupuncture analgesia. In our first experiment (3) we used 42 men aged 21 to 45 years, and we delivered brief bursts of constant current dental stimulation to them through a hand-held probe. Each dental stimulus consisted of a 0.1-sec burst of electrical pulses at a preset current level. In a preliminary session with each subject, we determined the threshold current required to elicit a sensation. This value was used to set the levels of current used in the experiment proper. During testing, one of the central incisors of the subject was used, and a continuous jet of air was delivered through the probe in order to keep the tooth dry.

Four levels of stimulation were selected for presentation during a signal detection task, and each was delivered 75 times, the presentation order of the four stimuli being random. To adjust the task to each subject, we chose stimulus intensities of zero, threshold minus 1 μA, threshold plus 1 μA, and threshold plus 3 μA. Each stimulus had to be rated by the subject on a seven-point scale ranging from "nothing" through "strong pain." After determining the settings for the stimulator, we gave each subject 100 practice trials. On another day he returned for 300 base-line trials, and on a third day he was given his second major testing session with analgesic treatment.

The design of the first experiment involved the comparison of three groups. On their third visit, subjects in the first group received acupunctural stimulation at the *ho-ku* point on the hand. A 20-min induction period preceded testing, and stimulation continued throughout the testing session. The second group received inhalation of 33% nitrous oxide in oxygen during a 20-min induction period before testing. A nasal mask was used and subjects were trained to maintain nasal breathing. The third group served as a control. All subjects were tested in two different sessions so that the treatment groups received a preliminary base-line test session (second visit) and a treatment session (third visit). The control subjects received two base-line sessions.

We observed a significant decrease in sensory sensitivity to pain in response to both acupuncture stimulation and 33% nitrous oxide inhalation. The amount of decrease was roughly equal for the two groups. Similarly, there were significant increases in response bias in both groups, so that subjects became less willing to report noxious stimulation as painful, even when they perceived it. Control subjects showed no change across sessions on either of the variables. This study demonstrated that acupuncture can have an analgesic effect, but the sensory changes observed were quite small and it would seem that psychological factors were equally or perhaps more important.

We undertook the second experiment (5) to determine if: (a) we could confirm our original findings; (b) the location of the acupuncture needles was important; and (c) it was necessary to penetrate the skin to achieve an analgesic effect. The second experiment was similar to the first one in procedure, and the control and acupuncture groups were the same. Sixty subjects were divided into four groups of 15 each including an acupuncture group and a control group, as well as a placebo-acupuncture group, and a group that received electrical stimulation at the *ho-ku* point through a surface electrode that did not penetrate the skin (transcutaneous electrical stimulation, or TES). The placebo-acupuncture group received the insertion of the needle on the back of the fifth metacarpal of each hand, an area that does not correspond to a traditional acupuncture point.

This experiment replicated the findings of our first study. Acupuncture had a small but significant effect on sensory sensitivity to pain, and a significant increase in response bias was observed in acupuncture subjects. Interestingly, subjects receiving TES showed similar changes in both sensory sensitivity and response bias. The controls did not show any change on either sensory sensitivity to painful stimulation or response bias. Thus stimulation of an acupuncture site by a penetrating needle electrode and by a surface electrode resulted in a significant decrease in sensory sensitivity to pain and also in a significant increase in response bias, or reluctance to report noxious stimulation as painful.

These studies illustrate successful application of signal detection theory to the study of acupuncture analgesia. Our results are inconsistent with those reported by Clark and Yang (8), who employed radiant heat dolorimetry, in that they observed no changes in sensory sensitivity to pain. Their negative findings may be because of procedural variables, as their critics have suggested (4,9,11), or it may be that acupuncture has little effect on the perception of radiant heat pain. Our data are in agreement with that of Clark and Yang in showing that acupuncture results in a positive increase in response bias, i.e., an increase in reluctance to label noxious stimuli as painful. Pain threshold increases observed after acupunctural stimulation in various other laboratories probably reflect both sensory and psychological changes. More work is necessary before the relative importance of these two factors in acupuncture analgesia can be understood.

REFERENCES

1. Andersson, S. A., Erickson, T., Holmgren, E., and Lindqvist, G. (1973): *Brain Res.*, 63:393–396.
2. Berlin, F. S., Bartlett, R. L., and Black, J. D. (1975): *Anesthesiology*, 42:527–531.
3. Chapman, C. R., Gehrig, J. D., and Wilson, M. E. (1975*a*): *Anesthesiology*, 42:532–537.

4. Chapman, C. R., Gehrig, J. D., and Wilson, M. F. (1975*b*): *Science,* 189:65.
5. Chapman, C. R., Wilson, M. E., and Gehrig, J. D. (1976): *Pain* (*in press*).
6. Chiang, C. Y., et al. (1973): *Scientia Sinica,* 2:157.
7. Clark, W. C. (1974): *Anesthesiology,* 40:272–287.
8. Clark, W. C., and Yang, J. C. (1974): *Science,* 184:1090–1098.
9. Hayes, R. L., Bennett, G. J., and Mayer, D. J. (1975): *Science,* 189:65–66.
10. Holmgren, E. (1975): Doctoral thesis, University of Goteborg, Goteborg, Sweden.
11. McBurney, D. H. (1975): *Science,* 189:66.
12. Research Group of Acupuncture Anesthesia, Peking Medical College, Peking (1973): *Chin. Med. J.,* 3:151–157.
13. Swets, J. A. (1973): *Science,* 182:990–1000.

Advances in Pain Research and Therapy, Vol. 1,
edited by J. J. Bonica and D. Albe-Fessard.
Raven Press, New York © 1976.

Modulation of EEG and Unit Discharges of Deep Structures of Brain During Acupunctural Stimulation and Hypnosis of Rabbits

Chifuyu Takeshige, Chang Pin Luo, and Yasuo Kamada

Department of Physiology, School of Medicine, Showa University, Shinagawa-ku, Tokyo, Japan

Numerous reports suggest that acupuncture stimulation produces various electrophysiologic and humoral changes. This chapter summarizes a series of experiments done to shed further light on these effects. These include analysis of the electroencephalogram (EEG) and recording of unit discharge from brainstem during and after acupunctural stimulation or animal hypnosis in rabbits. We also studied the EEG changes in recipient animals on cross-circulation experiments and the effects of 5-hydroxytryptophan (5-HTP), para-chlorophenylalanine (PCPA), and midbrain electrical stimulation.

ELECTROENCEPHALOGRAM

When acupunctural stimulation was applied to rabbits, animals became quiet several minutes after the onset of stimulation, then they laid down extending the extremities, and the pupils were constricted. Under these conditions, EEG of the brainstem, diencephalon, and cerebral cortex recorded by chronically implanted electrodes changed as follows: (a) several minutes after onset of stimulation, the rhythm of EEG became slow; (b) slow waves appeared later; and (c) after stimulation was turned off these changes lasted for a long time. In the EEG analyzed by a frequency analyzer, which provides the successive changes of the integrated signals of δ, θ, α, and β waves for 5 sec, the integrated θ wave decreased several minutes after the onset of stimulation and then the δ wave increased. Those changes in EEG lasted for a time after stimulation was terminated. The duration of this post-stimulation effect depends on the stimulation time. Usually it lasts more than half of the stimulation time.

The following stimulus conditions were necessary to cause those changes in EEG by acupunctural stimulation: (a) stimulus frequency had to be low, 1 or 2/sec; (b) stimulus strength had to be moderate and sufficient to cause moderate muscle contractions. Moderate muscle stimulation caused EEG changes, whereas skin stimulation prevented them. Moreover, strong muscle stimulation did not cause EEG changes.

It was difficult to find a special part of the body where electric stimulation caused significant EEG changes. However, we found that the most peripheral parts of the extremities or the base of the ear are effective in producing changes in the EEG.

EEG changes similar to those produced by acupunctural stimulation were induced by pinching or pulling the ear of the rabbit. Under these conditions, animals laid down and developed myosis. We also noted that EEG changes during animal hypnosis were similar to those produced by acupunctural stimulation. Animal hypnosis was induced by inversion of the animal into a dorsal supine position. During animal hypnosis, pupils were constricted and it was possible to insert a hypodermic into the ear vein without anesthesia. When animals were placed in a hypnotic state, the rhythm of EEG slowed down and the slow wave appeared later. However, unlike the changes produced by the acupunctural stimulated state, the hypnotic-induced EEG changes lacked a latent period and aftereffect.

The changes of EEG during acupunctural stimulated states or animal hypnosis were somewhat different from the changes observed in the spontaneously appearing EEG with slow wave. In acupunctural stimulated states, the θ wave decreased before the δ wave increased. During spontaneous changes in the EEG, depression of θ wave occurred when δ wave increased.

CROSSED-CIRCULATION EXPERIMENT

The possibility that a humoral factor might be involved with production of EEG changes by acupunctural stimulation and by animal hypnosis has been examined by a crossed-circulation experiment in which carotid arteries and jugular veins of two rabbits were connected to each other. As shown in Fig. 1, δ and θ waves of donor and θ and α waves of recipient were recorded simultaneously. As soon as δ waves were increased and θ waves decreased in the donor by pinching the ear (*left record*) or by acupunctural stimulation (*right record*), θ waves decreased in the recipient and the aftereffect also appeared in the recipient. Similar changes in EEG and increase of δ wave in the recipient were also obtained when donor was placed in the state of animal hypnosis.

EFFECT OF 5-HTP

The importance of the brainstem raphe system for the occurrence of synchronization of EEG has been emphasized by Jouvet (1). We have investigated whether or not 5-hydroxytryptamine (5-HT) influenced the

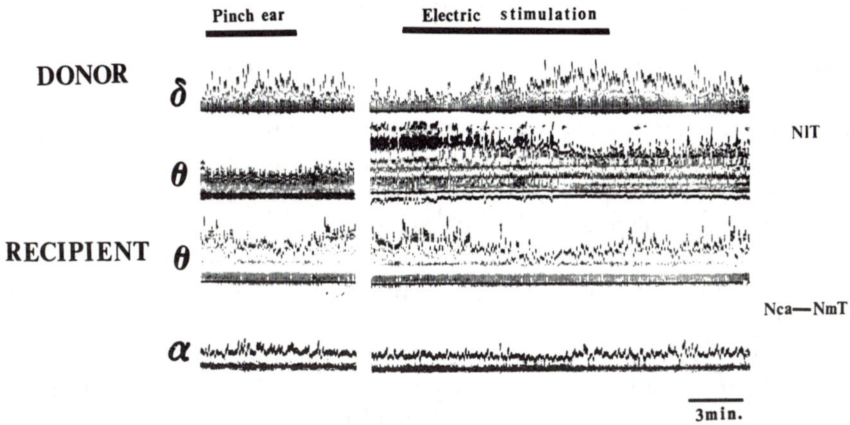

FIG. 1. EEG changes of recipient animal when acupunctural stimulation or ear pinch was applied to donor animal in crossed-circulation experiment. Simultaneous recordings of the integrated δ and θ waves of donor and θ and α waves of recipient. Durations of pinching ear (*left*) and acupunctural stimulation (*right*) are indicated by lines in the upper part of records.

Left record: When θ wave was decreased by pinching ear of donor, θ wave of recipient decreased correspondingly.

Right record: Acupunctural stimulation applied to donor animal caused reduction of θ wave and augmentation of δ wave several minutes after onset of stimulation. Reduction of θ wave in recipient occurred corresponding with reduction of θ wave in donor. After-effect also appeared in recipient as well as in donor.

EEG changes induced by acupunctural stimulation or by animal hypnosis by application of PCPA and 5-HTP.

Administration of 30 mg/kg of 5-HTP somewhat reduced the duration of hypnosis. However, the duration of hypnosis was markedly reduced after pretreatment with 300 mg/kg PCPA. Under these conditions 5-HTP prolonged the hypnosis markedly. These compounds also influenced the acupunctural stimulated states in a similar manner, i.e., acupunctural stimulation did not induce the slow EEG after treatment with PCPA and easily induced it after treatment with 5-HTP.

BRAINSTEM STIMULATION

It has been reported that the low-frequency stimulation of midbrain tegmentum and central gray substance, which were close to the serotonergic raphe system, led to EEG synchronization (2,3) and also caused an analgesic effect (4,5). In the present experiment the direct stimulation of these portions of the midbrain with 600-msec trains of 80-Hz acupunctural stimulator delivered at 1/sec induced reduction of θ wave and the subsequent increase of δ wave. Moreover, the "aftereffects" lasted for a long time, just like the effect of acupunctural stimulation.

UNIT DISCHARGES

As the next step in our investigation, we attempted to find in the medial portion within 3 mm of the midbrain some neurons that change the spontaneous firing rates during ear pinch or animal hypnosis in unrestricted and unanesthetized rabbits using tungsten microelectrodes. Three kinds of neurons that respond to ear pinch and to animal hypnosis were found.

The first type of neurons, which are often found in all portions of the medial midbrain, decreased the firing rates during ear pinch and animal hypnosis. This was confirmed by continuous integrator recordings and by interval histograms.

The second type of neurons increased the firing rates during ear pinch and decreased them during animal hypnosis (Fig. 2). These neurons are relatively frequent in the caudal medial part of the midbrain.

The third type of neurons decreased the firing rates during animal hypnosis and ear pinch. An aftereffect was observed in the firing rates. These neurons are mostly found in the rostral medial part of the midbrain.

These three kinds of responses are also found in the thalamus.

SUMMARY

The characteristic changes in EEG were induced by acupunctural stimulation, ear pinch, or electrical stimulation of midbrain, and these changes in

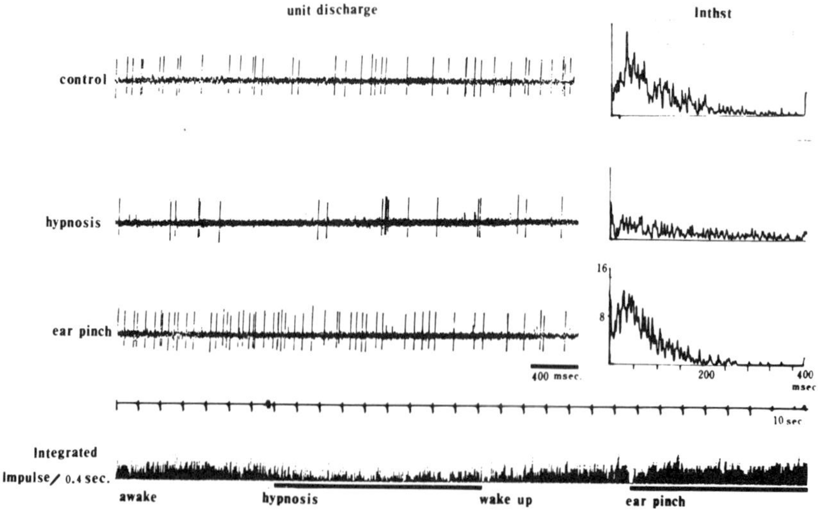

FIG. 2. Unit activity of medial caudal part of midbrain during animal hypnosis and ear pinch. Spontaneous unit discharges decreased during animal hypnosis and increased during ear pinch. Continuous integrated recordings for every 0.4 sec are shown at bottom. Lines indicate durations of animal hypnosis and ear pinch. Interval histograms (*right*) correspond to the unit discharges of control, hypnosis, and ear pinch.

EEG were also found in crossed-circulation animal experiments. Similar EEG changes were induced by animal hypnosis. 5-HTP modified the acupunctural stimulated states or animal hypnosis.

Different midbrain neurons were activated by the acupunctural stimulated states and by animal hypnosis. It is supposed that these midbrain neurons might be activated by acupunctural stimulation to produce analgesia.

REFERENCES

1. Jouvet, M. (1969): *Science,* 163:32–41.
2. Kostowski, W., Giacalone, W., Gartattini, S., and Valzell, L. (1969): *Eur. J. Pharmacol.,* 7:170–175.
3. Kuroki, T. (1958): *Folia Psychiatr. Neurol. Jpn.,* 12:317–340.
4. Liebeskind, J. C., Guilbaud, G., Besson, J., and Oliveras, J. (1973): *Brain Res.,* 50:441–446.
5. Mayer, D. J., Wolfle, T. L., Akil, H., Carder, B., and Liebeskind, J. C. (1971): *Science,* 174:1351–1354.

Advances in Pain Research and Therapy, Vol. 1,
edited by J. J. Bonica and D. Albe-Fessard.
Raven Press, New York © 1976.

Acupuncture Anesthesia and the Pain Threshold

Masayoshi Hyodo and Koichi Masayama

Department of Anesthesiology, Osaka Medical College,
Takatsuki City, Osaka, Japan

In our department of anesthesiology approximately 200 cases of various types of surgeries have so far been performed under acupuncture anesthesia. The rate of success with results obtained has been estimated at greater than 85% for the total cases.

All patients were anesthetized by *in situ* acupuncture needles at the proper acupuncture points according to the type of surgical operation; a positive-negative spike-like wave form low-frequency electrical current of approximately 3 Hz was conducted through the needles before and during all the operations. Although certain amounts of supplementary drugs were combined in some cases, we were able to confirm accurately definite anesthetic or analgesic effects of acupuncture for surgical procedures.

To clarify the many riddles of acupuncture anesthesia, we studied the relationship between the analgesic effect and the pain threshold using radiant heat stimulation.

METHODS

Nakahama has recently developed an excellently revised algesimeter modeled after Hardy's machine. Nakahama's algesimeter is compact, portable, and easy to operate. Before the skin is exposed to the radiant heat, the measuring spot is warmed to 35°C via the small heater installed near the window. The amount of radiant heat projected to the spot is readily calculated in calories per square centimeter per second by a self-contained digital computer. The accuracy, reliability, and reproducibility are of good order. It seems, therefore, that this apparatus can be recommended for practical as well as experimental research, among other things.

The pain threshold using this heat method is measured by either the duration of exposure time with a fixed heat dose or the heat dose given within a fixed duration of time.

To simplify the data, we set the duration of exposure at all sites at 2 sec for every measurement. As a ceiling point, we used the upper limit of the pain threshold, i.e., "unbearable" pain threshold, for each measurement.

All subjects were volunteers who did not have either central or peripheral nervous disorders.

RESULTS

Figure 1 shows a pair of standard Chinese needles inserted at bilateral *ho-ku* points in a 25-year-old man. Upon insertion of the needles the special sensation called *techi* (which means soreness, heaviness, numbness, and swelling) was elicited. At this point the needles were charged with a low-frequency electric current that was conducted for 50 min. The wave form is (+)(−) spike-like with approximately a 1-mm pulse length. The cycles were set at approximately 3 Hz. The strength of electrical power was adjusted to the maximum level that the subject could tolerate.

Ten or fifteen minutes after the conduction of electrical stimulation, the pain thresholds at various parts of the body began to increase gradually. Some differences in the degree of the rise were noted with respect to the parts of the body. The elevated pain thresholds reached their maximum levels in approximately 40 or 50 min. Even after the needle was removed the pain thresholds remained high. Similar tendencies were always observed in other subjects with the same low-frequency electric acupuncture (LFEA). The degree of the increase in pain threshold, however, was individually different.

When the level of pain threshold reached a certain height, analgesic effect by pinprick was also confirmed; consequently, prediction of the anesthetic effect is possible. It is also suggested that 15 or 20 min be allowed as an induction time for anesthesia; it is of no use to wait for more than 40 or 50 min.

The question arises as to how long the postanalgesic effect lasts. In a 50-

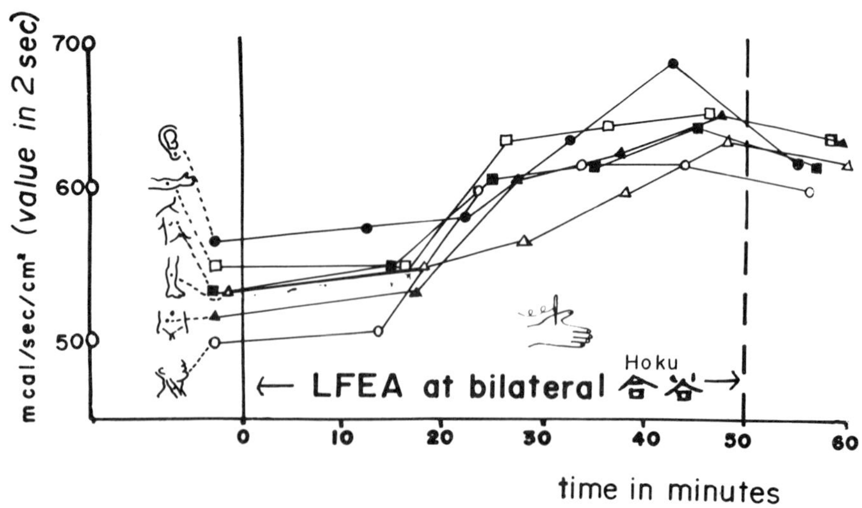

FIG. 1. Increase in pain threshold at various parts of the body by LFEA at *ho-ku* (28-yr-old male).

year-old man measurements were carried out during 3 hr after the cessation of acupuncture anesthesia. Rises at some parts of the body were still observed; these rises finally returned to their initial level after 16 hr. These prolonged rises account for the long-lasting postanalgesic effects observed clinically after surgical procedures.

Factors Influencing the Pain Threshold

When electrical current is not conducted through the needles, we found that the rises in pain threshold are not high enough to produce satisfactory anesthesia. Constant stimulation is required for maintaining and increasing the analgesic effect.

If the needles are inserted without obtaining the so-called *techi* sensation, rise in pain threshold is not expected, even with the conduction of low-frequency electric current.

Before the acupuncture needle was inserted, a local anesthetic drug was injected into the sites of the *ho-ku* points. Pain thresholds remained unchanged throughout the procedure.

These observations relate that proper acupuncture stimulation producing adequate nerve impulses are mandatory for obtaining anesthesia.

Instead of low-frequency electrical current, a direct current of 200 μA and 12 V was conducted in the same manner through the needles inserted at bilateral *ho-ku* points. Slight but insignificant rises in pain threshold were noticed.

The influence of tranquilization was investigated with the administration of 10 mg of diazepam in a 43-year-old woman. The changes in pain threshold at various parts of the body were minimal. However, when the same drug was given to the subject in combination with acupuncture anesthesia at the *ho-ku* points, even greater elevations in pain threshold were produced. Sedative drugs appear to enhance the effect of acupuncture anesthesia when properly administered.

Figure 2 shows the gradual increases in the pain threshold at various parts of the body with LFEA at the *ho-ku* points in an 18-year-old girl, who also received 30 mg of pentazocine intravenously. As a corollary to this, the pain thresholds notably increased (Fig. 3). Interestingly, the degree of the increases in pain threshold was nearly the same, the difference being the time it took to reach maximum levels.

Selection of the Points According to the Surgical Fields

The degree of the rise in pain threshold at a given part of the body differs according to the subject, even though the degree of stimulation remains the same.

With 10 subjects, the degree of the rise in pain threshold at the middle

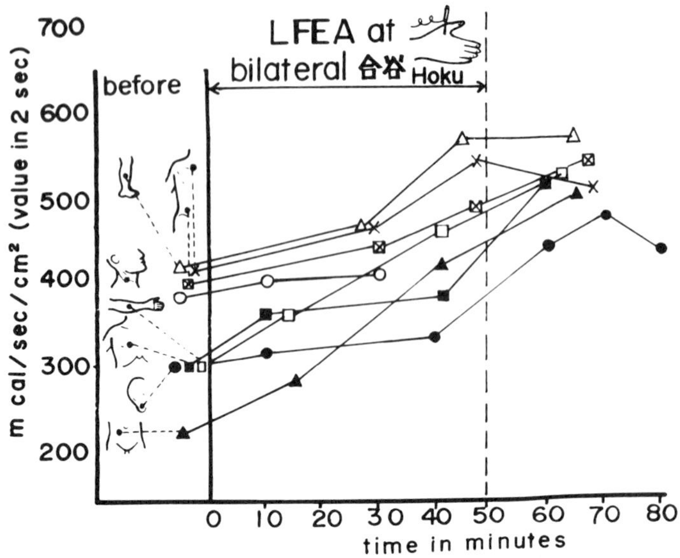

FIG. 2. Increase in pain threshold at various parts of the body by LFEA at *ho-ku* (18-yr-old female).

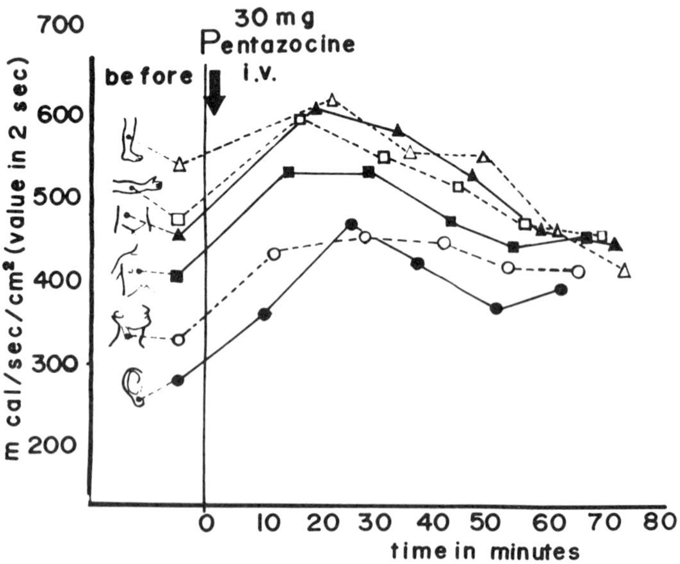

FIG. 3. Effect of pentazocine on pain threshold in an 18-yr-old female.

point of the forearm was measured using the same LFEA at the *ho-ku* points for 50 min (Figs. 4 and 5). The individual difference and the mean values of the rises are illustrated through plotting. Statistical analysis revealed in which parts of the body the rise in pain threshold is most or least prominent with LFEA at the *ho-ku* points (Fig. 5).

Likewise, the effects of raising the pain threshold have been investigated with the *tsu-sanri* point, which is also frequently used for acupuncture anesthesia. The rise in pain threshold on the earlobe was significantly greater; points on the abdomen ranked next.

Kuan-gen, the point located on the lower abdominal wall, exhibited the greatest rise in pain threshold for the abdominal region. Eight representative points routinely used for acupuncture anesthesia were examined in the same manner to determine the suitability of the corresponding surgical fields.

The correlation between the sites of the body and acupuncture points was also investigated. The rise in the pain threshold at the middle part of the forearm was greatest with LFEA at the *ho-ku* point. The *nai-kuan* point was ranked second in effect for the upper extremities (Figs. 6 and 7). The *ho-ku* and *kuan-gen* points were statistically significantly more effective than other points in raising the abdominal pain threshold (Fig. 7).

Table 1 shows the recommended acupuncture points according to surgical

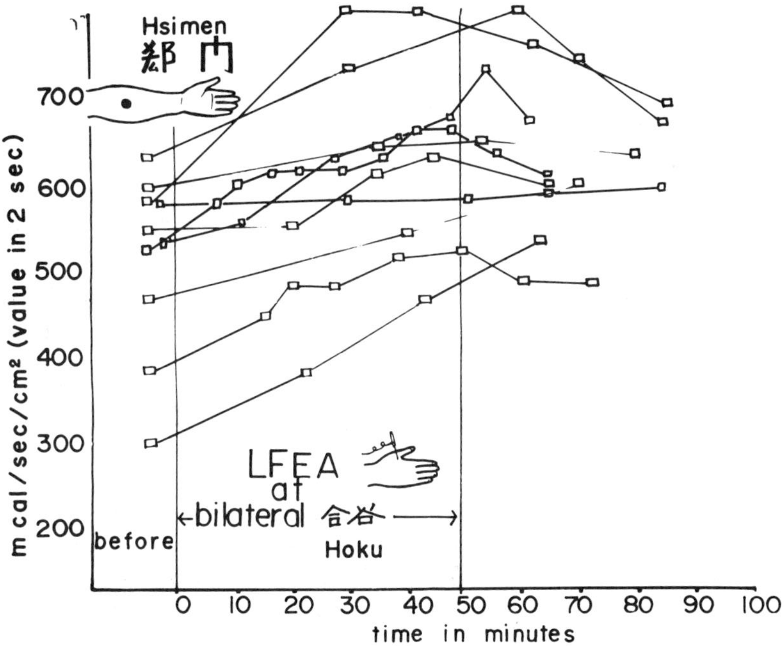

FIG. 4. Increase in pain threshold at Hsimen in the forearm by LFEA at *ho-ku*.

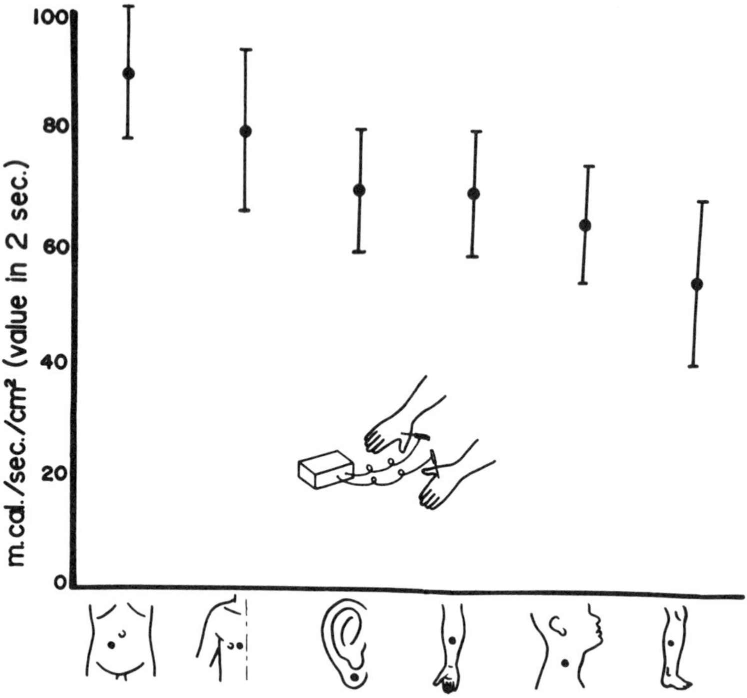

FIG. 5. Increase in pain threshold at various sites of the body (indicated by ●) by LFEA for 50 min at bilateral *ho-ku.*

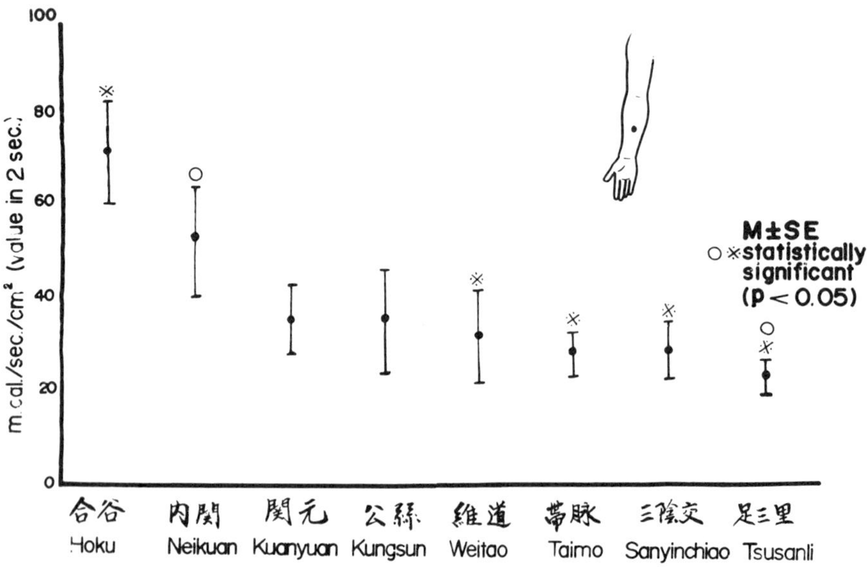

FIG. 6. Increase in pain threshold in the anterior part of the forearm (●) by LFEA in various acupuncture points.

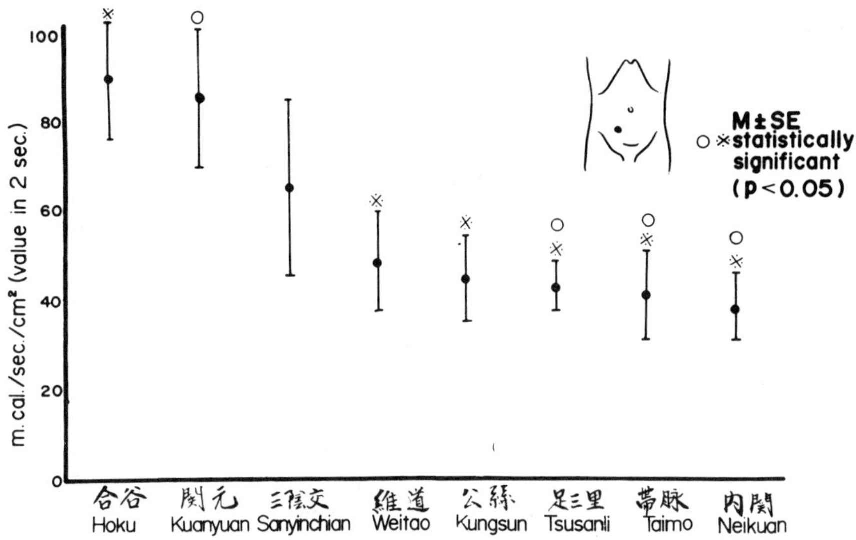

FIG. 7. Increase in pain threshold of skin in the right lower quadrant of the abdominal wall produced by LFEA in various acupuncture points.

fields. For example, if one wishes to undertake surgery of the head or face, the listed points should be taken in the order of *ho-ku, tsu-sanri,* etc.

Originally, in China the acupuncture points most suited to the corresponding surgical operations were empirically calculated. Through our experiments, the most suitable points according to the site of surgery have been statistically and scientifically determined. However, as the statistical analysis shows, clear-cut differences in the effect do not necessarily exist among the various acupuncture points being employed by physicians. Therefore, the acupuncture point listed for a given operation is the one we believe to be the most effective. Although the selection of the points for a given operation is different among physicians and hospitals, similarly good results are obtained.

Local Analgesic Effect

To investigate the local analgesic effect of acupuncture anesthesia, we measured the rise in pain threshold in the area between two electrical acupuncture needles inserted at short distances. With time, the rise in pain threshold at that region was found to be greater than that observed at more remote points. Our experiment indicates that the local analgesic effect is best produced mainly near the points of needle insertion.

It has been said that in such instances the acupuncture needle acts like regional anesthesia produced by local anesthetics. To test this hypothesis,

TABLE 1. *Recommended acupuncture points according to operative site*

Surgical field	Acupuncture points					
Head or face	Hoku	Tsusanli	Weitao	Neikuan	Kuanyuan		
Neck	Hoku	Weitao	Kungsun	Neikuan	Sanyinchiao	Taimo	
Upper extremity	Hoku	Neikuan					
Chest	Hoku	Sanyinchiao	Weitao	Kuanyuan			
Abdomen	Hoku	Kuanyuan	Sanyinchiao	Weitao	Kungsun	Tsusanli	Taimo
Lower extremity	Sanyinchiao	Kuanyuan	Hoku	Kungsun	Weitao	Neikuan	

we inserted an acupuncture needle in the infraorbital foramen near the infraorbital nerve. After low-frequency electric current was applied, the changes in the pain threshold were checked at several areas including the infranasal region innervated by the infraorbital nerve. We found an enhanced increase of the pain threshold in the region supplied by this nerve.

Rise in Aching Pain Threshold

For general and practical tests of the analgesic effect of acupuncture anesthesia, the pinprick method, which is crude and unreliable at best, is usually performed. In contrast, the radiant heat method is the best method for measuring pricking pain on body surfaces. The data presented herein should prove valuable for practical and theoretical use. Naturally, much remains to be solved. Pricking pain is only one aspect of the complex pain phenomenon. To investigate the analgesic effects of acupuncture anesthesia from the standpoint of deep aching pain, we used a coiled-spring pressure algometer in several subjects. Gradual increases in the pain threshold for aching pain along with individual differences during acupuncture anesthesia were also noted.

CONCLUSION

In order to clarify partially the mechanism of action of acupuncture anesthesia, we used a radiant heat method to investigate the analgesic efficacy of various acupuncture points in a large number of volunteers.

A newly devised and reliable algesimeter developed by Nakahama was used for these purposes. Useful clinical findings were obtained.

Advances in Pain Research and Therapy, Vol. 1,
edited by J. J. Bonica and D. Albe-Fessard.
Raven Press, New York © 1976.

Comparison of Transcutaneous Electrical Stimulation and Acupuncture in the Treatment of Chronic Pain

*Elisabeth J. Fox and **Ronald Melzack

**Department of Anesthesiology, Downstate Medical Center, Brooklyn, New York 11203; and **Department of Psychology, McGill University, Montreal, Quebec, Canada*

There is convincing evidence (5) that brief intense transcutaneous electrical stimulation (TES) at trigger points or acupuncture points provides an effective method for the relief of some forms of severe pathological pain. The duration of relief frequently outlasts the period of stimulation by hours, and occasionally by days or weeks, and the effect is significantly greater than that of placebo stimulation. The results resemble those of acupuncture stimulation for similar kinds of chronic pain (2). There is no evidence, however, that one procedure is superior to the other.

The purpose of the present study was to examine the relative effectiveness of both transcutaneous electrical stimulation and acupuncture in the same subjects, in terms of the magnitude and duration of pain relief.

METHODS

The subjects were 7 men and 5 women, whose ages ranged from 30 to 72 years, all of whom had a history of chronic low back pain. Six of them had already had one or more intervertebral discs removed, and two of them had had a spinal fusion in addition. Two patients, whose myelograms showed evidence of herniation of an intervertebral disc, had not been considered suitable for surgery. One patient had X-ray evidence of osteoarthritis of the lumbar spine. Three others had low back pain following injury, without any abnormal findings. All had failed to respond to conventional treatment and were referred to the Pain Treatment Centre at Montreal General Hospital.

Six patients received two treatments with acupuncture followed by two with TES. The remaining 6 received treatments in the reverse order. Treatments were given at weekly intervals, and each patient served as his own control.

Acupuncture was carried out by the insertion of a needle into points number 24, 26, and 62 on the bladder meridian (Fig. 1)—points commonly used for the treatment of backache, and two of which also correspond to

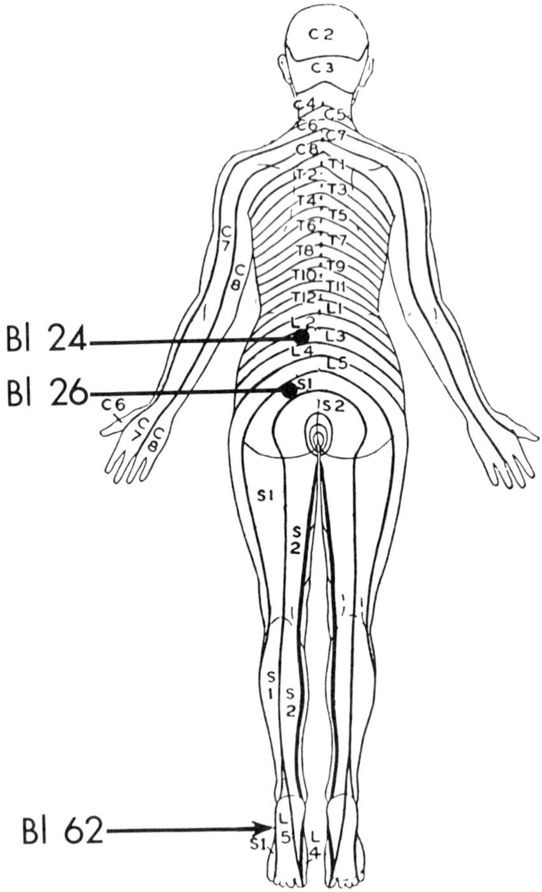

FIG. 1. Locations of acupuncture points Bl 24, Bl 26, and Bl 62 on the bladder meridian.

trigger points (6)—with strong manual rotation for 1 min at each point. Transcutaneous electrical stimulation was carried out by means of an EEG disc electrode applied for 10 min at each of the same points in succession, with an indifferent electrode placed at a distant site. The electrodes were attached to a custom-made stimulator having a variable output up to 35 V and producing 60 Hz sine wave trains at a variable rate. The voltage was raised to a level that was considered painful but not unbearable by the patient (5). An attempt was made to achieve, as far as possible, a comparable degree of pain with both acupuncture and TES.

The degree and duration of pain relief were measured by means of the McGill Pain Questionnaire, which was administered before and after each treatment, and by the McGill Home Recording Card (4). The two major indices measured by the questionnaire are the Pain Rating Index (PRI)—

which is the sum of the rank values of all the descriptive words chosen—and the Present Pain Intensity (PPI), which rates pain on a 1 to 5 scale: 1 = mild, 2 = discomforting, 3 = distressing, 4 = horrible, and 5 = excruciating. Percentage changes in PRI and PPI were calculated.

RESULTS

The results (Table 1) show that the mean percentage decrease in pain is greater for acupuncture than for TES. The two-tailed *t*-test, however, revealed no significant difference between the two forms of stimulation. Two other statistical tests were also applied, and neither revealed significant differences. Using PPI scores, we found that 6 patients showed greater relief with acupuncture, 4 with transcutaneous electrical stimulation, and 2 showed the same degree of relief with both. Using the PRI scores, we found that the mean decrease in pain was greater with acupuncture in 6 patients and greater with TES in 6 patients. In a further analysis, patients were classified in terms of mean pain relief of less than 33% and greater than 33%. Transcutaneous electrical stimulation produced more than 33% relief in 50% of patients using both PPI and PRI scores. Acupuncture produced more than 33% relief in 75% and 58% of patients using PPI and PRI scores, respectively. Thus acupuncture and TES of the same points both produce substantial pain relief, but neither procedure is statistically more effective than the other.

Most patients were relieved of pain for several hours, and some for 1 or more days. This is remarkable since stimulation lasted for only 3 min during acupuncture and 30 min during TES. Statistical analysis again failed to reveal any differences in duration between the two procedures.

The data showed clearly that acupuncture and transcutaneous electrical stimulation at acupuncture points produce significant pain relief (greater than 33%) in a substantial proportion of patients (50% to 75%). This has important clinical implications. Acupuncture has an aura of the mysterious and is widely regarded in Western medicine as quackery or, at best, a suspicious practice. It is becoming apparent, however, that there is nothing

TABLE 1. *Comparison of results produced by acupuncture (A) and TES*

	Mean percentage decrease				Mean duration of relief (hr)	
	PPI		PRI			
Treatment order	A	TES	A	TES	A	TES
A-T (6)	53	41	37	28	24	36
T-A (6)	61	51	61	38	55	10
Mean (12)	57	46	49	33	40	23

magical about meridians or the particular metal or angle of penetration of acupuncture needles (2). The folklore of acupuncture should not blind us, however, from recognizing its pain-relieving potential.

DISCUSSION

The present data suggest that acupuncture and TES both fall into the category of "hyperstimulation analgesia" and are simply methods of producing brief pain to relieve chronic intense pain (3). It is reasonable to assume that they have the same underlying mechanism. The most plausible explanation lies in the brainstem areas, particularly the central gray, which have been shown to be capable of inhibiting pain. Cells in these areas have large receptive fields and project to all levels of the spinal cord and brain. This system could act as a "central biasing mechanism." Thus intense peripheral stimulation would produce a predominantly small-fiber input that would give rise to pain but would also activate the central biasing mechanism, which would in turn inhibit pain signals from other areas (3).

The prolonged effects of stimulation require additional explanation. Livingston (1) and Melzack (3) have proposed that prolonged pathological pain may bring about changes in central neural activity, such as self-exciting neuron chains, representing memory-like processes. A brief intense input could disrupt such activity either by inhibition at the spinal level or indirectly by activation of the central biasing mechanism and consequent descending inhibition. Thus intense stimulation at one site could disrupt abnormal central neural activities initiated and maintained in the cord by pathology at a distant site. This disruption could long outlast the duration of the peripheral stimulation; and normal response activities following relief of pain could produce patterns of nerve impulses that would prevent the memory-like activity from recurring.

Since acupuncture and transcutaneous electrical stimulation are equally effective in relieving low back pain, the advantages and disadvantages of each merit consideration. The chief advantage of acupuncture is that the procedure is of short duration—only 3 min was required in this study. The method is, however, invasive and requires licensed practitioners with specialized training. Transcutaneous electrical stimulation, on the other hand, is noninvasive; and once the appropriate points are located, it can be administered by paramedical personnel or by the patient himself under supervision. It does, however, require a longer time and more frequent application to achieve the same results. When applied two or three times a week in 30-min sessions in a recent study (5), TES produced a mean pain decrease equivalent to that produced by acupuncture in the present study.

SUMMARY

In summary, the study shows that 50% to 75% of patients with low back pain obtained substantial relief for long periods of time with acupuncture or transcutaneous electrical stimulation, both methods being equally effective and probably having the same underlying mechanism of action. Consideration of the advantages and disadvantages of the two methods suggests that transcutaneous electrical stimulation is potentially the more practical since it can be administered under supervision by paramedical personnel.

ACKNOWLEDGMENTS

This research was supported by grant A 7891 from the National Research Council of Canada and was carried out at the Pain Treatment Centre of the Montreal General Hospital. We are grateful to the Johnson & Johnson Company for support provided to Dr. Fox, and to Mary Ellen Jeans, Paul Taenzer, and Ruth Beissel for their assistance.

REFERENCES

1. Livingston, W. K. (1943): *Pain Mechanisms.* Macmillan, New York.
2. Mann, F., Bowsher, D., Mumford, J., Lipton, S., and Miles, J. (1973): *Lancet,* 1:57–60.
3. Melzack, R. (1973): *The Puzzle of Pain.* Penguin Books, London.
4. Melzack, R. (1976): *Pain,* 1 (*in press*).
5. Melzack, R. (1976): *Pain,* 2 (*in press*).
6. Travell, J., and Rinzler, S. H. (1952): *Postgrad. Med.,* 11:425–434.

Advances in Pain Research and Therapy, Vol. 1,
edited by J. J. Bonica and D. Albe-Fessard.
Raven Press, New York © 1976.

Psychological Factors in the Effectiveness of Acupuncture for Chronic Pain

*Claire M. Hossenlopp, **Lillian Leiber, and †Benjamin Mo

*Departments of *Psychiatry, **Neurology, and †Anesthesiology, Edward J. Meyer Memorial Hospital, 462 Grider Street, Buffalo, New York 14215*

Since the recent reintroduction of acupuncture analgesia in the United States, there has been an ongoing controversy about the role played by psychological factors in the effectiveness of acupuncture as a type of pain treatment (see, for example, refs. 1,2). At a clinic using acupuncture for the treatment of chronic pain, we attempted to evaluate the effects on treatment outcome of demographic and pain-related variables and of a number of psychological factors that have been implicated in pain intensity, pain tolerance, and pain relief.

METHOD

Eighty-seven patients participated in the study. A description of the demographic and diagnostic characteristics of the patient sample is presented in Table 1. Most of the patients in our sample had had pain a long time and had previously tried a number of traditional therapeutic measures with no more than temporary success. The average pain duration for the sample was 10.6 years (range, 3 months to 48 years), and the average number of previous treatments tried was 1.7 (range, 0 to 5), not counting a wide variety of analgesic drugs. At the time of our initial contact, these patients were taking an average of 1.95 different pain and tranquilizing medications (range, 0 to 6), usually daily.

Procedure

Immediately before the first treatment, each patient completed an extensive questionnaire that was followed by a semistructured interview. The questionnaire and interview covered the following major areas:

The first area covered was *demographic information* such as age, sex, marital status, ethnic and religious background, employment, and living arrangements.

Second, to provide an indication of possible proneness to pain, we obtained information about *pain history and pain status,* including etiology, location, frequency, and chronicity of pain; past treatments for pain, includ-

TABLE 1. *Description of patient sample*

Sex	Men, 31%	Women, 69%			
Birthplace	Foreign, 15%	U.S., 85%			
Religion	Cath., 59%	Prot., 26%	Jew., 9%	Other, 6%	
Marital status	Married, 78%	Unmarried, 22%			
Age	25–44, 21%	45–64, 58%	65–85, 21%		
Education	3–8 yr, 20%	9–12 yr, 61%	13–18 yr, 19%		
Currently employed	Yes, 31%	No, 69%			
Diagnosis	Arthritis, 36%	Headache, 10%	Disc disease, 21%	Other, 11%	Unknown, 22%
Major pain location	Head and neck, 19%	Back or one joint, 33%	Multiple joints, 48%		

ing analgesics; current use of analgesic and tranquilizing medications; estimation of the degree to which pain interfered with life style, work, sleep, and social activities; and history of past medical illnesses and experience with pain.

In addition, patients made separate ratings of their usual pain intensity and the level of pain they were experiencing at the time of the interview on a 7-point scale from 0 (none) to 6 (unbearable). They rated their sensitivity to pain on a 7-point scale ranging from 0 (much less sensitive than average) to 6 (much more sensitive). The quality of the patient's pain was assessed by providing a list of 12 descriptors, e.g., throbbing, shooting (3), and patients were asked to check those adjectives that described their pain.

The third type of information we obtained was about *affective factors most consistently associated with pain: anxiety, depression, and anger.* We assessed these factors in two ways: clinically, on the basis of the patient's statements and behavior during the interview, and psychometrically, by the use of rating scales. All rating scales used were of the same format and consisted of a statement—e.g., "I feel downhearted and blue" —followed by a 5-point scale ranging from 0 (never) to 4 (most of the time). The published scales we used were modified to conform to this format. The Zung Depression Scale (6) was used to assess depression, and the State-Trait Anxiety Inventory (5) was used to assess trait anxiety.

Finally, *other emotional and attitudinal factors* reportedly associated with pain were assessed. These included suggestibility, internal-external control (4), faith and optimism, and attitudes toward physicians and medical care in general and expectations regarding the efficacy of acupuncture in particular.

The initial questionnaire and interview were followed by the patient's first treatment. The acupuncture was administered by an anesthesiologist trained in China, using the traditional Chinese acupuncture technique. The needles were inserted at points close to the sick meridians, ensuring that a sensation of *teh-chi* was obtained. The needles were twirled periodically for 5 to 10 sec as tolerated by the patient, and the twirling was repeated five or six times per session. Most patients came for two or three acupuncture sessions per week. The number of acupuncture treatments ranged from 1 to 33, with an average of 8. Although 9 patients discontinued after only one treatment, 48 patients underwent seven or more treatments.

The final stage of the study consisted of a telephone interview conducted with each patient 3 to 5 months after his last treatment. During the interview each patient was asked to give his current pain level, to estimate the amount of pain relief produced by the treatment, and to estimate any changes in work, social activities, and mood by comparison with his pretreatment level of functioning. Information was also obtained regarding the pain and tranquilizing medications the patient was taking at the time of the follow-up and about the patient's current attitudes toward acupuncture as a treatment modality.

RESULTS AND DISCUSSION

Percentage of Relief

Of the various indicators of therapeutic outcome we obtained, the most direct was the patient's own estimate of percentage of relief experienced at the time of the 3- to 5-month follow-up. In terms of relief obtained, the sample of patients could be divided into the following three groups: group 1, no relief—46%; group 2, 10% to 50% relief—23%; group 3, more than 50% relief—31%. Only 5 patients reported complete, i.e., 100%, relief of pain.

Factors Affecting Relief

Significant effects on treatment outcome were determined by one-way analyses of variance which tested the influence of each demographic, pain-related, and affective or attitudinal variable on percentage of relief obtained. Unless otherwise noted, all results reported below were statistically significant at or beyond the 0.05 level.

Demographic Variables

Of the demographic variables included in the study, only sex had a reliable effect on relief, with women obtaining, on the average, significantly more relief than men (36% versus 20%).

Pain-Related Variables

As can be seen from Figs. 1 and 2, patients whose pain was constant, intense, and disabling obtained less relief than patients whose pain was

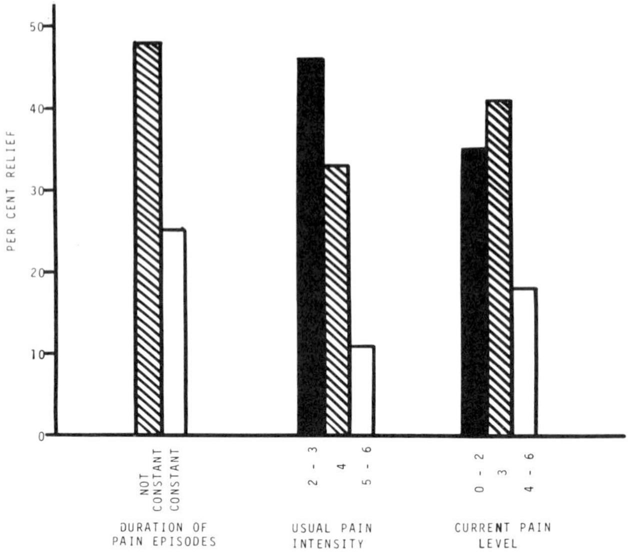

FIG. 1. Mean percentage of pain relief as a function of duration of pain episodes, usual pain intensity, and current pain level.

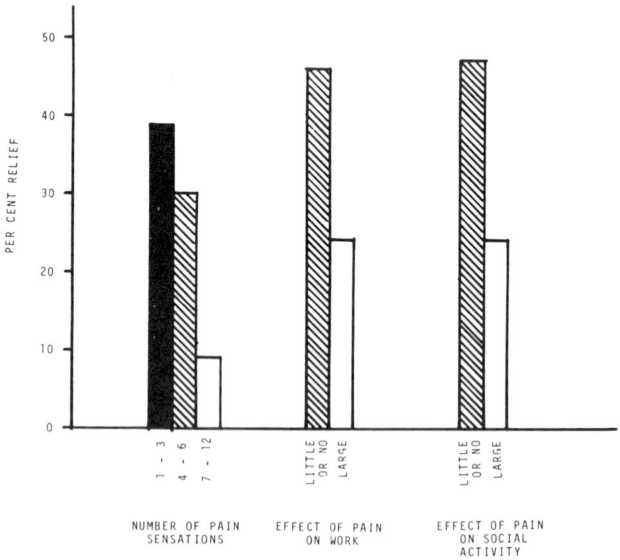

FIG. 2. Mean percentage of pain relief as a function of number of different pain sensations and of disruptive effects of pain on work and social activities.

mild, episodic, and less disruptive of work and social activities. There was also a tendency ($p < 0.10$) for patients who rated themselves as more sensitive to pain than the average to report less pain relief than those who rated themselves as less sensitive than the average.

Affective Variables

Figure 3 shows that moderate-to-severe depression, whether assessed clinically or psychometrically, was associated with significantly less pain relief than were relatively low levels of depression. Similarly, patients with high scores on the trait anxiety scale reported less relief than patients with low scores.

The effect of several other affective variables on percentage of relief obtained approached significance. Patients who acknowledged that their pain was increased by anxiety tended to obtain less relief than those whose pain was unaffected by anxiety ($p < 0.06$). Patients who appeared clinically to harbor substantial unexpressed anger obtained less relief than those who did not appear to harbor introjected anger ($p < 0.06$). And patients who scored high on the faith and optimism items tended to obtain more relief than low scorers ($p < 0.07$).

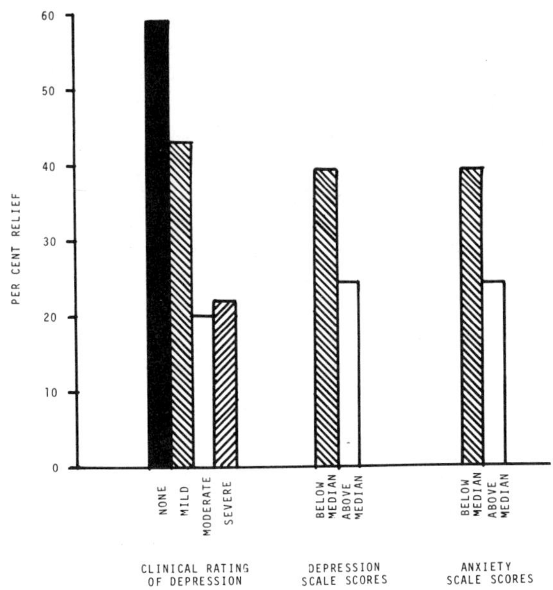

FIG. 3. Mean percentage of pain relief as a function of clinical rating of depression, depression scale scores, and anxiety scale scores.

Factors Unrelated to Treatment Outcome

In our study the number of acupuncture treatments was not related to percentage of relief reported 3 to 5 months after the conclusion of treatment. And, except for sex, none of the demographic variables had a significant effect on relief. Similarly, diagnosis, pain location, duration of pain over years, number of analgesics, and past medical history were unrelated to percentage of pain relief, as were measures of suggestibility, outcome expectations, and attitudes toward physicians.

Independent Effects of Pain-Related and Affective Variables

It is well known that protracted and severe pain can produce or exacerbate anxiety and depression. In order to determine if the patient's emotional state affected treatment outcome independently of his pain state, we divided the total sample into three groups on the basis of usual pain intensity, and each of these groups was further subdivided into those with low and those with high clinical ratings of depression.

The data of particular interest in Table 2 are the means, which reflect the significant interaction between usual pain intensity and clinical rating of depression ($p < 0.001$). As can be seen from Table 2, at a given level of pain intensity, patients with low ratings of depression obtained more relief than patients with high ratings of depression. These differences were statistically reliable for the low intensity group ($p < 0.001$) and for the medium intensity group ($p < 0.05$), but not for the high intensity group. These results indicate that although pain and depression may be related to each other, depression exerts an effect on treatment outcome over and above that produced by pain alone.

SUMMARY

In a study of 87 chronic pain patients who received an average of eight acupuncture treatments, almost one-half obtained no lasting relief and

TABLE 2. *Mean percentage of pain relief as a function of usual pain intensity and clinical rating of depression*

	Clinical rating of depression				
	Low (0 and 1)		High (2 and 3)		
Usual pain intensity	*N*	Relief (%)	*N*	Relief (%)	Mean relief (%)
Low (2 & 3)	14	65	9	17	41
Medium (4)	13	44	30	28	36
High (5 & 6)	4	28	17	8	18
Mean relief (%)		45		18	32

slightly less than one-third obtained more than 50% relief 3 to 5 months after completion of the treatment series. A negative view of these results would argue that acupuncture is a costly, time-consuming, and (for American patients) painful procedure that failed to produce any lasting relief in almost one-half of our chronic pain patients. A positive view of the same results would emphasize that of a sample of patients with chronic pain, who had not obtained significant relief with a variety of traditional forms of treatment, almost one-third obtained moderate-to-complete relief with acupuncture.

Our results indicate that the likelihood of therapeutic success was reduced if the patient's pain was constant rather than episodic, severe rather than mild, and if the pain interfered substantially with the patient's work and social activities. Therapeutic success was also less likely in patients with high levels of depression and anxiety. The fact that treatment outcome was strongly and negatively influenced by level of depression, independently of level of pain, suggests that patients seeking pain relief be routinely screened for anxiety and depression and that those patients with high levels of emotional distress be treated for their emotional distress before or at least simultaneously with the somatic treatment of pain.

ACKNOWLEDGMENT

We would like to thank Dr. Ross Markello for his help in facilitating the completion of this study.

REFERENCES

1. Chaves, J. F., Barber, T. X. (1973): *Hum. Behav.*, 2:19–24.
2. Kroger, W. S. (1973): *Am. J. Psychiatry*, 130:855–860.
3. Melzack, R., and Torgerson, W. S. (1971): 34:50–59.
4. Rotter, J. B. (1966): *Psycholog. Monogr.*, 80(1 Whole No. 609).
5. Spielberger, C. D., Gorsuch, R., and Lushene, R. E. (1973): *The State-Trait Anxiety Inventory*. Consulting Psychologists Press, Palo Alto, California.
6. Zung, W. W. K. (1965): *Arch. Gen. Psychiatry*, 12:63–70.

Advances in Pain Research and Therapy, Vol. 1,
edited by J. J. Bonica and D. Albe-Fessard.
Raven Press, New York © 1976.

Subjective and Objective Follow-up Assessment of Acupuncture Therapy Without Suggestion in 100 Chronic Pain Patients

Terence M. Murphy

Department of Anesthesiology and Anesthesia Research Center, University of Washington School of Medicine, Seattle, Washington 98195

The dilemma concerning acupuncture therapy for pain relief continues. Writers postulate various theories for its mechanism of action, ranging from yin and yang energy imbalance (7), through "gate theories" (4), to hypnosis (3), and beyond (1). Studies have established that an acupuncture treatment or series of treatments can result in subjective improvement in a certain percentage of patients for unspecified periods of time immediately after these treatments (2,6). However, we still do not know how long the claimed beneficial effects of acupuncture last with regard to the relief of chronic pain problems and if, in fact, the subjective relief that patients claim is complemented by appropriate objective changes in their pain symptomatology.

In this clinical study, therefore, acupuncture therapy was performed on 100 chronic pain patients to investigate the efficacy of acupuncture in the relief of the chronic pain syndrome in Western patients, and to study the maintenance of this relief either with or without subsequent treatments. It was also planned to see if the reduction in pain complaints was complemented by corresponding reduction in analgesic medication intake and in improvement in activity of those functions that pain had prevented the patient from undertaking.

METHOD

We studied 100 adult chronic pain patients sent by referring physicians to the Pain Clinic specifically for acupuncture therapy. It was required that the pain had been present for at least 6 months and had been unresponsive to conventional therapy. A recent examination by the referring physician and a confirmed diagnosis were required, and this diagnosis was often reconfirmed before treatment was begun. In an attempt to reduce the influence of suggestion and the charismatic effect of this novel (to Westerners) therapy, it was administered in a "matter-of-fact" fashion in a conventional procedure room without any Oriental embellishments (acupuncture charts, mannequins, etc.), and at no stage was any suggestion given to the patient. All patients were told that this was a technique of, as yet, unproven worth in North America that might be applicable to chronic pain states, but that we did not know whether it would help them.

The patients were acupunctured in the area of their pain, i.e., in this study no attempts were made to involve ourselves in the "meridian" theories of acupuncture. Although these theories remain to be tested, it proved almost impossible, even with the assistance of a "master acupuncturist," to build any convenient protocol into a system as elaborate and nebulous as the meridian theory. "Acupuncture points" (points of decreased electrical resistance) were sought by means of a neurometer (5) in the area where the pain existed. Needles were inserted in these points, and, because of the ubiquitous mention of the *ho-ku* point in almost all acupuncture literature, a needle was inserted at this point also in the first dorsal interosseus muscle of the hand ipsilateral to the pain site (or both hands if pain was bilateral). Usually a total of 2 to 6 needles was used for each treatment. The needles were then stimulated for 20 min, both electrically and manually, and the patient decided which helped best. Each patient was offered three trials at weekly intervals before abandoning the therapy.

The effects of acupuncture were measured rather simply. The patient kept a subjective daily record of pain, and the pain was given a value of from 0 to 10 (with 0 equal to no pain, and 10 equal to pain sufficient to drive the patient to suicide). Each patient also kept a medication record, i.e., a daily record of the tablets and pills he took. In addition, an activity record was maintained, whereby he kept a daily diary of his various activities, i.e., that time of the day spent sitting, reclining, going to work, etc. The patient kept these three records for a control period of 1 week before therapy and then throughout the acupuncture therapy. The average pain level (on a 0 to 10 scale) of the patient for the week prior to therapy was determined, and subjective pain relief was acknowledged if this average pain level was reduced by at least 30% after therapy. Subjective pain relief was noted after the first, second, and third acupuncture treatments.

RESULTS

After the first treatment, 80% of these 100 patients showed subjective pain relief by the above criteria, i.e., they declared their pain to be at least 30% better than before the treatment, and some even claimed dramatic or miraculous cures. However, by the time of the third acupuncture visit, only 15% maintained subjective improvement, the remaining initial successes by this time having become failures. Of the 15% who obtained pain relief, 11% could fairly predictably be maintained with partial but not complete subjective pain relief provided they were acupunctured at somewhere between a 2- to 4-week interval, but their pain was never really cured. With subsequent therapies in this group, attempts were made to vary the acupuncture technique, e.g., electrical compared to manual stimulation, insertion in "points" detected by neurometer, compared to insertion in other points at random. Subjective relief was obtained irrespective of acupuncture technique or points used. A small group (4 out of the 100 patients) received acupuncture treatments and claimed subjective relief for up to 6 months between treatments without need for further acupuncture therapy. Apart from some temporary dramatic results after the first treatment, at no stage did any of the patients involved in this study show any objective response to acupuncture therapy, medication intake was not altered on any long-term basis, nor was activity improved. Only 2 of the original group of patients failed to complete the three trials, and on attempted follow-up it was discovered that one had set himself up as an acupuncturist in a different state. (The other had opened a health spa.) Both declined to return any follow-up information. The results are summarized in Table 1.

There were no complications attributable to the acupuncture therapy in over 400 acupuncture treatments.

TABLE 1. *Short- and long-term results of acupuncture in 100 patients*

Diagnosis	Patients (no.)	No relief	Short-term relief	Long-term relief	"Cures"
Head pain					
Postherpetic neuralgia V	1	0	1	1	1
Atypical face pain	1	0	1	1	
Occipitofrontal headache	8	0	8	1	
Metastatic cancer	1	1	0	0	
Neck pain					
Cervical arthritis	6	1	5	1	
Painful torticollis	1	0	1	0	
Shoulder pain					
Myofascial syndrome	13	0	13	7	1
Upper extremity pain					
Brachial plexus injury	2	2	0	0	
Rheumatoid arthritis	2	1	1	0	
Trunk pain					
Posthoracotomy neuralgia	2	2	0	0	
Postherpetic neuralgia	1	1	0	0	
Myofascial syndrome	14	0	14	2	1
Low back pain	26	4	22	2	1
Abdominal scar pain	4	2	2	0	
Lower extremity					
Phantom limb pain	2	0	2	0	
Peripheral neuropathy	5	4	1	0	
Ischemic pain	1	1	0	0	
Psychogenic pain at miscellaneous sites	10	1	9	0	
Total	100	20	80	15	4

DISCUSSION

Had this study been terminated after the first acupuncture treatment, it would have produced results similar to those of studies claiming a high success rate in treating pain with acupuncture (6). However, the longer term follow-up presented a much more dismal success rate with only four potential "cures." One of these patients, after a 2-year period when he needed only three acupuncture treatments, has now failed to obtain prolonged relief and requires acupuncture every 3 to 4 weeks, thus joining the second group of successes, namely, 11% who claim partial subjective relief with acupuncture and enthusiastically continue to receive it. This group requires acupuncture every 2 to 4 weeks and does not show any objective changes in analgesic medication intake or activity levels as a result of this claimed pain relief. Another patient, an apparent "cure" who enthusiastically applauded the benefits of acupuncture at the 6 and 12 months' follow-up contact, is now attending a local arthritis clinic where he tells the doctors that acupuncture helped him only for 2 weeks. This illustrates that the veracity of patient reporting is inconsistent and a blight on all studies based on subjective assessment alone.

Considering objective assessment, acupuncture failed in every case to provide evidence of improvement. No patient decreased his analgesic medication and no patient increased his activity from control levels. It should be mentioned, however, that not all patients showed abnormally decreased activity before treatment. However, all patients were taking some form of analgesic medication. Even the "cures" persisted in their pretreatment analgesic regimen. The only factor common to the patients treated successfully is that 11 of these 15 patients had a pain site in either the shoulder or the head and neck; however, patients in a comparable sized group with pain in similar sites were failures. One could speculate that patients with pain in the arm, shoulder girdle, or head and neck would be more likely to obtain symptomatic improvement from acupuncture than patients with pain elsewhere.

This study did not compare acupuncture with other therapies, but this group of patients by definition had failed to be improved by other treatments, and maybe one should be grateful for any success rate. Therefore, this benign therapy is worth a try in such patients.

SUMMARY

In 100 chronic pain patients receiving acupuncture as described above, without "suggestion," the initial highly successful symptomatic relief after the first treatment proved short-lived. There was partial symptomatic relief in 11% of the patients over a longer period of 6 months to 2 years, provided that acupuncture was repeated on a regular basis. Only 4 patients had long-lasting relief of symptoms. No patients demonstrated objective improvement from this therapy. There was no apparent "specificity" with regard to the point needled. No complications occurred.

REFERENCES

1. Chapman, C. R. (1975): *Anesthesiology,* 43:501–506.
2. Kepes, E. R., Chen, M., and Schapira, A. (1973): In: *Proceeding of N.I.H. Acupuncture Research Conference,* edited by H. P. Jenerick. D.H.E.W. Publication No. 74–165, pp. 8–10.
3. Kroger, W. S. (1972): *J.A.M.A.,* 220:1012.
4, Mann, P. L., and Chen, C. H. (1972): *Dis. Nerv. Syst.,* 33:730.
5. Matsumoto, T. (1973): *Acupuncture for Physicians.* Charles C Thomas, Publisher, Springfield, Illinois.
6. Spoerel, W. E., and Leung, C. Y. (1974): *Can. Anaesth. Soc. J.,* 21:221–229.
7. Veith, I. (Trans.-Ed.) (1972): *The Yellow Emperor's Classic of Internal Medicine.* University of California Press, Berkeley.

Advances in Pain Research and Therapy, Vol. 1,
edited by J. J. Bonica and D. Albe-Fessard.
Raven Press, New York © 1976.

A Critical Evaluation of Acupuncture in the Treatment of Chronic Pain

Edith R. Kepes, Melanie Chen, and *Max Schapira

*Montefiore Hospital and Medical Center, and *Morrisania Hospital, Albert Einstein College of Medicine, 111 East 210th Street, Bronx, New York 10467*

Acupuncture has been used in China for 1,000 years to cure diseases and alleviate pain. The practice has gained popularity in Western countries during the past two decades, spreading to the United States after the partial lifting of the bamboo curtain in 1972.

Many Western-trained physicians (4) believe that the effect of acupuncture is similar if not identical to the therapeutic effect of hypnosis. Although acupuncture and hypnosis may be unrelated phenomena, the ceremonial effect of the Chinese needle, the stimulator, and the mannequin with meridians in the room is not dissimilar to hypnotic induction.

This study, done at Montefiore Hospital and Medical Center, New York, attempted to answer the following questions in the treatment of chronic pain with acupuncture: What is the importance of acupuncture points? Which painful diseases respond to acupuncture? Do the therapeutic results differ when acupuncture is administered by Chinese or Caucasian physicians? What is the relationship between results and hypnotizability?

METHOD

The 199 subjects for this investigation were patients over the age of 18 suffering from chronic pain. They were referred to us after their own physicians completed a diagnostic work-up and unsuccessful trials of conventional therapies for pain. These individuals were divided into four groups in a random fashion.

In group 1 (49 patients) acupuncture needles inserted into classic acupuncture points were stimulated manually. The points used were those recommended in the Chinese textbooks *Principles of Acupuncture* (5) and *Handbook of Acupuncture Therapy* (2).

These books were translated into English for us by one of the co-authors, Dr. Chen.

In group 2 (49 patients) acupuncture needles inserted into classic acupuncture points were stimulated electrically for 20 min. A transisterized electrical stimulator Model 626, manufactured in the People's Republic of

China, was used. This device has been described by Babich (1). A pulse frequency of 2 Hz was used with a voltage strong enough to be felt, but below the individual patient's pain threshold.

In group 3 (51 patients) acupuncture needles inserted into placebo points were stimulated manually.

Figure 1 shows on a mannequin the four selected points, which as can be seen, are at a considerable distance from all classic meridians.

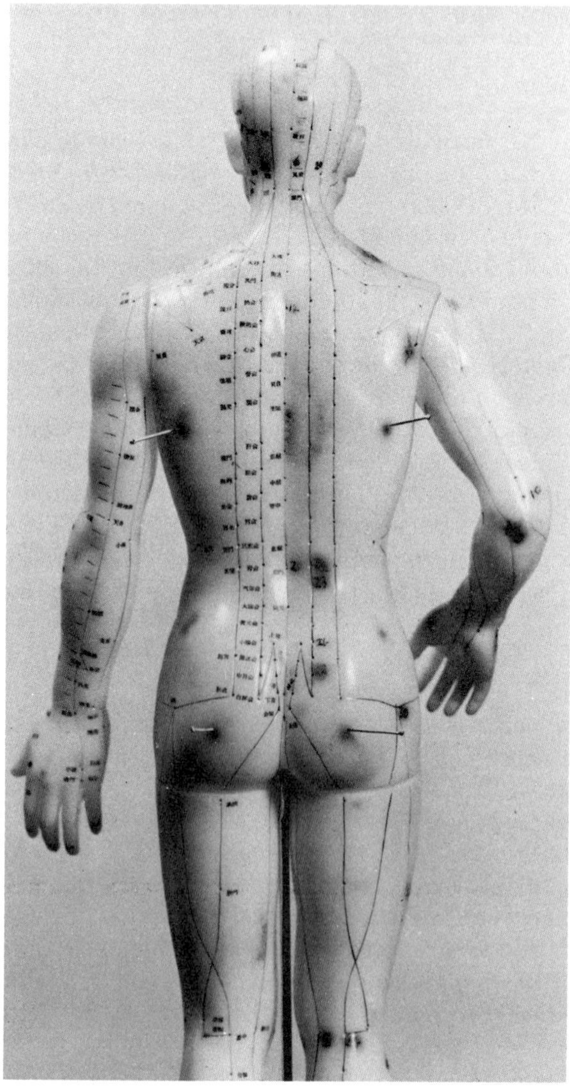

FIG. 1. Mannequin showing classic acupuncture meridians and 4 placebo points (needles).

In group 4 (50 patients) acupuncture needles inserted into placebo points were stimulated electrically as in group 2.

Patients were questioned about the sensation of the needle puncture, and the presence of *techi* (numbness, heaviness, soreness) was observed.

Before the second and subsequent visits, an interviewer unaware of the type of treatment received, assisted the patient in filling out a questionnaire. Response to treatment was classified as: pain-free, much less pain, little less pain, no change, or more pain. If there was improvement, the patient continued in his original group. An individual who achieved no benefit was moved into another group. The patient was discharged after four visits if there was no improvement with any of the four methods, or after two to eight visits if there was improvement or complete pain relief.

Before discharge, the patients were tested for their hypnotic induction profile by the "eye-roll levitation method" described by Spiegel (6,7). Patients were divided into five groups: from 0 (not hypnotizable) to 4 (highly hypnotizable).

The pertinent information obtained and the results of every treatment were recorded on a form suitable for computer processing.

RESULTS

A total of 199 patients received 1,054 treatments. The computer analysis of the results are as follows.

In 1,054 treatments there was no statistically significant difference in the therapeutic result between the four groups. Excellent-to-good results were obtained in 19.2% to 26.9% of patients, fair in 29.1% to 39% of patients, and none in 34% to 51.6% (Table 1).

The last acupuncture treatment in 199 patients (Table 2) showed excellent-to-good results in 21.2% to 25%, fair results in 20% to 31.8%, and no change in 46.8% to 55% of patients. Again there is no statistically significant difference in the therapeutic results of the four groups.

TABLE 1. *Results of all acupuncture treatments*

Treatment	Excellent	Good	Fair	0 or Worse	Total
A[a]	12 (4.8)[b]	49 (19.4)	95 (37.7)	96 (38.1)	252 (100)
A+E	10 (2.4)	101 (24.5)	151 (36.6)	151 (37.5)	413 (100)
P	7 (4.6)	22 (14.6)	44 (29.1)	78 (51.6)	151 (100)
P+E	10 (4.2)	53 (22.3)	94 (39.5)	81 (34.0)	238 (100)
Total	39 (3.7)	225 (21.3)	384 (36.4)	406 (38.5)	1,054 (100)

[a] A, acupuncture points—manual stimulation; A+E, acupuncture points—electrical stimulation; P, placebo points—manual stimulation; P+E, placebo points—electrical stimulation.

[b] Figures in parentheses indicate percentage of all cases.

TABLE 2. *Result of last acupuncture treatment*

Treatment	Excellent	Good	Fair	0 or Worse	Total
A[a]	3 (6.4)[b]	7 (14.9)	14 (29.8)	23 (48.9)	47 (100)
A + E	1 (1.2)	17 (20.0)	27 (31.8)	40 (47.1)	85 (100)
P	1 (5.0)	4 (20.0)	4 (20.0)	11 (55.0)	20 (100)
P+E	3 (6.4)	8 (17.0)	14 (29.8)	22 (46.8)	47 (100)
Total	8 (4.0)	36 (18.1)	59 (29.6)	96 (48.2)	199 (100)

[a] A, acupuncture points—manual stimulation; A+E, acupuncture points—electrical stimulation; P, placebo points—manual stimulation; P+E, placebo points—electrical stimulation.
[b] Figures in parentheses indicate percentage of all cases.

The results of treatment obtained in patients with pain caused by somatic (e.g., arthritis, myositis) or neurogenic (e.g., neuritis, radiculitis, neuralgia) diseases were comparable. Pain caused by ischemia had the poorest result (Table 3).

The results of our Chinese doctor, Dr. Chen, were similar to those of the two Caucasian physicians (Table 4).

Because 62 patients did not keep their last appointment when this test was performed, only 137 out of 199 patients had their hypnotic profile tested.

TABLE 3. *Result of last treatment by diagnosis*

Diagnosis	Excellent	Good	Fair	0 or Worse	Total
Pain of somatic origin	4 (3.0)[a]	18 (13.6)	44 (33.3)	66 (50.0)	132 (100)
Pain of neurogenic origin	2 (3.5)	17 (29.8)	14 (24.5)	24 (42.1)	57 (100)
Pain of ischemic origin	2 (2.0)	0 (0)	1 (10.1)	7 (70.0)	10 (100)
Total	8 (4.0)	35 (17.5)	59 (29.6)	97 (48.7)	199 (100)

[a] Figures in parentheses indicate percentage of all cases.

TABLE 4. *Result of last treatment by physician*

Physician	Excellent	Good	Fair	0 or Worse	Total
Kepes	1 (1.2)[a]	13 (15.1)	29 (33.7)	43 (50.0)	86 (100)
Chen	4 (7.4)	14 (25.9)	12 (22.2)	24 (44.5)	54 (100)
Schapira	3 (5.1)	9 (15.3)	18 (30.5)	29 (49.1)	59 (100)
Total	8 (4.0)	36 (17.6)	59 (29.6)	96 (48.2)	199 (100)

[a] Figures in parentheses indicate percentage of all cases.

TABLE 5. *Result of last treatment as related to hypnotizability*

Score	Excellent	Good	Fair	0 or Worse	Total
0+1	1 (1.5)[a]	8 (12.3)	17 (26.1)	39 (60.0)	65 (100)
2	1 (2.9)	7 (20.5)	10 (29.4)	16 (47.0)	34 (100)
3+4	2 (5.3)	9 (23.6)	13 (34.2)	14 (36.8)	38 (100)
Total	4 (2.9)	24 (17.5)	40 (29.1)	69 (50.3)	137 (100)

[a] Figures in parentheses indicate percentage of all cases.

For the hypnotic test, patients scoring 0 and 1 were classified as poor, those scoring 2 as good, and those scoring 3 and 4 as excellent hypnotic subjects.

Individuals scoring 3 and 4 had excellent-to-good pain relief in 28.9%, fair in 34.2%, and none in 36.8% treatments.

In contrast, those who scored 0 and 1 had excellent-to-good pain relief in only 13.8%, fair results in 26.1%, and none in 60% (Table 5).

Paired t-test, however, was only marginally significant, $p < 0.1$.

DISCUSSION AND CONCLUSION

There are numerous reports from China, Italy, France, Switzerland, Austria, and England about acupuncture's excellent analgesic and curative effects in patients suffering from acute and chronic pain. It is difficult to evaluate these reports since the experimental design does not conform to the present-day standards for the evaluation of a new drug or therapeutic technique. In order to do research on new forms of therapy, one has to separate the bias on the part of the therapist and the bias of the patient from the actual effect of a new method. This is difficult to do with acupuncture. The publicity given by press, radio, and television to acupuncture in the United States has preconditioned our population to the same extent as people in China who believe in acupuncture because of their cultural heritage. We have met few patients who did not believe in its efficacy before their first experience with acupuncture treatment.

Contrary to current opinion, in our experience the feeling of *techi* is not so significant in therapy for chronic pain. It is usually experienced on points that correspond to classic acupuncture points and only rarely on areas distant from meridians. We have found that not every patient is able to feel *techi* even if the correct point is stimulated. Others claim to feel it even if the needle is inserted at distant points. Visitors to China (F. F. Foldes, *personal communication*) report that in the selection of patients for surgery with acupuncture, those individuals who in the preoperative indoctrination were unable to experience *techi* were considered unsuitable for acupuncture analgesia.

Although our interviewer was unaware of the treatment received, the acupuncturist knew whether placebo or acupuncture points were stimulated. This undoubtedly must have introduced some bias into the experimental design.

In spite of these deficiencies, we can conclude from our data that in the treatment of chronic pain the location of the acupuncture needle has no bearing on the therapeutic result. Western-trained physicians, whether of Oriental or Caucasian background, have similar therapeutic successes. Because of the variety of conditions treated in this study, no definite conclusion can be drawn as to which types of pain respond best to acupuncture. However, it does appear that pain owing to ischemia has the poorest result.

Patients who are hypnotizable subjects have higher therapeutic success than nonhypnotizable subjects. These findings are in agreement with those of Katz (3) who concluded that acupuncture and hypnosis, although not identical, are parallel phenomena.

It is also worth noting that our therapeutic results are similar to results obtained in the treatment of pain with any form of placebo therapy.

We believe acupuncture, in spite of these observations, can be useful. We consider it a harmless, frequently effective therapeutic modality in chronic pain. Nevertheless, it is harmless only if patients are carefully screened by physicians using appropriate Western diagnostic methods, and if strict sterile techniques are used.

ACKNOWLEDGMENT

We are greatly indebted to Dr. Nina Elias for assistance in evaluation of the results to and Dr. Herbert Levine for statistical analysis.

REFERENCES

1. Babich, A. M. (1973): *Am. J. Chin. Med.,* 1:341–350.
2. Department of Acupuncture (Ed.) (1971): *Handbook of Acupuncture Therapy.* Chinese Traditional Medical College.
3. Katz, R. L., Kao, C. Y., Spiegel, H., and Katz, G. Y. (1974): *Advances in Neurology, Vol 4: International Symposium on Pain,* edited by J. J. Bonica, pp. 819–825. Raven Press, New York.
4. Kroger, W. S. (1973): *Am. J. Psychiatry,* 130:855–860.
5. Department of Acupuncture, (Ed.) (1972): *Principles of Acupuncture.* Chinese Traditional Medical College.
6. Spiegel, H. (1972): *Am. J. Clin. Hypn.,* 15:25–28.
7. Spiegel, H. (1973): *Manual for Hypnotic Induction Profile.* Soni Medica, New York.

Advances in Pain Research and Therapy, Vol. 1,
edited by J. J. Bonica and D. Albe-Fessard.
Raven Press, New York © 1976.

Acute and Chronic Pain—a Study of the Comparative Values of Acupuncture Therapy

Elizabeth A. M. Frost, Cher Y. Hsu, and *Donald Sadowsky

*Departments of Anesthesiology and *Dentistry, Albert Einstein College of Medicine, Bronx, New York 10461*

Acupuncture has been advocated as a successful mode of therapy for many pain syndromes (1,8,9). Travelers to the East have returned with enthusiastic reports of the use of acupuncture instead of conventional anesthetics for many major and minor surgical procedures (5,7,11). Reports from China have also cited the efficacy of acupuncture as an anesthetic modality (10). Its successful use in all types of chronic pain syndromes has been documented in many countries (6).

Over the past 2 years, three studies have been instituted at our hospital to test the value of acupuncture for pain relief. The first program involved testing acupuncture and local anesthesia in dental practice and attempting to correlate any effectiveness with suggestibility. The second protocol was set up to study the effect of acupuncture for postoperative pain relief. Both of these studies dealt with acute pain. The third program was a study of the value of acupuncture in various chronic pain syndromes in an outpatient setting.

All the subjects in the study were treated at a large municipal hospital in New York City, and we can thus assume that the patient population was reasonably standardized.

DENTAL ANALGESIA

METHOD

Patients coming to the dental clinic with similar bilateral dentoalveolar disease in either the mandible or maxilla requiring equivalent procedures were considered potential candidates for this study. As usual, these patients were appraised of their dental condition, and recommendations for treatment were made. In all, 12 patients met the study criteria, were informed of their dental needs, given a brief description of the planned study, and subsequently agreed to volunteer.

A second objective was to attempt to determine in a simple and direct way whether suggestibility or hypnotizability could be correlated with the efficiency of acupuncture as an analgesic method (13). Patients were asked to demonstrate their ability to look upward on signal while closing their eyelids (eye roll sign) (14). This test, which is scored on a 0 to 4 scale according to the amount of sclera visible between the lower eyelid and the lower edge of the cornea, has been found to correlate highly (75%) with hypnotic trance capacity.

Conventional local anesthesia was used on one side, and attempts were made to induce acupuncture analgesia on the other side. The sides were alternated with every other patient. The points chosen were those already described in Western and Chinese literature for production of anesthesia in the face and mouth (large intestine 4 and 11 with some jaw points). Mild stimulation of the 32-gauge stainless steel needles was continued for at least 20 min. With reference to the procedures performed with both conventional and acupuncture analgesia techniques, each subject was asked to rate pain according to the following scale: 0, no discomfort; 1, slight discomfort; 2, some pain; 3, moderate pain; 4, a lot of pain.

Scalar values were assigned to these answers so that statistical tests could be used in an attempt to find out if there were significant differences in pain perception between these two modalities. The acupuncturist—Eastern or Western—was also varied.

RESULTS

The suggestibility test showed that of the 12 patients, 2 were extremely suggestible, 2 reached the 75% mark, 2 were only moderately hypnotizable, and 6 appeared to be resistant to trance-like states (Fig. 1).

One patient requested that the stimulation be stopped and the needles removed after 10 min. The remaining 11 patients tolerated the needling well. However, when attempts were made after 20 min of continued stimu-

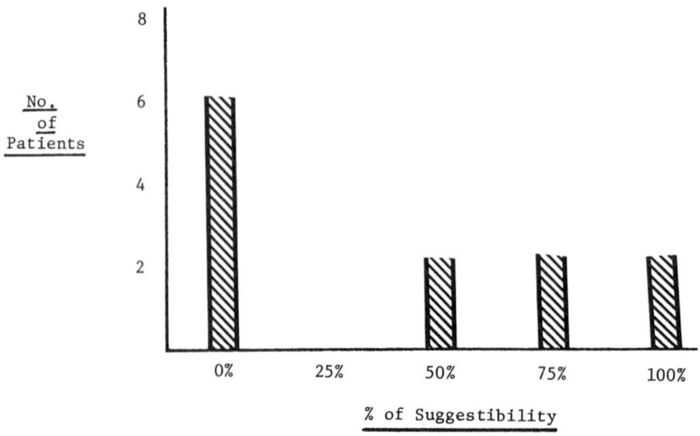

FIG. 1. Results of eye roll test.

lation to remove teeth, 9 of the patients complained of severe pain and asked for local anesthesia. Of the remaining 3 patients, 2 stated that they felt moderate but tolerable pain and 1 had no complaints. This last patient had been rated zero on the hypnotizability scale and had been treated by a Western physician.

POSTOPERATIVE PAIN

Method

Fifty patients treated with acupuncture for acute postoperative pain relief in the recovery room of a large municipal hospital were evaluated as to: (a) amount and duration of subjective pain relief; (b) changes in respiratory parameters such as tidal volume, vital capacity, FEV 1, 2, or 3, and arterial blood gas estimations; and (c) changes in all other commonly monitored vital signs.

Preoperative and postoperative attempts were made to exclude placebo reactors.

Comparison was made within the same three categories with 50 patients treated with conventional narcotics for postoperative pain relief. A control group of 30 patients who had comparable surgical procedures but who did not complain of pain and therefore received no analgesic therapy was also studied.

The acupuncture group was examined in addition as to physical status (ASA classification), race, sex, anesthetic agents and technique employed, type and duration of surgery, site of needling (peripheral or nose and ear), type of needle stimulation, and ethnic background of the acupuncturist.

Results

Acupuncture therapy afforded an average of 30% pain relief, which is within the placebo effect (Fig. 2). No patients obtained 100% pain relief. It proved time consuming but not particularly distressing to the postoperative patient. Statistical analyses of the data from all the parameters measured were not significant, with the only exception that none of the 6 black patients in the acupuncture group achieved any pain relief (Fig. 3). We were obliged to resort to conventional narcotic therapy in 44 of the patients studied.

CHRONIC PAIN

Method

One hundred patients with chronic pain problems were studied as to amount and duration of pain relief.

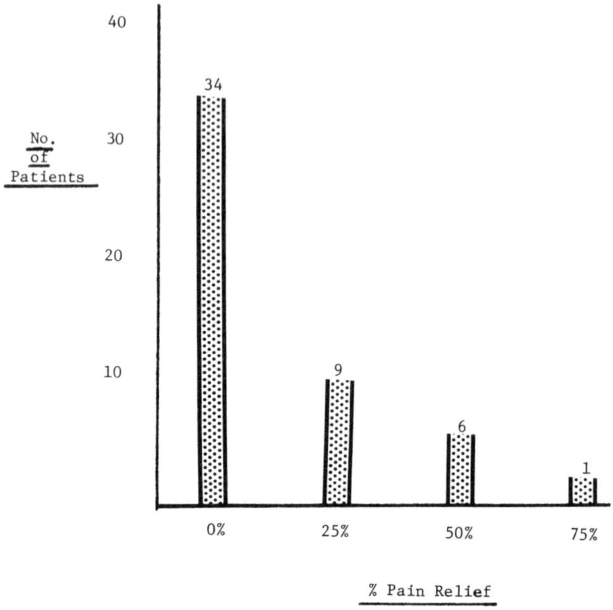

FIG. 2. Summary of pain relief.

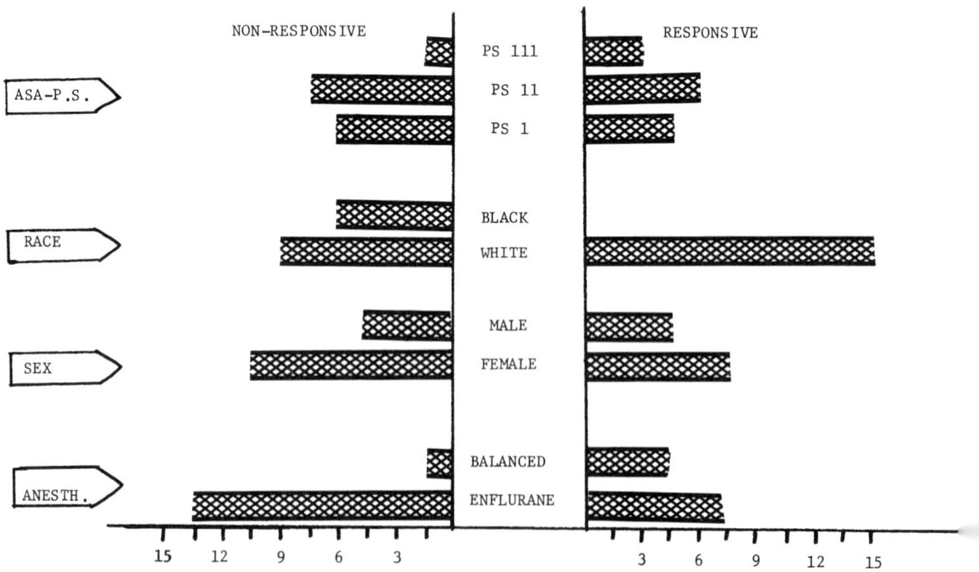

FIG. 3. Effects of other factors. PS, physical status.

TABLE 1. *Patient groups*

Group no.	Pain syndrome	Patients (no.)
1	Migraine headaches	18
2	Chronic low back pain	36
3	"Frozen" shoulder	14
4	Painful knee	9
5	"Tennis" elbow	12
6	Miscellaneous—wrist, neck, ankle	11

The patients were selected in that they met several criteria. They had all complained of pain, fluctuating in level of intensity, for at least 1 month; none of them had been treated surgically for the pain; no tissue destruction had been evidenced; and physical examinations had all been essentially negative.

Patients were grouped according to the site of pain (Table 1).

Results

The 18 patients in the first group ranged in age from 25 to 65. They all complained of severe headaches of several years' duration. Complete physical examination (including in two instances inpatient hospital work-up) in each case had revealed no abnormalities. Basic laboratory work such as complete blood counts, urinalysis, serum electrolytes, electrocardiograms, and chest X-rays were also all normal. The pattern of treatment in each case was to stimulate points in the hands and feet and combine these with local head points. The loci we used were large intestine 4 on the hands and stomach 44 and liver 3 on the feet with gallbladder 20 and governing vessel 19 on the head. Each patient required only three treatments, and we used mild electrical stimulation for approximately 15 to 20 min at each sitting. Improvement in terms of decreased number and severity of migraine attacks and decrease in amount of medication required was estimated at 77% over a 3-month period. After that time, there was an increasing incidence of return of headaches (Table 2).

Group 2 was made up of 36 medical or paramedical personnel—mostly women—between the ages of 20 and 50. They had all complained of low

TABLE 2. *Acupuncture for migraine*

Patients (no.)	Points used	Estimated improvement after 3 months
5	Stomach 44	75%
9	Liver 3, large intestine 4	90%
4	Gallbladder 20	50%

backache of variable duration from several weeks to several months. In each instance, lumbosacral X-rays had been negative.

We decided to use points other than those classically described and we added to the traditional governing vessel 26 and small intestine 6 other points along the bladder meridian (51, 54, 56, and 60).

Over an average of four treatments with electrical stimulation for approximately 20 min, pain relief was estimated at 70% over 3 months.

In the other four groups of patients—14 with stiff shoulders, 9 complaining of painful knees, 12 with a "tennis" elbow syndrome, and a miscellaneous group of 11—a similar pattern was seen. The overall pain relief was approximately 70%, and the duration of effect before symptoms returned averaged 4 months.

CONCLUSIONS

Acupuncture therapy would appear to have limited application in the treatment of acute pain in our patient population. However, in selected patients with long-standing pain syndromes, it has proven beneficial over a significant time interval.

We could postulate different pathways for acute and chronic pain. We have, for example, demonstrated that needling hand points in a boy with a transection of the cord at the C_1 level (4) (demonstrated at post mortem) resulted in reproducible analgesia in a chronic decubitus ulcer of his head. This would suggest pain pathways outside of the central nervous system. It is also possible that the careful selection of patients in the chronic pain group eliminated nonreactors.

Interesting also is that aspirin, a weak analgesic, potently blocks the production of prostaglandin E_2 and F_2 (2,3). A potent narcotic like morphine, on the other hand, has been shown to inhibit only partially a neuronal component of prostaglandin E_1 and E_2 stimulation (12). The inhibition produced is dose related but only at low concentration.

It is possible, therefore, that acupuncture, like aspirin, exhibits an anti-prostaglandin effect. Further evidence that acupuncture exerts its effect by humoral influence is seen by the reversal of acupuncture analgesia by naloxone (15).

REFERENCES

1. Bull, G. M. (1973): *Lancet,* 2:47–418.
2. Collier, H. O. J. (1971): *Nature,* 232:17–19.
3. Ferreira, S. M., Moncada, S., and Vane, J. R. (1973): *Br. J. Pharmacol.,* 49:86–97.
4. Frost, E. A. M., and Hsu, C. Y. (1975): 2nd Pain and Acupuncture Symposium, Hahnemann Medical College, Philadelphia.
5. Gordon, J. B. (1972): *J.A.M.A.,* 222:1310–1311.
6. Haller, J. S., Jr. (1973): *N.Y. State J. Med.,* 73:1213–1221.
7. Katz, A. M. (1974): *Am. J. Cardiol.,* 34:250–253.

8. Kerr, N. W. (1973): *Br. Dent., J.,* 134:201–204.
9. Mann, F. (1962): *Acupuncture, The Ancient Chinese Art of Healing.* Random House, New York.
10. Peking Acupunctural Anesthesia Coordinating Group (1972): *Peking Rev.,* 7–8:17–20.
11. Rosen, S. (1972): *N.Y. J. Dent.,* 43:144–6.
12. Sanner, J. (1971): *Ann. N.Y. Acad. Sci.,* 180:396–409.
13. Spiegel, H. (1963): *Am. J. Clin. Hypn.,* 6:1–5.
14. Spiegel, H. (1972): *Am. J. Clin. Hypn.,* 15:1, 25–28.
15. Sullivan, W. (1975): *N.Y. Times,* June 22, p. 26.

Advances in Pain Research and Therapy, Vol. 1,
edited by J. J. Bonica and D. Albe-Fessard.
Raven Press, New York © 1976.

Acupuncture for Acute Postoperative Pain Relief

Elizabeth A. M. Frost, Young I. Kim, Cher Y. Hsu, and Louis R. Orkin

Department of Anesthesiology, Albert Einstein College of Medicine, Bronx, New York 10461

Postoperative pain is subjective and an extremely variable phenomenon (10). Thus objective manifestations become very difficult to quantify. An approach to postoperative pain relief bypassing the general depressant effects of the drugs commonly employed would seem worthy of evaluation. Moreover, the commonest analgesic, morphine, at an optimum intramuscular dose of 10 mg/70 kg body weight (beyond which there is no commensurate increase in analgesic effect) affords only 75% relief of steady wound pain (7).

Pain does not, however, invariably follow surgery. Papper et al. (8) reported that even after thoracic and abdominal operations approximately 20% of patients did not complain of pain. Beecher (1) and his associates found that the average incidence of placebo relief in the postoperative period is between 30% and 40%. Personality variations contribute greatly to the degree of postoperative pain experienced (9). Delirium, due in its broadest aspects to cerebral hypoxia (5), also contributes greatly to differences in pain interpretation (4). Thus with so many intangible variables, it is hardly surprising that many therapeutic maneuvers (hypnosis, charisma, macumba, intravenous procaine, or scotch whisky) relieve patients of pain.

The principles for investigation of a new treatment (acupuncture), like those for investigation of a new drug, must clearly include predictable relief in each patient who has actual pain (not responsive to placebos). The relief must be compared to a recognized analgesic in the same patient or in a similar group. If the new treatment fails to offer adequate relief, subsequent treatment should demonstrate pain relief with a proven approach.

A preliminary study in 12 postoperative patients did not offer great promise of pain relief with acupuncture, but enthusiastic verbal reports from China (A. Topping, *personal communication*) and sustained worldwide interest (2,3) in this modality prompted the continued study which we now report.

METHOD

Fifty patients consented to be subjects in the study. All patients were visited the evening before surgery by the same physician (Y.I.K.) so that

TABLE 1. *Patient groups*

Group	Patient (no.)	Points used	Types of surgery
A	12	General body points	3, Abdominal 7, Head and neck 2, Breast
B	18	Face and ear points	12, Intra-abdominal 6, Breast
C	20	Large intestine 4, pericardium 5, gate of spirit	7, Intra-abdominal 5, Head and neck 8, Breast

the initial contact could be extended into the recovery room. There was no selection of the patients other than informed consent. All patients received general anesthesia, and those who had balanced anesthesia (relaxant-narcotic N_2O) had reversal therapy before entering into the experimental mode. Thus all patients were awake and oriented. All had complained of pain and asked for relief. Blood pressure, pulse, tidal volume, respiratory rate, forced vital capacity, minute volume, and arterial blood gas analyses were recorded in each patient immediately before needle insertion.

Acupuncture was performed with sterile stainless steel 32-gauge needles. The needles were stimulated electrically with the Electro-Therapeutic Apparatus, Model G805, Shanghai, China. In 10 patients the needles were manipulated by hand.

In the first 12 patients (group A), acupuncture points were located on the

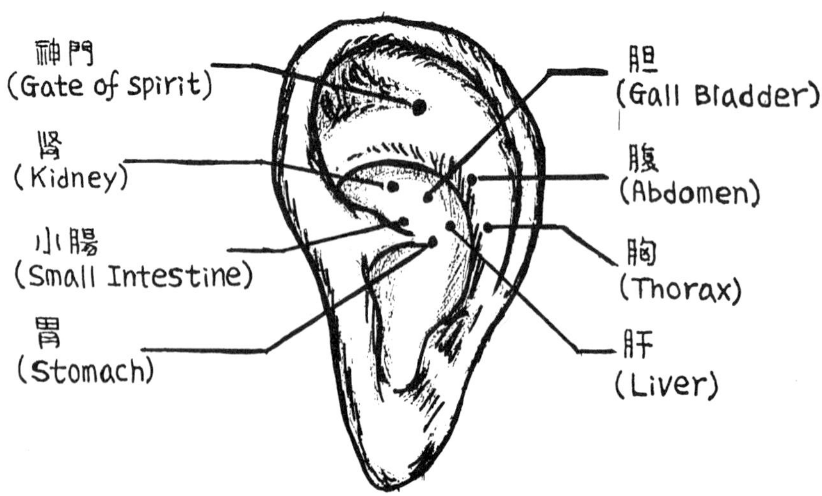

FIG. 1. Ear points.

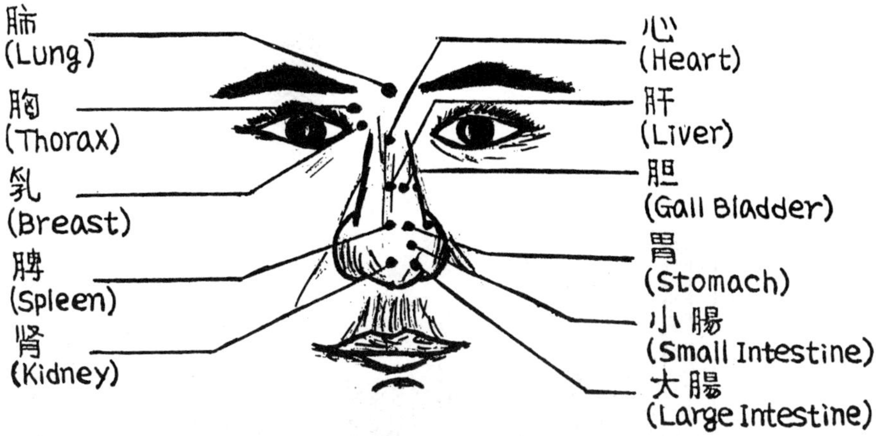

FIG. 2. Face points.

body by identifying those points on the meridians possessing low resistance (6). In 18 patients, group B, the sites for acupuncture were in the ear or on the face. These sites were selected because they were not covered by the dressings or monitoring equipment, offered a firm seat for the needles, and had been reputed to be effective areas in the Chinese literature.

In group C, points in the ear were combined with forearm points, a combination recorded as successful at the Bischko clinic in Vienna (C. Hsu, *personal communication*) (Table 1). With ear points it is not necessary to obtain a warm, tingling, heavy sensation, or *ti chi.* In the ear (Fig. 1) one needle is inserted first in the point designated gate of spirit, and then another needle in the site corresponding to the operative area. About the face (Fig. 2) the needle is first inserted at the lung point and then in a specific point determined by the localization of the pain. Acupuncture stimulation was maintained in 30 patients for the full 30 min but was stopped in 8 other patients because of persistent surgical pain.

The results estimated by the patient for subjective effect and the objective measurements were compared and analyzed by the unpaired *t*-test.

RESULTS

The first 12 patients studied were divided into three groups. Three patients, who had had intra-abdominal surgery, were needled at spleen 6 and 4 and at stomach 36 bilaterally. Two patients had no pain relief but the third, who had a subdiaphragmatic gunshot wound, felt better and coughed on request. Seven patients had surgery of the head and neck. They received acupuncture at large intestine 4 and 11, stomach 44, and pericardium 6. None of the patients volunteered that the pain was relieved, although 1 who had had an

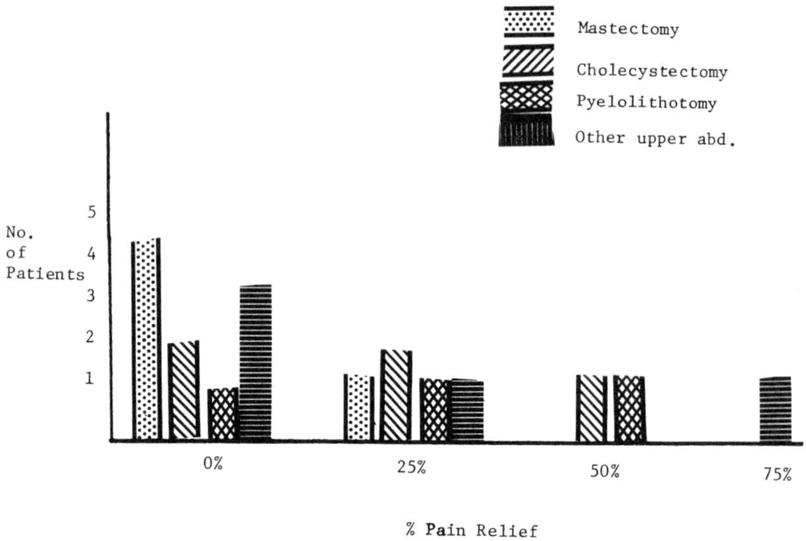

FIG. 3. Breakdown of group B.

orbital reconstruction appeared sedated and needed no other medication. The remaining 2 patients, operated on for breast nodules, had no pain relief whatsoever with needles at tri-heater 5 and heart constrictor 6. In none of the patients was there objective improvement in tidal volume, forced vital

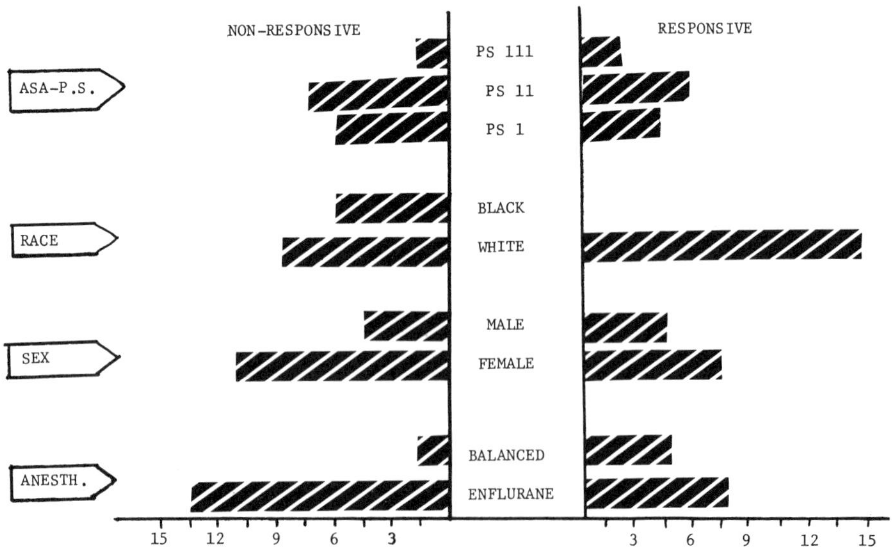

FIG. 4. Effects of other factors.

TABLE 2. *Effects of age and length of operation*

Result	Age (yr)	Length of operation (min)
Nonresponsive	42.7 ± 17.13	135 ± 72.08
Responsive	45.5 ± 16.90	98 ± 27.64

capacity, FEV 1, 2, or 3, arterial blood gas analyses, or any other vital signs.

The distribution and pain relief of the 18 patients in group B are shown in Fig. 3. None had complete relief of pain and 10 had no relief. There was no trend for relief after any specific operation. Again in the three categories—pain relief, changes in respirator parameters, and changes in other vital signs—there was no significant improvement. Similarly, in the 20 patients in group C, pain relief was minimal and no consistent changes in other parameters were obtained.

The patients were reclassified according to physical status (ASA Classification), race, sex, and type of anesthesia received (Fig. 4). None of the 6 black patients had any relief, but there were no other trends. Subclassification by the age of the patient or the duration of surgery (Table 2) did not appear to influence the results. The overall amount of pain relief achieved is shown in Fig. 5. Table 3 compares respiratory parameters measured in

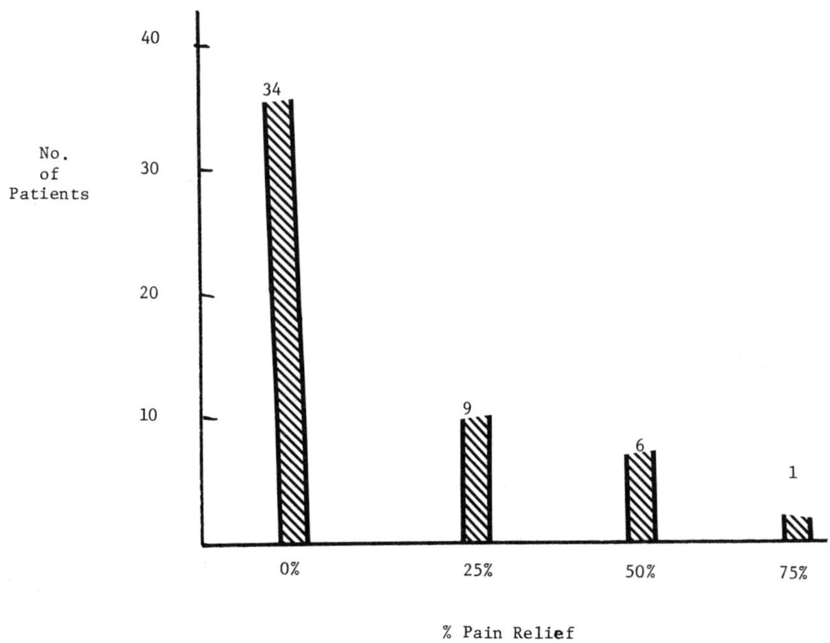

FIG. 5. Summary of pain relief.

TABLE 3. *Respiratory measurements*

Parameter	Nonresponsive (N=34)		Responsive (N=16)		Meperidine (N=50)	
VT mean %[a]	0.4	↓	2.0	↑	5.4	↓
Freq. mean %	5.9	↑	5.0	↑	5.6	↓
VC mean % (0.1)	0.1	↓	16.0	↑	.2	↓
MV mean %	4.1	↑	3.9	↑	0.8	↓
pH	0.019	↑	0.04	↑	.01	↑
$PaCO_2$ mean mm Hg	3.3	↓	3.4	↓	.7	↓

[a] VT, tidal volume; VC, vital capacity; MV, minute ventilation.

patients not having pain relief, in patients having 25% or more pain relief, and in 50 patients treated with conventional narcotics. There was no evidence that patients having an effect from acupuncture experience a laudatory effect on ventilation or arterial blood gas content. Mild hyperventilation is to be expected with pain. In the 50 control patients, the depressive ventilatory effect of meperidine is evident even with the small dose of 25 mg. The only improvement that can be implied is a 1 in 10 possibility that the vital capacity is improved. Since patients do not ordinarily breath with their entire vital capacity, there is no reflection of this improvement in the other measurements. The patients who failed to respond to acupuncture were given meperidine with good pain relief. Unfortunately, respiratory studies could not then be performed as we had simultaneously shown.

A second control group of 30 patients who had not complained of pain and who had therefore received no analgesic therapy were also studied as to changes in respiratory parameters and other vital signs on two occasions, 1 hr apart. No significant changes were found in the two sets of values obtained, and they were directly comparable with the figures obtained in the acupuncture group.

DISCUSSION

The need for a nondepressive nonpharmacological analgesic approach to pain relief is known to every member of the surgical team. All known analgesics produce respiratory depression, which cannot be divorced from the therapeutic effect. No such effect is seen with acupuncture, but the analgesic effect is indefinite and unpredictable. The technique itself is time consuming but not particularly distressing to the postoperative patient. If the patient is to be treated, it is a most expensive approach that would have advantages in only a small select group of patients. Unfortunately, it is extremely difficult to select the group that will respond. If the end results cannot be controlled or estimated, the failure of response can be harmful to the patient's psyche, the physician's estimation of the problems, and the patient-doctor relationship.

Our failure to obtain optimum results may be related to our patient population or to the skill of the several acupuncturists (both Eastern and Western) involved. We cannot admit to the latter. Others may yet suggest other acupuncture points. Our patient population is selective by virtue of our activity being centered in a large municipal hospital. It is striking, for example, that black patients were slow to volunteer for the study, and those few who did failed to respond favorably.

We are forced to conclude that acupuncture is of extremely limited value for postoperative pain relief in our population group.

REFERENCES

1. Beecher, H. K. (1959): *Measurement of Subjective Responses,* pp. 65–67. Oxford University Press, New York.
2. Cheng, S. B., and Ding, L. K. (1973): *Nature* (*Lond.*), 242:559.
3. Dimond, E. G. (1971): *J.A.M.A.,* 218:10, 1558.
4. Drummond, G. B. (1975): *Br. J. Anaesth.,* 47:130–140.
5. Eckenhoff, J. E., Kneale, D. H., and Dripps, R. D. (1961): *Anesthesiology,* 22:667–681.
6. Frost, E., and Orkin, L. (1973): *D.H.E.W.* Publication No. 74–165.
7. Lasagna, L., and Beecher, H. K. (1954): *J.A.M.A.,* 156:230–234.
8. Papper, E. M., Brodie, B. B., and Rovenstine, E. A. (1952): *Surgery,* 32:107–109.
9. Parbrook, G. D., Steel, D. F., and Dalrymple, D. G. (1973): *Br. J. Anaesth.,* 45:21.
10. Wallace, P. G. M., and Norris, W. (1975): *Br. J. Anaesth.,* 47:113.

Advances in Pain Research and Therapy, Vol. 1,
edited by J. J. Bonica and D. Albe-Fessard.
Raven Press, New York © 1976.

Effect of Acupuncture in Tension Headache and Brainstem Reflexes

V. Johansson, S. Kosic, O. Lindahl, L. Lindwall, and L. Tibbling

Regionsjukhuset, 581 85 Linköping, Sweden

This chapter reports a broad-based investigation of acupuncture, conducted as a joint project by the Departments of Neurology, Orthopaedics, Otorhinolaryngology, and Psychiatry at the medical school, and the Departments of Statistics and Electronics at the University of Linköping. The component studies were planned by the Department of Statistics and designed as double-blind, randomized experiments with control groups.

METHODS

An examination was made of the effect of acupuncture on tension headache (33 patients) and brachialgia (26 patients) and on formation reticularis (20 subjects). Electrical conductivity and temperature at acupuncture points were also determined. In this study the Chinese technique of acupuncture without electrical stimulation was used. The treatment was carried out by a fully trained and experienced specialist.

The placebo therapy consisted of the same kind of acupuncture treatment given by the same person, but the needles were then inserted systematically 1 cm distant from the actual acupuncture point. Neither the patient nor the physician appraising the results knew to which group the patient belonged. Contact between the patient and the acupuncture specialist was of short duration, and there was no form of conscious mental influence—hypnosis, for example.

The typical sensation that the patient is said to experience when the needle is inserted in the acupuncture point is, so far as we could ascertain, not particularly regular or characteristic. In any case it was unknown to the patients in this study, who therefore cannot have been aware of any difference between the true and the placebo treatments.

In the examination of the temperature and electrical resistance of the acupuncture points, we marked a large number of such points on the skin with circles, and next to each of them a false point was marked at a distance of 3 mm. A record of the true and false points was made. Technicians then measured temperature and electrical resistance for each point. The values obtained for the true and false points were then compared and submitted to statistical analysis.

The horizontal eye movements were registered by electronystagmography to test the effect of acupuncture on the reticular formation. The subject was submitted to an angular acceleration of 40°/s^2 to a speed of 120°/s in complete darkness with open eyes, and the postaccelerative nystagmus pattern was recorded. The speed for the slow nystagmus phase, which is a reflection of the inner ear stimulation plus the central habituation mechanisms, the amplitudes of the nystagmus beats, and the nystagmus frequency were calculated for 10 repeated experiments on each subject, and the collected data were then evaluated statistically.

RESULTS

The results of the study can be summarized as follows: Over a period of 8 weeks' observation, acupuncture had a significantly better effect on tension headache than placebo acupuncture. The level of significance was 1%. In brachialgia with no sign of specific cause of the symptoms, there was no significant difference between the effects of true and placebo acupuncture.

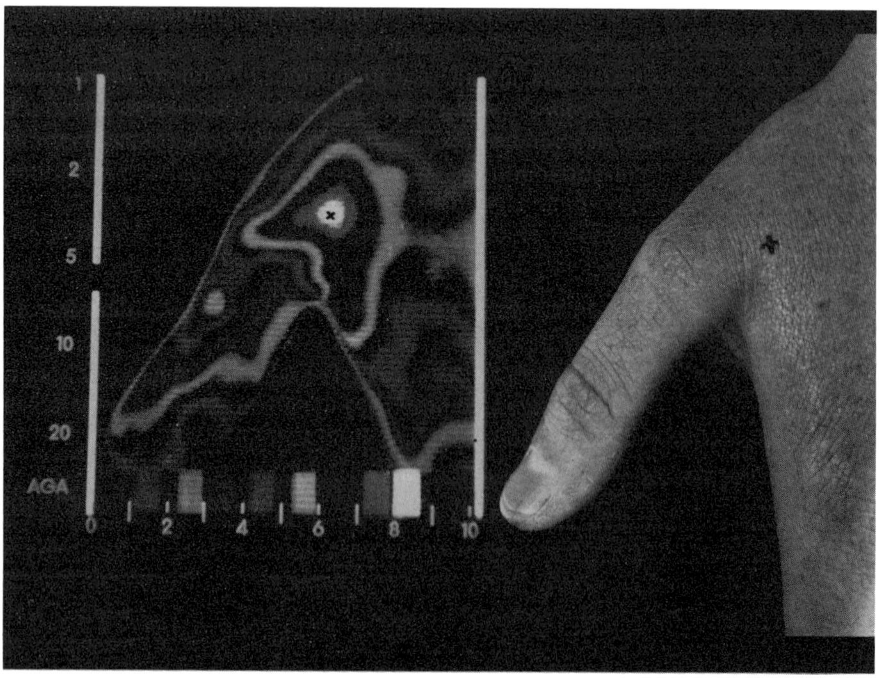

FIG. 1.

The series was, however, fairly small and does of course not prove that acupuncture treatment is ineffective in this disease. In the subjects with formatio reticularis, there was a significantly greater activation on the arousal part of the reticular formation for the acupuncture than for the placebo points. A similar effect may be observed after the administration of certain drugs, such as neuroleptics.

The temperature was considerably higher at the acupuncture points than at the false points 3 mm distant ($p < 0.001$). The electric resistence was lower at the acupuncture points than at the points 3 mm distant in all but 1 of the 42 cases. The difference was highly significant ($p < 0.00001$).

The acupuncture points can easily be localized by means of a color thermovision (Fig. 1).

CONCLUSIONS

It would seem justified to deduce from the results of this study that acupuncture points differ physically from the surrounding skin, and that acupuncture can exert a therapeutic effect. This effect cannot be accounted for by any suggestive mechanism such as hypnosis, by a peripheral change in the pain threshold, or by anesthesia, such as has been demonstrated in connection with surgical operations. The observed effect on the patient's symptoms persists over a long period.

In our opinion there is every reason to take acupuncture seriously and to conduct further research with the purpose of examining the useful application of this form of treatment and finding the mechanisms underlying its therapeutic effect.

ACKNOWLEDGMENT

This investigation was supported by the Bank of Sweden Tercentenary Foundation.

Advances in Pain Research and Therapy, Vol. 1,
edited by J. J. Bonica and D. Albe-Fessard.
Raven Press, New York © 1976.

Neurophysiological Basis for the Hypothalamic Lesion and Stimulation by Chronic Implanted Electrodes for the Relief of Intractable Pain in Cancer

David Fairman

Center of Oncologic Neurophysiopathology, University of Buenos Aires, Buenos Aires, Argentina

This chapter is based on 15 years of research, clinical studies, and surgical experience for the relief of pain produced by malignant tumors in a consecutive series of 575 patients. We have classified our series of patients in two groups according to the target selected. In a first group of 521 cases (Table 1) our target has been at the level of the thalamic intralaminar nucleus and the adjacent area of the centrum medianum (4–6, 8). In a second group of 54 patients (Table 2) our target has been the periventricular nucleus at the level of the hypothalamus (7,9).

The purpose of this chapter is to discuss the neurophysiological basis for the hypothalamic lesion and to present a new hypothesis. This hypothesis suggests that the hypothalamic periventricular nucleus modulates both the inhibitory and excitatory influences of synaptic transmission of pain impulses by blocking the pathways connecting the brainstem reticular formation to the different areas of the cerebral cortex which underlie conscious experience of pain.

MATERIAL AND METHODS

In all these cases a well-defined lesion of a predetermined size was produced by using a stereotactic apparatus and technique published in detail in 1959 (3). All the patients, except 25, were operated on under local anesthesia with minimal sedation. Electrical stimulation studies were performed before the lesion by inserting a bipolar electrode 0.8 mm in outer diameter with an interpolar distance of 0.5 mm.

The rate at which the stimulus is delivered, the duration of its application, the number of volts, and other factors have been shown to make considerable difference. Our optimal parameters when electrically stimulating the hypothalamus with square wave pulses have been 1 to 4 V, 10 to 20 cps, 1 msec for 3 to 6 sec. We developed the idea of performing repetitive stimulation sessions through chronic implanted electrodes in the hypothalamic periventricular nucleus, observing that pain relief was obtained outlasting the

TABLE 1. *Stereotactic thalamic tractotomy*

Site of carcinoma	Cases	
	Number	Percent
Lung	260	50
Head and neck	104	20
Uterus	78	15
Breast	52	10
Gastrointestinal tract	27	5
Total	521	100

TABLE 2. *Hypothalamotomy*

Site of carcinoma	Cases	
	Number	Percent
Lung	32	60
Head and neck	11	20
Uterus	5	10
Breast	4	7
Gastrointestinal tract	2	3
Total	54	100

stimulus for different extents of time without necessity in some cases of performing the lesion itself.

RESULTS

Satisfactory relief of pain, i.e., no pain at all or some tolerable pain no longer requiring narcotic analgesics, was obtained in 70% of all the patients. The pain relief lasted for the complete period of survival, which ranged between 2 and 12 months with an average duration of 6 months. Unsatisfactory results, consisting of no pain relief or partial relief but still requiring analgesics, or temporary remission with recurrence of pain, was obtained in 30% of the patients. There was a 10% incidence of complications consisting in hyperthermia or hemiparesis accompanied by a certain degree of mental obnubilation. These complications were reversible and the patient recuperated completely within 8 or 10 days of the operation. There was no operative mortality. The absence of sensory disturbances was a constant finding in all cases in which pain was alleviated. Before and after surgery thorough sensory examinations were carried out, which disclosed no change in tactile, thermal, or pain sensitivity.

DISCUSSION

The aim of the different investigators has been to find the correct target point where a lesion could act satisfactorily to alleviate pain. From a review of the literature, it appears that stereotactically applied destruction of the principal thalamic nuclear terminus of the spinothalamic tract (VPL, VPLo, or Hassler's V.c.a.e. and V.c.p.e.) has failed to produce the panacea for pain relief that was originally envisioned. Hecaen et al. (11) apparently were the first to report thalamic pain relief after a lesion produced at the centrum medianum. (CM).

Mark et al. (14) obtained alleviation of pain by resorting to extensive lesions in the region of the lamina medullaris interna. Spigel and Wycis (17) stated that a lesion produced in the region of the intralaminar nuclei and perhaps also in the CM if combined with lesions of the lateral spinothalamic and quintothalamic tracts or their terminations in the nuclei VP may be effective in relieving pain.

Only a few cases of surgical lesions placed in the human hypothalamus have been reported. Spigel and Wycis (16) performed stereotactic lesions at the lateral hypothalamic area in cases of schizophrenia. Sano (15) reported a procedure designated as posteromedial hypothalamotomy in patients with aggressive or restless behavior. The first report in the literature (7) of producing a lesion in the hypothalamus for the relief of intractable pain in patients with malignant tumors was presented in 1971.

We developed the idea of surgically attacking the hypothalamus in cancer patients with intractable pain by elaborating a working hypothesis based on the correlations between our above-mentioned experience and the following phylogenetic and neurophysiological facts. From the phylogenetic standpoint, the archithalamus—which includes the thalamic intralaminar nucleus—is closely related to the hypothalamic periventricular system belonging to the upper brainstem reticular formation. The latter receives the impulses of the unmyelinated fiber pathways mediating poorly localized sensations through the old paleospinothalamic tract. According to Arvanitaki (1), the brainstem reticular formation can have a rhythmic activity originating at the cellular level, that is, an ontogenic activity. Our theory is based on the fact that the hypothalamus is the correlation center of the autonomic nervous system, which integrates at all levels with the sensory motor and motor sensory systems, playing an essential role in the mechanism of pain. Moreover, our model is consistent with the studies of Gellhorn (10), who asserted that the hypothalamus could be the coordinating center of the whole brainstem reticular system and, therefore, the primary regulator of cortical activity and consciousness. Moreover, Bard and Mountcastle (2) have shown that the hypothalamus plays an important role in affectivity, including motivation and emotion, which—as is well known—are essential components of pain sensation.

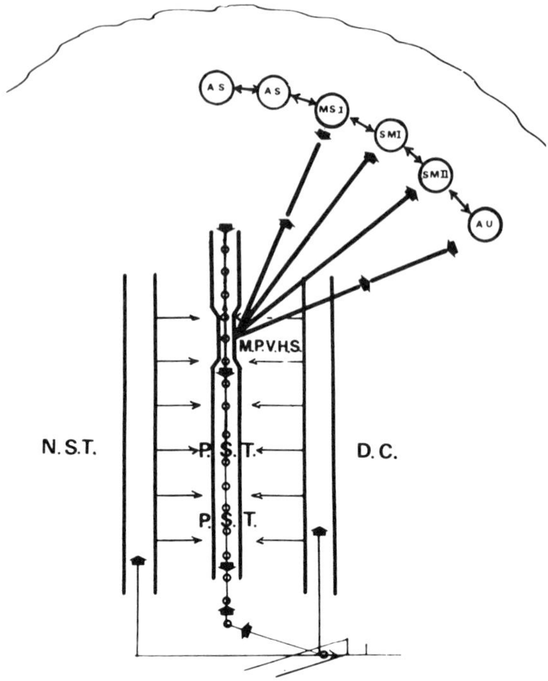

FIG. 1. Schematic diagram of modulating periventricular hypothalamic blocking system. N.S.T., neospinothalamic tract; P.S.T., paleospinothalamic tract; D.C., dorsal column; SMI, sensory motor I; SMII, sensory motor II; AS, associated areas; AU, autonomic area; M.P.V.H.S., modulating periventricular hypothalamic system.

Our hypothesis is consistent with the fact that from the anatomical standpoint the hypothalamus constitutes an area of convergence of the neuronal circuits, which are more circumscribed here than at any other level (Fig. 1). Consequently, the hypothalamus becomes the elective target that enables a strategic attack by a small, circumscribed lesion or by repetitive stimulation by chronically implanted electrodes, resulting in the effective blocking of pain impulses.

Magoun (13) has shown that efferent sensory, efferent motor, and autonomic volleys of fibers converge at the upper and lower brainstem reticular formation. Livingston (12) pointed out the possibilities that these volleys of fibers of different origin share at this level the same neuronal circuits.

These concepts support our theory which postulates that a dynamic competition for the use of the same neuronal circuits between the pattern of pain impulses and the pattern of impulses elicited by adequate stimulation results in the effective blocking of the pain impulses. In other words, the concept of the modulating periventricular hypothalamic blocking system explains why stimulation of the hypothalamic area provides the means for blocking the pathways that connect the periventricular hypothalamic structures to the different areas of the cerebral cortex. These areas underlie the conscious experience of pain.

The interpretation of each state of conscious experience of pain involves a dynamic process, i.e., integration of different cerebral functions including behavior, memory, attention, and affectivity. This integration results from the dynamic interaction exerted through transcortical and corticosubcortical connections, which function always as a dynamic unit.

ACKNOWLEDGMENT

This work was supported by the Universal Organism for Scientific Research.

REFERENCES

1. Arvanitaki, A. (1943): *Arch. Int. Physiol.,* 54:508–531.
2. Bard, D., and Mountcastle, V. B. (1948): *Res. Publ. Assoc. Res. Nerv. Ment. Dis.,* 27:362–404.
3. Fairman, D. (1959): *Am. J. Roentgenol.,* 81:1001–1005.
4. Fairman, D. (1966): *Confin. Neurol.,* 27:67–70.
5. Fairman, D. (1967): *Confin. Neurol.,* 29:146–152.
6. Fairman, D. (1970): *Confin. Neurol.,* 32:341–344.
7. Fairman, D. (1972): *Avicenum Czech. Med. Pr.,* 525–528.
8. Fairman, D. (1973*a*): *Cancer,* 31:700–706.
9. Fairman, D. (1973*b*): *J. Surg. Oncol.,* 79–84.
10. Gellhorn, E. (1952): *Pfluegers Arch.,* 255:75–92.
11. Hecaen, H., Talairach, J., David, M., and Dell, M. B. (1949): *Rev. Neurol.,* 81:917–919.
12. Livingston, R. B., French, J. D., and Hernandez-Peon, R. (1953): *Fed. Proc.,* 12:89–90.
13. Magoun, H. W. (1952): *Arch. Neurol. Psychiatr.,* 67:145–154.
14. Mark, V. H., Ervin, F. R., and Yakovlev, P. I. (1963): *Arch. Neurol.,* 8:528.
15. Sano, K. (1970): *J. Neurosurg.,* 33:689–707.
16. Spiegel, E. A., and Wycis, H. T. (1962): In: *Stereoencephalotomy (Thalamotomy and Related Procedures), Part II.* Grune & Stratton, New York.
17. Spiegel, E. A., and Wycis, H. T. (1966): *Confin. Neurol.,* 27:7–17.

Advances in Pain Research and Therapy, Vol. 1,
edited by J. J. Bonica and D. Albe-Fessard.
Raven Press, New York © 1976.

Microneurosurgical Treatment of Trigeminal Neuralgia by Selective Juxtapontine Rhizotomy of the Portio Major Sparing the Intermediate Fibers

Carlo A. Pagni and Paolo E. Maspes

Neurosurgical Clinic, University of Milan, Milan, Italy

In 1929 Dandy (1) reported that patients who presumably had had a total juxtapontine trigeminal rhizotomy still felt touch and pinprick over the entire face or large areas of it. He assumed that some fine sensory rootlets, he called them "accessory," must have escaped surgery.

Recently Jannetta and Rand (8,9) reconsidered the matter by studying the trigeminal root at the pons with an operating microscope with 10 to 15 times magnification, thus providing many anatomic details that escape the naked eye. They identified three parts in the root: (a) so-called portio minor, or motor root, (b) so-called portio major, or sensory root; and, (c) a group of small fibers that leave the portio major to enter the pons separately between the sensory and motor roots; some other fibers run from the sensory root and join the motor root to enter the pons anteriorly and caudally to the motor fibers. They called all these "intermediate fibers."

Jannetta and Rand (6,9) suggested that intermediate fibers convey tactile sensation and portio major conveys pain sensation, a concept embraced by Provost and Hardy (13). Jannetta (6) reported that "partial to *complete* section of the portio major at the pons with complete preservation of the intermediate fibers *in five* patients with trigeminal neuralgia" gave relief of pain and "mild hypalgesia to analgesia in the facial area corresponding to the portio of the nerve section. But in this same area perception of light touch was strikingly preserved. The corneal reflex also remained normal."

Thus the performance of the section of the portio major sparing the intermediate fibers raised the hope of reaching the following goals: (a) abolishing tic douloureux, sparing facial sensation and corneal reflex, and thus avoiding the risk of keratitis; (b) possibly avoiding postoperative paresthesia and painful anesthesia by reducing facial sensory loss. The following is a report of our results with this procedure.

MATERIAL AND METHODS

Juxtapontine trigeminal rhizotomy with the aid of the operating microscope was performed in 29 patients (20 women and 9 men) with severe intractable trigeminal neuralgia. There were no operative deaths. Ages of the patients ranged from 26 to 75 years.

The 29 patients had previously been unrelieved by medical treatment with carbamazepine (all cases), acupuncture (3 cases), peripheral anesthetic blocks (nearly all cases), alcoholic or phenolic blocks and avulsion of peripheral branches (9 cases), alcoholic block or electrocoagulation of the gasserian ganglion (3 cases), and Frazier's subtemporal rhizotomy (6 cases).

Surgical Approach and Operative Observations

In 11 patients we employed the *transtentorial subtemporal approach* (2,9). Four transitory complications (because of reclination of the temporal lobe with edema, section of veins) occurred: dysphasia, hemianopsia, seizures, and mental confusion. At long-term follow-up 2 patients still displayed temporal EEG abnormalities, and 1 had had two epileptic seizures. Root abnormalities were not observed except in 1 patient in whom many small arteries covered the root but did not cause distortion or compression.

Dandy's posterior fossa approach was employed in 18 patients. Four transitory complications were observed: nystagmus, hypoacusia, unsteadiness, and gastric bleeding. Unsteadiness and hypoacusia persisted at long-term follow-up in 1 patient. The following root abnormalities were observed in this group. In 2 cases a loop of an elongated vessel provoked compression and distortion of the root near the pons; when freed by dissection it left a groove on the root surface. In 3 cases a large arterial branch was firmly attached to the root; when dissected it assumed a new position. In 5 cases dense arachnoidal membranes surrounded the root, resulting in 3 in a true anulus fibrosus constricting the root. Two patients who had previously submitted to alcoholic block of the gasserian ganglion were found to have root disease. Rootlets were not separated but coalesced, giving the root a homogeneous gelatinous appearance. In 6 patients the root seemed free of abnormalities.

Intermediate fibers were identified in only 13 out of 29 cases (45%), either as small bundles entering the pons outside the sensory portion (12 cases), or as anastomotic bundles between the sensory and the motor portion (1 case). Intermediate fibers were identified in 2 patients out of the 9 who had previously submitted to rhizotomy or alcohol block and electrocoagulation of the gasserian ganglion (22%), but these fibers were observed in 11 out of 20 cases who had not undergone any previous surgical procedure on the ganglion and root (55%).

Our data compare with those of Gudmundsson et al. (5) who, on the basis of autopsy studies, stated that intermediate fibers are present in only 50% of the nerves. Therefore (see also ref. 12), intermediate fibers do not seem to be a constant anatomical feature of the trigeminal root at the pons.

The extent of the root section varied in various case groups. *Total rhizotomy* was performed in 15 cases. The whole sensory component of the root was divided, whether or not intermediate fibers had been identified. In 2 cases the motor root was accidentally damaged. In 5 cases a *partial rhizotomy* was performed, in which 66% to 75% of the root was divided. In these cases the intermediate fibers were not identified or were identified unclearly. *Selective rhizotomy* was performed in 9 cases. The whole portio major was sectioned, the intermediate fibers being completely spared. Clinical results of only these 9 cases are reported in this chapter.

EFFECTS OF SELECTIVE RHIZOTOMY OF THE PORTIO MAJOR SPARING THE INTERMEDIATE FIBERS

Pattern of Sensory Loss. Possible Functional Meaning of the Intermediate Fibers

Complete section of the portio major with preservation of the intermediate fibers gave the following sensory alterations. First, perception of pricking pain was abolished in the whole trigeminal area in 6 cases; in 2 cases some perception of pinprick was preserved mainly in the first and second branch territory. Second, thermal sensibility was abolished in 1 case. In 8 cases there was marked reduction all over the trigeminal area, with better preservation of sensibility in the upper part of the face. Third, there was some impairment of tactile sensibility in all the patients. In each case light touch sensation was reduced throughout the trigeminal area, with a more-or-less extensive area of total loss of perception. Usually the most severe touch alterations were referred to the lower part of the face, touch perception being preserved better in the upper part or in the first branch territory (5 cases). Nevertheless, in 1 case the area of most marked sensory loss was localized around the eye.

The reported data suggest the "intermediate fibers" are not mode-specific fibers for light touch. Clear separation between thermoalgesic and tactile afferent rootlets does not seem to exist in the trigeminal root. The usual better preservation of tactile, thermal, and painful perceptions in the upper part of the face seems to confirm that intermediate fibers are aberrant nonspecific fibers commonly contributing to the first branch as anatomical and electrophysiological studies showed (4,5). Anyway, the hypothesis that even some of the intermediate fibers have been damaged at operation in our cases cannot be forgotten; and that could explain the discrepancy between our observations and those of Jannetta (6).

It is interesting to report that in 15 cases submitted to total division of the root including (when identified) the intermediate fibers, the outcome was tactile, thermal, and pain anesthesia all over the trigeminal territory; in 2 cases only some perception of very strong tactile stimuli was preserved in the first and third branch (anastomosis with the portio minor?).

Preservation of the Corneal Reflex and Occurrence of Keratitis

In the series submitted to selective section of the portio major, the corneal reflex was normal in 2 cases, reduced in 1 case, and abolished in 6 cases. None had keratitis. The corneal reflex was abolished in all the 15 patients submitted to total rhizotomy; 4 of them had keratitis.

Effect on Neuralgic Pain

At 1 to 6 years follow-up, neuralgia was abolished in all the patients, including those submitted to selective rhizotomy (9 cases) and those submitted to total (15 cases) or partial (5 cases) rhizotomy. Two patients referred occasionally to sudden nonpainful sensations like "jumps" under the skin of less than 1 sec duration in some part of the face.

The conclusion seems reasonable that selective rhizotomy of the portio major sparing the intermediate fibers can produce long-lasting relief from neuralgia. The question obviously arises if the spared intermediate fibers might eventually be a sufficient substratum for recurrence of pain: only longer follow-up might answer this.

Postoperative Paresthesia and Painful Anesthesia

Paresthesia in the denervated area is the most common sequel of trigeminal rhizotomy (10,11,14). Paresthesias are not mentioned after juxtapontine selective rhizotomy (6,12,13); yet in our series they were a common complaint. All 9 patients referred to paresthesia in the denervated area. Three described it as "numbness" and "not annoying paresthesia"; they were very happy with the result. Four patients referred to "annoying paresthesia," but they too were happy with the result because the new sensations were not painful and were preferable to the previous neuralgic pain. Two patients complained bitterly of "painful anesthesia" and were very disappointed with the result.

Occurrence of paresthesia was even higher in the group of 15 patients submitted to total rhizotomy: 3 patients had only numbness and were very pleased with the result; 4 patients referred to "annoying paresthesia" but were nonetheless happy; 7 patients were unhappy owing to "painful anesthesia."

Owing to the high occurrence of paresthesia, even the section of the portio major sparing the intermediate fibers, as in every kind of posterior rhizotomy, must be rejected as the first step in treatment of trigeminal neuralgia. It must be considered only after trials with more conservative techniques have failed (10).

POSSIBLE ADVANTAGES OF MICROSURGICAL TECHNIQUE IN TRIGEMINAL NEURALGIA

Approaching the trigeminal root via the posterior fossa sometimes allows discovery of an organic lesion responsible for neuralgia (e.g., a small tumor, an arteriovenous malformation) which usually escapes clinical-neuroradiological investigations. That has been well known since Dandy's observations (14). Recently Jannetta (7,9) extended this concept, suggesting that even compression-distortion of the root because of arterial loops (usually superior cerebellar artery) or other causes (e.g., veins, arachnoidea) might be responsible for neuralgia. These findings, none of which has ever been noted in patients not affected by trigeminal neuralgia, are treatable only with the aid of the surgical microscope.

In our series such abnormalities have been observed in 10 out of 18 cases operated on by the posterior fossa approach. However, in our patients the posterior root was eventually divided at operation. In Jannetta's series (7), these abnormalities were treated in 60 patients by decompression of the root without section: neuralgia was abolished (see also ref. 3). This might be the new avenue open to microsurgical technique to cure trigeminal neuralgia: it might possibly attain the ideal aim of therapy, i.e., abolition of pain without any sensory loss.

REFERENCES

1. Dandy, W. E. (1929): *Arch. Surg.,* 18:687–734.
2. Dogliotti, A. M. (1936): *Atti 43rd Congress of the Society of Italian Surgeons,* 539 pp.
3. Duplay, J., Chiarelli, J., Grellier, P., Roche, J. L., and Rosset, M. J. (1974): *Neurochirurgie,* 20:593–598.
4. Emmons, W. F., and Rhoton, A. L., Jr. (1971): *Surg. Forum,* 19:440–441.
5. Gudmundsson, K., Rhoton, A. L., Jr., and Rushton, J. G. (1971): *J. Neurosurg.,* 35:592–600.
6. Jannetta, P. J. (1967): *J. Neurosurg.,* 26:159–162.
7. Jannetta, P. J. (1975): First World Congress on Pain, Abstr., p. 95.
8. Jannetta, P. J., and Rand, R. W. (1966*a*): *Anat. Rec.,* 154:362.
9. Jannetta, P. J., and Rand, R. W. (1966*b*): *Bull. Los Angeles Neurol. Soc.,* 31:93–99.
10. Maspes, P. E., and Pagni, C. A. (1974): In: *Recent Advances on Pain. Pathophysiology and Clinical Aspects,* edited by J. J. Bonica, P. Procacci, and C. A. Pagni, pp. 201–255. Charles C Thomas, Publisher, Springfield, Illinois.
11. Pagni, C. A. (1976): In: *Progress in Neurological Surgery, Vol. 7,* edited by H. Krayenbühl, P. E. Maspes, and W. H. Sweet. Karger, Basel.
12. Pertuiset, B., Philippon, J., Fohanno, D., and Khalil, M. (1972): *Rev. Neurol.,* 126:97–106.
13. Provost, J., and Hardy, J. (1970): *Neurochirurgie,* 16:459–470.
14. White, J. C., and Sweet, W. H. (1969): *Pain and the Neurosurgeon.* Charles C Thomas, Publisher, Springfield, Illinois.

Advances in Pain Research and Therapy, Vol. 1,
edited by J. J. Bonica and D. Albe-Fessard.
Raven Press, New York © 1976.

Microsurgical Lumbosacral Ganglionectomy Technique, Anatomic Rationale, and Surgical Results

Carroll P. Osgood, Manuel Dujovny, and Ronald Faille

Department of Neurological Surgery, University of Pittsburgh School of Medicine, Veterans Administration Hospital, Pittsburgh, Pennsylvania 15240

Sensory rhizotomy for chronic pain syndromes remains a controversial procedure because of the discouraging long-term success rates reported in most series (3,6,7,15). We suspect that the sensory ganglion itself is an important "way station" in the transmission of nociceptive stimuli in many chronic pain syndromes. We have developed a microsurgical ganglionectomy technique based on the anatomic study of 400 cadaver lumbosacral roots and ganglia using the operating microscope. This microganglionectomy technique has proved reliable in our clinical series of 18 cases, and good-to-fair pain relief has been achieved for 15 of these patients (longest follow-up, 16 months).

MATERIAL AND METHOD

A Zeiss OPM 1, with a 250-mm objective, was used in the dissection of over 400 lumbosacral root ganglia and their meninges. After the lamina is exposed, the lateral lamina edge is shaved inferiorly (3 mm) with a Hall drill (Fig. 1). Yellow ligament and epidural fat are then removed over the ganglion area using curets and a fine Kerrison rongeur at 10×. Then at 16×, the dural ganglion capsule is opened longitudinally by a 5-mm incision. A microspatula is then used to lift the ganglion up away from the dural septum overlying the motor root. A 4-mm metal clip is applied to the bifid sensory root 2 mm proximal to the ganglion, and the dorsal root immediately distal to this clip is divided. The ganglion corpus is then peeled laterally up and away from the dural septum protecting the motor root. Another metal clip is then placed across the distal ganglion, just beyond the exit of the dorsal division, and the ganglion is divided just proximal to this clip (Fig. 2).

Our 18 clinical procedures have been done using an identical anatomic approach, and these cases are summarized in Table 1. Selective root blocks (at the ganglion level) were done preoperatively under X-ray control in all cases as part of the routine patient selection process. Small amounts of relatively nondiffusing local anesthetic (1%), tetracaine, 15 mg, were used for each root. Patients who did not experience good pain relief after repeated root blocks were not considered ganglionectomy candidates.

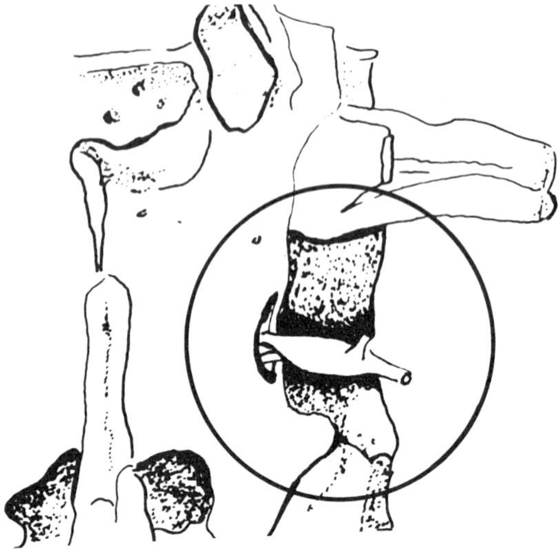

FIG. 1. Small amount of lateral lamina removed to expose left-sided lumbar ganglion.

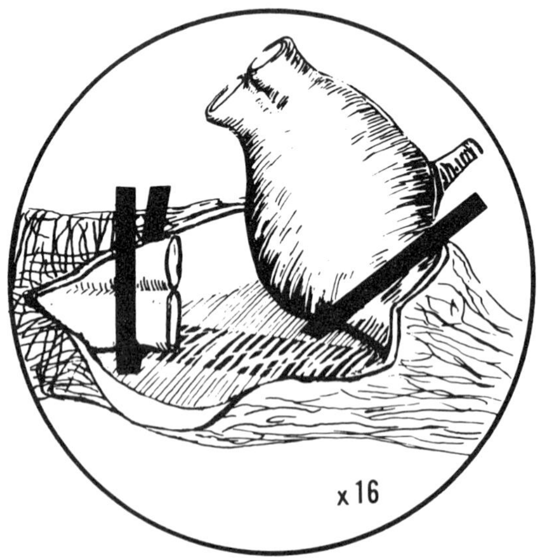

FIG. 2. Distal sensory root (bifid) divided and ganglion corpus reflected laterally. Note motor root (dark) protected by dural septum under sensory ganglion.

TABLE 1. *Summary of data on patients treated with anatomic approach*

Patient/ Age/Sex	Cause of pain	Duration and nature of pain	Previous procedures for pain relief	Ganglionectomy level	Length follow-up (mo)	Results
VH/51/M[a]	WW II injury, R sciatic nerve, retained mortar fragments	10 yr; deep aching pain posterior thigh	Exploration & partial resection sciatic nerve neuroma 2 times	R:L_4, L_5, S_1	10	Good; occasional dysesthesias inside R leg with urination
HB/37/M	GSW L upper chest	2 yr; deep aching & burning pain around wound in upper posterior chest wall	Electrical percutaneous intercostal blocks; local excision scar	L:T_{3-5}	8	Good
FB/48/M	L thoracotomy for hiatal hernia	2 yr; burning pain in thoracotomy scar	Alcohol blocks of intercostal nerves attempted elsewhere	L:T_{8-10}	4	Fair
BM/46/M	BK amputation L leg, post-traumatic osteomyelitis	4 yr; phantom limb pain in addition to local severe stump pain	Stump neuromas excised 6 times	L:L_5, S_1	16	Poor; phantom pain persists; stump pain improved; some pins & needles dysesthesias
GS/48/M	L_{4-5} HNP removed on L	1.5 yr; R sciatica low back pain	Multiple nerve blocks; negative interspace exploration L_{4-5}, L_5-S_1	R:L_5, S_1	14	Fair; good relief of original pain; now with intermittent dysesthesias inside of R leg, increased by urination; evacuating rectum; postural edema R foot
HL/57/M	Traumatic paraplegia L_1 level	2 yr; pain L flank, back, and L abdomen	None	T_{12}, L_1, L_2	6	Good

TABLE 1. (*Continued*)

Patient/ Age/Sex	Cause of pain	Duration and nature of pain	Previous procedures for pain relief	Ganglionectomy level	Length follow-up (mo)	Results
AS/48/M	WW II GSW R femoral nerve 2 in. below inguinal ligament	Deep aching throbbing pain R anterior thigh; hypersensitivity of R upper thigh	Excision of scar & neuroma from R femoral nerve 10 yr & 1 yr previously	R:L_{1-4}	7	Poor; only slight relief of deep thigh pain but hypersensitivity relieved; postural edema R foot
WS/27/M	GSW L abdomen flank, immediate laparotomy	Aching and burning L_4, foot distribution on L	None for pain	L:L_4	6	Good
BC/28/F	Status post L_5-S_1, lumbar discectomy & reexploration	Burning, aching pain down lateral aspect of R leg & foot	None aside from disc surgeries	R:S_1	10	Fair; some leg pain persists; ambulation much improved
BB/33/F	Status post L_{3-4} lumbar discectomy on L, and reexploration; von Recklinghausen's disease	2 yr; deep aching pain anterior L thigh	None aside from disc surgeries	L:L_{3-4}	2	Good
SI/30/F	Status post L_{4-5} & L_5-S_1 discectomy and reexploration	1 yr; deep aching pain down lateral aspect R leg	None aside from disc surgeries	R:S_1	2	Good
JH/34/M	Status post L_{4-5} discectomy, reexploration, lateral mass fusion; clinical EMG evidence of L_4-L_5 radiculopathy	Burning and electric-like pains down anterolateral aspect R leg and foot	None aside from disc surgeries and fusion	R:L_{4-5}	3	Good

MW/66/F	L_{4-5} & L_5-S_1 discectomies and reexploration	2 yr; burning, aching pain posterolateral aspect R leg and foot; clinical & EMG evidence of L_5 and S_1 radiculopathy	None	R:L_5, S_1	8	Poor; some relief original pain; now with significant, electric-like dysesthesias
GP/50/M	Clinical EMG evidence of C_8, T_1 denervation; suspected occult malignancy	1 yr; deep pain L ulnar distribution in hand and forearm	None	L:C_8, T_1	6	Good
RR/32/M	Traumatic division L brachial plexus & subclavian artery	Severe aching pain entire left hand; clinical & EMG findings revealed complete denervation L upper extremity	Exploration L brachial plexus revealed total disruption of all elements at clavicular level; extensive scarring & neuroma formation	L:C_6-T_1	2	Good
MM/57/F	Carcinoma sole R foot; excision large area plantar skin R foot	Severe, deep pain on ambulation in R foot; hypersensitivity entire sole R foot	None	R:L_5, S_1, S_2	1	Good
CB/34/M	Status post L_{4-5} chymopapain injection and subsequent L_{4-5} discectomies	1 yr; dull, deep aching pain down lateral aspect L leg; foot drop	None	L_5	2	Fair; significant back pain and some R leg pain persist
NS/49/M	Status post L_{4-5} lumbar discectomy 4 yr previously; reexplored L_{4-5} and L_5-S_1 previously	2 yr; deep and burning pains dorsolateral aspect R foot	None	S_1	3	Good

[a] M, male; F, female; R, right; L, left; GSW, gunshot wound; BK, below knee; HNP, herniated nucleus pulposus.

RESULTS

Additional cadaver microdissection revealed that two layers of dura could be separated just proximal to the ganglion but not over the ganglion itself. Within 2 mm of the ganglion, the arachnoidal trabeculae became extremely adherent to the dorsal root, often effectually sealing off the subarachnoid space. We have not encountered intra- or postoperative CSF leakage to date.

Extradural veins were evident on most dural root sleeves and were particularly prominent over the lower sacral roots and filum terminale. Smaller venous channels passed from these through the dura, to communicate with the two small veins generally present on the sensory bundle and the single small vein usually present on the motor root. A single large vein, less than 2 mm in size, drains the anterior aspect of the conus medullaris and arises from T_{11} to L_3 segments among the motor roots. We observed this anterior medullary vein to travel with an L_1 or L_2 motor root in 18% of our dissections.

The length and shape of the ganglia were quite variable. The upper lumbar ganglia (L_1 and L_2) were round and domeshaped, much like thoracic ganglia. The lower lumbar and sacral ganglia, however, had an elongated, oval shape up to 20 mm in length. The largest ganglia were those on lumbar roots 4 and 5 and sacral root 1. Sacral roots 3 and 4 had the smallest ganglia, and the sacral 5 and coccygeal roots were so small generally that their ganglia could not be consistently identified even at 25×. Only 12% of the lumbosacral ganglia proved to be completely bifid, with a dural septum dividing the ganglion into two distinct hemiganglia. In all cases, the sensory elements of each root consisted of two easily separable bundles as they entered their respective dural root sleeves and approached the ganglion. This division was maintained through the ganglion itself in only a minority of cases.

The distal dorsal root and its ganglion were always separated from the ventral root by a thick septum consisting of a double layer of dura. This septum began at a variable distance from the common dural sac (0 to 7 mm).

A small artery 0.2 to 0.6 mm in size was noted on most roots running on the horizontal dural septum between motor and sensory elements. In a few instances (15% of L_1 and L_2 roots), a much larger artery greater than 1 mm in diameter was noted to enter the ventral root sleeve dural proximal to the ganglion and run alongside the motor root toward the conus. These vessels were probably identical to the major radicular arteries described by Adamkiewicz, and they can be protected by careful microsurgical technique.

DISCUSSION

Foerster (5) in 1932 stated: "A single dermatome is represented not only in the totality of the corresponding root but in every single filament of the root. When all filaments except one of each of a number of roots are cut, no anesthesia results. Each of the corresponding dermatomes preserves its sensibility." There is then strong presumptive clinical evidence for suspecting that many rhizotomy failures may be because of incomplete division of all the pertinent sensory fascicles. Our own dissections (4) demonstrate a high percentage of significant intradural bridging fascicles connecting adjacent lower lumbar and upper sacral roots.

The surgeon who hopes to relieve leg or pelvic pain by sectioning only one or two roots would seem to have the odds often stacked against him. In fact, perhaps it is surprising that rhizotomy success rates are as good as they are. In addition to the numerous extramedullary sensory anastomoses, there may well be an anatomic substrate for sensory overlap at cord level in the medial and lateral tracts of Lissauer (8–11,13,14).

Coggeshall and co-workers (1,2) have recently found significant numbers of unmyelinated fibers in the ventral lumbosacral roots of the cat, rhesus monkey, and human. They estimate that approximately half of these unmyelinated fibers (cat) arise from cells in the dorsal root ganglion, whereas the other half are efferents from the spinal cord. Peripheral receptive fields have been found for these ventral root unmyelinated fibers, which include viscera, skin, and joints. The intensity of stimulation required for the firing of many of these fibers was such that they might be considered nociceptive. These ventral unmyelinated nociceptor fibers would not be interrupted by conventional intradural or extradural rhizotomy techniques (10,15). This may be another reason for the discouraging rhizotomy success rates reported previously (7). Our ganglionectomy technique, however, might be expected to interrupt many if not all of the ventral root unmyelinated afferents by removing their cell bodies.

Smith (12) has reported satisfactory clinical results using ganglionectomies for chronic thoracic pain syndromes. He did not use the operating microscope, however, and excised a ventral root segment as well as the ganglion. This would result in unacceptable motor deficits in the lumbosacral area where the motor roots are much larger and more important. We have not had significant postoperative motor loss to date. Our failure rate is already 17%, and only time will tell if microganglionectomies will yield better clinical results than the established intra- or extradural rhizotomy techniques.

ACKNOWLEDGMENT

We gratefully acknowledge the assistance of Ms. Aphia A. Abdou, Medical Illustration Department, Veterans Administration Hospital, who drew these illustrations.

REFERENCES

1. Coggeshall, R. E., Clifton, G. L., Vance, W. H., and Appelbaum, M. L. (1975): *Anat. Rec.,* 181:334.

2. Coggeshall, R. E., Appelbaum, M. L., Facem, M., Stubbs, T. B. III, and Sykes, M. T. (1975): *Brain,* 98:157–166.
3. Echols, D. H. (1969): *J. Neurosurg.,* 31:335–338.
4. Faille, R., Osgood, C. P., Dujovny, M., and Aull, W. (1976): *In preparation.*
5. Foerster, O. (1933): *Brain,* 56:1–39.
6. Loeser, J. D. (1972): *J. Neurosurg.,* 36:745–750.
7. Onofrio, B. M., and Campa, H. K. (1972): *J. Neurosurg.,* 36:751–755.
8. Ransom, S. (1913): *J. Comp. Neurol.,* 23:259–281.
9. Ransom, S. (1914): *J. Comp. Neurol.,* 24:531–545.
10. Scoville, W. B. (1966): *J. Neurosurg.,* 25:94–95.
11. Sindou, M., Quoex, C., and Baleydies, C. (1974): *J. Comp. Neurol.,* 153:15–26.
12. Smith, F. P. (1970): *J. Neurosurg.,* 32:574–577.
13. Snyder, R. L. (1975): *Anat. Rec.,* 181:485.
14. Szentagothai, I. (1964): *J. Comp. Neurol.,* 122:219–239.
15. White, J. C., and Kjellberg, R. N. (1973): *Neurochirurgia,* 16:141–170.

Advances in Pain Research and Therapy, Vol. 1,
edited by J. J. Bonica and D. Albe-Fessard.
Raven Press, New York © 1976.

Neuroadenolysis for Diffuse Unbearable Cancer Pain

Guido Moricca

Department of Anesthesiology, Regina Elena Institute, Via Regina Elena 291, Rome, Italy

In some patients it is extremely difficult to relieve cancer pain with nerve block or a neurosurgical procedure that produces analgesia in a limited part of the body. This is especially true in patients with diffuse multiple areas of pain. The relief of pain sometimes obtained in hormone-dependent tumors by additive or, better, ablative hormonal therapy or by the radioactive inactivation of the pituitary gland suggested to me the possibility of using a new kind of analgesic block: neuroadenolysis, or chemical hypophysectomy, achieved by the injection of alcohol into the pituitary gland.

Before applying this new procedure *in vivo,* we carried out studies on cadavers. The needle was inserted via the transnasal trans-sphenoidal route with the aid of successive radiographs as a guide in directing the needle into the sella. When the suitable position was reached, an ethanol solution tinted with methylene blue was injected. It was found that both the pituitary gland and its stalk assumed a bluish color because of the methylene blue injected. A bluish color was found even in the seat of the hypophysis, which had already been removed.

METHODS

Techniques

The technique has been described in detail elsewhere. Special needles are inserted through the nostril and gently hammered cranially and posteriorly until the floor of the pituitary fossa is reached and pierced and the gland is penetrated.

In the absence of an image intensifier, we carefully evaluate the position of the needles through X-ray control at each step of their introduction and, without any stereotactic apparatus, at their final position. Absolute alcohol, 0.6 to 2.0 ml according to several parameters, is injected into the gland.

We believe that by using two or more needles it is possible to get a more uniform and widespread diffusion of the neurolytic agent into the gland, thereby achieving a better effect.

The treatment is routinely repeated with a single needle from 4 to 15 days later in order to inject alcohol into other areas of the gland and obtain a more complete result. In hormone-sensitive tumors we usually perform further treatments after a due interval of time for therapeutic purposes. In 16% of the cases, such additional neuroadenolyses were required because pain had not been relieved. With this technique we treated randomly selected patients with diffused and/or associated bone, lung, liver, lymph node, and brain metastases caused by hormone-dependent and hormone-independent tumors. All of the patients suffered from multiple severe pain.

RESULTS

From 1963 until June 1975, neuroadenolysis was performed on 1,026 patients. Of the total number of patients, 828 underwent a second, 318 a third, and 200 a fourth or more treatment. Consequently, a total of 2,372 neuroadenolyses have been done. It is interesting to note that the interval of time between the successive treatments increases almost exponentially. It must be pointed out that this happens in patients who have reached a very advanced stage of disease, for whom all conventional therapies proved at this point to be useless, and whose condition was regarded as hopeless.

All of the patients were checked for pain relief, and in some physiologic disturbances and the behavior of the metastases were monitored. The results obtained were very satisfactory, particularly in regard to pain, which was strikingly relieved in all kinds of cancer. Only 1 patient did not benefit at all and 15 derived only partial relief. In 125 patients a good relief of pain occurred only after the third neuroadenolysis. In 885 cases pain relief was complete, immediate, and long lasting.

It is interesting to note that in more than 30% of the advanced hormone-dependent tumors, various data such as clinical findings, X-ray tests, lymphographies, and scintiscanning and histological findings showed an improvement or at least an arrest of the neoplastic disease.

Complications

Obviously the technique is not wholly free of complications, but I think that in most cases it would be more proper to speak of consequences rather than complications. Thus the very frequent diabetes insipidus, hypoadrenalism, hypothyroidism, and lowering of libido are closely and directly linked to inactivation of the pituitary. In all the cases we treated, serious complications—except cephalalgia, which is common but disappears spontaneously within 24 to 36 hr—were unusual. Complications included rhinorrhea, palpebral ptosis, diplopia, and hemianopsia. However, all these complications were transient. As for the occurrence of other phenomena such as hyperthermic crises, hyperphagia, and anhydrosis, we think that they should be considered as intermediate side effects. For instance, from one view, the hyperthermic crises are a complication, but they are a natural consequence caused by the involvement of their respective hypothalamic center. The same is true for the cases of hyperphagia and anhydrosis sometimes observed.

DISCUSSION

We believe that neuroadenolysis offers definite advantages over other procedures that aim at controlling diffused, severe cancer pain for several reasons. First, the equipment is simple and inexpensive. Second, the technique is easy to perform. As it is possible to insert into the sella even six to ten needles without complications, it is obviously quite simple to insert just one or two. Moreover, contraindications are practically nonexistent: neuroadenolysis can be performed on poor-risk patients, and it permits control of unbearable diffuse cancer pain with a single block. Third, neuroadenolysis can be repeated without limitations because of time and/or technical factors. And repeated neuroadenolyses increase the likelihood of a more complete inactivation and destruction of the gland.

These results can be compared with the effects produced by the so-called radioactive hypophysectomy, which, generally speaking, produces inadequate pain relief. These inadequate results of the radioactive treatment are a consequence of several factors. The main difficulty lies in the exact positioning of the pellets—which is obviously directly linked to the question of dosimetry. Therefore, in order to avoid complications, operators sometimes have to fall short of the required dosage, but this in turn prevents them from achieving the destruction of the pituitary and bringing about the desired therapeutic effects. The implantation of additional radioactive material is limited by difficulty in properly positioning the pellets because of the presence of previous material and because further implantation increases the incidence of accidents and/or complications.

The effects of the neurolytic agents are obtained through at least three mechanisms: (a) compression produced by injection—because the pituitary is located in a practically inexpansible space, compression causes subcapsular necrosis; (b) direct chemical action on the cells with subsequent dehydration; and (c) action on the vessels with thrombosis followed by cellular necrosis.

These findings may well explain the results on the evolution of advanced hormone-dependent tumors if we consider the correlations that exist between the hypothalamic-hypophyseal system and the target organs.

On the other hand, the diffusion of alcohol into the gland and the involvement of the pathways between the pituitary, the hypothalamus, and the thalamus might explain the analgesic effects even in absence of hormone dependency.

SUMMARY

In summary, neuroadenolysis is, first, a valid weapon against diffuse, so-called intractable pain caused by all kinds of cancer. Second, in advanced hormone-sensitive tumors it is in all respects a therapy of particular interest because it may be effective in very poor-risk patients for whom any major procedure is contraindicated.

Advances in Pain Research and Therapy, Vol. 1,
edited by J. J. Bonica and D. Albe-Fessard.
Raven Press, New York © 1976.

Mode of Action by Which Pituitary Alcohol Injection Relieves Pain

John Miles and Sampson Lipton

Regional Department of Medical and Surgical Neurology,
Walton Hospital, Liverpool 9, England

The value of pituitary ablation in relieving pain owing to hormonally dependent tumors is well established. It is known to be effective with all of the many different techniques practiced. Morrica (2) developed the transphenoidal alcohol injection for achieving pituitary ablation and reported its amazing efficiency in relieving pain in more than 600 patients in 1974. We (1) have applied this technique to patients suffering pain due to advanced neoplasia of all forms when the pain was not easily amenable to standard treatment such as cordotomy.

Although we have been unable to reproduce Morrica's almost total efficiency, approximately one-third of the patients have obtained excellent relief and one-third some relief. Our technique has been somewhat different from Morrica's, tending to be less "aggressive," and this might account for the difference in results.

As this method was equally effective with tumors not usually considered to be hormonally dependent, we were eager to determine the reason for pain relief. In an attempt to localize the site of injection accurately, we injected iophendylate (Myodil®) or meglumine iocarmate (Dimer X®) immediately before the alcohol. In 20% of our cases we were surprised to see the contrast material passing up from the pituitary fossa along the expected path of the stalk, along the floor of the third ventricle, and in many instances eventually breaking through into the third ventricle cavity.

This suggested to us the possibility that the pain relief might be because of direct hypothalamic injury. Sano (3) obtained good relief of pain in 50% of his patients by destroying the posterior hypothalamus by a stereotaxic approach from above. A study was therefore designed in an attempt to correlate radiological and histological tracking in the pituitary gland and hypothalamus.

METHOD

In autopsy cadavers and before intracranial examination, we performed a standard transnasal, transphenoidal puncture of the pituitary fossa. A 50/50 mixture of India ink and iophendylate or meglumine iocarmate was injected under X-ray screening control. Films were taken before and at the completion of injection. The skull was then opened and the pituitary gland removed intact and in continuity with the rest of the brain. The hypothalamus and pituitary were then examined macroscopically, and after fixation they were further examined by means of a sagittal section. Serial sections of the pituitary, its stalk, and the hypothalamus were then made for microscopic histological examination.

RESULTS

Radiological Tracking

In all cases contrast was seen, on screening, to be in the pituitary gland. The concluding radiograph showed persisting contrast in the subarachnoid space in 12 instances and in the pituitary gland in 13 cases. (On two occasions radiography was unsatisfactory for technical reasons and no concluding comment could be made.) In one instance dye tracked into the stalk area. In 5 cases the contrast spread up into the third ventricle. Once this spread had occurred, and this could be at any time during the injection, each increment seemed to go directly up into the ventricle. In two instances air also passed up into the ventricle. In three instances contrast was seen to have passed into the venous system. This spread occurred either into the basal veins running back to the great cerebral vein, or via the petrosal sinus to the transverse sinus.

Histological Tracking

In all but one instance India ink was seen in the gland itself. Usually this was free along the needle track but diffuse tissue spread was common. Vessels, particularly those in the fibrous tissue between the lobes and in the region of the pars intermedius, frequently contained the dye in their lumina and walls.

In every case the stalk contained dye. In two instances it was free in tissue planes, but in all cases, dye was in the vessels, particularly the large peripheral portal vessels, and their walls. In 13 cases dye was seen in the sections of the hypothalamus. The vessels in the subarachnoid space most regularly and most heavily contained the dye, but so also did the vessels within the hypothalamus right up to the immediate subependymal layer. In two instances dye was seen free in tissue planes in the hypothalamus. India ink was seen on the ependymal cells in 5 cases.

CONCLUSION

Fluid injected into the pituitary gland can spread rapidly and at distance from this site. It seems likely that the main spread is via the lumen of blood vessels, but rupture through the walls can also occur. This rupture could occur locally within the gland or at a distance such as in the hypothalamus. The main route from the gland to the hypothalamus seems to be via the portal vessels.

Injury to the hypothalamus by direct fixation with alcohol or indirectly by thrombosis and infarction could result in interference with pain perception or with the suffering of pain. This is presumably because of interruption of the hypothalamic-thalamic connections.

REFERENCES

1. Lipton, S., and Miles, J. B. (1975): *Presented for publication.*
2. Morrica, G. (1974): In: *Advances in Neurology, Vol. 4: International Symposium on Pain,* edited by J. J. Bonica, pp. 707–714. Raven Press, New York.
3. Sano, K. (1973): Presented to Symposium Sur la Doleur, Sept. 24 and 25, Paris.

Advances in Pain Research and Therapy, Vol. 1,
edited by J. J. Bonica and D. Albe-Fessard.
Raven Press, New York © 1976.

Headache: Disruption of Pain Modulation

Federigo Sicuteri

Department of Clinical Pharmacology, University of Florence, Viale Morgagni 85, Florence, Italy

Nociception, which includes pain sensation, is the function of an ancestral multiintegrated apparatus, the nociceptive system (NCS), which informs the organism of what to avoid in one's surroundings through a punitive "pain education." To complete its etiological defensive function, NCS involves several servomechanisms of impressive efficiency such as vocalization, aggression, escape, emotion, and memory. Undoubtedly one of the most important and active servomechanisms of the NCS is the mnemonic one: strong pain, even if occasional and unique, engraves an indestructible engram on the memory. The child who has burned his hand in playing with fire for the first time memorizes the pain sensations and avoids touching fire with any part of his body for the rest of his life. The recurrence of the same painful stimulus provokes the psychoaffective responses, recalls the corresponding engrams, and concludes in the progressive deformation of the nociception and its integrated functions. Thus acute pain, defensive in nature, when repeated can deteriorate the personality.

In human pathophysiology, no function is known to be exempt from disorder or frank disease; the nociceptive function is no exception to this rule. The NCS, particularly at the brain level, can be affected by gross (structural) injury or functional (biochemical) damage. As a general rule, the disorder of a system manifests itself through qualitative and quantitative alterations of its specific functions. In the NCS, a gross or biochemical affection manifests itself through a qualitative and/or quantitative disruption of the ratio between stimulus and pain. The distinction between physiological pain (expected responses to acute noxious stimulation and consequent activation of a normal NCS) and pathologic pain (spontaneous pain, or the exaggerated propensity to trigger algogenic sensations deformed in their usual physiognomy) is rational and essential.

Central pain is a well-known pathologic condition defined by Riddoch (23) as being "spontaneous pain and painful overreaction to objective stimulation resulting from lesions confined to the substance of the central nervous system." This definition was applied to "organic" central pain, secondary to lesions owing to aneurysms, cysts, tumors, inflammation, and traumata, among others. Recently, I introduced the possibility of central pain owing to local functional disorders, particularly chemical in nature, concerning those mediators involved in the central integration of pain (30). According to this concept, an organic lesion, the substrate of "organic" central pain, is substituted by a functional (biochemical) one.

In my thesis, the general concept of a reversible or irreversible biochemical lesion (20) is applied to the central portion of the NCS. Consequently, migraine and correlated essential headache (EH) are hypothesized to be among the most important examples of biochemical central dysnociception, a term signifying a disorder of nociception (33) (Fig. 1). Because of its anatomic substrate, organic central pain is usually constant in duration and characterized by localization of abnormal peripheral sensations. In contrast, functional central pain usually fluctuates in duration and localization according to its chemical mechanisms. If this new interpretation corresponds to facts, EH must be considered the "pain disease" per antonomasia, since it is correlated with a central biochemical dysnociception.

DOES HEADACHE HAVE CHARACTERISTICS OF CENTRAL PAIN?

The conventional theory considers pain in EH as peripheral in nature, the nociceptors being stimulated in a mechanical or vascular (41) or biochemical (28) way. The view of vasodilatation as a mechanical stimulus in EH must be discarded because spontaneous or provoked vasodilatation *per se* is not painful. Only by provoking vasodilatation through the administration of drugs such as histamine and bradykinin which are also powerful pain-producing agents can one provoke headache (29). Vasodilatation, when it develops, may be an adjunctive component when the sensitive threshold is locally lowered. On the other hand, the term "vascular" is popular and used widely, but one that generates ambiguities and confusion. The pain could be provoked peripherally by biochemical mechanisms following local release and concentration of pain-producing substances such as neurokinin (2), kinins, histamine, and particularly 5-hydroxytryptamine (5-HT) (26,28).

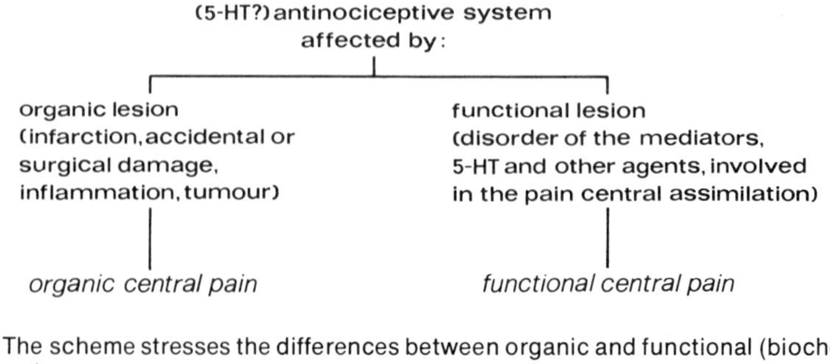

FIG. 1. The scheme stresses the differences between organic and functional (biochemical) central pain.

The possibility of potentiation among these vasoneuroactive substances both in pain (36) and on vascular receptors (43,44) is of interest. These substances could also be responsible for the formation of slight local subcutaneous edema in the painful region. Ache in EH does not exhibit the characteristic of peripheral (physiologic) pain. In fact, it is not too localized except when additional peripheral stimuli such as the pulsation of particularly sensitive vessels localize the pain. An extrastimulus, for instance, touch, jolting, or the administration of pain-producing substances such as kinin, histamine, or kallikrein (29), provokes a painful reaction that can last many minutes or hours. Such long-lasting overreaction is typical of central pain. An emotion or exposure to cold or heat may exacerbate a preexisting headache, and the exacerbation may last many hours. The hyperesthesia, or frank pain, can involve not only the conventional regions of the head but can also extend to the neck and shoulders, which is sometimes diagnosed as rheumatism or arthritis. Such extension of hyperesthesia or frank pain is quite difficult to attribute to a massive release of vasoneuroactive substances in peripheral tissues. Thus the paresthesia, dysesthesia, or pain in an arm or the trunk (hemicrania comitata) these patients complained of can be reasonably explained only through a central mechanism.

The most persuasive considerations about the central mechanism of pain in EH are the conditions able to increase the ache after a long latency. EH sufferers can have immediate and retarded pain reactions. The immediate reactions are induced by three factors: jolting, vasomotion (from different origins, physical and psychic included), and chemical agents (kinin, histamine, or allied substances). The delayed reactions may occur many hours or a day after an emotional or physical stress or intercourse. The delayed reactions can be most reasonably explained by changes in biochemical economy of the brain with late reverberation on the biochemical control of central nociception.

Of interest is nitroglycerin, which may provoke an immediate reaction, usually moderate, and a delayed reaction, sometimes in the form of a furious, long-lasting, and devastating attack long after the vasomotor reactions provoked by the drug have been exhausted. Reserpine (17,27) is also able to provoke a delayed reaction in only metabolic doses, amounts that are not able to modify vasomotility.

5-HT PAIN MODULATION: ITS DISRUPTION IN EH

Similar to other nervous functions, nociception is activated by the intervention of chemical mediators that act in different parts of the NCS to produce excitation or inhibition. In animal studies 5-HT appears to play a role as a modulating mediator in the central integration of pain. When the 5-HT concentrations are reduced by electrical microlesions (12) or specific drugs such as para-chlorophenylalanine (PCPA) (40) in those discrete areas involved in central nociception, animals become more sensitive to noxious stimuli. Morphine also apparently needs a physiologic 5-HT turnover in some areas of the brain in order to exhibit its analgesic activity (25). 5-HT precursors, particularly 5-hydroxytryptophan, are able to correct the dysnociception in 5-HT–deficient animals and the loss of analgesic activity from morphine (8,40).

In normal humans disruption of 5-HT pain modulation by depleting 5-HT cerebral reserves by PCPA is not apparently possible because of the toxic effects of PCPA. Not even in patients with excessive extracerebral 5-HT turnover, such as in carcinoid patients, is PCPA, even when given in high doses and for a long period of time, able to provoke painful manifestations (5). In contrast, in migraine and EH sufferers, in whom a precarious 5-HT turnover in discrete areas of the brain is hypothesized, PCPA provokes in approximately 20% of the cases circumscribed or systemic extra-head painful conditions, which resolve themselves within a few days after discontinuation of PCPA (30).

Another indirect evidence of the fragility of 5-HT brain turnover in EH is the slight aphrodisiac effect PCPA displays in EH sufferers (33), although in normal volunteers and in carcinoid patients (5) this sex stimulation does not appear. In EH sufferers with sexual deficiency, the administration of PCPA and testosterone appears strongly aphrodisiac in 30% of the patients. Because 5-HT in animals is the inhibiting mediator on the testosterone receptors of the brain mating centers (9), the aphrodisiac effects of PCPA in EH sufferers indirectly support the thesis of a precariousness of 5-HT turnover in this common dysnociception. The monoamine oxidase inhibitors are not considered as stimulators of sexuality; on the contrary, sometimes they provoke a loss of libido. When phenelzine or pargyline is administered during PCPA treatment in sexually deficient EH sufferers, sexual stimulation is experienced by approximately one-third of the patients (35). This seems to indicate that a clear shift between norepinephrine and 5-HT is able to sensitize the sexual receptors in the brain to plasma testosterone.

In Parkinson's disease a deficiency of brain 5-HT is believed to exist even if the administration of 5-HT precursors is unable to improve the clinical features of the disease (42). Treatment with PCPA in a patient with Parkinson's disease has provoked hyperalgesia and hyperesthesia, which promptly disappeared after stopping PCPA (42). If brain 5-HT concentrations in this disease are really decreased, the dysnociception provoked by PCPA must be considered as further evidence suggestive of the disruption of the central modulation of pain. Biochemical investigations are of some help, supporting a generic implication of monoamines, 5-HT in particular, in EH. Following my first suggestion of changes in 5-HT turnover during migraine attack (38), others have pointed out oscillations in

5-HT platelet concentration, as well as in urinary excretion of 5-HT and its metabolites (4,16). Of particular interest for the central theory are the investigations of 5-HT turnover carried out in cerebrospinal fluid (15,21).

INFLUENCE OF CONDITIONS OR FUNCTIONS ON EH

It is well known that emotion, physical stress, sleep, fever, menstruation, pregnancy, sexual intercourse, and other conditions modify EH, aggravating or improving the clinical picture. The peripheral theory, either mechanical (vascular) or biochemical, is unable to provide consistent interpretation for these EH modifying conditions. On the other hand, if one considers this problem within the perspective of the central pain theory of EH, some persuasive correlations can be seen. In the majority of conditions capable of influencing EH, monoamines, in particular 5-HT, have recently been implicated. Directly or indirectly 5-HT is involved in the control of sleep, estrus, emotion, sexual activity, thermoregulation, and other functions (3,10,11,14,18). Thus it appears that these basic functions directly or indirectly controlled by serotoninergic neurons can reverberate on the contiguous 5-HT antinociceptive system which, as previously mentioned, is involved in EH (32).

Menstruation can be considered a typical example: the attacks in the menstrual period arise in a high frequency. Menstrual migraine appears to be precipitated by the withdrawal of estrogen (39). On the other hand, animal study suggested that more than a peripheral action of hormones must play a role in the fluctuations of brainstem monoamines (19). Indirectly, the mood changes, fluid retention, sleep modification, and other factors that frequently disturb women in the premenstrual period clearly indicate the involvement of brainstem monoamines. This is further evidence of the involvement of the 5-HT antinociceptive system.

ANTIMIGRAINOUS DRUGS AND CENTRAL PAIN MODULATION

Ergotamine conventionally acts as an analgesic in the migraine attack by constricting the dilated and pulsating cranial arteries. Our opinion is that this is a complementary effect and not necessarily the essential mechanism, and that the antimigrainous action of ergotamine is localized in the nociceptive system in the brain. Our group has demonstrated that ergotamine in man, in low concentrations such as those expected in plasma after therapeutic administration, facilitates 5-HT on the venomotor receptors. The same 5-HT potentiation demonstrated at the periphery may also happen at the center in the brain (37). Methysergide, a classic antimigrainous agent, acts as antiserotonin when used in high nontherapeutic concentrations. However, it acts as proserotonin, namely, it potentiates 5-HT, when small amounts are given to produce plasma levels similar to those achieved with therapy. The painful spasm of the superficial vein of the legs observed in a few EH sufferers treated with small amounts (2 to 4 μg/kg) of oral methysergide wholly depends on the 5-HT potentiation which, in experiments on the human vein "*in vivo*," may reach high intensity. 5-HT facilitation in the same test of local venospasm "*in vivo*" in man is also observed with small amounts of LSD-25. This drug is able to improve EH as well as phantom limb pain when given in nonhallucinogenic doses. Because of its capacity to cross the blood-brain barrier and to concentrate in the nervous system, and in view of the small doses (0.05 μg/kg) used, its analgesic activity is thought to be at the brain level (7).

Also, different antiserotonin drugs such as GC-94, with structures different from those of lysergic methysergide and LSD-25, are able to potentiate 5-HT both in animals and in man (1) when administered in doses to achieve the same plasma levels as after oral administration of clinical doses (Fig. 2). Pizotifen, an active antimigrainous drug without vasoactive property, does not modify catecholamine uptake, although it strongly inhibits that of serotonin (24). Other details about the mechanisms of antimigrainous drugs are contained in a recent critical review by Fanchamps (6).

In conclusion, some drugs such as ergotamine and antiserotonin agents exhibit a specific analgesic activity in migraine and other forms of essential headache. The conventional hypothesis that the therapeutic activity is because of vasoconstriction (ergotamine) and antiserotonin peripheral activity (methysergide) must be reconsidered. This is especially compelling in view of recent results which suggest that the primary site of action is on the central NCS, probably by potentiating the pain-modulating capacity of 5-HT (Fig. 3).

In support of 5-HT deficiency in pain modulation in the mechanism of EH are the benefits from a diet supplemented with 5-HT precursors such as l-tryptophan or 1,5-hydroxytryptophan (31) which, unlike 5-HT, cross the blood-brain barrier and enrich the brain in 5-HT. The use of benserazide, a peripheral inhibitor of the decarboxylase which facilitates the concentration of 5-HT precursors in the brain, provides the same benefit with smaller doses of tryptophan and 5-hydroxytryptophan.

Because they condition the lives of many millions of people, migraine and other essential headaches are one of the most important problems of medicine. They can be considered as "pain disease" by antonomasia because pain without consistent objective cause dominates the clinical picture. EH may be considered as one of the most common disorders of the NCS. This disorder is apparently nonorganic but rather functional or biochemical in nature. Many animal and human observations suggest 5-HT as the important factor in EH. It is hypothesized that a deficiency of the turnover of brainstem 5-HT disrupts central pain modulation and thus facilitates pain in that part of the body, such as the head, endowed with

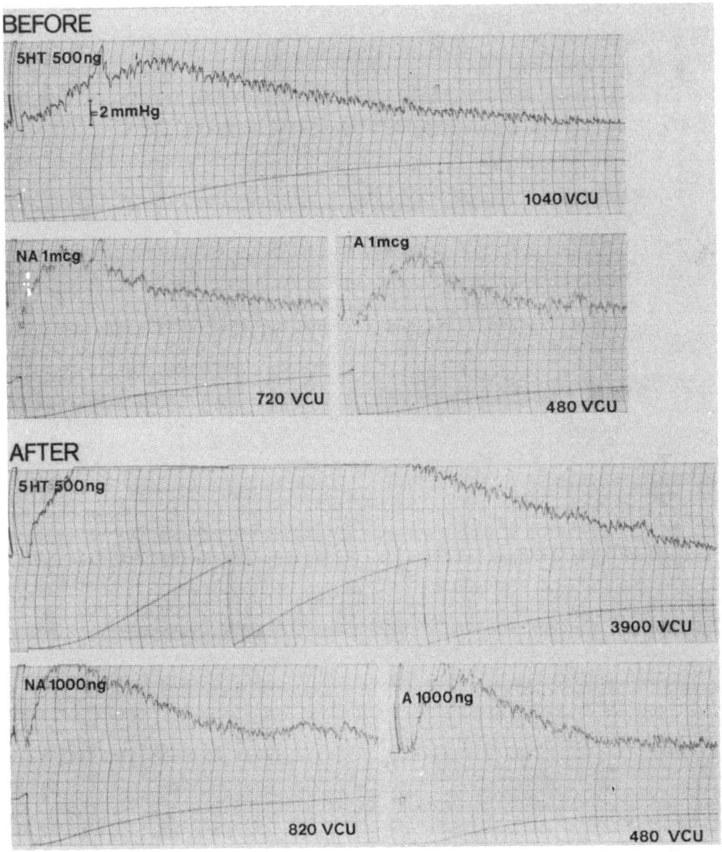

FIG. 2. Antiserotonin drugs, when tested in amounts roughly similar to those expected or proved (as in the case of the figure) in plasma following clinical doses, do not antagonize but facilitate 5-HT. The serotonin vascular reactivity, evaluated in man, *in vivo,* in venoconstrictive units (VCU), appears enhanced, following therapeutic doses of the antiserotonin drug Org. GC 94; the venoreactivity to catecholamines is not modified.

sensitivity and exposed to mechanical factors, such as jolting. Other functions and conditions particularly pertinent to the limbic system—e.g., emotion, sleep, fever, sex, menstruation, and pregnancy—may interact with EH, aggravating or improving the clinical picture (27,28,34).

The implication of the limbic system in migraine has recently been reconsidered (22). Daily or occasional headache by itself is a cause of deterioration of the personality with consequent social inactivity and neurosis. Biochemical pharmacological data (particularly in urine, platelets, and cerebrospinal fluid) are in agreement with a discrete involvement of 5-HT turnover in EH. Further evidence is provided by the facility of aggravating or improving the clinical picture through use of drugs that intervene in some

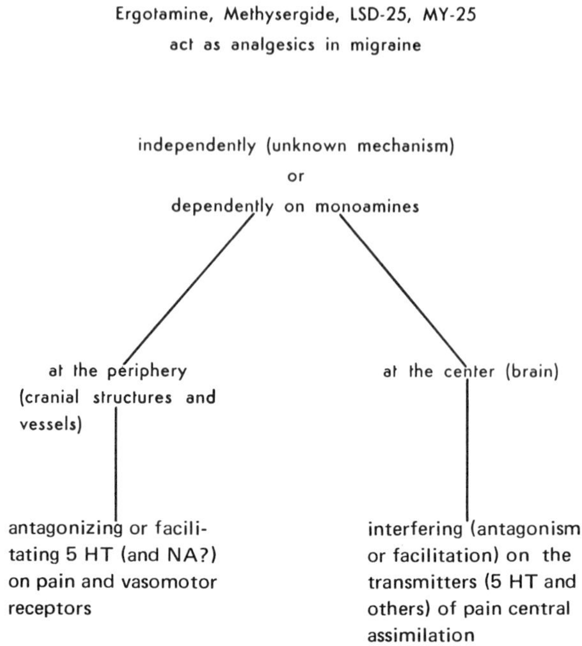

FIG. 3. It is difficult to affirm that the antimigraneous drugs act simply because of their vasoconstrictive (ergotamine) and antiserotonin (methysergide) properties; in this figure the possible mechanisms of these drugs are pointed out.

way in the synthesis, storage, release, and receptorial activity of 5-HT. For the majority of these drugs capable of crossing the blood-brain barrier, a hypersensitivity or reduced tolerance is observed. In contrast, parenteral administration of large doses of serotonin, which does not cross the blood-brain barrier, is well tolerated by EH sufferers. Moreover, small intravenous doses of reserpine (e.g., 1 to 2 μg/kg) or fenfluramine, both of which decrease 5-HT brain turnover, can precipitate a headache crisis with nervous reactions that are much more intense than those experienced by normal (control) subjects.

Serotonin precursors such as l-tryptophan and 5-hydroxytryptophan are able to improve EH, probably by increasing the 5-HT concentration, particularly if given with a decarboxylase inhibitor such as benserazide or carbidopa; and this effect continues for long periods. The incongruity between this sort of "proserotonin" therapy with conventional treatment with antiserotonins is only apparent. We have demonstrated in man and subsequently others have shown in animals that when clinical doses of ergotamine, methysergide, or Org. GC. 94 are given, facilitation of 5-HT action on the vascular receptors can be noted. Therefore, the concept of functional (biochemical) central pain of EH can no longer be considered a working hypothesis but must be recognized as a theory supported by facts. Peripheral events such as vasomotility and increased permeability of the capillary bed must be considered not essential but rather as accessory responses. In fact, they could also be provoked by local microvascular processes secondary to the painful condition from central disruption of pain modulation.

SUMMARY

As an alternative to the conventional thesis of peripheral (vascular or chemical) causation, I emphasize the probability that essential headache is due to central disruption of pain modulation. Animal and human studies provide evidence that central pain can be caused not only by well-known organic lesions but also by functional disorders of those biochemical systems that participate in the integration of pain input at the brain levels. Specifically, pain could be owing to a deficiency of the turnover of 5-hydroxytryptamine, which normally acts as a pain-inhibiting mediator. Clinical, biochemical, and pharmacological studies suggest that there also exists a serotonin defect in EH sufferers. An especially strong suggestion is in the reciprocal involvement of EH with ancestral functions such as emotion, sleep, appetite, vomiting, thermoregulation and sex, all of which are directly or indirectly controlled by serotonin. The apparent incongruency of the benefit from both antiserotonin drugs (such as ergotamine, methysergide, Org. GC. 94, and LSD-25 in nonhallucinogenic doses), and naturally occurring substances (such as l-tryptophan) with proserotonin activity provides further support for the 5-HT central deficiency theory, since human and animal investigations show a 5-HT facilitation from the antiserotonins when given in clinical amounts. If this thesis finds further support, EH will become the "pain disease" for antonomasia, thus acquiring the right of a well-defined nosological position.

REFERENCES

1. Anselmi, B., Chafik, M. L., Del Bianco, P. L., Galli, P., Lamar, J. C., Schönbaum, E., Sicuteri, F., and Van der Veen, F. (1975): *International Symposium on Clinical Pharmacology of Serotonin,* edited by F. Sicuteri and E. Schönbaum. Karger Press, Basel. (*In press.*)
2. Chapman, L. F., Ramos, A. O., Goodell, H., Silverman, G., and Wolff, H. G. (1960): *Arch. Neurol.,* 3:223.
3. Coppen, A. J., and Lewis, G. P. (1961): *J. Neurochem.,* 7:155.
4. Curran, D. A., Hinterberger H., and Lance, J. W. (1965): *Brain,* 88:997.
5. Engelman, K., Lovenberg, W., and Sjoerdsma, A. (1967): *N. Engl. J. Med.,* 277:1103.
6. Fanchamps, A. (1975): *Headache,* 15:79.
7. Fanciullacci, M., Franchi, G. C., Perez-Acuna, F., and Sicuteri, F. (1975): In: *Vasoactive Substances Relevant to Migraine.* Charles C Thomas, Springfield, Illinois.
8. Fennessy, M. R., and Lee, J. R. (1970): *J. Pharm. Pharmacol.,* 22:930.
9. Gessa, G. L., Tagliamonte, A., Tagliamonte, B., and Brodie, B. B. (1970): *Nature,* 227:616.

10. Gong, S. N., and Rogers, K. J. (1971): *Proc. Br. Pharmac. Soc.,* Aug: 646.
11. Greengrass, P. M., and Tonge, S. R. (1971): *J. Pharm. Pharmacol.,* 23:897.
12. Harvey, J. A., and Lints, C. E. (1965): *Science,* 148:250.
13. Hilton, S. M., and Schain, R. J. (1961): *J. Physiol. (Lond.),* 157:46.
14. Jouvet, M. (1969): *Science,* 163:32.
15. Kangasniemi P. (1975): *International Symposium on Clinical Pharmacology of Serotonin,* edited by F. Sicuteri and E. Schönbaum. Karger Press, Basel. (*In press.*)
16. Kangasniemi, P., Sonninen, V., and Rinne, V. K. (1972): *Headache,* 15:69.
17. Kimball, R. W., and Friedman, A. P. (1961): *Recent Adv. Biol. Psych.,* 3:200.
18. Malmnas, C. O., and Meyerson, B. J. (1971): *Nature,* 232:398.
19. Meyerson, B. J. (1964): *Acta Physiol. Scand.* [*Suppl.*], 241:5.
20. Peters, R. A. (1963): *Br. Med. Bull.,* 25:223.
21. Poloni, M., Nappi, G., Bono, R., Arpesella, M., Tenconi, M. T. (1975): *International Symposium on Clinical Pharmacology of Serotonin,* edited by F. Sicuteri and E. Schönbaum. Karger Press, Basel. (*In press.*)
22. Raffaelli, E., and Menon, A. D. (1975): *Headache,* 15:69.
23. Riddoch, G. (1938): *Lancet,* 1:1093.
24. Salzmann, R., and Kalberer, F. (1973): In: *Background to Migraine,* vol. 5, p. 63. Heinemann, London.
25. Samanin, R., Gumulka, W., and Valzelli, L. (1970): *Eur. J. Pharmacol.,* 22:930.
26. Sicuteri, F. (1959): *Int. Arch. Allergy,* 15:300.
27. Sicuteri, F. (1960): In: *International Symposium on Mediatori Chimici, Funzione Nervosa e Circolo Cerebrale,* edited by F. Sicuteri. Fidenza, Italy.
28. Sicuteri, F. (1967): In: *Research and Clinical Studies in Headache,* vol. 1, p. 6. Karger Press, Basel.
29. Sicuteri, F. (1970): In: *Handbook of Experimental Pharmacology: Bradykinin, Kallidin, and Kallikrein,* edited by G. Erdos, vol. XXV, p. 482. Springer Verlag, Berlin.
30. Sicuteri, F. (1971): *Pharmacol. Res. Commun.,* 3:4.
31. Sicuteri, F. (1972): *Pharmacol. Res. Commun.,* 4:213.
32. Sicuteri, F., Anselmi, B., and Del Bianco, P. L. (1973): *Psychopharmacologia,* 29:347.
33. Sicuteri, F. (1974): *Pharmacol. Res. Commun.,* 4:6.
34. Sicuteri, F., Anselmi, B., and Fanciullacci, M. (1974): In: *Advances in Neurology, Vol. 4,* edited by J. Bonica, p. 383. Raven Press, New York.
35. Sicuteri, F., Del Bene, E., and Fonda, C. (1975): *International Symposium on Clinical Pharmacology of Serotonin,* edited by F. Sicuteri and E. Schönbaum. Karger Press, Basel. (*In press.*)
36. Sicuteri, F., Fanciullacci, M., Franchi, G. C., and Del Bianco, P. L. (1960): *Life Sci.,* 4:409.
37. Sicuteri, F., Franchi, G. C., and Fanciullacci, M. (1974): *Second Congress Hung. Pharmacol. Soc.* (Abstr.), 1:28.
38. Sicuteri, F., Testi, A., and Anselmi, B. *Int. Arch. Allergy,* 19:55.
39. Somerville, B. W. (1972): *Neurology,* 22:824.
40. Tenen, S. S. (1967): *Psychopharmacologia,* 10:204.
41. Tunis, M. M., and Wolff, H. G. (1952): *Am. J. Med. Sci.,* 224:565.
42. Van Woert, M. H., Ambani, L. M., and Levine, R. J. (1972): *Dis. Nerv. Syst.,* 33:777.
43. Weiner, R., and Altura, B. M. (1967): *Proc. Soc. Exp. Biol. Med.,* 124:494.
44. Zweifach, B. W. (1966): In: *Hypotensive Peptides,* edited by G. Erdos, N. Back, and F. Sicuteri, p. 451. Springer Verlag, Berlin.

Advances in Pain Research and Therapy, Vol. 1,
edited by J. J. Bonica and D. Albe-Fessard.
Raven Press, New York © 1976.

Possible Monoamine Mediation of the Analgesic Activity of Ergotamine and Other Lysergic Derivatives in Migraine

Giancarlo Franchi, Marcello Fanciullacci, Paolo Galli, and Federigo Sicuteri

Headache Center, Department of Clinical Pharmacology, University of Florence, Italy

The mechanism of the pain of migraine which is its most characteristic symptom is still undefined. According to the earlier classic vascular theory (13), pain develops from vasodilatation. Subsequently, the biochemical hypothesis evolved which attributes the pain to a release of biological substances (mainly serotonin and kinins) stimulating the vessels' nociceptors and other painful head structures (8). As a consequence of this hypothesis, antiserotonin therapy was proposed by Sicuteri (7). However, more recent evidence suggests the genesis of pain in migraine to be central in nature (10): i.e., a disorder of the biochemical mechanism which controls the nervous structures involved in the central modulation of pain input.

Indirect evidence suggests that serotonin may play an important role in this mechanism. A monoamine deficiency, particularly of serotonin, can occur at the central level in migraine and other types of essential headache. Consequently, a supersensitivity phenomenon at the serotonin central receptors level develops, such as occurs when the specific mediator is deficient (1,9,12). Besides its important clinical implication of treatment with 5-hydroxytryptophan (5-HT) and tryptophan precursors, this central hypothesis suggests a reconsideration of the ergotamine and methysergide mechanism in migraine.

According to traditional opinion, ergotamine interrupts the migraine attack through vasoconstriction. The therapeutic mechanisms of methysergide and ergotamine were subsequently attributed to their antagonistic effect on peripheral 5-HT receptors. On the other hand, the plasma concentration of these lysergic derivatives, which are able to antagonize serotonin in experimental studies, is much higher than that reached after their administration for therapeutic purposes. In fact, when therapeutic doses of ergotamine and methysergide are administered in man, the blood concentration of these drugs cannot exceed the range of 50 ng/ml of blood plasma.

In view of these considerations, we undertook to study the action of therapeutic concentrations of ergotamine and methysergide on 5-HT reactivity in man. The study entailed the use of the venoconstriction test (VCT) which uses the vein wall as 5-HT substrate *in vivo.*

METHODS AND RESULTS

The study was carried out in normal volunteers and untreated migraine patients referred to the Department of Clinical Pharmacology of the University of Florence. After obtaining informed consent and using the technique previously described (11), we placed the subjects or patients on a bed and a superficial vein of the back of the hand was orthodromically cannulated with a thin needle provided with a rubber membrane. The needle was connected to an infusion pump and to a pressure transducer. The pump was refilled with saline, methysergide bimaleate, or ergotamine tartrate solutions. Through the needle's rubber membrane, 5-HT, methysergide, or ergotamine, diluted in 1 ml of saline, was acutely injected. The solutions were infused at the speed of 0.5 ml/min. Local venous pressure changes were quantified by connecting the pressure transducer to an automatic computer. Venoconstriction was evaluated arbitrarily in venoconstriction units: 1 unit was defined as an increase of 1 mm Hg/sec of local venous pressure. Usually the threshold dose of serotonin in most of the cases ranged between 250 and 1,000 ng.

The volunteers were divided into four groups of 5 subjects each. In one such group, the 5-HT threshold dose was determined and then 10 ng of methysergide was acutely administered. Subsequently, the same threshold dose of serotonin was repeated every 10 min for 2 hr. The acute administration of methysergide enhanced the venospastic reaction of the threshold dose of 5-HT within 15 min. Such facilitation lasted approximately 30 min.

In another 5 subjects a dose of methysergide equal to the threshold dose of serotonin was acutely administered. Successively the threshold dose of serotonin was repeatedly injected every 10 min for a 2-hr period. At this dose, methysergide completely inhibited the venospasm by serotonin for 30 min. This antagonistic effect gradually disappeared, and 45 min after the methysergide injection a facilitation of the 5-HT venoconstriction occurred. Finally, after 75 min serotonin exhibited the same effect as in basic conditions (Fig. 1). This phenomenon was observed in all 5 subjects.

In the third group of subjects the saline infusion was replaced with an infusion of methysergide at a rate of 0.5 ng/0.5 ml/min, and in another 5 subjects with an infusion of ergotamine at a rate of 5 ng/0.5 ml/min. During the infusion of both these drugs, the threshold dose of serotonin was repeated every 10 min. The slow infusion of methysergide induced a facilitation of 5-HT venospastic threshold effect: this facilitation was evident 30 to 60 min from the start of the infusion and disappeared 30 min after the end. The slow infusion of ergotamine did not modify the basal tonus of the vein. The sensitivity to serotonin tested during the first phase of

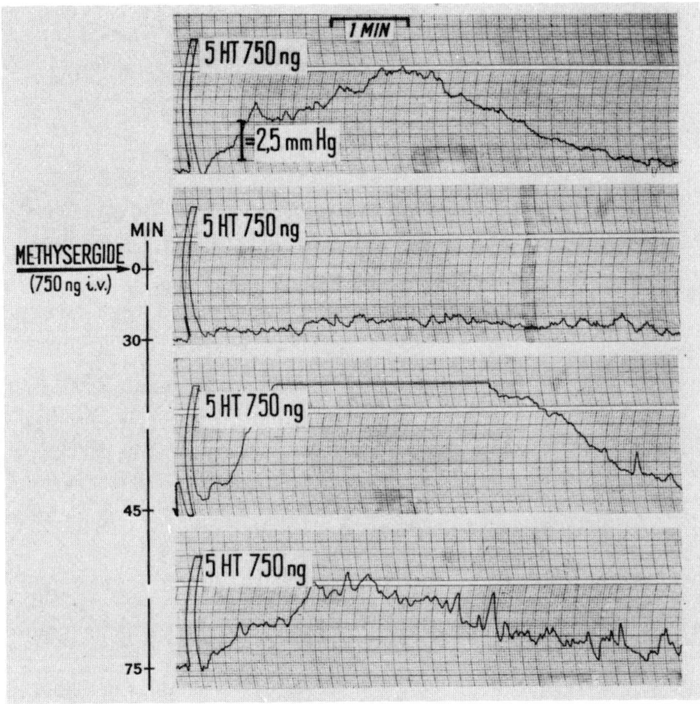

FIG. 1. Administration of methysergide at the same dose at which serotonin provokes an initial inhibition of 5-HT venospastic activity. Successively the facilitation of venoconstriction appears.

the saline infusion also remained unchanged during the first 20 min of the ergotamine infusion. Successively, an increased sensitivity appeared and it was maintained during the remainder of the ergotamine infusion, as well as 40 to 60 min thereafter during a subsequent infusion of saline alone. Thus a gradual return to the basic sensitivity to 5-HT was registered. This phenomenon was observed in 4 of the 5 subjects (Fig. 2).

COMMENT

The present results, previously referred to in a preliminary report (3), are the first demonstration in man of the facilitation of 5-HT venoconstriction by ergotamine and methysergide. Some experimental data demonstrate that ergotamine interferes with the turnover of vasoactive amines such as norepinephrine and 5-HT. Ergotamine inhibits the reuptake of neuronally liberated norepinephrine into storage sites in animals (6) and the uptake of 5-HT in blood platelets isolated from healthy subjects (5). The 5-HT potentiation by methysergide is supported by research in an isolated animal artery preparation (4).

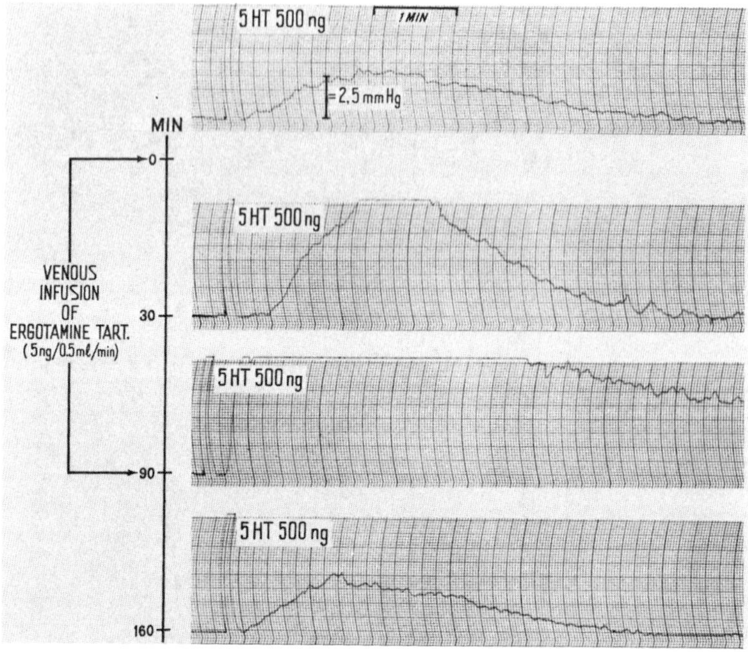

FIG. 2. Infusion of ergotamine at the indicated dose by itself does not induce changes in local venous pressure. After 20 min of this drug infusion, a facilitation of 5-HT venospastic activity appears.

5-HT facilitation by methysergide seems to acquire a peculiar importance in the interpretation of one of the side effects of this ergot compound and also in its therapeutic mechanism of action.

It is known that in a few migraine sufferers, methysergide provokes constriction of arteries of the inferior and superior limbs. Because methysergide is not in itself a vasoconstrictor agent, the norepinephrine potentiation of this drug could explain the vasoconstriction (2).

The present results also suggest still another interpretation of the adverse effect of methysergide, that is, a facilitation of serotonin.

In conclusion, this study in man demonstrates that ergotamine and methysergide in clinical dosages potentiate 5-HT venospasm. Therefore, these ergot compounds seem to achieve a proserotonin therapeutic effect in migraine rather than an antiserotonin one. From the present findings we may extrapolate that the analgesic properties specifically exhibited in migraine by ergotamine, methysergide, and correlated drugs may be owing to a potentiation of 5-HT in the nervous structures involved in pain modulation.

REFERENCES

1. Cannon, W. B., and Rosenblueth, A. (1969): *The Supersensitivity of Denervated Structures.* The Macmillan Company, New York.
2. Dalessio, D. J., Camp, W. A., Goodell, H., and Wolff, H. G. (1961): *Arch. Neurol.,* 4:235.
3. Fanciullacci, M., Franchi, G., Perez-Acuna, F., and Sicuteri, F. (1975): In: *Vasoactive Substances Relevant to Migraine,* edited by S. Diamond, D. J. Dalessio, J. R. Graham, and J. L. Medina. Charles C Thomas, Publisher, Springfield, Illinois.
4. Fozard, J. R. (1973): In: *Background to Migraine,* edited by Cumings, pp. 150–169. Heinemann, London.
5. Lingiaerde, O., Jr. (1970): *Eur. J. Pharmacol.,* 13:76.
6. Pacha, W., and Saltzmann, R. (1970): *Br. J. Pharmacol.,* 38:439.
7. Sicuteri, F. (1959): *Int. Arch. Allergy,* 15:300.
8. Sicuteri, F. (1960): *Emicrania e Mediatori Chimici,* edited by Mattioli. Fidenza, Italy.
9. Sicuteri, F., Anselmi, B., and Del Bianco, P. L. (1973): *Psychopharmacologia,* 29:347.
10. Sicuteri, F., Anselmi, B., and Fanciullacci, M. (1974): In: *Advances in Neurology, Vol. 4: International Symposium on Pain,* edited by J. J. Bonica, pp. 383–394. Raven Press, New York.
11. Sicuteri, F., Del Bianco, P. L., Fanciullacci, M., and Franchi, G. (1964): *Boll. Soc. Ital. Biol. Sper.,* 40:1148.
12. Tenen, S. S. (1967): *Psychopharmacologia,* 10:204.
13. Wolff, H. G. (1938): *Trans. Assoc. Am. Physicians,* 53:193.

Advances in Pain Research and Therapy, Vol. 1,
edited by J. J. Bonica and D. Albe-Fessard.
Raven Press, New York © 1976.

Hypnotic Treatment of Post-Traumatic Headache

Claes Cedercreutz, Raimo Lahteenmaki, and Jukka Tulikoura

Hamina Hospital, Hamina, Finland

In 1969 we started to investigate the possibilities of curing post-traumatic headaches with hypnosis. We sent a letter to all patients with skull injuries who had been at our hospital between 1965 and 1969 asking them if they suffered from headaches and offering them free hypnotic treatment. A total of 161 patients replied and of these 34% had headaches. This is similar to the 32% incidence reported by Brenner et al. (1) and the 30% incidence reported by Zetterholm (2).

In Finland, with a population of 5 million, 7,000 patients with skull injuries are treated in hospitals yearly. This means that the number of patients suffering from post-traumatic headaches increases by 2,300 per year. Later we also offered treatment to all patients with skull injuries seen at our polyclinic and all who were admitted to our hospital but had not been able to obtain relief. Consequently, a total of 140 consecutive cases were collected for the study methods. Patients were hypnotized from one to ten times. Each session lasted 20 to 30 min, and the suggestions were repeated several times. It seems necessary to use the same words as the patient does when he describes pain. In many cases in which the patient described pain as sensations of burning and stinging, only the burning sensations disappeared when I did not use the word stinging. At the following session I used the proper word and the sensation disappeared.

An average of three to four sessions of hynposis was sufficient to produce persistent complete or partial relief. The hypnotic sessions were given at intervals of 1 week to enable us to see how the treatment worked. Relapses occurred usually during the month after the last hypnosis. If the patient was free from symptoms or his condition was ameliorated 1 month after treatment, the result was usually permanent.

RESULTS

Results of treatment shown in Table 1 indicate that 70 patients or 50% of the group remained symptom-free, 20% were improved, and 30% had no lasting effect or no effect at all. A correlation can be seen between the state or depth of hypnosis achieved and the incidence of relief. The observation time was 1 year and 10 months.

TABLE 1. *Results of treatment in relation to state of trance*

State of hypnosis	Total relief	Symptom-free	Ameliorated	No effect
Deep	19	13	0	6
Medium	65	38	20	7
Light	36	19	8	9
No response	20	0	0	20
Total	140	70	28	42

CONCLUSIONS

Our experiences suggest that the results will be better if hypnotic treatment can be begun immediately after trauma than after, say, 6 months. Among patients treated immediately after skull injury, many would be cured of their headache even without treatment. Among patients who have suffered from headaches for as long as 6 weeks, few could be relieved without hypnotic treatment. On the basis of these experiences, we plan to pursue hypnotic therapy vigorously soon after development of post-traumatic headache.

ACKNOWLEDGMENT

This work was aided by research grants from "Signe and Ane Gyllenberg's Foundation."

REFERENCES

1. Brenner, C., Friedman, A., Merroy, H., and Denny-Brown, D. (1944): *J. Neurosurg.*, 1:379–390.
2. Zetterholm, S. (1947): *Acta Psychiatr. Scand. Suppl., 45.*

Advances in Pain Research and Therapy, Vol. 1,
edited by J. J. Bonica and D. Albe-Fessard.
Raven Press, New York © 1976.

An Investigation into the Psychogenic Bases of the Temporomandibular Joint Myofascial Pain Dysfunction Syndrome

Ernest W. Small

Department of Oral Surgery, School of Dentistry, and Department of Surgery, School of Medicine, University of North Carolina, Chapel Hill, North Carolina 27514

In recent years much attention has been devoted to the temporomandibular joint (TMJ) pain/dysfunction syndrome and to the anatomy, physiology, and pathology of the joint in the professional literature (1,4,5,7–12,16). This chapter reports an investigation into the incidence of psychogenic factors underlying the TMJ syndrome. The TMJ syndrome is a perplexing group of symptons characterized by deep pain in the side of the face elicited by limited movement of the lower jaw and accompanied by noise from the joint. In many patients there are no discernible, consistent clinical findings to explain the symptoms on the basis of altered anatomy or physiology. It has been postulated that psychogenic factors are the consistent basis for this syndrome. The treatment for patients with organic disease differs from that for patients with functional bases. The former treatment may be of long duration and considerable expense. The treatment for functional pain is quite different if recognized as such. Counseling of some patients to help them gain insight into their problem may be all required for relief.

The purpose of this study was to evaluate two personality inventories as aids in the diagnosis of psychogenic factors in the etiology of the TMJ syndrome and in differentiating patients with psychogenic bases for their complaint. The personality inventories used in this study have been the subject of many articles in the literature (2,3,6,14,15).

METHODS AND PROCEDURES

Fifty consecutive patients referred for diagnosis and treatment of TMJ syndrome were studied. No restrictions on age or sex were imposed. Twenty-six patients were women, ages ranging from 14 to 54 years, and 24 were men ranging from 19 to 47 years of age.

The Minnesota Multiphasic Personality Inventory (MMPI) is a psychometric instrument designed ultimately to provide, in a single test, scores on all the more important aspects of personality. This study used four MMPI validity scales plus the usual ten clinical scales: Hypochondriasis, Depression, Hysteria, Psychopathic Deviation, Masculine/Feminine Interest, Paranoia, Psychasthenia, Schizophrenia, and Hypomania. The Taylor Manifest Anxiety Scale (TAS) was used in this study. The TAS contains a selected group of 45 items in the 550 statements of the MMPI. Form N2 of the Cornell Index (CI) was also used. The 101 questions were scaled: Fa for fear and inadequacy, Dep for depression, NA for nervousness and anxiety, NC for neurocirculatory symptoms, SR for startle reactions, PS for psychosomatic symptoms, HY for hypochondriasis and asthenia, GI for gastrointestinal symptoms, SS for sensitivity and suspiciousness, and TP for troublesome psychopathy.

The same sequence was followed for each patient. After initial clinical examination and completion of a TMJ history, the patient was referred for TMJ roentgenography and administration of the MMPI, CI, and TAS by the clinical psychologist. All roentgenographic films of the joints were read as normal by radiologists. On return but before the results of the personality studies were available, all patients were treated with a fixed regimen.

The treatment consisted of patient-applied heat to the TMJ area, soft diet, limitation of mouth opening to 2 cm, tongue exercises to strengthen the suprahyoid musculature, a technique developed to prevent yawning, mild analgesics and muscle relaxants, and, most importantly, counseling of the patient to help him gain some insight into the problem he is possibly creating. Evaluation of treatment effectiveness was predicated on the finding of persistent pain relief.

The statistical technique for examining the frequency data in the study was chi square (χ^2). Chi square was used to compare the 50 patients on the basis of their physical findings both as a total group and as a group evidencing the neurotic triad of the MMPI. A further statistical analysis was performed using the *t*-ratio or *t*-test of the significance of the difference between sample means on the MMPI, the CI, and the TAS: i.e., the means of the "normal" patients compared to the means of the "abnormal" patients.

RESULTS

The pertinent physical findings noted in the clinical examination and the TMJ history are summarized as follows. Of the 26 women patients with pain located in the face, ears, jaw, head, or TMJ and accompained by tenderness in 22 cases, 3 had constant sharp pain, 10 had constant dull pain, 3 had intermittent sharp pain, and 10 had intermittent dull pain. Among this group 9 had limited motion, 13 had unilateral chewing, 14 had joint noise, 10 had the Bruxer-Clencher test, 23 had thruster, and 10 had voluntary "popper." Of the 24 men patients with similar pain locale accompanied by tenderness in 17 cases, 1 had constant sharp pain, 7 had constant dull pain, 7 had intermittent sharp pain, and 9 had intermittent dull pain. Among this group 15 had limited motion, 11 unilateral chewing, 17 joint noise, 10 Bruxer-Clencher test, 15 thruster, and 13 voluntary "popper." The chi square test found a significant difference to the 0.01 level in patients exhibiting the pattern of thrusting, tenderness to palpation, and the experience of dull pain as compared to those with the pattern not thrusting, non-tenderness to palpation, and sharp pain. A negative correlation was found in the incidence of clenching and bruxing.

On the basis of the MMPI profiles, CI scores, and TAS scores, the clinical psychologist determined the personality characteristics of the 50 patients. Ten of the patients were categorized as "normal" in their personality integration. The remaining 40 patients were categorized as "abnormal." These two groups were then labeled "normal" group and "abnormal" group. The physical findings and the TMJ history were not made available to the clinical psychologist, nor were the personality findings made known to the treating clinician. The personality characteristics are summarized in Tables 1 and 2.

The difference in the total CI mean scores for the "normal" and "abnormal" patients was significant to the 0.01 level of significance on the basis of the *t*-test.

The 10 "normal" patients had a mean TAS of 7.30, whereas the "abnor-

TABLE 1. *Summary of personality characteristics of 26 female temporomandibular joint pain patients evidenced by MMPI and CMI*

No.	Characteristics	Age	TAS	CMI	Neurotic Triad
1	Poor appetite, paranoid	37	24	27	yes
4	Schizoid	39	14	17	yes
6	Depression	36	12	8	no
7	Severe anxiety, paranoid	50	25	27	yes
9	Severe anxiety, poor appetite	14	27	26	no
14	Loner, anxiety	31	24	19	yes
16	Poor appetite, paranoid	39	25	46	yes
18	Hostility, instability	41	11	6	yes
19	Hostility, instability	37	16	11	yes
20	Instability	16	6	0	no
21	Schizoid, paranoid, depressed	34	41	61	no
22	Normal	45	11	2	yes
24	Anxiety, depression	27	22	15	no
26	Confused identity	21	10	5	yes
27	Passive insecurity	29	22	17	yes
28	Confused identity, passive	14	8	7	yes
30	Instability	16	25	18	no
32	Inconsistent, seclusive	22	16	5	yes
35	Inadequate	54	13	10	no
36	Disabling anxiety	39	31	55	no
37	Normal	47	7	1	yes
38	Passive insecurity	34	10	2	no
39	Anxiety, poor appetite	45	21	11	yes
41	Anxiety, poor appetite	31	29	16	yes
47	Pathologically anxiety-free	20	8	3	no
49	Schizoid	25	23	16	yes

NOTE: TAS indicates the score on the Taylor Anxiety Scale of the Minnesota Multiphasic Personality Inventory. CMI indicates the score total on the Cornell Medical Index. The Neurotic Triad indicates elevation of Scales 1 and 3 with relative depression of Scale 2 of the MMPI.

TABLE 2. *Summary of personality characteristics of 24 male temporomandibular joint pain patients evidenced by MMPI and CMI*

No.	Characteristics	Age	TAS	CMI	Neurotic Triad
2	Normal	37	18	6	no
3	Liability, instability	21	12	25	no
5	Depressed instability	20	15	4	no
8	Anxiety	28	11	11	yes
10	Hyperactivity-Normal	20	6	5	yes
11	Normal	21	5	2	yes
12	Normal	31	5	5	no
13	Anxiety, Seclusiveness	22	25	13	yes
15	Depressed anxiety	24	24	9	no
17	Marked defensive anxiety	21	3	2	yes
23	Depressed psychosomaticism	36	20	15	yes
25	Hysterical hostility	21	7	13	yes
29	Depressed anxiety	37	19	11	no
31	Severe schizoid, hostility	20	34	26	no
33	Depression	46	15	14	no
34	Normal	38	5	1	no
40	Poor appetite, anxiety	20	20	8	yes
42	Severe anxiety	19	29	11	no
43	Hyperactivity, paranoid	39	9	1	yes
44	Normal	32	6	3	no
45	Neurotic anxiety	23	16	20	no
46	Hostility, seclusiveness	24	7	3	yes
48	Normal	21	5	7	yes
50	Normal	47	5	3	yes

NOTE: TAS indicated the score on the Taylor Anxiety Scale of the Minnesota Multiphasic Personality Inventory. CMI indicated the score total on the Cornell Medical Index. The Neurotic Triad indicates elevation of Scales 1 and 3 with relative depression of Scale 2 of the MMPI.

TABLE 3. *Results of treatment in 26 female temporomandibular joint pain patients*

Patient	Pain Duration	Response to Past Treatment	Past Treatment	Results of Current Treatment
1	15 years	unfavorable	equilibration	good response- free of pain
4	2 years	unfavorable	splints	good response- free of pain
6	1 month	unfavorable	analgesics	good response- free of pain
7	3 weeks	-	no treatment	good response- free of pain
9	9 months	-	no treatment	good response- free of pain
14	1 year	unfavorable	analgesics	good response- free of pain
16	3 days	unfavorable	analgesics	good response- free of pain
18	2 months	slight improvement	equilibration	good response- free of pain
19	"years"	unfavorable	equilibration	good response- free of pain
20	1 month	-	no treatment	good response- free of pain
21	"years"	unfavorable	loss of all teeth	good response- free of pain
22*	1 month	-	no treatment	good response- free of pain
24	9 months	unfavorable	analgesics	good response- free of pain
26	"years"	-	no treatment	good response- free of pain
27	3 months	unfavorable	splints	good response- free of pain
28	6 months	-	no treatment	good response- free of pain
30	4 weeks	-	no treatment	good response- free of pain
32	18 months	-	no treatment	good response- free of pain
35	6 months	-	no treatment	good response- free of pain
36	1 year	-	no treatment	good response- free of pain
37*	6 months	unfavorable	equilibration	poor response- persistent pain
38	5 years	unfavorable	analgesics	good response- free of pain
39	4 months	unfavorable	analgesics	good response- free of pain
41	7 years	some alleviation	equilibration	good response- free of pain
47	6 months	unfavorable	equilibration	good response- free of pain
49	18 months	-	no treatment	good response- free of pain

*Indicates patients categorized as "normal" by the Clinical Psychologist.

TABLE 4. *Results of treatment in 24 male temporomandibular joint pain patients*

Patient	Pain Duration	Response to Past Treatment	Past Treatment	Results of Current Treatment
2*	1 month	unfavorable	analgesics	required surgery to free of pain
3	2 years	unfavorable	analgesics	good response- free of pain
5	"years"	unfavorable	analgesics	good response- free of pain
8	3 weeks	unfavorable	analgesics	good response- free of pain
10*	1 year	unfavorable	bite adjustment	fair response- slow pain relief
11*	18 months	-	no treatment	required surgery to free of pain
12*	6 years	unfavorable	splints	required prostheses for relief
13	1 year	unfavorable	analgesics	good response- free of pain
15	2 months	unfavorable	analgesics	good response- free of pain
17	1 year	some improvement	bite adjustment	good response- free of pain
23	6 months	-	no treatment	good response- free of pain
25	3 weeks	unfavorable	analgesics	good response- free of pain
29	6 months	unfavorable	analgesics	good response- free of pain
31	3 months	unfavorable	analgesics	good response- free of pain
33	3 days	-	no treatment	good response- free of pain
34*	5 weeks	-	no treatment	required prostheses for relief
40	2 weeks	unfavorable	analgesics	good response- free of pain
42	7 months	unfavorable	analgesics	good response- free of pain
44*	"years"	-	no treatment	required surgery to free of pain
45	3 years	-	no treatment	good response- free of pain
46	4 months	unfavorable	bite adjustment	good response- free of pain
48*	5 months	-	no treatment	good response- free of pain
50*	2 years	unfavorable	bite adjustment	required surgery to free of pain

*Indicates patients categorized as "normal" by the Clinical Psychologist.

mal" group showed a mean TAS score of 18.23. The difference in the TAS mean scores of the "normal" group and the "abnormal" group was significant to the 0.01 level on the basis of the *t*-test.

Group personality scores were analyzed after the clinical psychologist had assigned each patient to a group. It is noted that the neurotic triad on the MMPI did not differentiate the two patient groups.

An analysis using the *t*-test was done on the differences in the mean scores of the "normal" and "abnormal" groups on all of the subscales of the MMPI. The only significant difference (0.05) in the means of the two groups was found in the F scale, a validity scale of the whole inventory. A high F score means an invalid MMPI. It is to be noted that the norms are six to seven significant responses to the 64 items in the scale. The "abnormal" group mean F scale was 4.97, whereas the "normal" group mean was 2.7. These low F scores indicate rational, relatively pertinent records showing response conformity. The results of treatment are shown in Tables 3 and 4. It was found that all patients who were considered "abnormal" on the basis of the MMPI, CI, and TAS responded to the conservative, noninvasive treatment and were rendered free of pain.

CONCLUSIONS

On the basis of the MMPI profile, the TAS, and the CI scores, a clinical psychologist characterized 50 consecutive TMJ pain syndrome patients as "normal" or "abnormal" in personality characteristics. On the basis of response to conservative treatment—counseling, corrective exercises, and noxious habit inhibition—we divided the patients into two categories.

Forty-three responded to the conservative treatment and became free of pain. Of the remaining 7 patients, 4 responded to surgery, 1 to prostheses, and 1 failed to respond. All 40 "abnormal" patients and 3 "normal" patients responded to conservative therapy.

From the findings it is concluded that psychogenic factors played a major role in the etiology of the TMJ syndrome in the patients with "abnormal" personality characterizations inasmuch as 100% of them responded to conservative treatment.

It appears that the MMPI, CI, and TAS were excellent instruments to differentiate a group of patients who had facial pain of a functional nature from those who may have had organic causes. Although the MMPI ranges and means did not distinguish the groups, the individual profiles can be expected to have aided the clinical psychologist in distinguishing the "normal" and "abnormal" patients.

There appears to be some basis to infer that other factors played a major etiologic role in the 10 patients characterized as "normal," since only 30% of this group responded to conservative treatment. The findings of this study suggest that further investigation is warranted into the field of personality testing in patients presenting with facial pain owing to other than obvious clinical causes.

REFERENCES

1. Berry, D. C. (1967): *Br. J. Oral Surg.,* 24:223.
2. Brackbill, G., and Little, K. B. (1954): *J. Consult. Psychol.,* 18:433.
3. Coleman, W., and Collett, D. M. (1959): *Rev. Educ. Res.,* February:58.
4. Friedman, A. P. (1966): *Dent. Clin. North Am.,* 10(3):545.
5. Gerry, R. G. (1966): *J. Prosthet. Dent.,* 16:316.
6. Hathway, S. R., and McKinley, J. C. (1951): *Minnesota Multiphasic Personality Inventory Manual,* pp. 1–31. Psychological Corporation, New York.
7. Husted, E. (1968): *Dent. Clin. North Am.,* 12(3):601.
8. Merritt, H. H. (1968): In: *Facial Pain and Mandibular Dysfunction,* edited by L. Schwartz and C. M. Chayes, p.v. W. B. Saunders, Philadelphia.
9. Miller, C. W. (1952): *J. Am. Dent. Assoc.,* 44:387.
10. Moulton, R. E. (1968): In: *Facial Pain and Mandibular Dysfunction,* edited by L. Schwartz and C. M. Chayes, p. 318. W. B. Saunders, Philadelphia.
11. Perry, H. T., Jr. (1968): *J. Prosthet. Dent.,* 19:291.
12. Sicher, H. (1968): *Oral Anatomy,* p. 497. C. V. Mosby, St. Louis.
13. Stemmer, A. L., op. cit., p. 1163. Cameron, B. M. (1967): *Am. J. Orthopsychiatry,* 9:7.
14. Taylor, J. (1953): *Psychol. Abs.,* 27(7):28.
15. Weider, A., Wolff, H. F., Brodman, K., Mittelmann, B., and Wechsler, D. (1948): *Cornell Index Manual,* Psychological Corporation, New York.
16. Whinery, J. G. (1968): *J. Oral Surg.,* 26:110.

Advances in Pain Research and Therapy, Vol. 1,
edited by J. J. Bonica and D. Albe-Fessard.
Raven Press, New York © 1976.

Sensory Loss and Prolonged Remission of Tic Douloureux After Selective Alcoholic Gasserian Injection

Arthur Ecker

407 University Avenue, Syracuse, New York 13210

"It is an unexplained fact that sensory denervation of the face cures tic douloureux" (13). Yes, but how much of the half-face must be denervated, how completely, and for how long? These old questions have become even more pertinent since trigeminal root "decompression" with little sensory loss has frequently relieved tic douloureux (TD) (1), albeit with a high rate of early recurrence (17).

Total deafferentation of the painful area, with freedom from pain, can be produced temporarily by neurectomy of a peripheral trigeminal branch or of the half-face permanently by destruction of the entire gasserian ganglion or root (3–5,11,12). Partial section of the trigeminal sensory root, the Frazier operation (10), was expected to produce permanent anesthesia of the lower two-thirds of the face. In fact, it produces an unpredictable pattern (16) of hemifacial anesthesia of uncertain duration (2,16,17). Nevertheless, it relieves TD in most patients for 5 years (17). No correlation has been found between remission of TD and the actual anesthesia produced by the Frazier operation (16), blunt trauma to the root, or "decompression" (1).

In selective corneal-sparing alcoholic destruction of the trigeminal root with the Ecker-Perl method (6–8,14,15), the immediate goal is total anesthesia and analgesia of the painful area (PA). The resulting mucocutaneous anesthesia often diminishes within a day or two, and yet tic douloureux is usually relieved for many years (6). Our sensory examinations and follow-up studies permit the present report which deals with the questions: Does the degree of sensory deficit in the PA a day or two after injection correlate with remission of TD for several years? Is a recurrence of TD related to further recovery of sensory function?

CLINICAL MATERIAL

Over a period of 21 years, 322 successive cases of classic TD (312 patients with 10 having bilateral pain) resistant to medication (diphenylhydantoinate sodium and/or carbamazepine) have been treated by the Ecker-Perl method of selective alcoholic gasserian injection which consisted of a partial rhizolysis. In more than 90% of cases, at the time of injection we produced anesthesia and analgesia of the PAs that lasted 25 min after the final injection.

This treatment has produced no death, no permanent masticator muscle paralysis, no significant visual loss, nor any other major permanent complication except for a few cases of anesthesia dolorosa. Corneal sensation was preserved in approximately 85% of the cases; superficial keratitis developed in 4% and produced in a single case a diminution of visual acuity to 20/60. Regardless of the level of sensation 1 to 2 days after injection, we repeat the injection only if severe TD persists. This completion of the original procedure within 2 months was required in 28 (9%) of the cases.

In our entire series the rate of pain relief of severe persistent TD in any trigeminal division until death or at least 7 years is 77% or, in the same trigeminal division 78%. Among 104 patients followed for more than 7 years, 63 remained pain-free for 7 to 10 years, 22 for 11 to 14 years, and 9 for 15 to 18 years. Of the other 10 patients, pain recurred before 11 years in 8 and before 14 years in 2.

METHODS

Technique of Injection

The patient is awake and supine. Local anesthesia precedes the insertion of a 21-gauge lumbar puncture needle. Radiographs are used to position the head and to select a precise entry point in the skin and a precise target within the skull. The needle passes vertically downward, outside the oral mucosa, and through the center of the foramen ovale so that its tip lies on the target (Fig. 1) exactly 4 mm beyond the posteromedial border of the foramen ovale and 2 mm above the base of the skull at the petrosphenoid junction. Whether or not cerebrospinal fluid is obtained, the injected alcohol will enter Ferner's ganglionic sinus (9) where the juxtaganglionic rootlets are arrayed as in the peripheral divisions and also are the thinnest, most widely spread, and least intertwined. Usually not more than 0.05 ml of absolute alcohol is injected at one time; 0.10 ml is the median total quantity required. A partial rhizolysis results.

Frequent sensory examinations are made and recorded. If necessary, the head's attitude is altered, re-injection is made, and/or an adjustment is made in the needle's depth, direction, or tip orientation. The immediate goal is anesthesia and analgesia of the trigger and PAs for 25 min after the last injection as well as our inability deliberately to precipitate TD. If any unfavorable event develops, the procedure is discontinued at once. It may be completed or repeated on another day.

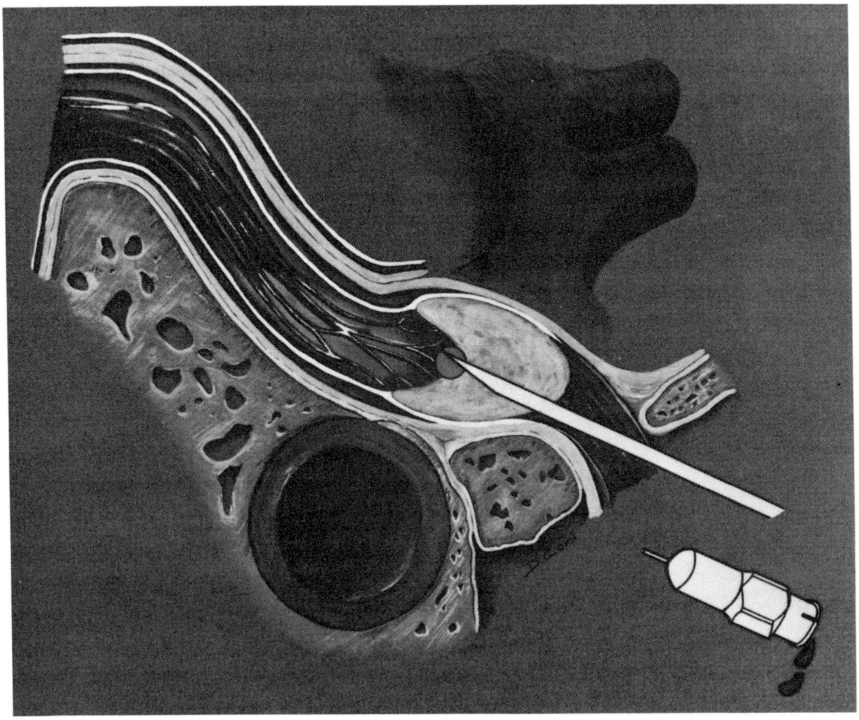

FIG. 1. Vertical section, right middle fossa, in plane of needle through foramen ovale, mandibular division, gasserian ganglion, triangular plexus, compact portion of trigeminal sensory root, and anterior surface of petrous bone containing the carotid artery. Small gray circle is the target (see text). Medial two-thirds of the gasserian ganglion is seen from above. Head was positioned to permit vertical descent of the needle.

Testing of Sensation

On each half of the face, we test eight areas for light touch and seven for sharp point (6). For the cornea, only a wisp of cotton wool is used (Fig. 2A). For the forehead, cheek, upper and lower lips, upper and lower alveolar processes, and tongue: to test for light touch we brush lightly a cotton swab 1 to 2 cm; to test for sharp point sensation we roll gently a pointed rotating metal wheel on the skin or mucous membrane for 1 to 2 cm (Fig. 2B). We always test the healthy side first, and the patient considers the sensation to be normal or 100%; then we test the corresponding area of the affected side; the patient reports this sensation as a percentage of the normal. It is recorded semiquantitatively. In each case the author personally tested sensation before injection, repeatedly during injection, after 1 to 2 days, and subsequently years later.

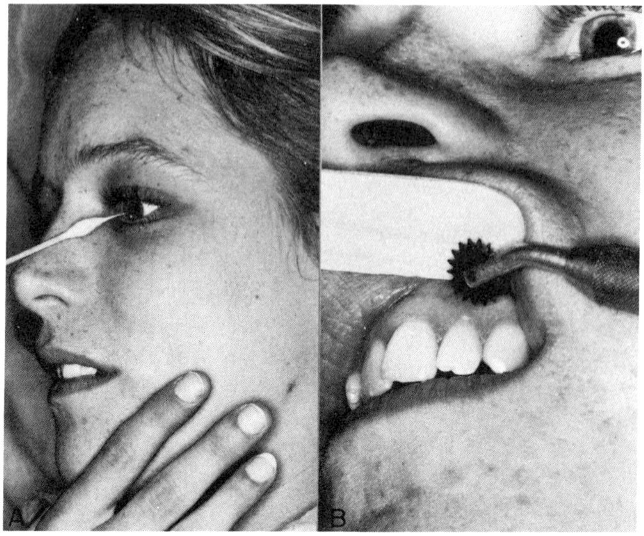

FIG. 2. A: Wisp of cotton testing corneal sensation. Patient's fingers indicate degree of sensation. **B:** Rotating metal wheel testing sharp point sensation on gingiva.

RESULTS

The present study is based on injection and follow-up of 248 patients after 2 to 21 years. The immediate goal was achieved in over 90% of cases. At 1 to 2 days after injection, the number of patients with each degree of loss of sharp point sensation in the PA is shown in Table 1: the number with loss of light touch sensation is almost identical.

At every level of sensory deficit there was a recurrence rate of severe persistent TD of 10% within the first 2 years, 6% in the third and fourth years, 4% in the fifth and sixth years, and 4% at 7 to 13 years after injection.

TABLE 1. *Results after alcoholic gasserian injection*

Loss of sensation of sharp point, painful area at 1–2 days		Remission tic douloureux for 7 years	
Degree of loss	No.	No.	%
None or minimal	23	20	86
Moderate	21	17	80
Marked	42	32	76
Complete	162	134	83
Total	248	203	81

The data also reveal that there is no correlation between the degree of early loss of sharp point sensation and 7-year remission of severe persistent TD. Study of degrees of loss of light touch sensation yield almost identical results. Naturally, patients prefer to retain sensation in the face, provided TD does not recur.

Of 23 patients who had slight or no loss of sensation to sharp point 1 to 2 days after injection, 20 were free from recurrent severe persistent TD until death or for at least 7 years; but 15 of these 20 had some area of complete loss of sharp point sensation in an adjacent region, 14 in the oral cavity.

Among 32 reexamined patients who had had complete anesthesia and analgesia in the PA 1 to 2 days after injection and were still free from pain 1 to 18 years (median 7.5 years) after injection, 22 had persistent complete or marked loss of sensation and in 10 sensory loss was moderate to mild.

Of the 248 patients in this study, 63 had recurrent severe TD from less than 1 year to 13 years (median 3 years) after injection. Reexamination revealed that in the PA, compared with the state 1 to 2 days after injection, there was less sensory loss in 56, the same sensory loss in 5 (complete loss in 1, minimal to none in 4), and more sensory loss in 2. At recurrence, there was practically normal sensation in more than half the cases and complete loss in the PA in 9%. In 6 cases of recurrent TD despite persistent complete anesthesia and analgesia in the PA (5 upper jaw, 1 lower jaw), there was considerable sensation in the adjacent lip.

SUMMARY

Of 248 patients with classic tic douloureux and with follow-up after injection 2 to 21 years ago, 203 (81%) had persistent relief of TD until death or for at least 7 years. One to two days after selective trigeminal rhizolysis (Ecker-Perl method) the sensory deficit in the painful area was minimal in 23 (9%), moderate in 21 (8%), marked in 42 (17%), and complete in 162 (65%). The level of sensation to light touch and to sharp point was not relevant to the risk of recurrence or to the time of recurrence. The same conclusion was reached in studies after other methods of partial destruction of the trigeminal sensory root (1,16,17).

Of 39 pain-free patients with complete anesthesia in the PA 1 to 2 days after injection who were examined years later, complete or marked sensory deficit in the painful area had persisted in 26 (67%). But recurrences appeared up to 13 years after treatment, decreasing in frequency with time. At recurrence in 63 patients, there was partial recovery of sensation in 56 (89%) and complete recovery to normal state in 38 (60%). In short, for prolonged relief, early sensory recovery is irrelevant but late sensory recovery indicates likelihood of recurrence. Therefore, this study shows that the meaning of late sensory status of a patient depends on comparison with the early status.

ACKNOWLEDGMENT

We acknowledge the help of Roslyn Freudenthal, Ph.D., Biostatistical Consultant.

REFERENCES

1. Bohm, E., and Højeberg, S. (1960): *Acta Chir. Scand.,* 120:233–236.
2. Burmeister, H. (1960): *Arch. Klin. Chir.,* 295:175–185.
3. Carmichael, E. A., and Woollard, H. H. (1933): *Brain,* 56:109–125.
4. Cushing, H. (1904): *Johns Hopkins Med. J.,* 15:213–232.
5. Davies, H. M. (1907): *Brain,* 30:219–276.
6. Ecker, A. (1974): *N.Y. State J. Med.,* 74:1586–1592.
7. Ecker, A., and Perl, T. (1958): *Neurology,* 8:461–468.
8. Ecker, A., and Perl, T. (1963): *Acta Radiol.,* 1:901–912.
9. Ferner, H. (1970): In: *Trigeminal Neuralgia,* edited by R. Hassler and A. E. Walker. W. B. Saunders Co., Philadelphia.
10. Frazier, C. H. (1925): *Arch. Neurol. Psychiatr.,* 13:378–384.
11. Haertel, F. (1912): *Arch. Klin. Chir.,* 100:193–292.
12. Harris, W. (1926): *Neuritis and Neuralgia.* Oxford University Press, London.
13. Penman, J. (1968): In: *Handbook of Clinical Neurology, Vol. 5,* edited by P. J. Vinken and G. W. Bruyn. North Holland Publishing Co., Amsterdam.
14. Perl, T., and Ecker, A. (1959): *Am. J. Roentgenol.,* 82:830–839.
15. Perl, T., and Ecker, A. (1969): *Acta Radiol.,* 9:38–48.
16. Rasmussen, P. (1965): *Facial Pain.* Munksgaard, Copenhagen.
17. White, J. C., and Sweet, W. H. (1969): *Pain and the Neurosurgeon,* pp. 202,228,230. Charles C Thomas, Publisher, Springfield, Illinois.

Advances in Pain Research and Therapy, Vol. 1,
edited by J. J. Bonica and D. Albe-Fessard.
Raven Press, New York © 1976.

Contributions of Physical Anthropology to Understanding the Aches and Pains of Aging

William S. Hunter

Department of Internal Medicine, Kaiser-Permanente Medical Center, San Francisco, California 94115

Among the aches and pains of aging, a considerable portion are of locomotor origin. Physical anthropology, specifically phylogenetic anatomy, provides a number of explanations for pains in this category and suggests simple, safe methods of treatment.

In discussing this topic, I would like to mention two important historical figures. Half a millenium ago Leonardo da Vinci, in the course of his self-education in anatomy, conceived the world's first movable skeletal model. And soon afterwards, also in Florence, Borelli was a founding member of the first modern scientific institute in Europe, the Academia del Cimento. He conducted the world's first study of human gait: On Animal Movement.

ANTHROPOLOGICAL EXPLANATIONS FOR CERTAIN LOCOMOTOR PAINS: A WORKING HYPOTHESIS

Approximately 20 years ago in my clinical practice, I observed that a number of patients had undergone inappropriate removal of ovaries or appendices because of abdominal pain that represented strain of three muscles: the coccygeus and piriformis, which line the back of the pelvis, and the obturator internus, which lines the front of the pelvis (5). The anatomy texts suggested that these muscles are involved in the mechanics of the hip and sacroiliac joints. Such pain, if not associated with anatomic or physiologic anomalies, could often be eliminated by correcting postural abnormalities. Yet no heed was paid in any medical text to the contribution of postural abnormalities to abdominal pain.

This neglect was the more remarkable because standards for efficient stance still in use today were determined in Germany before the Franco-Prussian War in attempts to develop a more efficient foot soldier (12). In seeking to identify the center of gravity of the head, trunk, and extremities, it was arbitrarily determined that a carpenter's plumb line dropped from the external ear canal should cross the tip of the shoulder, the greater trochanter, and pass in front of the lateral malleolus (6). Recent French work has

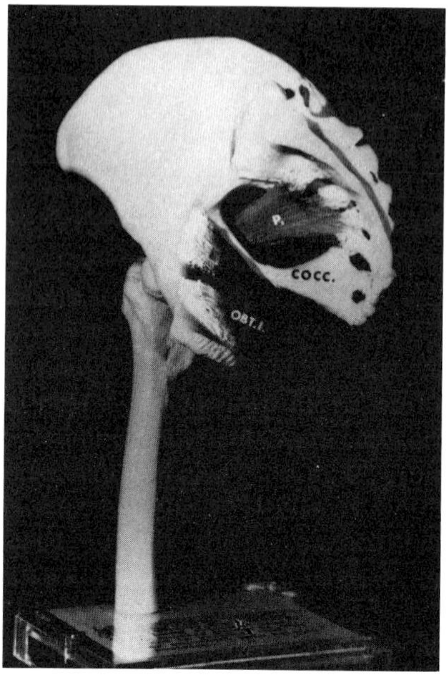

FIG. 1. Obturator internus (OBT. I.), piriformis (P.), and coccygeus (COCC.) muscles seen from inside the pelvis.

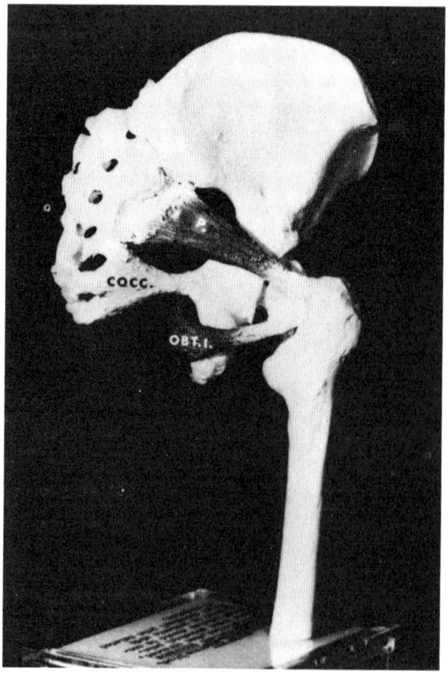

FIG. 2. Same muscles as in Fig. 1 viewed from outside the pelvis.

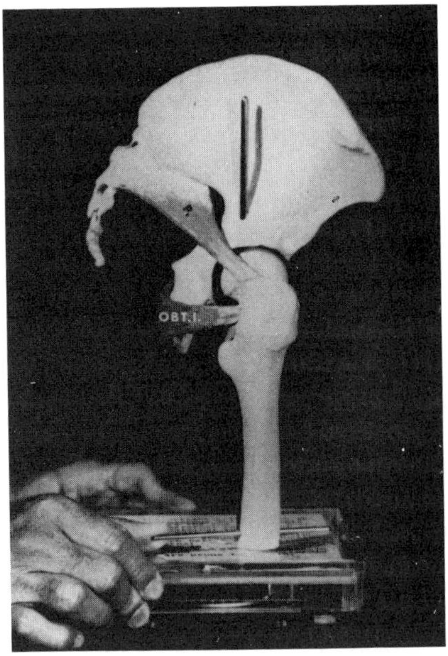

FIG. 3. Sacroiliac joint—resting.

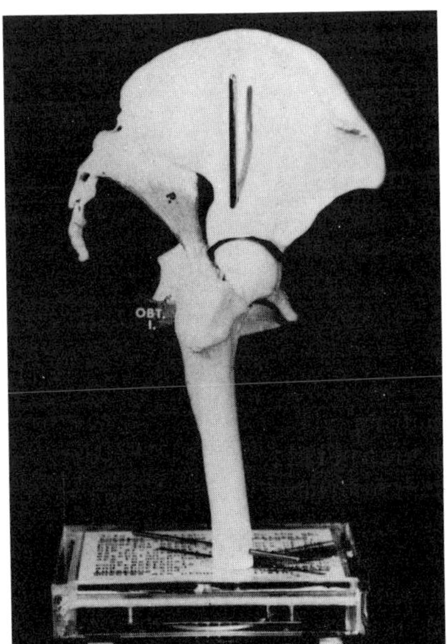

FIG. 4. Sacroiliac joint with weight bearing showing movement of the sacrum around a transverse axis being restrained by the coccygeus muscle.

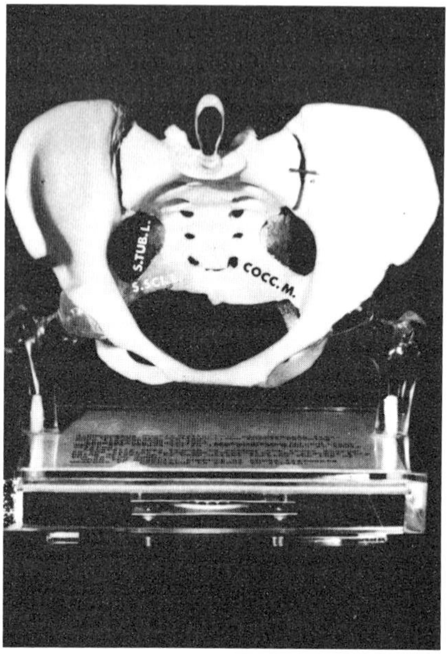

FIG. 5. Obturator internus and piriformis muscles acting as external rotators of the hip around a vertical axis. COCC. M., coccygeus muscle; S.TUB. L., sacrotuberous ligament; S.SCI. L., sacrosciatic ligament.

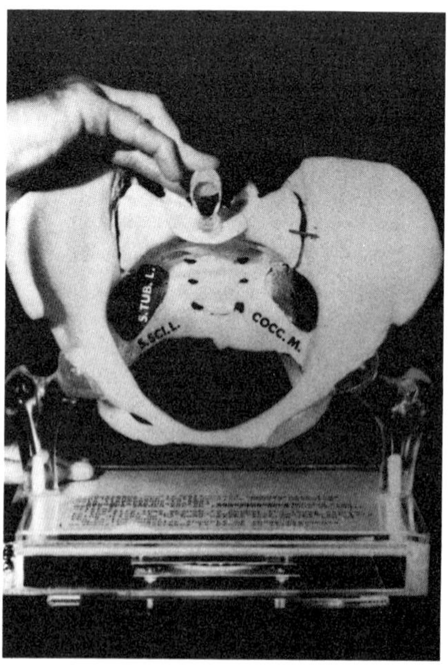

FIG. 6. Same as Fig. 5.

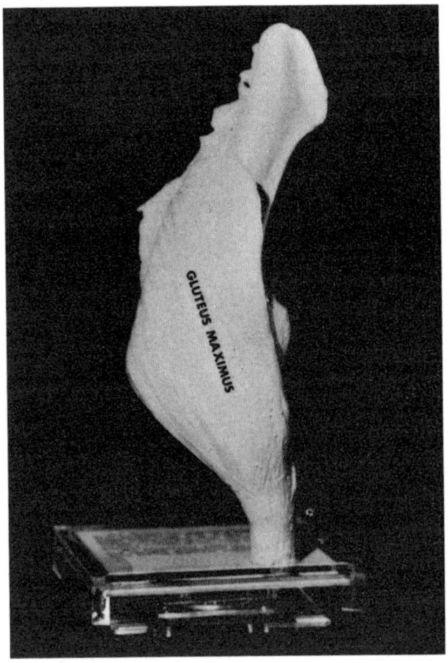

FIG. 7. Gluteus maximus in the chimpanzee.

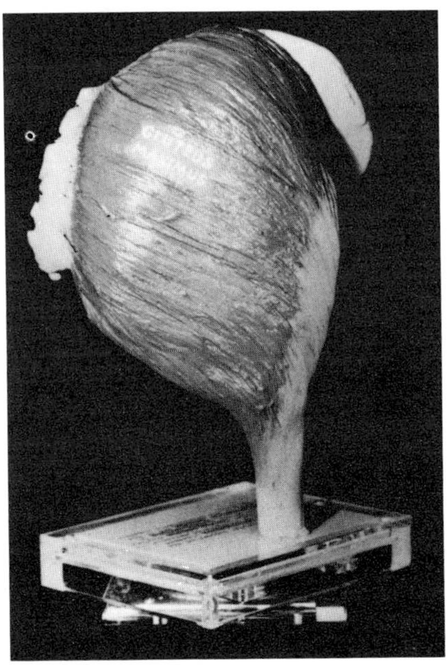

FIG. 8. Gluteus maximus in man. The muscle is much larger than that in the chimpanzee and is rearranged so that it bolsters the sacroiliac joint and acts on the hip joint as an extensor and external rotator.

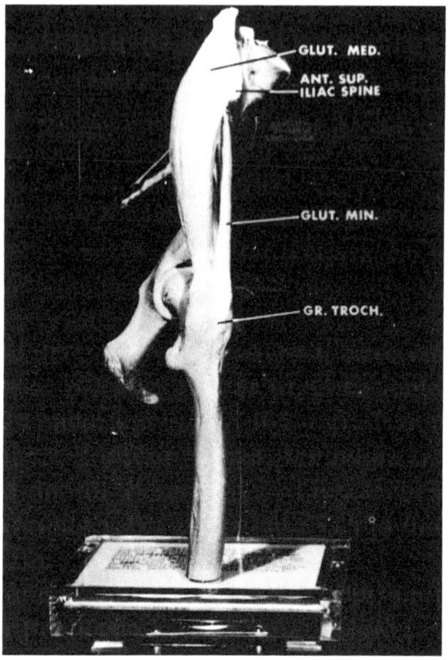

FIG. 9. Gluteus medius (GLUT. MED.) and minimus (GLUT. MIN.) in the upright chimpanzee. (GR. TROCH., greater trochanter).

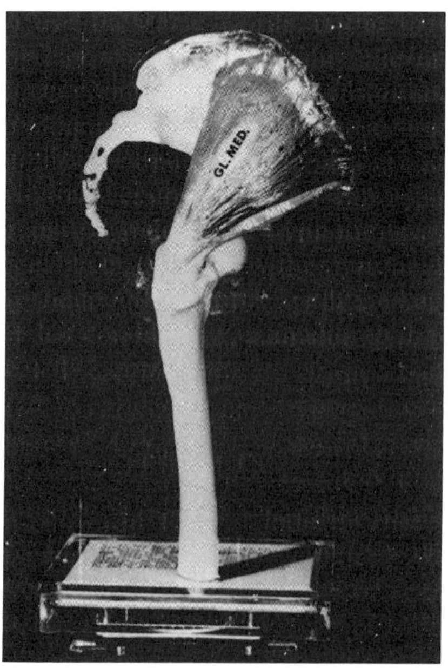

FIG. 10. Gluteus medius and minimus in upright man brought half way from the vertical as seen in the chimp to the horizontal plane so they can act as internal rotators (the only ones) of the hip in normal gait.

established that normal, efficient gait is not simply falling forward and recovery, but involves rotation at the lower ankle joint, the hip, the spine, especially in the area of the floating ribs, and the shoulder girdle (3).

I found it of clinical value to consider as a working hypothesis that deviations from the standards for efficient stance occur and increase with aging because the human locomotor system as it has evolved from our anthropoid ancestors has certain major defects. Investigation of this concept was pursued with Dr. Adrienne Zihlman, with the advice of Professor S. L. Washburn, at the University of California at Berkeley. The work included construction of models that permitted anatomic comparisons among man and other primates.

Evolutionary Development of Human Posture

In his evolutionary drive to dominate the other animals, man has concentrated on certain limited functions. He has attempted to develop a locomotor system that enables him to get up off the ground and walk slowly for long distances, leaving the arms free to handle lightweight tools (S. L. Washburn, *personal communication*). To accomplish this, he has acquired major antagonistic muscle groups of unequal strength. The external rotators of the hip overpower its internal rotators; in the shoulders the opposite occurs: the longitudinal spinal muscles overpower the abdominal muscles so that efficient spinal alignment is lost. In brief, unless we pay particular attention, we tend as we become older to become splay-footed, round-shouldered, and pot-gutted. The posture of an old man and that of an upright chimpanzee are strikingly similar: the head juts forward, the palms face backward, the back is bent, and the feet toe out. This similarity suggests that at least in certain respects, degeneration of man's locomotor system is reversion to an earlier phase in its evolutionary development. I shall describe some of these changes, starting with the foot.

By raising and lowering the longitudinal arch (a structure found in none of the apes) and by contraction and relaxation of the posterior tibial muscles, man can transfer his weight from one foot to the other with much less expenditure of energy than is required for leaning the trunk from side to side. To facilitate this movement, the tendons of insertion of the posterior tibial and long peroneal muscles cross the sole of the foot to form a "stirrup," an arrangement also seen in no other primate. With aging, loss of rotation at the lower ankle joint is one cause of repeated painful swelling of the knee.

Motion in the upper ankle joint is predominantly dorsi- and plantar flexion of the foot. It has long been observed that man's heel bone is much larger than that of other anthropoids; less appreciated is his need for an extensile calf muscle to keep the heel bone on the ground during most of the weight-bearing phase of gait. The most common cause of night calf cramps, a frequent complaint of the elderly, is loss of extensibility of the calf.

Man seems to be trying to evolve a knee joint that is more nearly a hinge than is that of the chimpanzee; the knee of the chimpanzee permits much more torsion.

Recent human evolution has seen a great increase in the mass of the gluteus maximus muscle (4,9), as well as a change in its shape and position to bolster the sacroiliac joint—of obvious importance in maintaining a superimposed vertical vertebral column. The human quadriceps femoris has also increased markedly in weight. Like the gluteus maximus, the quadriceps femoris uses the fascia lata—a structure found in no other primate (1)—as a tendon of insertion. In addition, the human patella enables the quadriceps femoris to insert into the tibia at an angle that is closer to 90° than in other anthropoids, greatly enhancing the effective force of the muscle. The fascia lata absorbs the lateral component of body force transmitted across the hip and femoral neck.

Having rearranged the locomotor apparatus of the feet and legs to support an upright trunk, man has taken further evolutionary steps to stabilize vertebral alignment. Back muscles have been moved to a more lateral position (2,11). The rectus abdominis has been converted from a single long muscle to a series of short ones by the introduction of transverse fibrous striations into the muscle (8).

The three muscles that, when strained, accounted for the abdominal pain in my patients are essential to human gait and stance. The coccygeus is part of the sacroiliac joint. In the erect chimpanzee, the gluteus medius and minimus are vertical and so incapable of acting as hip rotators. Man, by tipping the pelvis forward, has brought the gluteus medius and minimus muscles into a more horizontal position where they can act as internal rotators of the hip. Because they are so much stronger than the internal rotators, the external rotators, gluteus maximus, obturator internus, and piriformis, are prone to contraction, rotating the lower extremity into a toed-out position. These shortened external rotators are prone to strain, which may cause abdominal pain as the first forewarning of hip degeneration years before X-ray changes occur. This cause of lower abdominal pain may be detected during rectal or vaginal examination, when the pain of the strained muscle is reproduced by the pressure of the examiner's finger against each of these muscles in turn. In addition to causing abdominal pain, loss of rotation at the hip joint with aging is another frequent cause of painful swelling of the knee.

There has been controversy as to whether or not movement occurs in the sacroiliac joint; but all reported research on cadavers and living subjects that I have found has led to the conclusion that there is movement throughout life in most women, and during the first half of life in men, in this joint (7 and M. F. Ivanitsky, *personal communication*). In old people, it was my clinical impression that the sacrum has moved to a position more horizontal than that which it occupies in earlier human life. This impression was verified by X-rays of the pelvis viewed laterally in a series of more than 100 patients of various ages. This change of position must occur in episodes that are not always painless. Because the sacrum is set into the pelvis on a beveled plane, it can change position only if the iliac wings separate.

Loss of lumbar lordosis and accentuation of the thoracic hump with age cause increasing wedging of lower lumbar intervertebral discs, setting the stage for disc protrusion.

TREATMENT

Although abdominal strengthening is probably the most frequently recommended exercise in posture clinics, the locomotor function of the abdominal wall remains overlooked in clinical medicine. Rehabilitative exercises are almost never prescribed for the patient who has undergone a surgical assault on the abdominal wall; yet many of my patients have experienced the onset of abdominal pain after such an operation. The tendency to overlook the locomotor function of the abdominal wall may reflect the concept that the vertebrae are comparable to the roadway of an upright suspension bridge: the cable is represented by the longitudinal muscles; the uprights supporting the cables, by the vertebral spines (10). This concept has placed great emphasis on strengthening the back muscles of patients with back pain. Kummer, a comparative anatomist, has shown that what this concept overlooks is that the uprights are fixed into the rock under the water; and that in the human, this rock is the abdominal wall (8).

Pain in the lower abdomen that is traced to age-related loss of strength in the intrapelvic muscles may be treated by exercises directed specifically to the coccygeus, obturator internus, and piriformis.

Exercises to relieve low back strain and lumbar disc pain are directed to strengthening the abdominal wall and gluteus maximus muscles to resist separation of the iliac wings.

For the pain associated with hip joint degeneration, foreshadowing femoral neck fracture, it would appear important to maintain the strength of the gluteus maximus and quadriceps femoris muscles. Climbing stairs two at a time is simple and effective.

Night cramps and pain in the knee caused by tightness of the calf are treated by stretching the calf muscles until they permit dorsiflexion of the foot to 30° beyond the 90° angle. The calves are heated by standing before a heater or soaking them in a hot bath. The patient then stands at arm's length from a door, palms on the door, heels on the floor, and pushes the pelvis forward until a pull is felt in the calves. Maintaining this position 30 sec to 1 min, a dozen times in succession, causes a rapid increase in the range of motion of both the upper and the lower ankle joints.

CONCLUSIONS

My search to understand the relations between anthropologic changes and pains caused by degenerative changes has proved rewarding in approaching patients suffering from pain of locomotor origin. It is obvious that multidisciplinary work is needed to clarify these relationships. The clinical observations suggest that coordinated efforts by workers in the disciplines of physical medicine, anthropology, neurology, and engineering would hold much promise for clarifying our understanding of and our capacity to deal effectively with a substantial portion of the aches and pains of aging.

SUMMARY

The clinical observation that lower abdominal pains incorrectly attributed to ovarian or appendiceal disease were in fact owing to strain of muscles lining the pelvis, and that they could often be relieved by correcting postural abnormalities led to inquiry into phylogenetic anatomy for explanations of such pains. Human stance and gait demand development of muscles and tendons lacking or rudimentary in other anthropoids. Characteristics of man's stance and gait as his locomotor system degenerates with age suggest reversion to an earlier evolutionary stage. Maintenance of human posture as muscles weaken may cause strain and pain. Definition of specific structures accounting for specific pains enables one to outline rational and effective therapy. Clinical results imply that pooling of information by physical anthropologists, physicians, neurologists, and engineers could lead to further definition of the causes of locomotor pains of aging and to more appropriate therapy.

ACKNOWLEDGMENTS

I gratefully acknowledge the following: Arthur Steindler, late head of the Orthopedics Department at the University of Iowa, for advice about who is doing research of practical value on the locomotor system, all of whom will be mentioned here; Donald Stilwell of the Department of Anatomy at Stanford for access to the third largest collection of skeletons in the United States; Vern Inman, head of the Department of Orthopedics of the University of California in San Francisco, for access to his collection of translations of foreign research on the locomotor system made preliminary to his research on the development of artificial limbs; Elmer Belt of Los Angeles for access to his research into Leonardo da Vinci's work on the locomotor system, a most interesting da Vinci library; Harvey Billig of Los Angeles for his ideas about mobilization of the human body; Florence and Henry Kendall of the Department of Physical Medicine at the Children's Hospital in Baltimore for their ideas about posture and pain; Charles Lowman, late head of the Orthopedics Hospital in Los Angeles, for similar help. M. Ivanitsky, head of the Department of Anatomy of the Central Institute of Physical Education of the U.S.S.R., for the gift of five books describing the work of his institute; Janet Travell for, among many other things, her research on trigger points, and for interesting the Defense Department in the translation of Dr. Ivanitsky's text; and to Dr. Philip Lee, former director of H.E.W. and chancellor of the medical school of the University of California in San Francisco, for interesting the National Library of Medicine in translating the others; E. Hintszge, former head of the Department of Anatomy at Bern, for the opportunity to study Strasser's anatomical models and for the gift of five volumes of Strasser's and R. Fich's anatomy texts; Benno Kummer of the Department of Anatomy at Cologne for his volume on mammalian anatomy; Sidney Garfield and the National Institute of Medicine for grants for construction of anatomical models by Harry Richardson; the Ducroquets in Paris for their incomparable hospitality and research on gait; M. R. Francillon of Zurich for his hospitality and introduction to the electromyography research on gait; Sherwood Washburn of the Department of Anthropology of the University of California in Berkeley and Adrienne Zihlman of the same department (now at University of California in Santa Cruz) for hours of thought, dissection, and advice; my wife for her forebearance; Ruth Strauss for her writing ability; and others too numerous to mention.

REFERENCES

1. Bluntschli, H. (1913): *Verh. Anat. Ges.*, 27:43–46.
2. Broca, P. (1870): *Ordre des Primates Parallèle Anatomique de l'Homme et des Singes,* p. 171. Reinwald, Paris.
3. Ducroquet, R., Ducroquet, J., and Ducroquet, P. (1968): *Walking and Limping. A Study of Normal and Pathological Walking,* translated by W. S. Hunter and J. Hunter, pp. 76–80. J. B. Lippincott Co., Philadelphia.
4. Fick, R. (1925): *S.-B. Dtsch. Akad. Wiss., Kl. Phys.-Math. Wiss.*, 6, 11:162–197.
5. Hunter, W., and Zihlman, A. L. (1970): *Clin. Orthop.*, 71:279–280.
6. Kendall, H. O., Kendall, F. P., and Boynton, D. A. (1952): *Posture and Pain,* p. 10. Williams & Wilkins Co., Baltimore.
7. Klein, G. (1891): *Z. Geburtshilfe Perinatol.*, 21:74–118.
8. Kummer, B. (1959): *Bauprinzipien des Säugerskelettes,* pp. 43–46. George Thieme Verlag, Stuttgart.
9. Preuschoft, H. (1963): *Anthropol. Anz.*, 26:308–317.
10. Tschachmachtschjan, H. (1919): *Morph. Jb. (Leipzig)*, 44:297–370.
11. Vallois, H. V. (1928): *Ann. Sci. Nat. Zool.,* Series 10, 11:1–65.
12. von Meyer, G. H. (1873): *Die Statik und Mechanik des menschlichen Knochengerüstes,* pp. 192–194. Wilhelm Engelmann, Leipzig.

Advances in Pain Research and Therapy, Vol. 1,
edited by J. J. Bonica and D. Albe-Fessard.
Raven Press, New York © 1976.

Electrogenic Nature of Palpable Bands and "Jump Sign" Associated with Myofascial Trigger Points

David G. Simons

Veterans Administration Hospital, Long Beach, California 90801; and Department of Physical Medicine and Rehabilitation, University of California, Irvine, California 92664

Myofascial pain syndromes are a common source of pain that is frequently disregarded because of difficulty in locating the trigger point or trigger area responsible for the pain. Objectively, both active and latent trigger areas are characteristically found at one point along a rope-like band of muscle that is identifiable by a particular palpation technique. This technique of palpation may produce a "jump sign" (J. Travell, *this volume*) that commonly responds more vigorously to palpation of more active trigger areas. Also objectively, both kinds of trigger points are commonly associated with some weakness and reduced range of motion of an affected muscle group. Subjectively, both active and latent trigger points consistently evidence localized exquisite tenderness to digital palpation. However, only an active trigger point is responsible for clinical pain that the patient may describe as constant or intermittent, present at rest, or associated with muscular activity. Pain is referred to remarkably constant areas which, depending on what muscle contains the trigger point, may be local or remote parts of the body (15,16). Usually only an active trigger point will respond to sustained pressure by producing pain in its reference zone. This typical referred pain pattern is frequently produced when either an active or a latent trigger point is penetrated by a needle.

The term "jump sign," as used by Travell (*this volume*), indicates a finger-like dimpling, or slow, circumscribed twitch of the skin overlying the band of muscle fibers that are responding to palpation of that band of muscle. The "jump sign" looks and feels as if the mechanical stimulus of palpating the band has elicited a transient contraction of just those fibers in the band of muscle. In some muscles it may also be seen as a twitch of the body segment activated by that muscle. Muscles such as the pectoralis major, latissimus dorsi, extensor digitorum communis, gluteus maximus, and peroneus longus are likely to show jump signs.

The nature of this band, and to some its very existence, remain controversial. The anatomical nature of the trigger area and its neurophysiological relation to the band are unknown. The tender palpable band associated with the myofascial pain syndrome has previously been identified as fibrositis or fibrositic nodules (7,13), commonly as muscular (10) or nonarticular rheumatism (12), and as myogelosis (9) or muscle hardenings (6). Both light microscopic (2,8) and ultramicroscopic (1,4) changes have been reported which, in only a few cases, fully account for the palpable changes in muscle consistency.

Electromyographically, motor unit action potentials (MUAPs) were reported in association with pain into a deltoid muscle reference zone (17). Elliott (3) reported bursts of motor unit activity in response to deep palpation; the relation to trigger zones or reference zones was not clear. Electromyographic examination of muscles at rest specifically in the region of the trigger zone showed no motor unit activity (5).

The localized twitch (14) of the jump sign suggests the contraction of a localized band of fibers in response to palpation. The author has reported the visible contraction of localized bands, palpated in a dog muscle that was widely exposed for muscle biopsy (11).

To determine whether the mechanical stimulation of firm, brisk palpation induces localized motor unit activity characteristic of transient contraction, we studied palpable bands containing trigger points in different muscles in 3 people. Subjects were two volunteers, a man 52 and a woman 73 years old without pain complaints (latent trigger points), and a 46-year-old male patient with a chronic right rotator cuff tear and rest pain over the deltoid muscle.

METHODS

A Teca TR-4 electromyograph using one or two channels and direct-print photographic recording was used with small Teca surface electrodes at active sites and a 2×3 cm plate for the ground. A 3.9-cm Teflon®-coated monopolar electromyogram needle was inserted intramuscularly.

RESULTS

Quadriceps

Three tender palpable bands of the quadriceps femoris were identified most likely in the vastus lateralis, rectus femoris, and the vastus medialis muscles (Fig. 1) in the male volunteer. The central band was approximately 14 cm long. The shorter adjacent bands were nearly parallel to and 4 cm to either side of it. The needle was placed in the proximal end of the central band and the other active electrode was placed near it. Voluntary contraction produced normal 200- to 600-μV MUAPs with the needle tip in the palpable band (Fig. 1A). Motion artifact with a few isolated MUAPs was produced by gently tapping the needle (Fig. 1H). Snapping palpation was used to

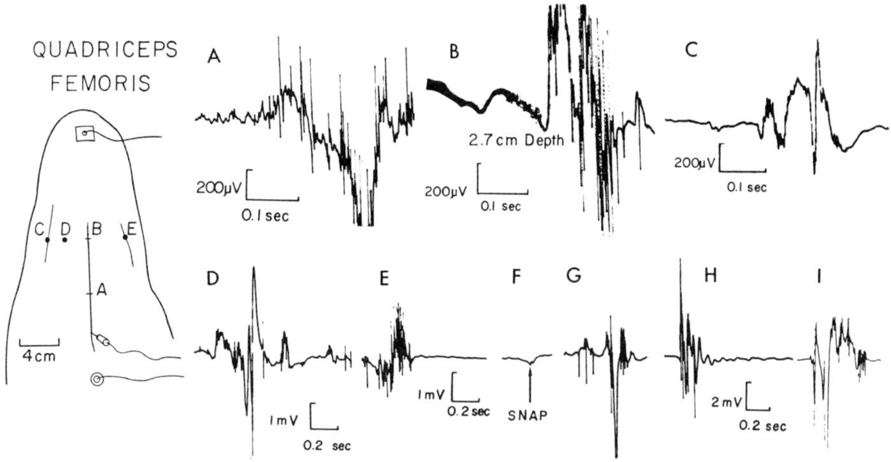

FIG. 1. Quadriceps femoris responses. **A:** Voluntary contraction. **B:** Snap at **A,** needle in band. **C:** Snap at **A,** needle out of band. **D:** Snap at **B,** in same band. **E:** Snap at **C,** in another band. **F:** Snap at **D,** between bands. **G:** Snap at **E,** in another band. **H:** Tap on needle. **I:** Tendon tap response. Calibrations for **F, G,** and **I** same as for **E.**

stimulate the monitored band 4 and 9 cm from the needle, to stimulate the two adjacent bands, and to stimulate similarly the intervening muscle that was free of a palpable band. Mechanical stimulation at point A (Fig. 1) produced a burst of 500-μV MUAPs which lasted 0.2 sec and were superimposed on motion artifact (Fig. 1B). After the needle was withdrawn 5 mm, snapping palpation at point A produced a similar motion artifact but less than 100-μV potentials which appeared and sounded like remote MUAPs (Fig. 1C). Reinserting the needle 5 mm restored the previous response as in Fig. 1B. Snapping palpation at point B in the same band produced a less-intense MUAP response (Fig. 1D) with potentials of amplitude and configuration similar to those in Fig. 1B.

Palpation of adjacent bands produced approximately 0.2-sec bursts of MUAPs (Fig. 1E and G). Palpation of intervening band-free muscle elicited no such response (Fig. 1F). Tendon tap responses (Fig. 1I) show the expected synchronized response, then more isolated discharges.

Deltoid

One active and one latent trigger area was identified in parallel palpable bands approximately 4 cm long lying 2.5 cm apart in the right middle deltoid. Pressure on band A reproduced the shoulder pain (active trigger area). Simultaneous recordings were made from needle electrodes placed near the trigger area in each band (Fig. 2). Both bands responded to voluntary contraction with similar motor unit activity patterns (Fig. 2A). Snapping

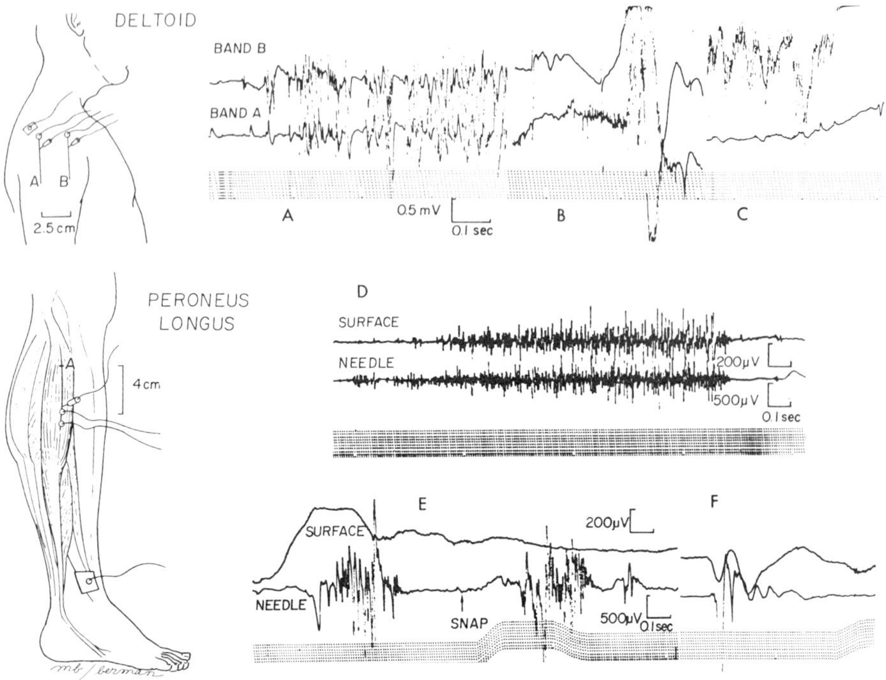

FIG. 2. Deltoid responses. **A:** Voluntary contraction. **B:** Snap of band **A**. **C:** Snap of band **B**. Calibrations for **B** and **C** same as for **A**. Peroneus longus responses. **D:** Voluntary contraction. **E:** Snap at **A**. **F:** Snap beside band.

palpation of first one and then the other band produced some motion artifact in both records, most marked in the snapped band. Band A responded to palpation (Fig. 2B) with intermittent bursts of motor unit activity for 0.35 sec preceding the motion artifact, and continuously through the motion artifact for a total duration of 0.5 sec. A burst of MUAPs appeared in band B 0.35 sec later and for only 0.1 sec. Snapping of band B (Fig. 2C) generated a sustained burst of MUAPs that preceded motion artifact for 0.4 sec and continued into motion artifact. Band A showed no response during the evoked electrical activity of band B.

Peroneus Longus

A palpable band 5 cm long associated with a latent trigger point was identified at point A in the left peroneus longus muscle of the other normal volunteer (Fig. 2). A needle electrode was inserted into the band near its distal end. Surface electrodes beside the needle recorded more widespread electrical activity of the muscle. Gain was adjusted so that voluntary activity generated responses of similar amplitude (Fig. 2D). The region of the trigger point in the band was stimulated by snapping palpation 4 cm proximal to the needle. Bursts of MUAPs appeared in the band throughout a period of 1.0 to 1.4 sec while none appeared on the surface electrode (Fig. 1E). Jump sign responses (eversion twitch of the foot) were seen during the audible burst of motor unit activity. Palpation of adjacent band-free muscle produced motion artifact without motor unit action potentials (Fig. 2F). A response suggesting a differentiated galvanic skin response appeared on the surface electrodes. Slow snaps of 1.0- to 1.5-sec duration produced less intense and more scattered motor unit activity than fast snaps of 0.25- to 0.5-sec duration. Motor unit responses gradually disappeared after dozens of stimulations over a period of 45 min.

DISCUSSION

Consistently, early palpations of sufficient vigor revealed MUAP responses when the tip of the monitoring electromyographic needle was within a few millimeters of the center of the same palpable band. This was consistent with the specific response of bands of canine muscle fibers to palpation (11) and with the "jump sign" observed in man (J. Travell, *this volume*). In some cases the band was palpable when no electrical activity was observed. Palpation of one band often elicited electrical response from another band in the same muscle group. The electrical response to palpation appeared to be specific to the fibers within a palpable band, and to be absent in band-free portions of the muscle. Palpation of band-free muscle produced no electrical response. These observations show that palpable bands of at least some muscles may exhibit a hyperirritable response to mechanical stimulation that can produce transient motor unit activity in it and adjacent bands. Clinically, one frequently encounters bands that respond only when snapped vigorously. Failure to recognize this characteristic could readily account for the difficulty some individuals encounter when trying to locate these bands. It could also account for some of the controversy associated with their nature and existence.

Two features suggest a hyperirritable spinal reflex phenomenon: the increased motor unit response with increasingly vigorous palpation and the simultaneous activation of adjacent palpable bands. Although muscle spindles immediately come to mind for the afferent limb, the close association with pain calls for consideration of other muscle afferents. A localized myotonic response may contribute to the contraction.

Once located, the palpable band is useful because it provides objective indication of the location and sensitivity of the trigger point within the band, and provides a good landmark for injecting the trigger point. The decreasing vigor of electrical response with repeated mechanical stimulation recalls the use of massage and *Shiatzu* (thumb pressure) as treatment.

CONCLUSIONS

Hyperirritable areas (latent and active trigger points) were located along palpable bands of muscle. Snapping palpation of such a band resulted in a transient burst of MUAPs which were restricted to the vicinity of a palpable band. The "jump sign" appears to be the result of this transient burst of MUAPs. The palpable characteristics of the bands associated with trigger points appear, at least in part, to be generated by the process of palpation.

REFERENCES

1. Awad, E. A. (1973): *Arch. Phys. Med. Rehabil.*, 54:449–453.
2. Brendstrup, P., Jespersen, K., and Asboe-Hansen, G. (1957): *Ann. Rheum Dis.*, 16:438–440.
3. Elliott, F. A. (1944): *Lancet*, 1:47–49.
4. Fassbender, H. G., and Wegner, K. (1973): *Z. Rheumatol.*, 32:355–374.
5. Kraft, G. H., Johnson, E. W., and LeBan, M. M. (1968): *Arch. Phys. Med. Rehabil.*, 49:155–162.
6. Lange, F., and Eversbusch, G. (1921): *Munch. Med. Wochenschr.*, 68:418–420.
7. Llewellyn, L. J., and Jones, A. B. (1915): *Fibrositis.* Heinemann, London.
8. Miehlke, K., Schulze, G., and Eger, W. (1960): *Z. Rheumatol.*, 19:310–330.
9. Schade, H. (1919): *Z. Gesamte Exp. Med.*, 7:275–374.
10. Schmidt, A. (1916): *Munch. Med. Wochenschr.*, 63:593–595.
11. Simons, D. G., and Stolov, W. C. (1976): *Am. J. Phys. Med.*, 55:65–88.
12. Smythe, H. A. (1972): In: *Arthritis and Allied Conditions, Ed. 8*, edited by J. L. Hollander and D. J. McCarty, pp. 874–884. Lea & Febiger, Philadelphia.
13. Stockman, R. (1920): *Rheumatism and Arthritis.* W. Green, Edinburgh.
14. Travell, J. (1952): In: *Connective Tissues; Transactions of the Second Conference*, edited by C. Ragan. Josiah Macy, Jr., Foundation, New York.
15. Travell, J. (1955): *N.Y. State J. Med.*, 55:331–339.
16. Travell, J. (1967): *Headache*, 7:23–29.
17. Travell, J., Berry, C., and Bigelow, N. (1944): *Fed. Proc.*, 3:49.

Advances in Pain Research and Therapy, Vol. 1,
edited by J. J. Bonica and D. Albe-Fessard.
Raven Press, New York © 1976.

Myofascial Trigger Points: Clinical View

Janet Travell

Department of Medicine, George Washington University School of Medicine, Washington, D.C. 20037

BASIC CONCEPTS

Clinical studies on many hundreds of patients (16–22,27,29,32–35,38,39) show that chronic painful states of obscure causes often depend on feedback cycles from myofascial trigger points and their pain reference zones (Fig. 1). Symptoms long outlast precipitating events, owing to perseverating reflex patterns and continuing mechanical stresses on affected somatic structures. When injured, most tissues heal, but skeletal muscles "learn"; they readily develop habits of guarding that limit movement and impair circulation. Chronic pain, stiffness, and dysfunction of muscles result.

Myofascial structures, like viscera, refer pain in predictable patterns (7,14,19,21,22,34,35) which do not follow a simple segmental distribution (26) but which are specific for a given site of origin. This constancy of myofascial pain distribution enables one to use the patterns of referred pain, once they have been learned, to locate trigger points responsible for the pain.

In these clinical entities, neurological deficits are not observed unless a muscle that harbors a trigger point entraps a peripheral nerve. Then inconsistent sensory and motor signs may confuse the diagnosis. Trigger point pain is deep and aching, whereas ischemic-compression nerve pain is prickling, tingling, and numbing.

THE TRIGGER POINT: ACTIVE AND LATENT WITH RESPECT TO PAIN

A trigger point in a skeletal muscle is identified by localized deep tenderness in a palpably firm band of muscle [muscle hardening (9)]; and at the point of maximum deep hyperalgesia by a positive "jump sign" (21), a visible shortening of that part of the muscle which contains the band. To elicit the jump sign most effectively, one must place the relaxed muscle under moderate passive tension and snap the band briskly with the palpating finger. This procedure evokes local pain and perhaps a secondary jump by the patient.

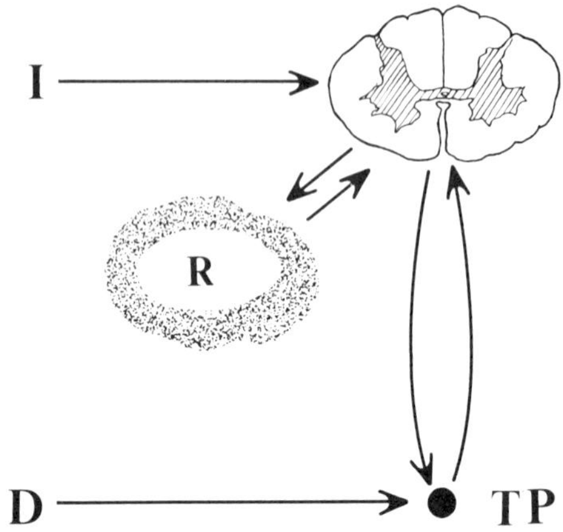

FIG. 1. Theoretical pathways of separate feedback cycles which link trigger point (TP, ●) and its pain reference zone (R) with the CNS. Relationship of trigger point with reference zone remains the same whether noxious stimuli act directly (D) on the trigger point or indirectly (I) through the spinal cord. It is evident that afferent inputs from trigger point and reference zone may summate in pain perception and may reinforce each other's efferent discharges.

Induction of referred pain during sustained pressure on the trigger point is reported by the patient if the trigger point is actively causing episodes of referred pain and its threshold to mechanical stimulation is relatively low. In the case of *latent* trigger points, however, which are clinically asymptomatic with respect to pain, induction of referred pain is not reported during similar sustained pressure. A latent trigger point does exhibit deep tenderness and a positive jump sign on vigorous snapping; referred pain may also be evoked by accurate insertion of a needle into the point.

The muscle which contains a trigger point, even a latent one, is further identified by the presence of weakness on active contraction, without atrophy over long periods, and by some degree of restricted motion at the joint or joints traversed by the apparently shortened muscle. Although its identification is in part subjective, the trigger point is actually a physical sign, disclosed primarily on physical examination.

Normal muscle does not contain trigger points, is not tender to ordinary pressure, and does not give a jump sign. With advancing age, many people who do not complain of pain to a physician have accumulated unsuspected latent trigger points; these may persist for years after seeming recovery from an injury. Nevertheless, these dormant trigger mechanisms predispose to attacks of musculoskeletal pain. Latent trigger points are readily activated by minor stresses such as periods of immobility, overstretching of muscles, overuse in repetitive movement or prolonged static effort, and chilling during fatigue. Simple strains are more likely to activate latent trigger points after alcohol ingestion and during convalescence from infectious illness.

COINCIDENTAL PATHOPHYSIOLOGY

Nerve root compression owing to discogenic disease may activate trigger points in the segmental distribution of pain. This fact may explain the post-disc syndrome of continuing pain when surgery was successful but the debris of referred myofascial pain was not cleared away.

Remote lesions in joints, and also chronic visceral disease and dysfunction, may provide the noxious feedback which perpetuates trigger points (14); the somatic component of cardiac pain is a clear example (16,17,19, 30,31). The converse is also true of somatovisceral reflexes from trigger points which may reinforce and perpetuate a dysfunctional disorder of a viscus, for example, a cardiac ectopic rhythm (12,24). Emotional stimuli of psychogenic tension and conversion hysteria (27) may also serve as the major perpetuating factor in some myofascial pain syndromes.

Uncorrected hypothyroidism and estrogen deficiency, hyperuricemia, a chronic focus of infection, mild anemia, low potassium or calcium reserves, low "normal" (not optimal) blood levels of ascorbic acid with diminished vitamin C content of the adrenal cortex, and vitamin B deficiencies with impaired vibratory perception constitute systemic factors which appear to predispose to chronicity of trigger points. Their causes, direct and indirect (Fig. 1), are almost always multiple (23).

PAIN REFERENCE ZONE

In pain reference zones of trigger points actively causing pain, one observes diffuse deep tenderness; increased motor unit activity at rest during induction of referred pain, but no such increased activity in muscles nearby but outside the reference zone (25); and vasomotor, secretory, and other autonomic changes (19). Vasoconstriction, pallor, sweating, and coldness of the skin may be evident during intense referred pain; vasodilatation is observed at once after extinction of the responsible trigger point by local injection.

Latent trigger points, in the absence of referred pain, may be associated with diffuse "soreness" in related reference zones.

Secondary outpost, or satellite, trigger points eventually develop in reference zones of chronically active trigger points and give rise to overlapping patterns of pain. Thus trigger points in the sternal division of the sternocleidomastoid muscle (21,22) refer pain to the sternum and are often associated with satellites in the sternalis muscle on the front of the sternum. These, in turn, refer pain deep beneath the sternum and across the upper pectoral regions. Outposts may then develop in the pectoralis major muscles and refer pain and "soreness" into the breast (mastalgia) and, further, diffusely in the pectoral area, the front of the shoulder, and the ulnar distribution of the upper extremity. The chain reaction initiated perhaps by a neck strain now mimics the pain of coronary artery disease.

Another mechanism for the chain reaction of referred pain is reflex splinting of muscles that function together as a myotatic (mechanical) unit. Parallel or semiparallel lines share the work with that muscle which contains the primary trigger point and tend to develop secondary trigger points with the passage of time. In the patient who complains of long-standing pain, the most acute and intense referred pain pattern is likely to derive from the trigger point which was added last in the chain.

EXTINCTION OF TRIGGER POINTS

Local treatment of myofascial pain syndromes must be directed primarily at trigger points where pain originates, rather than at reference zones where pain is felt. Therapy is based on dry needling and injection of active trigger points, or stimulation of the overlying skin representation of affected muscles by a vapocoolant spray or other kinds of counterirritation. For all types of trigger point therapy, the goal is restoration of normal resting muscle length and a full range of motion, achieved first by passive stretching during the period of action of the therapeutic modality, and finally by active effort under a light load.

Spray-Stretch Procedure

The intermittent application of intense cold was found (5) to be the most effective counterirritant for relief of experimentally induced deep pain. On-and-off ice massage (11) is useful at times. In my hands, the light application of a vapocoolant spray over affected muscles by a special technique (Fig. 2), with simultaneous passive stretching of these muscles (11,18,22), often obtains dramatic benefit. This noninvasive therapeutic method influences deep and inaccessible trigger points by neurogenic reflex effects from the skin (33). It also permits treatment of numerous muscle groups within a relatively short time. If certain precautions are taken to avoid sudden quick overstretching and direct cooling of underlying muscle by excessive cold (Fig. 2), the risk of severe afterpain, sometimes seen after local injection of trigger points, is minimized. Lowering of skeletal muscle temperature has been shown to cause deleterious changes (10): a delay in the development of twitch tension, a decrease in its peak, delay in relaxation, and a marked decrease in the frequency of stimulation necessary to produce tetanic fusion.

I have not used ethyl chloride spray in approximately 20 years. I prefer a fluoromethane spray mixture (Fluori-Methane Spray®, calibrated nozzle; composition: 15% dichlorodifluoromethane and 85% trichloromonofluoromethane). The liquid, as propelled from the bottle, is sterile but not bactericidal. The fine-calibrated nozzle delivers a jet stream which induces intense spot cooling and contrast with the normal skin temperature; a nozzle which delivers a mist is much less effective. This spray mixture has advan-

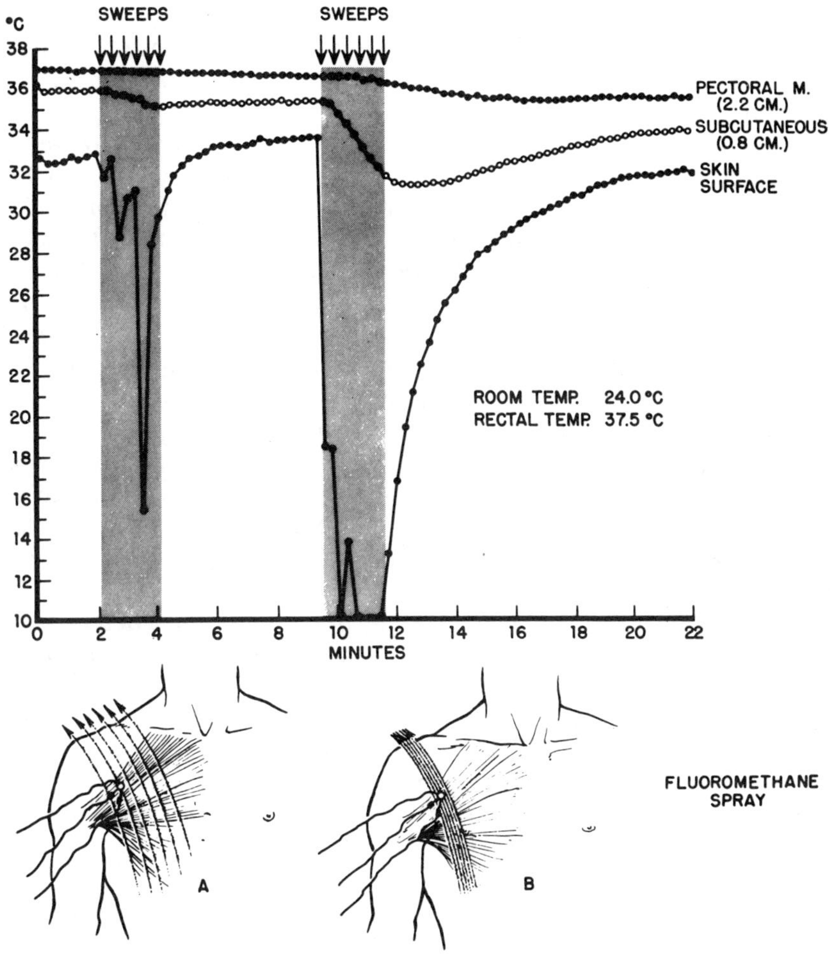

FIG. 2. Degree of muscle cooling by correct and incorrect techniques of applying Fluori-Methane Spray®. Temperatures were recorded by a tier of 3 needle electrodes from: (1) pectoral muscle (*upper line*) at a depth of 2.2 cm; (2) subcutaneous tissue (*middle curve*) at a depth of 0.8 cm; and (3) skin surface (*bottom curve*). Fluoromethane jet stream was applied in 6 slow, even sweeps in one direction during 2 min. In **A** (*left half of graph*), sweeps covered adjacent skin areas and only 1 sweep traversed the tier of electrodes. In **B** (*right half of graph*), all 6 sweeps traversed the same path directly over the 3 electrodes. When a given skin area was covered only once **(A)** by the jet stream, the fall in muscle temperature was negligible, 0.2°; but muscle temperature dropped 1.5° in **B,** starting during jet stream application and continuing during rewarming of the overlying subcutaneous tissue.

tages over ethyl chloride in that it is not flammable or explosive, it is not a general anesthetic, and it has slightly less cooling power (39). Ethyl chloride is too cold as usually applied (3). With proper instruction of the patient and a sound diagnosis, the physician can safely dispense Fluori-Methane Spray for home use. It must be kept in mind that if inhaled, as from an aerosol asthma spray, fluoromethane gas is absorbed from the lungs and appears briefly in the bloodstream (13), and under conditions of hypoxia it may be toxic. Urticaria owing to cold allergy was observed in only 1 patient, in the region sprayed with ethyl chloride.

The spray-stretch procedure is carried out as follows. After active trigger points are identified and the extent of restricted motion is noted, voluntary relaxation is encouraged by proper support of the part and instruction of the patient. The jet stream of the spray is directed at an acute angle with the skin over the affected muscle and is applied in one direction, from the trigger point toward its reference zone, in slow, even sweeps over *adjacent* skin areas. Sweeps travel at a rate of approximately 10 cm (4 inches) per second. In this manner, a given area of the skin is covered by the spray only once or perhaps twice; six sweeps over the same skin area are too many and may cool the muscle underneath (Fig. 2).

It is not desirable to frost the skin. Extinction of trigger points does not require refrigeration anesthesia of the surface, as originally suggested (8); nerve conduction block by cold occurs at approximately 10°C or below. This level of cooling is not reached by the correct application of the vapocoolant (Fig. 2).

During the unhurried, rhythmic spraying, passive stretching of the specific muscle is applied with steady, gradually increasing force, holding the stretch at a tolerably painful point which does not induce reflex contraction of the muscle or general guarding. Skin and subcutaneous temperatures require approximately 5 min to rewarm (Fig. 2). During this time, hot, moist packs are applied to the sprayed region while the spray-stretch procedure is carried out on another area of the body, to which hot packs are also applied.

Spraying may be repeated for any given area several times after adequate rewarming. The range of passive and active motion is tested before and after each procedure and serves as a guide to the response to therapy. Spray application should be carried out not only over identifiable trigger points, but also over related reference zones to eliminate their feedback and potential satellite trigger points.

If spray-stretch fails, even with repeated trials, direct needling and injection of trigger points may still permanently relieve pain and restore lost mobility.

The chief causes of failure of the correct spray-stretch procedure are inability to secure full muscle length because of bone or joint abnormalities, and probably a subordination of the reflex mechanisms of trigger point pain to fibrosis or some other pathology in the muscle itself.

Trigger Point Injection

In my experience, dry needling and physiologic saline injection of trigger points have proved effective (16,28) but much more painful to the patient than is the injection of a local anesthetic into trigger points of comparable irritability. Furthermore, in concentrations less than those required for nerve conduction block, local anesthetics have other actions that may be beneficial (4): they markedly lengthen the relative refractory period of peripheral nerves and limit the maximum frequency of impulse conduction.

For purely fascial trigger points, as in joint capsules, ligaments, and bursae, I inject a corticosteroid compound with a local anesthetic, usually procaine. For trigger points within skeletal muscles, I prefer procaine hydrochloride in 0.5% solution made isotonic with sodium chloride and with added bacteriostatic material that is nonirritant and that preferably has some local anesthetic effect, for example, benzyl alcohol or chlorobutanol (20). Details of local injection procedures (22,29,35) have been amply described in the literature, modified somewhat by each physician.

My preference for procaine is based on its high record of safety for local injection and on the versatility (6) of its pharmacological actions. In addition to its effects on peripheral nerves, it is a vasodilator (1) and it relaxes muscle directly through a curare-like action. Furthermore, it has been recently shown (2) that procaine and its degradation product, para-aminobenzoic acid, can restore the spherical shape of "irreversibly" sickled red blood cells by mediating the flux of trapped calcium ions through the cell membrane. It is also known (15,36,37) that the caffeine rigor of skeletal muscle, which is due to binding of calcium ions, is blocked by procaine.

SUMMARY

The important role of myofascial trigger points in musculoskeletal pain, their etiology, and specific techniques for their extinction have been presented. These conditions are among the most important causes of painful disability. Their importance stems partially from their frequency. Perhaps more importantly, many physicians fail to recognize and treat them, but if these conditions are promptly diagnosed and effectively treated patients are spared prolonged disability.

REFERENCES

1. Altura, B. M., and Altura, B. T. (1974): *Anesthesiology,* 41:197–214.
2. Baker, R., Powars, D., and Haywood, L. J. (1974): *Biochem. Biophys. Res. Commun.,* 59:548–556.
3. Borken, N., and Bierman, W. (1955): *Arch. Phys. Med.,* 36:288–290.
4. Condouris, G. A. (1966): *Pharmacologist,* 8:187.
5. Gammon, G. D., and Starr, I. (1941): *J. Clin. Invest.,* 20:13–20.
6. Harrison, G. G. (1971): *Br. Med. J.,* 3:454–456.
7. Kellgren, J. H. (1938): *Br. Med. J.,* 1:325–327; and *Clin. Sci.,* 3:175–190.
8. Kraus, H. (1941): *J.A.M.A.,* 116:2582–2587.
9. Kraus, H. (1973): *N.Y. State Med. J.,* 73:1310–1314.
10. Maclagan, J., and Zaimis, E. (1957): *J. Physiol.,* 137:89–90.
11. Mennell, J. M. (1975): *J.A.O.A.,* 74:1146–1158.

12. Mennell, J. M., and Travell, J. (1974): *Spray-Stretch for Relief of Pain and Muscle Spasm.* Scientific Film.
13. Paterson, J. W., Sudlow, M. F., and Walker, S. R. (1971): *Lancet,* 2:565–568.
14. Sinclair, D. C., Weddell, G., and Feindel, W. H. (1948): *Brain,* 71:184–211.
15. Strobel, G. E. (1971): *Lancet,* 1:40.
16. Travell, J. (1949): *Miss. Valley Med. J.,* 21:13–21.
17. Travell, J. (1951): *Circulation,* 3:120–124.
18. Travell, J. (1952*a*): *Arch. Phys. Med.,* 33:291–298.
19. Travell, J. (1952*b*): In: *Connective Tissue (Transactions of the Second Conference),* edited by C. Ragan, pp. 86–125. Josiah Macy, Jr., Foundation, New York.
20. Travell, J. (1955*a*): *J.A.M.A.,* 158:368–371.
21. Travell, J. (1955*b*): *N.Y. State J. Med.,* 55:331–340.
22. Travell, J. (1960): *J. Prosthet. Dent.,* 10:745–763.
23. Travell, J. (1967): *Headache,* 7:23–29.
24. Travell, J. (1969): *Office Hours: Day and Night,* pp. 248–304. World Publishing Company, New York.
25. Travell, J., Berry, C., and Bigelow, N. H. (1944): *Fed. Proc.,* 3:49.
26. Travell, J., and Bigelow, N. H. (1946): *Fed. Proc.,* 5:106.
27. Travell, J., and Bigelow, N. H. (1947): *Psychosom. Med.,* 9:353–363.
28. Travell, J., and Bobb, A. L. (1947): *Fed. Proc.,* 6:378.
29. Travell, J., and Travell, W. (1946*a*): *Arch. Phys. Med.,* 27:537–547.
30. Travell, J., and Rinzler, S. H. (1946*b*): *Proc. Soc. Exp. Biol. Med.,* 63:480–482.
31. Travell, J., and Rinzler, S. H. (1948*a*): *Am. Heart J.,* 35:248–268.
32. Travell, J., and Rinzler, S. H. (1948*b*): *Can. Med. Assoc. J.,* 59:333–338.
33. Travell, J., and Rinzler, S. H. (1949): *Fed. Proc.,* 8:339.
34. Travell, J., and Rinzler, S. H. (1952): *Postgrad. Med.,* 9:425–434.
35. Travell, J., Rinzler, S. H., and Herman, M. (1942): *J.A.M.A.,* 120:417–422.
36. Weber, A., and Herz, R. (1969): *J. Gen. Physiol.,* 52:750, 760 ff.
37. Weed, R. I., LaCelle, P. L., and Merrill, E. W. (1969): *J. Clin. Invest.,* 48:795–809.
38. Weeks, V. D., and Travell, J. (1955): *J. Pediatr.,* 47:315–327.
39. Weeks, V. D., and Travell, J. (1957): *AMA Scientific Exhibits Volume,* pp. 318–322. Grune & Stratton, New York.

Advances in Pain Research and Therapy, Vol. 1,
edited by J. J. Bonica and D. Albe-Fessard.
Raven Press, New York © 1976.

Treatment of Chronic Low Back Pain and Sciatica: Comparison of Caudal Epidural Injections of Bupivacaine and Methylprednisolone with Bupivacaine Followed by Saline

Harald Breivik, *Per E. Hesla, István Molnar, and Bjørn Lind

*Departments of Anesthesiology and *Neurology, University of Oslo, Akershus Central Hospital, N-1474 Nordbyhagen, Norway*

Patients suffering from low back pain and sciatica have been treated with epidural anesthesia for nearly five decades (2,6,8,12) and with epidurally applied steroids with or without local anesthetic solutions for two decades (1–5,7,9–11,14–17). The large number of reports concluding that such epidural medication gives relief to many patients suggests that the technique may be useful. However, only a few well-controlled studies have been performed: in acute and subacute cases a majority of patients benefit, and it has been shown that epidurally applied steroids alone (7) and epidural anesthesia without steroids (2,6) and with steroids (2) are about equally effective in relieving the pain and shortening the time the patient is unable to work because of pain.

In chronic cases a smaller proportion of patients are helped by epidural medication, and it appears that epidural steroids may be more effective than epidural anesthesia in these patients (2,15). Some authors feel that epidural anesthesia is more effective when given with a large volume of solution (6,8,12). We have previously made similar observations: a few patients with chronic low back pain and sciatica were dramatically relieved by epidural anesthesia followed by a large volume of saline. The present study was, therefore, undertaken to compare in a controlled way the effects of epidural anesthesia followed by a large volume of saline with those of an epidurally applied local anesthetic solution and a steroid on patients with chronic low back pain and sciatica.

MATERIAL AND METHODS

Thirty-five patients with incapacitating chronic low back pain and sciatica unresponsive to conservative treatment for several months to several years were studied. Eleven patients had previously undergone surgery for prolapsed intervertebral discs. Thirty-two patients had radiculography with metrizamide[1] before the injections showing arachnoiditis in eight, prolapsed disc in eight, no abnormality in eleven, and inconclusive findings in five (Tables 1 and 2).

The patients were admitted to the neurologic ward for evaluation before

TABLE 1: PRIMARY injection: BUPIVACAINE and DEPOTMETHYLPREDNISOLONE

Radiculo-graphy	Norm?		Norm	Norm?	Norm	Prol	Norm	Prol	Arach	Prol	Arach	Norm?	Norm?	Norm?	Prol	Arach
Surgery									x2	x1	x1					x2
Injections	1	1	2	3	3	3	3	3	3	3	2	3	3	3	3	3
PAIN-RELIEF	+	+	+	+	+	+	+	+	+	-	-	worse	worse	-	-	-
OBJECTIVE IMPROVEM.	-	-	+	+	+	+	+	-	+	-	-	-	-	-	-	-
									SUBSEQUENT inj. of BUPIVACAINE and SALINE							
Injections												1	1	1	3	3
PAIN-RELIEF												-	worse	+	-	-
OBJECTIVE IMPROVEM.												-	-	+	-	-
Working	+	-	+	+	+	+	+	+	+	-	-	-	-	+	-	-
Obs. time months	18	18	13	12	10	11	8	3	3	19	12	20	16	9	3	3
Relapse after mos.	9				7	6								6		

N = 16. Eight women, eight men. 30 - 63 years old.
Prol = prolapsed disc. Arach = arachnoiditis. Norm? = probably not normal

the treatment, and the first caudal epidural injection was usually given while the patient was in the hospital. Subsequent injections were given in the outpatient clinic. The anesthesiologists gave each patient up to three caudal epidural injections at weekly intervals.

According to a list of random numbers, the patients were given either 20 ml bupivacaine 0.25% with 80 mg depotmethylprednisolone (Depo-Medrol®) or 20 ml bupivacaine 0.25% followed by 100 ml saline. If there was no improvement 3 weeks after the last injection, up to three injections of the alternative type were given. All patients received similar regimens of medical and physical therapy. The patients, as well as the neurologist who evaluated the results of treatment, were unaware of the type of injection given. The results were evaluated according to the effects on severity of pain, hypo- or anesthesia, Lasègue's test, paresis, spinal reflexes, and sphincter disorders. Considerable relief was defined as significant diminution of pain and/or paresis to a degree which enabled the patient to return to work or to be rehabilitated to other work.

[1] Nyco, Oslo, Norway.

TABLE 2: PRIMARY injection: BUPIVACAINE followed by SALINE

Radiculography		Norm	Norm	Prol	Prol	Norm	Norm	Norm	Arach	Prol	Arach	Arach	Arach	Norm	Prol	Norm	Arach	Norm	
Surgery									x2		x1	x1	x1		x1		x2		x2
Injections	3	2	2	3	1	3	1	3	3	3	3	3	3	3	3	2	3	2	2
PAIN-RELIEF	+	+	+	+	+	–	worse	–	–	–	–	–	–	–	–	–	–	worse	–
OBJECTIVE IMPROVEM.	+	+	+	+	+	–	–	–	–	–	–	–	–	–	–	–	–	–	–
									SUBSEQUENT inj. of BUPIVACAINE and DEPOTMETHYLPREDNISOLONE										
Injections									3	3	2	3	3	2	3	3	3	3	2
PAIN-RELIEF									+	+	+	+	+	+	+	+	–	–	–
OBJECTIVE IMPROVEM.									+	+	+	+	–	–	–	+	–	–	–
Working	½	+	+	+	+	–	½	–	+	+	+	+	+	+	+	+	–	–	–
Obs. time months	17	14	9	3	3	3	12	12	16	9	9	8	7	5	3	4	8	7	3
Relapse after mos.	2									5									

N = 19. Ten women, nine men. 30 – 61 years old.

Prol = prolapsed disc. Arach = arachnoiditis. Norm = normal

RESULTS

Tables 1 and 2 show the age and sex distribution, radiculography findings, numbers and types of injections, and observation times of the patients. Table 1 shows the results of the 16 patients who received bupivacaine and depotmethylprednisolone as their primary injection. Nine patients (56%) had considerable pain relief, six with objective neurologic signs of improvement. Two patients temporarily had more pain, five patients had no change in their pain. Five of the seven patients who did not improve had subsequent injections of bupivacaine followed by saline, one with less pain and objective signs of improvement. Radiculography showed prolapsed disc in 2, arachnoiditis in 1 (previous laminectomy), and inconclusive or normal findings in 6 of the 10 patients who improved. In the 6 patients who did not improve, radiculography showed herniated discs in 2, arachnoiditis in 2 (previous laminectomies), and inconclusive findings in 2 (Table 1).

Table 2 shows the results of the 19 patients who received bupivacaine followed by saline as their primary injection. Five (26%) had considerable pain relief with objective neurologic signs of improvement. Radiculography showed prolapsed disc in 2 and normal findings in 2 of these patients. Fourteen patients had no lasting pain relief. Of these, 11 subsequently received injections of bupivacaine and depotmethylprednisolone; 8 (73%) experienced considerable pain relief (and objective signs of improvement were present in 5 of these 8 patients). Radiculography showed prolapsed disc in 2 of these

8 patients, arachnoiditis in 4 (all of whom had previously had laminectomy), and normal findings in 2. Among the 6 patients who did not improve, radiculography showed normal findings in 4 patients and arachnoiditis in 1 (previous laminectomy).

Five patients who did not improve after the primary injections for various reasons did not get the alternative type of injections. The final results in 24 patients after the primary and alternative injections were: 6 (25%) improved after bupivacaine followed by saline, and 17 (63%) improved after bupivacaine and depotmethylprednisolone. This difference is statistically significant ($\chi^2 = 5.942; p < 0.05$). Of all 35 patients, 23 had considerable relief and 21 could return to their previous occupation or be rehabilitated to other work. Six patients had relapse after 2 to 9 months (Tables 1 and 2), three of whom then had surgical removal of prolapsed intervertebral discs.

DISCUSSION

Caudal epidural injections of bupivacaine followed by saline gave 25% of the patients in this study subjective pain relief and objective improvement from their chronic low back pain and sciatica. This is approximately the same success rate as Swerdlow and Sayle-Creer (15) obtained in chronic and recurrent cases injected epidurally (lumbar or caudal) with lidocaine and saline. Caudal epidural injections of bupivacaine and depotmethylprednisolone gave 63% pain relief and 41% objective improvement in our double-blind study. This again is of the same order of magnitude as the success rate of Swerdlow and Sayle-Creer (15) in their open study of chronic cases. The difference between the results of the two types of injections in our study is statistically significant ($p < 0.05$).

One important finding in our study is that 5 of 8 patients with arachnoiditis after previous surgery for prolapsed intervertebral disc had relief after bupivacaine and depotmethylprednisolone, whereas none of 6 patients with arachnoiditis had any benefit from bupivacaine and saline.

Since as many as 25% of our patients treated with bupivacaine and saline had definite subjective and objective improvement, and because the success rate of those patients who received bupivacaine and depotmethylprednisolone after a series of bupivacaine and saline was 73%, compared to 56% in those who received bupivacaine and depotmethylprednisolone as their primary treatment, we will not dismiss bupivacaine and saline as an ineffective treatment. Rather, our future approach to these chronic low back pain and sciatica patients will be to offer them one or two injections of bupivacaine and saline first, and then give bupivacaine and depotmethylprednisolone if no relief ensues from the former.

Swerdlow and Sayle-Creer (15) found no difference in results between lumbar and caudal epidural injections. The lumbar epidural approach has the advantage of fewer technical failures, but it has the disadvantage of severe headache in the occasional patient who gets a dural puncture. Moreover, the lumbar epidural space may be difficult to locate in patients who previously have had surgical removal of prolapsed intervertebral discs.

The mechanism of action of epidurally applied steroids in low back pain and sciatica is probably through its anti-inflammatory effects, which reduce the swelling and irritation in and around compressed nerve roots (13). This hypothesis is supported by our finding that several patients with radiculographically verified arachnoiditis had pain relief and objective signs of improvement.

The beneficial effect of epidural anesthesia and saline may be merely a placebo effect or may act through breaking a "pain-muscle-spasm-ischemia-pain" cycle (16). Whether or not an additional effect is obtained by injecting a large volume of saline and thus possibly breaking epidural and perineural adhesions (8,16) is still a matter of conjecture.

SUMMARY AND CONCLUSIONS

Thirty-five patients with chronic low back pain and sciatica were treated in a double-blind trial with caudal epidural injections of either bupivacaine and depotmethylprednisolone or bupivacaine followed by saline. Patients with no improvement after three injections were subsequently treated with the alternative type of injection. Pain relief and objective neurological improvement sufficient to enable the patient to return to work or to be rehabilitated to other work was obtained in 63% of those who received bupivacaine and depotmethylprednisolone and in 25% of those who received bupivacaine followed by saline ($p < 0.05$). These results confirm the findings of previous studies that epidural medication should be offered to patients with incapacitating low back pain and sciatica where surgical intervention is not indicated. If one or two epidural injections of bupivacaine and saline do not give significant relief, up to three injections of bupivacaine and methylprednisolone should be given.

ACKNOWLEDGMENT

Depotmethylprednisolone (Depo-Medrol®) was supplied through the courtesy of The Upjohn Company, Oslo, Norway.

REFERENCES

1. Barry, P. J. C., and Hume Kendall, P. (1962): *Ann. Phys. Med.,* 6:267–273.
2. Béliveas, P. (1971): *Rheumatol. Rehabil.,* 11:40–43.
3. Burn, J. M. B., and Langdon, L. (1970): *Rheumatol. Rehabil.,* 10:368–374.
4. Cappio, M. (1957): *Reumatismo,* 9:60–70.
5. Cho, K. O. (1970): *Am. Surg.,* 36:303–308.
6. Coomes, E. N. (1961): *Br. Med. J.,* 1:20–24.
7. Dilke, T. F. W., Burry, H. C., and Grahame, R. (1973): *Br. Med. J.,* 1:635–637.

8. Evans, W. (1930): *Lancet,* 2:1225–1229.
9. Gardner, W. J., Goebert, H. W., and Sehgal, A. D. (1961): *Trans. Am. Neurol. Assoc.,* 86:214–215.
10. Goebert, H. W., Jallo, S. J., Gardner, W. J., and Wasmuth, C. E. (1961): *Anesth. Analg.,* 40:130–134.
11. Harley, C. (1967): *Ann. Phys. Med.,* 9:22–28.
12. Kelman, H. (1944): *Am. J. Surg.,* 64:183–190.
13. Lindahl, O., and Rexed, B. (1950): *Acta Orthop. Scand.,* 20:215–225.
14. Mahner, A. (1960): *Zentralbl. Chir.,* 85:625–635.
15. Swerdlow, M., and Sayle-Creer, W. (1970): *Anaesthesia,* 25:341–345.
16. Warr, A. C., Wilkinson, J. A., Burn, J. M. B., and Langdon, L. (1972): *Practitioner,* 209:53–59.
17. Winnie, A. P., Hartman, J. T., Meyers, H. L., Ramamurthy, S., and Barangan, V. (1972): *Anesth. Analg.,* 51:990–1003.

Advances in Pain Research and Therapy, Vol. 1,
edited by J. J. Bonica and D. Albe-Fessard.
Raven Press, New York © 1976.

Lower Abdominal and Pelvic Pain in Women

*Eamonn de Valera and **Hugh Raftery

**Department of Obstetrics and Gynaecology, University College; and **Saint Luke's Hospital, Dublin, Ireland*

Chronic lower abdominal pain and backache are very common complaints in women, especially during the reproductive years. These pains are seldom visceral in origin, although they are often so ascribed. In the minority of cases in which there is a visceral cause—gastrointestinal or genitourinary—this can usually be diagnosed without difficulty. In most cases no such visceral cause is found, and frequently, after a series of investigations with negative results, the pains are labeled psychosomatic or neurotic and no effective treatment is given.

For some years we have been interested in these cases and have found two common organic causes: (a) nerve entrapment in the abdominal wall and (b) internal pelvic ligamentous strains. Both of these are characteristically worse premenstrually and during pregnancy and the puerperium. We theorize that this may be because of two factors: (a) fluid retention with tissue edema, possibly due to prolactin secretion; and (b) relaxation of the pelvic joints and ligaments by the action of relaxin secreted by the corpus luteum or placenta.

This chapter briefly describes the diagnostic features and treatment of these two common causes of lower abdominal and pelvic pain in women.

NERVE ENTRAPMENT

The cause of the pain is the nipping of the thoracic and upper lumbar nerves as they emerge through the rectus sheath (1,2). The pain is chiefly abdominal but may radiate through the posterior division of the nerve causing some backache, which is seldom severe.

Diagnosis

A diagnosis of nerve entrapment should always be considered in cases of chronic lower abdominal pain and discomfort. Visceral and spinal causes for such symptoms are readily excluded by a careful history and physical examination, backed by appropriate investigations. A maneuver which helps in making a tentative diagnosis is made by getting the patient to tense the

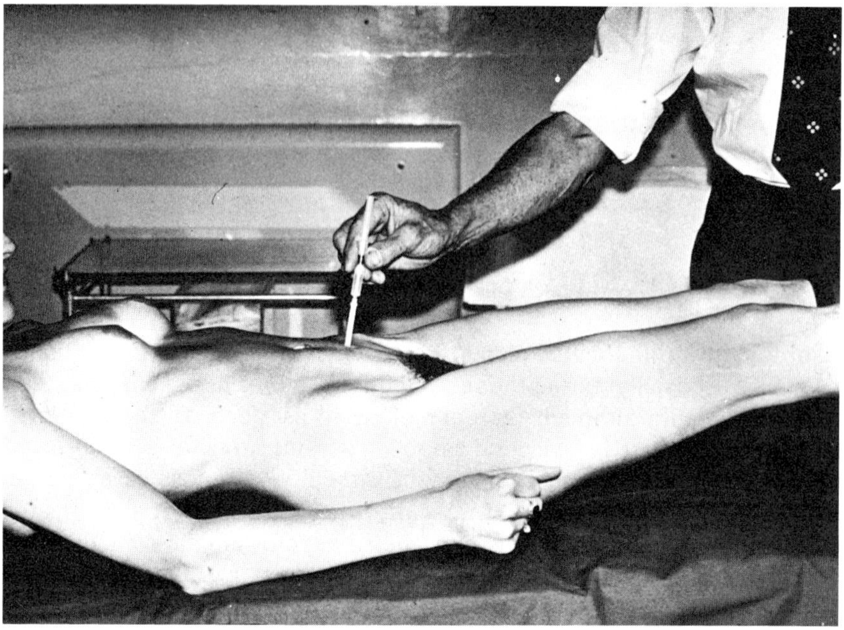

FIG. 1. Nerve entrapment. Note tensed abdominal muscles, with legs extended and shoulders raised. Pressure with probe along outer edge of rectus muscle to identify site of entrapment.

abdominal wall by raising the shoulders and extending the lower limbs (Fig. 1), and then by pressing the outer side of the rectus muscle with a blunt probe. This maneuver dramatically exacerbates existing pain or, if absent, incites it intensely. When the abdominal wall is relaxed, the pain is relieved and becomes more diffuse. It is noteworthy that patients with abdominal pain are usually asked to relax rather than tense the abdominal wall during examination. Consequently, a correct diagnosis is usually missed. The tentative diagnosis is confirmed with a diagnostic block consisting of injection of a small amount (1 to 2 ml) of local anesthetic (e.g., 1% lidocaine) on the nerve as it emerges from the sheath.

Treatment

The treatment is injection of the nerve at the same site (as it emerges from the sheath) with a small quantity—usually less than 0.5 ml—of 6% aqueous phenol. The precise location of the injection at the point of entrapment is critical and requires skill and patience, especially in obese women. Pain is usually relieved, but some residual tenderness, lasting approximately a week, is common at the injection site. Assessment of the results in 50 consecutive patients 6 months after block revealed that 31 (62%) were still free of pain and another 10 (20%) were improved but not completely free of pain. In many patients repeated injections are needed to achieve complete cure.

The only complications that occurred after this treatment were occasional small hematomas. Early in the series there were three instances of chemical peritonitis when too large an injection was given in thin women. All recovered without special treatment.

INTRAPELVIC LIGAMENTOUS STRAIN

Posterior sacroiliac and iliolumbar strains are another common cause of pain in the lower abdomen. These are effectively treated by injections of local anesthetics and corticosteroids with or without physiotherapy. Diagnosis in such cases depends on the demonstration of localized tender areas by palpation. In our experience internal pelvic ligamentous strains are much more common and are usually not diagnosed. These conditions can be diagnosed only by vaginal examination.

Figure 2 shows the common sites of intrapelvic ligamentous strains. They are numbered 1 to 4 in the order of their observed frequency. The symptoms vary with the location of the strain. When the strain is posterior—i.e.,

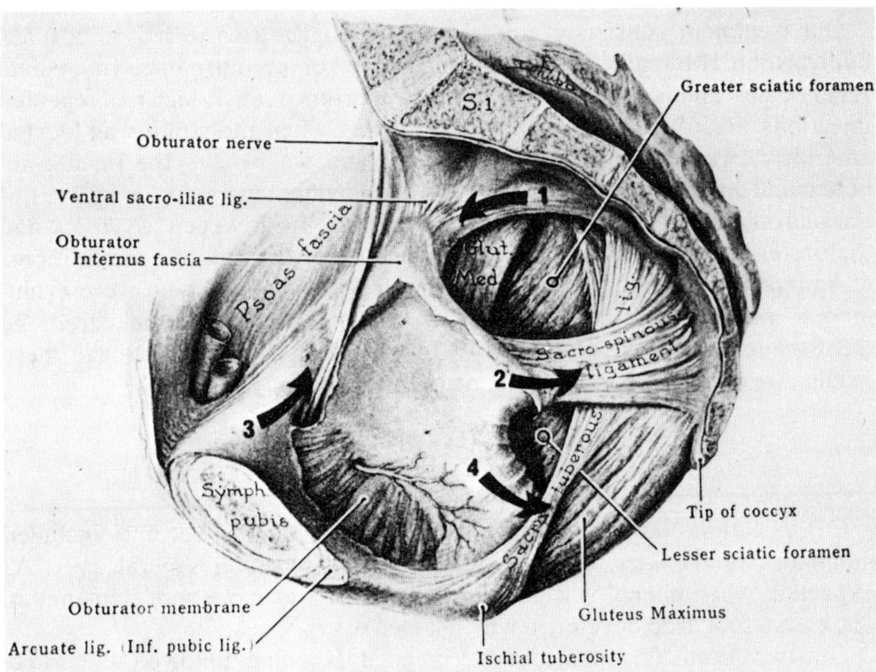

FIG. 2. Principal areas of tenderness found in internal pelvic ligamentous strain, numbered in order of frequency of occurrence.

sacroiliac, sacrospinous, or sacrotuberous (sites 1, 2, and 4)—the pain is felt chiefly in the back. When the strain is on the lateral pelvic side wall (site 3), the pain is more often referred to the iliac fossa or upper part of the thigh.

Diagnosis

Intrapelvic ligamentous strain is diagnosed by vaginal examination, which is much more accurate than rectal examination. The pelvic side walls and the sacroiliac joints are carefully palpated, as are the sacrospinous ligaments. In such cases an extremely tender and often sharply localized trigger area is found. Pressure on this area evokes the characteristic pain of which the patient complains. The same vaginal examination will rule out gross visceral causes for pain. In these conditions two etiologic factors stand out: (a) pregnancy and childbirth, and (b) examination under anesthesia in the lithotomy position especially when muscle relaxants are used.

Treatment

Our treatment consists of injection of the trigger area with 5 ml of 0.5% bupivacaine (Marcaine®) containing 25 mg of prednisolone. Immediate relief occurs and is encouraging, but the recurrence rate is high and repeated injections are often required. In a few cases when the strain was located anteriorly, we used 6% aqueous phenol and we believe the results are better and longer lasting. If, however, the ligamentous strain is in front of the sacroiliac joint near the lumbosacral plexus, the great pelvic vessels, and the ureter, we avoid phenol injection because of the risk of complications.

Among 88 consecutive patients treated with injection who were evaluated 6 months after interruption, 42 (47%) were considered cured, 29 (33%) were improved, and 17 (29%) were unimproved. To achieve these results, we had to give more than one injection in many patients.

Complications

Complications after intrapelvic injection with bupivacaine included numbness of the legs, but this effect disappeared after several days. As expected, when phenol was used the numbness was more persistent, and in one case a foot drop developed which lasted over a week.

On two occasions considerable vaginal bleeding followed the injection, but no active treatment was required. An ischiorectal abscess developed in one patient when an inexperienced operator perforated the rectum. Fortunately, the patient recovered completely with a good result.

SUMMARY

Nerve entrapment and internal pelvic ligamentous strain are among the most frequent causes of chronic lower abdominal pain and backache in women, especially during reproductive life. Because of the probable hormonal background, such pains are often cyclic in intensity and consequently they are usually misdiagnosed as visceral instead of musculoskeletal disorders. A correct diagnosis requires that a musculoskeletal cause be considered, a proper vaginal and musculoskeletal examination done, and diagnostic blocks correctly used. Definitive therapy consists of injection of aqueous phenol or bupivacaine and prednisolone. Repeated injections are often required for prolonged relief.

REFERENCES

1. Kopell, H. P., and Thompson, W. A. L. (1963): *Peripheral Entrapment Neuropathies*, p. 1. Williams & Wilkins, Baltimore.
2. Mehta, M., and Ranger, I. (1971): *Anaesthesia*, 26:3.

Advances in Pain Research and Therapy, Vol. 1,
edited by J. J. Bonica and D. Albe-Fessard.
Raven Press, New York © 1976.

Predictive Factors in the Treatment of Low Back Pain by Surgical Intervention

*E. M. Waring, **Gary M. Weisz, and †Stewart I. Bailey

*Departments of *Psychiatry, **Psychology, and †Orthopaedic Surgery, Victoria Hospital, London, Ontario, Canada*

The influence of personality and neurotic illness on pain tolerance and pain expression is widely accepted (3,6,7). The low back pain "loser" is a patient that orthopedic surgeons recognize as having personality and neurotic problems which have a profound influence on treatment efficacy (8). Pace (4) recently advocated that all candidates for low back pain surgery undergo preoperative psychological testing to assist in determining which patients will receive pain relief.

Using the Minnesota Multiphasic Personality Inventory (MMPI), Hanvik (2) identified a "conversion-V" profile which distinguished cases of presumed psychogenic backache from cases with clear organic disease. In this profile the hysteria (Hs) and hypochondriasis (Hy) scales are elevated, the depression (D) scale is relatively low, and there is a mild rise on the psychasthenia (Pt) scale. Phillips (5) and Wiffling and associates (9) have confirmed the above and in addition found that patients with less-neurotic symptomatology recover more quickly. Wiltse and Rocchio (10) carried out a large-scale study on 130 low back pain patients admitted for chemonucleolysis. They found that the best predictors for functional (activities of daily living) success of chemonucleolysis were the Hs and Hy scales of the MMPI. This could be very helpful to the orthopedic surgeon, particularly when no organic abnormality is evident.

This study attempted to determine if routine psychological assessment of all low back pain patients admitted to a busy orthopedic service would be clinically useful to the surgeon. In addition, the General Health Questionnaire (GHQ) (1), a 60-item, self-administered rating schedule that has been used in general practice settings as a screening instrument for discovering nonpsychotic emotional illness, was assessed for its predictive screening value. It was hypothesized that the MMPI and the GHQ would be better predictors of operative success than the clinical judgment of orthopedic surgeons.

METHOD

A consecutive series of low back pain patients electively admitted to a general hospital orthopedic surgery department was studied. Each patient received the MMPI and GHQ within 48 hr of admission. Demographic data on all subjects were also collected.

The research psychologist, psychiatrist, and the orthopedic surgeons involved in the treatment of these patients were blind to the results of the MMPI and GHQ. The patients were treated totally on the basis of the surgeon's clinical judgment. The orthopedic surgeons treating each case rated the patient preoperatively as to how good a candidate for surgery he was from both an organic and an emotional standpoint.

Six months postoperatively the surgeon rated each patient on the organic and functional-emotional outcome of surgery. The MMPI and GHQ scores plus demographic data and physician's preoperative ratings were all correlated with physician's postoperative ratings of operative success in order to examine their usefulness in predicting operative outcome.

RESULTS

Thirty-four patients admitted to Victoria Hospital's orthopedic department with low back pain being considered for surgery were studied. The age range was 24 to 68 with a mean of 40.4 years, and there were 20 men and 14 women. Seventeen were classed as laborers and 13 as nonlaborers; no occupational data were available on four patients. The mean duration of symptoms for the present episode of back pain prior to hospitalization was 55 weeks, and the mean number of previous surgical interventions for low back pain was 0.75. Many of these patients had clear objective physical signs and positive radiological evidence of organic disease.

Correlation coefficients were calculated between all predictive factors and treatment outcome and are shown in Table 1. It should be noted that the MMPI Hs and Hy scales had no predictive value. The D scale had a small, nonsignificant correlation with organic outcome.

With respect to operative success from an organic standpoint, the physician's preoperative organic ratings were the best predictor, yielding a significant correlation of 0.46. The only other meaningful predictor was whether or not the patient was receiving Workmen's Compensation for his disability. This factor yielded a significant correlation of 0.39. In predicting operative success from a functional-emotional standpoint, the physician's preoperative emotional rating was also a useful predictor, yielding a positive significant correlation of 0.45. The most useful predictor, however, was whether or not the individual was receiving Workmen's Compensation for his disability. This factor yielded a significant correlation of 0.60.

The GHQ was not a useful predictor of operative success. In supplementary analyses various cutting scores (i.e., 12, 20, 25) for the GHQ were used, but no support for the hypothesis that this instrument can be useful in the prediction of operative outcome was obtained.

An additional analysis was performed in which the "good" outcome

TABLE 1. *Prediction of operative outcome*

Predictor	Organic outcome	Functional outcome
Age	0.06	0.23
Sex	−0.05	−0.13
Occupation	0.24	0.18
Education	0.20	0.30
Duration of symptoms	0.09	0.23
Previous admissions for back – surgical	0.25	0.21
Previous admissions for back – nonsurgical	−0.24	0.13
Previous admissions for non-back – surgical	0.18	0.17
Previous admissions for non-back – nonsurgical	−0.09	−0.27
Back pain in family	0.06	−0.01
Workmen's Compensation	0.39[a]	0.60[b]
Physicians preoperative rating – organic	0.46[c]	0.42[a]
Physicians preoperative rating – emotional	0.39[a]	0.45[c]
Physicians preoperative rating – overall	0.46[a]	0.44[c]
GHQ	0.22	−0.09
MMPI – Hs	0.04	−0.15
MMPI – D	0.21	−0.01
MMPI – Hy	0.08	−0.16
MMPI – Pd	0.05	−0.20
MMPI – Pa	0.04	−0.04
MMPI – Pt	0.05	−0.08
MMPI – Sc	0.11	0.08
MMPI – Ma	0.25	0.03
MMPI – Si	0.12	−0.04

[a] Significant at 0.05 level.
[b] Significant at 0.001 level.
[c] Significant at 0.01 level.
Pd, psychopathic deviate; Pa, paranoia; Sc, schizophrenia; Ma, mania; Si, social introversion.

patients were separated from the "poor" outcome patients on both organic and functional-emotional postoperative ratings. Of particular interest was the finding that for good functional outcome patients, the MMPI mean *t*-scores were 62.1 for Hs, 61.7 for D, and 60.6 for Hy. For poor functional outcome patients ($N = 5$), the mean MMPI *t*-scores were 63.8 for Hs, 55.0 for D, and 63.4 for Hy. It can be noted that the "conversion-V" emerges with the poor functional outcome patients because of the reduced D scale score.

DISCUSSION

In this study, the MMPI and GHQ were not useful in predicting surgical outcome. The findings of Wiltse and Rocchio (10) that MMPI Hs and Hy scale elevations were better predictors of operative success than surgeon's preoperative ratings was not confirmed. The surgeons' ratings of the patients were the most accurate predictors of eventual surgical outcome. In addition, the situational factor of whether or not the patient was receiving Workmen's Compensation was a significant predictor of both organic and functional outcome.

The discrepancy between these results and those of previous studies may in part be a function of our smaller sample size. However, it is more likely a function of a difference in sample selection. Wiltse and Rocchio (10) stated that they were treating subjective symptoms. Thus in their study no patient had severe organic illness which would complicate evaluation of chemonucleolysis. The findings of the present study might be expected with an acute sample of orthopedic patients with a high proportion or organic disease (2). The finding of a "conversion-V" on a small number of poor functional outcome patients also suggests support for previous findings (2,10).

It should also be noted that in our sample the surgeon had already made a decision about admitting these patients to the hospital. Presumably, he had already eliminated many patients with a poor prognosis for surgery by the use of his own judgment.

Finally, a high degree of intercorrelation of the MMPI scales raises methodological questions regarding the usefulness of traditional psychological tests for the present purposes. The authors' attempt to replicate Wiltse and Rocchio's use of the stepwise multiple linear regression analysis (10) produced conflicting results of doubtful clinical validity. The authors will discuss the above methodological questions more fully in a future publication and suggest that specific tests to assess factors predictive of operative success should be developed empirically.

REFERENCES

1. Goldberg, D. P. (1972): *Detection of Psychiatric Illness by Questionnaire,* Maudsley Monograph. Oxford University Press, London.
2. Hanvik, L. H. (1949): *J. Consult. Psychol.,* 15:350–353.
3. Merskey, H. (1965): *J. Psychosom. Res.,* 8:405–19.
4. Pace, B. (1974): *The Medical Post,* Nov. 12.
5. Phillips, E. L. (1964): *Curr. Pract. Orthop. Surg.,* 2:165–176.
6. Stengel, E. (1965): *Br. J. Psychiatry,* 111:795–802.
7. Sternbach, R. A. (1968): *A Psychophysiological Analysis.* Academic Press, New York.
8. Sternbach, R. A. (1973): *Psychosomatics,* 14:226.
9. Wiffling, F. J., Klonoff, H., and Kofan, P. (1973): *Clin. Orthop.,* 90:153–160.
10. Wiltse, L. L., and Rocchio, P. D. (1975): *J. Bone Joint Surg.,* 57-A:4, 478–483.

Advances in Pain Research and Therapy, Vol. 1,
edited by J. J. Bonica and D. Albe-Fessard.
Raven Press, New York © 1976.

Interdependence of Low Back Pain and Psychiatric Symptomatology

A. Spring, R. Wittek, and R. Wörz

Nervenkrankenhaus Günzburg, 887 Günzburg, West Germany

Painful organic diseases are frequently associated with psychological disturbances. But little is known about psychological alterations if the physical causes of pain are removed. Therefore, we examined patients with low back pain and sciatica caused by lumbar disc herniation pre- and postoperatively.

METHODS

Thirty-five patients were tested. No special selection method was used. The average age was 38 years (range 20 to 59 years). The indications for operation were neurological disturbances, long-lasting pain, and typical myelographic findings. The kind of anesthesia and surgical procedure were virtually the same for each patient. In 18 cases the disc L_4-L_5 was removed, in 12 cases L_5/S_1. In the remaining cases disc L_3-L_4 was removed, and two lower lumbar discs were removed in one operation.

The patients were examined 10 weeks after the operation for the first time. Another examination will be done in 1 year. In all cases there were no myelographic signs of relapse. The neurological deficits were improved in all patients substantially or disappeared. Therefore, we believe that it is valid to compare the psychological development of our patients.

Several psychological tests were applied, and the following were evaluated for this first study: Reduzierter Wechsler Intelligence Test, Benton Test, Maudsley Medical Questionary (MMQ), Befindlichkeitsskala (BS)—behavior scale, and Beschwerdenliste (BL)—list of complaints (the last two tests are elaborated at the Max Planck Institute in Munich). The intensity of pain and the reduction of pain after the operation were evaluated by rating scales [corresponding to the "visual analogue scale" defined by Huskisson (2)]. The actual, maximal, and average pain intensity were estimated by the patient. For this study we used the data of the average pain and distinguished between low back pain and sciatica. Detailed explorations were performed to detect neurotic, depressive, and other psychiatric symptoms.

RESULTS

Using a rough simplification of the characteristics less and more pain, psychiatric amelioration, and psychiatric deterioration, we recorded three typical patterns. In the first group the results of a 21-year-old man were representative (Fig. 1). The post-treatment subjective pain estimates for the low back pain and sciatica were obviously decreased, whereas the psychological test results—BS, BL, and MMQ—were almost the same. The psychiatric results did not change. This group consisted of 9 patients (26%).

The second group is represented by a 43-year-old man (Fig. 2). The low back pain improved and the sciatica disappeared. Scores on all psychological tests were greatly reduced, and the psychiatric statement improved. This was the largest group: 14 patients or 40% of those tested.

In the third group of 11 patients (31%), reduction of pain was reported. But the scores on the BS and MMQ tests increased. The BL showed nearly the same results or even more complaints. In the case of a 37-year-old woman presented in Fig. 3, the BL decreased atypically. All patients of the third group showed psychological disorders such as irritability, indecisiveness, inability to concentrate, and misery or depressive mood. They seemed to be more neurotic or depressive than they had been preoperatively. Only 1 patient (3%) had more pain and seemed to be more neurotic than preoperatively.

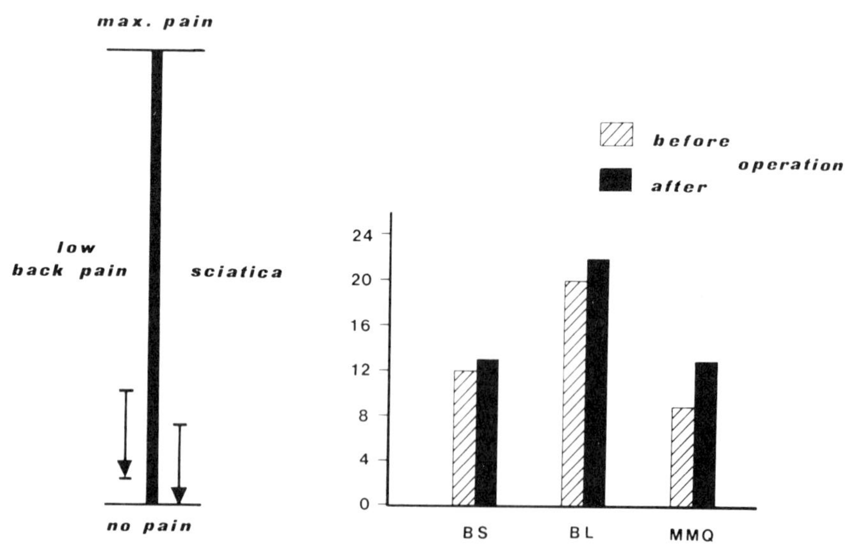

FIG. 1. Rating scale for pain and results of psychological tests pre- and postoperatively in a 21-year-old man. Example of less pain and the same psychological results postoperatively. **Left:** Rating scale for pain (original size 20 cm) estimates for low back pain and sciatica. Base of the arrow indicates preoperative pain intensity, arrowhead signifies postoperative pain intensity. **Right:** Ordinate, scores on the psychological tests.

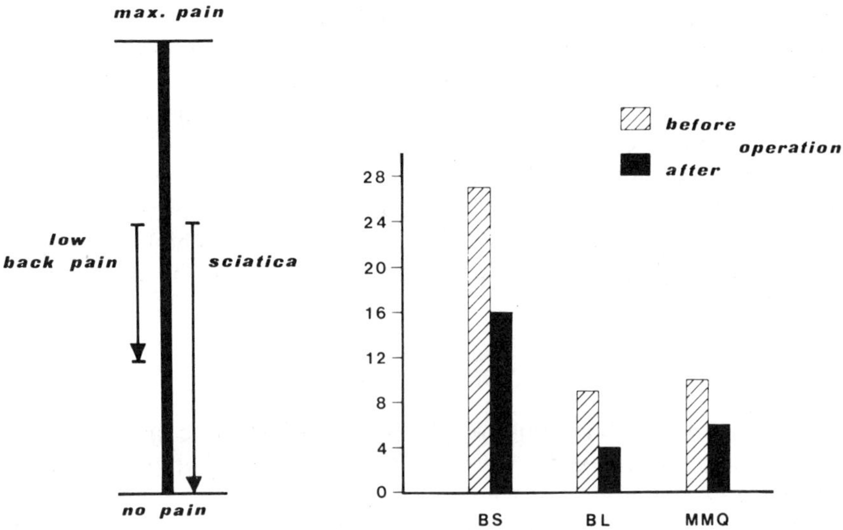

FIG. 2. Rating scale for pain and results of psychological tests pre- and postoperatively in a 43-year-old man. Example of less pain and psychological amelioration. (For further explanation, see Fig. 1.)

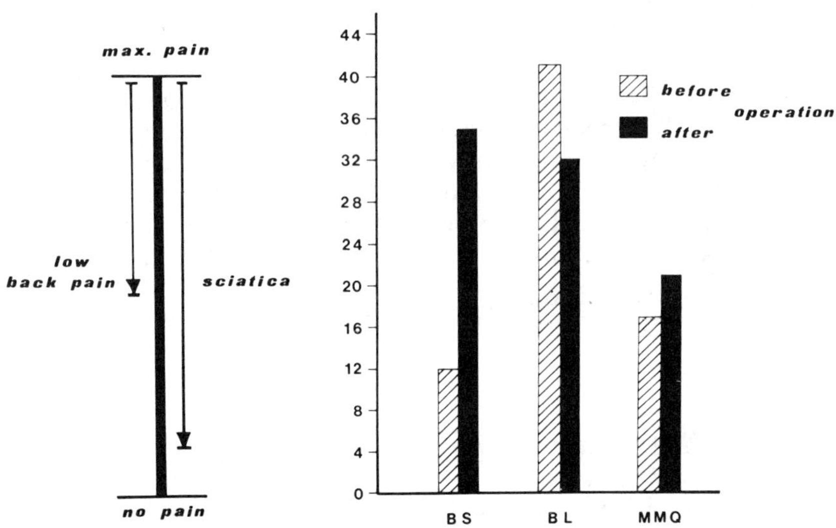

FIG. 3. Rating scale for pain and results of psychological tests pre- and postoperatively in a 37-year-old woman. Example of less pain and psychological deterioration. (For further explanation, see Fig. 1.)

It was striking that 12 or more than 30% of our patients complained postoperatively about new pain syndromes or other symptoms which had no organic cause. The new pain syndromes were located on other regions of the body, in some cases in the contralateral leg. The new pain was less intense than the previous one. It is evident that the new complaints came mostly from the group with psychiatric deterioration (7 of 11 patients). Patients with unchanged psychiatric behavior seemed also to be at risk of developing new symptoms or neuroticisms (4 of 9 patients). In the group showing psychiatric improvement, only 1 patient developed a new pain syndrome.

DISCUSSION

The objective amelioration of the neurological state postoperatively seems to be a psychological stress for many patients. The patients appear to be more neurotic or depressive than before. Transformations to other or the same somatic signs and symptoms develop if there is a concealed neurosis. The neurosis is no longer represented in somatic symptoms caused physically.

These findings correspond with the reports of Bond (1) and are in contrast with those of Sternbach et al. (3). We believe that neurotic traits often persist or intensify after pain-relieving procedures. The good results of Sternbach et al. (3) may be explained by the psychological treatment and rehabilitation program which all patients received.

The consequence for neurosurgical intervention is that the indication for operations must be restricted to patients with neurological and corresponding myelographic findings. Patients with long-lasting low back pain and without radicular syndromes should undergo psychological testing preoperatively. Patients with neurotic signs and symptoms run the risk that the psychiatric symptomatology will persist or even increase after the pain-relieving operation. Therefore, all patients should participate in a postoperative pain rehabilitation program (3,4). It is insufficient to remove only the causes of pain surgically. Psychological disorders must be treated in cooperation with the psychologist and psychiatrist to obtain good results.

SUMMARY

Psychological tests and psychiatric explorations were performed in 35 patients with low back pain and sciatica pre- and postoperatively. Three typical reaction patterns were evaluated after the operation: less pain and the same psychological statement, less pain and psychiatric amelioration, and less pain but psychiatric deterioration. Some patients complained about new pain syndromes or other symptoms in other regions of the body. The consequences for neurosurgical intervention are discussed.

REFERENCES

1. Bond, M. R. (1973): *J. Psychosom. Res.,* 17:257–263.
2. Huskisson, E. C. (1974): *Lancet,* 9:1127–1131.
3. Sternbach, R. A., and Timmermans, G. (1975): *Pain,* 1:177–181.
4. Stimson, B. B. (1947): *Psychosom. Med.,* 9:210–212.

Advances in Pain Research and Therapy, Vol. 1,
edited by J. J. Bonica and D. Albe-Fessard.
Raven Press, New York © 1976.

Modulating Effect of Secondary Gain on the Low Back Pain Syndrome

Bernard E. Finneson

Low Back Pain Clinic, Crozer Chester Medical Center, Upland, Chester, Pennsylvania 19013

FINANCIAL ASSISTANCE FOR OCCUPATIONAL DISABILITY

The world is becoming progressively more responsive to the individual who becomes physically disabled and is rendered occupationally dysfunctional. The usual method of dealing with such problems in modern industrial societies is to provide monetary assistance in the form of either regular-interval payments or a lump sum settlement. When blame for the causative factor can be attributed to a financially responsible party, the monetary assistance is almost always significantly greater. Two common examples are disability arising from an occupational hazard that can be attributed to an employer, and that owing to an accident that can be blamed on the negligence of a financially responsible individual or organization. In contrast, when blame or fault cannot be attributed to outside parties, financial assistance is usually provided either by privately "self-obtained" disability insurance or, more frequently, by various governmental agencies in the form of a subsistence allowance; in the latter instance assistance is invariably much less. The more generous financial assistance plans related to "fault or blame" which involve regular-interval payments differ in numerous respects, but in almost all plans payments are terminated when the disability ends.

WORK-ETHIC PRINCIPLE

The payment of monies is universally recognized as a reward for positive action. Worker and professional alike consider their salary or fee an acknowledgment of their worth in performing a job or service. When financial assistance is rendered to a disabled individual, implicit in this plan is that the recipient is rewarded or paid for his disability. Such a concept is at odds with the fundamental work-ethic principle, which extols the diligent worker and denigrates the individual who is unable to function because of disability or disinclination.

SECONDARY GAIN

With increasing usage of systems involving generous financial aid for disability, clinicians are able to perceive a significant prognostic difference in patients who are receiving or hope to receive such aid in comparison with patients suffering from an identical syndrome who are not in a position to be compensated for their illness. It is evident that the patients receiving financial aid are disabled for significantly longer periods of time. The term secondary gain has developed increasing use and generally refers to the financial rewards associated with disability. Rewards other than financial compensation must also be considered such as preferential or less-hazardous working conditions, the sympathy and concern of family and friends, or the opportunity to withdraw from an unpleasant or unsatisfactory life role.

SPECIAL CHARACTERISTICS OF THE LOW BACK PAIN SYNDROME

The following features of the low back pain syndrome merit consideration. First, the causative factors of low back pain syndrome are often attributed to direct or indirect trauma, which tends to eventuate in a large percentage of secondary gain situations. Second, those patients who do not readily respond to the usual conservative measures are often referred to orthopedists and neurosurgeons who are surgically oriented and tend to seek a surgical solution to what may be a nonsurgical problem. Third, the long-term outcome of surgery is more disappointing than the published statistics indicate. Finally, the patient who has not responded satisfactorily to surgery is often treated with additional surgical procedures, frequently resulting in increased physical disability superimposed on the original low back dysfunction.

Low back pain may be contrasted to headache, another common pain syndrome. Headaches are less frequently attributed to trauma and so are less likely to fit into a secondary gain situation. Headaches are usually managed by medically oriented physicians who are inclined to treat the problem as a psychosomatic illness. This point of view is in accordance with the general cultural acceptance of associating headaches with tension or "nerves."

SECONDARY GAIN VERSUS NON-SECONDARY GAIN

Because of the unique features discussed above, the low back pain syndrome presents a special problem in relationship to secondary gain. Between 1961 and 1970, 623 patients with low back pain were successfully treated by nonsurgical measures. Of these, 324 patients without secondary gain averaged a total disability interval of 16 days for the specific episode, whereas 281 secondary gain patients averaged 36 days of total disability (3).

Between 1961 and 1970, 72 out of 1,000 patients with herniated lumbar discs treated surgically were classified as having had unsatisfactory results. This number included 657 non-secondary gain patients, of whom 34 or 5% had unsatisfactory results; in 343 secondary gain patients, 38 or 11% had unsatisfactory results (2).

MALINGERING VERSUS CONDITIONED RESPONSE

Initially it was thought that the bulk of these secondary gain problems were attributable to malingering. However, when many of the suspected malingerers were observed surreptitiously, evidence of low back dysfunction could be seen. Although some malingerers will invariably be found in a secondary gain situation, it is felt that a significant number of patients undergo a conditioned response related to the secondary gain which results in prolongation of symptoms. The psychosomatic aspects of the low back pain syndrome and the generally accepted specialty referral patterns relating to the management of the syndrome cause it to be specifically vulnerable to the inherent weaknesses built into the secondary gain system.

This results in a number of problems. The cost of a compensation program is adversely skewed and possibly endangered by the increasing payments of monies for this particular syndrome. For example, in the Commonwealth of Pennsylvania between the years 1971 and 1973, although only 9% to 11% of all industrial accidents were classified as "low back injuries," 30% to 40% of compensation payments were for low back pain (1). As the compensation laws become increasingly liberal, the financial problems become more acute. Although the maintenance of a fiscally viable and balanced compensation program is of considerable importance, as physicians our primary concern is the patient; and in this situation the greatest disservice is to the patient. The individual with a low back pain syndrome who is coerced by the compensation system to defer returning to the job becomes enmeshed in a situation with progressively more restrictive courses of action. To defend his prolonged absence from work he may be coerced to submit to studies or even surgery, which may further aggravate his low back dysfunction. The decision to perform these diagnostic studies or surgery is based as much on his prolonged absence from work as on the actual symptoms or physical findings.

RECOMMENDATIONS

I recommend the following: (a) perhaps most importantly, general recognition and acceptance of the adversely modulating effect of secondary gain on the low back pain syndrome; (b) broad-based statistical analysis from various medical centers obtaining long-term results on patients with low back pain syndrome and comparing these results in patients with and without secondary gain; (c) sociological and psychological studies of the factors causing prolongation of disability with secondary gain; and (d) modification of compensation laws and insurance plans to encourage reentry of low back pain patients into economic society with financial rewards favoring gainful employment rather than continued disability.

REFERENCES

1. Bureau of Vocational Rehabilitation, Commonwealth of Pennsylvania, Harrisburg.
2. Finneson, B. E. (1973): *Low Back Pain*. J. B. Lippincott Co., Philadelphia.
3. Low Back Pain Clinic, Crozer-Chester Medical Center, Chester, Pennsylvania.

Advances in Pain Research and Therapy, Vol. 1,
edited by J. J. Bonica and D. Albe-Fessard.
Raven Press, New York © 1976.

Role of Sympathetic System in Reflex Dystrophies

Paolo Procacci, *Fabio Francini, Massimo Zoppi, Marco Maresca, and *Lorenza Giovannini

*Pain Center, Medical General Clinic, and *Institute of Human Physiology, University of Florence, Florence, Italy*

A prominent role of the sympathetic nervous system in the pathogenesis of the reflex dystrophic pain syndromes is generally admitted. This concept was first proposed by Leriche in 1916 (6) and subsequently was supported by his clinical observations and those of others (2,7).

Livingston in 1943 (8) proposed a pathophysiological mechanism of the reflex sympathetic dystrophies in his well-known hypothesis of a "vicious circle," in which noxious stimulation in the periphery from disease forms a circle of periphery-CNS-periphery. Subsequently, many writers studied these syndromes (1,4,5) and some proposed modification of this hypothesis. However, the sequence and the mechanism of the modifications that occur in the structures involved in the vicious circle still remain a subject of controversy. Even from a clinical and nosographic point of view, the concept of reflex sympathetic syndromes does not yet have a clear definition. According to the opinion of most investigators, an abnormal sympathetic reflex activity is present not only in the classic post-traumatic reflex dystrophies like major and minor causalgia, but also in many diseases differently classified, as in some vascular diseases of the limbs like erythromelalgia, Raynaud's disease, occlusive arterial diseases, and some rheumatic diseases, for example, myofascial pain syndrome with "myalgic" or trigger spots.

In order to study the mechanisms of the vicious circle, we investigated in neurodystrophic patients before and after sympathetic block: (a) the afferent function, examined as cutaneous pain threshold; and (b) the efferent sympathetic function, observed as variations of the skin potentials.

MATERIAL AND METHODS

Our study was carried out on 27 normal subjects, 24 men and 3 women between 19 and 50 years of age, and on 42 hospitalized patients, 29 men and 13 women between 21 and 70 years of age. All the patients had sympathetic reflex dystrophy of the upper or lower limb. Two had major causalgia, eleven had minor causalgia, and twenty-nine patients had minor reflex dystrophies consequent to: crush injuries (4), gunshot wounds (2), fractures (8), contusions (13), and frostbite (2). The symptoms were present or prevalent in one limb. In most patients we observed myalgic spots, often with the well-known characteristics of the "trigger points" (2).

In every patient we induced a reversible chemical block of the sympathetic chain ipsilateral to the affected limb with 5 to 10 ml of 0.5% bupivacaine (Marcaine®). The blocks were induced at the level of the stellate ganglion (C_7-T_1) for the upper limb, and the second, third, and fourth lumbar sympathetic ganglia for the lower limb. All the blocks were carried out at the same hour of the day (8 A.M.). The duration of the block lasted from 6 to 9 hr.

In 30 patients we determined the cutaneous pain threshold using a special thermal dolorimeter based on the original method proposed by Della Corte et al. (3). The tests were performed in every subject at prefixed intervals: (a) before the block; and (b) 15 min and 1, 3, 6, 12, 24, and 48 hr after the block.

In 12 patients we observed the variations of the skin electrical potentials measured between a surface disk unpolarizable electrode (8 mm in diameter) and a subcutaneous stainless steel needle electrode 0.4 mm in diameter insulated except for the distal 2 mm. The potentials were amplified by means of a high-impedance amplifier (DC, 500 cps). In order to investigate the reflex sympathetic activity, we applied different stimuli: sudden acoustic nonpainful stimuli; and electrical square wave stimuli (0.5 msec; 200 cps) in series lasting 20 msec, applied with disk unpolarizable electrodes on different areas of the upper and lower limbs. The stimulating apparatus was assembled with a stimulus insulation unit. In every test these stimuli were applied at intervals of 30 sec. The electrical stimulation was applied in the limb ipsilateral to the block, in the contralateral one, and in another limb.

RESULTS

The clinical effect of the sympathetic block was reduction or complete disappearance of pain and paresthesias and of the trophic disorders. We noted that the "trigger points" became less painful to pressure or completely disappeared, even in the limb contralateral to the block.

Cutaneous Pain Threshold

Before the sympathetic block the threshold of the affected limb was generally higher or lower than that of the contralateral one. After the sympathetic block we observed a sequence of damped oscillations of the threshold values, both in the limb ipsilateral to the block and in the contralateral one. The periods of the oscillations of the contralateral limb were directly correlated ($p < 0.001$) to those of the ipsilateral limb. After the last oscillation, the threshold of both limbs tended to the same value (10). These oscillations were much wider than those we observed in the phases of the circadian and circatriginthan rhythms of the pain threshold (9).

Skin Potentials

Normal Subjects

We observed two patterns of variations of the skin potentials: (a) a generalized variation of the skin potential present in the four limbs after sudden and unusual stimuli [this response shows habituation and represents a diffuse sympathetic activation (alarm reaction)]; and (b) a variation of the skin potential present only in the stimulated limb and in the contralateral one. This response does not show habituation and represents a segmental sympathetic activation. The responses observed in (a) and (b) were synchronous and of the same amplitude (Fig. 1a).

Subjects with Sympathetic Dystrophies

Before the block we observed the same patterns of variation of the skin potential as in normal subjects, but with the following differences. The first response was different in amplitude in the affected limb in respect to the others. The second response, i.e., the variations of the skin potential in the stimulated affected limb and in the contralateral one, was irregular in shape, prolonged in time, and of lower amplitude than the response observed in normal subjects (Fig. 1b).

Immediately after the sympathetic block we observed disappearance of

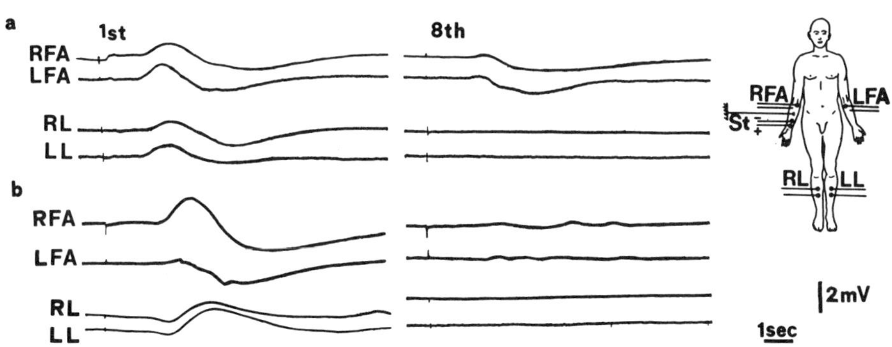

FIG. 1. a: Healthy subject: 1st stimulus, variation of the cutaneous potential is present in every limb; 8th stimulus, variation is present only in limb ipsilateral to the stimulation and in contralateral one but not in the lower limb. **b:** Subject with a reflex dystrophy of the right upper limb: 1st stimulus, variations are present in every limb; 8th stimulus, only small variations are observed. St, stimulating electrodes. Recording electrodes: RFA, right forearm; LFA, left forearm; RL, right leg; LL, left leg.

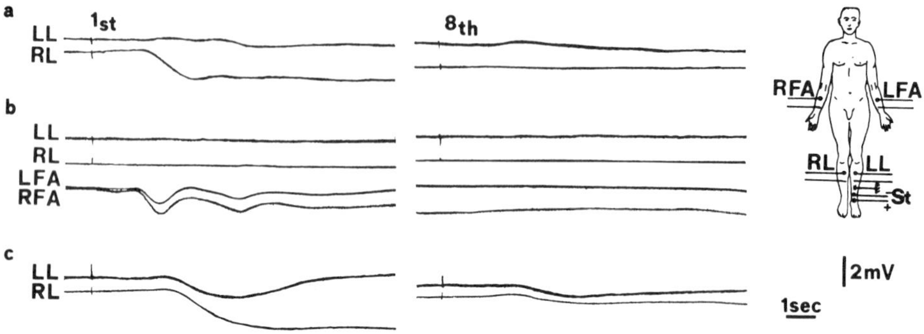

FIG. 2. Subject with a reflex sympathetic dystrophy of the left lower limb. Variations of the cutaneous potentials: **a:** before block of the left sympathetic chain (L_2-L_4); **b:** 1 hr after block; **c:** 48 hr after block. Abbreviations same as in Fig. 1.

the skin potential variations not only in the limb ipsilateral to the block but also in the contralateral one. The other two limbs showed normal responses (Fig. 2a and 2b).

Approximately 48 hr after the block we observed that both the general (type 1) and segmental (type 2) responses showed a pattern similar to that observed in normal subjects (Fig. 2c).

DISCUSSION

The analysis of our results suggests that:

First, the sympathetic system controls, through rapidly and slowly acting mechanisms, the cutaneous pain threshold, both in the dystrophic limb and in the contralateral one, through a feedback loop involving skin → afferent input → CNS → sympathetic output → skin. This is suggested by the damped oscillations of the threshold itself.

Second, the afferent discharge of a limb controls the contralateral sympathetic output through central mechanisms. This is suggested by the resetting of the thresholds of the two limbs 48 hr after the block.

Third, the sympathetic output, as reflected by the variations of the skin potentials, is modified in reflex dystrophies and reset 48 hr after the block.

The results propose, in modern neurophysiological terms, an interpretation of the classic hypothesis of the "vicious circle" and of the therapeutic effects of the sympathetic block.

REFERENCES

1. Bonica, J. J. (1953): *The Management of Pain.* Lea & Febiger, Philadelphia.
2. Bonica, J. J. (1957): *J.A.M.A.*, 165:732–738.
3. Della Corte, M., Procacci, P., Bozza, G., and Buzzelli, G. (1965): *Arch. Fisiol.*, 64:141–170.

4. De Takats, G. (1965): *Med. Clin. North Am.,* 49:117–129.
5. Gross, D. (1974): In: *Advances in Neurology, Vol. 4: International Symposium on Pain,* edited by J. J. Bonica, pp. 93–104. Raven Press, New York.
6. Leriche, R. (1916): *Presse Med.,* 24:178–180.
7. Leriche, R. (1949): *La Chirurgie de la Douleur,* Ed. 3. Masson et Cie., Paris.
8. Livingston, W. K. (1943): *Pain Mechanisms,* Macmillan, New York.
9. Procacci, P., Della Corte, M., Zoppi, M., and Maresca, M. (1974): *Chronobiologia,* 1:77–96.
10. Procacci, P., Francini, F., Zoppi, M., and Maresca, M. (1975): *Pain,* 1:167–175.

Advances in Pain Research and Therapy, Vol. 1,
edited by J. J. Bonica and D. Albe-Fessard.
Raven Press, New York © 1976.

Phantom Pain Relief by Focal Destruction of the Substantia Gelatinosa of Rolando

Blaine S. Nashold, Jr., *Bruno Urban, and David S. Zorub

*Department of Surgery, Division of Neurosurgery, and *Department of Anesthesiology, Duke University Medical Center, Durham, North Carolina 27710*

Complete avulsion of the roots of the brachial plexus is a disabling injury with pain appearing within a few hours and plaguing the patient for the rest of his life. Of 50 patients with brachial plexus avulsion studied at Duke Medical Center, 67% developed intractable phantom pain (6). The pain is of central origin, yet its site of origin within the CNS and the pathophysiology responsible for its genesis are still unknown. In the past, surgical treatment has not been uniformly satisfactory and has included amputation of the arm, high cervical cordotomy, mesencephalic tractotomy, and, more recently, electrical activation of the dorsal columns (2,5). We proposed coagulating the substantia gelatinosa of Rolando in the dorsal root entry zone on the basis that the central pain may originate from the deafferent neurons in the zone of injury. Four patients with intractable pain after avulsion of the brachial plexus have been treated and have experienced significant short-term relief after selective focal coagulation of the cervical cord substantia gelatinosa.

METHODS

Clinical Material

R. L., a 45-year-old man, sustained avulsion injury in 1973 with a complete motor and sensory deficit in the arm and intractable pain (Table 1). Electrical stimulation of the dorsal columns for 6 months did not relieve the pain, nor did a bilateral cingulotomy. In March of 1975, focal coagulations were carried out in the dorsal root entry zone area between C_5 and T_1 with immediate and significant relief of pain which has persisted.

In a motorcycle accident in 1973, A. T., a 20-year-old man, sustained traumatic avulsion of the brachial plexus associated with spinal fractures at T_{6-7} and a head injury. He had a complete motor and sensory deficit in the arm with intractable pain referred to the hand, first and second digits, and radial aspect of the arm. Because of the pain he developed severe drug addiction and psychological deterioration. A myelogram revealed

TABLE 1. *Clinical data of 4 patients with brachial plexus avulsion*

Patient	Age	Date of trauma	Trauma	Clinical findings	Treatment	Results	Follow-up
R. L.	45	1973	Avulsion of brachial plexus	Left arm pain	Amputation	No relief	
				Horner's syndrome	DCS[a]	No relief	
				Abnor. myelogram	Cingulotomy	No relief	
					SG lesions	50% relief	6 mo
A. T.	20	1973	Avulsion of brachial plexus;	Arm pain			
			Fracture T_6-T_7;	Horner's syndrome	Psychiatric therapy		
			Head injury	Drug addiction			
				Abnor. myelogram	SG lesions	60% relief	1 yr
J. S.	30	1974	Avulsion of brachial plexus	Arm pain	TCS	No relief	
				Horner's syndrome	DCS—percut.	Partial relief	
				Abnor. myelogram	SG lesions	80% relief	6 mo
L. Y.	40	1956	Avulsion of brachial plexus	Arm pain	TCS	No relief	
				Horner's syndrome	DCS	No relief	1 mo
				Abnor. myelogram	SG lesions	80% relief	

[a] DCS, dorsal column stimulation; SG, substantia gelatinosa; TCS, transcutaneous stimulation.

arachnoidal cysts at C_6, C_7, and T_1. Surgical exploration of the cervical cord between C_5 and C_6 confirmed the complete avulsion of the sensory roots, and six focal coagulations carried out on the dorsal root entry zone were followed by 60% relief of pain with discontinuance of narcotic drugs and improvement in the psychological state for 1 year. Postoperatively he complained of numbness in both legs which cleared.

J. S., a 30-year-old man, sustained traumatic avulsion of the brachial plexus in December of 1974 with complete motor and sensory deficit, severe pain in the right arm, and Horner's syndrome. Myelography revealed extradural defects at C_6 and C_7. Treatment of the pain by transcutaneous stimulation provided no relief, and dorsal column stimulation resulted in only partial relief. The cervical cord was surgically explored from C_6 to T_1 with six coagulations of the dorsal root entry zone, and this was followed by 80% relief for 6 months.

L. Y., a 40-year-old man, sustained a brachial plexus injury as the result of a bicycle accident in 1956, and he experienced total motor and sensory loss with severe pain in the arm for 20 years. A myelogram revealed evidence of the avulsed roots. Dorsal column stimulation resulted in no relief of pain. Surgical exploration of the cervical cord from C_6 through T_1 revealed evidence of atrophy and complete avulsion of both motor and sensory nerve roots. Fifteen focal coagulations carried out from C_5 through C_7 in the substantia gelatinosa resulted in immediate significant relief of burning pain for the first time in 20 years. A postcoagulation deficit occurred with weakness of the ipsilateral leg and mild dysfunction of the dorsal column, but this gradually disappeared.

Two patients (R. L. and L. Y.) developed transient postoperative complications. R. L. complained of vague change in sensation in his legs. However, on neurological examination, aside from hyperreflexia in the legs, only a minimal disturbance of position sense could be detected and it cleared. He ambulated normally with no motor weakness. L. Y. developed definite motor weakness of the ipsilateral leg, but this improved rapidly over a 2-week period. He also complained of a sensation in the leg and numbness up to the midthorax. Neurological examination revealed a normal appreciation of pinprick and pain on that side of the body and a minimal reduction of vibratory sense in the ipsilateral leg, which the patient sometimes interpreted as a burning sensation. There was minimal incoordination of heel-to-shin testing on the ipsilateral side.

It was interesting that both patients complained of some alteration in sensation with minimal objective changes in sensation, and those present were mainly related to transient dorsal column and corticospinal dysfunction. These symptoms were probably owing to lesion encroachment or edema of the adjacent dorsal columns on the nearby corticospinal pathways. The incoordination of the ipsilateral leg could be a temporary

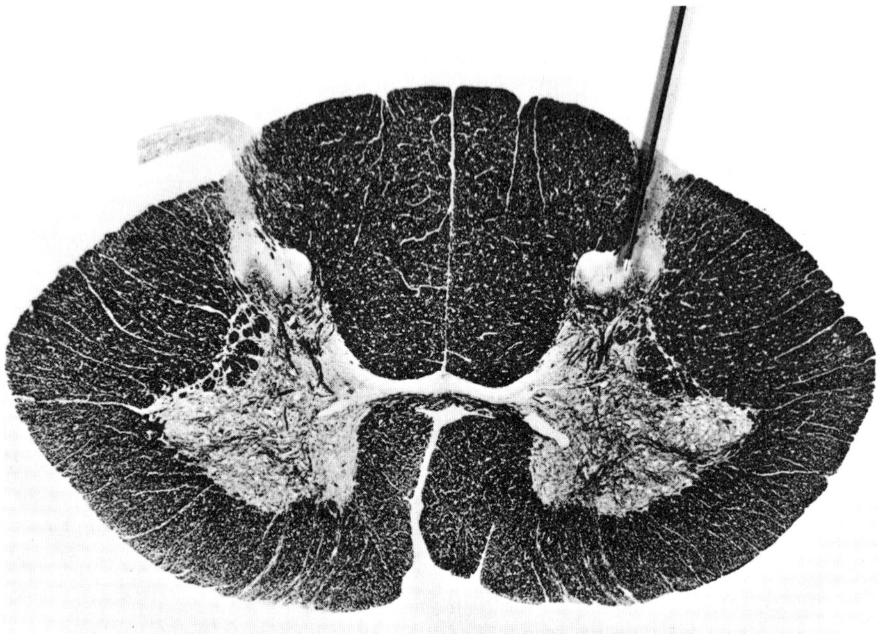

FIG. 1. Cross section of cervical cord indicating angle of entrance of coagulating needle.

change in the spinocerebellar pathway whose cells originate in the dorsal root entry zone.

Surgical Technique

The cervical cord was exposed through a laminectomy at the level of the avulsion injury (C_5 through T_1). When the dura was opened, the cord was usually deformed and shrunken on the side of the injury with absence of the dorsal roots and in some cases the ventral roots as well. The operator uses magnifying loupes to identify the cord structures, and the electrode is introduced lateral to the intermediolateral sulcus at a 20° angle into the cord for a distance of 3 to 4 mm (Fig. 1). The electrode is the type used for percutaneous cordotomy and is hand-held.

The sites for coagulation on the avulsion side correspond to the origin of the filaments composing the dorsal root on the normal side. A Radionics coagulator is used to produce the lesion at 75 mA for 15 sec. Coagulation of the cord tissue results in a small, whitish zone of coagulated tissue around the electrode measuring approximately 1 to 2.5 mm. The points of the coagulation are spaced approximately 1 to 2 mm apart or at the same interval of distance between each of the filaments of a normal dorsal root. The coagulations were carried out mainly between C_5 and C_6 since the pain was referred to these dermatomes in the denervated limb.

DISCUSSION

Does pain begin in the dorsal horn? This question has fascinated numerous authors and was recently examined in detail by Crue et al. (1), who postulate "a set of command neurons in the dorsal horn that can signal pain." It is not possible to examine fully all the evidence in this brief communication except to reemphasize the importance of the dorsal root entry zone as I believe we have demonstrated in patients with brachial plexus avulsion.

Our observations give no specific clues as to the exact neural substrate responsible for the pain. Theoretically, the avulsion of the dorsal root would remove the inhibiting effect of the large myelinated afferents on the small substantia gelatinosa and pericornual cells, as already proposed by Melzack and Wall (4). The release of inhibition may allow these cells to become hyperactive or overactive via the spinoreticular and spinothalamic pathways, resulting in central pain.

The possibility of chronic deafferentation of spinal cord interneuronal pools as a source of pain should also be considered. Loeser and Ward (3) have demonstrated chronic deafferentation of the spinal cord neurons and recorded spontaneous hyperactivity of these cells in the dorsal horn. Another possible explanation for pain relief in our patients could simply be the combined destruction of the neurons responsible for the spinothalamic and spinorecticular tracts.

Neurosurgeons who treat pain are all too familiar with reports of initial relief followed by later failure, and we recognize that a longer period of observation in our group of patients is needed before our method can be considered a specific treatment modality. On the other hand, we would like to reemphasize the importance of the dorsal root entry zone as a possible source for the phantom pain in brachial avulsion. In an effort to answer this question more directly, we feel that an animal model of the avulsion injury could be devised and studied neurophysiologically. Hopefully, such an experimental model might give further clues as to the neurological basis of central pain.

REFERENCES

1. Crue, B. L., Jr. (Ed.) (1975): *Pain Research and Treatment.* Academic Press, New York.
2. Falconer, M. A. (1953): *Br. Med. J.,* 1:299–304.
3. Loeser, J. D., Ward, A., Jr., and White, L. E., Jr. (1968): *J. Neurosurg.,* 29:48–50.
4. Melzack, R., and Wall, P. D. (1965): *Science,* 150:971–979.
5. Nashold, B. S., Jr., Wilson, W. P., and Slaughter, D. G. (1969): *J. Neurosurg.,* 30:117–126.
6. Zorub, D. S., Nashold, B. S., Jr., and Cook, W. A., Jr. (1975): *Surg. Neurol.,* 2:347–353.

Advances in Pain Research and Therapy, Vol. 1,
edited by J. J. Bonica and D. Albe-Fessard.
Raven Press, New York © 1976.

Mechanisms of Ischemic Pain in Peripheral Occlusive Arterial Disease

P. Arcangeli, V. Digiesi, *O. Ronchi, B. Dorigo, and V. Bartoli

*Departments of Internal Medicine and *Neurology and Psychiatry, University of Florence, Florence, Italy*

The pain in muscular structures of the calf which is produced by exercise or walking and disappears quickly with rest is the leading symptom of atherosclerosis obliterans of the lower limbs, commonly designated intermittent claudication. A history of constant or nocturnal rest pain is strongly suggestive of severe arterial disease and often connotes either a distal level of occlusion or an extensive degree of obstruction.

In previous reports attention has been focused mostly on the level of arterial occlusion, on the methodology for measuring blood flow through the collateral arteries at rest and after exercise or ischemia, and on disease progression or improvement. Some studies deal also with metabolic demands and involvement of the muscular tissue during ischemia. A review of medical literature reveals, moreover, few reports on the clinical impairment of the muscles and of afferent function in arteriosclerosis obliterans of the lower limbs (2–4,6,13).

The work described here was performed to evaluate the importance of impairment of the muscles and of afferent function in the mechanisms of intermittent claudication and rest pain (ischemia pain) in peripheral arterial disease.

MATERIAL AND METHODS

A total of 58 patients (96 limbs) were examined in a period of 18 months: at the initial visit a complete history was elicited and physical examination and routine blood analyses were performed.

To document arterial disease accurately, we included in the follow-up procedure, in order of performance: (a) palpation of femoral, tibial, and pedidial pulses and auscultation or phonoarteriography of major arteries (abdominal aorta, iliac, and superficial femoral); (b) morphoscillography; (c) venous occlusion plethysmography; and (d) arteriography when possible.

The tactile threshold was measured in the lower limbs with von Frey's hairs; the cutaneous pain threshold was determined on the top of the foot, on the lateral area of the calf, and on the thigh using radiant heat as pain stimulus (7); the vibratory perception threshold was determined with a pallesthesiometer on the medial malleolus (11). Limb ischemia was produced by placing a 12 cm wide pneumatic cuff with a pressure of 200 to 250 mm Hg around the thigh so that the lower border of the cuff was approximately 7 cm above the patella. Before the test, care was taken in each case to keep the limb raised for 30 to 60 sec and then the cuff was inflated rapidly to a pressure of 200 to 250 mm Hg, which was maintained for 20 min. Paresthetic and painful sensations arising during the compression stage were examined. The maximal conduction velocity of motor nerve was measured in the lateral popliteal nerve (cap. fib.-ankle) derivation with a needle electrode.

The presence of myalgic spots on the foot, calf, thigh, and buttock was diagnosed on palpation as tender localized muscular areas (5,9,12) and because of appearance of the "jump sign" (10). The presence of trigger points in the myofascial structure of the calf (triceps surae) and buttock (gluteus medius, tensor fasciae latae) was diagnosed when spontaneous pain in a target zone of the foot, buttock, or thigh was reproduced or intensified by firm digital pressing on the tender spot in gastrocnemius, soleus, gluteus medius, or tensor fasciae latae muscles, according to Travell (12) and Arcangeli et al. (2).

It was possible to classify patients according to the following criteria: (a) level of main arterial occlusion (aortoiliac, femoropopliteal, tibial); (b) age of onset of the clinical symptoms; (c) occurrence of intermittent claudication, rest pain, and impending or actual gangrene; (d) presence or absence of diabetes mellitus, chronic alcoholism, intervertebral disc lesion, and other diseases potentially damaging the nerves.

RESULTS AND COMMENT

The observations made from this study are summarized in the following paragraphs.

The pain or other discomforts and the paresthesias arising during the walking are mostly localized in the calf (81.2%) (Table 1).

At the muscular level, it is always possible to find in limbs with rest pain and impending or actual gangrene, and frequently in those with intermittent claudication, myalgic or trigger areas in the muscles of buttock, thigh, calf, and foot. Often the myalgic spots are located in the triceps surae and tibialis anticus muscles. When the terminal aorta, common iliac, or hypogastric arteries are stenosed or occluded, myalgic or trigger points can be present in the buttock muscles (gluteus medius and tensor fasciae latae) (Fig. 1).

The reference zone of trigger area (Fig. 2) of the soleus is in the heel and the sole of the foot; of gastrocnemius muscle in the inferior hind portion of the thigh, in the calf, and in the heel; of tibialis anticus in the top of the foot as far as the big and second toes; of gluteus medius in anus region and

TABLE 1. *Site of pain during walking in the lower limbs of patients with peripheral arterial disease*

Site	Limbs (No.)	%
Calf	36	37.5
Calf and foot	17	17.7
Calf and thigh	10	10.4
Calf, buttock, thigh, and foot	9	9.4
Calf, thigh, and buttock	6	6.2
Foot	4	4.2
Thigh	1	1.0
Buttock	1	1.0
No pain	11	11.5
Unknown	1	1.0

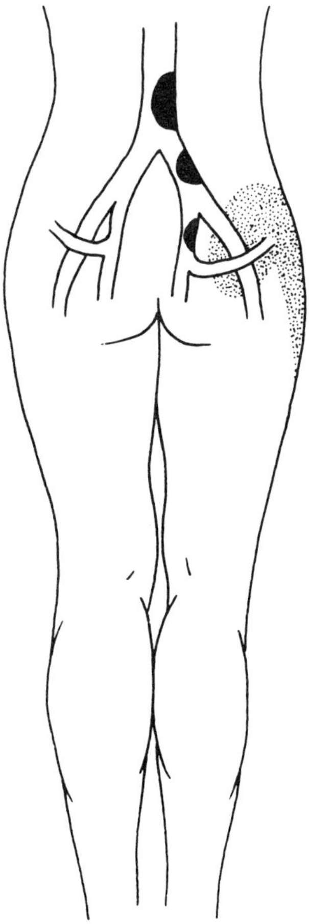

FIG. 1. Myalgic areas in the muscles of the buttock when the terminal aorta, common iliac, or hypogastric arteries are stenosed or occluded.

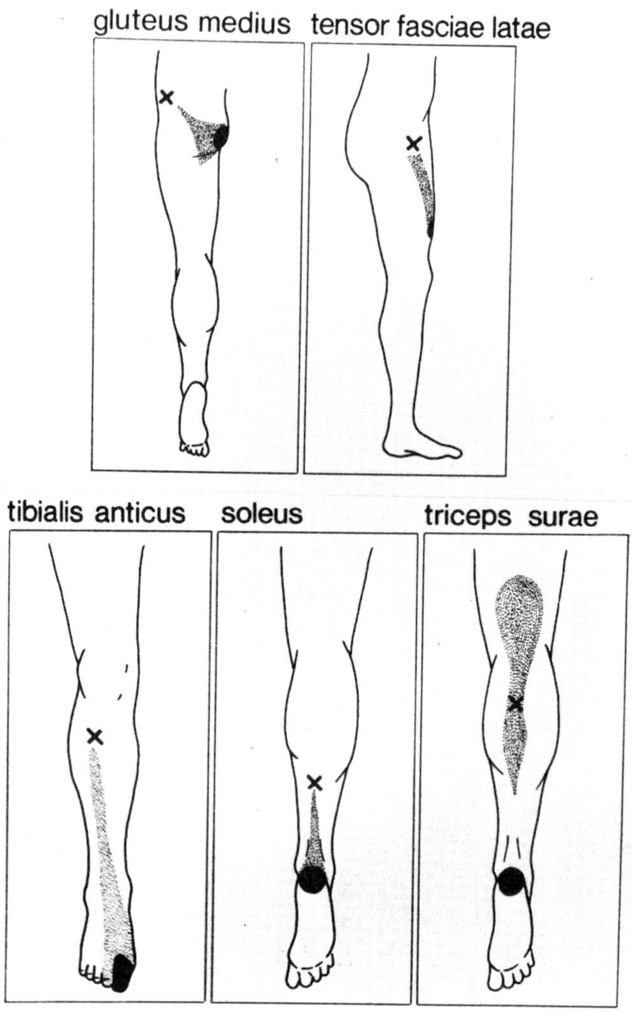

FIG. 2. Reference pattern of pain (*black and stippled*) associated with trigger areas (x) in muscles of buttock and leg in patients with peripheral occlusive arterial disease.

gluteofemoral fold; and of tensor fasciae latae in the thigh over fascia lata.

The tactile threshold is increased in the foot or in the calf in approximately 20% of the patients and in the thigh in 12.8% of cases. The cutaneous pain threshold is increased in the foot or in the calf in 33.3% and in the thigh in 30.8% and is decreased in the foot in 4.7% of patients. These findings demonstrate that the alterations of the senses of touch and pain are more frequent in the distal sites of the limbs. The vibration perception threshold is increased in 34.9% of patients.

During ischemia of the lower limb the tingling sensation is reduced in 79.7% and increased in 7.6% of cases, and painful sensations are felt in

43.4%. Ischemia of the limb causes the onset of pain in those sites where there are myalgic areas or painful processes (e.g., cutaneous phlogosis, phlebitis, osteoarthritis). When trigger areas are present, ischemia causes pain in the reference zone of these areas.

The maximal motor nerve conduction velocity (MCV) of lateral popliteal nerve, measured in 91 limbs, was less than 40 m/sec in 12 (13.2%), and from 40 to 45 m/sec in 29 subjects (31.9%) (Table 2). In most of these cases, diabetes mellitus, chronic alcoholism, or lumbar disc lesions were associated with arteriosclerosis obliterans.

No relationship was demonstrated between reduced MCV and stage of disease, level of obstruction, or age of patient. Nevertheless, repeated measurements in a subject during progression of disease show a significant reduction of motor nerve conduction velocity. In another case, with unilateral arterial occlusion and chronic alcoholism the MCV was more reduced in the ischemic than in the normal limb.

The concomitant or subsequent appearance of pain in other muscles of the limb during walking or exercise is possible when one or more of the following conditions are present:

First, as regards pain in the foot (at various sites, including the forefoot, heel, sole, or top of the foot, big and second toe, and ankle): (a) severe ischemia (peak flow of reactive hyperemia in the calf less than 10 ml/100 ml tissue per minute); (b) diversion phenomenon, according to Hyman and Winsor (8) and Allwood (1): during exercise, in patients with occlusion of the main arteries of the lower limbs, sometimes the volume flow of blood is redistributed to different tissues of the calf and foot; the skin of the foot pales, and after the pallor the patient experiences paresthesias and pain in the foot and in the calf; (c) myalgic spots in myofascial structures (fibromyositis of small foot muscles; plantar fasciits); (d) ankle, midtarsal arthritis; (e) trigger areas in calf muscle (triceps surae and tibialis anticus), but not all patients with trigger points in calf muscles experience pain at foot level during walking.

Second, as regards pain in the buttock and thigh: (a) severe stenosis or

TABLE 2. *Maximal motor nerve conduction velocity of lateral popliteal nerve in subjects with peripheral occlusive arterial disease*

	Only arterial disease		Arterial disease and diabetes		Arterial and other diseases		Total	
MCV	No.	%	No.	%	No.	%	No.	%
Under 40 m/sec	3	3.3	4	4.4	5	5.5	12	13.2
40–45 m/sec	11	12.1	10	11.0	8	8.8	29	31.9
Under 45 m/sec	14	15.4	14	15.4	13	14.3	41	45.1

TABLE 3. *Calf blood flow and myalgic spots in subjects with peripheral arterial disease*[a]

Case	Leg	Level of main occlusion	Reactive hyperemia peak flow[b]	Myalgic spots				Symptoms and signs
				Buttock	Calf	Tibialis anticus	Foot	
C.F. 60 yr	R	Aortoiliac	8.52 after 156 sec	+++	+++	+++	+++	Gangrene of forefoot
+ diabetes mellitus	L	Aortoiliac	18 after 20 sec	0	+−−	+−−	+−−	IC
F.F.	R	Common iliac	13.36 after 108 sec	+++	+++	+++	0	IC (WD 150 m)
53 yr	L	Popliteal	18.20 after 23 sec	0	+±−	+±−	0	No pain
C.V. 69 yr	R	Iliac and femoral	8.74 after 238 sec		+++	+++	++±	IC (WD 100 m)
+ chronic alcoholism	L	Femoral	9.27 after 203 sec		+++	+++	++±	IC (WD 100 m)

[a] R, right; L, left; IC, intermittent claudication; WD, walking distance.
[b] Flow is measured as ml/100 ml tissue per minute.

TABLE 4. *Walking distance, calf blood flow, and myalgic spots in subjects with intermittent claudication*

Case	Level of main occlusion	Leg	Reactive hyperemia (peak flow)[a]	Myalgic spots: Buttock	Myalgic spots: Calf	Myalgic spots: Tibialis anticus	Myalgic spots: Foot	Walking distance
B.R. 66 yr	Aortoiliac	R	19.32 after 24 sec	0	0	0	0	2 km (L)
		L	16.33 after 31 sec	±−−	±−−	0	0	
P.A. 60 yr	Right iliac and femoral	R	16 after 9 sec	++−	++±	++±	0	150 m
V.P. 54 yr	Bilateral common iliac	R	25.30 after 27 sec	+++	+++	0	0	150 m (R)
		L	40 after 17 sec	0	+±−	0	0	
F.N. 73 yr	Left femoro-popliteal	L	15.39 after 58 sec	0	±−−	0	0	> 1 km
F.A. 44 yr	Right femoral	R	14.88 after 32 sec	0	±−−	0	0	1 km
A.M. 65 yr	Left femoro-popliteal	L	23.10 after 28 sec	0	+++	+−−	0	200 m
C.A. 70 yr	Bilateral femoro-popliteal	R	20.10 after 67 sec	0	+±−	0	0	250 m (L)
		L	8.60 after 66 sec	0	++−	0	+++	

[a] Flow is measured as ml/100 ml tissue per minute.

occlusion in the abdominal aorta, common iliac, hypogastric or femoral artery (causing pain primarily in the thigh); (b) trigger or myalgic areas in the muscles of the buttock (gluteus medius and tensor fasciae latae) and myalgic areas in the thigh (vastus medialis, adductor group).

Some patients with extensive aortoiliac or femoral obstruction initially experience pain in the calf, followed by pain or distress in the thigh and/or buttock or foot, and then muscular block and severe muscular weakness of the entire lower limb. Thus walking must be promptly interrupted.

The occurrence of myalgic spots in the lower limbs and the severity of limb ischemia are often parallel (Table 3): in the same patient myalgic or trigger areas were prevalent in the limb where the hyperemic blood flow was reduced. But in some subjects walking distance was related more to the severity of myalgic spots than to the decrease of the calf blood flow (Table 4).

Lack of intermittent claudication with occlusive arterial disease is possible when limb ischemia is moderate and myalgic spots are absent or very light. Seven subjects of this series did not complain of pain or other distress during exercise or walking. In a patient with femoral obstruction, intermittent claudication arose when myalgic areas appeared in the calf and foot, although the calf blood flow during reactive hyperemia was almost unchanged. Injection of procaine in the myalgic areas lengthened the walking distance.

The severity and the early development of pain or other distress in intermittent claudication are therefore related to reduced blood flow; site of arterial obstruction; occurrence and number of myalgic spots and/or trigger areas; nerve lesions; and concomitant soft tissue or articular rheumatism.

SUMMARY

We examined 58 patients (96 limbs) with peripheral arterial disease in order to study impairment of muscles and afferent function as mechanisms of intermittent claudication and rest pain.

The pain arising during the walking is mostly localized in the calf. The concomitant or subsequent appearance of pain in other muscles of the limb is possible when some morbid conditions are associated with arterial occlusion. Very important is the presence of myalgic and trigger areas in myofascial structures of buttock, thigh, calf, and foot.

Tactile, vibratory, and pain thresholds are frequently impaired. Maximal conduction velocity of lateral popliteal nerve was less than 45 m/sec in 45.1% of limbs examined.

Pain and other distress of intermittent claudication are therefore related to: reduced blood flow; site of arterial occlusion; occurrence and number of myalgic or trigger points; nerve lesions; and concomitant soft tissue or articular rheumatism.

REFERENCES

1. Allwood, M. J. (1962): *Clin. Sci.,* 22:279–286.
2. Arcangeli, P., Corradi, F., and D'Ayala Valva, G. (1964): *Rass. Neurol. Veg.,* 18:167–238.
3. Arcangeli, P., Corradi, F., and D'Ayala Valva, G. (1965): *Acta Neuroveg.,* 27:511–545.
4. Bolletti, A., Dorigo, B., Zoppi, M., Pampanini, A., Voegelin, M. R., Bartoli, V., and Procacci, P. (1971): *Minerva Cardioangiol.,* 19:506–512.
5. Bonica, J. J. (1953): *The Management of Pain.* Lea & Febiger, Philadelphia.
6. Boyd, A. M., Ratcliff, A. H., Jepson, R. P., and James, G. W. H. (1949): *J. Bone Joint Surg.,* 31B:325–355.
7. Della Corte, M., Procacci, P., Bozza, G., and Buzzelli, G. (1965): *Arch. Fisiol.,* 64:141–170.
8. Hyman, C., and Winsor, T. (1959): *Am. J. Cardiol.,* 4:566–571.
9. Ibrahim, G. A., Awad, E. A., and Kottke, F. J. (1974): *Arch. Phys. Med. Rehabil.,* 55:23–28.
10. Kraft, G. H., Johnson, E. W., and LaBarr, M. M. (1968): *Arch. Phys. Med. Rehabil.,* 49:155–162.
11. Steiness, I. (1957): *Acta Med. Scand.,* 158:327–335.
12. Travell, J. (1951): In: *Connective Tissues. Transactions of the Second Conference,* edited by C. Ragan. J. Macy, Jr., Foundation, New York.
13. Travell, J., Baker, S. J., Hirsch, B. B., and Rinzler, S. H. (1952): *Fed. Proc.,* 11 (1):164.

Advances in Pain Research and Therapy, Vol. 1,
edited by J. J. Bonica and D. Albe-Fessard.
Raven Press, New York © 1976.

Therapeutic Effect of the Polypeptide Aprotinin on Intermittent Claudication and on Pain at Rest in Patients with Peripheral Arterial Occlusive Disease

V. Digiesi, V. Bartoli, and B. Dorigo

Department of Internal Medicine, University of Florence, Florence, Italy

Aprotinin (Trasylol®), a basic polypeptide extracted from bovine lung with a molecular weight of 6512, is composed of 58 amino acids of 16 different types. The amino acid sequence is the same as that found in the pancreatic trypsin inhibitor (7) discovered by Kunitz. Pharmacologic actions ascribed to aprotinin (4,5,9) include: (a) inhibition of plasma kallikreins; (b) stabilization of lysosomal membranes; (c) inhibition of lysosomal cathepsins; (d) prevention of the activation of proteolytic enzymes in pancreatic homogenates (i.e., trypsin, chymotrypsin); and (e) reduction of the rate and quantity of pancreatic enzyme secretion.

During ischemia, an activation of kallikreins (8) and an increase of tissue proteolysis by activation of protein-hydrolyzing lysosomal enzymes (1) are hypothesized. Moreover, the specific activity of some lysosomal enzymes, and particularly of cathepsins, is increased in gastrocnemius muscle of patients with obstruction of the arteries of the lower limbs (2).

On the basis of the above-mentioned effects of aprotinin on plasma kallikreins, proteolytic activity, and lysosomal enzymes, we undertook this investigation to determine the effect of this polypeptide on intermittent claudication and on pain at rest in patients with peripheral arterial disease.

MATERIALS AND METHODS

This study group consisted of 20 male patients with peripheral arterial disease; the age range was 39 to 74 years and the mean age was 64 ± 3.1 years. The control group consisted of 10 subjects of similar age who were apparently healthy and had normal arterial circulation. All patients in the study group had intermittent claudication, 5 also had pain at rest, and 2 had trophic lesions. The effect of aprotinin on pain, skin sensibility, and calf blood flow was examined.

In a first group of 5 patients and 5 normal controls, the effect of the polypeptide, given i.v. just before the test in a single dose of 100,000 KIU diluted in 10 ml of 0.9% NaCl, was studied on the initial pain limit walking tolerance (only in patients with arterial disease), on tactile, cutaneous pain and vibratory threshold, and on basal resting calf blood flow measured before and after the treatment. As control, the effect on the same tests of 10 ml of 0.9% NaCl was examined.

In a second group of 15 patients and 5 normal controls, the polypeptide was given i.v. twice a day for a week in a single dose of 100,000 KIU diluted in 10 ml of 0.9% NaCl. As control, 10 ml of NaCl 0.9% was given i.v. twice a day for a week to one-half of the group before and to the other half after the administration of the polypeptide. Before and after the treatment, the following parameters were examined: (a) tactile, cutaneous pain and vibratory thresholds; (b) calf basal resting and reactive hyperemia blood flow; and (c) pain at rest, initial pain limit walking tolerance, and myalgic and "trigger" areas located in the gastrocnemius, soleus, or tibialis anticus muscle in patients with peripheral arterial disease. The methods used were the same as those referred to in another chapter of this volume (V. Digiesi et al.).

The initial pain limit walking tolerance, i.e., walking distance to the first symptom of pain, was determined on a treadmill (speed, 3 km/hr). The walking distance and sensory thresholds were measured on different days. In comparing the results obtained with aprotinin and the equivalent volume of diluent (0.9% NaCl), we used Student's *t*-test.

RESULTS

In tactile, cutaneous pain and vibratory thresholds, no variations were observed in normal controls or in patients with arterial disease after administration for a week of a single dose or many doses of both aprotinin and NaCl 0.9%.

Table 1 shows the values (mean ± SE) of the calf blood flow. No significant difference was observed between the values obtained with aprotinin and those with NaCl 0.9%. Also, in normal controls no variations were observed.

TABLE 1. *Effect of aprotinin on calf blood flow and on walking distance to the first symptom of pain in patients with peripheral arterial disease*

	No. of subjects	Variation of calf blood flow (ml/100 ml tissue/min)		Increase of walking distance (meters)
		Basal resting	Reactive hyperemia	
Aprotinin				
100,000 kiu	5	0.47 ± 0.44[a]	–	16.2 ± 3.72[b]
NaCl 0.9%	5	0.34 ± 0.33	–	1.8 ± 0.37
Aprotinin				
200,000 kiu/7 days	15	0.31 ± 0.11[a]	0.28 ± 0.46[a]	69.7 ± 11.8[b]
NaCl 0.9%/7 days	15	0.33 ± 0.13	0.29 ± 0.38	2.3 ± 1.2

[a] Does not differ significantly from the corresponding value after NaCl.
[b] Differs significantly from the corresponding value after NaCl ($p < 0.005$).
Data are given as mean ± SE.

There was a significant increase ($p < 0.005$) in the initial pain limit walking tolerance both after a single dose of aprotinin (+16.2 ± 3.72 meters) and after administration twice a day for a week (+69.7 ± 11.8 meters). The pain at rest in myalgic and "trigger" areas located in the muscles of the lower limbs decreased, sometimes markedly, in all the patients examined after receiving aprotinin; in contrast, after the administration of NaCl 0.9%, there was a slight improvement in only one case.

DISCUSSION

The results of the present study demonstrate that aprotinin increases the initial pain limit walking tolerance and decreases the intensity of pain at rest in the myalgic and "trigger" areas of patients with peripheral arterial disease. The mechanism of the favorable effect of this polypeptide on pain cannot be owing to the increase of calf blood flow because this was unchanged. Also, the hypothesis that this treatment could influence the mechanism of perception of painful stimuli may be discarded because the pain thresholds were unvaried. It seems reasonable to suggest that aprotinin acts on biochemical mechanisms that cause the ischemic pain (Fig. 1).

Kinins are likely to be in part responsible for pain that arises during ischemia. Indeed, it is known that decrease of pH, developing during ischemia and muscular exercise in man (6), inhibits kininase, the enzyme that inactivates the kinins (3). Moreover, during ischemia, an activation of kallikreins (8) is hypothesized.

Although the true mechanism is still unknown, it is probable that aprotinin inhibits kininogenases (9), particularly killikreins locally activated by decrease of tissue pH during ischemia and proteolytic activity, and simultaneously stabilizes lysosomal membranes.

SUMMARY

Twenty patients with peripheral arterial disease and ten normal controls were submitted to i.v. injection of aprotinin in order to examine its effects on lower limb pain, lower limb sensibility, and calf blood flow.

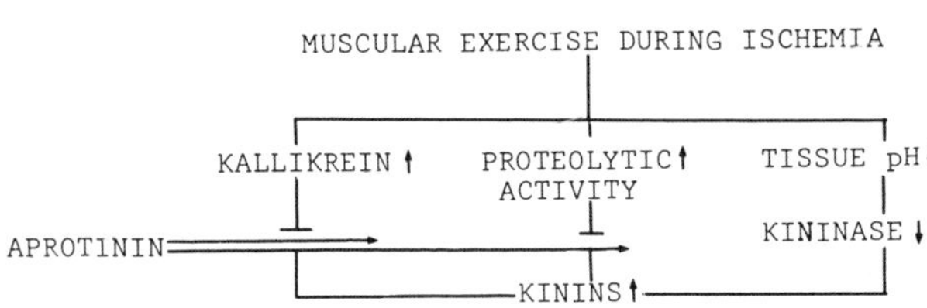

FIG. 1. Hypothesis of the mechanism of the effect of aprotinin on the ischemic pain of patients with peripheral arterial disease.

Aprotinin is able to increase the initial pain limit walking tolerance and to decrease the intensity of pain at rest of myalgic or "trigger" areas. No variation is observed on skin sensibility or on calf blood flow.

The favorable effect of the examined polypeptide on ischemic pain can be attributed neither to increase of calf blood flow nor to influence on perception of painful stimuli. It seems, therefore, logical to suggest that aprotinin acts on biochemical mechanisms that cause the ischemic pain. Presumably it inhibits kininogenases and tissue protein-hydrolyzing enzymes activated during ischemia.

REFERENCES

1. Arcangeli, P. (1965): *Riv. Crit. Clin. Med.,* 65:263–343.
2. Digiesi, V., Nassi, P., Castigli, E., Cicchi, P., Ramponi, G., and Arcangeli, P. (1974): *Boll. Soc. Ital. Biol. Sper.,* 50:532–536.
3. Edery, H., and Lewis, G. P. (1961): *J. Physiol.,* 160:20P.
4. Glenn, T. M., Herlihy, B. L., and Lefer, A. M. (1973): *Arch. Int. Pharmacodyn. Ther.,* 203:292–304.
5. Haberland, G. L. (1970): In: *Shock: Biochemical, Pharmacological and Clinical Aspects,* edited by A. Bertelli and N. Back. Plenum Publishing Corp., New York.
6. Hermansen, L., and Osnes, J. B. (1972): *J. Appl. Physiol.,* 32:304–308.
7. Kassel, B., Radicevic, M., Ansfield, M. J., and Laskowsky, M. (1965): *Biochem. Biophys. Res. Commun.,* 18:255–258.
8. Stock, W., and Isselhard, W. (1972): *Vasc. Surg.,* 6:255–262.
9. Trautschold, I., Werle, E., and Zickgraf-Rudel, G. (1967): *Biochem. Pharmacol.,* 16:59–72.

Summary of Workshops and Other Symposia

Advances in Pain Research and Therapy, Vol. 1,
edited by J. J. Bonica and D. Albe-Fessard.
Raven Press, New York © 1976.

Workshop on Data Banks

Chairman: Richard G. Black

University of Washington School of Medicine, Seattle, Washington 98195

This sparsely attended conference addressed itself to Data Collection systems and their practice and philosophy as applied to the problem of chronic pain. The paucity of information concerning the epidemiology, clinical management, and natural history of the individual with chronic pain as a primary health problem has been noted by Dr. Bonica. This session was dedicated to investigating current and future methodology for providing meaningful information in these areas.

Papers and discussion were presented by Dr. T. C. Chen, a statistician of the National Institute of Neurological and Communicative Disorders and Stroke, National Institutes of Health; Dr. R. J. Evans, an anesthesiologist and director of the Pain Clinic at the University of Toronto; and Dr. R. G. Black, assistant director of the University of Washington Pain Clinic at Seattle.

Dr. Chen emphasized the theoretical fundamentals of data collection systems, discussing problems in the areas of the nature of the data sought, the sources of the data, and their processing. He went on to suggest an approach to developing a data base, using a pilot study for experience prior to correction of data content and running of a long-term data collection system. Collaborative work between researchers, clinicians, system analysts, and statisticians was anticipated, as well as development of extensive computer software.

Dr. Evans described the Toronto experience of 11 years of pain data collection using a pain record chart, punched cards, and a computer. His study, comprising 2,000 patients, has led Dr. Evans to conclude that this type of data has much to offer in identifying patterns of pain in specific groups and analysis of new or current treatments. The educational benefits of such a data bank were noted to include better patient care through better physician and student access to wider international experience and current knowledge as well as better insight into pain mechanisms and their management.

Attempts at data collection in the highly service-oriented Seattle pain clinic were explained by Dr. Black. The current approach using a mark sense data-collection form, which is part of an anesthetic record, looks promising in that it offers economy and compliance in acquisition of the data at the clinical level.

Much enthusiasm was demonstrated by all present; unfortunately, future plans were clouded by problems in funding a clearly defined data base for chronic pain on which to proceed.

Ten Years' Experience with a Computerized Pain Data Retrieval System

Ramon J. Evans

Irene Eleanor Smythe Pain Clinic, Toronto General Hospital, and University of Toronto School of Medicine, Toronto, Ontario, Canada

A pain clinic was established in 1965 by the University of Toronto to investigate difficult pain problems from all aspects, with the ultimate hope of improving general management. In reviewing the literature, it became apparent that much of the information was shallow and imprecise, with variations proportional to the special interest of the subspecialist concerned. We therefore elected to devise a standard legible system to follow, one that could be transferred to punch cards for computerization. Thus we felt we could review data from time to time, produce a "pain data bank," and reduce the necessity for reviewing the hospital records. At the same time, it was felt that the role of the computer in research, teaching, and standards of care might be evaluated. We appreciated at the outset that no system is perfect, and that certain aspects of pain management are not "computerizable," e.g., religious beliefs, personal, family, and physicians' judgments and attitudes. The data collected were to be used initially for a retrospective analysis of results of conventional therapies, in the hope that factual data might be more meaningful and might promote research approaches to individual patient treatment.

Working with an informal interdisciplinary team, we constructed our pain record chart (Fig. 1) in an endeavor to collect what we felt would be significant data. The contents of this chart includes the following. Each patient is assigned a clinic code number to ensure privacy, for which only relevant data are recorded. We feel that our chart can be partly completed by a secretary, and, with a little practice, the remainder can be completed in approximately 15 min. Subjective clinical fact places strong reliance on a patient's history, which may be a disadvantage; but the advantages must be weighed against the participating physician's ability to assess the facts correctly and objectively, as there is no consistent teaching or approach to pain control.

The collected data are transferred to a code index form from a self-designed program. Examples of the columns are as follows. We use 70 columns at present, but can add to these, which is the great advantage of a computer program. The coded forms are then given to a keypunch operator for input to a time-shared computer. In order to complete the code index form, a careful editing of the record is required; without rigid definitions or categories, inconsistencies will occur. Quality control of facts relating to pain is helped by continuity of care; therefore, close follow-up and adherence to programming is essential.

In a cosmopolitan city such as Toronto, and with modern methods of transportation, the geographic variations and epidemiological studies are complex, and patterns of disease and complaints are irregular. It is therefore important to have a number large enough to be computed, in order to analyze data satisfactorily. We have found that approximately 50% of our patients have pain associated with malignant disease, and this forms the major part of our program of 2,000 patients at present.

Pain Clinic Record

Patient Code No. ______

AGE: 18	EYES 19	SEX 20	HAIR 21	PERSONALITY 22	MISC. 23	24
01 DECADE	01 BLUE	01 MALE	01 FAIR	01 NORMAL	01 ALCOHOLIC	01 IN PAIN
02 10	02 BROWN	02 FEMALE	02 DARK	02 ANXIOUS	02 DRUG ADDICT	02 NO PAIN
03 20	03 GREY		03 RED	03 OBSESSIONAL		
04 30	04 GREEN		04 GREY	04 DEFENSIVE		
05 40	05 OTHER		05 BALD	05 MANIAC		
06 50			06 OTHER	06 SCHIZOID		
07 60				07 IMMATURE		
08 70				08 PSYCHOPATHIC		
80				09 HYSTERICAL		
				10 DEMENTED		
				11 DEPRESSED		
				12 SENILE		

INSURANCE DETAILS. P/S.P./Pr.

INVEST. 17
11 pH & GASES
10 HAEMOGLOBIN
09 W.B.C.
08 E.S.R.
07 PL. PROTEINS
06 F.B.SUGAR
05 URIC ACID
04 CALCIUM
03 POTASSIUM
02 URINALYSIS
01 CSF.

HOSP. NO.

02 OUT PATIENT 16
01 HOSPITALISED

DATE

X-RAYS 15
15 CHEST
14 SKULL
13 NECK
12 SPINE
11 ABDOMEN
10 ARMS
09 HANDS
08 LEGS
07 FEET
06 PELVIS
05 IVP.
04 GIT.
03 BA.EN.
02 GBV.
01 ANGIOGRAM

PATIENT NO. INT. CODE NO.:

SURNAME: MR./MRS./MISS FIRST NAME:

ADDRESS: TEL. NO. FAMILY DR.:

OCCUPATION: REFERRED BY:

CLIN. DIAGNOSIS: DATE DIAGNOSED:

OPERATIONS & DATES:

CHIEF COMPLAINTS: PREVIOUS T'TMENTS:

SOCIAL HIST: M/S/W/D CHILDREN REL. SMOKES M/E ALCOHOL S/E

FAM. HIST: T.B., THYROID, DIAB., EPIL., PSYCH., LUES, PARALYSIS, OTHER

PAST HIST:

SITE 01
NEURECTOMY
RHIZOTOMY
CORDOTOMY – CERVIC.
– THORAC.
– LUMB.
HYPOPHYSECTOMY
LOBOTOMY
P.V. SYMPATHETIC
P.V. SOMATIC
CAUD. SYMPATHETIC
CAUD. SOMATIC
SP. SYMPATHETIC
SP. SOMATIC
CERVICAL PLEXUS
BRACHIAL PLEXUS
LUMBAR PLEXUS
TRIGGER POINT
THALAMOTOMY
LEUCOTOMY
EXTRADURAL
SUBARACHNOID
OTHER

PRETREATMENT RECORD

LYMPH GLANDS: AXILL., S. CLAV./JUGULAR/ INGUINAL, OTHER

TEMP. N/E, ANAEMIC, CLUBBING, RASHES, NOURISHMENT G/A/P, OEDEMA, JAUNDICE, THYROID, BREASTS R/L, APPEARANCE

R.S. U.R.T.I., COUGH, HICCOUGH, ASTHMA, PNEUMONITIS, PLEURISY, EMPYEMA, EMPHYSEMA, ABSCESS, N.A.D., OTHER

E.N.T.

THERAPY NOTES

POST TREATMENT RECORD

AGENT 02
TRANQUILLIZERS
HYPNOTICS
NARCOTICS
ANALGESICS
ANALEPTICS
LOCAL ANAES.
ALCOHOL
PHENOL
I.V. SOLN.
RADIOTHERAPY
– X-RAYS
– COBALT
CHEMOTHERAPY

WEIGHT 14
LBS.
03 GAIN
02 STEADY
01 LOSS

COMPLICATIONS 13
10 PARESIS
09 PARALYSIS
08 HAEMORRHAGE
07 SHOCK
06 PARAESTHESIA
05 HYPERAESTHESIA
04 INCONT. BOWELS
03 INCONT. BLADDER
02 BLOOD DYSCRASIA
01 OTHER

HISTORY 12
03 RELIABLE
02 VAGUE
01 LANGUAGE DIFFIC.

C.V.S. PREV. DIS., FUNC. CAP. 1, 2, 3, 4
SHOCK, HYPERTENSION, FIBRILLN., P. /M.
J.V.P.N/E B/P , ECG.

A.S. APPETITE G/A/P, DISTENSION,
BOWELS R/C, NAUS./VOM., ASCITES,
L/K/S PALP., HERNIAL ORIF., RECTAL,
VAG. EXAM.

G.U. FREQUENCY, DYSURIA, HAEMATURIA,
PNEUMATURIA, NOCTURIA, INCONT., URGENCY,
RESIDUAL CCS.

OBST. PARA: TOXAEMIA, OTHER
MENARCHE , MENSES , MENOPAUSE
DISCHARGES

C.N.S. CR. NERVES FUNDI: R/L
TONE POWER
CO-ORDN. SENSATION PP/LT

REFLEXES R: B.T.S.K.A.PL. ABD
L: B.T.S.K.A.PL. CREMASTERIC Ⓡ Ⓛ

EEG.

SKEL. SYST.

DEFORMITY
TENDERNESS
DIM. R.O.M.
WASTING
S.L.R. - R. L.
SPRINGS < RA R.L. / LA L.L.

AGENT 02
(CONTINUED)
SURGERY
E.C.T.
PSYCHOTHERAP
PHYSIOTHERAPY
HORMONES
COMBINATIONS
PLACEBO
OTHER

OPERATOR
DR.

ANAESTH. C
SEDATION
LOCAL ANAESTH
GEN. ANAESTH.
OTHER
NIL

RESULTS 04
EXCELL.
GOOD
POOR
NO CHANGE

1 MON.
2 MOS.
3 MOS.
4 MOS.
5 MOS.
6 MOS.
6 to 12
12 to 24
24 to 36

SITE OF PAIN 11	CLASSIFICATION 10	PAIN 09	DURATION 08	SEVERITY 07	IN'FERENCE WITH SLEEP 06	TESTS
12 MULTIPLE	11 OTHER	03 SUPERFICIAL	03 DAYS	03 MILD	03 YES	05 OTHER
11 HEAD & NECK	10 CIRCULATORY	02 DEEP	02 MONTHS	02 MODERATE	02 NO	04 AMYTAL
10 THORAX	09 PSYCHOGENIC	01 UNKNOWN	01 YEARS	01 SEVERE	01 UNKNOWN	03 P.G.R.
09 BREAST	08 ORGANIC					02 DERMOMETER
08 U. ABDOMEN	07 PER. NERV./SYST.					01 K.D.T.
07 L. ABDOMEN	06 SYMP. DYSKINESIA					
06 PERINEUM	05 MALIGNANCY					
05 ARM R/L	04 INFLAMMATORY					
04 LEG R/L	03 POST TRAUMATIC					
03 BACK	02 DEGENERATIVE					
02 EYE R/L	01 POST OPERATIVE					
01 E.N.T.						

INVESTIGATIONS 17

DATE	HB.	W.B.C.	E.S.R.	PL. PROT.	K^+	$CA.^{++}$	URIN-ALYSIS	C.S.F.	pH	PCO_2	PO_2	TCO_2	B.E.

ADDITIONAL POST TREATMENT RECORD

FIG. 1. Pain record chart.

BENEFITS OF A COMPUTER PROGRAM

In this age of superspecialization and an explosion of knowledge, no one person can be expected to know, let alone keep abreast of, international literature or events.

Continuing education and language barriers are a constant concern to us all; by collection of data in digit form, however, a wider experience can be collated, up-to-date knowledge can be more easily obtained, and analyses by independent groups become more meaningful.

Up to this time, the major output of our program includes the following.

A. Patient Care
   1. Learning the incidence of intractable pain in malignant disease (0.1–0.2%).
   2. Learning the primary sites of tumor most likely to cause intractable pain.
   3. Learning the patterns of pain associated with tumors at these primary sites, for example, the carcinoma of cervix story.
   4. Learning the outcome of various modes of treatment, with concomitant improvement in quality of care; for example, earlier percutaneous cordotomy, fewer phenol nerve blocks, extenuating radiotherapy, which has encouraged
   5. New diagnostic examinations and therapeutic regimens, for example, inferior vena cavography, thermography, lymphography, percutaneous cordotomy.
   6. Reduces dilemmas of treatment: The student, physician, patient, and family can be better informed.
   7. Colleague acceptance
   8. Lessened demand for chronic care beds

B. Teaching
   1. We have been able to give accurate facts related to pain to undergraduates, postgraduates, and paramedical personnel, without traditional misconceptions or bias.
   2. We can review our own experience and update our knowledge.
   3. Through improved factual information, judgment—the basic "art of medicine"—can be compounded with scientific expertise to improve patient care and public relations.
   4. We can compare alternative treatment programs in different hospitals within the city.
   5. Undesirable side effects or complications of specific regimens can be put in perspective so that esoteric and common problems are given correct emphasis.

C. Research
   1. Accurate, easily retrievable, factual information is recorded.
   2. The time-consuming task of searching hospital records has been avoided.
   3. Epidemiological data, useful in formulating future plans, has improved patient care, for example, paraaortic radiation in Stage III carcinoma of cervix.
   4. Clinical assessment has been correlated to devise new diagnostic/therapeutic principles and regimens.
   5. As a learning/teaching tool, it has made statements more meaningful.
   6. *Pharmacological efficacy* and data give precise data, rather than impressions.

SUMMARY

A review of 10 years' experience with 2,000 patients in a computer pain data retrieval system is presented, with comments on the limitations and advantages of the system. In the past, isolated expert observers, intuition, and previous experience in similar circumstances have been the mainstays of pain management, but with an orderly factual approach it is hoped that the quality of patient care will improve.

It is concluded that computerized pain data have much to offer in rendering data readily available in a standard, international digit language for patient, student, and physician. Patterns of pain may be identified within specific groups, and analysis of data initiates new investigations or treatment, which improve the quality of patient care.

There is a need for international collaboration to build banks of pain data in digit form on a shared international basis; the benefits may be summarized as follows.

1. Good patient care, through student/physician access to wide international experience and up-to-date knowledge.
2. Continuing education can be enhanced through international collaboration.
3. There is no language barrier.
4. Time can be conserved by preventing the need for library or hospital chart searches.
5. "Pain data banks" may initiate greater understanding of pain mechanisms, and provoke a more aggressive approach to its management.

Pain Data Center, Epidemiology, and Statistics

Ta-Chuan Chen

National Institute of Neurological and Communicative Disorders and Stroke, National Institutes of Health, Bethesda, Maryland 20014

Chronic pain is a complex health problem the resolution of which requires the joint effort of related scientific disciplines. The development of a pain data center that would consist of a data bank on pain which would serve as the information pool for research and clinical investigations on pain, and an operating unit which would assume the basic function of systematic planning, collection, processing, and retrieval of data on pain seems to be a necessary prerequisite to the promotion and the facilitation of research on, and clinical investigations of, pain. Collecting clinical data through a cooperative system would have the advantage of saving cost and time by reducing duplication of effort, and providing investigators and clinicians of related disciplines with a broad and comprehensive source of information on pain. However, such problems as how to make use of the data, how to avoid bias in the collection, and how to maintain the quality of the data, etc., must be resolved before such a system can be usefully established.

This paper describes some of the problems, approaches, and plans relating to the development of a pain data center as well as the potential use of the data for preliminary epidemiological and clinical studies on pain.

PROBLEMS

Relating to Data Collection

What do we expect to learn from the data? What problems are to be investigated with the data?

What kinds of data would provide sufficient information for the investigations intended? What kinds of data can be collected without special effort or burdening the patients?

What kinds of patients are to be involved in the data collection? (Patients admitted by pain clinics, hospital pain units and/or private physicians?)

What are the standards for recording and reviewing these data?

Relating to the Cooperative Data-Collection System

What are the qualifications of the participating units in the cooperative system? (Depends on the completeness of examination, diagnosis, evaluation, and treatment of pain used by each participating unit.)

How to maintain cooperation and consistency among participating units in the collection and recording of data? (Complete cooperation and willingness to adopt a standard system of recording and reviewing data is necessary.)

How to maintain the quality of the data, and to maintain consistency of recording over time? (Some data quality control system must be developed for this purpose.)

Relating to the Central Processing and Service Unit

What shall the primary goal of the central unit be? A comprehensive data center, or a data source information center?

If the latter, what kinds of data should be indexed, filed, and stored in the data center?

After the goals and functions are established, what services should be expected from the data center?

APPROACH

It would be wise at the beginning to concentrate on a few relatively clearly defined chronic pain syndromes in the data collection system.

Preparatory Phase

For each pain syndrome:

List problems to be studied and questions to be answered using the data.
List data items and definitions required.
Design appropriate charts and forms for data recording.
Establish standards and procedures for data recording.
Develop a data coding and data entry system.
Develop computer indexing, retrieval, and reporting systems.

Pilot Study Phase

Develop a pilot data center to investigate the workability and feasibility of the data collection and computer system proposed in the preparatory phase, to determine problems and points to be improved.

Design a small-scale study requiring the stored data (e.g., evaluation of some pain assessment questionnaire) to check the coordination and consistency among participating units and the data retrieval and reporting service.
Estimate, using the pilot study results, the costs and the most efficient way of operating a data center on a normal basis.
Design on the basis of pilot study experience the most appropriate administrative and organizational structure of a data center (size of staff, positions, responsibilities, etc.)

Normal Operation Phase

Increase the number of data-collection participants. Expanding the pilot study to a full-scale operation.

Develop annual and special summary reports of data collected.
Develop information services, regulations, and procedures for users. (Planning pain-related clinical data collection for specific clinical and epidemiological studies.)

PLANS

Design of Data Pool

Organize a work team including researchers, clinicians, system analysts, and statisticians to:

1. Develop a preliminary protocol of a list of questions and problems expected to be studied with the data. Define the problems and questions. Provide a detailed list of data items and information to be collected for the purpose of study. Classify data into those recordable in an ordinary pain clinic set-up and those which would require specific perhaps costly procedures. Categorize the data information to be recorded.
2. Submit the list of questions and problems and the list of data categories and items, etc., to a selected team of pain research scientists and clinicians in major related disciplinary areas for review of their appropriateness, and for comments, revisions, and modifications.
3. Obtain and compile feedback from the reviewers, that is, their comments, additional questions, problems, and data items, etc.
4. Develop charts and forms for data recording. Design instruction sheets for standard recording and specifications.
5. Submit revised list of problems, questions, data item, categories, charts, forms, etc., to the selected team for further review, comments, and corrections.
6. Obtain and compile additional feedback from reviewers.
7. Finalize design of charts, forms, standards, and standard procedure of data recording.
8. Prepare a report of the work for a presentation or publication in some journal such as *Pain*.

Development of Computer "Software" System

Organize a work team including researchers, clinicians, system analysts, computer programmers, and statisticians, and so forth, to:

1. Develop data coding and verifying systems.
2. Develop a data processing and retrieval system suitable for an individual participating unit.
3. Develop an indexing, searching, processing, and retrieval system for the data center.
4. Develop computer programs for indexing, storage, retrieval, tabulating, and reporting of the data information.

Computer Hardware Facilities

1. Investigate computer equipment necessary for the operation of a central coordinating and data source information system, its cost, maintenance, and personnel required to operate the facility.
2. Evaluate the computer equipment necessary for the operation of a comprehensive data center (if decided), its cost, maintenance costs, and the personnel required to operate the facility.

Pilot Study

1. Time required to conduct the pilot study: approximately 3 years.
2. Number of participating units: 3–5.
3. The staff required in the data unit of each participating clinic consists of one part-time physician to supervise data recording and review charts and forms to maintain the quality and standards of data; and one part- or full-time coding, keypunch, and data-processing computer aide.
4. Establish contract for the use of a computer system for the pilot central unit.
5. Determine the feasibility of the data collection and recording procedures and system consistency among participating units for data collection and recording.
6. Test the suitability of the central processing and retrieval system under actual operating conditions.

USE OF DATA AND THEIR LIMITATION

1. The data must be used constantly for various retrieval of information and for studies. (A data center should not merely be a huge storage of data with no definite purpose.)

2. The generality of the inferences made and the information drawn from the data are subjected to the limitation of the kind of data collected and to the characteristics of the patient group from whom the data were obtained.

3. Results of studies using clinical data of the pain data center should generally be regarded as suggestive and less definitive. For certain kinds of studies, the conclusions should be verified and confirmed further by a well-designed study.

4. Potential use of the data for preliminary epidemiological and clinical studies employing statistical techniques can be:

Clinical definition and classification of chronic pain syndromes.

Case finding of various chronic pain syndromes. (Estimation of incidence and prevalence of chronic pain in general and specific syndromes in particular, validity depends on the representativeness of the patient group.)

Etiological factors, which may be responsible for certain chronic syndrome pain, or formulation of etiological hypotheses for further investigations.
Health care statistics of chronic pain patients (cost and indirect cost.)
Investigation of psychological, sociological, and environmental influences on chronic pain patients.
Investigation of some questionnaire for the assessment and evaluation of pain.
Investigation of correlations among various clinical and psychological pain reactions.
Investigation of the efficiency of matching experimental pain to the pathological pain as a method of measuring severity of pain.

Workshop on Taxonomy of Pain

Aaron Ganz

National Institute of Dental Research, National Institutes of Health, Bethesda, Maryland 20014

Approximately 25 individuals attended this workshop. After the chairman briefly described the purpose of the workshop and some general aspects of the pain taxonomy problem, Dr. Edward Driscoll, National Institute of Dental Research (NIDR), reported on the workshop on Oral-Facial Pain held under NIDR auspices in Bethesda, Maryland on November 18–19, 1974. This workshop–conference was held to examine problem areas in the diagnosis and treatment of orofacial pain, with special emphasis on problems of definition and classification. Pain syndromes were divided into four major categories based on their primary site of origin: neurological, musculoskeletal, vascular, and psychogenic. Following a general session, four working groups were established to examine each of the above categories in depth and to develop a preliminary classification system for each category. A final general session was held in which each group reported on its progress and during which a number of related general topics (such as the development of a computer-based system for pain data information storage) were discussed. Some progress was made despite the difficulty and complexity of the task. Problems of overlap were considerable, and difficulties emerged in attempting to integrate the individual category classification structures into a meaningful overall classification system. Greatest progress was made by the group that dealt with the neurologic category.

At the Florence workshop meeting, it was not possible to delve into the substantive issues involved in pain taxonomy. Strong support was expressed from the floor for the importance of the problem and for the objective of continuing efforts to develop a generally acceptable pain taxonomy, including a standardized terminology. The current state of confused terminology and absence of an acceptable pain classification system has resulted in major communication problems, which confound the reporting and evaluation of pain research results, particularly in clinical pain research. Appreciation was expressed to NIDR for its pioneering effort in pain taxonomy, and strong encouragement was provided to NIDR to continue these efforts. Finally, NIDR was designated to serve as the focal point for continued information dissemination and coordination on an international basis as an official activity of the IASP. It was clear from the discussion that the difficulties of this task should not be underestimated. A progress report on these efforts will be presented at the next World Congress on Pain at Montreal in 1978.

Introduction to Symposia

J. J. Bonica

During the First World Congress on Pain, two symposia were held in Florence, one on Friday evening, September 5, and the second on Monday evening, September 8. I was pleased to be chairman of each of these sessions because it gave me an opportunity to interact with some of the most experienced and distinguished investigators of analgesics and sedatives—drugs that constitute the most important method of managing pain today.

Although not an integral part of the Congress, I believe it was most appropriate to hold these symposia in conjunction with this first major meeting on pain. One of the purposes of the International Association for the Study of Pain, the sponsor of the Congress, is to promote dissemination of new information through various mechanisms. One means is to encourage meetings that will bring together scientists, physicians, and other health professionals from different disciplines to exchange scientific information, and another is through its publications. Pursuant to these purposes, a summary of each of the two meetings is included in this monograph.

Symposium on Nefopam HCl (Acupan®): A New Analgesic

Chairman: J. J. Bonica
University of Washington, Seattle, Washington

Co-chairman: W. T. Beaver
Georgetown University, Washington, D.C.

Participants:
J. R. Aluja-Deu *Hospital Juarez, Mexico City, Mexico*
J. W. Bellville *University of California, Los Angeles, California*
A. Cohen *Peninsular Testing Corporation, Miami, Florida*
G. E. Cronheim *Riker Laboratories, Northridge, California*
L. de Thibault *University of Ghent, Ghent, Belgium*
W. Forrest *Stanford University, Palo Alto, California*

Sponsored by Riker Laboratories, a subsidiary of the 3M Company.

M. M. Gassel *San Francisco, California*
R. W. Houde *Sloan-Kettering Institute, New York, New York*
D. C. Kvam *Riker Laboratories, St. Paul, Minnesota*
O. N. Ré *Riker Laboratories, Northridge, California*
A. Sunshine *New York University Medical Center, New York, New York*

Bonica: Ladies and gentlemen. I am pleased to be chairman of this symposium and to have Dr. Beaver as my co-chairman. On our behalf and on behalf of the panelists, we welcome you to what I hope will be a very informative session. As you are all aware, the purpose of this symposium is to discuss the data derived from some of the investigations done to date on a promising new analgesic compound, which formerly had a generic name of fenazoxine, but which now has the generic name of nefopam. The drug was developed by Riker Laboratories, which has given it the trademark of Acupan®. In compliance with FDA regulations in the United States, Riker has submitted this drug to very thorough laboratory and clinical studies carried out by highly competent individuals. It is therefore most appropriate to begin this symposium by having Dr. Osvaldo Ré, Director of Medical Services of Riker, give a brief overview of the history of the compound, the rationale for its early development, and also some of the material on a few of the earlier studies that will not be presented in any detail tonight.

SUMMARY OF PRESENTATIONS

Ré: I would like to present a brief summary of some of the pharmacological actions of this compound, as well as some of its therapeutic applications. The compound was synthesized in the early 1960s at Riker Laboratories in California. During the years 1964 through 1966, the early pharmacology as well as the necessary toxicological studies to make it possible to be studied in the clinic were carried out. In 1966, the compound was introduced into the clinic, and the first metabolic and safety studies, as well as the first exploratory trials for therapeutic applications, were carried out. At the same time, teratological investigations as well as pharmacologic and toxicologic studies were continued in the laboratory. In 1971, simultaneously at three centers, in Madrid, Athens, and San Francisco, a team headed by Dr. Fernandez, Dr. Diamantoupolos, and Dr. Gassel (all of whom are here with us today) defined the analgesic propensities of this compound quite clearly. In 1973, we undertook expanded clinical trials, and Dr. Sunshine in New York, Dr. Forrest in Palo Alto, and Dr. Cohen in Miami confirmed the analgesic effects of this drug. More recently, Dr. Aluja-Deu in Mexico City, as well as some other investigators in Mexico and in Germany, have further documented the analgesic effects of this compound. Nefopam hydrochloride stands alone as a chemical entity, as well as in its pharmacological actions, in the field of analgesia. It's not related chemically or pharmacologically to any other analgesic available.

[This paper was also presented during the regular sessions of the Congress. Please refer to the full paper elsewhere in this book for the rest of the presentation.]

Sunshine: Dr. Sunshine presented two papers. The first study concerned an evaluation of nefopam versus morphine, parenterally. This paper was presented during the regular sessions of the Congress, a full report of which can be found elsewhere in this book. Briefly, results of this study showed 20 mg nefopam as approximately equivalent to 12 mg of morphine. Onset and duration of action of both drugs were similar. The second study involved a double-blind comparison of 325 and 650 mg aspirin, 30, 60, and 90 mg nefopam, and placebo: Comparison of 30 and 60 and 90 mg Acupan® with aspirin demonstrated that the mean onset of activity seems to be quicker for Acupan® than for aspirin. These data suggest a relative potency of 10, meaning that Acupan® is 10 times as potent as aspirin on a per-milligram basis.

Aluja-Deu: The objective of this clinical trial was to compare the analgesic effects of nefopam in doses of 20 mg with pentazocine in doses of 30 mg every 6 hr by using a double-blind non-crossover method. Both analgesics were used in a series of 60 patients suffering from severe and acute pain; all patients had some orthopedic disease or were admitted for orthopedic surgical procedures. Nefopam provided a faster onset of relief than did pentazocine, and it was found to be as potent as pentazocine with the advantage of showing fewer and milder unwanted effects.

Gassel: During studies in our neurophysiological laboratories, patients in pain recorded a decrease in discomfort and showed clinical improvement concomitant with, and in spite of, facilitation of flexion and stretch reflexes. The full therapeutic effect was manifested at a time when the patients, as well as normal subjects, reported a decrease in the pain associated with a regular and invariable shock to the dorsum of the foot used to evoke the flexion reflex. Subsequent experiments with normal volunteer subjects by means of a new experimental technique and with patients in pain led this investigator to believe that nefopam was a potent analgesic effective by oral and parenteral administration and prompted the clinical trial for the report of this evening. In the double-blind crossover study of the analgesic effects of intramuscular doses of nefopam (20 mg), pethidine (50 mg), and saline placebo in 20 patients, nefopam and pethidine were found to be equally effective and statistically superior to placebo. A double-blind randomized study was also made of orally administered nefopam (60 mg) 3 times a day for 3 days and placebo 3 times a day for 3 days, in 80 patients. Nefopam was distinctly superior to placebo in analgesic effectiveness, both in initial single dose and in maintaining therapeutic benefit for the duration of a 3-day trial. Dr. Gassel concluded that nefopam is a potent analgesic of novel structure and unique physiological properties.

Forrest: These are the same data presented at the National Academy of Science meeting 2 years ago. This study was designed for a population of postsurgical patients, and the hope was that all patients would take all four medications, so they would receive 5 and 10 mg morphine, and 10 and 20 mg nefopam in randomized fashion. As it turned out, 12 patients completed all 4 medications, 11 completed 3, and a smaller number took 2 meds and 1 med. The analysis proposed as the appropriate approach for these data, takes into account position effects. Each group of patients was evaluated—those who completed 4 meds, those who completed 3, those who completed 2, and those who only took one—as individual groups on which bioassays are done, and the data are then pooled by Bennett's method. And if all four of these are pooled—those patients who got 4 medications, those patients who got 3, those patients who got 2, and those patients who got 1—a potency of approximately 0.2 with wide limits is obtained, taking into account the position effects.

Cronheim: Dr. Cronheim presented data which were obtained by Dr. Schietzel at the Radiation Clinic of the University Clinic in Essen, West Germany. Unfortunately, Dr. Schietzel could not attend this symposium. Forty patients with moderate chronic pain attributed to various forms of cancer, mostly with metastases, were included in a double-blind 10-day study comparing the analgesic efficacy of Acupan® with that of pentazocine. The doses of 60 mg Acupan® and 50 mg pentazocine, given 3 times daily for 10 days, were purposely held on the low side so as to accentuate any possible difference. The morning predrug pain was uniform throughout the study, thus demonstrating the chronic character of the pain. The SPIDs after the drug are 1.3 to 1.5 for pentazocine, and 2.3 to 2.9 for Acupan®, indicating substantial analgesia with both compounds. Patients on pentazocine showed a high incidence of sleepiness, whereas on Acupan® there was some incidence of sweating and peripheral vasodilatation. Gastrointestinal disturbance in the form of nausea occurred with the same frequency after both drugs. The investigator made the additional comment that the side effects after Acupan® were almost always mild, whereas in about 50% of the cases on pentazocine, they were classified as moderate.

Bellville: Dr. Bellville's paper was also presented during the regular sessions of the Congress; a full report can be found elsewhere in this book. The data showed little, if any, respiratory depression with the therapeutic doses of nefopam as compared with significant depression induced by morphine.

Cohen: In anticipation of widespread clinical use, a study of possible interactions of nefopam with eight other analgesics, tranquilizers, and antiinflammatory medications, when administered concomitantly, was undertaken. Each regimen consisted of 60 mg nefopam, in combination with 650 mg aspirin, 5 mg diazepam, 60 mg phenobarbital, 65 mg propoxyphene, 60 mg codeine, 50 mg pentazocine, 25 mg indomethacin, 50 mg hydroxyzine pamoate, and placebo. All medications were prepared in capsules of identical color and shape. Drug combinations were administered three times daily, and subjects were monitored daily. Serum levels of nefopam showed not unexpected variations between individuals in a given treatment regimen. Because of the large variation within the groups, a Mann-Whitney U-test was used to compare each group with the nefopam–placebo regimen. This test indicated no significant differences between the placebo regimen and the other eight regimens. Further analysis did show significant differences between serum levels for day 3, hr 2 and 4 versus day 1, indicative of continued drug absorption. Hence, these data suggest no defect in nefopam bioavailability due to the drug combinations tested.

Clearly, a higher incidence of side effects was detected in regimens nefopam–codeine and nefopam–pentazocine. The data suggest a simple additive effect in that these drugs, like nefopam, are central-acting analgesics. The lower incidence found with diazepam and phenobarbital, drugs with a central nervous system profile opposite to nefopam, might have resulted from a cancellation of side effects. This speculation deserves further study.

Thibault de Boesinghe: This panelist carried out an Acupan® study in cancer patients, with bone metastases, some of them with pathological fractures. The time between the intramuscular injection of 20 mg and the onset of analgesia was between 15 and 20 min. In seven cases, pain completely disappeared; in 22 cases, pain was diminished, the patients feeling that the pain was tolerable there was no necessity to give additional drugs. In three cases, there was only a slight effect; in two cases, there was no effect. These patients did not respond to morphine either. Side effects were mild—nausea and perspiration. A study with 10 patients with injections three times a day, 20 mg, intramuscularly was in progress. The only side effect seen was perspiration. Sometimes Acupan® is combined with tranquilizers so that pain is controlled throughout the day. The conclusion was that 20 mg of Acupan® parenterally is a very good analgesic. Orally, 90 mg is preferred, and no side effects were observed with this dosage.

Beaver: Dr. Beaver presented the results of the first 16 patients who have completed a study comparing graded doses of intramuscular nefopam, 7½ and 15 mg in one series, and 15 and 30 in a second series, with 4 and 8 mg intramuscular morphine. In this study, each patient received two doses considered by Dr. Forrest as optimal for postoperative pain. The preliminary data on only 16 patients showed a significant slope for the relative potency assay, and the best estimate of relative potency is 0.37. This puts it only slightly less than 0.5 or so that Dr. Sunshine arrived at in the same comparison, and somewhat above Dr. Forrest's initial estimate, and somewhat below his estimate when he revised his method of analyzing the data. Dr. Beaver concluded that these relative potency estimates all fall into a reasonably close range.

Kvam: To answer the question as to whether or not Acupan® is a narcotic antagonist, Dr. Kvam tested the drug in animals and found that it did not antagonize morphine in any of the analgesic tests, nor did it precipitate morphine abstinence in addicted monkeys or in rats.

DISCUSSION

Question: What about its performance in the standard animal screening tests for analgesic activity?

Kvam: It is active in certain of the common analgesic screening procedures. It is inactive in the tests that detect narcotic-like activity, such as radiant heat procedures, the tail-flick procedure, hot plate, etc.

Gassel: Lack of activity in some preclinical testing is explained on the basis that withdrawal and tail tests, are in fact, just simple flexion reflexes. The flexion reflex is particularly facilitated by this drug to mask the potential analgesic effects.

Black: I have questioned this drug's addicting and habituating properties.

Ré: We haven't had any such evidence so far . . . we have given this drug to normal volunteers for 3 months at the maximum oral dose on a blind basis versus placebo in an attempt to quantify the response after 3 months of therapy; we found no differences between those who took placebo and those who took drug. Admittedly, this is not a study fully intended to answer your question, but it suggests lack of abuse potential.

Houde: With regard to the question of abuse liability, this is a problem that is not really settled at this time. Apparently, this drug does not produce dependence of the morphine type; but whether or not it produces abuse, whether it has abuse liability in that it may produce euphoria or at least the feeling of well-being, is not known. This is one thing on which drugs are evaluated in terms of whether they should or should not be regulated.

Pepeu: It was mentioned that the drug interferes with cathecholamine uptake and that there was a mild central nervous system stimulation effect. Can we suspect a mild amphetamine-like effect in your drug?

Ré: In my opinion, this kind of a stimulation is more of an atropinic nature—the kind of excitation that one would get with atropine or with other anticholinergic drugs, or perhaps even like caffeine. I don't think it's an amphetamine effect.

Pepeu: On the other hand, you mentioned that among the side effects was sweating. Sweating is certainly not an atropinic effect. So, I wonder if you have any encephalographic recording showing the typical atropine-like pattern?

Ré: No, we don't have those kinds of data. This effect is probably weak and only detectable in the way of side effects; and when I mentioned dry mouth and blurred vision, I was just referring to two of the side effects we've seen. We have had some few cases of urinary retention, for example. I don't know if we can make a definite association between that and the use of the drug. So, in an attempt to categorize the drug, my overview of its pharmacology would be that it is indeed a weak anticholinergic. Now, we don't have any encephalograms to document this further. Sweating may be a premonitory manifestation of vasomotor effects.

Question: In relation to this, because depression is one of the important characteristics of chronic pain, I wonder if anyone has looked at the antidepressant effects of this drug and compared it to the traditional antidepressants in cancer patients, for example.

Ré: When the drug was synthesized, one of the pharmacological actions that was characterized through the screening procedures was one of antidepressant activity. And so it was tested as a psychotropic agent and it was found to be a weak central nervous system stimulant.

Bonica: If you can get this effect in a patient with chronic pain, he is going to get relief and he also gets elevation of mood, which is a very important attribute. Let me say that I have seen a lot of patients with chronic pain, and even when they get relief, if they have a prognosis whereby the pain is going to persist, they are going to have it for a long period of time; even though they, at that moment feel better, they still have the depression. I think you have to use something besides a true analgesic, for example, an antidepressant.

Dam: . . . About the atropine-like effect, does it increase pulse rate? Does it depress the blood pressure? What is the action on the myocardium? I'm interested in it because I might try it on myocardial infarction.

Ré: In the clinic, we've seen occasional tachycardia and transient increase in blood pressure. So, I think that this kind of sympathetic–anticholinergic activity emerges from time to time but, certainly, it dosen't seem to pose a practical problem.

Bonica: Ladies and gentlemen. I believe it is time to end this interesting discussion. We have heard some well-designed studies, comparisons with standards of reference, aspirin, placebos, etc. Acupan® shows some therapeutic efficacy and I'm impressed by the literature I have read and what we have heard this evening about the lack of, or at least much less, respiratory, circulatory, central nervous system effects, and possibly no dependence.

Symposium on Recent Studies on Narcotic–Tranquilizer Interaction in the Relief of Acute Pain

Chairman: John J. Bonica *University of Washington School of Medicine*
Participants: William T. Beaver *Georgetown University School of Medicine*
William H. Forrest, Jr. *Stanford University School of Medicine*
Lawrence M. Halpern *University of Washington School of Medicine*
Thomas G. Kantor *New York University Medical Center*
John E. Stambaugh, Jr. *Jefferson Medical College, Thomas Jefferson University*

INTRODUCTION

Ladies and gentlemen, on behalf of the participants and the sponsor, I welcome you to this symposium. As you are aware, the purpose of this evening's meeting is to discuss some recent studies on the interaction of hydroxyzine and other so-called tranquilizers and narcotics for the relief of acute pain. The symposium is being sponsored by the Pfizer Company, which manufactures hydroxyzine under the tradename of Vistaril®, and which has supported much of the research to be described this evening.

We all appreciate that the quest for a better pain reliever began thousands of years ago. Since 1806, when Sertuner synthesized morphine and the subsequent discovery of salicin by Le Roux, which eventually led to the development of acetyl-salicylic acid and other non-narcotic analgesics, there has been an ever-increasing, indeed, frenetic search for the perfect analgesic without side effects. The material to be presented this evening will be briefly summarized in the proceedings of the World Congress and published separately.

SUMMARY OF PAPERS

Dr. Beaver, under the topic "Interaction of Narcotics and Mood-Altering Drugs: A Brief Historical Review," discussed the investigation of the interaction of drugs not usually considered analgesics with the classic analgesics.

Since the isolation of morphine—the classic analgesic—many research efforts have been made to overcome its disadvantages by finding an agent that would be equi-analgesic, but without its undesirable side effects. This quest has taken many directions, including development of new analgesic compounds, the addition of other compounds to narcotics, or the combination of narcotics with mood-altering drugs. But evaluating the results of these efforts is a problem: well-controlled studies are lacking, and interrelating studies of acute and chronic pain are not feasible.

It has been said, in a general way, that any drug that makes people less anxious or that sedates them may have a place in the treatment of pain. However, this has not proved true. Two studies, one using chlorpromazine and morphine and the other using promethazine and morphine, found neither agent to relieve pain or enhance the analgesic effectiveness of morphine. Lack of either analgesia or potentiation of narcotic analgesic effect has also been demonstrated with triflupromazine. However, a study comparing metrotrimeprazine and morphine showed that phenothiazine to be half as potent an analgesic as morphine.

Studies with the minor tranquilizer hydroxyzine have suggested potentiation when used concomitantly with narcotics. A study by Momose evaluating pentazocine and hydroxyzine substantiated this effect, whereas another study by Sunshine suggested that hydroxyzine not only enhanced the analgesic activity of morphine, but seemed to have analgesic activity of its own.

Dr. Beaver concluded that owing to the heterogeneous nature of tranquilizers, further research is necessary on an individual basis.

Dr. Forrest ("The Bioassay of Morphine and Morphine Plus Hydroxyzine in Postoperative Pain") presented an interim report of an almost completed study that was designed as a four-point bioassay, comparing 5 and 10 mg morphine alone with 4 and 8 mg morphine combined with 100 mg hydroxyzine (for a total of four treatments). So far, he had studied 65 postoperative patients who received a total of 142 medications. All patients were interviewed by trained nurse-observers pre-operatively and postoperatively at 30- and 45-min intervals, for up to six observations. The two subjective response variables used were pain relief and pain intensity.

The total TOTPAR pain relief score results, remarked Dr. Forrest, reflect a positive dose-response curve. Furthermore, they showed that one can double the effect of morphine by adding 100 mg hydroxyzine. As far as side effects were concerned, up to that point in the study, the additive sedative effects were not large, and there were no instances of nausea following therapy with hydroxyzine alone or combined with morphine.

Dr. Beaver ("A Comparison of Analgesic Effects of Morphine, Hydroxyzine, and Morphine plus Hydroxyzine in Postoperative Pain"), prompted by the findings of Momose and Sunshine, designed a double-blind study to evaluate the analgesic effects of 8 mg morphine, 100 mg hydroxyzine, a combination of the two, and placebo. The methods used were similar to those of the Forrest study except that each of the 96 patients received only one dose of the four possible test medications. Standard subjective scaling was employed and questions were asked hourly by a full-time nurse-observer. The design was the classic 2×2 factorial, intended to analyze for interaction between treatments given together.

Dr. Beaver showed that the combination appeared to have a greater analgesic effect than either drug alone. An unexpected finding was that hydroxyzine alone had analgesic effect statistically equivalent to that of 8 mg morphine.

Dr. Beaver also looked into the variables of tension–anxiety. The patients were given a tension–anxiety questionnaire at the time of drug administration and 2 hr later. Relief of tension–anxiety closely paralleled that of pain relief. The only side effects that occurred frequently were those related to sedation, but these did not create any significant problem.

Dr. Beaver concluded that because hydroxyzine in his study unequivocally demonstrated a potent analgesic effect, further investigation of this agent and its congeners seems worthwhile.

Dr. Kantor ("Studies of Orally Administered Narcotics, Ataractics, and Combinations of the Two") discussed studies on oral pain relief and the problems inherent in such studies.

The first study he referred to was one that evaluated the analgesic effects of meprobamate (200 mg) and its combination with aspirin (325 mg). The patient population was similar to those studied by Dr. Beaver and Dr. Forrest. Surprisingly, 200 mg meprobamate resulted in less pain relief than did placebo. But with the combination of aspirin and meprobamate, the relief of pain was comparable to that seen with placebo. Aspirin seems to have "rectified" the algesic activity of meprobamate.

The second study tested the combined use of 50 mg meperidine with 100 mg hydroxyzine, and 100 mg meperidine with 100 mg hydroxyzine against 50 and 100 mg meperidine alone, and placebo. Fifty mg meperidine was not effective orally, although 100 mg meperidine was clearly effective. However, 100 mg hydroxyzine did not seem to augment its analgesic effect. Hydroxyzine alone was not statistically different from placebo.

Dr. Kantor then expanded on this apparent discrepancy in the action of parenteral and oral medications and brought up several possible reasons, including dosage and bioavailability, especially applicable to hydroxyzine. He also discussed possible modes of action of the minor tranquilizers, including modulation of the perception of pain, particularly with sedatives, as well as possible interference with the internuncial pools, a special feature of the carbamates.

Dr. Stambaugh ("Pharmacokinetic Studies of the Interactions Between Meperidine and Other Drugs"), who developed a pharmacokinetic model system in order to study the interaction of meperidine with other drugs, discussed the importance of such systems and their role in future studies. The inclusion of pharmacokinetic data in a study would permit better conclusions as to patient variation, closer approximation of therapeutic and toxic dosages, and more valid predictions of potentially toxic clinical situations.

Based on earlier work by Mather and Tucker, Dr. Stambaugh developed a sensitive assay of meperidine with a precision of 98% and a sensitivity of 10 ng/μl. Thus, it was possible to assay meperidine given in the normal therapeutic dosage range. In addition, Stambaugh measured the levels of the major metabolites of meperidine in the urine. By studying these levels, he could predict closely any changes in the metabolism of meperidine.

Prompted by a report on meperidine metabolic alterations caused by oral contraceptives, alterations considered similar to those caused by MAO inhibitors—namely, a reduction in meperidine excretion and an increase in normeperidine formation—he studied the effects of oral contraceptives on meperidine metabolism in 12 volunteers. There was no change in *n*-demethylation of meperidine. Meperidine and normeperidine excretion in both groups was identical.

The next investigation explored the interaction between meperidine and phenobarbital in 12 medical students. The findings showed that phenobarbital had no effect on serum meperidine levels. However, there was a definite decrease in urinary excretion of meperidine and an increase in normeperidine when phenobarbital was given, indicating enhancement of a *n*-demethylation of meperidine.

Among investigations of other potential interactions, Dr. Stambaugh referred to his study of hydroxyzine and meperidine. Using the same model system, six volunteers were administered placebo or hydroxyzine in doses of 25, 50, or 100 mg, intramuscularly, in combination with meperidine, intramuscularly. There was no significant difference in meperidine serum levels with or without hydroxyzine, and there were no changes in the cumulative excretion of meperidine or normeperidine in urine.

Dr. Halpern ("Theories of Pain Transmission and Perception"), reviewed several fundamental theories on the physiological aspect of pain, and examined some of the ways these theories can be applied to managing pain. He also discussed the problems involved in the management of acute, chronic–benign, and chronic–malignant pain.

Among the theories that form the basis of our understanding of pain, Dr. Halpern mentioned "specificity," "pattern," and the most recent one, the gate concept of Melzak and Wall, which perceives pain as "a multidimensional space comprising several sensory and affective dimensions."

During the discussion following the presentations, some important points were raised. Dr. Bonica remarked on the important physiological and psychological differences one sees between patients with acute pain and those with chronic. To the question as to whether there is any parallelism between enhancement of analgesia and side effects, Dr. Beaver commented that with sedatives, hypnotics, or tranquilizers there is no necessary correlation between analgesia and side effects.

Based on partial results of his study, Dr. Forrest believed that there were indications that hydroxyzine decreased the side effects of nausea and vomiting (given in combination with 8 mg morphine). Dr. Beaver also found a reduction in nausea and vomiting after hydroxyzine.

In answer to a question on possible respiratory depressant effects with hydroxyzine, Dr. Beaver quoted a study by Dr. Bellville. In that study, 100 mg hydroxyzine administered alone produced mild respiratory depression. This was statistically significant compared to placebo, but was unlikely to be of clinical significance in patients with normal respiratory function. However, pentazocine had a considerable respiratory depressant effect. The combination of the two was additive, and Dr. Beaver pointed out that by reducing the dose of pentazocine and adding hydroxyzine, one would expect respiratory depression to be less of a problem than with the larger dose of pentazocine alone. Dr. Bonica concluded that the overall profile of the studies presented suggests that, when given parentally in combination with narcotics, hydroxyzine does potentiate analgesia.

The complete proceedings of the symposium were published in a special report as a supplement to the January 1976 issue of *Hospital Practice*.

Subject Index

Advances in Pain Research and Therapy
Volume 2

INTERNATIONAL SYMPOSIUM ON PAIN OF ADVANCED CANCER

Advances in Pain Research and Therapy
Volume 2

International Symposium on Pain of Advanced Cancer

Editors

John J. Bonica, M.D., D.Sc., F.F.A.R.C.S.
President of the International Association for the Study of Pain
Professor of Anesthesiology
Director of Pain Center
University of Washington
Seattle, Washington

Vittorio Ventafridda, M.D.
Director
Division of Pain Therapy and Rehabilitation
Istituto Nazionale per lo Studio e la Cura dei Tumori
Milano, Italy

Associate Editors

B. Raymond Fink, M.D.
Secretary of the International Association for the Study of Pain
Professor of Anesthesiology
University of Washington
Seattle, Washington

Louisa E. Jones, B.S.
Executive Secretary and Treasurer, International Association for the Study of Pain
Editor, Research Publications
Department of Anesthesiology
University of Washington
Seattle, Washington

John D. Loeser, M.D.
Associate Professor of Neurological Surgery
Member of Pain Clinic
University of Washington
Seattle, Washington

Raven Press ▪ New York

Raven Press, 1140 Avenue of the Americas, New York, New York 10036

Made in the United States of America

International Standard Book Number 0–89004–2705
Library of Congress Catalog Card Number 78–55811

This Volume is Dedicated to

Dr. Ing. Virgilio Floriani
and
Signora Loredana Floriani

Two wonderful human beings whose magnificent personal attributes and extraordinary sense of humanitarianism are a constant source of admiration and inspiration.

Preface

This monograph contains the scientific papers presented and discussions held at the International Symposium on Pain of Advanced Cancer held in Venice, Italy on May 24–27, 1978. This symposium, sponsored by the Floriani Foundation of Milan, Italy and under the auspices of the International Association for the Study of Pain, L'Union International Contre Le Cancer, and the three most important Italian agencies against cancer, was attended by nearly 500 scientists, physicians, and other health professionals representing several dozen disciplines from 22 countries. This was, without doubt, the largest gathering of people interested in cancer pain ever held anywhere.

The primary goal of this symposium was to help rectify the serious deficiencies that exist in the current management of pain of advanced cancer by bringing together outstanding authorities from different disciplines to discuss virtually every aspect of the topic. The objectives of the symposium were: (1) to discuss the importance and magnitude of cancer pain, its mechanisms, and the physiologic, psychologic, and sociologic impact it has on the patient, the family, and society; (2) to evaluate all of the methods that may be used to relieve cancer pain within the framework of our current knowledge and human resources; (3) to critically analyze deficiencies that exist and to suggest how they may be eliminated; (4) to suggest some future directions that research might take to improve current methods and develop new methods of cancer pain therapy. These objectives were achieved and the results are presented in this monograph.

The reader's attention is called to the introductory remarks by Albino Cardinal Luciani, then Patriarch of Venice, who 3 months later was elected Pope John Paul I.

Part I of the volume contains a discussion of the importance and magnitude of cancer pain as a serious national and world health problem and a comprehensive overview of the anatomic, neurophysiologic, biochemical, psychologic, and behavioral aspects of nociception and pain in general. This serves as a background for the material in Part II, which includes discussion of etiology and mechanisms of cancer pain and its psychologic, emotional, psychosocial, sociologic, and nursing aspects.

The subsequent five sections contain reports intended to evaluate all of the methods currently being used to relieve cancer pain including various anticancer modalities, psychologic techniques, and sociologic strategies, systemic analgesics and related drugs, nerve blocks, ablative neurosurgical procedures, and neurostimulating techniques. Each of these sections contains a number of reports dealing with different agents or techniques. Each report was written by a person who is nationally or internationally recognized as an expert in the specific field. Most of these reports contain an evaluation of the efficacy, advantages, limitations, side effects, and complications of each particular technique or method based upon the personal experience of the author and review of the recent literature.

The contents of the next three sections are intended to integrate the preceding material into discussions of the clinical management of patients with pain due to cancer in one of several body regions which are among the most frequent and most difficult problems to deal with: head and neck; brachial plexus and chest; abdominal viscera and perineum. Each of these three sections includes a brief description of the incidence of pain in that particular part of the body and a summary of the efficacy and limitations of the most important modalities used for its relief. These are followed by a section that contains discussions of the basic principles of continuing and terminal care of cancer patients with special emphasis on the management of pain and a description of the organization and function of St. Christopher's Hospice by two highly qualified and experienced individuals: Dr. R. Twycross and Dr. C. Saunders. Also in the same section, Dr. G. Ford presents important facts about the incidence of cancer and cancer pain and its treatment within the framework of the British National Health Service. The last section contains prepared and spontaneous comments on future needs, goals, and directions regarding the research, teaching, and patient-care in the field of cancer pain. Most of the comments in this section were based on the information presented during the preceding 4 days.

We believe that the contents of this volume will be of significant interest to many health professionals, but especially to surgical, medical, and radiation oncologists, algologists (dolorologists), psychologists, psychiatrists, clinical pharmacologists, neurosurgeons, anesthesiologists, social workers, nurses, theologians, and all others who have the serious responsibility of managing patients with cancer pain. The information contained herein should give basic scientists and clinical investigators an insight into the great voids in our knowledge about basic mechanisms and, it is hoped, should stimulate further research efforts in this area. In view of the great paucity of information on the basic principles of managing cancer pain in oncology textbooks or other sources of information, the book should prove useful to teachers and students alike. Finally, proper application of the information about the various therapeutic modalities should markedly enhance the capability of physicians and other health professionals to provide most, if not all, patients with cancer pain with optimal pain relief. We hope that in this and other ways the book will help to improve and sustain the quality of life in patients with cancer—a responsibility that remains one of the most important obligations and laudable objectives of all health professionals involved in the care of these patients.

John J. Bonica
Vittorio Ventafridda
October 1978

Acknowledgments

On behalf of all of the speakers and participants of the symposium and all of the millions of patients suffering from cancer pain, the editors wish to express sincerest thanks, great appreciation and, indeed, gratitude to Mr. and Mrs. Virgilio Floriani of the Floriani Foundation for their generous support of the symposium on which this volume is based. Mr. and Mrs. Floriani and the Board of Directors of the Foundation deserve warmest congratulations and commendation for their foresight and perspicacity for proposing the development of a major international meeting to discuss the pain of advanced cancer. As is emphasized throughout the book, effective pain relief and the prompt management of the patient with advanced cancer related thereto is one of the most urgent problems of modern society.

On behalf of the Floriani Foundation and the speakers and registrants of the symposium, we express appreciation to His Excellency Giovanni Leone, then President of the Republic of Italy, for the High Patronage and the moral support provided the symposium and to Albino Cardinal Luciani for taking time out of his extremely busy schedule to attend and give the opening remarks. We also wish to express appreciation to other members of the Honorary Committee. The senior editor is especially delighted to acknowledge the presence of a dear friend, Princess Yana Alliata di Montereale, at the opening ceremonies. Having had that important meeting held on the beautiful island of St. Giorgio was a fitting tribute to her late father, Count Vittorio Cini, a magnificent human being, great philanthropist, and a truly Renaissance man.

The auspices of five professional societies or institutions helped to assure the success of the symposium, and for this the editors thank them most sincerely.

L'Union International Contre le Cancer
The International Association for the Study of Pain
L'Associazione Italiana per lo Studio del Dolore
Lega Italiana per la Lotta Contro i Tumori
L'Istituto Nazionale per lo Studio e la Cura dei Tumori

The development and running of such a large, comprehensive, scientific program and the highly successful outcome of the symposium were made possible only by the contributions of many, many individuals to whom we wish to acknowledge our indebtedness. The senior editor wishes to express sincere thanks and appreciation to members of the Scientific Program Committee for the help given in the development of a scientific program which made the symposium highly successful and productive. We also wish to express great appreciation and indebtedness to the members of the Organizing Committee for their time and effort in taking care of the hundreds of details required for the arrangements of the facilities needed for the scientific program on the island of St. Giorgio and the social activities for the speakers, their spouses, and the participants. These made it possible for us to run the impressively full and very comprehensive program on time and without a single flaw or problem. Among the members of the Organizing Committee several people deserve special recognition for their contributions.

First and foremost is Signora Loredana Floriani, not only for her enthusiastic support of the symposium, but equally important for her extremely active participation in the planning of the conference, in the development of the local arrangements, and in providing valuable help during the meeting. It is virtuously admirable that, considering her position in the Floriani Foundation, she put aside national tradition and worked long hours alongside the staff managing the registration desk and taking care of every need mentioned by speakers and participants alike. Signora Floriani's personal touch and involvement made the social events memorable experiences. Her infectious smile, warm personality, her unusual ability to exude friendship and other attributes that make her a magnificent human being greatly facilitated the onerous tasks of both editors.

In a similar fashion, Mr. Virgilio Floriani worked long hours during the development and running of the program and for several weeks after the symposium. The reader's attention is called to his introductory remarks because they reveal some of the unusual characteristics of this man and his unusual interest in the welfare of people and his compassion for patients with cancer pain. It is worth noting that through his brilliant mind, his interest and expertise as an electronics engineer, and through his own personal herculean efforts, Mr. Floriani rose from virtual poverty after World War II to head one of the most important industrial complexes dealing with electronics in the world. In addition to the financial support which made the symposium possible, his personal involvement, planning, and running of the 4-day meeting, and taking care of the most menial tasks and his unremitting enthusiastic support were critical to the success of the conference and to the publication of this monograph.

We also express very special thanks to Ms. Wanda Segre, secretary of the Floriani Foundation, for coordinating all of the activities of the Organizing Committee and for personally taking care of many of the details during the development and running of the symposium. She also coordinated the translation of a number of papers into English and carried out innumerable other tasks in an extremely efficient and very cooperative manner.

Ms. Louisa Jones, Executive Secretary and Treasurer of the International Association for the Study of Pain and editor of the Department of Anesthesiology of the University of Washington, helped the senior editor coordinate the development of the scientific program, was responsible for the editing and printing of the program and book of abstracts, and also helped the members of the Organizing Committee during the symposium. During the past several months, she has expended an unusual amount of time and effort in collating and editing all of the typed manuscripts and galley and page proofs for this volume. For these and other efforts on this project, we express our thanks and gratitude, Ms. Jones.

The editors also wish to acknowledge their appreciation and thanks to Drs. B. R. Fink and John Loeser for their editorial assistance; to Ms. Rosita Walsh, administrative secretary to the senior editor, for her invaluable help during the long and arduous process of planning the scientific program and editing this volume; to Ms. Linda Hipps and Juanita Cooke for typing of the edited manuscripts; and to Ms. Virginia Martin of Raven Press for her invaluable help in the publication of the volume.

Contents

PART 1. BASIC CONSIDERATIONS

PART 2. MANAGEMENT OF PAIN OF ADVANCED CANCER

Systemic Analgesics and Related Drugs

Nerve Blocks

Contributors

Page numbers refer to chapter opening page, or panel discussion page.

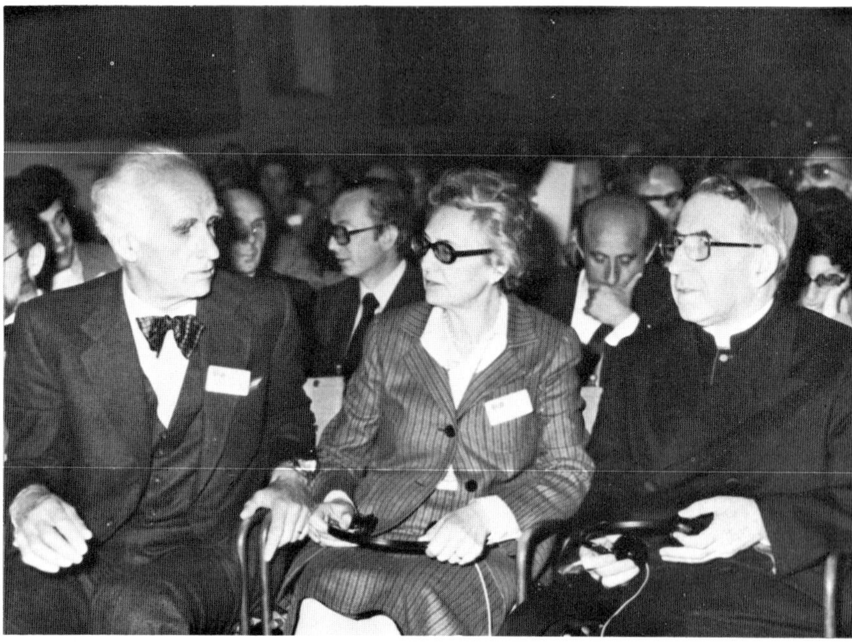

FIG. 1. *Left to right:* Ing. Virgilio Floriani, Mrs. Loredana Floriani, Albino Cardinal Luciani.

Introduction to Venice Symposium

Dr. Ing. Virgilio Floriani

One evening in the spring of 1977, Professors Maggi, Ventafridda, and Barbi, Dr. Motta, my son Marco, my wife, and myself met in Milano. We had recently formed the FONDAZIONE FLORIANI and we were examining the possible activities needed to fulfill the aims defined in the bylaws of the Foundation. The topic of pain, especially in the cancer patient, appeared not to have attracted sufficient attention in the past. Doctors tend to consider pain a secondary factor. The primary aim, the fundamental one in which they spent all their energy, is the cure and elimination of the disease. But the statistics tell us that in Italy alone there are more than 250,000 patients suffering from cancer and nearly 110,000 die annually from this disease. Of this latter group about 65 to 80% suffer such severe pain that it gravely affects both their quality of life and their relationship with their family and society.

We asked ourselves: Couldn't this be the subject of an international symposium? The answer was positive. But to have success, we had to stimulate the interest of a certain number of scientists of international renown from different disciplines with interest and expertise in this neglected field of medicine. In order to ensure that this would occur, it was necessary that the task be undertaken by a leading exponent in this field who was well-known and respected by other world scientists and clinicians. Professor Ventafridda suggested Professor John J. Bonica of Seattle.

In May 1977, while my wife and myself traveled in the United States, we went to Seattle and met Professor Bonica. We described to him our intention. We had no problem in convincing him to undertake such a task. I believe that we were favored in obtaining a positive response by the good reasons mentioned above, by Professor Bonica's long and intense interest in cancer pain, and also by the fact that he is of Italian origin and the symposium would be taking place in Venice—on the beautiful island of St. Giorgio. The symposium took place in May 1978, and this volume includes all the proceedings. The speakers were, in their essence, scientists: For them Nature is objective, its laws are unchangeable. The truth (or knowledge) obtains its origins from the systematic comparison between logic and experience, and this ensures a progressive character to knowledge itself.

The presentations, together with the discussions, took place before nearly 500 doctors and scientists from many countries; the publication of the proceedings and their diffusion constitute a further milestone in the fight against cancer pain. This was the aim that we had looked for. As it was foreseeable, such a symposium placed us face-to-face with a subject which is so complex that we were able to deal with it only in broad terms. Medicine as a true science—the study, the knowledge of the human body, the cure of its diseases—is a conquest of modern western civilization. Although its beginnings go back several millenia, it has been only since the time of Galileo that medicine has had a truly scientific basis. In the relatively short period of 300 years it has made many advances, especially during the past three or four decades, when more biomedical knowledge has been acquired than in all of the preceding period of human history. This has instilled great faith and confidence in the generations of our time, for many diseases which heretofore killed or disabled millions of people throughout the world have been eliminated or sufficiently controlled.

Although we still have not understood all of the mysteries of cancer, significant progress has been made in its therapy and some forms of this disease, if properly treated, in time can be cured. Since it is likely that the impressive momentum of biomedical research and new discoveries consequent thereto will continue at an even greater pace, we should have great faith that eventually this dreadful group of disorders given the generic term of *cancer* will be conquered. In the meantime, we must continue and indeed increase our efforts to assure patients with cancer that they will continue to enjoy the quality of life. To achieve this, we must effectively relieve the pain that is often associated with cancer, especially in the late phases of the disease. We may affirm that with the means we have today 70 to 80% of the patients with cancer pain could be relieved of the pain completely or it could be reduced to a tolerable level. Although progress has been made in this field, as attested by the papers presented in this volume, unfortunately it appears that heretofore the knowledge we already have has not been applied in the most effective way and often not at all. Consequently, innumerable patients with cancer continue to suffer and die with their pain unrelieved.

The presentations and discussions made during the 4-day symposium make it impressively clear, even to me as a layman, that we must mount a multipronged program suggested by Professor Bonica and emphasized by many others. We must disseminate the information already available and encourage all physicians and health professionals who assume the serious responsibility of caring for patients with cancer pain to apply it promptly and correctly. It is also clear that there must be a marked increase in research on all aspects of cancer pain in order to eliminate the voids of knowledge that currently exist. Only with new knowledge can we develop new drugs and modalities that will relieve pain more effectively without side effects and complications so that *all* patients with recurrent or inoperable cancer will enjoy a quality of life until their death.

To achieve the "total" answer to the problem of pain, to the doubts and apprehensions and suffering that it provokes, and to the fear of knowing that death is rapidly approaching requires many, many changes. For one thing, persons from many different disciplines must participate in this total effort of patient-care, research, and teaching. In addition to basic scientists, physicians, and other health professionals, there must be involvement of philosophers, theologians, and other men of culture. From this type of team effort will come the knowledge, the expertise, the hope, and the faith which will help patients with cancer, not only by relieving their pain, but also by giving them faith and hope that they will live the rest of their life in comfort and in the company of their family and friends.

Finally, and most importantly, the scientists, physicians, and other health professionals must have the moral and financial support from society, and the national, provincial, and municipal governments, as well as from the private sector. One of the most important reasons for organizing and supporting this symposium by the FLORIANI FOUNDATION has been to make the people more aware and appreciative of the serious nature of cancer pain as a major national and world health problem and to generate greater interest and support by various governmental and private agencies within and without Italy. The Board of Directors of the FLORIANI FOUNDATION hopes that this objective has been achieved. We will await with great anticipation for greater and more active involvement by all concerned in this noble cause.

Editor's Note

Almost exactly 3 months after Albino Cardinal Luciani, then Patriarch of Venice, made the following remarks as the first speaker at the official opening ceremony of the International Symposium on Pain of Advanced Cancer, he was elected Pope John Paul I. The feeling of extreme pride and pleasure by all those concerned with the symposium to have had such a great personality participate in the meeting was abruptly replaced 33 days later by immense grief and a sense of great loss. Mr. and Mrs. Floriani and other members of the Board of the Floriani Foundation, and members of the Scientific Program Committee, and the editors of this monograph take this opportunity to express great grief and distress at this tragically premature death of a man who in 34 days captured the imagination of the world and won the affection of millions—Catholic and non-Catholic alike—with his unprecedented humility, great humor, and winning smile.

On the basis of the remarks summarized here and his performance throughout his priestly life, it is apparent that he was intensely interested in the welfare and the rights of the individual, particularly those who were poor or ill—characteristics that caused him to be called "the Pastoral Pope." Moreover, in private conversation with the senior author at the time of the symposium, Cardinal Luciani expressed intense interest in patients with cancer pain and other chronic pain syndromes and his willingness to vigorously support future efforts by all those individuals involved in pain research and therapy and all those agencies interested in this field. We are confident that, had he lived, he would have lent his inestimably valued support and influence as Pope to "the cause of pain"—the current worldwide movement to markedly increase pain research and teaching and thus improve the lot of those who suffer cancer pain and other painful syndromes. In view of this and his many other attributes, the death of Pope John Paul I must be viewed as an immeasurable loss, not only to Catholics but all of the people of the world.

Remarks by Cardinal Albino Luciani

We are on the island of St. Giorgio, but thanks to its owner, the late, great philanthropist Count Cini, its name has been changed to "the Island of Hope." I sincerely wish that the results of this symposium will give great hope to patients affected with pain of advanced cancer.

I have been asked to say a few words on human suffering and its relief. In this world people ask you professors of medical research: "Please ease my pain, heal me with your expert knowledge and skill, help medicine take further steps forward toward the cure of cancer." In this same world people ask me other kinds of questions: "Why these pains that destroy the best part of the human being? Why must children and innocents suffer? If it is true that God exists, God our Father, how can we reconcile his Divine Providence with so many things that seem so out of place?" These questions hurt the heart of those who ask them and mine also because I have no clear, definite, and convincing answer to give, but only elements, bits and pieces of answers. I usually say: "I understand you, it is only human to have such problems." Christ on the cross cried: "God, why have you abandoned me?" And Christ said "no" to those who wanted to solve the problem of pain with "religious mathematics." He encountered the blind man and immediately His disciples asked him: "Master, who has sinned? He or his parents, that he was born blind?" And Jesus answered: "He has not sinned, nor have his parents."

Pilatus had ordered some Galileans killed; a tower fell in the same day killing 18 people. The disciples were tempted to apply "religious mathematics," but Jesus said: "Do you think that those Galileans were more sinners to have suffered such a fate? No, I tell you. Or do you think that the 18 killed were more guilty than all the inhabitants of Jerusalem? No, I tell you." The Bible thus shows us that the good are not always rewarded in this world, nor the bad punished. So? So we must remember that human life, to quote Cronin, is an adventure in two worlds. We begin here, but the conclusions are in the other world.

The Bible says: "The souls of the just are in God's hands. The foolish thought them dead, their end was considered a disaster, their departure from us a downfall; but they are in peace, their hope is full of immortality." Hope and faith in a future life are the first element for my answer.

When we think of Paradise we can understand a little about suffering that is not directly wanted but only permitted by the Lord, who wishes only well for His children. This even if He does not want to interfere with miracles, to modify the course of nature that He himself has created with its own laws.

Even Christ in the Gethsemane Garden at the beginning prayed the Father to remove the "chalice of pain," and only after having prayed and received courage was He able to add: "Thy will, not mine, be done." And it is not Christ's pain, as such, that saved us, but the patience, the love, the obedience with which He accepted pain. And here we have another element to answer our question on human suffering. If pain is accepted and mastered, it can help to teach us the way to become better persons.

I repeat these are only "bits and pieces" of answers, and I want to underline the fact that Christ has taught us more about how to endure our pain and other people's pain than why we must suffer, and He has shown us that he loves those who suffer.

When Jesus tells the story of the Good Samaritan who helped the man who had been robbed and beaten by the thieves, He ended saying: "Go and do the same." He even made Himself and the sick man one, saying: "I was sick and you visited me, you have done it to me." Many have taken these words seriously.

But Christ's pains give us precious indications toward understanding the behavior of sick people during their illness. In the Gethsemane Garden He wanted to try to undergo the horrors of suffering as if to tell us: "I shall open the way; I will not be so surprised if also you will be afraid of pain; only try to imitate me."

"The Lord our Father," Jesus once said, "knows what you need even before you ask Him." And when Jesus is afraid He calls to his Father, asks, and obtains the necessary force and faith.

Many sick Christians, taking example from Christ, pray to have the strength to accept and bear pain with courage and resignation. Sometimes passive resignation of pain becomes an active offering of sufferings to God.

But Christ did not overlook even the smallest remedies. In the Gethsemane

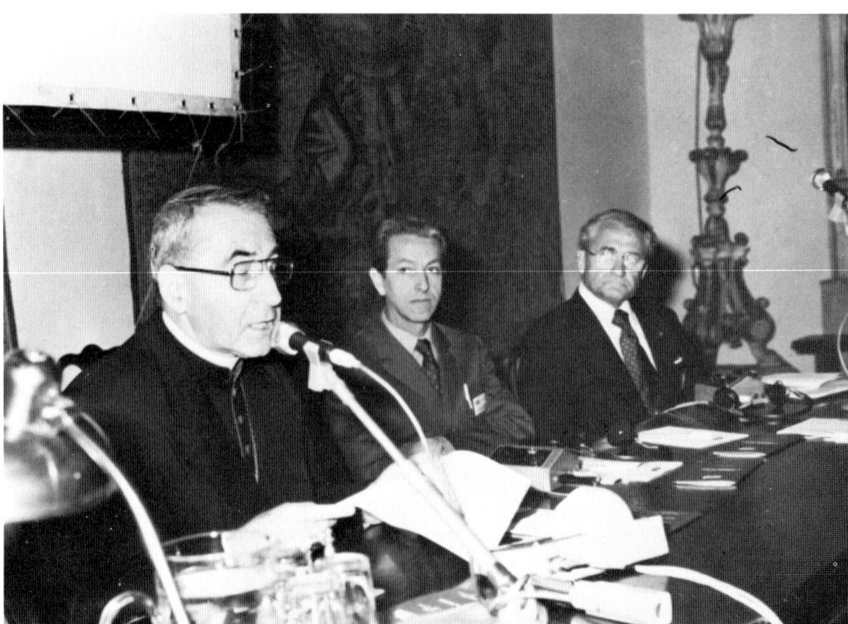

FIG. 1. *Left to right:* Albino Cardinal Luciani, Prof. Carlo Morpurgo, Prof. John Bonica.

Garden He looked for comfort from His disciples, and He was very sad when He found them sleeping because they were tired. This goes to prove that when people suffer they need their dear ones near; they don't want to be left alone, but they need understanding and love; they must be able to talk to people who can encourage them and comfort them.

Patients must be allowed to have visitors and to keep each other company. Hospitals must be technically and clinically well equipped, but they must also favor visits to patients and train their personnel to be kind and helpful with the ailing. Charles Fleury wrote that the way men are treated when sick and dying is a clear indication of the degree of civilization of an age and government.

The few things I have said are only "crumbs" of a Christian philosophy that can be found in the works of Seneca, St. Augustine, Boezio, Pascal, and Peguy and others. Our great writer Alessandro Manzoni exemplified very well this philosophy when he wrote: "Sufferings do often come because of our mistakes, but even the most innocent conduct cannot keep them away and when they do come, with or without our fault, faith in God makes them less unbearable or makes them useful for a better life."

Finally, as emphasized 21 years ago by His Holiness Pope Pius XII, the patient is not required by Christian or moral law "to will suffering for its own sake."[1] Physicians should use all their knowledge, skills, and energies to apply the best means at their disposal to relieve the pain of advanced cancer.

---

[1] *Editor's Note:* The following are excerpts of the address His Holiness Pope Pius XII made on February 24, 1957 (and alluded to by Cardinal Luciani and Professor Bucalossi (p. 670)) in reply to three questions concerning the religious and moral aspects of pain therapy which were submitted by the President of the Italian Society of Anesthesiologists at the time of the IX National Congress held in Rome, Italy, October 15–17, 1956. In response to the first question, "Is there a universal moral obligation to refuse analgesia and to accept physical pain in a spirit of faith?" Pope Pius stated, ". . . there is no obligation of this kind. Man, even after the Fall, retains the right of control over the forces of Nature, of employing them for his own use, and consequently of deriving benefit from all the resources which it offers him either to suppress or avoid physical pain." Although Pope Pius acknowledged the value of physical pain and suffering to help persons grow to maturity and rise "to the highest point of Christian heroism" and that under certain circumstances it must be accepted, he also stated that "the Christian, then, is never obliged to will suffering for its own sake." Indeed, he emphasized that pain is one of the forces that produces "harmful effects and prevents a greater good." In discussing the use of pain-relieving therapy for those who are dying from incurable cancer, he stated, "To declare that the dying have a greater moral obligation than others—whether from Natural Law or from Christian teaching—to accept suffering or to refuse its alleviation, is in keeping neither with the nature of things nor with the source of Revelation. . . . The growth in the love of God—does not come from the sufferings themselves which are accepted, but from the intention in the will supported by grace. This intention, in many of the dying, can be strengthened and become more active if their sufferings are eased, for these sufferings increase the state of weakness, physical exhaustion, check the ardour of the soul and sap the moral powers instead of sustaining them. On the other hand, the suppression of pain removes any tension in the body and mind, renders prayers easy and makes possible a more generous gift of self." He emphasized the responsibility of the doctor to provide pain-relief by stating, "The doctor who accepts (the responsibility of providing analgesia) . . . is seeking in accordance with the Creator to bring suffering under man's control and to do so makes use of the conquest of science and of technical skills."

Introduction

Emilio Ambrogio

Direttore Generale dei Servizi di Medicina Sociale (General Director of Social Medicine Services) of the Republic of Italy

Hon. Tina Anselmi, Minister of Health, was supposed to be present. Unfortunately, she was unable to come and I am here to represent her. The Minister sends her regards and wishes to thank the Floriani Foundation for sponsoring this symposium. The presence of the Italian Health Department witnesses the interest that this initiative has for the Health Ministry.

Assistance toward those who suffer from advanced cancer pain is not only a problem that regards treatment to reduce pain but it involves the deepest aspects of the human soul. It is necessary to create for the dying patient an atmosphere not of pitiful solitude but of full life and of dignified acceptance till the end. In this sense, the most recent studies give great importance to the quality of terminal assistance. And, according to the World Health Organization, this assistance should become part of the tasks of the health services of each nation.

Currently, an increasing number of patients prefer to return home to die in their own bed. This is a natural request and it should not be considered as a way to get rid of the patient and to free a bed, but as a solution that permits the patient to enjoy the comfort and companionship of his family and friends. Therefore, it is necessary to give to the medical and paramedical staff an adequate preparation to provide terminal care at the home of the patient. Although this request involves contact with specialized cancer centers and general hospitals, it is essential that in complying with the patient's wishes we must ensure adequate relief of pain.

The Ministry of Health of the Republic of Italy recognizes its moral, social, professional, and economic obligations to patients with cancer pain and will use whatever resources it is able to muster to fulfill these obligations. With the help of the biomedical scientific community and the health professions we can and should develop an overall national plan to support research by scientists and teaching of physicians so that patients with pain of advanced cancer will be effectively relieved of their suffering. The departments of pain therapy should be given greater national, provincial, and municipal governmental support to fulfill their important missions. These include not only the carrying out of various therapeutic modalities for the relief of pain within the hospital but also the instructing of nurses, social workers, and other paramedical personnel in providing effective psychologic support and relief from suffering to the patient and the family in the home environment.

Advances in Pain Research and Therapy, Vol. 2,
edited by J. J. Bonica and V. Ventafridda.
Raven Press, New York © 1979.

Importance of the Problem

John J. Bonica

Department of Anesthesiology, University of Washington, Seattle, Washington 98195

The proper relief of pain of advanced cancer is one of the most pressing and most important issues of modern society. This importance stems from several facts: (a) Cancer pain afflicts hundreds of thousands and, indeed, millions of people throughout the world annually. In addition to the severe physiologic, emotional, affective, and economic impact of pain in general, cancer pain has special attributes and significance to the patient and family. (b) All too frequently cancer pain is inadequately managed and, consequently, the patient ends his or her last weeks and months or even years of life in great discomfort, suffering, and disability which precludes "a quality of life" that is vital to these patients. (c) The drugs and other therapeutic modalities available at the present time, properly administered, are effective in relieving the pain of most patients.

In this presentation I will attempt to indicate the magnitude of cancer pain, the deficiencies that currently exist which all too often preclude effective relief, and the reasons for these deficiencies. I hope this will serve as a framework or background for the discussion that follows. Following long tradition throughout the world, we will use "cancer pain" generically to include pain caused by any neoplastic disease or occurring as a consequence of therapeutic intervention for neoplastic disease or both.

MAGNITUDE OF THE PROBLEM

For reasons that will be given below, the magnitude of the problem of the pain associated with cancer throughout the world cannot be defined with any accuracy. However, one can gain some insight by citing statistics about the incidence of cancer and deaths consequent to this dreadful disease in Italy and in the United States. I have been informed that in Italy each year about 250,000 patients develop cancer and there are nearly 110,000 deaths from the disease (31). In the United States, the figures are 700,000 new cases of cancer diagnosed and nearly 400,000 deaths from cancer annually (2). This rate of one death per 645 persons makes cancer second only to heart disease as a killer of Americans. Of these deaths, over 23% are due to cancer of the lung, about 13% to lesions of the large intestines, 8.5% to carcinoma of the breast, about 5% to cancer of the prostate or uterus and ovary, 4% to stomach cancer, and 4% to cancer of the bladder and kidney. Realizing that the incidence of oncologic disease and each specific type varies in different countries, these figures suggest that, throughout the world, well over 5 million people die each year from cancer.

INCIDENCE OF CANCER PAIN

Cancer is not usually painful at its onset or during the early phases of the disease, and a significant percentage of patients are cured through surgical, radiation, or anticancer modalities. However, many of the patients with recurrent or metastatic cancer eventually develop pain which becomes progressively more severe and finally develops into a relentless suffering that greatly aggravates the physiologic and psychologic deterioration of the patient caused by the disease itself. Although there are no data from large-scale national epidemiologic studies on the incidence and severity of cancer pain, the data from several surveys of small groups of patients in specific hospitals suggest that moderate to severe pain is experienced by about a third of the patients with the intermediate stages of the disease and by 60 to 80% of the patients with advanced cancer.

Wilkes (33) reported that among nearly 300 patients admitted to a 25-bed unit in an English provincial city which is especially interested in caring for the dying patient, pain was the major symptom in 58%; it occurred in 82% of the patients with cervical cancer, 75% of patients with gastric cancer, and 45 to 60% of patients with cancer of the lungs, rectum, and breast. Twycross (30) reviewed the records of the patients admitted consecutively to St. Christopher's Hospice, the well-known facility for the care of advanced malignant disease in London. About 500 patients are admitted each year and, through an outpatient and domiciliary service, an equal number are supported at home. He reported that more than 80% of the inpatients received diamorphine for severe pain at some time of their hospital stay.

Another very important series of surveys has been carried out by Foley, Houde, and their co-workers (15) at the Memorial Sloan-Kettering Cancer Center. In one survey of 540 inpatients, pain was experienced by 85% of patients with primary bone tumors, 80% with cancer of the oral cavity, 75% of males and 70% of females with cancer of the genital urinary system, 52% of patients with breast cancer, 45% of patients with cancer of the lung, 20% of patients with lymphoma, and only 5% of patients with leukemia. In a subsequent survey of 397 patients, about 38% had pain related to cancer, but the figure rose to 60% among the terminally ill patients in the hospital.

In another survey carried out in Britain, Parkes (26) found that among patients managed in the hospital, 37% had moderate pain and 22% had severe pain, whereas of the group cared for in the home, 21% had moderate pain, and 50% had severe pain. In still another British study, Cartwright and associates (12) found that 87% of patients who died from cancer had pain prior to death.

Pannuti and associates (25) report that of 290 patients with advanced specific tumors admitted to their service, 64% had moderate to severe pain. The incidence of pain in patients with specific tumors was as follows: 68% with breast cancer, 59% with cancer of the prostate, 58% with intestinal tumors, 57% with lung tumors, 55% with kidney tumors, and 47% with head and neck tumors. Molinari (22) reports that more than 50% of patients with head and neck tumors at the National Cancer Institute in Milan have severe pain especially in the advanced stages.

PHYSIOLOGIC AND PSYCHOLOGIC EFFECTS OF CANCER PAIN

Usually the physiologic and psychologic impact of cancer pain on the patient is greater than that of nonmalignant chronic pain which is now generally considered a major health problem (9). The physical deterioration is much more severe because these patients have greater problems through lack of sleep, lack of appetite, nausea, and vomiting. Moreover, their pain threshold and pain tolerance decreases, possibly in part because of depletion of endorphins. As a result of persistent noxious stimulation, patients with persistent cancer pain develop anxiety and reactive depression, and many have hypochondriasis, somatic preoccupation with disease conviction, somatic focusing, and a tendency to deny life problems unrelated to their physical problem. This cluster of psychologic factors, which Pilowsky, Chapman, and Bonica (27) have labeled "abnormal illness behaviors" is characteristic of chronic pain regardless of etiology.

Many patients with cancer pain, knowing that the causative factors are unremovable, cannot give meaningful purpose to the pain and develop feelings of hopelessness and despair. These, like the sleeplessness, spiral to greater proportion as the patient is subjected to surgical operations, chemotherapy, or radiation therapy, and other anticancer modalities. Each time the patient may experience hopefulness but, if the therapy fails, this is followed by disappointment, gradually increased bitterness, and resentment. Many of these patients become more and more preoccupied with the pain and gradually lose interest in social activities: The pain becomes their central focus and dominates their lives.

The social effects of the uncontrolled cancer pain are equally devastating. Many patients develop interpersonal problems with members of their family, friends, and the community. The fact that most patients with advanced cancer have to stop working poses not only an economic but also an emotional stress and a feeling of dependency and uselessness. The physical appearance and behavior produced by the patient's pain and suffering stress the family emotionally; this, in turn, is perceived by the patient and consequently aggravates the pain and suffering. Some patients with severe intractable pain become so discouraged and desperate as to contemplate suicide. (7) The psychologic and psychosocial aspects of cancer pain are discussed in more detail in later chapters.

CURRENT STATUS OF CANCER PAIN CONTROL

Various sources of information suggest that, like chronic pain in general, cancer pain is improperly managed. A study carried out by Marks and Sachar (20) of Montefiore Hospital in New York revealed that many physicians prescribed inadequate amounts of analgesics for patients with cancer pain (and other medical disorders) and that of the amount prescribed, most patients actually received only about 20 to 25% of the (inadequate) amount prescribed. Consequently, in most patients, moderate to severe pain persisted after narcotic therapy. The reason for the inadequate therapy will be discussed in a later section.

Parkes (26) surveyed 276 patients with cancer pain and found among the hospital patients who had severe to very severe pain during the preterminal stage it remained unrelieved during the terminal stage of the disease. Moreover, in 65 cancer patients managed in their homes, 30% had severe to very severe pain which was unrelieved during the terminal phase of the disease.

Additional evidence that many patients with cancer pain are improperly managed is provided by the hundreds of letters received by the National Committee on the Treatment of Intractable Pain, a non-profit organization in the United States with the primary goal of effecting better pain control in patients with advanced cancer (28). Virtually every letter describes one or more relatives who spent the last few months with severe, excruciating cancer pain which remained unrelieved until their death. Although admittedly these are anecdotal reports, the fact that the committee has hundreds of such letters on file suggests that a not-insignificant number of patients who die from cancer spend the terminal part of their lives with unrelieved severe pain. Finally, I have observed hundreds of cancer patients in many medical centers throughout the world who had moderate to severe pain which was unrelieved by the therapy being used.

In view of the great advances in biomedical scientific knowledge and technology, and especially the great amount of interest in cancer research and therapy, why is cancer pain so poorly managed? Serious consideration of this important question during the course of the past quarter-century suggests that it is because of neglect of the problem of pain (in contrast to the cancer) by investigators, teachers in colleges, research institutions, and national and international cancer agencies (5,6,11). Consequently, there are great voids in our knowledge, and whatever knowledge is currently available is improperly applied. Let us consider these two issues.

REASONS FOR INADEQUATE PAIN RELIEF

Lack of Knowledge

There still exist great voids in our knowledge of the basic mechanisms and physiopathology of cancer pain. It is true, of course, that in the century and a half since the reports of Majendie (19), Bell (4), and Mueller (23) stimulated the first truly scientific study of pain, a vast amount of information has become available about pain, especially during the last decade (9,32). Unfortunately, most of this information has not been so beneficial to patients with cancer pain as one might anticipate or as many people believe. This less-than-optimal payoff from the many research efforts, in turn, has been due to the fact that until recent years no attention was paid to the application of new knowledge and technology to the study of chronic pain syndromes in general and cancer pain in particular (6).

In the past, many basic scientists working in the isolation of the animal laboratory were not concerned with clinical pain. As a result of the fragmented, independent research efforts on artificially induced acute pain, hypotheses and concepts were developed which, though reasonable for the times and the scientific data available, were not relevant to chronic pain. Moreover, as pointed out by Melzack (21), pain research and theory remained conceptually stagnant for over a century. Thus, we have little or no scientific information on the exact mechanisms by which cancer and other disease states produce chronic pain. To be sure, many speculations have been proposed, but hard scientific supporting data are lacking.

The relatively small number of clinicians interested in the study of cancer pain and other pain syndromes have consistently faced the frustrating problem of the inability to quantify the pain, let alone study its mechanisms. The fact that pain is a subjective and very personal experience which cannot be seen, touched, or measured by persons other than the individual who has it, has presented almost insurmountable problems to the study of its phenomena in patients. This is especially relevant to patients with cancer where the pain and suffering have special emotional and psychologic substrates. Consequently, clinicians have borrowed the hypotheses of basic scientists developed from acute pain experiments in animals to explain cancer pain and other pain syndromes. On the basis of these hypotheses, therapeutic modalities were developed and applied, some of which are not only ineffective but, not infrequently, produce serious complications of their own.

Another reason for the voids in our knowledge of cancer pain has been the lack of sufficient scientifically trained persons working on this problem. Related to this has been the meager amount or total lack of funds for research or research training in this field. Consequently, there has existed a vicious circle of inadequate scientific manpower → inadequate number of grant applications submitted to the research agencies → inadequate amount of funds budgeted for pain research and research training → discouragement of scientists to pursue cancer pain research and causing them to investigate other areas → inadequate scientific manpower.

Again, I want to emphasize that these problems related to inadequate research on chronic pain in general and cancer pain in particular have existed not only in undeveloped and developing countries, but even in the highly developed, scientifically advanced, and affluent countries. I will mention the situation in the United States where about $1 billion will be spent this year for cancer research by the National Cancer Institute (NCI) and other federal, state, and municipal agencies and by voluntary agencies, private institutions, and the pharmaceutical industry. These funds support the research of hundreds of thousands of scientists, technicians, physicians, and other health professionals who are investigating the cause, prevention, and treatment modalities of every form of cancer. However, until recently, research on *cancer pain* per se, which from the viewpoint of the patient and his family is one of the most important aspects of this dreadful disease, was virtually nonexistent. Analysis of a computer printout for the period 1971 to 1975 revealed that NCI spent a total of nearly $2.5 billion to support its program and of these *only* $560,000 was spent for cancer pain research. This averages about $112,000 annually, which represents 0.022% of the annual budget for those years of the major federal agency which supports cancer research. Fortunately, through the interest and efforts of Dr. Diane J. Fink, Director of the Division of Cancer Control and Rehabilitation, and some of her associates, a pain-control program was mounted some three years ago. As a member of the committee that reviewed applications for cancer pain research and therapy, I have been greatly disappointed by the totally inadequate number of meritorious proposals submitted to the Institute. This reemphasizes the point made that there is an obvious lack of scientific manpower interested in carrying out pain research.

Another impressive and distressing aspect of this whole problem is the fact that there are no accurate data on the incidence and magnitude of cancer pain. Again using NCI as an example, we note that it has a biometry branch and an epidemiologic branch, which carry out very detailed epidemiologic studies on the incidence of every kind of cancer, and have the most sophisticated computer system for data which is stored and easily retrieved. The efforts of these two branches have produced accurate information on every aspect of cancer, including detailed information on the most infrequent types of cancer. However, at the time of this writing, the Institute has no data on the incidence, magnitude, and cost of the *pain* associated with malignant disease. This neglect of epidemiologic studies pervades the entire network of cancer hospitals, cancer centers, and agencies.

Fortunately, things are beginning to improve in the United States in regard to funding for cancer pain research and therapy. In 1976 the NCI spent

$330,000 (more than double the amount spent in 1975), and it spent $661,000 in 1977. In addition, the Institute supported hospice projects and rehabilitation programs which included pain therapy (14).[1] Moreover, the office of the President of the United States has manifested significant interest in cancer pain.

Inadequate Application of Current Knowledge

The second major group of reasons for deficiencies in managing patients with cancer pain has been the improper or inadequate application of knowledge currently available for the care of these patients. The reasons for this include: (a) lack of organized teaching of medical students and physicians and other health professionals in the management of cancer pain, (b) the progressive trend toward specialization, (c) the inability or unwillingness of some practitioners to devote the necessary time and effort to provide optimal pain relief, and (d) the meager amount of published information on the proper treatment of cancer pain.

Review of curricula of the medical schools in the United States reveals that few, if any, teach students the basic principles of the use of narcotics and other therapeutic modalities that effectively relieve cancer pain. Indeed, I have been impressed that many physicians in residency training for specialization in surgical, medical, and radiation oncology receive little or no teaching about the proper management of cancer pain. Usually, the senior house officer, who has vague and scanty information about cancer pain and its proper control, teaches the junior house officer how to deal with the problem in a rather empirical way and passes on some of the misconceptions that will be mentioned below.

Lack of interest in the problem of pain by oncologists is further attested by the fact that very little, if any, information about the proper management of pain is found in the oncology literature, voluminous as it is. Of the many textbooks on various aspects of cancer, only a few deal with the problem of pain-management and then do so in a totally inadequate manner. For example, review of seven of the most important textbooks and monographs on the management of cancer published in English reveals the following facts: Of the two recently published books on surgical oncology, one does not mention pain at all (24), whereas the other devotes one sentence to the problem (29). In a 408-page manual for practitioners published by one of the state chapters of the American Cancer Society (ACS), there is no mention of pain (3), and in another published by the Committee on Professional Education of the International Union Contre Le Cancer (UICC) pain-management is disposed of in 1½ pages (13). In one of the best-known and most widely read books on cancer diagnosis and treatment, pain is mentioned in

[1] Subsequent to, and probably partly as a result of, this Symposium, NCI has initiated major programs in the evaluation of pain management teams and epidemiology studies.

connection with each tumor, but its treatment is not considered at all (1). In another 819-page book on clinical oncology, 2½ pages are devoted to pain (18). Finally, in the most comprehensive 2,000-page volume on cancer medicine, only 13 pages are devoted to the problem of pain and its control (17). A recent survey of the same types of books published in Italy and other European countries reveals that the same problems exist in those countries.

As a result of this lack of education of students and graduate physicians and other health professionals, the pain of cancer is treated in an empirical manner. Insufficient knowledge or lack of consideration of the various mechanisms and types of cancer pain and the associated physiologic, emotional, and behavioral responses is partly responsible for mismanagement of the pain. A related reason is the lack of personnel with the interest and expertise in the proper application of these modalities. Consequently, most practitioners rely on narcotic analgesics which, while very useful and having a definite role in the control of pain in cancer, for a variety of reasons are often misused.

In a small percentage of patients, potent narcotics are used initially for mild pain which could be relieved by non-narcotic analgesics alone or combined with sedatives or psychotropic drugs. The practice of some physicians to "snow the patient under" because the patient has recurrent or metastatic cancer denotes a lack of understanding of the problem (10). Because it is difficult to estimate the length of life in individual cases, such false humanitarianism may potentiate the depressant effects of the disease, and the patient will have narcotic-induced anorexia, nausea, and vomiting, which will aggravate the physiologic effects of the cancer. Even patients with terminal cancer should *not* be subjected to excessive narcotic analgesics and the consequent respiratory depression and stupefaction which preclude the "quality of life" that these patients deserve.

At the other end of the spectrum, many, if not most, patients with moderate to severe pain of advanced cancer are given inadequate amounts of narcotics. The very high incidence of undertreatment of cancer pain is due to inadequate knowledge of the pharmacology of these drugs and, particularly, to serious misconceptions among physicians, nurses, and other health professionals about the "risk of addiction." As part of the study previously mentioned, Marks and Sachar (20) surveyed 102 physicians in training in two major hospitals and found that because of inadequate knowledge most physicians underestimated the effective dose range of narcotics, overestimated duration of their action, and had an exaggerated opinion of the dangers of addiction. Apparently, this problem of inadequate knowledge and misconception about addiction is widespread because many others have reported similar findings. The findings of Parkes (26) and Cartwright and associates (12) have been cited.

This misconception about the problem of "addiction" is further aggravated by the fact that narcotic drugs are carefully monitored by federal and state governments, and physicians in prescribing such medication and pharmacists in filling such prescriptions follow strict regulations in handling these drugs. Thus, tight government control, clinicians' lack of understanding of the pharmacology of narcotics and other drugs that may be used as adjuncts, and the physicians' and nurses' concern about addiction have provided a milieu which has prevented adequate management of pain in patients with cancer.

In some patients, systemic drugs are not sufficiently effective and other modalities need to be used alone or in combination with drugs. These include nerve blocks and neurosurgical interruption of pain pathways and some of the old and newer psychologic techniques which have been shown to be effective in helping or totally relieving cancer pain. Unfortunately, for the aforementioned reasons, the efficacy, indications, and advantages, as well as the limitations, disadvantages, and complications of these other therapeutic modalities, are not known or applied by most practitioners and even by many oncologists. Consequently, in most patients who could be more effectively relieved by one of these procedures or a combination of two or more of these, these other therapeutic modalities are not considered or, if they are considered, this is done too late. Related to this is the lack of personnel with interest and expertise in the proper application of these other therapeutic modalities.

RECOMMENDATIONS FOR IMPROVEMENT

I believe that more effective management of patients with cancer pain requires a multipronged attack consisting of:

1. *Much greater research efforts* which should include: (a) comprehensive epidemiologic studies on the incidence and magnitude of cancer pain with each type of tumor; (b) study of the neurophysiologic and biochemical and physiopathologic mechanisms of cancer pain; (c) evaluation of the efficacy of the methods currently used to relieve cancer pain; and (d) the development of new therapeutic modalities;
2. *Intensive educational programs* for medical students and other health professionals, as well as physicians in practice, including: (a) knowledge about the causes and mechanisms of pain; (b) the efficacy, indications, limitations, and complications of current methods of pain relief; and (c) specific guidelines about proper management of these patients;
3. *Intensive educational campaigns* for the public, patients, and families, as well as federal agencies;
4. *Provision of better sources of information* through the oncologic literature, books and special articles, and brochures on cancer pain.

Future research should provide much new information on the exact biochemical, neurophysiologic, and psychologic substrates of chronic pain in general and cancer pain in particular. Once such information is available, we can use the vast amount of knowledge and technology now available in chemistry, pharmacology, and biochemistry to develop agents that can act in an exquisitely specific way to prevent or promptly terminate the various biochemical and neurologic factors that act at molecular and cellular levels to produce pain. Such new agents would produce complete relief without any side effects. Moreover, future studies should permit more specific definition of the impact of various emotional, psychologic, sociologic, and environmental factors on cancer pain and how this information could be applied more effectively in its relief.

Until we acquire new information, we should be able to effectively use the knowledge currently available to do a much better job in relieving the suffering and pain of cancer. To achieve this goal, it is necessary for the health professionals responsible for the care of cancer patients to consider the neurophysiologic, biochemical, and psychologic substrates of nociception and pain in general and then consider how these are affected by various types of cancer and cancer therapy in causing pain. In other words, we need to consider the possible causes and mechanisms of cancer pain. Moreover, it is necessary to consider within the framework of current knowledge what role psychologic, emotional, environmental, and sociologic factors play in causing suffering and pain in cancer patients. All of these aspects will be considered in this volume.

Once these are defined, it is essential to evaluate the efficacy, indications, and advantages as well as the limitations, disadvantages, and complications of the various therapeutic modalities available at the present time. These considerations will be the subjects of the following chapters. In addition to considering the mechanism, we will evaluate in detail the various therapeutic modalities that are being used in the relief of certain specific cancer pain syndromes. Finally, one of the most important aspects of the problem of cancer pain is continuing and terminal care. We are fortunate in having three outstanding authorities who have pioneered or have important roles in the development of these programs in Britain.

All these discussions and considerations will make it obvious that optimal care of the patients with pain of advanced cancer requires the efforts of health professionals from various disciplines working as members of cancer-pain therapy teams (6,8). A team of this type should be part of every comprehensive cancer center. Such a team should be composed of basic scientists and clinicians with special interest and expertise in chronic pain in general and cancer pain in particular who would devote the time and effort to evaluate carefully each patient with severe cancer pain and determine what is the best method or methods of relieving the pain. I will discuss this issue in more detail later.

I close this introductory section by again expressing the hope that this volume will help to improve the care of patients with pain of advanced cancer. I exhort everyone to exert maximum effort in pursuing vigorously each of the specific objectives I mentioned earlier. Hopefully, this will help us to achieve our ultimate goal—optimal pain-relief for all patients with cancer pain.

REFERENCES

1. Ackerman, L. V., and Del Regato, J. A. W., editors (1970): *Cancer Diagnosis, Treatment and Prognosis,* 4th ed., p. 783. Mosby, St. Louis.
2. American Cancer Society (1978): *Cancer Facts and Figures.* American Cancer Society, New York.
3. American Cancer Society—Massachusetts Division (1968): *Cancer: A Manual for Practitioners,* p. 408. American Cancer Society, Boston.
4. Bell, C. (1811): *Idea of a New Anatomy of the Brain Submitted for the Observations of His Friends.* Strahan & Preston, London.
5. Bonica, J. J. (1959): Management of Cancer Pain. *GP,* 10:35–43.
6. Bonica, J. J. (1978): Cancer pain: A major national health problem. *Cancer Nurs. J.,* 4:313–316.
7. Bonica, J. J. (1976): Cancer pain: A national health problem. Presentation to C.C.G.R. Committee, National Cancer Institute, June 28, 1976.
8. Bonica, J. J. (1974): Organization and function of a pain clinic. In: *Advances in Neurology, Vol. 4,* edited by J. J. Bonica, pp. 433–443. Raven Press, New York.
9. Bonica, J. J., and Albe-Fessard, D., editors (1976): *Advances in Pain Research and Therapy, Vol. 1.* Raven Press, New York.
10. Bonica, J. J. (1953): *The Management of Pain.* Lea & Febiger, Philadelphia.
11. Bonica, J. J. (1954): The management of pain of malignant disease with nerve blocks. *Anesthesiology,* 15:134 (March) and 280–301 (May).
12. Cartwright, A., Hockey, L., and Anderson, A. B. M. (1973): *Life Before Death.* Routledge & Kegan Paul, London.
13. Committee on Professional Education of U.I.C.C. (1973): *Clinical Oncology (A Manual for Students and Doctors),* p. 322. International Union Against Cancer. Springer-Verlag, Berlin.
14. Fink, D. J. (1978): Personal communication to J. J. Bonica, August 1.
15. Foley, K. M. (1979): Pain syndromes in patients with cancer. In: *Advances in Pain Research and Therapy, Vol. 2,* edited by J. J. Bonica and V. Ventafridda. Raven Press, New York.
16. Ford, G. (1979): Terminal care from the viewpoint of the National Health Service. In: *Advances in Pain Research and Therapy, Vol. 2,* edited by J. J. Bonica and V. Ventafridda. Raven Press, New York.
17. Holland, J. F., and Frei, E., III, editors (1973): *Cancer Medicine,* p. 2018. Lea & Febiger, Philadelphia.
18. Horton, J., and Hill, G. J., II, editors (1977): *Clinical Oncology,* p. 819. W. B. Saunders, Philadelphia.
19. Majendie, F. (1822): Experiences sur les fonctions tes racines des nerfs rachidiens. *J. Physiol. Exp. Pathol.,* 2:276–279.
20. Marks, R. M., and Sachar, E. J. (1973): Undertreatment of medical inpatients with narcotic analgesics. *Ann. Intern. Med.,* 78:173–181.
21. Melzack, R. (1973): *The Puzzle of Pain.* Basic Books, New York.
22. Molinari, R. (1979): Therapy of cancer pain in the head and neck. In: *Advances in Pain Research and Therapy, Vol. 2,* edited by J. J. Bonica and V. Ventafridda. Raven Press, New York.
23. Mueller, J. (1826): *Zur Vergleichenden Physiologie des Gesichtssinnes des Menschen und der Thiere nebst einem Versuch über die Bewegungen der Augen und über den Menschlichen Blick.* Cnobloch, Leipzig 32:462.
24. Najerian, J. S., and Delaney, P., editors (1976): *Advances in Cancer Surgery,* p. 608. Stratton Intercontinental Medical Book Corp., New York.

25. Pannuti, F., Martoni, A., Rossi, A. P., and Piana, E. (1979): The role of endocrine therapy for relief of pain due to advanced cancer. In: *Advances in Pain Research and Therapy, Vol. 2,* edited by J. J. Bonica and V. Ventafridda. Raven Press, New York.
26. Parkes, C. M. (1978): Home or hospital? Terminal care as seen by surviving spouse. *J. R. Coll. Gen. Pract.,* 28:19–30.
27. Pilowsky, I., Chapman, C. R., and Bonica, J. J. (1977): Pain, depression and illness behavior in a pain clinic population. *Pain,* 4(2):183–192.
28. Quattlebaum, J. (1978): President of the National Committee for the Treatment of Intractable Pain. Personal communication.
29. Raven, R. W., editor (1977): *Principles of Surgical Oncology,* p. 510. Plenum Medical Book Co., New York.
30. Twycross, R. G. (1974): Clinical management with diamorphine in advanced malignant disease. *Int. J. Clin. Pharmacol.,* 93:184–198.
31. Ventafridda, V. (1978): Incidence of cancer in Italy. Personal comment.
32. Wall, P. D., and Gutnick, M. (1974): Ongoing activity in peripheral nerves: The physiology and pharmacology of impulses originating from a neuroma. *Exp. Neurol.,* 43:550–593.
33. Wilkes, E. (1974): Some problems in cancer management. *Proc. R. Soc. Med.,* 67:23–27.

Advances in Pain Research and Therapy, Vol. 2,
edited by J. J. Bonica and V. Ventafridda.
Raven Press, New York © 1979.

Neurophysiology of Nociception, Pain, and Pain Therapy

Manfred Zimmermann

II. Physiologisches Institut, Abteilung Zentralnervensystem der Universität, Im Neuenheimer Feld 326, 6900 Heidelberg, GFR

What is commonly labeled by the word *pain* covers a wide range of subjective phenomena from the perception of an experimental noxious stimulus (e.g., heating the skin), to the most severe and excruciating chronic or recurrent pain in patients with, e.g., terminal cancer, thalamic syndrome, or trigeminal neuralgia, all of which may profoundly alter the personality traits of the patient. Most of what we know on nervous mechanisms refers to experimentally induced pain, whereas knowledge of the physiologic basis of chronic pain remains to be elucidated.

Many new results have come from animal experiments. We conclude from the observation of motor, vegetative, and behavioral expressions (such as flexor-reflexes, blood pressure increases, tachypnea, vocalization) that some sort of behavioral state occurs in higher mammals which corresponds to pain in man, since all these nocifensive reactions of animals also are concomitants of human pain-perception and behavior. This suggests that the basic nervous system mechanisms involved are similar in all higher mammals, including man.

This chapter is aimed at giving a short outline only of the neurophysiologic basis for pain. A number of recently published comprehensive review articles and monographs are available (4,5,6,12,16,20,21,25,27,31,33,42,44,47).

PERIPHERAL ENCODING AND CONDUCTION OF PAIN INFORMATION: NOCICEPTORS AND NOCICEPTIVE AFFERENTS

Afferent Fibers

In most cases pain is produced by the excitation of specialized receptors, the nociceptors, or of their afferent fibers. The existence of such nervous elements was deduced, about 50 years ago, from experiments using electrical stimulation of skin nerves (Fig. 1): nocifensive reactions (in animals) and pain sensations (in man) occurred when the stimulus strength was above

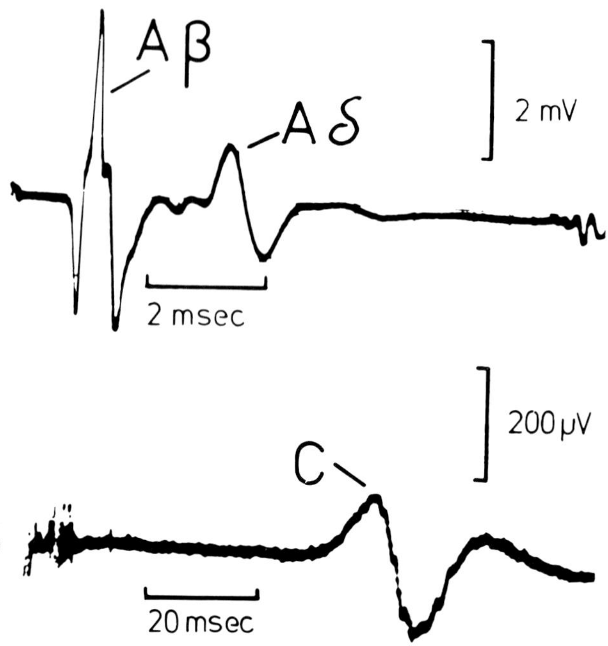

FIG. 1. Compound action potential after electrical stimulation of a cutaneous nerve (sural of the cat) displayed at two vertical gains and sweep speeds to show the three main fiber components. Conduction distance was 70 mm. The table indicates the functional types of afferents in each fiber class. Aβ. sensitive mechanoreceptors; Aδ. sensitive mechanoreceptors (hairs), cold receptors, mechanosensitive nociceptors; C. sensitive mechanoreceptors (hairs), warm receptors, mechanosensitive nociceptors, heat nociceptors, polymodal nociceptors.

threshold for the thin myelinated (Aδ, or Group III) fibers; when stimulus strength was sufficient to recruit nonmyelinated C-fibers (or Group IV afferents) the pain was increased and was of a burning quality.

Through research initiated by the pioneer work of Zotterman in 1939 (46), the existence of specialized nociceptors has been well established, especially during the last decade. However, not all of the Aδ- and C-afferents have nociceptive functions; there are also low-threshold mechanoreceptors and thermoreceptors in these fiber classes (see table in Fig. 1); in addition a large proportion of C-fibers in all nerves are sympathetic efferent fibers. Nociceptors are ubiquitous in practically all organs. I have estimated that about half of the afferent fibers entering the spinal cord via the dorsal roots are nociceptive.

Nociceptors

Best known are the nociceptors of the skin, based on single-fiber studies in animals. Recently nociceptors have been investigated in man by recording

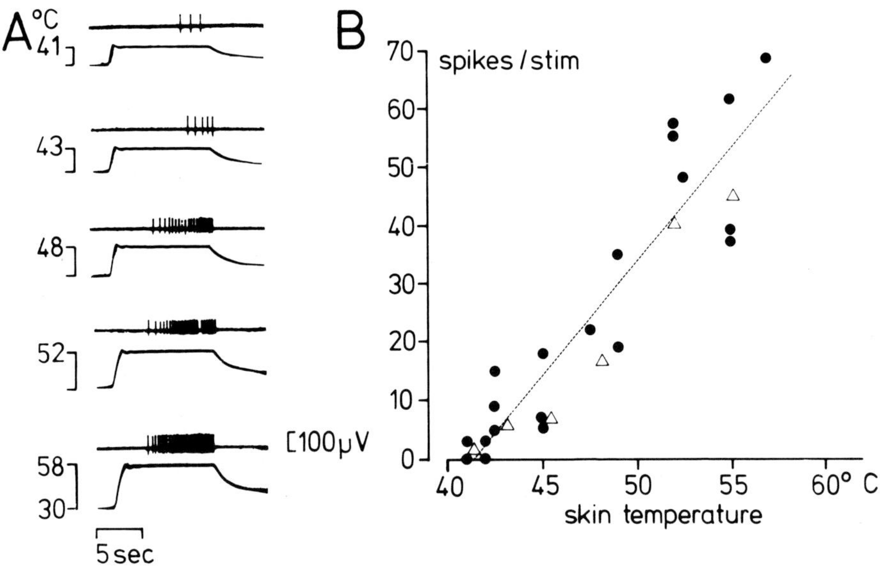

FIG. 2. Discharges of a single cutaneous C-fiber to noxious heating of the skin. **A:** Oscilloscope displays of nerve impulses (*upper trace*), recorded synchronously with skin temperature (*lower trace*); a controlled radiant-heat source was directed to the receptive field of the fiber on the hind foot of the cat. **B:** Relationship between skin temperature and no. of impulses per 10 sec of heat stimulation (●) or during the last 4 sec of heat (△). Conduction velocity of fiber was 0.6 m/sec. (From Beck et al., ref. 3, with permission.)

from single C-fibers with percutaneous microelectrodes (47). Fig. 2 shows an example of, a nociceptor of the cat's foot responding to noxious heat, i.e., when the skin temperature reached a level near 45°C. The response, i.e., the number of impulses per 10-sec heating, was linearly related to the temperature beyond threshold. This suggests that the nociceptor not only signals the mere presence of a noxious stimulus, but that it transmits information on stimulus intensity which is encoded in the impulse frequency.

These electrophysiologic findings on single nociceptors are in accordance with psychophysical measurements in human subjects: the threshold for heat pain is around 45°C skin temperature; various levels of skin temperature above this threshold can be well discriminated by the subject [cf. the psychometric Dol-scale according to Hardy et al. (15)].

The most common excitants of nociceptors in skin, muscles, tendons, ligaments, and visceral organs are strong mechanical deformation, chemical substances released by pathological processes (see below), and ischemia. The majority of nociceptors respond to various excitants, e.g., mechanical, thermal, chemical; these are called polymodal nociceptors.

Knowledge of visceral and muscle nociceptors is less advanced than that of cutaneous nociceptors. Some visceral mechanoreceptors respond to distention combined with contractions of the smooth-muscle wall of hollow organs (32); this mechanism most probably is involved in spasmodic colic pain. Since muscle nociceptors, including cardiac nociceptors, can be excited by chemical substances, it is thought that muscle and cardiac pain are mediated by chemical mediators such as bradykinin (see below).

MECHANISMS FOR CHRONIC PAIN

Noxious stimuli impinging on the skin, such as those used in the laboratory for the investigation of pain (Fig. 2), can be terminated quickly in daily life by an appropriate behavioral response (escape, avoidance). Therefore they usually do not result in a chronic pain state. However it is the persistence which makes pain a most urgent problem in medicine. Some basic physiologic mechanisms of chronic pain will be considered here.

Compression of Nerves

Excitation of nerves takes place not only at the sensory end-organ; nerve impulses can also be elicited anywhere along the sensory fiber in the nerve trunk by electrical stimulation or by local mechanical distortion. Persistent compression (e.g., by dislocation of vertebral discs, by the carpal ligaments) often produces ongoing discharges in afferent fibers which are perceived as paresthesias or pain and are localized by the patient in the innervation territory of that nerve. Some neuralgias which are characterized by irradiation of pain to the territory of a peripheral nerve or dorsal root may have such an origin.

A long-lasting compression, which also might produce some local ischemia of the nerve, eventually can result in a conduction block, which is preferential for $A\beta$-fibers (i.e., tactile afferents). This has been shown in experiments on man and animals. The persistence in these cases of ongoing activity in nociceptive afferents, and the absence of concomitant discharges in tactile afferents, might be the reason why the resulting pain is particularly disagreeable.

Chemical Excitation and Sensitization of Nociceptors

Pathologic alterations of the skin and viscera, e.g., trauma or inflammations, are accompanied by release or enhanced production of chemical substances such as KCl, serotonin, bradykinin, prostaglandin E. Each of these endogenous chemicals can either excite or sensitize nociceptors depending on their local concentrations. They are called algogenic substances (22). Such chemical influences on nociceptors have been reported to occur in the skin (2), in muscle (24,29,30), and in the viscera (18,26). Their increased production during muscle ischemia, particularly in cardiac ischemia (38), has been suggested to be a causal link in ischemic pain, e.g., angina pectoris.

Most probably several of the algogenic substances liberated upon tissue injury combine to excite nociceptors. The time-course of endogenous production and decomposition of the algogenic substances usually is slow, resulting in a long-term excitation of nociceptors.

In moderate tissue injury the concentrations of algogenic chemicals often are not sufficient to excite the nociceptors. However, they can produce sensitization in these cases, i.e., enhancement of responses and/or decrease of threshold of a nociceptor to another adequate stimulus. It is tempting to assume that sensitization of nociceptors by various endogenous chemicals is the physiologic basis for states of increased pain sensitivity which accompany pathologic conditions such as inflammation or sunburn: hyperalgesia and hyperpathia.

The involvement of prostaglandin E in sensitization and excitation of nociceptors during inflammation provides a plausible explanation for the peripheral analgesic effect of acetylsalicylic acid (aspirin): this drug is an inhibitor of prostaglandin synthesis (8). In the presence of acetylsalicylic acid the concentration of this local hormone is greatly reduced and likewise its facilitatory effect upon nociceptors. Thus, in pain involving prostaglandin E, acetylsalicylic acid and similarly acting drugs (e.g., indomethacin) can produce analgesia.

Regenerating Nerves

Nerve transections (e.g., by traumatic lesions, amputations, or neurosurgical transections) induce a powerful stimulus for the fibers of the proximal stump to regenerate. Such sites often are sources of severe pain, particularly when a neuroma has developed. Can this pain arise at the sprouts of the regenerating fibers? Experiments have been conducted recently in rats in which a neuroma was induced by placing the proximal stump of the cut sciatic nerve into a plastic cap (9,40). In such preparations ongoing impulse activity was found in Aδ- and C-fibers (Fig. 3); this was initiated at the fiber sprouts in the neuroma. No such ongoing activity occurred in Aβ-fibers. It is tempting to assume that many of the spontaneously active Aδ- and C-fibers previously had nociceptive endings, so that the impulse flow in these fibers would be interpreted by the central nervous system (CNS) as coming from a noxious stimulus.

Two additional results emerged from these investigations on experimental neuroma (Fig. 3): the ongoing impulse discharge was enhanced by perfusion of the neuroma with noradrenaline (norepinephrine), and suppressed by electrical stimulation of the nerve fibers. The effect of norepinephrine is circumstantial evidence that sympathetic efferents might exert some stimulatory action on nociceptive fibers in the neuroma, a mechanism which had been claimed to operate in causalgia, a pain syndrome that often occurs in patients with a neuroma (see also p. 19).

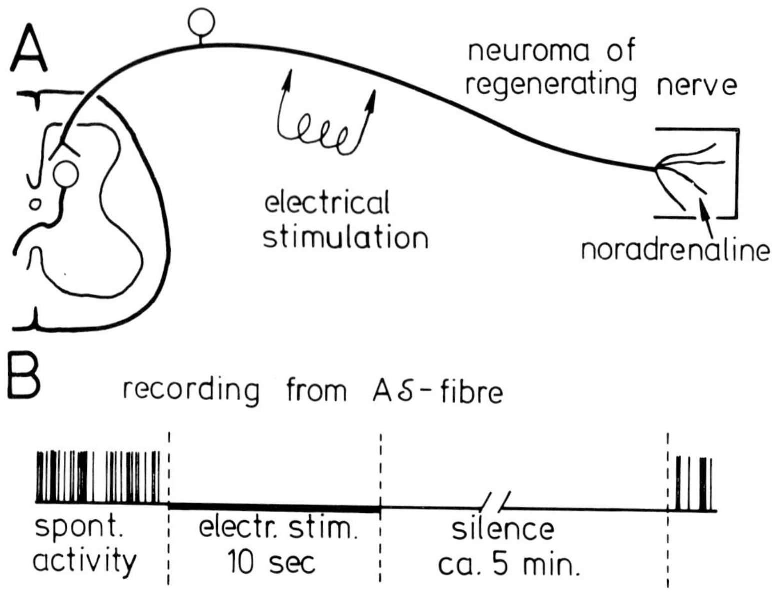

FIG. 3. Properties of nerve sprouts in a neuroma (schematic). **A:** A neuroma had been induced in transected rat nerves by putting a plastic cap over the proximal stump. Afterwards the nerve was prepared for stimulation, recording, and perfusion of the neuroma. **B:** Spontaneous activity in Aδ-fibers arising in the neuroma could be silenced for a long time by a short period of repetitive electrical nerve stimulation. Schematic drawings according to results by Wall and Gutnick (40).

A short period (e.g., 10 sec) of repetitive electrical stimulation of the nerve at a strength above threshold for the single fiber under study completely stopped the ongoing discharge for several min (Fig. 3B). This is a possible foundation for analgesia produced by transcutaneous nerve stimulation in amputees. Apart from this peripheral analgesic action the stimulation will elicit inhibitory processes in the CNS (see below, Inhibition of Spinal Neurons by Afferent Nerve Stimulation).

When a regenerating nerve reaches its peripheral innervation territory (e.g., in the skin), hyperpathia can be observed in patients (37). This situation has been simulated in animal experiments (11). When the sprouting fibers had reached the skin, nociceptors having similar functional characteristics to those in normal skin immediately developed. However, the threshold to noxious heating was significantly reduced by 4°C in the regenerated C-nociceptors, which might account for hyperpathia to thermal stimuli in patients with regenerated nerves.

Implications of Motor and Sympathetic Reflexes in Chronic Pain

Usually motor and sympathetic reflexes to noxious stimuli are aimed to counteract the noxious effect; they can be considered as negative feedback mechanisms to protect the organism from injury (e.g., flexor reflex, hyperemia of an injured organ). However, such reflexes might sometimes function as a positive feedback; i.e., they increase rather than decrease the effect of a noxious stimulus (Fig. 4).

A motor reflex, for example, initiated by a cutaneous or visceral pain stimulus might set up activity in muscle or tendon nociceptors by the muscle contraction (Fig. 4A). This in turn can increase the motor reflex, which eventually will lead to a self-sustained reflex muscle spasm and, concomitantly, to ongoing pain.

Such a vicious circle is also possible in the case of sympathetic reflexes (Fig. 4B). Positive feedback might be considered as causative in the clinically well-known syndrome of sympathetic reflex dystrophy. The sympathetic effector then enhances rather than decreases the excitation of the nociceptors. Several mechanisms can account for such a deleterious effect: vasoconstriction and ischemia; vasodilatation and increase in vascular permeability, thus changing the extracellular fluid environment; contracture of smooth muscle surrounding the nociceptor; direct action of locally released neurotransmitters, neuromodulators; and algogenic chemicals (e.g., norepinephrine, substance P, serotonin, bradykinin, prostaglandin). These adverse effects of sympathetic efferent influences, although apparent from many clinical observations, still lack a physiologic foundation. A systematic investigation of these problems is highly desirable.

Therapeutic actions should be aimed to interrupt the positive feedback or self-excitation loop, either by a regional analgesic block in the afferent or efferent branch of the reflex, or by activating inhibitory systems in the CNS. Local anesthesia of the afferent nerve yields pain-relief which often outlasts, by days or even weeks, the duration of pharmacologic action of the anes-

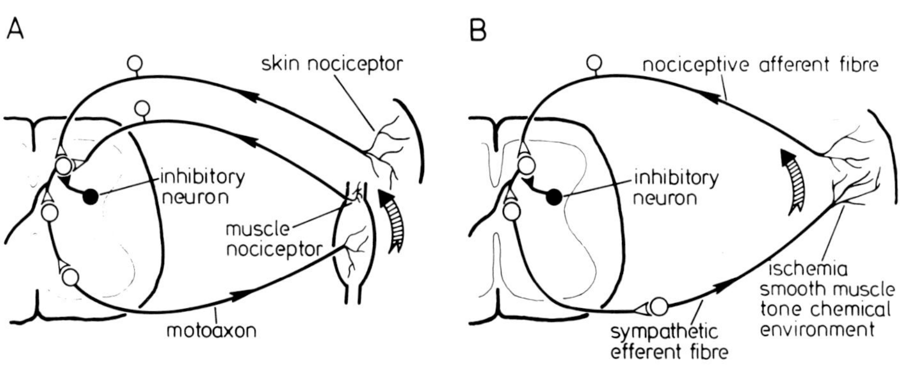

FIG. 4. Hypothetical mechanisms of self-excitation of nociceptors by spinal reflexes (schematic). **A:** Motor reflex induced by skin or/and muscle nociceptors, the contraction acting as a stimulus on muscle nociceptors. **B:** Sympathetic reflex evoked by nociceptors; various sympathetic effector mechanisms are indicated, which can enhance the excitability of the nociceptors.

thetic. This enduring pain-relief lends support to the assumption that the pain really was of the self-sustaining type. Another method of interrupting the positive feedback loop is to activate neuronal inhibition in the spinal cord, as indicated in Fig. 4 (see below).

CENTRAL NERVOUS SYSTEM MECHANISMS OF PAIN AND ANALGESIA

The physiology of nociception and pain is much more complex in the CNS than it is in the peripheral nervous system. A center for pain, comparable to the mapped projections of tactile, visual, and auditory senses onto the cortex, does not exist. Afferent input from nociceptors sets up activity in many subsystems of the CNS. Some of the subsystems and a typical example of related functions are listed below.

Spinal cord:	Motor and sympathetic reflexes
Brain stem:	Control of circulation and respiration, reticular activating system
Hypothalamus:	Homeostasis; release of hormones from the pituitary
Limbic system:	Affective-motivational components of behavior
Neocortex:	Cognitive components of behavior

These CNS subsystems are involved in all of the various behavioral states of a subject; therefore, we argue that pain behavior may be based upon a characteristic pattern of activity in, and interaction among, these brain parts.

This general concept implies that it might be inappropriate to search for central neurons which are specifically related to nociceptive afferents, but not to others. Presumably any central neuron will share in many different functions. In principle, information about noxious stimuli can be extracted from a population of neurons, none of which is specifically excited by such stimuli (45). So, the investigation of the physiology of pain should emphasize these questions: (a) In which neurons can information be found on noxious peripheral events, irrespective of whether or not a particular neuron has additional non-noxious inputs; and (b) are there neuronal mechanisms by which this pain-related information in the central neurons can be modified?

The best-studied examples of neurons yielding answers to these questions are the dorsal horn neurons in the spinal cord (Fig. 5). Here are the central terminals of the Aδ- and C-fibers from nociceptors in the skin, viscera, and muscles. Noxious information received by the dorsal horn neurons is dispensed to contribute to spinal motor and sympathetic outflow, some pathophysiologic implications of which have been emphasized above (Fig. 4). Long axons of some dorsal horn neurons ascend to the brain, e.g., in the anterolateral tract (41), transection of which (cordotomy) may give pain-relief. However, there are additional spinal ascending pathways to

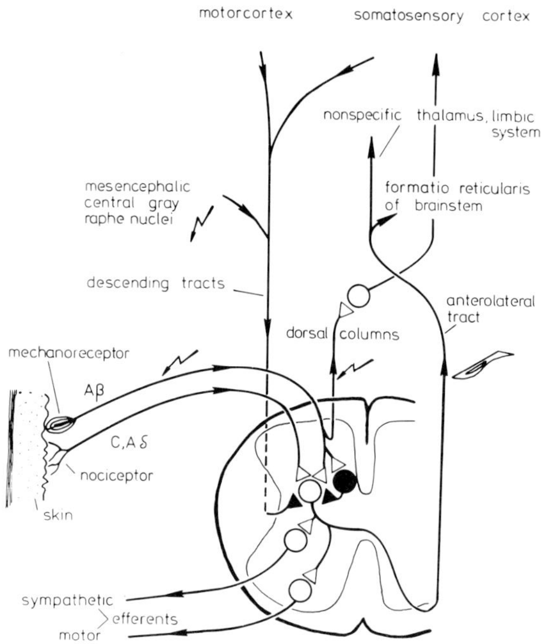

FIG. 5. Functional diagram of the dorsal horn neuron (highly schematic). Afferent fibers synapse onto dorsal horn neurons, which in turn conduct their impulses to segmental motor and sympathetic efferents and to ascending tracts. The dorsal horn neuron can be inhibited; inhibitory synapses and neuron drawn in black. Voltage arrows indicate sites where stimulation can produce inhibition of the dorsal horn neuron; the scalpel indicates cordotomy for pain-relief.

carry pain information, which explains why pain can persist or recur after a cordotomy. Many brain areas, e.g., those mentioned above, may be reached by the pain information transmitted through the ascending pathways, mainly via the brainstem reticular formation and the nonspecific thalamic nuclei (Fig. 5). Tactile skin stimuli, on the other hand, activate mechanoreceptors which project, via the dorsal columns, to the specific somatosensory system in the thalamus and cortex.

However, sensory systems generally are not organized as one-way streets for excitatory impulse traffic. As is indicated in Fig. 5, some segmental and suprasegmental descending inhibitory influences can affect information flow through the dorsal horn neuronal system. Some details of these modulatory mechanisms, which might be regarded as representative for neuronal interactions in pain neurophysiology, will be considered below.

Dorsal Horn Neuronal Responses to Noxious Skin Stimuli

Radiant heat applied to our skin is very painful when the skin temperature is above 45°C. We know that such controlled heating is a practically selective stimulus for nociceptive Aδ- and C-afferents in the cat's hind foot (3). We used radiant heat as a purely noxious stimulus to study the functional characteristics of the neuronal circuitry in the dorsal horn.

About 50% of lumbar dorsal horn neurons respond vigorously to skin-heating (Fig. 6). Varying the intensity of the heat stimulus resulted in a linear relationship between skin temperature and mean discharge frequency, which is quite similar to that found in the C-nociceptors (Fig. 2B). However, there were differences between the discharges of C-nociceptors and spinal neurons: (a) The discharge frequencies were higher by a factor of 10, indicating considerable convergence of many C-fibers to each neuron. (b) The dorsal horn neuronal discharges displayed a build up of responsiveness during repetitive electrical C-fiber stimulation, which indicates temporal facilitation to occur in the synaptic transmission. (c) The discharge frequency slowly decayed within 10 to 100 sec after cessation of the heat stimulus (Fig. 6). These temporal features can be explained by assuming that a synaptic transmitter is involved which has slow kinetics of release, post-

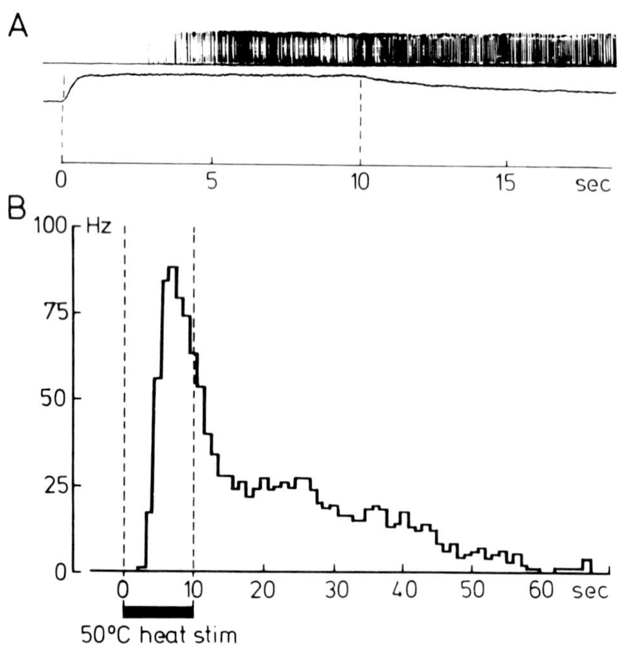

FIG. 6. Impulse discharge of a single dorsal horn neuron in the cat's spinal cord to noxious heat stimulation of the skin. **A:** Oscillographic record of nerve impulses (*upper trace*) and of the skin temperature (*lower trace*), when heating to 50°C, 10 sec in duration, was performed on a 1-cm^2 skin area of the footpad. **B:** Same discharge plotted as histogram, i.e., impulse frequency vs. time, during and after heat stimulation. The period of heating is indicated by the vertical broken lines. (From Dickhaus et al., ref. 10, with permission.)

synaptic action, and inactivation. These and other results hint at substance P, a polypeptide contained in small-diameter primary afferents, to be the synaptic transmitter (17).

These neuronal characteristics correlate with psychophysiologic phenomena of pain sensation. First, the intensity of a painful stimulus can be judged by the subject, based on the frequency modulation in nociceptors (Fig. 2B), whose coding principle obviously is preserved at the synaptic relay to the dorsal horn neurons. The temporal facilitation of neuronal responsiveness corresponds to enhancement of pain when stimulation is repeated at certain rates. The long afterdischarge of the neurons to noxious heat is reminiscent of aftersensations that often are felt subsequent to a painful stimulus.

Descending Control of Spinal Pain Transmission

It is well established now that in all sensory systems the ascending information is modulated by centrifugal influences from the brain. In the somatosensory system such backward modification is exerted via pathways descending in the white matter of the spinal cord. Such descending controls originate in the cortex, the diencephalon, and the brainstem (Fig. 5). In the context of pain, brainstem systems are of great importance. Inhibition of nociceptive messages in dorsal horn neurons has been reported to originate in the mesencephalic periaqueductal gray (PAG), in some of the raphe nuclei which contain serotonergic descending neurons, in the locus coeruleus (noradrenergic neurons), and in parts of the reticular formation.

An example is given in Fig. 7. Spinal neuronal responses to standardized noxious stimulation are shown as histograms in B and C. Repetitive electrical stimulation of the PAG was performed before and during the heat-response in C: This discharge clearly was inhibited to less than ⅓ of the control (B). The particular site of stimulation in the PAG is shown in Fig. 7A, along with effective electrode placements from other experiments.

When this procedure was repeated to a series of heat stimuli at varying heat intensities, the relationship between discharge frequency and skin temperature, i.e., the characteristic line of intensity coding, was affected as shown in Fig. 7D: A decrease in slope to typically less than 50% of control occurred, whereas the threshold remained the same. The inhibitory system arising in the PAG thus may be interpreted as controlling the gain of pain transmission in the spinal dorsal horn (7). There are other descending inhibitory systems which do not change the slope, but produce a shift, of the intensity-coding line to higher thresholds and lower discharge frequencies. Thus, the interactive network of spinal and brainstem neurons might provide a functional system of great dynamic capabilities.

The descending brainstem systems have been characterized also in terms of

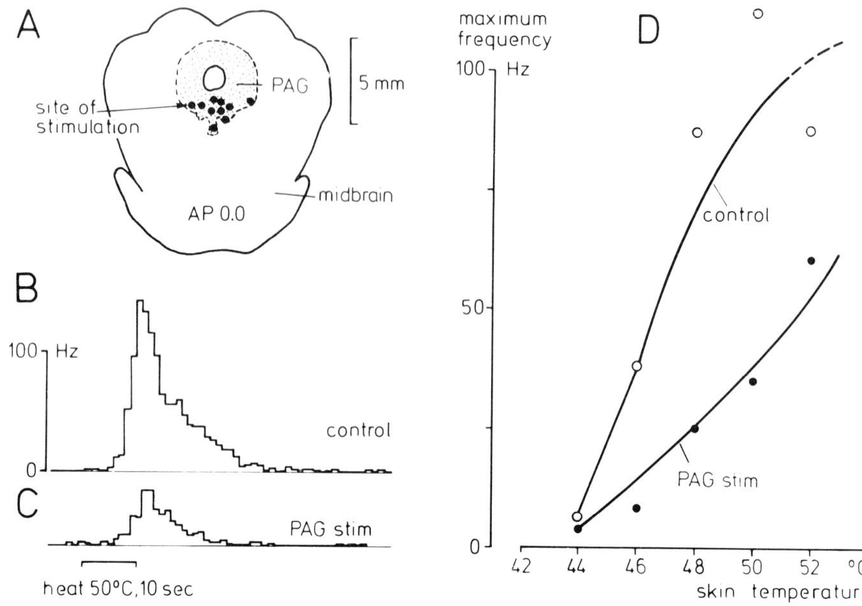

FIG. 7. Descending inhibition of cat's spinal neuron by stimulation in the midbrain. **A:** Histological confirmation of sites in the periaqueductal gray (PAG) of the midbrain (at stereotaxic coordinates AP 0) where stimulation produced inhibition in the spinal cord. **B:** Discharge of a dorsal horn neuron in the lumbar spinal cord to noxious heat (50°C, 10 sec) applied to the receptive field on the pad. **C:** Same heat stimulus; however, repetitive electrical stimulation was given before and during recording of the heat-evoked discharge to the site labeled by arrow in A. Parameters of PAG stimulation were: square impulses 300 μA, 0.1 msec in duration, 100-Hz trains during 0.1 sec, trains repeated at 3 Hz. **D:** Peak frequency of heat-evoked discharges is plotted against the temperature of the skin-heating, under control conditions (○) or during PAG stimulation (●). Data from Carstens et al. (7).

neurochemistry. Thus, serotonin and various neuropeptides have been identified to play a role as neurotransmitters or neuromodulators in these systems (12,27,31). A dramatic advance in this field was the discovery of endogenous opiate-like peptides, the enkephalins and endorphins (13,23, 35). The endogenous opiates and morphine both are suggested to activate the descending inhibitory system via the same neuronal receptors (42). Details of neurochemical knowledge will be presented in the following chapter by Benedetti.

In the behaving animal, analgesia or hypalgesia can be produced by electrical stimulation (25), and by microinjection of morphine (42) in the brainstem. Also, in human patients brainstem stimulation has been used for treatment of severe pain (1,34).

The antinociceptive effects are suggested to be due to descending inhibition in the spinal cord and, possibly, also to inhibitory influences ascending to more rostral brain areas (Benedetti, *this volume*).

Inhibition of Spinal Neurons by Afferent Nerve Stimulation

It is a general principle of nervous system function that any sensory inflow not only excites nerve cells, but also produces inhibition. Inhibition is a stabilizing factor in nervous system function. Nociceptive afferents too are subject to, and produce, inhibition.

The inhibition normally operating in the spinal dorsal horn (Fig. 5) can be enhanced by intentional afferent stimulation, as has been shown in animal experiments: Neuronal responses to noxious skin-heating were partially or totally suppressed during repetitive electrical stimulation of afferent cutaneous nerves (Aβ strength) or of the dorsal columns (14). The inhibition ceased immediately at the end of the stimulation period, which lasted a few seconds.

A longer time-course of inhibition was observed when the periods of electrical nerve stimulation were prolonged to several minutes (Fig. 8). The discharges to noxious skin-heating (50°C, 10 sec), plotted as histograms

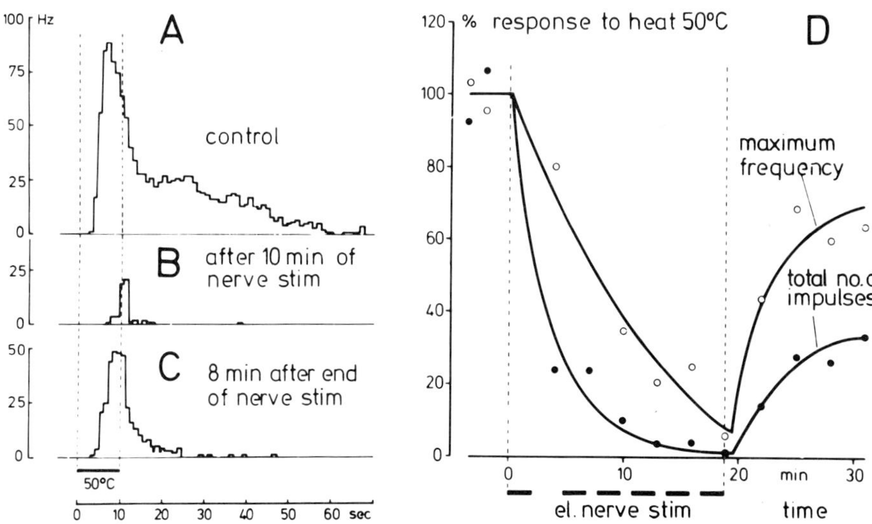

FIG. 8. Inhibition by repetitive, cutaneous A-fiber stimulation of responses in a spinal neuron of the cat evoked by noxious heat stimulation of the skin. **A:** Histogram of the discharge of a lumbar dorsal horn neuron evoked by heating (50°C, 10 sec) the cutaneous receptive field on the hind footpad. **B:** Same heat stimulus as in A was applied, being however preceded by a total of 10 min of repetitive (50 Hz) electrical stimulation of the A-fibers of the posterior tibial and superficial peroneal nerves. **C:** Response to the heat stimulus (as in A) 8 min after cessation of electrical A-fiber stimulation amounting to 12 min totally. **D:** Time-course of peak discharge (○) and total no. of impulses (●) per heat-evoked response of the dorsal horn neuron, during and after the electrical A-fiber stimulation; repeated 2-min periods of electrical nerve stimulation indicated below abscissa. Discharge measures were relative to control values recorded before the period of electrical nerve stimulation. (From Dickhaus et al., ref. 10, with permission.)

(A to C), revealed a considerable suppression even when the repetitive electrical nerve stimulation (50 Hz, Aβ strength) was restricted to the period between the noxious heat stimuli produced at a 3-min rate (as indicated by bars under the time scale in Fig. 8D). Thus, after nerve stimulation amounting to a total of 10 min, the discharge to heat stimulus was reduced to a few percent of control (Fig. 8B). It should be pointed out that the inhibition affected predominantly the afterdischarge to the noxious stimulus, which is suggested to contribute to the aftersensation and therefore will make pain of this type so disagreeable.

After the end of the electrical stimulation, the responsiveness of the neuron to noxious heat slowly recovered (Fig. 8C, D). In a systematic study of this type, time-courses of between 10 sec and more than 10 min were found for the build-up and decay of inhibition. In practically all cases, however, inhibition considerably outlasted the period of electrical stimulation, which has so far not been previously reported (10).

Concerning the neuronal mechanisms involved in these slow alterations, several possibilities might be proposed: (a) The observed time-courses (Fig. 8D) might reflect the turning on and off of inhibitory system(s), being of spinal or/and of supraspinal origin, or (b) alterations in the extra- and intra-cellular ionic compositions (e.g., of K^+), which in turn affect membrane transport mechanisms and, hence, membrane excitability (10,43).

The inhibition in Fig. 8 is reminiscent of hypalgesia produced by transcutaneous nerve stimulation and by stimulation through acupuncture needles in man, where stimulation periods of 10 to 30 min have often been required for the hypalgesia to develop fully. Both these methods of hyperstimulation in human patients presumably have common mechanisms, one of these being the suppression of dorsal horn neurons reported here.

SUMMARY AND CONCLUSIONS

Pain sensations usually are based upon activity in nociceptive afferents. Although there is considerable knowledge on nociceptors, both from man and animals, the key mechanisms of chronic pain are only poorly understood. In this regard, systematic investigations in man and animals are required in these fields:

1. Effects on nociceptors of a variety of endogenous chemicals produced in diseased organs; of particular interest are the basic properties and chemical modifications of nociceptors in the deep organs, e.g., viscera, muscles, tendons, and bones.

2. Excitability conditions of nociceptive fibers in regenerated nerves and freshly reinnervated organs; how can the formation of a neuroma be prevented after nerve lesions?

3. Motor and sympathetic reflexes that act upon nociceptors, thus establishing a positive-feedback, self-excitatory loop to maintain chronic pain.

Although there is impressive evidence in patients for such phenomena, we do not know why such reflexes develop.

In the CNS no pain center exists. The cognitive, affective, motivational, and vegetative dimensions of pain-perception and behavior presumably are based on a complex pattern of activity in, and interactions of, many central nervous functional subsystems. Some basic neuronal mechanisms that might be related to pain and analgesia have been studied in the spinal dorsal horn neurons of animals. However, we are far from having a coherent picture of central pain physiology. The following problems need to be investigated intensively:

4. The neurophysiology of supraspinal CNS. Since nociceptive responses presumably are affected by anesthesia, waking, unrestrained animals should be used, enabling correlations of the electrophysiologic and behavioral responses to noxious stimuli.

5. The dorsal horn physiology, including the afferent and descending inhibitory effects, should be studied in animal models for chronic pain, e.g., induced inflammations of skin or joints. The results of such studies, even when conducted under anesthesia, would be more relevant for the understanding of pain and analgesia in man than the present work using acute noxious stimuli, such as pinching or heat.

6. The gap between the neurophysiologic and neurochemical (pharmacological) approaches should be narrowed, e.g., by relating microelectrophysiologic and microelectrophoretic studies with the histochemical identity of the neuron under study.

7. Studies in man, healthy subjects and patients, should be intensified. A great repertoire of methods is available, such as psychophysiologic measurements, EEG, evoked potentials, EMG, microneurography, diagnostic microelectrode recordings during stereotaxic operations and cordotomies.

The future study of pain physiology will require the use of chronic pain in animals. There are, however, enormous ethical objections, since it is difficult to design appropriate experiments and prevent inducing suffering in animals (36,39). A competent multidisciplinary committee should elaborate guiding principles for such work.

ACKNOWLEDGMENTS

The author wishes to thank Frau Ursula Nothoff for typing and bibliographical assistance, Frau Almuth Manisali for graphics, and Dr. E. Carstens for improving the English.

REFERENCES

1. Adams, J. E. (1976): Naloxone reversal of analgesia produced by brain stimulation in the human. *Pain,* 2:161–166.
2. Beck, P. W., and Handwerker, H. O. (1974): Bradykinin and serotonin effects on various types of cutaneous nerve fibres. *Pflügers Arch.,* 347:209–222.

3. Beck, P. W., Handwerker, H. O. and Zimmermann, M. (1974): Nervous outflow from the cat's foot during noxious radiant heat stimulation. *Brain Res.,* 67:373–386.
4. Bonica, J. J. (editor) (1974): *Advances in Neurology, Vol. 4.* Raven Press, New York.
5. Bonica, J. J., and Albe-Fessard, D. (editors) (1976): *Advances in Pain Research and Therapy, Vol. 1.* Raven Press, New York.
6. Boivie, J., and Perl, E. R. (1975): Neural substrates of somatic sensation. In: *International Review of Physiology, Vol. 3: Neurophysiology I,* pp. 303–411; edited by C. C. Hunt. Butterworths, London.
7. Carstens, E., Yokota, T., and Zimmermann, M. (1979): Inhibition of spinal neuronal responses to noxious skin heating by stimulation of the mesencephalic periaqueductal gray in the cat. *J. Neurophysiol.* (*in press*).
8. Collier, H. O. J. (1971): Prostaglandins and aspirin. *Nature,* 232:17–19.
9. Devor, M., and Wall, P. D. (1976): Type of sensory nerve fibre sprouting to form a neuroma. *Nature,* 262:705–708.
10. Dickhaus, H., Pauser, G., and Zimmermann, M. (1978): Hemmung im Rückenmark, ein neurophysiologischer Wirkungsmechanismus bei der Hypalgesie durch Stimulationsakupunktur. *Wien. Klin. Wochenschrift,* 90:59–64.
11. Dickhaus, H., Zimmermann, M., and Zotterman, Y. (1976): The development in regenerating cutaneous nerves of C-fibre receptors responding to noxious heating of the skin. In: *Sensory Functions of the Skin in Primates,* edited by Y. Zotterman, S. 415–425. Pergamon Press, Oxford, New York, Toronto, Sydney, Paris, Frankfurt.
12. Fields, H. L., and Basbaum, A. I. (1978): Brainstem control of spinal pain-transmission neurons. *Ann. Rev. Physiol.,* 40:217–248.
13. Goldstein, A. (1976): Opioid peptides (endorphins) in pituitary and brain. *Science,* 193:1081–1086.
14. Handwerker, H. O., Iggo, A., and Zimmermann, M. (1975): Segmental and supraspinal actions on dorsal horn neurons responding to noxious and non-noxious stimuli. *Pain,* 1:147–165.
15. Hardy, I. D., Wolff, H. D., and Goodell, H. (1952): *Pain Sensations and Reactions.* Williams & Wilkins, Baltimore.
16. Hassler, R. (1960): Die zentralen Systeme des Schmerzes. *Acta Neurochir.* (*Wien*), 8:353–423.
17. Henry, J. L. (1976): Effects of substance P on functionally identified units in cat spinal cord. *Brain Res.,* 114:439–451.
18. Hick, V. E., Koley, J., and Morrison, J. F. B. (1977): The effects of bradykinin on afferent units in intra-abdominal sympathetic nerve trunks. *Quart. J. Exp. Physiol.,* 62:19–25.
19. Horeyseck, G., and Jänig, W. (1974): Reflexes in postganglionic fibres within skin and muscle nerves after noxious stimulation of skin. *Exp. Brain Res.,* 20:125–134.
20. Iggo, A. (editor) (1973): *Somatosensory System. Handbook of Sensory Physiology, Vol. II.* Springer Verlag, Berlin, Heidelberg, New York.
21. Janzen, R., Keidel, W. D., Herz, A., and Steichele, C. (editors) (1972): *Pain: Basic Principles—Pharmacology—Therapy.* Georg Thieme Verlag, Stuttgart.
22. Keele, C. A., and Armstrong, D. (1964): *Substances Producing Pain and Itch.* Edward Arnold Ltd., London.
23. Kosterlitz, H. W. (editor) (1976): *Opiates and Endogenous Opioid Peptides.* North-Holland, Amsterdam.
24. Kumazawa, T., and Mizumura, K. (1977): Thin-fibre receptors responding to mechanical, chemical and thermal stimulation in the skeletal muscle of the dog. *J. Physiol.* (*Lond.*), 273:179–194.
25. Liebeskind, J. C., and Paul, L. A. (1977): Psychological and physiological mechanisms of pain. *Annu. Rev. Psychol.,* 28:41–60.
26. Lim, R. K. S. (1970): Pain. *Annu. Rev. Physiol.,* 32:269–288.
27. Mayer, D. J., and Price, D. D. (1976): Central nervous system mechanisms of analgesia. *Pain,* 2:379–404.

28. Mayer, D. J., Price, D. D., and Rafii, A. (1977): Antagonism of acupuncture analgesia in man by the narcotic antagonist naloxone. *Brain Res.,* 121:368–372.
29. Mense, S. (1977): Nervous outflow from skeletal muscle following chemical noxious stimulation. *J. Physiol.* (*Lond.*) 267:75–88.
30. Mense, S., and Schmidt, R. F. (1977): Muscle pain: Which receptors are responsible for the transmission of noxious stimuli? In: *Physiological Aspects of Clinical Neurology,* edited by F. Clifford Rose, pp. 265–278. Blackwell Scientific Publications, Oxford, London, Edinburgh, Melbourne.
31. Messing, R. B., and Lytle, L. D. (1977): Serotonin-containing neurons: Their possible role in pain and analgesia. *Pain,* 4:1–22.
32. Neil, E. (editor) (1972): *Enteroreceptors. Handbook of Sensory Physiology, Vol. III/1.* Springer Verlag, Berlin, Heidelberg, New York.
33. Price, D. D., and Dubner, R. (1977): Neurons that subserve the sensory-discriminative aspects of pain. *Pain,* 3:307–338.
34. Richardson, D. E., and Akil, H. (1977): Pain reduction by electrical brain stimulation in man. *J. Neurosurg.,* 47:178–194.
35. Snyder, S. H. (1977): Opiate receptors and internal opiates. *Sci. Am.,* 236:44–56.
36. Sternbach, R. A. (1976): The need for an animal model of chronic pain. *Pain,* 2:2–4.
37. Sunderland, S. (1968): *Nerves and Nerve Injuries.* Livingstone, Edinburgh and London.
38. Uchida, Y., and Murao, S. (1974): Excitation of afferent cardiac sympathetic nerve fibers during coronary occlusion. *Am. J. Physiol.,* 226:1094–1099.
39. Wall, P. D. (1975, 1976): Editorials in *Pain,* 1:1–2 (1975) and *Pain,* 2:1 (1976).
40. Wall, P. D., and Gutnick, M. (1974): Ongoing activity in peripheral nerves: The physiology and pharmacology of impulses originating from a neuroma. *Exp. Neurol.,* 43:580–593.
41. Willis, W. D., Trevino, D. L., Coulter, J. D., and Maunz, R. A. (1974): Responses of primate spinothalamic tract neurons to natural stimulation of hind limb. *J. Neurophysiol.,* 37:358–372.
42. Yaksh, T. L., and Rudy, T. A. (1978): Narcotic analgetics: CNS sites and mechanisms of action as revealed by intracerebral injection techniques. *Pain,* 4:299–359.
43. Zimmermann, M. (1975): Neurophysiological models for nociception, pain and pain therapy. In: *Brain Hypoxia—Pain: Advances in Neurosurgery, Vol. 3,* edited by H. Penzholz, M. Brock, J. Hamer, M. Klinger, and O. Spoerri, pp. 199–209. Springer-Verlag, Berlin, Heidelberg, New York.
44. Zimmermann, M. (1976): Neurophysiology of nociception. In: *International Review of Physiology, Vol. 10, Neurophysiology II,* edited by R. Porter, pp. 179–221. University Park Press, Baltimore.
45. Zimmermann, M. (1977): Encoding in dorsal horn interneurons receiving noxious and non noxious afferents. *J. Physiol.* (*Paris*), 73:221–232.
46. Zotterman, Y. (1939): Touch, pain and tickling: An electrophysiological investigation on cutaneous sensory nerves. *J. Physiol.* (*Lond.*), 95:1–28.
47. Zotterman, Y. (editor) (1976): *Sensory Functions of the Skin in Primates.* Pergamon Press, Oxford.

Advances in Pain Research and Therapy, Vol. 2,
edited by J. J. Bonica and V. Ventafridda.
Raven Press, New York © 1979.

Neuroanatomy and Biochemistry of Antinociception

Costantino Benedetti

Department of Anesthesiology, University of Washington School of Medicine, Seattle, Washington 98195

Professor Zimmermann has, in the preceding chapter, effectively and extensively reviewed the peripheral and central nociceptive system and has alluded to antinociceptive mechanisms. Now I would like to give an overview of the presently known systems which are involved in the modulation of pain and, in particular, a system which is located in the central nervous system (CNS) and is activated either by endogenous morphine-like substances (enkephalins or endorphins), or by exogenous opioids.

In 1965, after many years during which pain research received very little scientific attention, Melzack and Wall (30) published the Gate Control Theory. Even if the original hypothesis of the Gate Control Theory has to be modified, it nonetheless had a great impact, because in the following years many researchers turned their attention to a neglected area of research—pain (64).

ELECTRICAL STIMULATION ANALGESIA

In 1968, Reynolds reported his experience with electrical stimulation of specific areas of the rat brain (39). By implanting electrodes in the periaqueductal gray (PAG) of rats and electrically stimulating them after the animals had recuperated from the original neurosurgery, he was able to induce, in some animals, sufficient analgesia to allow the performance of laparotomies. Following surgery, when the electrical stimulation was discontinued, Reynolds noted that residual skin analgesia remained for a few minutes, but within 5 min, vigorous, aversive responses to painful stimulation had returned.

In 1971, Mayer et al. (29) repeated this experiment in more detail and under more-controlled experimental conditions. They found that electrical stimulation of subcortical loci could indeed cause profound analgesia without apparent accompanying motor or motivational deficits, and the majority of animals appeared to have no impaired response to visual, auditory, or tactile stimuli. In fact, some were hyperreactive to light touch. The animals were analgesic not only to mechanical noxious stimuli, but also to other noxious events, and the analgesia outlasted brain stimulation by 30 sec to 5 min. In light of these observations, the investigators postulated that the electrical brain stimulation activated an endogenous neurophysiologic system that blocked or at least decreased noxious input.

In a similar experiment, Samanin and Valzelli (43), showed that stimulation for 1 hr of the dorsal raphe nuclei before the subcutaneous injection of morphine markedly enhanced the analgesic effect of this drug, while lesions of the nucleus raphe medianus antagonized morphine analgesia. These authors further observed that the analgesic effect paralleled the increase of 5-hydroxyindoleacetic acid (a metabolic by-product of serotonin) in the forebrain. This finding was in agreement with the results of Aghajanian et al. (2), who had previously demonstrated that electrical stimulation of raphe nuclei, in the vicinity of the central gray, released serotonin in brain synapses.

ROLE OF NEUROTRANSMITTERS

In an attempt to elucidate the interrelationship of pain modulation and serotonin, Tenen (50) lowered the serotonin concentration in rats and reported that these experimental animals developed hyperalgesic behavior, which could be reversed by injecting replacement doses of the serotonin precursor, 5-hydroxytryptophan. Sicuteri et al. (45) inadvertently induced similar hyperalgesia in humans suffering from migraine or other headaches by administering, for headache therapy, parachlorophenylalanine, an inhibitor of tryptophan hydroxylase which causes decrease of serotonin synthesis. They found that 20% of the patients developed hyperalgesia which lasted for 5 to 10 days after the discontinuation of the drug, a period consistent with the usual duration of action of the drug. However, normal subjects did not show this response (44).

The further demonstration that the decrease of serotonin concentration caused a reduction of the analgesia elicited by morphine or other opioids (49) led Akil and Liebeskind (3) to study the roles which the three cerebral monoamines (norepinephrine, dopamine, and serotonin) might play in analgesia. They found that the simultaneous depletion of all three neurotransmitters severely inhibited not only the analgesic effect of morphine, but also the effect of electrical stimulation at specific brain sites. The original level of analgesia could be restored by injection of the precursor of either serotonin (5-hydroxytryptophan) or dopamine (L-dopa). Selective depletion of serotonin reduced the analgesia, whereas elevation of its concentration at the synaptic cleft enhanced it. Pimozide (which blocks dopamine receptors) decreased the analgesia, while apomorphine (a dopamine-receptor stimulator) or L-dopa increased it. On the other hand, depletion of only norepinephrine enhanced the analgesic action of these substances, whereas its increase caused reduction of the analgesic state. If the norepinephrine level was depressed and the dopamine elevated, the analgesic effect was particularly potentiated. Therefore, it appears that dopamine and serotonin are necessary neurotransmitters to facilitate the analgesia whereas norepinephrine depresses it. In accordance with this result is the recent report by Wang (59), who found that 100 to 200 μg of serotonin administered in the lumbar subarachnoid space of rats produced profound analgesia lasting up to 40 min. Behavioral and morphological observation fail to show any adverse reaction.

Bonica (8), in 1953, had already reported that patients suffering from chronic pain sometimes improved after treatment with amphetamines; and since this drug probably acts on the serotonin receptors of the brain, this observation is also in accordance with the above findings. Recently, it has been clinically demonstrated that 10 mg of dextroamphetamine almost doubles the analgesic effect of 12 mg of morphine, while at the same time it decreases the respiratory depression and the lethargy caused by the opioid (14).

SIMILARITIES BETWEEN OPIOID ANALGESIA AND STIMULATION-INDUCED ANALGESIA

The observations that (a) morphine action is dependent on the availability of serotonin and on the integrity of certain raphe nuclei, and (b) electrical stimulation of the dorsal raphe nuclei enhances morphine's action and increases serotonin by-product in the forebrain, suggested that both periventricular electrical stimulation and morphine activated a similar inhibitory mechanism. Akil, Mayer, and Liebeskind (6) reported that analgesia induced by electrical stimulation of PAG was reduced, like morphine analgesia, when the raphe nuclei were lesioned or when the brain level of serotonin was lowered (4). They further observed that a pure opioid antagonist like naloxone reversed the analgesic effect of electrical stimulation (5). All these data strongly indicate that morphine and brain electrical stimulation are very similar in action and that both activate the same nociception-suppressing descending system. The system appears to be tonically active at least in some animal species, since lesioning of the raphe nuclei leads to hyperalgesia in the animals.

OPIATE RECEPTORS

In the early 'seventies other laboratories were actively investigating the mode of action of morphine with particular attention to the mechanism of addiction. In 1973, Pert and Snyder (36) isolated opiate receptors from the synaptosomal fraction of brain homogenate and more specifically from the synaptic membrane. These structures are proteolipid and have a characteristic chemical and physical configuration which makes them stereospecific and bind only the active opioid isomers in a manner similar to the action of a proper lock and key (15). Opiate receptors are present only in the vertebrates (35), and they are distributed in different areas of the body including the brain, spinal cord, and gastrointestinal tract. In both human and lower primates the brain contains the highest concentration of receptors (25). The amygdala, hypothalamus (parts of the limbic system which largely mediate emotional behavior), corpus striatum, caudate nucleus, periaqueductal gray, and thalamus are the areas most heavily endowed. The grey matter of the spinal cord also contains opiate receptors and most of them are located in the substantia gelatinosa. The cerebellum is devoid of opiate receptors whereas the cerebral cortex has a low concentration of them (36). It has been hypothesized that the combination of the opioid agonist with the receptor causes membrane changes that initiate the pharmacologic response, an event which does not occur when an antagonist binds to the receptor.

DISCOVERY OF ENDOGENOUS OPIOIDS

The existence of receptors in the brain which would bind with a substance found in the opium poppy, is certainly a peculiar occurrence. Researchers began to believe that the exogenous opiate must activate a neuromodulation system that is normally mobilized when an endogenous substance, similar in action to morphine, binds to the receptors specific to that substance. In 1975, both Terenius (56) and Hughes (20) independently succeeded in isolating a substance from the brain which had actions similar to opioids and these actions were reversible by naloxone. These findings indicated that endogenous substances with opiate-like actions do indeed exist.

These reports were soon confirmed by other investigators. Cox et al. (11) reported the isolation of a morphine-like substance from the pituitary gland, and Pasternak et al. (34) were able to isolate a similar substance from rat brain. Hughes et al. (21), shortly afterward, reported that the substance was a peptide of molecular weight of about 900 daltons and he termed it *enkephalin.* A few months later, Hughes and colleagues (22) again reported the identification of two related pentapeptides with potent opioid agonistic activity from pig-brain homogenate. The two peptides were identical except for the fifth amino acid, which was either methionine or leucine. These authors also reported that the amino acid sequence of met-enkephalin is identical to the 61–65 amino acid fraction of β-lipotropin, a polypeptide hormone of 91 amino acids from pituitary glands of sheep, pig, and man as represented in Fig. 1. Other fractions of this same molecule contain the amino acid sequence of other brain peptides such as β Melanocyte Stimulating Hormone (β-MSH) and part of ACTH. Subsequently, numerous other investigators have reported the isolation, structure, synthesis, and mode of action of various morphine-like substances.

Bradbury et al. (9) studied the effects of other fragments of β-lipotropin hormone. They found the 61–91 sequence of amino acids had opioid agonist

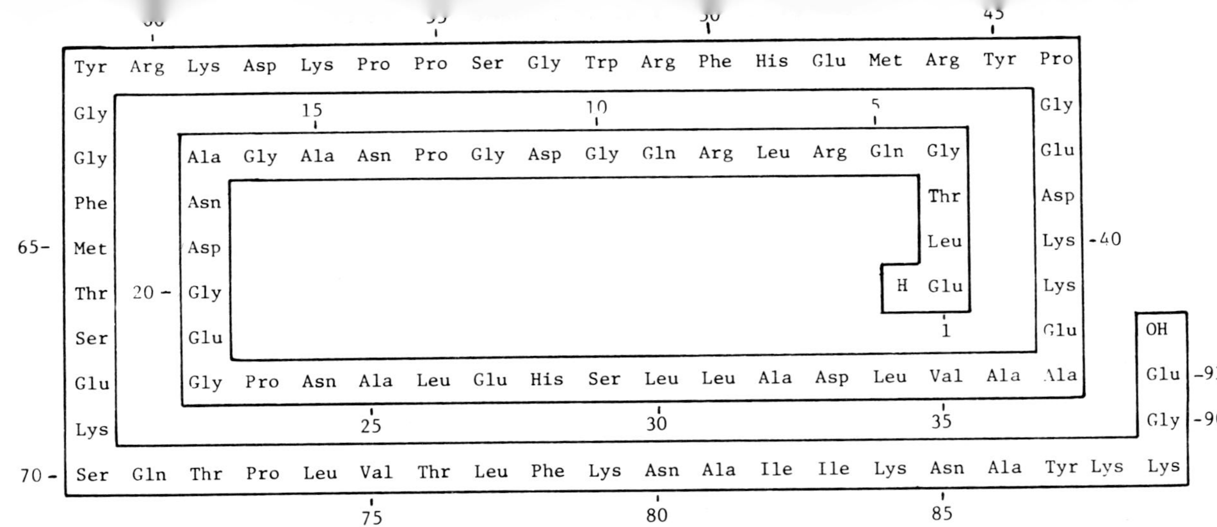

Ala : Alanine
Arg : Arginine
Asn : Asparagine
Asp : Aspartic acid
Gln : Glutamine
Glu : Glutamic Acid
Gly : Glycine
Ile : Isoleucine
His : Histidine
Leu : Leucine
Lys : Lysine
Met : Methionine
Phe : Phenylalanine
Pro : Proline
Ser : Serine
Thr : Threonine
Trp : Tryptophan
Tyr : Tyrosine
Val : Valine

FIG. 1. Amino acid sequence of pituitary human β-lipotropin hormone (β LTH). Sequence 1–55 represents α-lipotropin hormone, 41–58 β Melanocyte Stimulating Hormone (β-MSH), 61–65 met-enkephalin, 61–76 α-endorphin, 61–77 γ-endorphin and 61–91 β-endorphin. The amino acid sequence 47–53 is common to ACTH, β MSH and α-lipotropin hormone. This sequence has been shown to have opioid analgesia antagonistic activity.

activity. Cox, Goldstein, and Li (10) tested the entire β-lipotropin hormone molecule and found it devoid of opioid activity, whereas they confirmed that the 61–91 fragment had about the same potency as met-enkephalin. They elected to call this compound *β-endorphin* (endogenous-morphine) in contrast to another fragment 61–76 described by Guillemin et al. (17) and named *α-endorphin.*

Soon thereafter met-enkephalin and other endorphins were produced synthetically and tested on experimental animals. It became apparent that met-enkephalin is more potent than leu-enkephalin and that both are soon inactivated, probably by amino peptidase, since their half life is less than 1 min. β-endorphin is more resistant to plasma inactivation, and it can be injected intravenously to cause analgesia up to 2 to 3 hr (57). Lately, a synthetic enkephalin analog has been produced which shows effects even after oral intake (41). The cross-tolerance between these various endogenous ligands with morphine has been noted. Abstinence symptoms caused by discontinued administration of morphine soon disappear after injection of endorphin. Also, chronic administration of the endorphins causes tolerance and withdrawal symptoms after removal of the drug or reversal by naloxone (58).

From *in vitro* studies using both endogenous and exogenous opioids, multiple receptors have been demonstrated. In addition to the receptors which bind the classic morphine-like substances, others have been identified which show preferred selectivity for opiate peptides and naloxone has less affinity for these receptors. Different tissues have different populations of these receptors, but their distribution in the body and in particular in the CNS is not yet known (27,46,53).

Of similar importance to the discovery of endogenous opioids was the realization that endogenic antagonistic substances exist. Initially, Winter and Flataker (62) had demonstrated that ACTH reduced the analgesic effect of morphine. This work was confirmed and extended by Paroli (33), who found that the antagonistic effect of ACTH was dose-related. Zimmermann and Krivoy (63) have reported that not only ACTH, but also β-MSH has an antagonistic effect on morphine analgesia.

Terenius et al. (51,54) tested these earlier observations in an *in vitro* preparation of opioid receptors. They found that antagonistic activity of ACTH, β-MSH and other smaller peptides was dependent on the presence of the amino acid sequence Met-Glu-His-Phe-Arg-Trp-Gly (47–53 of β-lipotropin hormone) which is common to the above-mentioned hormones and lipotropin hormone (Fig. 1). This sequence is essential for the antagonistic effect and these peptides show affinity to the opiate receptors, which, however, is not so marked as the affinity of the endorphins. Wiegant et al. (61) have recently confirmed the antagonistic effect of this peptide on opioid analgesia in an animal model. This peptide does not possess any intrinsic analgesic properties; however, it can elicit non-analgesic effects in rats, such as excessive grooming, which is also seen with low doses of morphine. This could indicate that this peptide has both agonistic and antagonistic properties.

NEUROANATOMY AND NEUROPHYSIOLOGY OF ANTINOCICEPTION

By means of immunohistochemical analysis, attempts have been made to study the distribution of these polypeptides. It is interesting to note that β-endorphin is located mostly in the pituitary gland and hypothalamus (19) and, in particular, in the same cells which contain ACTH and it is released concomitantly with this hormone (18). In contrast, the enkephalins and in particular met-enkephalin, have a much wider distribution. Met-enkephalin, in fact, is located not only in the brain, but also in the spinal cord, in the nerve plexi of the gastrointestinal tract, and more recently has been found also in the exocrene cells of the stomach and intestine (37).

In the spinal cord it appears that met-enkephalin is located in interneurons of the substantia gelatinosa and/or in the proprioceptive afferents (19), since its level does not change after cordotomy. Immunohistochemical analysis also shows that there is a strict relationship between met-enkephalin and substance P, an excitatory peptide that is necessary for transmission of noxious impulses from the periphery to the higher centers of the brain (24). The demonstration of opiate receptors on the superficial laminae of the dorsal horn and their marked decrease after dorsal rhizotomy suggest their presynaptic localization on primary nociceptive afferents (26). The binding of enkephalin or morphine to these receptors apparently inhibits the release of substance P, preventing the synaptic transmission of noxious impulses (23).

While enkephalin acts on the segmental level of the spinal cord, other antinociceptive descending systems have now been established. Descending substance P pathways have been identified (19), and they may also be involved in the analgesia created by electrical stimulation of mesencephalic brain areas. Substance P, being a stimulating neurotransmitter, may activate the enkephalin neurons in the dorsal horn causing the release of this peptide (19). This is substantiated by the fact that small quantities of substance P given intraventricularly or systemically causes a naloxone-reversible analgesia (28,48).

Another descending antinociceptive system has been known for the last few years. This system is either activated by the electrical stimulation of the periaqueductal gray, or by the action of morphine-like substances (Fig. 2). Neurons in the ventrocaudal area of the gray matter surrounding the aqueductus cerebri make synaptic contact with a cluster of nerve cells which are located ventrally to the fourth ventricle and form the nucleus raphe magnus (42). All these neurons have high concentration of met-enkephalin, substance P, and opiate receptors (19). These neurons send their axons centrif-

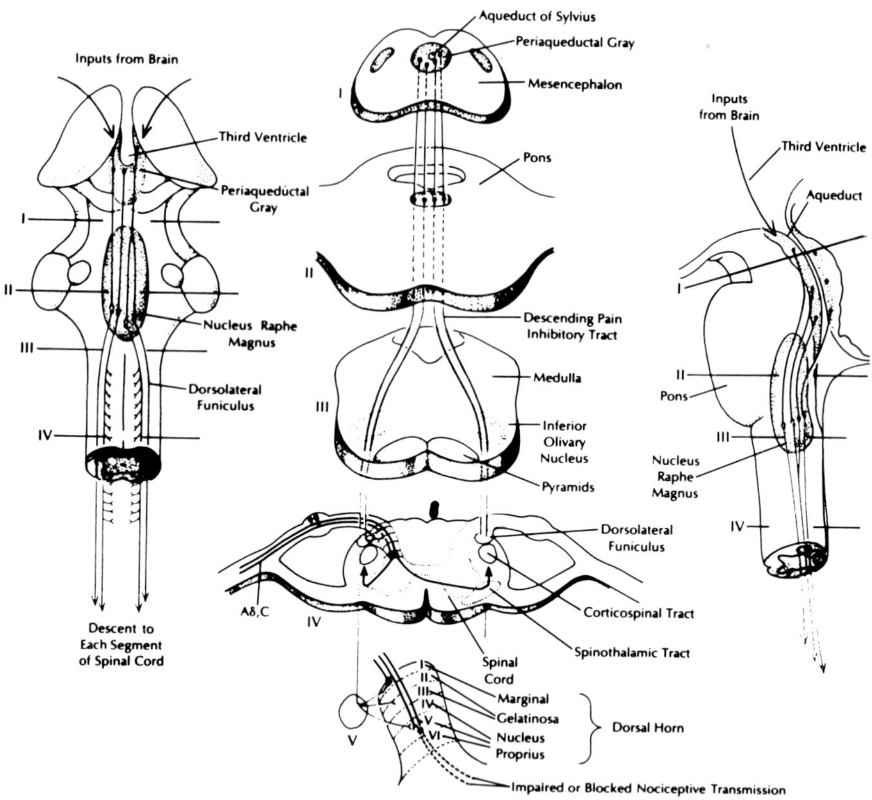

FIG. 2. Schematic drawing of the neuroanatomy of the descending inhibitory system activated by opioids and electrical stimulation of periaqueductal gray. [Courtesy of Dr. John J. Bonica: Pathophysiology of pain. *Hosp. Pract.* (Special Report), January 1978, p. 9.]

ugally in the dorsolateral funiculus just lateral and posterior to the motor axons which form the pyramidal tract and enter the dorsal horn at various levels of the spinal cord (7). These axons, which release serotonin at their synaptic terminals (4,12,16), make contact with nerve fibers located in laminae I, II, and V. This serotonergic system probably inhibits transmission of noxious impulses by axo-axonic influence on the primary nociceptive neurons in the dorsal horn (13,38). It should be noted at this point that some neurons in other raphe nuclei (raphe medianus and dorsalis) send their axons rostrally to innervate many regions such as the hypothalamus, hippocampus, corpus striatum, septum, and cortex (31). Their involvement in pain-modulation is not yet defined, but they appear to contain dopamine and norepinephrine as neurotransmitters, which have been shown to be involved in the modulation of pain (3).

SUMMARY

The data now available indicate that morphine analgesia mimics the action of endogenous morphine-like substances, termed *enkephalins* and *endorphins* and that electrical stimulation of specific areas of the brain causes their release. Strong evidence suggests that a peptide included in ACTH and β-MSH molecules acts as an endogenic opioid antagonist, at least for analgesia.

Since β-endorphin is located mainly in the pituitary-hypothalamic area and the enkephalins are located in other parts of the central nervous system, it appears that at least two major endorphin-releasing systems exist (52). One which is located in the pituitary gland may exert a prolonged hormonal activity owing to the long half-life of β-endorphin (57). The other, where met-enkephalin is the major modulator, acts both in a direct and indirect manner. Direct inhibition occurs when the enkephalin, released by the interneurons of the substantia gelatinosa cells (probably the same cells of the Gate Control Theory), binds to the opiate receptors located at the synapse of the nociceptive afferents and prevents the release of substance P and therefore, nociceptive transmission. Strong experimental evidence indicates that these enkephalin neurons are activated whenever axons descending from the upper centers of the central nervous system or primary proprioceptive afferents secrete substance P at the synaptic junction. Indirect modulation occurs when the neurons of the periaqueductal gray release endorphin. This substance activates a descending inhibitory system which includes neurons located in the nucleus raphe magnus. Their axons run in the dorsolateral funiculus and make axo-axonic synapses with the peripheral nociceptive afferents as they enter the dorsal horn. The release of serotonin at this junction causes nociceptive inhibition.

The observation that dopamine is directly involved in the modulation of pain and that this neurotransmitter is not present in the spinal cord suggests that the analgesic mechanism of endorphins and morphine may involve other inhibitory systems located in the brain. Further research will be needed to elucidate both this mechanism and the pathways of the norepinephrine system which appear to counteract morphine analgesia. Since changes of psychologic state alter the concentration of certain hormones and of neurotransmitters implicated in the endorphin system, it seems plausible that different psychologic states may activate or deactivate this mechanism of pain-modulation.

IMPLICATIONS FOR CANCER PAIN

Having briefly reviewed the endorphin antinociceptive system, let us consider what implications it may have in relation to cancer patients suffering severe pain.

In addition to the fact that the tumors produce noxious stimuli by causing inflammation of the surrounding areas, destruction of tissue, compression of nerve roots, obstruction of a hollow viscus and pressure, the above information suggests that these patients may possibly be hyperalgesic. This can be explained by multiple biochemical mechanisms. In fact, Terenius and Wahlström (55) and Sjölund et al. (47) have found that endorphins in the cerebrospinal fluid (CSF) are decreased in patients suffering from both chronic and cancer pain. Other substances are also implicated. As Dr. Chapman will emphasize in the paper that follows, the majority of patients suffering from a chronic illness, or knowing or suspecting affliction by a neoplastic disease, develop varying degrees of depression and are continuously under abnormal psychologic and physical stress. Distress is known to produce an increase in secretion of ACTH and norepinephrine, substances which act as antagonists at different levels of this antinociceptive system, as previously described. In addition, there are strong indications that depression is accompanied by diminished levels of serotonin, and recent preliminary observations in our institution seem to indicate that depressed patients are usually affected with chronic pain and experience a decrease in pain threshold. Both the decreased amount of serotonin and the increased amount of ACTH and norepinephrine will contribute to hyperreactivity of cancer patients to noxious input.

The ability to change or improve this psychologic state either by pharmacologic means or by psychotherapy will possibly help relieve the pain sensations of the patient. This is possibly the mode of action of amphetamines as observed and reported by Bonica (8) for treatment of some chronic pain states. Drugs used to block pituitary activities, as reported in this volume by Pannuti, and chemical hypophysectomy, developed by Moricca (32) to relieve diffuse cancer pain in terminal patients, may very well affect this endogenous antinociceptive system by altering the interdependent concentrations of the agonist and antagonist substances in favor of the agonist.

Direct application in the clinical setting of pure experimental techniques has also been reported. Richardson and Akil (40) and Adams (1) inserted electrodes in the periventricular gray matter of patients suffering from intractable chronic pain, and they were able to induce a pain-free state by electrical stimulation of this area. The analgesia ensued after 1 to 2 hr of stimulation and outlasted it for about 20 hr. Levels of morphine-like substances increase after the electrical stimulation and naloxone reverses this type of analgesia (personal communication with Akil).

CONCLUSION

To conclude, I would like to emphasize that this new area of biologic research will help us to understand how pain is modulated and possibly help us to explain the individual variation of pain-sensitivity in health and disease. It will also help to explain different psychologic disorders, since preliminary indirect observations seem to indicate that the endorphins are implicated in certain psychiatric conditions (60).

However, an enormous research effort is still needed to elucidate fully how the nervous system modulates noxious input under different situations, and to find therapeutic modalities which will activate these or other yet-unidentified autoanalgesia systems. The discovery of endorphin-selective receptors may yet enable us to develop pure analgesics without the undesirable side effects caused by the presently known narcotics (52).

REFERENCES

1. Adams, J. E. (1976): Naloxone reversal of analgesia produced by brain stimulation in the human. *Pain,* 2:161–166.
2. Aghajanian, G. K., Rosecrans, J. A., and Sheard, M. H. (1966): Serotonin release in forebrain by stimulation of midbrain raphe. *Science,* 156:420–423.
3. Akil, H., and Liebeskind, J. C. (1975): Monoaminergic mechanisms of stimulation-produced analgesia. *Brain Res.,* 94:279–296.
4. Akil, H., Mayer, D. J. (1972): Antagonism of stimulation-produced analgesia by p-CPA, a serotonin synthesis inhibitor. *Brain Res.,* 44:692–697.
5. Akil, H., Mayer, D. J., and Liebeskind, J. C. (1976): Antagonism of stimulation-produced analgesia by naloxone, a narcotic antagonist. *Science,* 191:961–962.
6. Akil, H., Mayer, D. J., and Liebeskind, J. C. (1972): Comparaison chez le rat entre l'analgésie induite par stimulation de la substance grise periaqueducale et l'analgésie morphinique. *C. R. Acad. Sci.* [*D*] (*Paris*), 274:3603–3605.
7. Basbaum, A. I., Clanton, C. H., Fields, H. L. (1976): Opiate and stimulus-produced analgesia: Functional anatomy at a medullospinal pathway. *Proc. Natl. Acad. Sci. USA,* 73:4685–4688.
8. Bonica, J. J. (1953): *The Management of Pain.* Lea & Febiger, Philadelphia, p. 532.
9. Bradbury, A. F., Smyth, D. G., Snell, C. R., Birdsall, N. J. M., and Hulme, E. C. (1976): C fragment of lipotropin has a high affinity for brain opiate receptors. *Nature,* 260:793–795.
10. Cox, B. M., Goldstein, A., and Li, C. H. (1976): Opioid activity of a peptide [β LTH (61–91)], derived from β lipotropin. *Proc. Natl. Acad. Sci. USA,* 73:1821–1823.
11. Cox, B. M., Opheim, K. E., Teschemacher, H., and Goldstein, A. (1975): A peptide-like substance from pituitary that acts like morphine. *Life Sci.,* 16(12): 1777–1782.
12. Dahlström, A., and Fuxe, K. (1965): Experimentally induced changes in the intraneuronal amine levels of bulbospinal neuron systems. *Acta Physiol. Scand.* (*Suppl. 64*), 247:5–36.
13. Fields, H. L., Basbaum, A. I., Clanton, C. H., and Anderson, S. D. (1977): Nucleus raphe magnus inhibition of spinal cord dorsal horn neurons. *Brain Res.,* 126(3):441–53.
14. Forrest, W. H., Brown, B. W., Brown, C. R., Defalque, R., Gold, M., Gordon, H. E., James, K. E., Katz, J., Mahler, D. L., Schroff, P., and Teutsch, G. (1977): Dextroamphetamine with morphine for the treatment of postoperative pain. *N. Engl. J. Med.,* 296(13):712–715.
15. Goldstein, A., Lowney, L. I., and Pal, P. K. (1971): Stereospecific and nonspecific interactions of the morphine congener levorphanol in subcellular fractions of mouse brain. *Proc. Natl. Acad. Sci. USA,* 68(8):1742–1747.
16. Guilbaud, G., Besson, J. M., Oliveras, J. L., and Liebeskind, J. C. (1973): Suppression by LSD of the inhibitory effect exerted by dorsal raphe stimulation on certain spinal cord interneurons in the cat. *Brain Res.,* 61:417–422.
17. Guillemin, R., Ling, N., and Burgus, R. (1976): Endorphines, peptides, d'origine

hypothalamique et neurohypophysaire á activité morphinomimétique. Isolement et structure moléculaire de l'α-endorphin. *C. R. Acad. Sci.* [*D*] (*Paris*), 282:783–785.
18. Guillemin, R., Vargo, T., Rossier, J., Minick, S., Ling, N., Rivier, C., Vale, W., and Bloom, F. (1977): β-endorphin and adrenocorticotropin are secreted concomitantly by the pituitary gland. *Science,* 197:1367–1369.
19. Hökfelt, T., Ljundahl, A., Terenius, L., Elde, R., Nilsson, G. (1977): Immunohistochemical analysis of peptide pathways possibly related to pain and analgesia: Enkephalin and substance P. *Proc. Natl. Acad. Sci.,* 74:3081–85.
20. Hughes, J. (1975): Isolation of an endogenous compound from the brain with pharmacological properties similar to morphine. *Brain Res.,* 88:295–308.
21. Hughes, J., Smith, J., Morgan, B., and Fothergill, L. (1975): Purification and properties of enkephalin-the possible endogenous ligand for the morphine receptor. *Life Sci.,* 16(12):1753–1758.
22. Hughes J., Smith, T. W., Kosterlitz, H. W., Fothergill, L. A., Morgan, B. A., and Morris, H. R. (1975): Identification of two related pentapeptides from the brain with potent opiate agonist activity. *Nature,* 258:577–579.
23. Jessell, T. M., and Iversen, L. L. (1977): Opiate analgesics inhibit substance P release from rat trigeminal nucleus. *Nature,* 268:549–551.
24. Konishi, S., and Otsuka, M. (1974): The effects of substance P and other peptides on spinal neurons of the frog. *Brain Res.,* 65:397–410.
25. Kuhar, M. H., Pert, C. B., and Snyder, S. H. (1973): Regional distribution of opiate receptor binding in monkey and human brain. *Nature,* 245:447–450.
26. Lamotte, C., Pert, C. B., and Snyder, S. H. (1976): Opiate receptor binding in primate spinal: Distribution and changes after dorsal root section. *Brain Res.,* 112: 407–412.
27. Lord, J. A. H., Waterfield, A. A., Hughes, J., and Kosterlitz, H. W. (1977): Endogenous opioid peptides: Multiple agonists and receptors. *Nature,* 267:495–499.
28. Malick, J. B., and Goldstein, J. M. (1977): Substance P: Analgesia following intercerebral administration in rats. *Fed. Proc.,* 36:994.
29. Mayer, D. J., Wolfle, T. L., Akil, H., Carder, B., and Liebeskind, J. C. (1971): Analgesia from electrical stimulation in the brainstem of the rat. *Science,* 174: 1351–1354.
30. Melzack, R., and Wall, P. D. (1965): Pain mechanisms: A new theory. *Science,* 150:971–978.
31. Messing, R. B., and Lytle, L. D. (1978): Serotonin-containing neurons: Their possible role in pain and analgesia. *Pain,* 4:1–21.
32. Moricca, G. (1976): Neuradenolysis for diffuse unbearable cancer pain. In: *Advances in Pain Research and Therapy, Vol. 1,* edited by J. J. Bonica and D. Albe-Fessard, pp. 863–869. Raven Press, New York.
33. Paroli, E. (1967): Indagini sull effetto antimorfinico dell' ACTH, Relazioni con il corticosurrene ed i livelli ematici degli 11-OH steroidi. *Arch. Ital. Sci. Farmacol.,* 13:236–237.
34. Pasternak, G. W., and Snyder, S. H. (1975): Identification of novel high affinity opiate receptor binding in rat brain. *Nature,* 253:563–565.
35. Pert, C. B., Aposhian, D., and Snyder, S. H. (1974): Phylogenetic distribution of opiate receptor binding. *Brain Res.,* 75:356–361.
36. Pert, C., and Snyder, S. (1973): Opiate receptor: Demonstration in nervous tissue. *Science,* 179:1011–1014.
37. Polak, J. M., Sullivan, S. N., Bloom, S. R., Facer, P., Pearse, A. G. E. (1977): Enkephalin-like immunoreactivity in the human gastrointestinal tract. *Lancet,* 1:972–74.
38. Proudfit, H. K., and Anderson, E. G. (1974): New long latency bulbo-spinal evoked potentials blocked by serotonin antagonists. *Brain Res.,* 65:542–546.
39. Reynolds, D. V. (1968): Surgery in the rat during electrical analgesia induced by focal brain stimulation. *Science,* 164:444–445.
40. Richardson, D. E., and Akil, H. (1977): Pain reduction by electrical brain stimulation in man. *J. Neurosurg.,* 47:178–83.

41. Roemer, D., Buescher, H. H., Hill, R. C., Pless, J., Bauer, W., Cardinaux, F., Closse, A., Hauser, D., and Huguenin, R. (1977): A synthetic enkephalin analogue with prolonged parenteral and oral analgesic activity. *Nature,* 268:547–549.
42. Ruda, M. A. (1976): Autoradiographic examination of the efferent projections of the midbrain central grey in the cat. Ph.D. Thesis, University of Pennsylvania.
43. Samanin, R., and Valzelli, L. (1971): Increase of morphine-induced analgesia by stimulation of the nucleus raphe dorsalis. *Eur. J. Pharmacol.,* 16:298–302.
44. Sicuteri, F. (1976): Headache: Disruption of pain modulation. In: *Advances in Pain Research and Therapy,* Vol. 1, edited by J. J. Bonica and D. Albe-Fessard, pp. 871–880. Raven Press, New York.
45. Sicuteri, F., Anselmi, B., and Del Bianco, P. L. (1973): 5-hydroxytryptamine supersensitivity as a new theory of headache and central pain: A clinical pharmacological approach with p-chlorophenylalanine. *Psychopharmacologia,* 29: 347–356.
46. Simantov, R., and Snyder, S. H. (1976): Morphine-like peptides, leucine enkephalin and methionine enkephalin: Interactions with the opiate receptor. *Mol. Pharmacol.,* 12:987–998.
47. Sjölund, B., Terenius, L., and Eriksson, M. (1977): Increased cerebrospinal fluid levels of endorphins after electroacupuncture. *Acta Physiol. Scand.,* 100:382–384.
48. Stewart, J. M., Getto, C. J., Neldner, K., Reeve, E. B., Krivoy, W. A. and Zimmermann, E. (1976): Substance P and analgesia. *Nature,* 262:784–785.
49. Tenen, S. S. (1968): Antagonism of the analgesic effect of morphine and other drugs by p-chlorophenylalanine, a serotonin depletor. *Psychopharmacologia,* 12: 278–285.
50. Tenen, S. S. (1967): The effects of p-chlorophenylalanine, a serotonin depletor, on avoidance acquisition, pain sensitivity and related behavior in the rat. *Psychopharmacologia,* 10:204–19.
51. Terenius, L. (1975): Effect of peptides and amino acids on dihydro-morphine binding to the opiate receptor. *J. Pharm. Pharmacol.,* 27:450–451.
52. Terenius, L. (1978): Endogenous peptides and analgesia. *Annu. Rev. Pharmacol. Toxicol.,* 18:189–204.
53. Terenius, L. (1977): Opioid peptides and opiates differ in receptor selectivity. *Psychoneuroendocrinology,* 2:53–58.
54. Terenius, L., Gispen, W. H., and DeWied, D. (1975): ACTH-like peptides and opiate receptors in rat brain: Structure-activity studies. *Europ. J. Pharmacol.,* 33: 395–399.
55. Terenius, L., and Wahlström, A. (1975): Morphine-like ligand for opiate receptors in human CSF. *Life Sci.,* 16(12):1759–1764.
56. Terenius, L., and Wahlström A. (1975): Search for an endogenous ligand for the opiate receptor. *Acta Physiol. Scand.,* 94:74–81.
57. Tseng, L. F., Loh, H. H., and Li, C. H. (1976): β-endorphin as a potent analgesic by intravenous injection. *Nature,* 263:239–240.
58. Tseng, L. F., Loh, H. H., and Li, C. H. (1976): β-endorphin: Cross tolerance to and cross physical dependence on morphine. *Proc. Natl. Acad. Sci. USA,* 73(11): 4187–9.
59. Wang, J. K. (1977): Antinociceptive effect of intrathecally administered serotonin. *Anesthesiology,* 47:269–271.
60. Watson, S. J., Berger, P. A., Akil, H., Mills, M. J., Barchas, J. D. (1978): Effects of naloxone on schizophrenia: Reduction in hallucinations in a subpopulation of subjects. *Science,* 201:73–75.
61. Wiegant, V. M., and Gispen, W. H. (1977): ACTH-induced excessive grooming in the rat: Latent activity of $ACTH_{4-10}$. *Behav. Biol.,* 19(4):554.
62. Winter, C. A., and Flataker, L. (1951): The effect of corticosterone, desoxycorticosterone and adenocorticotrophic hormone upon the responses of animals to analgesic drugs. *J. Pharmacol. Exp. Ther.,* 103:93–105.
63. Zimmermann, E., and Krivoy, W. (1973): Antagonism between morphine and

the polypeptides ACTH, $ACTH_{1-24}$ and β MSH in the nervous system. *Prog. Brain Res.*, 39:383–394.
64. Zimmermann, M. (1976): Neurophysiology of nociception. In: *International Review of Physiology. Neurophysiology II., Vol. 10,* edited by R. Porter, pp. 179–221. University Park Press, Baltimore.

Advances in Pain Research and Therapy, Vol. 2,
edited by J. J. Bonica and V. Ventafridda.
Raven Press, New York © 1979.

Psychologic and Behavioral Aspects of Cancer Pain

C. Richard Chapman

Departments of Anesthesiology, Psychiatry and Behavioral Sciences and Psychology, University of Washington School of Medicine, Seattle, Washington 98195

Pain often emerges as a severe problem for patients with advanced cancer. Viewed from the biologic perspective, it is an aversive sensory experience that signals progression of disease, and it is best controlled by destroying pain pathways or by administering analgesic medications. From the viewpoint of behavioral science, however, pain is part of the total human response to the sickness. In part, pain reflects the way in which the patient experiences the pathologic process, what the disease means to him, and how this meaning affects his interaction with others. Both perspectives offer valuable approaches to the management of the suffering patient, but it is the biologic that dominates current medical practice. The purpose of this chapter is to offer a conceptual framework for the management of cancer patients in pain that encourages the integration of biomedical with biosocial therapies.

THE BIOMEDICAL MODEL

Engel (4) has recently described the biomedical model of sickness that determines current medical practice. This model, which has the status of a dogma in contemporary Western medicine, holds that disease is deviation from the norm of measurable biologic variables. Within the model, psychologic and social aspects of illness are irrelevant. As applied to pain-management, the model requires that pain be viewed as a by-product of disordered biochemical or neurophysiologic processes that exist independently of behavioral and social factors. Recent acknowledgment of the epidemic occurrence of chronic pain disorders (1) suggests that the biomedical framework, despite its many brilliant achievements, has failed to solve the problem of persistent pain.

A fundamental limitation of the biomedical model is that it must construe pain problems as arising consequent to disease and that such troubles will subside when the disease is cured or controlled. This perspective is not incorrect but rather incomplete. Contemporary theories of pain emphasize that sensation, emotion, and meaning are intrinsic parts of the experience (2,11). In developing the McGill Pain Questionnaire, Melzack and Torgerson distinguished among the sensory, affective, and evaluative dimensions of pain. The biomedical model lags behind contemporary concepts of pain and current directions in pain research. Furthermore, as Fordyce (5) and others have emphasized, learning processes can occur when illness behavior is reinforced, and social factors such as financial compensation can sometimes force patients into situations where illness behavior supports the vested interests of the patient better than well behavior. In such cases, pain complaints may persist when the noxious sensory barrage disappears. When this occurs, as it sometimes does in patients who have chronic pain without malignancy, the biomedical model becomes entirely inappropriate in patient care.

PSYCHOLOGIC FACTORS IN CANCER PAIN

The literature indicates that psychologic disturbances are important in almost all kinds of medical disorders, as well as in cancer-related pain problems. Stoeckle, Zola, and Davidson (16), studied psychologic distress in medical patients. In reviewing the literature in this area they noted that in most accounts of office medical practice between 5 and 40% of patients

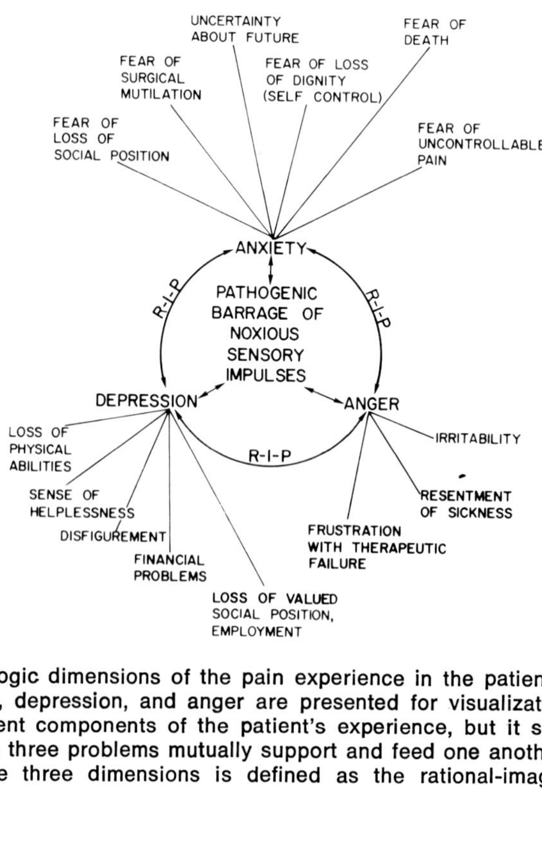

FIG. 1. Psychologic dimensions of the pain experience in the patient with advanced cancer. Anxiety, depression, and anger are presented for visualization purposes as three independent components of the patient's experience, but it should be recognized that these three problems mutually support and feed one another. The relationship among the three dimensions is defined as the rational-imaginative process (R-I-P).

showed a notable amount of basic psychiatric illness. When the concept of psychologic distress was expanded to include stress disorders, psychiatric complaints, and psychosomatic problems, the figure rose to as high as 70% or more. Indeed, in all forms of significant sickness, psychologic problems can arise which reflect the physical distress occasioned by the disease and the impact of disease on the life-style of the patient. When the diagnosis of cancer is made known to the patient, the situation becomes even more complicated. The patient is confronted with the realization that he has a dreaded and possibly terminal disease. Responses of fear, resentment, anger, and frustration are likely to occur. All of these factors enter into the experience of pain and contribute to the patient's pain behavior.

Figure 1 presents a model for the pain associated with advanced cancer. The basic building-block of this pain experience is the barrage of noxious sensory impulses that arises in diseased or damaged tissues. While the nociceptive barrage may be a by-product of neoplastic disease, for the patient with advanced cancer it may be generated by other sources as well. Iatrogenic disease, for example, is not uncommon in individuals who have been operated on multiple times, subjected to radiation or chemotherapy, and given other powerful drugs. In addition, painful neurologic disorders may occur consequent to cancer therapy. Herpes zoster, for example, commonly afflicts patients subjected to immunosuppressant therapies. This disease is exquisitely painful in its onset and throughout its course. In addition, post-herpetic neuralgia may remain as a severe and debilitating problem for an indefinite length of time. The problem is further complicated since the patient's invalid status may lead to severe changes in activity levels, postural changes, and other stresses that may generate pain of muscular origin.

Anxiety

The barrage of noxious sensory impulses gives rise to the conscious experience of pain only after it has been filtered by attentional mechanisms at higher central levels and amplified by various other psychologic factors. One of the principal contributors to the pain experience for the cancer patient is anxiety. Once the patient knows that he has cancer, there is a fear or a sense of dread of the death experience. In addition, patients fear the loss of social position that is a consequence of increasing invalidism, possible loss of control with the progression of the metastatic process and increased medication, and possible surgical mutilation.

Much of the fear experience that characterizes the cancer patient is a function of uncertainty, a factor that has been linked to anxiety and its associated physiologic arousal patterns in the psychologic literature (10). Chronic anxiety is known to result in disturbed autonomic and endocrine function, and it may lead to a variety of well-known psychosomatic symptom complexes such as tension headache, peptic ulcer, or spastic colon. Psychiatric patients with anxiety problems tend to have a large number of pain complaints (3). The presence of nociceptive impulses feeds the cancer patient's anxiety state because it may signal the spread of a disease to a new area. In turn, anxiety has an impact on attentional mechanisms so that the patient becomes hyperreceptive to noxious signals that may indicate changes in the disease process. Anxiety and nociception coexist reciprocally, as though in a vicious circle, as indicated by the bi-directional arrow in Fig. 1. Indeed, many patients experience intense fear with any ache or pain associated with normal living, because such sensations could possibly be symptoms of spreading disease.

Depression

As the patient becomes more and more disengaged from his normal social functioning and increasingly dependent on care-providers and the medical establishment, a sense of helplessness develops. As the disease progresses and reaches advanced stages, the patient typically evolves from repeated bouts of feeling helpless to a general theme of hopelessness and despair. Such depression can be increased by financial problems that face his family because of his inability to work and his mounting medical costs. A sense of self-grief is often evident in these patients, as well, since they undergo a severe loss of valued social position and employment status, and they lose certain physical abilities associated with good health. Many, especially women, suffer grief consequent to surgical disfigurement associated with breast amputation, limb amputation, or facial surgery. Biologic changes associated with depression are well documented in the psychiatric literature. Current theories hold that environmentally precipitated depression may be associated with the depletion of critical neurotransmitter substances such as serotonin. Such biochemical disturbances alter the body's ability to modulate pain states, as Dr. Benedetti described in the previous chapter. Von Knorring (17), Singh (15), and others have shown that pain may emerge as a major complaint in depressed psychiatric patients, even if there is no other specifiable organic disease.

Anger

Because patients perceive and interpret their own suffering and the losses associated with the progress of the disease, many tend to respond with anger, which takes different forms. It is not uncommon for patients to ask, "Why me?" Resentment and bitterness may develop over time as patients develop a sense of hopelessness. Such anger is consequent, in part, to frustration with therapeutic failure. Repeatedly, the patient finds that he is given hope by his physicians only to learn that yet another failure has occurred and the disease has again eluded treatment. When anger is turned inward, it feeds depression. This is represented by the bi-directional arrows connecting the depression and anger parts of Fig. 1. In addition, physiologic changes during anger, similar to those associated with anxiety, may help contribute to information-processing of noxious sensory input. Anger may feed anxiety when the patient begins to fear further frustrations that may provoke him to anger or irritability.

It must be emphasized that the anxiety, depression, and anger described in Fig. 1 are not necessarily abnormal or neurotic responses. Such reactions to the incredible stress of terminal disease are best considered normal and reasonably appropriate when considered from the patient's perspective. Of course, many patients have neurotic tendencies, and these will lead to heightened problems with certain aspects of the psychologic response pattern. Such problems need to be dealt with psychotherapeutically.

Thought Processes

Figure 1 includes a factor that represents the dynamic interrelationship among anxiety, depression, and anger, which is labeled the rational-imaginative process (R-I-P). This process involves the patient's rational interpretation of his problem within his own framework of understanding and the interaction of this interpretation with his imagination about therapeutic outcome and progress of the disease. In brief, the concept represents ongoing thought processes, and it is through such thinking mechanisms that anxiety states help to feed mood disturbances, and vice versa.

While most contemporary therapy is aimed at the pharmacologic control of anxiety and mood disturbance, manipulation of the rational-imaginative processes may provide a viable alternative. The patient's thinking processes are sensitive to information provided by health-care professionals, and, indeed, anger, anxiety, and depression may respond to counseling or proper psychotherapeutic intervention. More importantly, in the cancer patient, prophylactic psychotherapeutic control of such problems can be achieved.

ILLNESS, DISEASE, AND PAIN

Basic Concepts

One of the most useful conceptual schemes for dealing with the problem of cancer-pain management can be derived not from a psychologic framework, but from anthropology. This framework has been most clearly articulated for medical practice by Kleinman and his associates (9). These investigators have offered a conceptual distinction between disease and illness which may be usefully applied to the cancer patient. A *disease* is defined within this context as an abnormality in the function or structure of body organs and systems. It involves the malfunction or maladaptation of certain biologic processes in the patient. In contrast, *illness* is construed as the patient's personal reaction to the disease and associated discomfort. Illness may take a variety of forms depending on the cultural factors that govern the perception of, the classification of, and the explanation of the sickness experience. From the viewpoint of the behavioral scientist, illness refers to the way sick persons perceive, experience, and explain their diseases. Such reactions reflect not only the evaluation of the individual, but also the reactions of the family, the patient's immediate social network, and the culture.

Illness, as defined by Kleinman et al. (6,7,8,9), incorporates the beliefs and attitudes about the sickness held by the patient as well as by his family and his peers. Patients behave, during sickness, in ways that are consistent with the conceptualizations they hold about their problems. They present their symptoms, including their pain complaints, in a way that is rationally related to their illness concerns, interpretations of symptoms, and personal beliefs. To the extent that the patient depends on his doctor for an explanation of what is wrong, the doctor assigns a set of illness-behavior expectations to the patient, and by so doing, determines that patient's social role behavior. But as Kleinman et al. (9) have noted, there is often a discrepancy between the perspective of the health-care professional and that of the patient, his family, and his friends. Indeed, there may be a significant conflict or divergence in beliefs, attitudes, and interpretation among these people for an important health problem. Such conflicts result in poor patient-compliance, searches for quack and folk remedies, and general frustration for both doctor and patient.

The Physician's Perspective

From the viewpoint of the anthropologist, the physician behaves as he does because he has been socialized according to the biomedical model. Trained to maintain the biomedical perspective, physicians and other health-care professionals share a unique "medical" subculture that differs from attitudes toward disease shared by the rest of society. Furthermore, they share a language of technical terms that can be unintelligible to others outside of the medical subculture. Even when the patient strives to understand the physician's perspective on a disease problem, he may be stymied by a language barrier. It is not surprising, therefore, that the patient and the doctor often construe the sickness experience in very different ways.

In general, the physician focuses intensely on disordered biologic processes and looks for ways of applying modern technology so that these destructive trends can be stopped or reversed. In contrast, the patient is concerned with the ways in which the disease and its treatments alter his normal life and social identity. Illness problems involve disturbances in normal daily routine, limitation of activities, psychologic stress experiences such as anxiety, frustration, or a sense of hopelessness, and possible loss of position in the society due to disease-inflicted limitations.

Patient's Perspective

For the cancer patient there are often illness concerns related to fear of death, disturbance of family life, and fear of the unknown course of the disease and uncontrollable pain. Patients need help with these and other illness problems. Further difficulties include changes in premorbid social status and social role, sanctioning of a certain kind of sickness role, financial troubles related to the onset of disease, problems related to family stresses that have grown out of the sickness episode, and problems related to the patient's and the family beliefs about the cause and significance of the sickness.

Most patients expect help from the medical community in dealing with these difficulties. Indeed, such issues may elicit more concern from the patient than the physical symptoms that are so critical to the doctor. In other cases, the patient and his family do not even realize that these problems need attention. Identifying illness problems is an important step in helping such patients and their families, and the long-term consequences for the family of dealing with such problems before death occurs are particularly beneficial. Family crises often emerge after the prolonged illness, suffering, and death of a family member with cancer, but this can be averted in most cases if illness problems are faced and solved while the patient is still living.

Rationale for a Behavioral Perspective

The implication of the medical anthropologic framework for the management of the cancer patient is that both disease and illness problems need to be recognized and managed. The importance of applying all the advantages of medical technology to the problems faced by the cancer patient cannot be denied, but the perspective of medicine has been limited by the biomedical model so that the illness problems surrounding cancer have not been properly appreciated and dealt with in the majority of cases.

In addition, the biomedical model is unable to account for the perceptual complexity of pain. Just as the physiology of vision cannot explain the perceiver's appreciation of a masterful painting, the physiology of pain is inadequate to account for the nature of the pain associated with terminal cancer. Perception is a psychologic experience that involves more than information transmission in the nervous system.

PATIENT BELIEFS AND CANCER PAIN

The Explanatory Model

The rational-imaginative process in Fig. 1 emphasizes the importance of patient beliefs and attitudes in determining the nature of the pain experience.

Kleinman (7) has emphasized that both patients and their families hold explanatory models (EMs) for the occurrence of sickness. These models are systems of beliefs and attitudes that express the lay understanding of the cause, the course, and the nature of the sickness problem. It also incorporates the way that these individuals assign meaning or significance to the problem, as well as the treatment goals that they maintain. Patient EMs are conceptual schemes that derive partly from the patient's culture, his educational experiences, and his family history. In general, American and western-European folk models for disease are rough approximations of the biomedical model held by the physician, but sometimes these approximations are rather poor. It is common to observe in the United States, for example, that patients suffering with a herniated disk will explain that "My back went out" or "I slipped a disk."

In the clinical encounter, the doctor generally explains his model for the disease process to the patient and his family, but it is sometimes presented in a technical idiom which cannot be understood by patients. This is particularly problematic if there is a socioeconomic or cultural difference between the physician and the patient. Often, little or nothing of value is communicated in such an interchange. The author recalls once meeting a poorly educated American black lady from the rural south, who explained that her mother had come down with "Smilin' Mighty Jesus," which was all she could derive from the term *spinal meningitis*.

In the management of cancer pain, the patient's EM is an extremely important factor because it determines his understanding of the situation, his hopes for the future, and his fears for what is yet to come. Some of the suffering observed in patients with advanced cancer is due to the confusion and uncertainty in the patient's thinking and his inability to understand the doctor's EM. In some instances there is a marked discrepancy between the patient and family EMs, which further stresses the patient. Sometimes, and particularly in ethnic subcultures, family members will interpret the disease in terms of a folk medicine or a religious explanation, criticizing the patient for his dependence on physicians and the health-care establishment.

A Cultural Comparison

A fundamental EM cultural contrast in the management of the cancer patient centers around the issue whether or not the victim should be told that he has cancer. Broadly speaking, there are substantial culturally based differences in practice among the various countries of the world. For convenience, it is interesting to compare the United States with Italy. In the United States, most patients are told when cancer is diagnosed. Although there are exceptions to this rule, it is generally considered to be the patient's "right" to know his diagnosis. This news comes as a blow to most patients, and the effects on the patient's psychologic well-being are profound. Most American physicians make strong efforts to explain the patient's situation as best they can; that is, there is an effort to fit the patient's EM to the physician's EM. All too often, unfortunately, this is a failure. The popularity of diet therapies and folk remedies of all sorts bears a silent testimonial to this problem. Recently, for example, the infatuation of American patients with the drug Laetrile led to a public demand that became a major issue in American medical ranks (12,13).

A contrast in cancer-patient management can be observed in Italy where in most instances the patient is not told that he has cancer when it is diagnosed. Usually the family is informed, and doctors elicit their help in actively seeking to mislead the patient into believing that he does not have a malignant disease. The physician and the family both go to great lengths to help the patient develop an EM for his problem that excludes any possibility of cancer, even if the patient is admitted to a cancer hospital. On a covert level the patient may or may not believe what he is told, but on a more overt level he is forced to cooperate in acknowledging that his disease problem is not that of cancer. Whether or not the patient's true beliefs follow the dictates of the family and physician is of little consequence socially, because the patient will not engage in behaviors inconsistent with the beliefs given him by family and authorities.

It would be meaningless to cite the relative advantages of these two patient-management practices, for they are cultural behavior patterns rather than therapeutic strategies. The contrast, however, serves to illustrate the central importance of the patient's EM in the cancer experience.

CONSIDERATIONS FOR PAIN DIAGNOSIS AND THERAPY

Kleinman (8) has suggested that medical-care delivery could be improved by: (a) including a parallel evaluation of illness and disease problems in diagnosis; and (b) undertaking both illness and disease interventions. Table 1 provides parallel lists of cancer-pain–related illness and disease problems. While the listing is incomplete and only suggestive, it illustrates how such an approach might be developed. This approach could be employed in a problem-oriented medical record.

Saunders (14) has provided an example of how important the first item on the illness-problem list can be. She described a 54-year-old woman with advanced carcinoma of the cervix and metastasis to the vulva. Pain was a major complaint. A few days after admission the patient confided a preoccupation with guilt and her beliefs that her disease was related to past sins which had cut her off from God. The chaplain was called, and he was able to successfully allay her fears. As a result she spent her last days in a "tranquility and acceptance that never failed to the end and compelled admiration from us all." Such illness interventions clearly have a place in the care of the dying patient.

TABLE 1. *Considerations in cancer pain diagnosis*

Illness problems	Disease problems
Conflicting beliefs about the cause, nature, significance of the sickness	Metastatic progression
Family distress	Iatrogenic surgery
Loss of social position, status	Therapy-related disease (such as herpes zoster)
Financial difficulties	Side effects of radiation, chemotherapy
Unsatisfactory communication with care-givers	
Fear of death	

Illness and disease interventions should be planned jointly and listed for formulation and recommendation as suggested in Table 1. Some illness interventions may be carried out by the primary care physician but others may require other health-care specialists or expert services from the community such as legal assistance. The best approach is that of a multidisciplinary team that diagnoses and plans comprehensive treatment for pain problems.

The following concerns are basic illness interventions that would benefit most cancer patients with pain (based on Kleinman) (8):

1. presentation in simple language of the physician's EM for the disease and the pain
2. comparison of patient and physician EMs with negotiation between the two viewpoints
3. family therapy
4. financial counseling and planning assistance
5. ongoing monitoring of noncompliance or dissatisfaction with medical care
6. counseling aimed at resolving fears of death and dying.

By allaying the psychologic distresses of anxiety, depression, and anger, these interventions can substantially contribute to the control of suffering and the complaint of pain in the patient with advanced cancer.

FINAL CONSIDERATIONS

Pain is a complex perceptual experience that cannot be reduced to a problem of disturbed physiology in the cancer patient. The impact of prolonged major disease on the psychologic well-being of the patient is enormous, and the stresses imposed on his family by his invalidity add to his burden. The beliefs that the patient holds about the disease, its course, the cause of pain, and his future contribute intimately to the moment-to-moment perception of painful disorders.

The dichotomy between illness and disease discussed previously is in some ways an artificial one. It is important to acknowledge that most therapeutic interventions have an impact on both disease and illness. Placebo treatment, for example, is an illness intervention presented in the disguise of a disease intervention. But to the extent that the placebo rallies the patient's resources or resistance to disease, it becomes a disease therapy. Conversely, nerve blocks, surgical procedures, and other straight-forward disease interventions often have an incidental impact on patient attitudes and beliefs, thus affecting illness. Nonetheless, the dichotomy may serve a useful purpose in the management of cancer pain, since its use helps ensure that illness needs are not unnoticed, untreated, or inappropriately treated by disease interventions. Furthermore, the dichotomy, if employed in diagnosis, can help guarantee that the patient's illness problems will be directly and aggressively dealt with rather than incompletely and incidentally treated, as they are at present in many settings. Pain is often the focus of the patient's enormous suffering, and management of the dying cancer patient in pain must require treatment of both organic disease processes and illness behavior problems.

REFERENCES

1. Bonica, J. J., and Albe-Fessard, D. (1976): Preface. In: *Advances in Pain Research and Therapy, Vol. 1,* pp. v–vi. Raven Press, New York.
2. Chapman, C. R. (1977): Sensory decision theory methods in pain research: A reply to Rollman. *Pain,* 3:295–305.
3. Delaplaine, R., Ifabumuyi, O. I., Merskey, H., and Zarfas, J. (1978): Significance of pain in psychiatric hospital patients. *Pain,* 4:361–366.
4. Engel, G. L. (1977): The need for a new medical model: A challenge for biomedicine. *Science,* 196(4286):129–136.
5. Fordyce, W. E. (1976): *Behavioral Methods for Chronic Pain and Illness.* C. V. Mosby Company, St. Louis.
6. Kleinman, A. (1978): Clinical relevance of anthropological and cross-cultural research: Concepts and strategies. *Am. J. Psychiatry,* 135(4):427–431.
7. Kleinman, A. M. (1975): Explanatory models in health care relationships, In: *Health of the Family* (National Council for International Health Symposium), pp. 159–172. NCIH, Washington, D.C.
8. Kleinman, A. M. Recognition and management of *illness* problems: Therapeutic recommendations from clinical social science. *Massachusetts General Hospital Series on Psychiatric Medicine,* (*in press*).
9. Kleinman, A., Eisenberg, L., and Good, B. (1978): Culture, illness and care: Clinical lessons from anthropological and cross-cultural research. *Ann. Intern. Med.,* 88:251–258.
10. Mandler, G. (1975): *Mind and Emotion.* John Wiley & Sons, Inc., New York.
11. Melzack, R., and Casey, K. L. (1968): Sensory, motivational and central control determinants of pain. A new conceptual model. In: *The Skin Senses,* edited by D. Kenshalo, pp. 423–443. Charles C. Thomas, Springfield, Ill.
12. Moertel, C. G. (1978): A trial of Laetrile now. *N. Engl. J. Med.,* 298(4):218–219.
13. New York Academy of Medicine (1977): Statement on Amygdalin (Laetrile). *Bull. N.Y. Acad. Med.,* 53(9):843–846.

14. Saunders, C. (1976): Control of pain in terminal cancer. *Nurs. Times,* 72(29): 1133–1135.
15. Singh, G. (1968): The diagnosis of depression. *Punjab Med. J.,* 18:53–59.
16. Stoeckle, J., Zola, I. K., and Davidson, G. (1964): The quantity and significance of psychological distress in medical patients. *J. Chron. Dis.,* 17:959–970.
17. Von Knorring, L. (1975): The experience of pain in depressed patients. *Neuropsychobiology,* 1:155–165.

Discussion

Part I. Basic Considerations

J. Bonica and C. Morpurgo (Moderators)

Vignali (Massa): Dr. Benedetti, why don't endorphins produce addiction?

Benedetti (Seattle): As I mentioned in my paper, endorphins do produce addiction exactly as morphine does. So far we cannot see this substance as the "all-healer" for easing pain.

Meglio (Rome): Is it possible to measure beta endorphin in body fluids? How? If it has been done in humans, what are the relative concentrations of the drugs?

Benedetti: We can measure endorphins in the cerebrospinal fluid. A solution is made with receptors together with a solution of radioactive morphine. Then we let this solution react with organic liquids, and we measure how much of the isotopic morphine is taken away from the receptors. These tests have been carried out also on humans, and it is interesting that patients affected by cancer and suffering chronic pain have a reduced concentration of these endorphins or similar substances in the spinal fluid.

Questioner: Man can acclimatize to hot climates in 6 to 8 weeks. Is there any evidence that man can acclimatize to chronic pain?

Bonica (Seattle): I would like to answer that question both as one who has observed patients with chronic pain over the past 30 years and one who has himself suffered pain for the past 12 years or so. I think, if anything, the individual becomes more sensitive and probably there is a gradual decrease of the endorphins which help the individual to cope with the pain. So, the earlier the therapy, the better for the patient and the less chance of complications.

Zimmermann (Heidelberg): Not only is there a lack of adaptation to chronic pain, often there is recurrence of chronic pain after a treatment which is successful initially. So, pain seems to be a sensory system which is very difficult to interfere with because it is basically important for life.

Procacci (Florence): Do endogenous substances always produce a sensitization or a modulation sometimes positive, sometimes negative?

Zimmermann: Concerning your first question, there are experimental findings in man and animals that with manipulations which normally produce a sensitization of receptors, the sensitization is sometimes preceded by a period of desensitization, a period of reduced sensitivity, and it might be that this is also due to the early stage of action of some endogenous substances which are released in response to noxious stimulus, such as bradykinin or serotonin.

Bricolo (Verona): As one of your slides has shown us, there would appear not to be a specific central point for the pain reception. Such a hypothesis is in contrast with that recently reported by Kitahata and his group when testing bulbar cells which respond to pain stimulation. If there is no pain center in the CNS, treating pain is a critically difficult problem for neurosurgeons.

Zimmermann: Thank you for this very basic and important question: Are there neurons in the central nervous system that are specific and specifically related to a noxious stimulus? In animal experiments, there have been found some neurons, for example, in the spinal cord, that respond specifically to a noxious stimulus, but the majority of neurons that respond to noxious stimulation also respond to other forms of afferent input. And this is quite expected in the nervous system. The motor output that can be activated by a command for movement or by a command for speech can also be activated by a nociceptive input, and so there must be in the nervous system a mixing up of several modalities which determine behavior. So from this standpoint, it must be expected that the most relevant information concerned with pain is contained in the activity of nerve cells that are not only related to a noxious stimulus. Of course, there are some bypasses, for example, the spinothalamic tract where the information on noxious stimulus or on a pain state in the periphery is transmitted high up to the brain; and at this strategic site, one can produce pain-relief by a cordotomy. But, the spinothalamic or anterolateral tract is not only concerned with pain; that is also well established. And the assumption that in the central nervous system there is no pain tract and no nucleus specifically involved in pain does not exclude that a neurosurgical procedure is successful in removing pain because there is a strategic site through which all the pain related information must go.

Bonica: When one considers that cordotomy will relieve pain for many months; and then, despite the fact that analgesia still persists, the pain recurs, one has to consider that perhaps some of the other systems are also involved.

Advances in Pain Research and Therapy, Vol. 2,
edited by J. J. Bonica and V. Ventafridda.
Raven Press, New York © 1979.

Pain Syndromes in Patients with Cancer

Kathleen M. Foley

Department of Neurology, Memorial Sloan-Kettering Cancer Center, New York, New York 10021

INTRODUCTION

Pain complicating cancer is often a difficult and frustrating clinical problem. A wide variety of complex pain problems in patients with cancer is encountered in a cancer hospital where, since the treatment available is often palliative and noncurative, the assessment and treatment of pain assumes the utmost importance. Pain in the patient with cancer may be caused by any of the pathophysiologic alterations which affect the general population and does not necessarily imply recurrent or persistent cancer. To facilitate appropriate diagnostic and therapeutic approaches for such patients, some knowledge of the common and uncommon causes of pain in patients with cancer and their clinical presentation is essential.

Existing data assessing the prevalence of pain in patients with cancer come predominantly from terminal-care facilities, where 50 to 60% of terminal patients are reported to have pain (8). These data do not report the incidence of pain in patients undergoing active therapy for cancer and do not attend to the causes of the pain. Therefore, we undertook to (a) assess the prevalence of pain in cancer patients and (b) define the common pain syndromes in patients with cancer.

Prevalence

Between January 1974 and December 1977, 3,424 (9%) of the 36,800 admissions to Memorial Sloan-Kettering Cancer Center (MSKCC), a 561-bed active cancer center, had pain of sufficient magnitude and complexity to require consultation from the Pain Service. This 9% figure represents patients with difficult diagnostic or therapeutic pain problems which the oncologists had had trouble in either assessing or treating.

Such a figure obviously underestimates the overall incidence of pain. To estimate the true incidence of pain in hospitalized patients with cancer, we surveyed the entire inpatient cancer population during a 1-week period (4). Postoperative pain was not included in this study. Of 540 patients evaluated,

TABLE 1. *Types of cancer associated with pain: adult group (143)*

Type	No. pts.	% Total pts.[a]
Breast	46	52
Lung	30	45
Bone	6	85
Oral cavity	12	80
GI	20	40
GU—Male	10	75
Female	14	70
Lymphoma	4	20
Leukemia	1	5

[a] % total pts. admitted with tumor type.

156 (29%) had pain which required the use of analgesic drugs. Primary cancers associated with pain in adults are presented in Table 1. When the number of patients with pain for each tumor type were compared with the number of patients in-hospital at that time with the same tumor type, the percentage of patients with specific types of cancer and pain could be demonstrated. Eighty-five percent of patients with primary bone tumors and 52% of patients with carcinoma of the breast had pain, whereas only 5% of the patients with leukemia had pain. In children, 13 of 39 (33%) had pain. The types of cancer associated with pain in the pediatric group revealed a high incidence of primary bone tumors, with 8 of the 13 pediatric patients having this cancer diagnosis.

A second study was undertaken in 1977. Pediatric postoperative and noncancer patients were excluded from the study; 420 patients were personally questioned, and 397 agreed to a full interview. Data about the severity of their pain, onset, nature, specific pain syndrome, primary tumor, and previous and concurrent therapy were recorded. Of the 397 patients interviewed, 152 (or 38%) complained of pain; 39 of these 397 were terminal, and 23 of the 39 (or 60%) had significant pain.

Based on these two surveys and other clinical experience we have attempted to classify according to etiology specific pain syndromes occurring in patients with cancer in order to facilitate diagnosis (Table 2). The pain syndromes fit into three major groups, according to etiology: (a) 77% of patients in this series had pain caused by tumor invasion or compression of pain-sensitive structures (bone, nerve, and hollow viscus); (b) 19% had pain caused by or associated with cancer therapy; and (c) 3% had pain unrelated to their cancer or their cancer therapy. Before considering these syndromes, certain general principles should be adhered to closely in the evaluation and treatment of patients with pain and cancer.

TABLE 2. *Pain syndromes in patients with cancer*

- I. Pain associated with direct tumor involvement
  - A. Tumor infiltration of bone
    - 1. Base-of-skull metastases
      - a. jugular foramen
      - b. clivus
      - c. sphenoid sinus
    - 2. Vertebral-body metastases
      - a. subluxation of the atlas
      - b. C_7-T_1 metastases
      - c. L_1 metastases
      - d. sacral metastases
  - B. Tumor infiltration of nerve
    - 1. peripheral neuropathy
    - 2. brachial, lumbar, sacral plexopathy
    - 3. meningeal carcinomatosis
    - 4. epidural spinal-cord compression
  - C. Tumor infiltration of hollow viscus
- II. Pain associated with cancer therapy
  - A. Pain occurring post-surgery
    - 1. post-thoracotomy pain
    - 2. post-mastectomy pain
    - 3. post-radical neck pain
    - 4. phantom-limb pain
  - B. Pain occurring post-chemotherapy
    - 1. peripheral neuropathy
    - 2. post-herpetic neuralgia
    - 3. steroid pseudo-rheumatism
    - 4. aseptic necrosis of bone
  - C. Pain occurring post-radiation therapy
    - 1. radiation fibrosis of the brachial plexus and lumbar plexus
    - 2. radiation myelopathy
    - 3. radiation-induced peripheral-nerve tumors
- III. Pain unrelated to cancer or cancer therapy
  - A. Diabetic neuropathy
  - B. Cervical- and lumbar-disc disease
  - C. Rheumatoid arthritis

Evaluation of Pain in Patients with Cancer

Clarification of the Pain Complaint

A careful history of the pain complaint can often provide the diagnosis. One must attempt to elicit a clear description of the onset of pain, its characteristics, the referral pattern, and exacerbating and relieving factors. Further information about the associated signs and symptoms can often clarify the diagnosis: e.g., in a patient complaining of severe back pain exacerbated by lying down, the associated complaint of difficulty in urinating would suggest the diagnosis of epidural spinal-cord compression.

Examination of the Site of the Pain

There is no substitute for a careful physical and neurologic examination to provide objective data and to substantiate the clinical history. The neurologic examination is particularly useful in differentiating local pain from referred pain and peripheral-nerve involvement from plexus or cord involvement. For example, in a patient with low-back pain and radicular symptoms, reflex changes may suggest root rather than plexus disease.

Use of the Appropriate Diagnostic Tools

Since the diagnosis of metastatic disease may be elusive, the limitations of the available diagnostic procedures should be recognized by the physician ordering such studies. Plain X-rays are a useful screening procedure, but a normal study should not overrule a strong clinical impression of bony metastases. There must be a 40 to 60% change in bone density to detect changes on X-ray, and pain can occur with lesser changes. The bone scan provides a more sensitive method for demonstrating abnormalities often 3 to 4 months before changes appear on plain films. Plain X-rays are inadequate to assess certain areas of the body where bone shadows overlap, such as the base of the skull, C_7-T_1 area, and sacrum. Tomography is necessary to discern bony changes in such areas. Computerized transaxial tomography (CT scan) allows for even further detailed visualization of soft tissue and bone and is rapidly becoming the procedure of choice to evaluate the retroperitoneal, paravertebral, pelvic, and skull-base areas. Cisternal and lumbar myelography and cerebrospinal fluid (CSF) cytologic evaluation are other diagnostic procedures which can further help to delineate the pain diagnosis. These diagnostic procedures should be personally reviewed with the specialist interpreting them to ensure adequate visualization of the area under study.

Evaluation of the Extent of Disease

A clear evaluation of the extent of metastatic disease may help to confirm the diagnosis of a specific pain syndrome. For example, in a patient with carcinoma of the colon, perineal pain and negative X-rays and the presence of a rising CEA antigen can suggest local nerve infiltration as the etiology of pain. It is important to remember that the incidence of second primary tumors is increased in patients with a past history of cancer, and in patients in whom the presentation is atypical or the response to therapy different from predicted, needle biopsy or surgical exploration should be performed to establish a tissue diagnosis.

Early Treatment of Cancer Pain

Establishing an accurate diagnosis is the key to providing appropriate therapy, and a cooperative patient is necessary to facilitate this workup. Generally analgesics are the mainstay of therapy, and adequate pain-control will allow the patient to undergo the necessary diagnostic procedures. In patients with epidural spinal-cord compression or diffuse, painful bony metastases, high-dose steroids dramatically relieve their pain, with a concomitant reduction in their analgesic-drug requirements.

SPECIFIC PAIN SYNDROMES IN PATIENTS WITH CANCER: PAIN ASSOCIATED WITH DIRECT TUMOR INVOLVEMENT

Tumor Infiltration of Bone

Pain from invasion of bone by either primary or metastatic tumor is the most common cause of pain in patients with cancer. The pain may be the presenting complaint, as for example in patients with multiple myeloma, or it may represent the first sign of metastatic disease, as occurs in patients with carcinoma of the breast. The patient may have his pain at the site of the lesion, e.g., rib pain, or the pain may be absent locally but referred to a distant area of the body, e.g., knee pain associated with metastatic hip disease. The characteristics of the pain vary with the site involved, but in general the pain is constant and usually grows progressively more severe. A detailed description of pain in metastatic bone disease is beyond the scope of this chapter. However, several important pain syndromes are often misdiagnosed because physicians are unfamiliar with the characteristic signs and symptoms. Some of these syndromes are considered below:

Metastases to the Base of Skull

The syndromes reported here all share two common features. Pain is the earliest complaint, often preceding neurologic signs and symptoms by several weeks to months, and documentation with plain X-rays is often difficult.

Syndromes

Jugular-foramen syndrome. Occipital pain, often referred to the vertex of the head and ipsilateral shoulder and arm, is an early presenting symptom. The pain is often exacerbated by head movement and associated with local tenderness over the occipital condyle. The patient's signs and symptoms vary with the cranial nerve involved, but can include hoarseness, dysarthria, dysphagia, neck and shoulder weakness, and ptosis. The neurologic examination can help to localize the lesion by determining the function of the IXth, Xth, XIth, and XIIth cranial nerves since involvement of all four of these nerves suggests jugular foramen and hypoglossal-canal involvement with secondary nerve dysfunction. The presence of a Horner's syndrome suggests sympathetic involvement extracranially but in close proximity to the jugular foramen.

Clivus metastases. Pain characterized by a vertex headache exacerbated by neck flexion is a common mode of presentation of this entity. Lower-cranial-nerve dysfunction (VIth–XIIth) usually begins unilaterally, but often progresses to bilateral lower-cranial-nerve dysfunction.

Sphenoid-sinus metastases. Severe bifrontal headache radiating to both temples, with intermittent retro-orbital pain, suggests this entity. The patient often complains of nasal stuffiness or a sense of fullness in the head, with a concomitant diplopia. The neurologic sign of unilateral or bilateral VIth nerve palsy helps further to suggest the diagnosis.

Diagnostic Workup

Base-of-skull metastases occur more commonly in patients with nasopharyngeal tumors, but can occur with any tumor type which metastasizes to bone. A lateral X-ray of the neck to assess the retropharyngeal space is an important aspect of the initial workup. Tomography of the skull and CT scan are the procedures of choice to delineate body changes and associated soft-tissue masses. At times, biopsy of the nasopharynx or sphenoid sinus may be necessary to establish the tumor diagnosis.

Differential Diagnosis

Primary nerve and bone tumors (e.g., meningioma, neurofibroma, or chordoma) are commonly associated with these syndromes and should be differentiated from metastatic disease. Meningeal carcinomatosis should be similarly ruled out by CSF cytologic evaluation.

Metastases to Vertebral Bodies

These syndromes share the common feature of pain as an early symptom which, if not accurately diagnosed, may lead to irreversible neurologic deficits, e.g., paraplegia.

Cervical Vertebrae

Subluxation of the atlas. Metastatic disease involving the odontoid process of the axis (C_1 vertebral body) can result in a pathologic fracture with secondary subluxation of it and resulting spinal-cord or brainstem compression. The early symptoms include severe neck pain radiating over the posterior aspect of the skull to the vertex, exacerbated by movement, particularly flexion of the neck. Neurologic signs include progressive sensory and motor signs beginning in the upper extremities with associated autonomic dysfunction. Neck-manipulation in these patients is dangerous, and tomography is generally necessary to confirm the diagnosis.

C_7-T_1 metastasis. Pain originating from metastatic disease to the C_7-T_1 vertebral bodies is usually localized to the adjacent paraspinal area and characterized by a constant, dull, aching pain radiating bilaterally to both shoulders. There may be tenderness to percussion over the spinous process at this level. With nerve-root compression, radicular pain in the C_7-C_8-T_1 distribution occurs most commonly unilaterally in the posterior arm, elbow, and ulnar aspect of the hand. The neurologic symptoms include paresthesias and numbness in the 4th and 5th fingers, with progressive hand weakness and triceps weakness. The presence of a Horner's syndrome suggests paravertebral sympathetic involvement. Metastatic bone disease at this level results from either hematogenous spread to bone or, more commonly, from tumor originating in the brachial plexus or paravertebral space and spreading along the nerves to the contiguous vertebral body and epidural space.

Diagnostic workup. Plain X-rays of the cervical and thoracic spine do not provide adequate visualization of the C_7-T_1 area because of overlapping cardiac and bony structures. Coned-down views, tomography, or CT scan, in that order, may be necessary to define the presence of metastatic disease. In patients with bilateral radicular symptoms or signs of spinal-cord dysfunction, myelography should be performed to rule out an associated epidural spinal-cord compression.

Lumbar

L_1 metastases. Dull, aching mid-back pain exacerbated by lying or sitting and relieved by standing is the usual presenting complaint. Radicular pain in a girdle-like manner anteriorly or to both paraspinal lumbosacral areas may also be present. Occasionally patients will have only pain referred to the sacroiliac joint and/or the superior iliac crest. Lack of knowledge of these referred points for L_1 disease leads to inappropriate X-rays of the sacroiliac joint and iliac crest, without visualization of the L_1 area.

Diagnostic workup. AP, lateral, and oblique views of the lumbar spine, bone scan, and tomography, in order, should be the diagnostic approach. Myelography may be necessary to define the presence of epidural disease.

Sacral metastases. Aching pain, beginning insidiously, in the low back or coccygeal region, exacerbated by lying or sitting and relieved by walking is the common clinical complaint. Increasing pain, with the neurologic signs and symptoms of perianal sensory loss, bowel and bladder dysfunction, and impotence help to localize the site of disease.

Diagnostic workup. Plain X-rays of the sacrum are usually inadequate. AP and lateral tomography of the sacrum and the CT scan are the most useful diagnostic procedures in evaluating metastatic disease in this region. A barium enema and IVP can also be helpful to define the presence of presacral tumors.

Differential Diagnosis

Degenerative disc disease, osteoporosis, and epidural spinal-cord compression are the common differential diagnoses to consider in patients with cancer and complaints of neck or back pain from metastatic bony disease.

Degenerative disc disease rarely occurs at the C_7, T_1 or L_1 areas, and this fact should suggest a need for further workup of pain complaints involving these areas. Osteoporosis can often mimic the signs and symptoms of metastatic bone disease. Radiographic differentiation of these two entities can also be difficult, particularly in the case of vertebral-body collapse. Bone scans are positive in both metastatic and osteoporotic vertebral-body collapse. Tomography and CT scanning have been more useful in delineating the nature of the collapse. Tomography in osteoporotic vertebral-body disease reveals intact vertebral-body bony plates and symmetrical bony collapse, in contrast to metastatic disease where the vertebral plates are eroded with associated pedicle destruction and asymmetric collapse of the vertebral body.

Epidural spinal-cord compression is associated with vertebral-body metastases in 85% of patients (5), and a careful neurologic history and examination can help to establish evidence of spinal-cord dysfunction. If there are signs of neurologic dysfunction, myelography should be performed to delineate the extent of epidural disease and to define the appropriate radiation portals.

Tumor Infiltration of Peripheral Nerve, Plexus, Root or Cord

Peripheral Nerve

Constant, burning pain with hypesthesia and dysesthesia in the area of sensory loss is the usual clinical presentation. Tumor compression of peripheral nerve proximally occurs most commonly in association with paravertebral or retroperitoneal tumor. The pain is radicular and unilateral, and a careful sensory examination can often delineate the site of nerve compression. Metastatic tumor in rib often produces intercostal nerve involvement. In this entity, pain is the earliest symptom, with progressive sensory loss distal to the site of nerve compression.

Brachial Plexus

Radicular pain in the shoulder and arm is the earliest presenting symptom. This syndrome, often referred to as the superior pulmonary sulcus or pancoast syndrome, results from tumor infiltration of the lower brachial plexus. It is characterized by pain radiating to the ipsilateral shoulder, posterior aspect of the arm and elbow, in a C_8-T_1 distribution. The neurologic symptoms of pain and paresthesias in the fourth and fifth fingers may precede objective clinical signs for several weeks to months. These paresthesias progress to numbness and weakness in a C_7, C_8, T_1 distribution. The supraclavicular and axillary regions may be normal. The presence of a Horner's syndrome suggests involvement of the sympathetic chain in the paravertebral space.

Diagnostic Workup

This should include a chest X-ray with apical lordotic views, coned-down views of the C_7-T_1 area, and a bone scan. In certain instances, tomography and CT scan are more sensitive to delineate a mass in this region. It is not uncommon for tumor to spread along the nerve root into the epidural space and, if epidural extension is suspected, myelography may be necessary to define the extent of tumor infiltration. This information is particularly useful in defining the ports for radiation therapy. Needle biopsy or surgical exploration may be necessary to ascertain a tissue diagnosis.

The differential diagnoses include brachial neuritis, rotator-cuff tear at the shoulder joint, cervical-disc disease, and radiation fibrosis. They are the common pain syndromes which are often misdiagnosed in patients who have brachial plexus tumor infiltration. Each of these syndromes has characteristic neurologic signs and symptoms and has been previously well described (1,13–15).

Lumbar Plexus Tumor Infiltration

This entity occurs most commonly in patients with genitourinary, gynecologic, and colonic cancers from local tumor extension into adjacent lymph nodes and bone. The pain varies with the site of plexus involvement and is generally of two types: radicular pain in an $L_{1,2,3}$ distribution to the anterior thigh and groin, or down the posterior aspect of the leg to the heel in an L_5-S_1 distribution. Referred pain without local pain may also occur and presents a more difficult diagnostic problem. L_1 pain has been discussed previously. Pain in the anterior thigh, lateral aspect of the calf or heel, and associated palpable local tenderness are often misinterpreted as suggesting local pathology. X-rays and bone scan of these tender areas are often taken without clear awareness that these pains represent referred pain from lumbar plexus tumor infiltration. The neurologic symptoms include paresthesias followed by numbness and dysesthesias, with progressive motor and sensory loss in a plexus distribution. The presence of asymmetric or absent reflexes on neurologic examination often suggests root involvement. The absence of palpable tumor in the pelvis or groin does not preclude the diagnosis.

Diagnostic Workup

Since nerves are not radio-dense, X-rays in general are often unhelpful in discerning tumor infiltration in nerve plexuses, and one must rely on changes in contiguous bony or soft-tissue structures to suggest tumor infiltration. Tomography and CT scanning are more appropriate to define soft-tissue masses or bony abnormalities in the lumbosacral and pelvic regions. Specific studies like lymphangiography and certain radionuclide scans (gallium scan in patients with Hodgkin's disease) may give the necessary added information to suggest the presence of tumor in adjacent lymph tissue. At times, all of these radiographic studies may be negative, and to ascertain the diagnosis, surgical exploration and biopsy may be necessary. As previously noted, tumor infiltration of the epidural space may occur from infiltration along contiguous nerve roots. Myelography may be required to rule out the extension of tumor from lumbar plexus into the epidural lumbar space, to allow for appropriate radiation ports to be established, and for adequate treatment to be given.

The differential diagnosis includes most commonly lumbar neuritis, postsurgical lumbar plexopathy, radiation fibrosis, and lumbar-disc disease. Each of these entities has a characteristic neurologic presentation and should be differentiated from tumor infiltration of the lumbar plexus.

Sacral Plexus Tumor Infiltration

Dull, aching midline pain with sensory loss beginning in the perianal area is the usual clinical presentation. This entity occurs more commonly in patients with colonic, genitourinary or gynecologic cancers. The sensory findings are initially unilateral, with progression to bilateral sacral sensory loss and autonomic dysfunction including impotence and bowel and bladder dysfunction.

Diagnostic Workup

Sacral tomography in the anterior-posterior plane and CT scan are the procedures of choice in evaluating this area. Neither procedure can delineate sacral nerves except to define pre- or postsacral masses and bony destruction in proximity to the sacral nerves. Surgical exploration or needle biopsy may be necessary to establish a tissue diagnosis.

The differential diagnosis includes posttraumatic neuromas in patients with previous local surgery, localized infection, radiation fibrosis, and a series of syndromes characterized as the tension myalgias of the pelvic floor.

Meningeal Carcinomatosis

This is a clinical entity in which there is tumor infiltration of the cerebrospinal leptomeninges with or without concomitant invasion of the parenchyma of the nervous system (10). Pain occurs in 40% of patients and is generally of two types: (a) headache with or without neck stiffness characterized by a constant pain; and (b) back pain most commonly localized to the low back and buttock regions. Pain results from traction on tumor infiltrated nerves and meninges.

Diagnostic Workup

Lumbar puncture is the procedure of choice to detect malignant cells in the cerebrospinal fluid (CSF) of such patients. An elevated CSF protein and low glucose concentration are often associated findings. In patients with low-back and buttock pain, myelography can be helpful to delineate tumor nodules along the nerves in the cauda equina.

The differential diagnosis varies with the site of neurologic involvement. However, in patients with known cancer, signs and symptoms of neurologic dysfunction at several levels of the neuraxis should suggest this possible diagnosis. Alternate considerations may include fungal meningitis, cauda-equina epidural tumor, and arachnoiditis.

Epidural Spinal-Cord Compression

Severe neck and back pain is the hallmark of this entity. Gilbert et al. (5) reviewed 130 patients with epidural spinal-cord compression and found that pain was the initial symptom in 96% of patients, and in 10% was the only symptom of this entity. The pain occurs from local bone or root compression and is generally of two types: (a) local pain occurring over the involved vertebral body; or (b) radicular pain occurring unilaterally in patients with cervical or lumbosacral compression, and bilaterally in patients with thoracic cord compression. The neurologic symptoms vary with the site of epidural disease and commonly include motor weakness progressing to paraplegia, a sensory level, and loss of bowel and bladder function. Eighty-five percent of patients in Gilbert's series had associated vertebral-body tumor.

Diagnostic Workup

Plain X-rays of the spine do not delineate the integrity of the epidural space, and lumbar and cisternal myelography are necessary diagnostic procedures to delineate the extent of the epidural block. It is imperative to define the full extent of epidural tumor to provide the appropriate treatment. Epidural tumor often extends beyond the level of associated vertebral-body metastasis and may be independent of bone disease, and these observations have supported the need for myelographic definition of the problem.

PAIN SYNDROMES ASSOCIATED WITH CANCER THERAPY

This category includes those clinical pain syndromes which occur in the course of, or subsequent to, treatment of cancer patients with the common modalities of surgery, chemotherapy, or radiation therapy. The onset of pain to the cancer patient who fears recurrent tumor and to the physician unfamiliar with the clinical presentation of these nonmalignant syndromes portends a serious clinical problem.

Postsurgery Pain

Postthoracotomy Pain

Pain in the distribution of an intercostal nerve following surgical injury or interruption occurs in a small percentage of patients undergoing thoracotomy. The incidence of this entity is unknown. Pain becomes evident 1 to 2 months following the surgical procedure and is characterized by a constant pain in the area of sensory loss with occasional intermittent shock-like pains. Dysesthesias in the scar area, with hypesthesia in the surrounding zone, are often prominent symptoms. Movement exacerbates the pain, and these patients may develop a concomitant frozen shoulder characterized by limitation of movement at the shoulder joint and disuse atrophy of the arm. Early recognition of this syndrome and its sequelae can often prevent the development of further shoulder limitation.

Diagnostic Workup

The diagnostic workup should include a careful history to delineate the onset of the pain as well as the appropriate radiographic views, including plain X-rays, tomography, or CT scan, to rule out recurrent disease. Disuse atrophy of the humerus has a characteristic appearance on plain X-rays which should not be confused with metastatic disease, although the bone scan is positive in this entity as well. We have observed several instances in which, because of the clinical symptoms of pain and limitation at the shoulder joint, the X-ray findings of the humerus were interpreted as metastatic disease and patients were radiated for disuse atrophy of the arm without evidence of metastatic disease.

Differential diagnosis includes tumor infiltration of the peripheral nerve, rib, chest wall or paravertebral space. Awareness of the postthoracotomy pain syndrome and a careful history are essential to early diagnosis.

Postmastectomy Pain

Pain in the posterior arm, axilla, and anterior chest wall in patients following radical mastectomy occurs from interruption of the intercostobrachial nerve, a cutaneous branch of T_1 nerves. The onset of pain is usually 1 to 2 months following the surgical procedure and is more common in patients with a complicated postoperative course of either excessive local swelling or infection. The pain is characterized as a tight, constricting, burning pain in the posterior arm and axilla which radiates across the anterior chest wall. There is usually no associated lymphedema of the arm. The pain is exacerbated by arm movement, and patients often posture the arm in a flexed position close to the chest wall. As occurs in postthoracotomy pain, a frozen shoulder may develop, producing a second problem of increased pain and limitation of movement at the shoulder joint.

Diagnostic Workup

The diagnostic workup should include a careful history to delineate the onset of the pain as well as the appropriate radiographic workup of plain X-rays, tomography, or CT scan to rule out recurrent disease.

The differential diagnosis includes tumor infiltration of the brachial plexus, but the clinical history should make the diagnosis.

Postradical Neck Dissection Pain

Pain following radical neck dissection occurs from surgical injury or interruption of the cervical nerves. The pain is characterized by a constant burning sensation in the area of sensory loss. Dysesthesias and intermittent shock-like pain may also be present.

Diagnostic Workup

This should include a careful history of the onset of pain and appropriate X-rays of the painful area to rule out recurrent disease. Recurrent tumor involving the cervical spine or base of the skull is the major differential diagnosis.

Phantom-limb Pain

Pain following surgical amputation of a limb is generally of two types: stump pain and phantom-limb pain. These painful clinical entities are separate from phantom-limb sensation, which occurs in all patients following limb amputation. The true incidence of phantom-limb pain in patients following amputation for cancer is unknown. The phantom-limb pain is usually characterized by a burning, cramping pain in the phantom limb, often identical in nature and location to preoperative pain. The underlying mechanisms of such pain are controversial (2).

Diagnostic Workup

This should include a careful definition of the phantom-limb pain, and etiological factors such as local stump pathology.

Postchemotherapy Pain

The group includes a series of pain problems which occur in cancer patients receiving chemotherapy. The major features of each of these entities is briefly described below.

Peripheral Neuropathy

Painful dysesthesias following treatment with the *Vinca* alkaloid drugs occur as part of a symmetrical polyneuropathy (11). Both vincristine and vinblastine are neurotoxic drugs in the doses required to achieve an antineoplastic effect. The dysesthesias are commonly localized to the hands and feet, and are characterized by burning pain exacerbated by superficial stimuli. In children, a more diffuse syndrome occurs from the use of these drugs. It is characterized by generalized myalgias and arthralgias, often beginning with jaw pain and progressing to a symmetrical polyneuropathy including cranial-nerve dysfunction.

Steroid Pseudo-rheumatism

This entity occurs from both rapid and slow withdrawal of steroid medications in patients taking these drugs for either short or long periods of time (12). The syndrome consists of prominent diffuse myalgias and arthralgias, with muscle and joint tenderness on palpation but without objective inflammatory signs. A sense of generalized malaise and fatigue is a common feature of this entity. These signs and symptoms revert with reinstitution of the steroid medication.

Aseptic Necrosis of Bone

Both aseptic necrosis of the humoral and, much more commonly, the femoral head are known complications of cancer therapy, specifically chronic steroid therapy (6). Pain in the shoulder or knee and leg are the common presenting complaints, with X-ray changes occurring several weeks to months after the onset of pain. Limitation of joint movements, with progressive inability to use the arm or hip functionally, is the natural history of this illness. It occurs most commonly in patients with Hodgkin's disease, although it can occur in any patient on chronic steroid therapy. The bone scan is the most useful diagnostic procedure and is usually positive before changes in the plain films appear.

Post-herpetic Neuralgia

This is a well-described clinical entity (9) characterized by pain which persists after the cutaneous eruptions from herpes zoster infection have cleared. In patients with cancer, herpes zoster infection commonly occurs in the area of tumor pathology or in the port of previous radiation therapy. The true incidence of post-herpetic neuralgia in patients with cancer is unknown, but it appears to be more common in patients who develop the infection after the age of 50. There are generally three types of pain: (a) a continuous, burning pain in the area of sensory loss, (b) painful dysesthesias, and (c) intermittent, shock-like pain.

Postradiation Therapy Pain

Radiation Fibrosis of the Brachial Plexus

Pain occurring in the distribution of the brachial plexus following radiation therapy (RT) occurs from fibrosis of the surrounding connective tissue and secondary injury to nerve (13,14). It may appear as early as 6 months or as late as 20 years following radiation treatments. It represents a difficult diagnostic problem in that it must be differentiated from recurrent tumor. The clinical symptoms include complaints of numbness or paresthesias in the hand, usually in a $C_{5\text{-}6}$ distribution. Pain occurs later in the course of this clinical entity and is often characterized as diffuse arm pain. Lymphedema in the arm and radiation skin changes and induration of the supraclavicular and axillary areas are often present. The neurologic signs include sensory changes in a $C_{5,6,7}$ distribution, with motor weakness most prominent in the deltoid and biceps muscles. These signs progress to the development of a painful, useless, swollen extremity. In contrast, tumor infiltration of the brachial plexus presents with pain as its earliest symptom, with sensory changes in a C_8-T_1 distribution and motor weakness beginning distally rather than proximally. The associated signs with radiation injury include evidence on X-ray of radiation injury to the lung, rib, or humerus. These findings may help to confirm a history of radiation injury in the absence of appropriate radiation data.

Radiation Fibrosis of Lumbar Plexus

Pain occurring in the leg from radiation fibrosis of the lumbar plexus represents a similar diagnostic problem of radiation injury versus recurrent tumor. Pain occurring late in the course of progressive motor and sensory changes in the leg is more common with radiation fibrosis but is not the most reliable clinical symptom. A previous history of radiation treatment and local skin changes or lymphedema of the leg with X-ray changes demonstrating radiation necrosis of bone may help to establish this diagnosis.

The diagnostic workup to differentiate nerve fibrosis from nerve infiltration by tumor should include plain X-rays of the area to delineate radiation changes in bone or evidence of recurrent metastatic disease. The CT scan has not been helpful in this differential diagnosis except to define an enlarging soft-tissue mass, representing tumor in the area in question or recurrent bony erosion. In certain instances, surgical exploration may be necessary, particularly in patients free of known metastatic disease, to determine further cancer management.

Radiation Myelopathy

Pain is an early symptom in 15% of patients with this entity (7). The pain may be localized to the area of spinal-cord damage or may be referred pain, with dysesthesias below the level of injury. Clinically, the neurologic symptoms and signs are that of a Brown-Sequard syndrome (ipsilateral motor paresis with contralateral sensory loss with a cervical or thoracic level) which progresses to a complete transverse myelopathy. The diagnostic workup should include careful plain X-rays of the spine and myelography, both of which are usually normal. Occasionally widening of the cord at the injured area may be noted. The differential diagnoses include intramedullary tumor, epidural spinal-cord compression, arteriovenous malformation, or a transverse myelitis.

Radiation-induced Peripheral-nerve Tumors

A painful, enlarging mass in an area of pervious irradiation suggests this entity. We have reported a series of 9 radiation-induced nerve tumors (7 malignant and 2 atypical schwannomas) occurring 4 to 20 years following RT (3). Seven of the 9 patients presented with pain and a progressive neurologic deficit, with a palpable mass involving the brachial or lumbar plexus. Surgical exploration and biopsy is necessary to establish this diagnosis. The important differential diagnoses include radiation fibrosis and recurrent tumor.

PAIN UNRELATED TO CANCER OR CANCER THERAPY

Approximately 3% of the pain syndromes which occur in cancer patients have no relationship to the underlying cancer or cancer therapy. Degenerative disc disease, thoracic and abdominal aneurysms, and diffuse osteoporosis are the most common noncancer pain syndromes observed. This category serves to emphasize the point that pain in a cancer patient does not necessarily imply recurrent or persistent disease, and it supports the thesis that a careful diagnostic evaluation in the cancer patient is necessary to define the specific pain syndrome before embarking on a therapeutic course.

REFERENCES

1. Cailliet, R. (1966): *Shoulder Pain.* F. A. Davis, Philadelphia.
2. Carlen, P. L., Wall, P. D., Nadvorna, H., and Steinbach, T. (1978): Phantom limbs and related phenomena in recent traumatic amputations. *Neurology,* 28:211–217.
3. Foley, K. M., Woodruff, J. M., Ellis, F., and Posner, J. B. (1975): Radiation-induced malignant and atypical schwannomas. *Neurology,* 25:354.
4. Foley, K. M., Roger, A., and Houde, R. W. (1978): Pain in patients with cancer: A quantitative reappraisal. *Proc. Am. Soc. Cancer Res.,* 19:357.
5. Gilbert, R. W., Kim, J-H., and Posner, J. B. (1978): Epidural spinal cord compression from metastatic tumor: diagnosis and treatment. *Ann. Neurol.,* 3:40–51.
6. Ihde, D. C., and DeVita, V. T. (1975): Osteonecrosis of the femoral head in patients with lymphoma treated with intermittent combination chemotherapy (including corticosteroids). *Cancer,* 36:1585–1588.
7. Jellinger, K., and Sturm, K. W. (1971); Delayed radiation myelopathy in man. *J. Neurol. Sci.,* 14:389–408.
8. Lipman, A. (1975): Drug therapy in terminally ill patients. *Am. J. Hosp. Pharm.,* 32:270–276.
9. Noordenbos, W. (1959): *Pain,* pp. 68–89. Elsevier, Amsterdam.
10. Olson, M. E., Chernik, N. L., and Posner, J. B. (1974): Infiltration of the leptomeninges by systemic cancer: A clinical and pathological study. *Arch. Neurol.,* 30:122–137.
11. Rosenthal, S., and Kaufman, S. (1974): Vincristine neurotoxicity. *Ann. Int. Med.,* 80:733–737.
12. Rotstein, J., and Good, R. A. (1957): Steroid pseudorheumatism. *Arch. Int. Med.,* 99:545–555.
13. Stoll, B. A., and Andrews, J. T. (1966): Radiation-induced peripheral neuropathy. *Br. Med. J.,* 1:834–837.
14. Thomas, T. E., and Colby, M. Y. (1972): Radiation-induced or metastatic brachial plexopathy: A diagnostic dilemma. *JAMA,* 222:1392–1395.
15. Tsairis, P., Dyck, P. J., and Mulder, D. M. (1972): The natural history of brachial neuropathy. *Arch. Neurol.,* 27:109–117.

Advances in Pain Research and Therapy, Vol. 2,
edited by J. J. Bonica and V. Ventafridda.
Raven Press, New York © 1979.

The Role of Cerebral Cortex in the Pain of Advanced Cancer

C. V. Morpurgo

Istituto Ortopedico G. Pini, Piazza Card. Ferrari 1, 20122 Milan, Italy

Pain has an important biologic function in the organism's defense against external and internal noxious events. However, when cancer is the noxious agent, pain often fails to signal the onset of the disease in time for successful therapy. On the contrary, it usually becomes intense and extremely difficult to treat in the advanced stages of cancer.

What role does the cerebral cortex play in such a situation? Our experimental and clinical observations suggest the following hypotheses: a) body areas with a small cortical representation have late onset of pain when cancer occurs; b) constant pain can induce an increase in the cortical representation of the affected area.

Moreover we have noticed that if the patient has had previous significant pain experiences in proximity of the body area affected by cancer, there is a high incidence of "incorrect" referred pain. In these particular cases the perception of the correct site of the noxious stimuli produced by the cancer will occur very late.

Recent neurophysiologic and psychophysiologic data have called attention to the structural changes taking place in the central nervous system (CNS) when the subject must cope with unusual situations (2,4,9). When repetitive unusual experiences occur during the period of growth, irreversible changes in the cortex can take place (10). The relative permanence of changes due to early experiences during initial developmental periods is well known to behavioral scientists. Recent findings indicate that this phenomenon also influences perceptual functions, including pain (7,11).

At birth only small parts of the cortex are committed to specific tasks. The rest will be shaped by experience. If part of this experience is repetitive and is related to the endeavours of the subject to adjust to the environment or to fight it, an increasing number of neurons become specified for that particular task so that the organism is able to accomplish it skillfully (5).

Some groups of neurons maintain functional flexibility; others are so highly specific that they can perform only a single task. After months or years these neurons, excited by nonspecific stimuli, will produce the perception of the specific stimulus that caused the changes in the brain.

The term *plasticity* is used by neurophysiologists to define the permanent modifications occurring in the functional units of the brain when excited by repetitive experiences relevant for the subject. Plasticity probably implies the strengthening of some synapses and the weakening of others in order to develop mechanisms that permit skillful performance of complex functions of the cortex (memory, recognition, decision, learning). We consider perception related to these high functions.

The plastic changes, when well consolidated, will become "unerasable" or irreversible.

Plasticity means flexibility to become specific. This can occur in relationship to unusual experiences: In this case plasticity will involve uncommitted units as well as neurons which in the normal individual are specified for a different task.

When specified by a long-lasting experience in the early stages of life (6,13) at which time plasticity is marked, the functions of a unit cannot be easily changed. However, in the adult, different experiences, even though stronger, will be ineffective because the flexibility of the system is markedly reduced.

Kittens exposed to repetitive noxious stimuli in a body part with small cortical representation have shown a dramatic change of the contralateral cortical representation as compared with the unaffected, opposite side (8). As pain experience continued, larger and larger areas of the cortex became involved and a higher number of neurons became specific to pain.

A second evaluation, after several months without any pain stimuli, revealed persistent alterations in the cortical map, as recorded at the end of the training. These data suggest that at the brain level the pain experiences produce complex mechanisms of perception, involving a large number of neurons and causing an abnormal sensitivity to noxious stimuli.

These changes in cortical projection seem to be supported by concomitant changes of the anatomic aspect of the posterior sigmoidal gyrus observed in the experimental animals.

A corresponding increase in the firing of pain neurons has been recorded by Albe-Fessard (1) in the thalamus in rats experiencing chronic pain due to unilateral deafferentation of the spinal cord from C5 to T2. Moreover, it has been demonstrated very recently that pain itself enhances the plasticity of the CNS. Unpublished findings by Spinelli (12) demonstrate that the training time necessary to alter the function of neurons in visual cortex in kittens can be dramatically reduced to $\frac{1}{30}$ by associating pain with visual stimulation. These observations suggest that the cortical representation of different parts of the body can be modified by the experience of the subject. In the same way the cortical projection of a region chronically affected by pain would be predicted to increase according to the intensity and duration of the noxious stimuli.

This means that a strong, long-lasting pain can produce dramatic, irreversible changes in the perceptual processes and induce an increase in the cortical representation of the affected areas. This will lead the patient to perceive pain differently than a naive patient who has not suffered persistent pain.

Meanwhile the affective and perceptual state of hypersensitivity produced by pain will render unbearable every sensation. So the patient will tend to isolate in a state of sensory deprivation in which pain alone influences the activity of the cerebral cortex. The start of a vicious circle (pain increases the perceptual mechanism → increased perception enhances the sensibility to pain, and so on) must be suspected when a patient tends to isolate himself and focuses all of his attention on pain. At this point, pain is no longer a useful warning signal, but becomes aggressive, unbearable, and difficult to handle. If the circle is not interrupted, pain will become intractable and predominant over all the other symptoms, aggravating the physical and psychic condition of the patient.

This is the end result when the problem of pain is not properly considered and treated promptly.

In order to compare the experimental data with clinical observations, we have reviewed all the patients admitted to the Centro Oncologico of the Istituto Ortopedico G. Pini of Milano. The total number is small because the activity of the section started only two years ago, but it is evident that cancer affecting parts of the body having a larger cortical representation will cause intense pain more frequently than cancer of the viscera with little or no cortical representation.

In agreement with the data presented at this meeting by Dr. Foley (3), 9 (60%) out of our 15 patients with cancer of the femur were resistant to simple treatment with analgesic and required combined therapy for pain relief. It was also noted that cancer and metastases affecting parts of the body well represented on the somatosensory cortex caused severe pain, whereas tumors of the viscera were often painless or produced very little pain. In 3 patients with a long history of pain, the visceral cancer gave rise to "incorrect" referred pain.

Of our group of patients, 50% were hospitalized with major pain problems and only 2 patients had no pain. Pain was severe in 22 of 40 patients who had somatic localizations of the cancer and in only 1 of 15 who had visceral lesions.

It will be important to study a larger number of patients to ascertain: (a) whether more intense pain occurs with lesions in parts with large cortical representation compared with lesions involving parts with small somatosensory cortical representation; (b) whether an earlier experience of pain plays any role in determining the characteristics of a subsequent cancer pain. (In one of our patients a long history of lumbar pain made it very difficult to discover a pancreatic cancer because of an incorrect referred pain, until the outset of the signs of metastatic compression of the right ileo-inguinal nerve).

In future investigations of the role of the cortex in cancer pain we should consider that: (a) Chronic pain can produce changes in the cerebral cortex affecting the mechanism of pain perception; (b) perception of chronic pain arising in the various parts of the body will vary depending on the extent of their cortical projection as predetermined by the genome and determined by repetitive pain experiences; (c) in a cancer patient without any interest in life, chronic pain should be promptly controlled to avoid its natural tendency to become intractable.

CONCLUSIONS

Clinical observations in agreement with experimental neurophysiologic and psychophysiologic data suggest that the cerebral cortex plays an important role in determining the modality of pain perception in patients with advanced cancer.

REFERENCES

1. Albe-Fessard, D. (1978): Personal communication.
2. Dunn, A. J. (1976): Biochemical correlates of training experiences: A discussion of the evidence. In: *Neural Mechanisms of Learning and Memory,* edited by M. R. Rosenzweig, and E. L. Bennett, pp. 311–320. The MIT Press, Cambridge, Mass., and London.
3. Foley, K. (1979): Pain syndromes in patients with cancer. In: *Advances in Pain Research and Therapy, Vol. 2,* edited by J. J. Bonica and V. Ventafridda. Raven Press, New York.
4. Hirsch, H. V. B., and Spinelli, D. N. (1970): Visual experience modifies distribution of horizontally and vertically oriented receptive fields in cats. *Science,* 168:869–871.
5. Hirsch, H. V. B., and Spinelli, D. N. (1971): Modification of the distribution of receptive fields orientation during development. *Exp. Brain Res.,* 13:509–527.
6. Hubel, D. H., and Wiesel, T. N. (1970): The period of susceptibility to the physiological effects of unilateral eye closure in kittens. *J. Physiol.* (*Lond.*), 206: 419–436.
7. Morpurgo, C. V., and Spinelli, D. N. (1976): Plasticity of pain perception. *Brain Theory Newsletter,* 2:14–15.
8. Morpurgo, C. V., and Spinelli, D. N. (1978): Unpublished data.
9. Pettigrew, J. D., Olsen, C., and Barlow, H. B. (1973): Visual experience without lines: Effect on developing cortical neurons. *Science,* 182:599–601.
10. Spinelli, D. N., Hirsh, H. V. B., Phelps, R. W., and Metzler, J. (1972): Visual experience as a determinant of the response characteristics of cortical receptive fields in cats. *Exp. Brain Res.,* 15:289–304.
11. Spinelli, D. N., Metzler, J., and Phelps, R. W. (1975): Neural correlates of visual experience in single units of cat's visual and somatosensory cortex. *Neurosci. Abstracts, Soc. for Neurosci., 5th Annual Meeting.*
12. Spinelli, D. N. (1978): Personal communication.
13. Wiesel, T. N., and Hubel, D. H. (1965): Extent of recovery from the effects of visual deprivation in kittens. *J. Neurophysiol.,* 28:1060–1072.

Advances in Pain Research and Therapy, Vol. 2,
edited by J. J. Bonica and V. Ventafridda.
Raven Press, New York © 1979.

Psychologic and Emotional Aspects of Cancer Pain

M. R. Bond

Department of Psychological Medicine, Southern General Hospital, Glasgow. G51 4TF

"Cancers are diseases and pain is a symptom." It is important to keep this statement in mind when discussing emotional aspects of painful malignant disease, because the development of a particular form of it, knowledge of its presence, and its significance to the sufferer produce changes in feelings and behaviour which are altered further by the presence of pain. Moreover, the state of emotion produced by the disease influences the severity of the pain and any changes in the former are reflected in the latter. The way in which an individual responds to illness, and in particular to one of the chronic and possibly painful and potentially fatal cancer group, is determined by his or her premorbid emotional characteristics, experiences of previous illness, and attitudes towards illness amongst members of the family and the cultural group to which he or she belongs.

It has been estimated that cancer is responsible for 20% of all deaths in the United States and other Western countries (22), including Britain. Approximately half the 30,000 who die from cancer each year in Britain have pain, of whom about a quarter experience severe pain at times. The pain is usually chronic but fluctuates in severity, being influenced by many factors, some physical and some psychologic, and it is the latter that are of particular interest and importance and yet so often neglected by those who care for the patient. This is surprising, for as Hanay (9) has pointed out, cancer is one of the most researched disease entities, and moreover it is one viewed with the greatest fear by the general public, one that affects many lives and families and one that is very expensive to Society.

EMOTIONS AND CANCER

The Role of Personality in the Development of Cancer

A considerable amount of time and energy has been devoted to examining the possibility that certain personality attributes predispose towards the development of cancer, a concept which, if it were correct and sufficiently specific, would have important implications for the prevention and treatment of this group of diseases.

Rassidakis and others (22) are of the opinion that certain premorbid personality characteristics are associated with the development of cancer and that these include early childhood conflicts and a sense of isolation through life, inability to express hostile feelings and difficulties in interpersonal relationships, and loss of a close relationship which produces depression and despair. In support of their view they quote Engel (7) who earlier reported that where circumstances in life lead to feelings of hopelessness, an organic illness may ensue. It is certainly true to say that in a situation of this kind, as after a bereavement, the incidence of all forms of ill-health amongst widows during the first year after their husband's death is significantly greater than in nonwidowed women of similar age.

The illness may be mental rather than physical for it has been shown by Brown et al. (5) that a depressive illness may occur where an individual develops feelings of helplessness and lowered self-esteem secondary to the loss of loved ones or important sources of value in life. Perris and Pierce (19) were critical in their analysis of the literature and stated that early attempts to find a "cancer type" rarely made it possible to distinguish among psychologic characteristics which might be causative factors, those which might be typical reactions to any serious disease, and those which showed purely accidental variations.

In a review dealing with possible psychologic precipitants of cancer, Surawicz (26) noted that early searchings for a "specific causogenic personality" were not fruitful insofar as many of the claims initially made have not been substantiated. However, it is accepted that individuals who adapt poorly to psychologic and physical stresses may develop one of several physical diseases, including cancer, and that prior to their onset, anxiety or the state of hopelessness and helplessness predominates.

Hanay (9) commented on another aspect of this issue and pointed out that life events of a stressful kind also determine the extent to which each person attends to his or her body and the nature of an individual's behavior when ill, that is, the way he or she perceives, evaluates, and acts upon messages and sensations of the body. In other words he noted that "illness behavior," the term first used by Mechanic (16), differs from person to person once an illness has been established.

Thus it seems that perhaps the individual who develops the cancer may well do so after a period of emotional stress which produces feelings of helplessness and hopelessness. The same emotional combination also produces depression—a state of mind which reflects capitulation and resignation and which is associated with increased levels of pain when present and a reduced ability to cope with it.

The General Emotional Effects of Cancer

Studies of the emotional characteristics of patients who have cancer reveal several interesting facts. First, those general to all patients with malignant disease; second, those specific to patients who also have pain. Chronic illness, whatever its form, is viewed with foreboding by most individuals, and cancer in particular is associated in the minds of many with pain, destruction, loss and often with death. Individuals are concerned not only about the eventual outcome of their illness but also with the possibility of further suffering, especially severe pain, before their lives end. Thus the disease brings with it a sense of helplessness, a feeling of total inability to control events, and a futility too, making life seem meaningless and bringing difficulties in tolerating pain which itself seems to have no biologic purpose and which is often referred to as "useless pain."

Specific anxieties arise and include fear of separation from the family and friends, loss of work, loss of life's goals, and the consequences of illness for others. Patients fear increasing dependency, loss of their faculties, and mutilation by surgery. In the case of carcinoma of the breast, a form of malignant disease of which members of the public are very aware and afraid and which is associated with severe pain at times in its later stages, Maguire (15) has shown that psychiatric morbidity begins as soon as the afflicted woman notices a breast lump. Amongst patients he studied 52% were moderately to severely anxious at this stage, and only 8% claimed they were free from all anxiety. A quotation from one of his patients crystallizes the reaction of women to the discovery that they have a breast tumour:

> I don't know whether it's me or not, but the feeling is just indescribable. Unless you've experienced it you just don't know. . . . I was so frightened. All I could think of was the children. If anything is going to happen to me they're so young, that's what I latched on to. . . . My feelings were indescribable. I think I touched absolute hell, I didn't want to die and I didn't know if I'd got cancer. It's the thing everyone dreads. At first you think it can't be happening to you. Then, by God— it is.

He also commented that patients have to live with the knowledge that they have a disease which is potentially fatal and deal with fears that it may recur after treatment and invade other areas of the body causing pain and other very unpleasant symptoms. They must also deal with the side effects or consequences of treatments themselves, which include mutilation, the production of anesthesia, baldness, failure of bladder function, and major disturbances of other kinds.

EMOTIONS AND CANCER PAIN

The General Emotional Effects of Chronic Pain

The presence of chronic pain whether arising from benign or malignant diseases causes individuals to become withdrawn, introspective, and neurotically depressed. Many exhibit hostility and anger, which is an important emotion, for as Pilowsky and Spence (21) have shown, those who suppress anger tend to have more affective disturbance than those who experience and express it. Pain also causes increased preoccupation with other physical symptoms; in other words it leads to hypochondriasis. Examination of the effects of chronic pain on personality as measured by the Eysenck Personality Inventory or the Minnesota Multiphasic Personality Inventory reveals that it causes an increase in levels of neuroticism (2,11,14,23) and that the level of neuroticism falls when pain is relieved (11,24).

As a consequence of debility and lessened mobility there is less contact with friends and a reduction in social activities. The pattern of coping behavior adopted by any given person varies depending upon his or her premorbid personality characteristics; for example, some become dependent upon their family and friends to an unnecessary extent, whereas others attempt to do more than is compatible with their physical and emotional state.

Emotional Changes in Patients with Cancer Pain

The difficulties imposed by the exhausting and stressful nature of painful malignant disease deter many from working with patients with this form of ill-health, and as a result there are relatively few papers dealing with the psychologic characteristics of cancer patients with pain. However available studies show that, as in the case of patients with chronic pain due to benign disorders, most sufferers from painful cancer have raised levels of neuroticism. However, Kissen and Eysenck (12) and Bond and Pearson (4) have reported that men with lung cancer and women with cancer of the cervix, respectively, who were pain-free, had extremely low levels of emotionality. Both groups argued this is due to operation of the mental mechanism of denial brought about by exposure of the patient to the intolerable stresses imposed by the illness they suffer. Further, Bond (3) notes that this is not a permanent change, for he has observed that low levels of neuroticism in some cancer patients with intractable pain rise after the pain is relieved by percutaneous cervical cordotomy. The scores of patients with high levels of neuroticism fell after operation, leaving an overall impression that personality factors are distorted by the presence of severe illness and pain and that in the case of the latter, some restoration in the direction of normality of personality is achieved if it is relieved.

Woodforde and Fielding (28) examined cancer patients with and without pain using the Cornell Medical Index and demonstrated that the former group were significantly more emotionally disturbed than the latter and that they responded least well to treatment of their cancer and died sooner. The main cause of emotional morbidity was found to be depression, although hypochondriasis and psychosomatic symptoms were also recorded. They were uncertain whether the depression was a primary or secondary event but commented that the combination of intractable pain and depression represents symptoms that indicate a state of helplessness, of inability to cope with the disease, damage to the body, and the threat to life, and that, as was stated earlier, this is a response to having a progressive and potentially fatal illness. The implication of these observations is that if each individual's confidence and self-esteem can be restored by the provision of appropriate and alternative goals, the level of suffering may be reduced. This has been reported by Goldfarb et al. (8) and Blumberg et al. (1), although their findings were not conclusive.

Regarding hypochondriasis, it is a state of mind in which there is absorption with physical and mental symptoms. Kenyon (10) suggests that the word *hypochondriasis* implies that "hypochondriacal traits, symptoms, ideas and fears should carry with them the implication that there is morbid preoccupation with mental and bodily functions or state of health." Pilowsky (20) takes the view that, in broad terms, hypochondriasis is a specific set of attitudes towards health and showed that cancer patients have higher levels of hypochondriasis than healthy people and nonhypochondriacal psychiatric patients. Raised levels of hypochondriasis in cancer patients with pain were recorded by Bond (2) in patients who also had high levels of neuroticism as measured by the Eysenck Personality Inventory. He also showed that the lowest levels of hypochondriasis were found in pain-free cancer patients who exhibited low levels of emotionality. Looked at in another way, the degree of pain and neuroticism irrespective of its form correlate highly—the more neurotic the patient, the greater is his or her pain. This relationship is well known and is fundamental to the psychologic and pharmacologic methods of pain-relief based upon reduction of emotional tension.

The Consequences of Physical Treatment upon Emotion in Cancer Patients

Physical treatments available for patients with painful malignant diseases include drugs of various kinds and in particular analgesics, surgery, radiation therapy, and the use of cytotoxic drugs. Each form of treatment has its hazards, and these are increased where multiple therapies are in use. It is not possible to comment in detail on all forms of therapy, and indeed there are relatively few papers in the literature dealing with the emotional consequences of the treatment of cancer and even fewer dealing with the specific emotional and social needs of patients receiving treatment and those who have had treatment (15).

Considering surgery, it is undoubtedly true that if successful in relieving pain and other symptoms this form of treatment lessens patients' emotional tensions and reactions to their disease. However it is often not appreciated that a considerable number of patients have persistent emotional symptoms, and unfortunately these may go unheeded. For example, Lee and Maguire (13) reported that after surgery for breast cancer as many as one-third of the patients had significant levels of anxiety and that marital problems and sexual difficulties actually increased in the year after operation. They also showed that the husbands of the women they studied exhibited an increased level of emotional disturbance matching that of their partner. Devlin et al. (6) made similar comments about patients undergoing surgery for anorectal cancer, noting the adverse emotional and social effects of colostomy. Thus it has been estimated that at least 1 in 4 patients who have had a mastectomy or surgery for rectal cancer develop depressive illness, anxiety neurosis, sexual problems, or marital difficulties.

In the case of radiation treatment, Peck and Boland (18) found that among 50 patients, 60% of whom had been told they had cancer, all arrived unprepared for their treatment and as a consequence they believed that radiation treatment was "bad news," that it was potentially dangerous and damaging and could actually cause cancer, and seldom believed that it would produce a cure. After treatment only a third felt it had improved their health; and whereas 60% had evidence of depression and anxiety beforehand, this increased to 80% immediately after treatment.

The Consequences of Staff-Patient Interactions upon Emotion and Pain

These observations lead naturally to a consideration of what individual patients feel about those who are responsible for treating them in terms of dealing with their anxieties and fantasies about the illness and treatment to be given. Mitchell and Glicksman (17) interviewed 50 patients and found that 52% of them were inadequately prepared for radiation therapy and that the patients did not believe that the referring doctor or technician who gave the treatment were people with whom they could discuss their worries and fears. Maguire (15) reports similar attitudes amongst women with breast cancer and comments from two of his patients summarize the feelings of many. One said, "I felt I had no right to burden them (the medical and nursing staff) with my worries. . . . I just put a face on it," and the other, "They didn't seem interested in what I really felt." It appears that only 5% of patients in this series were asked about their emotions after surgery, and it seemed that surgeons were unwilling to explore their patients' emotions and often failed to appreciate their depth if they were aware of any distress.

Careful studies of interactions between staff and patients on wards for cancer patients reveals that treatment transactions involving analgesics for pain are subject to the influence of culturally determined attitudes of both patients and staff to illness behavior. Indeed, the classic studies of Zborowski (29) supported by the work of Sternbach and Turskey (25) and Turskey and Sternbach (27) lead to the conclusion that the factor governing the behavior of individuals in pain seems to be the level of approval given by society for the public expression of emotions. British attitudes are reflected in recent work by Bond (3) on two groups of patients in Scottish hospitals. He found that irrespective of the source of their pain, all patients believed they should bear it as long as possible. Moreover, in another study it was found that patients' complaints of pain and requests for analgesics were not necessarily taken at their face value by nurses who, despite the evidence that potent drugs were required, tended to give ones of low potency without any attempt to provide emotional support either. On the other hand, independent decisions by nursing staff to give drugs often seemed to lead to the administration of powerful analgesics, indicating that they felt their judgment of patients' needs were more appropriate to the level of pain. It is not surprising therefore that they failed on many occasions to realize that the patients' complaints of pain have a more general purpose in that they signaled distress not only about physical discomfort, but emotional and social problems too.

To conclude, the emotions aroused by the presence of cancer are many and varied, and all are exacerbated by the presence of pain. This is well recognised, although not on the whole handled well by doctors and nurses other than those in special centers where specific training programs exist. Even less recognition and attention is paid to the persisting emotional difficulties of cancer patients, with and without pain, who have had treatment and who have emerged from hospital to live in the outside world. This is a matter which deserves close attention in the future.

REFERENCES

1. Blumberg, E. T., West, P. M., and Ellis, F. W. (1954): A possible relationship between psychological factors and human cancer. *Psychosom. Med.,* 16:277–290.
2. Bond, M. R. (1971): The relation of pain to the Eysenck Personality Inventory, Cornell Medical Index and Whiteley Index of Hypochondriasis. *Br. J. Psychiatry,* 119:671,678.
3. Bond, M. R. (1978): Unpublished data.
4. Bond, M. R., and Pearson, I. B. (1969): Psychological aspects of pain in women with advanced carcinoma of the cervix. *J. Psychosom. Res.,* 13:13–19.
5. Brown, G. W., Harris, T., and Copeland, J. R. (1977): Depression and loss. *Br. J. Psychiatry,* 130:118.
6. Devlin, H. B., Plant, J. A., and Griffin, M. (1971): Aftermath of surgery for rectal cancer. *Br. Med. J.,* 3:413–418.
7. Engel, G. L. (1962): *Psychological Development in Health and Disease.* Saunders, Philadelphia.
8. Goldfarb, C., Driesen, J., and Cole, D. (1967): Psychophysiologic aspects of malignancy. *Am. J. Psychiatry,* 123:1545–1552.
9. Hanay, C. H. (1971): Illness behaviour and psychosocial correlates of cancer. *Soc. Sci. Med.,* 11:223–228.
10. Kenyon, F. E. (1976): Hypochondriacal states. *Br. J. Psychiatry,* 129:55–60.
11. Kissen, D. M. (1964): The influence of some environmental factors on personality inventory scores in psychosomatic research. *J. Psychosom. Res.,* 8:145–149.
12. Kissen, D. M., and Eysenck, H. J. (1962): Personality in male lung cancer patients. *J. Psychosom. Res.,* 6:123.
13. Lee, E. G., and Maguire, P. (1975): Proceedings: Emotional distress in patients attending a breast clinic. *Br. J. Surg.,* 62:162.
14. Lovell, R. R. H., and Verghese, A. (1967): Personality traits associated with different chest pains after myocardial infarction. *Br. Med. J.,* 2:327–330.
15. Maguire, P. (1976): The psychological and social sequelae of mastectomy. In: *Modern Perspectives in the Psychiatric Aspects of Surgery,* edited by J. G. Howells, pp. 390–422. Brunner/Mazel, New York.

16. Mechanic, D. (1977): Illness behaviour, social adaptation, and the management of illness. *J. Nerv. Ment. Dis.,* 165:79–87.
17. Mitchell, G. W., and Glicksman, H. S. (1977): Cancer patients: Knowledge and attitudes. *Cancer,* 40:61–66.
18. Peck, A., and Boland, J. (1977): Emotional reactions to radiation treatment. *Cancer,* 40:180–184.
19. Perris, G. M., and Pierre, I. R. (1959): Psychosomatic aspects of cancer. *Psychosom. Med.,* 21:397–401.
20. Pilowsky, I. (1967): Dimensions of hypochondriasis. *Br. J. Psychiat.,* 113:89–93.
21. Pilowsky, I., and Spence, N. D. (1976): Pain, anger and illness behaviour. *J. Psychosom. Res.,* 20:411–416.
22. Rassidakis, N. C., Evotocritou, A., and Volidou, M. (1976): The psychopathology of cancer. In: *Modern Perspectives in the Psychiatric Aspects of Surgery,* edited by J. G. Howells, pp. 48–60. Brunner/Mazel, New York.
23. Sternbach, R. H. (1974): *Pain Patients, Traits and Treatments,* p. 17. Academic Press, New York.
24. Sternbach, R. H., and Timmermans, G. (1975): Personality changes associated with reduction of pain. *Pain,* 1:177–181.
25. Sternbach, R. H., and Turskey, B. (1965): Ethnic differences among housewives in psychophysical and skin potential responses to electric shock. *Psychophysiol.,* 1:241–246.
26. Surawicz, F. G., Brightwell, D. R., Weitzel, W. D., and Othner, E. (1976): Cancer, emotions and mental illness: The present state of understanding. *Am. J. Psychiatry,* 133:1306–1309.
27. Turskey, B., and Sternbach, R. H. (1967): Further physiological correlates of ethnic differences in responses to shock. *Psychophysiol.,* 4:67–74.
28. Woodforde, J. M., and Fielding, J. R. (1975): Pain and cancer. In: *Pain: Clinical and Experimental Perspectives,* edited by M. Weisenburg, pp. 332–336. The C. V. Mosby Co., St. Louis.
29. Zaborowski, M. (1952): Cultural components in responses to pain. *J. Soc. Issues,* 8:16–30.

Advances in Pain Research and Therapy, Vol. 2,
edited by J. J. Bonica and V. Ventafridda.
Raven Press, New York © 1979.

Pain in Children with Cancer

J. Gerald Beales

Department of Rheumatology, University of Manchester, Manchester, England

INTRODUCTION

The increasing attention which has, in recent years, been paid to cancer pain and its treatment has focused almost exclusively upon adult patients. Pain in children with cancer has attracted comparatively little interest. In the pediatric oncology literature, references to pain are surprisingly infrequent, and when pain is mentioned it is usually in terms of its implications for diagnosis rather than as a symptom demanding treatment in its own right. Pain on presentation is generally better described in the literature than pain in the later stages of childhood malignant disease.

To some extent, this relative neglect of the subject of pain in child cancer patients simply reflects the lack of study devoted to pain in children as a whole. In part, it may also be a result of a general belief that pain is less of a problem among children with cancer than it is among adults. For many children, cancer is, indeed, substantially painless. But, for many others, pain is an important and distressing feature of their disease. The excruciating intractable pain which afflicts a significant proportion of adult cancer patients does seem to be rare in children, but the pain of children with cancer is nonetheless often quite severe. Furthermore, it could be argued that, if a child has cancer, even relatively mild pain is serious and demands relief.

A child who must die has the right to do so with the absolute minimum of suffering. But even where the prognosis is less gloomy, the relief of pain is equally necessary. Improvements in cancer therapy are now creating a growing pool of children who will survive into adult life, and it is therefore important to ensure that the normal psychologic development of these children is disrupted as little as possible by the disease or the treatment. Continual pain can have emotional consequences which seriously interfere with such development, as well as reduce the child's willingness to cooperate with therapy. The minimization of pain is therefore an important requirement in any chronic childhood disease.

Pain is a complex phenomenon. It is the final product of several processes and is consequently capable of being acted upon at a number of levels and by numerous means. Anticancer radiotherapy or chemotherapy may remove pain by acting directly on the pathology from which pain-producing signals originate. Analgesics, or neurosurgery, can be used to interfere with the transmission of those signals to the brain. But the experience of pain is also influenced by processes which operate within the brain—by psychologic mechanisms—and the manipulation of these mechanisms is a potentially valuable means of reducing or avoiding pain. This is true not only of that pain which is considered to have psychologic origins, and is labeled "psychogenic," but also of pain which arises from a detectable physical insult produced by disease itself or the treatment of disease. There are reasons, which will be discussed later, for suggesting that some psychologic mechanisms involved in the perception of pain may be manipulated much more easily in children than in adults. Yet, this particular approach to the treatment of pain in children with cancer has seen very little systematic use. The aim here will therefore be to consider some of the precise psychologic factors likely to be involved in the pain experienced by children with malignant disease, and to suggest means by which these factors might be acted upon in order to avoid or relieve pain.

THE ROLE OF PSYCHOLOGIC INTERVENTION

The manipulation of psychologic mechanisms has a place in the treatment of all three basic types of pain encountered in child cancer patients. These are: pain which is directly attributable to malignant disease; pain produced by anticancer therapy; and pain which appears to have its immediate origin in the emotional rather than the physical state of the child.

Pain produced by tumor may be relieved for a time at least by direct action upon the malignancy. Bone pain, associated with skeletal destruction occurring in the primary bone tumors and histiocytosis X, and commonly in leukemia and neuroblastoma, often responds well to local radiotherapy. Headache caused by the raised intracranial pressure of brain tumor may disappear with the reduction of that pressure by surgical or chemotherapeutic means. In cases of intraspinal malignancy, pain resulting from compression of a nerve root may be relieved by surgical decompression.

Analgesics are required in order to relieve pain until specific anticancer therapy is able to exert its effect, where no such therapy is available, or where advancing disease no longer responds to therapy. In the later stages of childhood cancer, pain may become increasingly severe, and it may be necessary to resort to the more potent drugs (8). The value of psychologic intervention is likely to be in complementing the role of the analgesics.

Where a clear organic cause of pain is discernible, it is easy to assume that the pain is entirely and directly determined by the physical pathology. Yet the extent of physical pathology by no means always correlates with the severity of pain experienced. This appears to be particularly true of bone pain associated with skeletal destruction. Some children with extensive bone lesions deny pain altogether. Others, with several lesions, report pain from only one site. Toddlers with lower-limb involvement often present with a limp which is apparently unaccompanied by pain. But, in other cases, pain is reported before any lesion becomes radiologically detectable (7,9).

These variations may be the result of cerebrocortical mechanisms inhibiting pain-producing signals in some cases and augmenting them in others. There is convincing evidence that psychologic processes are capable of alleviating or blocking pain despite extensive injury (3). Such processes would also seem capable of producing pain from weak signals emanating from minimal tissue damage. Where pain is directly attributable to malignancy, the contribution of psychologic intervention may therefore be to reduce cerebrocortical augmentation of pain-producing signals and to encourage inhibition.

When a child who has previously suffered well-defined and well-localized pain begins to complain of vague, generalized pain in the absence of demonstrable organic pathology, the new pain is likely to be labeled "psychogenic." A common assumption is that pain of this kind is entirely a product of psychologic factors and has no organic origin. But it is possible that so-called "psychogenic" pain is the result of cerebrocortical augmentation of signals arising from damage so slight as to be undetectable by radiologic or other clinical means. It has been suggested (8) that if a new pain is abolished by tranquilizers alone, it is unlikely to indicate a metastatic lesion. But if tranquilizers exert their effect on pain by reducing psychologic augmentation of weak signals, this cannot be assumed. The origin of the signals may be innocent—the result of normal bodily wear and tear—but it may not. In the case of a child with cancer, the distinction between "organic" and "psychogenic" pain may be an inappropriate and a misleading one.

Psychologic augmentation of pain-producing signals, from whatever source, may be influenced by the use of drugs. But it may be acted upon more precisely through normal sensory channels: by talking to the child, in particular. Words can have a powerful effect, but they are capable of exerting their effect in either direction. They may reduce cerebrocortical augmentation of signals, or they may increase it. In fact, much of what is said to the child with cancer, by doctors, nurses, parents, or fellow patients, may unintentionally make his pain worse. What is said to the child often makes it likely that he will experience signals produced by minimal tissue damage as painful, or that he will suffer unnecessary pain as a result of therapeutic procedures.

Much of anticancer therapy is potentially painful. Vincristine frequently produces pain in the abdomen, jaw, or limbs (6,14). Bone-marrow aspiration, lumbar puncture, and venipuncture are regularly inflicted upon many children. In some centers, those procedures which are potentially most painful are conducted only under a general anesthetic, but this practice is by no means universal. Mennie (12) has complained that the measures taken to relieve pain during episodes of therapy are frequently inadequate or nonexistent. But the withholding of drugs is not the only means by which pain may be caused unnecessarily. As will be explained later, if one follows recommendations in the literature about what the child should be told prior to potentially painful therapy, the likelihood of his experiencing significant pain will probably be increased.

Because of the manner in which psychologic mechanisms involved in pain may be influenced, it is hardly possible for those concerned with the child to avoid acting upon them. It is not only the words which are said that may exert an effect: What is not said can also have an impact upon psychologic modulation of pain-producing signals. It has to be ensured, therefore, that the influence which is exerted is in the direction of avoiding or reducing pain, rather than increasing it.

PSYCHOLOGIC MECHANISMS THAT MAY MODULATE PAIN

Pain comprises a combination of sensation and negative affect (11). It occurs when physical insult gives rise to sensation and that sensation is experienced as unpleasant. If sensation is not unpleasant, there is no pain. Sensation and negative affect involve different areas of the brain and can be modulated independently. Pain may be relieved or avoided by inhibiting sensation or by reducing the extent to which sensation is experienced as unpleasant.

Removing or reducing the unpleasantness of a sensation may be accomplished to some degree by surgery or drugs, but it may be achieved with a greater degree of success and precision by purely psychologic means.

Studies of visual perception in man have indicated that the direction and degree of affect which become linked to particular sensation depend on the meaning which the object giving rise to that sensation has for the individual. If the object has pleasant associations for the individual, then simply seeing the object comes to be experienced as pleasant. Although different sensory modalities have their own specialized receptors and nerve pathways, it seems likely that they are influenced by similar psychologic processes. There is evidence to suggest that the pain experienced by patients with physical pathology depends to some extent on the meaning which that pathology has for them (10). If a certain injury becomes associated with actual attainment of some important goal, the sensation resulting from the injury may itself evoke no feeling of unpleasantness (3). Where, as is more usual, the pathology has unpleasant associations for the individual, the degree of negative affect linked with the sensation—and therefore the degree of pain—may be related to the extent of those unpleasant associations.

For example, in a study of children with juvenile chronic arthritis, it was found that older children associated their disease with considerably more frustration of their goals than did younger children (1). They also indicated more severe joint pain than did younger children. When the sensation and negative-affect components of pain were measured separately, the older children reported only slightly more sensation from their joints, but considerably more negative affect. Some of the younger children denied pain altogether: They claimed that the sensation which they experienced from their diseased joints was not at all unpleasant (2).

The unpleasantness of a sensation may therefore be partly dependent upon the extent to which the pathology it indicates has undesirable consequences for the child. But it may also depend upon whether or not the sensation is recognized as indicating pathology in the first place. A child has to learn that sensations of a particular kind indicate that there is something wrong with his body. Clearly, it is easier for him to link a sensation with physical damage if that damage is immediately visible—if it occurs at the body surface. Because it is much more obvious to them, younger children are primarily concerned with, and most disturbed by, insult to their body surface. They have little or no concept of their internal makeup, and little idea of what the implications may be if it goes wrong. Consequently, in younger children, cerebrocortical augmentation of the negative-affect component of pain is more likely to occur if the responsible injury is cutaneous than if it is internal. The older the child, and the greater the awareness of the possible sinister meaning of an internally originating sensation, the less this difference in the effect of psychological mechanisms upon negative affect might be expected to be.

The sensation component of pain is particularly influenced by the mechanisms of attention and distraction (10). If the individual's attention is focused upon certain signals, he will detect them more quickly, and at lower strengths than he would otherwise do. He might experience sensation from signals so weak that under normal circumstances they would not have impinged upon consciousness. Conversely, distraction of attention has the effect of raising the signal strength necessary to produce conscious sensation. Although many factors may influence the individual's state of attention or distraction at any particular time, there is likely to be an age difference here too. Younger children will be on the look-out for pain-producing signals if placed in a situation in which they anticipate damage to their body surface. Older children who have, or fear, internal pathology, may focus their attention on signals having an internal origin.

PSYCHOLOGIC INTERVENTION IN CHILD CANCER PAIN

In respect of *pain directly attributable to malignancy,* the principal aim of psychologic intervention should be to act on the meaning which the disease has for the child. It may be possible to reduce the negative-affect component of pain by reducing the unpleasant consequences associated with the disease. The younger the child, the easier such modification of meaning is likely to be.

There is a tendency to assume that cancer has only one real meaning for the child: death. And therefore it may be difficult to appreciate how the disease can be made less of a disaster for the patient. But studies have shown that young children either have little awareness of death or do not recognize its full implications (4,13). They may deplore their disease simply because it interferes with play and cuts them off from their friends. If they fear death at all, they may do so because they fear separation from the love and protection of parents.

It is important not to assume that children must inevitably share the reactions of adults to a potentially fatal disease. It should not be taken for granted that, if a child is dying, nothing else is of importance to him. All who are concerned with the treatment of the child with cancer should be fully aware of the child's own point of view and of the things which matter to him personally. Ensuring that there is minimal disruption of the child's play activities, that he is not separated prematurely from parents and friends, and that he is allowed to lead as normal a life as possible for as long as possible may go a considerable way to reducing the negative meaning which the disease has for him.

The older the child, the closer the concept of death approaches to that held by the adult, and the greater its importance may seem. But even where the implications of death are recognized, apparently trivial things may still be of importance to the patient, and interference with them may be a source of additional distress. With the older child, therefore, it is equally necessary to know how the patient himself views his cancer and to be aware of all the unpleasant associations which it has for him. It may well be possible to remove some of those associations quite easily: for example, by making it possible for the child to continue some favorite activity, or by paying particular attention to the protection of his self-esteem.

Death, however, is no longer the inevitable prognosis for all child cancer patients. Therefore, even in the case of the older child, it will not necessarily figure prominently in the patient's appraisal of his condition. Children who are not primarily concerned with death will react to their cancer in the same way as children with any chronic disease. Modifying the meaning of chronic disease to the patient is generally easier with children than with adults. The adult's interests, ambitions, and way of life are well established. Those of children are undergoing change, and because of their flexibility, they may be adapted to compensate for the restrictions on activities imposed by the disease. Younger children can be encouraged to develop alternative play interests; older children can be guided toward a career which is not incompatible with their physical condition.

Making it possible for a child with cancer to lead as normal a life as possible for as long as possible might also have specific impact on the sensory component of pain through the mechanism of distraction. If the child's attention is directed toward play or schooling, for example, he is less likely to become preoccupied with his disease and to focus upon his symptoms. Because of their greater appreciation of what is happening inside them, older children are particularly likely to be on the look-out for any signals indicating the spread of their cancer, and comparatively weak signals resulting from minimal tissue damage may therefore give rise to pain. If *pain unrelated to malignancy* or any other significant organic pathology does develop, it might perhaps be relieved by amending the child's interpretation of it. He may cease to concentrate his attention upon the pain if he is reassured that it has no sinister significance. Some pain of this kind might be avoided by reminding older children with cancer that their bodies are subject to the same normal wear and tear as those of other children, and that every internally originating signal does not indicate malignancy.

It was suggested earlier that much of the *pain caused by anticancer therapy* is avoidable: Painful treatment is often performed without adequate analgesia. Perhaps the reason for this is that medical personnel concerned with therapy are not always aware of the amount of pain which they are inflicting on their young patients. It is by no means easy to assess pain accurately in young children, whose ability to express their pain verbally may be limited or nonexistent. Crying may be attributed to fear rather than pain. Furthermore, it may be assumed that prolonged exposure to pain leads to a greater tolerance of it, so that a child who has had, for example, extensive skeletal lesions for some time may be thought to be inured to pain and unlikely to be distressed by anything inflicted on him in the course of treatment. This assumption, in fact, seems to be quite widespread, although, as Green (5) has pointed out, there is no evidence to support it.

It is particularly easy to underestimate pain caused by therapeutic procedures in children who fail to complain of pain despite extensive malignancy. It might understandably be concluded that if a child does not have pain despite considerable skeletal destruction or a large abdominal mass, he must have an exceedingly high "pain threshold," and therefore will be safe from pain as a result of venipuncture, or lumbar puncture, or having his dressings changed. But it is wrong to assume that a child has a single pain threshold which applies in all situations, for all types of physical insult. Because young children are more concerned about the body surface than what lies beneath it, they may be far more distressed by even a mild insult to the skin than by considerable subcutaneous pathology which is out of sight and consequently out of mind. Therefore, they may experience more pain from it. Because of the meaning which surface damage has for them—because they find it so unpleasant—the unpleasantness of the resultant sensation may be augmented.

Unnecessary pain may also be caused by focusing the child's attention on pain-producing signals during treatment episodes. It is now widely recommended in the pediatric oncology literature that, prior to painful therapy, the child should be informed that pain will be inflicted, in order to ensure that he continues to trust those responsible for his care. But the expectation of pain has the effect of allowing weaker signals to be experienced as conscious sensation, and pain may thereby be actually increased. However, the best of both worlds may perhaps be obtained by warning the child reasonably well in advance of possible pain, but attempting distraction during the treatment episode.

Pain resulting from therapy can often be reduced or even avoided altogether by the use of distraction. But when distraction is attempted during a potentially painful procedure, it is usually in an impromptu and unorganized way, with a junior nurse frequently taking the initiative. If it were used more systematically, with adequate preparation being made to ensure that the child's attention could be engaged in some pleasant activity at the time when pain might be caused, the child might be spared a great deal of suffering. Distraction is undoubtedly easier to achieve in children than in adult patients. Young children in particular will probably accept a game or story as perfectly valid in this situation and allow themselves to become absorbed in it. Adults tend to regard therapy as being so serious a matter that they may consider any attempt to draw their attention away from it as improper.

Of course, it is not always necessary to inform a child that pain might be caused by therapy for him to anticipate pain. The mere suspicion that something unpleasant is about to happen to him may encourage him to create a fantasy in which the level of damage inflicted on him far exceeds reality. The best way of avoiding such fantasies is to give the child as much accurate information about his treatment as he is capable of assimilating, given his age and level of intelligence. It should not be assumed that if a young patient does not ask for information, he does not want to know what will be done to him. It may be his fear which prevents him from asking.

The presence of a parent during treatment episodes may help to reduce the child's fear. But parents are not always encouraged to stay. Some clinicians claim that if a parent is present the child is inclined to exaggerate pain and is generally more difficult to handle. It is undoubtedly true that some parents can lead their child to feel pain, simply by demonstrating, with gasps and appropriate facial expressions, that they are already suffering on his behalf. But if parents are told of what will happen during therapy and warned not to communicate their own anxieties to the child, they can do much to ease his suffering.

The treatment of pain in children with cancer by the manipulation of psychologic mechanisms is not just a job for the doctor. *Everyone concerned with the care of the child has a contribution to make.* Parents are of importance, not simply for the reassurance they can provide during episodes of treatment, but also because they can play a considerable part in minimizing the unpleasant associations which the disease has for their child. During periods of remission, when the child is at home, they can do a great deal to distract the child's attention away from his disease and symptoms. However, parents cannot be expected to undertake this task successfully without guidance and support. Many will be naturally inclined to overprotect a seriously ill child, restricting his activities beyond those precluded by the cancer. Therefore, unless they are given proper help and advice, they may unintentionally increase the negative meaning which the disease has for the young patient, and so perhaps increase his pain through the augmentation of the negative-affect component. Unless warned of the specific dangers, they may pass on their own anxieties about the disease to their child and so make it more likely that his attention will be focused on signals which might indicate a worsening of his physical condition.

Ensuring that augmentation of pain by psychologic mechanisms is minimized, and that cerebrocortical inhibition of pain-producing signals is encouraged, is a full-time activity and a team responsibility. All social contact with the patient may have an influence, for good or ill, on the pain he experiences directly or indirectly as a result of his cancer. It is not enough simply to administer an analgesic to a child if, in the process of so doing, one says something to him which is likely to cause psychologic processes to exert their effect in the direction of increasing pain. Indeed, saying the right words in such a situation may sometimes be of greater value from the point of view of relieving pain than the actual drug administered.

Although it has been possible to suggest the likely identity of some of the psychologic mechanisms involved in the modulation of pain, and to indicate means by which those mechanisms could be manipulated, there is clearly a need for considerably more research in this area. The cerebral cortex has undoubted ability to increase, reduce, and abolish pain, but comparatively little effort has been made to understand, and thereby learn how to make use of, the means by which it can exert this control. Greater study here may produce results of real benefit to those who suffer pain—including children with cancer.

ACKNOWLEDGMENTS

I should like to express my gratitude to Drs. P. J. L. Holt, D. Pearson, and C. Bailey for their help during the preparation of this paper.

REFERENCES

1. Beales, J. G., Holt, P. J. L., Keen, J., and Mellor, V. (1979): Juvenile chronic arthritis: The child's perception of the disease. (*in preparation*)
2. Beales, J. G., Keen, J., and Holt, P. J. L. (1979): Juvenile chronic arthritis: Age and the experience of pain. (*in preparation*)
3. Beecher, H. K. (1959): *Measurement of Subjective Responses.* Oxford University Press, New York.
4. Burton, L. (1974): Tolerating the intolerable. In: *Care of the Child Facing Death,* edited by L. Burton. Routledge & Kegan Paul, London.
5. Green, M. (1967): Care of the dying child. *Pediatrics,* 40(3):492–498.
6. Heyn, R. M., Beatty, E. C., Jr., Hammond, D., Louis, J., Pierce, M., Mur-

phy, M. L., and Severo, N. (1966): Vincristine in the treatment of acute leukemia in children. *Pediatrics,* 38(5):82–91.

7. Jones, P. G., and Campbell, R. E., editors (1976): *Tumors of Infancy and Childhood.* Blackwell Scientific Publications, Ltd., Oxford.
8. Lane, D. M. (1973): Principles of total care—psychologic support. In: *Clinical Pediatric Oncology,* edited by W. W. Sutow, T. J. Vietti, and D. J. Fernback. The C. V. Mosby Co., St. Louis.
9. Marsden, H. B., and Steward, J. K., editors (1976): *Tumors in Children.* Springer Verlag, Berlin.
10. Melzack, R. (1973): *The Puzzle of Pain.* Penguin, New York.
11. Melzack, R., and Casey, K. L. (1968): Sensory, motivational, and central control determinants of pain: A new conceptual model. In: *The Skin Senses,* edited by D. Kenshalo. Charles C Thomas, Springfield, Ill.
12. Mennie, A. T. (1974): The child in pain. In: *Care of the Child Facing Death,* edited by L. Burton. Routledge & Kegan Paul, London.
13. Nagy, M. H. (1959): The child's view of death. In: *The Meaning of Death,* edited by H. Feifel. McGraw-Hill, New York.
14. Sutow, W. W., Berry, D. H., Haddy, T. B., Sullivan, M. P., Watkins, W. L., and Windmiller, J. (1966): Vincristine sulfate therapy in children with metastatic soft tissue sarcoma. *Pediatrics,* 38(1):465–472.

Advances in Pain Research and Therapy, Vol. 2,
edited by J. J. Bonica and V. Ventafridda.
Raven Press, New York © 1979.

Sociologic Effects of Cancer Pain

Margo McCaffery

Consultant in the Nursing Care of Patients with Pain, Santa Monica, California 90404

The sociologic perspective encompasses how the inner states of the individual affect his relationships and interactions with his social environment. People interact with many social environments, ranging from the family or significant others to the large, impersonal agencies and bureaucracies.

The problems the patient has with the community and large institutions are not my focus nor my area of knowledge. But problems exist in these areas and some are easily observed. As an example, the patient with cancer faces possible loss of his job and associated fringe benefits if the employer learns of the patient's diagnosis. This is illustrated by a woman with pain and suspected pancreatic or intestinal cancer who had been a top designer in the clothing industry for more than 30 years. She remained amazingly energetic and made every effort to hide her pain, but suspicions were aroused by her weight-loss. One afternoon she was fired without warning. Five people had to be hired to take the place of this one woman. Although her productivity would have decreased gradually, she could have been an asset to the company up until about 3 months prior to her death almost 2 years later.

Just as industry is learning that it is often less expensive to rehabilitate an alcoholic than to replace him, industry might also find some ways of benefiting from the skills of employees with cancer pain who may die and/or gradually reduce their working time. Certainly there is the need for education and exploration in this area.

My focus, however, is concerned with factors that may hamper the patient's relationships with significant others, especially his family and close friends. I have selected a few somewhat overlapping but seemingly significant factors:

1. differences between the patient's pain-related attitudes and behaviors and those expected of him by others,
2. role-change adjustments,
3. expressions of affects such as anger and depression, and
4. the fight between dependence and independence.

Anthropologic and sociologic studies have shown clearly that early in life people begin learning very specific and detailed cultural expectations regarding pain and that these expectations may differ greatly from one sociocultural group to another. These findings are clinically relevant, but not because they tell us how a person from a particular sociocultural group will respond to pain. Rather these studies reveal the myriad of attitudes and responses regarding pain that may be present to some extent in any person regardless of his cultural background. For example, Zborowski found that the Irishman was proud of being able to handle pain by himself and tended to go through a long period of struggling with his pain before he sought assistance from a physician (4). However, this response may be exhibited by a patient who does not possess an ounce of Irish blood. Further, his family and close friends, while seemingly members of the same sociocultural group, may have opposing views.

When significant others in the patient's environment do not share the patient's attitudes and beliefs about pain-related behavior, their interpersonal interactions may be severely damaged. People tend to view their learned responses to pain as correct and normal. Responses that are different from their own are often regarded as improper, abnormal, or wrong. Therefore, the family member or friend who differs from the patient regarding how to handle pain usually finds it quite difficult to be understanding, compassionate, or even tolerant of the patient's behaviors.

Arguments and social isolation are among the possible outcomes of differing pain-related beliefs. A previously described characteristic associated with the Irishman serves as an example. The spouse may believe that it is senseless to endure pain, especially when a disease such as cancer has been diagnosed, and that pain-relief should be sought immediately. The husband and wife may argue about these differences daily.

Consider the woman who cries easily about her pain and feels that this is a natural response that need not be suppressed. Friends who value minimal expression of pain may begin to avoid her for several reasons. For instance, they may want to spare her the embarrassment they believe she feels when she cries in their presence. On the other hand, if she feels that crying is childish and her efforts to control it are unsuccessful, she may fear that others will be disgusted or uncomfortable with her. Consequently she may impose her own social isolation.

The degree to which a person is expected to discuss and share his problems is also partially determined by cultural expectations. This is particularly significant for the patient with cancer pain, since discussion of death-related topics tends to be especially taboo.

One study showed that many patients with pain say they do not like to discuss their pain with others or are ambivalent about it. But usually the reason they give for this reticence is that they feel others are not interested in their pain. For example, one patient with metastatic cancer commented, "I don't feel anybody's really interested. . . . Oh, they're interested, but I mean, well not really. . . . They've got their problems too, probably, so I just feel, why burden them with mine." Patients with cancer pain seemed especially aware of the social stigma attached to complaining about pain. This study found that when patients do talk about their pain, the person they most frequently talk with is the spouse (1). When pain is of long duration and associated with cancer and death, the spouse obviously will have personal needs and at least occasionally will find it difficult to talk with the patient.

Role-change represents another area of disruption in interpersonal relationships. Illness and pain lasting only a few days will interfere with role-function. This problem is enormously increased when pain and illness are prolonged and lead to death.

Roles vary of course from person to person, but more importantly the patient's roles have varying significance to him and to those around him. Some roles are heavily invested emotionally, whereas other roles are of a more practical nature. For example, a man may find that cancer and pain prevent him from fulfilling his role as financial provider for himself and his family. This poses practical and serious economic problems for the entire family. But in addition to this, work may have been a very gratifying activity for the patient and a major contributor to a positive self-concept.

One study of patients with bone metastasis from breast cancer found that the necessary limitations on movement were extremely hard on women with young children. Mothering was a much more difficult role to relinquish than that of housekeeping (3).

When the patient is no longer able to function in a particular role, the activities associated with this role may have to be assumed by others. This may be depressing for the patient to witness, and it may impose a great hardship on those who must assume the patient's previous responsibilities. The husband who must now wash dishes and feed the children may become genuinely, although irrationally, resentful toward his ill wife.

Another factor that may hamper the patient's relationships with others is the effect of certain emotions associated with having cancer pain. A sociologist who was also in pain shared with me his experiences in this area. He felt that the anxiety, fear, depression, and other feelings elicited by pain tend to heighten the patient's interpretations of various situations. As a result the patient exacerbates and discolors minor events in social interactions. The patient is often angry and irritable and makes exaggerated responses to his environment. The other person involved in the interaction usually is not sophisticated enough to identify the part that pain plays in what the patient says or does. Hence, the response of the person with whom the patient interacts will tend to increase in intensity to match that of the patient. This often leads to a highly emotional climate. As the interaction continues, each person is responding with greater intensity and the process spirals upward.

He pointed out that in addition to the emotions associated with the illness and the pain, side effects from medications may further complicate interpersonal interactions. Among these side effects may be irritability, fatigue, drowsiness, confusion, weakness, and increased or decreased libido.

The previously discussed factors along with other factors contribute to the conflict between dependence and independence. Some patients struggle against depending upon others in meeting emotional and physical needs. Such patients may resent the assistance offered by others. Those who wish to help the patient may be hurt or baffled by the patient's response to their well-intentioned actions.

On the other hand, some patients are not threatened by certain degrees of dependence upon others. In this case the problem may be that the people upon whom the patient depends may find the situation too demanding. They may lack the time, interest, or energy to respond to the patient's dependency needs. The egocentricity that so often accompanies prolonged pain and illness may render the patient insensitive to these feelings (2). The balancing of the patient's needs for dependence and independence against the needs of others is clearly problematic regardless of which way the pendulum swings.

In summary, there are many factors related to cancer pain that may hamper the patient's relationships with others. There is no single solution to this. However, a simple but significant beginning might be to provide the patient and others close to him with counseling, perhaps by a nurse or social worker, for the purpose of identifying and discussing the basic dynamics of their interpersonal problems.

REFERENCES

1. Jacox, A., and Stewart, M. (1973): *Psychosocial Contingencies of the Pain Experience.* University of Iowa Press, Iowa City.
2. McCaffery, M.: *Nursing Management of the Patient with Pain,* 2nd ed. J. B. Lippincott, Philadelphia.
3. McCorkle, M. R. (1973): Coping with physical symptoms in metastatic breast cancer. *Am. J. Nurs.,* 73:1034–1038.
4. Zborowski, M. (1969): *People in Pain.* Jossey-Bass, Inc., San Francisco.

Advances in Pain Research and Therapy, Vol. 2,
edited by J. J. Bonica and V. Ventafridda.
Raven Press, New York © 1979.

Sociological and Nursing Aspects of Cancer Pain

Ada G. Rogers

Analgesic Studies Section, Sloan-Kettering Institute for Cancer Research, New York, New York 10021

Recorded history and anthropological discoveries have revealed that cancer has been prevalent in man and animals since the dawn of civilization. Until the 20th century, it was classified by many as an incurable disease. Even today, despite all the advances that have been made in its treatment, there are those including some health-care professionals who feel that cancer is an incurable disease, accompanied by intractable pain, ending only in death. We recognize that this is not true; not all cancer is incurable and in some cases, even when the disease is far advanced, pain may not be a problem. However, when one considers the history of cancer and its slow evolution, one can understand these attitudes.

Prehistoric man used rituals and superstitions as a weapon against cancer, and in some cultures this has prevailed up to the present time. Hippocrates the "Father of Medicine" recognized the disease, defined its grave prognosis, and named it *karkinos,* meaning "a crab." The name described the appearance of advanced breast cancer. The Latin word *carcinoma* is derived from the Greek *karkinos* (9). Although the Greeks had temple-hospitals where care was given primarily by priests, patients with cancer were removed to the seclusion of nearby woods, abandoned, and left to die. Conversely, the Romans did everything they could to effect a cure and the sick, even their slaves, were treated at home, nursed by the women of the household (10).

During the next 1,500 years, essentially the only advances made were in recognizing the different forms of cancer. Galen listed 61 types but included among them inflammation, swelling, and ulceration. In the 16th century, Giovanni Fillippo Ingrassia, Professor of Medicine and Anatomy at Naples and called the "Sicilian Hippocrates," extended the list to 287 varieties (9). The treatment and understanding of this "horrible" disease was still based on astrological charts, handwriting analysis, the use of strong odors, e.g., garlic and onions, "trapping the evil spirits," and "the evil eye." During this time, the care of the sick was under the auspice of religious groups, both Jews and Christians. This seemed appropriate, since disease and pain were thought of as punishment or atonement for sins. The monasteries had absolute control over their members, and their great purpose was the moral and spiritual discipline of the young and old, of the sick and well, of those who minister and those who were ministered to. Nursing was learned through practice and had special virtues. Because of the hard work and distasteful duties, it was considered to be an effective way for mortifying the flesh and developing humility, patience, and other Christian virtues. Some of these monasteries had a place for the shelter of travelers and these were called *hospices*. Religion continued its influence in the care of the sick.

The world's first cancer hospital was established at Rheims in France by Bishop Jean Godinet in the middle of the 18th century, but it was closed in 1778 because the public thought that cancer might be contagious. It was not until 1840 that French hospitals admitted cancer patients, but in separate blocks. In England at the end of the 18th century, a cancer ward was established at the Middlesex Hospital. However, little was done in the treatment of the cancer patient until 1851, when the first cancer hospital was founded. It was later called the Royal Cancer Hospital (4). In America, progress in the field of cancer was even slower.

Our first American institutions for care of the sick were a combination of municipal hospital, poorhouse, insane asylum, house of correction, and orphanage. Cancer patients were included among these. Bellevue Hospital in New York City was a classic example of this type of institution. The care-givers were prostitutes, drunks, and petty criminals. It took almost a hundred years to recognize that the care-giver should be trained and its trainees come from a better class. In 1873, one of the first nursing schools to use the Nightingale system was established at Bellevue. Since cancer had the stigma of venereal disease or some hereditary deficiency, the wealthy class were treated at home. They feared that if the presence of cancer were divulged, their families would be disgraced as well as their descendents.

The well-to-do class was responsible for establishing better hospitals, but unfortunately, they imposed their own ignorance and prejudices on the admission of cancer patients. In 1847, The New York Hospital admitted 1,022 patients with typhus fever, 177 with fractures, 280 with syphilis, but only 4 with cancer. If by accident, cancer patients were admitted, they were promptly discharged as "improper objects" or "disorderly" (4). A man who fought against the injustices to patients with cancer was Dr. James Marion Sims. Sims specialized in feminine ills, and he was responsible for the founding of the Women's Hospital in New York City. Sims and his colleagues, seeking a cure for uterine cancer, admitted women who were suffering from this disease into the hospital. The Lady Managers opposed this practice and for years there was constant opposition. Eventually, Sims gave up the fight and resigned his position; however, his dedication to this cause continued.

In a letter to his friend, John Parsons, who was John J. Astor's lawyer, he wrote: "A cancer hospital should be built on its own foundation wholly independent of all other hospitals. Its medical board ought to be men who go into it with zeal, determined not only to give temporary relief to human suffering, but to do something towards discovering better methods of treatment. It is time we turn a listening ear to the cries of humanity." The letter received widespread publicity in the New York newspapers and led to a meeting of a group who were a minority of the Board of Governors of the Women's Hospital who had sided with Sims. Out of this meeting came the basic plans and proposals for a cancer hospital. In 1884, the New York Cancer Hospital, the first hospital specializing in the treatment of cancer patients, was established in America. This should have ended public opposition, but it did not. The New York Cancer Hospital at West 105th Street and Central Park, was called by many "The Bastille."

In an attempt to lessen the stigma still attached to cancer, the name of the hospital was changed in 1888 to the General Memorial Hospital for the Treatment of Cancer and Allied Diseases. Owing to financial problems caused by insufficient public funds and the cost of cancer care, private surgical patients with benign disease had to be admitted. By 1913, only 10% of the cases handled involved cancer, and those patients were walled off from the others by a partition in two least-desirable wards away from the park, but a rebirth of Memorial was soon to come through the deep interest of Dr. James Douglas, who had lost a daughter to cancer, and the timeless devotion of Dr. James Ewing, who became President of the Medical Board. There were many changes over the next few years. In 1915, the word "General" was dropped from the name of the hospital. In 1917, with funds provided by Douglas, a new research laboratory was opened. In 1922, the X-ray extension was added; in 1923, a dental clinic was established; and in 1924, the outpatient extension was opened. In 1927, John D. Rockefeller, Jr. started making contributions of $60,000 a year for research and clinical development, and six clinical fellowships were established. Rockefeller's generosity did not stop there. He donated the site of the present Memorial Sloan-Kettering Cancer Center in 1936 (6).

The battle toward the conquest of cancer was on its way through treatment, research, and education. Nevertheless, the emotional impact on and reaction of every patient to this disease, and the effects on his family, friends, and even health-care professionals is still a problem that is not fully appreciated. In the last few decades, some efforts have been made to understand and cope with these problems. In 1969, Dr. Elizabeth Kübler-Ross (8) published a book entitled *On Death and Dying* in which she states that the patient goes through five emotional stages in the course of terminal disease: denial and isolation, anger, bargaining, depression, and acceptance. However, it is not uncommon to find that the patient may continue in one stage until the end, and this may also be true for his family, friends, and professional care-givers.

When pain is present it can emphasize the hopelessness of terminal disease, and inadequately controlled pain contributes to greater anxiety, fear, desperation, guilt, hostility, depression, and even attempted suicide. Old taboos still play a role: The religious beliefs that disease and pain are punishment for sins committed in this life or in another life, that we must suffer to attain a greater glory after death, and that cancer is contagious or hereditary and that we may be passing it on to our loved ones.

In addition to knowing one has cancer, the treatments may cause suffering. How often does the patient who has lost a part of his body have the opportunity to mourn openly for that loss and how well is he adjusting to disfigurement and/or changes in bodily functions? Some patients never verbalize their feeling of embarrassment, of being dirty and foul-smelling, uncomfortable, fearful, and socially unacceptable—they just go and hide and become anti-social and lonely.

To many Americans, the added financial burden of this illness is of considerable concern. The head of the household will worry about if and when he will be able to go back to work, and, indeed, whether or not his job will still be there when he is able to return. Financial problems are increased with multiple hospitalization, as his medical insurance may not cover the hospital and doctor bills. The housewife will be concerned about being able to care for her family and the home. One lovely lady was upset because she would not be able to cook for her husband; no one else had cooked for him for 30 years. She was afraid he would be angry with her and she would lose his love. Cooking for him is what she talked about, but there were many other things she could not do for him that she did not discuss. Sexual problems are seldom discussed, and yet, sexual activity is an important function that may be changed permanently. By and large, female patients will not discuss this aspect with male physicians and even many male patients may not. Wise (11) has stated that: "It has been observed that cancer patients with poor prognoses wish to have various forms of physical closeness with their spouses, if not direct genital intercourse." Consideration of these needs has been sadly neglected by the medical and nursing professions.

Nausea and vomiting, major changes in eating and sleeping habits, constipation, diarrhea, dehydration, weakness, metabolic, motor, or sensory changes may contribute to discomfort, fear, and anxiety. There are many other situations that the staff may be unaware of that may be causing distress: A patient with a language barrier who cannot communicate with the staff may feel that the staff is not concerned about him; changes in awareness of world and local events; changes in degrees of independent behavior and personal privacy; presence of unfamiliar machines and mechanical devices; inadequate explanations of treatments; unfamiliar or new staff members; presence of a severely ill or noisy roommate; and perhaps most important, hospital routines that are designed for the benefit of the staff and not the patient.

Patients need a feeling of friendliness around them and this is too often forgotten by the hospital staff. Staff-patient relations can be improved when patients feel free to call the staff by their first names. Some staff members object to this, believing that over-friendliness may result in a loss of objectivity. However, as one patient stated: "Good nursing and good doctoring is not destroyed because of first names. I like the intimacy—it makes me feel that the doctors and nurses care. After all, the hospital is another family and another life for me. I like to think that I am leaving a legacy of intimacy, that I am worth something here." Perhaps there would be better understanding of how the patient feels if we think of the patient as a member of our own family—mother, father, sister, brother, son, or daughter—and how we would want them to be treated. Most patients want to be known as "good patients," and many patients will not complain because they fear reprisal, particularly if a staff member has been abusive, hostile, and mean. Even patients who feel they are coping with the disease and treatment have confided that this is the one fear they have.

It was not too many years ago that the rehabilitation of cancer patients with or without advanced disease was thought of as foolish, ridiculous, and a waste of money. After all, these patients were going to die eventually, so why bother? Rehabilitation service in the United States before 1967 was only given if the patient was 18 months post-surgery, without evidence of metastases, and had full-time employment. This 18-month waiting period was exempt for part-time workers or housewives. Some funds were available from the vocational Rehabilitation Administration of the Department of Health, Education and Welfare. In 1972, accelerated federally supported programs were instituted for rehabilitation and counseling as part of an all-out attack against human cancer (7). Similar efforts were made in other countries.

Emphasis was placed on the team approach and the effort and supportive role of each member of the team. Change in attitude was directed toward the quality of life, hope, and the will to live. The services of psychiatrists, psychologists, social workers, dieticians, clergymen, physical therapists, occupational therapists, self-help groups, volunteers, and nurses all play an important role in these changes.

In the last two decades, nursing has had to take a new look at the care of patients with cancer to keep in step with the advances being made in the treatment of cancer. Today, schools and colleges of nursing have Cancer Nursing as part of their curricula. Cancer hospitals and cancer units have had to update their inservice education programs in order to ensure better patient care. The American Cancer Society has held two national conferences on cancer nursing (2) in the last 5 years, and each year the local divisions of the American Cancer Society as well as State Nurses Associations have workshops and/or symposiums to keep their nurses informed of the latest advances in cancer.

Cancer nursing is now a recognized specialty (2). The University of Pittsburgh, School of Nursing awards a Master's Degree in Cancer Nursing and the Oncology Nursing Society held its Third Annual Convention in Washington, D.C., April 5–7, 1978. *Cancer Nursing,* an international journal for cancer care, had its premier issue this past February. The Editor-in-Chief Rachel Ayers and Senior Editor Carol Reed-Ash (3) in a Message from the Editors wrote:

> Cancer is a part of the work of every nurse, and practitioner, teacher, administrator, researcher, and student alike face an exposure of knowledge associated with caring for people living with cancer. Every nurse from the experienced specialist who cares exclusively for cancer patients to the general practitioner who must coordinate cancer care with other equally important assignments, has a common need and cause—to learn, to explore new approaches, and to share their experiences, awareness and understanding of cancer nursing, advances in treatment, and the implications of research findings.

This is indicative of the importance being placed on cancer nursing and the advancement being made.

However, this is not the case when we speak of the role of the nurse in the management of pain due to cancer. There is lack of knowledge and understanding, and this is quite evident when, too often, you see and hear the nurses' negative responses to the patient who has pain. This aspect of the care of the patient with cancer has not been fully developed. There are nurses who have had the opportunity to become involved with patients with pain due to advanced cancer and they have responded with sensitivity and compassion to these patients but, unfortunately, their numbers are too few. Pain due to cancer presents special problems with which most nurses are unprepared to cope. The patient with cancer may be facing a life-threatening situation. If the cancer causes persistent pain or the pain reappears after definitive treatment, the patient may feel that the original treatment has failed and that he is doomed.

Although most patients will accept the temporary use of narcotics, many will reject their continuous use. Most patients are extremely concerned about taking too much medication. Many of them will suffer needlessly by refusing to take medications because of misunderstandings about the nature of addiction. This may be reinforced by the nurses, and this produces more anxiety and guilt. The nurse may withhold an analgesic in order to prevent addiction and may even tell the patient he is taking too much narcotic and that he will become a drug addict. When the nurse administers an analgesic, she sometimes acts as though she is doing the patient a favor. Some patients may feel that nobody believes he has pain.

Unfortunately, many nurses do not know the basic pharmacology of analgesics, and this is also true of some physicians. For example, some physicians will write orders for parenteral and oral narcotics in the same milligram dose, typically meperidine 50 mg i.m. or PO q. 4 to 6 hr prn. If the nurse is busy, she will probably give the oral form—it is easier. But, if at one time or another, the patient should receive the parenteral dose and reports good relief, the nurse and doctor will conclude that he just "likes" the injection. However, oral meperidine is only ¼ as potent as the parenteral dose and is about equivalent to 650 mg of aspirin. Also, meperidine is a relatively short-acting narcotic and may be effective for only 2 to 3 hr. In addition, the patient whose pain comes on suddenly, will prefer the injection since peak effect of most parenteral narcotics occurs within 1 hr, whereas peak of oral effect may occur as late as 2 hr after administration. The ratio of oral versus parenteral potency of narcotics will vary with the drug. Methadone is twice as potent by parenteral route; morphine 6 times as potent.

The continuous use of narcotics will inevitably produce tolerance. This is often confused with addiction.

The first sign of tolerance is that the duration of effect has lessened. Patients will request their medication before it is scheduled. These patients are labeled first "clock-watchers" and then "addicts" who have lost control of themselves. The tendency for the doctor is to order another narcotic, usually in an inappropriately low dose, or to order a less-potent drug. The patient then continues to complain of inadequate relief. After several changes of narcotics with the same results, both the nurse and doctor become frustrated. This leads to hostility toward the patient who is called "a chronic complainer," "a neurotic," and again, "an addict." Nobody believes that he has that much pain, and they are convinced that the patient's pain must be supratentorial or that he is overreacting. The next step often taken is to try to modify the patient's behavior rather than treat his pain. Very often, it is the nurse who will suggest to the doctor that the patient needs a tranquilizer or even a placebo.

In our experience, we have found that the addition of a tranquilizer or a sedative does not potentiate the analgesic effects of narcotics but instead will not only sedate the patient, but cause confusion and disorientation, and in some instances, may cause the patient to act in an irrational manner, especially if his pain is not being controlled.

By now, we all should understand the effects of a placebo. The patient who has confidence in his doctor and nurses, will almost always have a positive response to the placebo even when his pain correlates with demonstrated organic disease.

Since patients with cancer are often candidates for complications, one cannot assume that the cause of pain will necessarily be the same from day to day. Before giving an analgesic, the nurse should ask the patient if the pain is the same or if there has been some change. If there has been a change, she should obtain more information about it. Any new pain should be reported to the patient's physician as soon as possible. Some complications, if not treated promptly can lead to irreversible effects, such as cord compression.

There are times when the nurse should anticipate when the patient may require an analgesic. These times may be:

1. Before a patient is sent for a procedure that may be painful or uncomfortable and may require several hours (e.g., skeletal survey, scans, I.V.P., etc.). Patient may be unable to lie on a hard table because of pain and may refuse to complete the procedure. These patients are often sent back to the hospital floor with the notation that the patient was uncooperative. The nurse should be aware of the nature of these procedures and explain them to the patient, and she should encourage the patient to take his medication before the pain becomes unbearable so that the medication ordered would be most effective.
2. Before ambulation (if pain increases on movement or on sitting)
3. Before meals (if the patient's pain increases while he is eating or shortly after).
4. At bedtime (if the patient states the pain gets worse at night or he can't fall asleep even with sedation because the pain keeps him awake).

To be effective, a nurse must be aware and sensitive to all the problems that these patients may be facing. It is not enough just to know the disease process and the cause of pain. Her role as a care-giver requires understanding and a willingness to attend to even the little things.

Today, the public is more educated and is demanding better understanding of health-care services and that their rights and expectations, interests, needs, and concerns be recognized. Since 1913, the American Cancer Society has been involved in cancer control, public education, and services. In their 1978 publication, *Cancer Facts and Figures,* they discuss basic data, why early detection is vital, early detection and high-risk groups, the cancer checkup, cancer trends, treatment trends, and the function of the American Cancer Society in public education and information, professional education, service and rehabilitation, research, cost of cancer, and their sources of income and the allocation of ACS Funds.

Although it would be important to discuss all these aspects in more detail, two areas that warrant more emphasis are public education and information and costs of cancer.

The American Cancer Society allocated 30.2% of their 1976–1977 budget to research ($37,987,000) and the next highest figure, 16.7%, to public education ($20,973,000). Special emphasis is placed on projects involving person-to-person contact. A 1977 Gallup study indicated a broad receptiveness to that kind of cancer education. To help advance the person-to-person education concept, the Society now is using specialized volunteers who are individuals already trained professionally in certain skills that can be adapted to fighting cancer. Ex-smokers are leading Quit-smoking Clinics to help smokers "kick the habit." Nurses are teaching the breast self-examination (BSE) and encouraging women at or after menopause to have endometrial-tissue samplings taken.

Other programs include the new "Early Start to Good Health" in an attempt to introduce good health-habits to children in kindergarten through the third grade. During the annual ACS Cancer Crusade, volunteers made personal home visits urging individuals to protect themselves against cancer. Last year, local public education programs involving two-way communication reached more than 22.5 million people throughout the United States, and in conjunction with business and industry, 1.3 million workers.

It is difficult to estimate the impact of public-information programs. Surveys have shown, for example, that only one woman in three practiced breast self-examination (BSE), however, 9 out of 10 said they had heard of it and 36% were interested in learning. Teenage girls are smoking more. In this age group, it has increased by 5% from 1964 to 1975 to a level of 27%. The number who smoke a pack or more a day quadrupled. Teenage boys held steady at 30%. The Society's antismoking campaign through mass media has been accelerated with a new series of TV spots, new pamphlets, such special events as writing contests and no-smoking days. It is unfortunate that scare tactics may not always work; in fact, in many instances, the negative approach may actually defeat the purpose. The person who may have a cancer phobia may be too afraid to seek medical advice for he may think it is too late and nothing can be done anyway. On the other hand, a patient may go from doctor to doctor and be labeled a hypochondriac. In the last several years, many of our motion-picture films or films made for television have been based on those who have died of cancer rather than on those who have been cured of cancer or are living with cancer.

Although the American Cancer Society has issued a new booklet entitled *The Hopeful Side of Cancer*, in which they mention community and patient services that are available, this information and information of the costs of cancer is seldom conveyed to the public via the mass media. The total cost of cancer is now estimated to be, including earning loss, at over $18.9 billion a year in the United States. The Third National Cancer Survey of the United States Department of Health, Education and Welfare placed the average cost of cancer hospitalization in 1969 and 1970 at $2,529—about $90 a day—over a 28-day period. The Health Insurance Institutes' latest statistics show the average community-hospital costs per day for 1975 were $151, which would raise the 28-day cancer stay to $4,228. A 1973 study by Cancer Care, Inc. of New York City reported overall cancer expenses ranging from $5,000 to $50,000 with a median of $19,000 spent over 2 years (1). Because of inflation, the cost of hospitalization, physicians' services, drugs, treatments, nursing services, and equipment is even higher today. The public has no idea of these costs until it happens to them, and the health-care professionals know even less. Although prevention, early detection and public education are vital, the public should be better informed as to what can be done for the patient who has advanced cancer and pain. The patient expects to be treated as a whole human being; therefore, every effort should be made to look at him as a whole person—his social, cultural, and economic environment in and out of the hospital, social-psychological factors in his illness, and patient–professional health-care-team interaction (5). Our aim for the patient who has pain due to advanced cancer is an understanding of his suffering and, through understanding, relief.

ACKNOWLEDGMENTS

Supported in part by grants awarded by the National Institute on Drug Abuse (DA 01707–02).

I wish to thank Miss Julie Franchi and Mr. George Heidrich, R.N., B.S.N., for their assistance in the literature search and Miss Natalie M. Rogers for her assistance in the preparation of the manuscript.

REFERENCES

1. American Cancer Society (1978): *Cancer Facts and Figures.* American Cancer Society, New York.
2. American Cancer Society (1977): *Proceedings of the Second Nursing Conference on Cancer Nursing.* American Cancer Society, New York.
3. Ayers, R., and Reed-Ash, C. (1978): Message from the editors. *Cancer Nurs.,* Vol. I, No. I.
4. Butler, F. (1955): *Cancer Through the Ages: The Evolution of Hope.* Virginia Press, Fairfax, Va.
5. Chasca, N. (1977): Medical Sociology for Whom? *Mayo Clinic Proc.,* 52:813–818.
6. Considine, B. (1959): *That Many May Live.* Memorial Center for Cancer and Allied Diseases, New York.
7. Hardy, R. E., Cull, J. G. (1975): *Counseling and Rehabilitating the Cancer Patient, No. 964: American Lecture Series.* Charles C Thomas, Springfield, Ill.
8. Kübler-Ross, E. (1969): *On Death and Dying.* The Macmillan Company, New York.
9. Shinkin, M. B. (1977): *Contrary to Nature.* United States Department of Health, Education and Welfare, Public Health Service, National Institute of Health, Washington, D.C.
10. Time-Life Books (1966): *Great Ages of Man: A History of the World's Culture.* Time-Life Books, New York.
11. Wise, T. (1978): Sexual functioning in neoplastic disease, *Med. Aspects Hum. Sexuality,* 12(1):16–31.

Discussion

Part I. Basic Considerations (continued)

K. Foley and G. Martino (Moderators)

Chapman (Seattle): Dr. Beales, to what extent are the parents' beliefs and fears about the child's disease likely to become a factor in the developing pain of the child?

Beales (Manchester): The parents' attitudes are of vital importance because how the child interprets what is going on inside his own body is greatly influenced by learning, and he is very much dependent upon other people's telling him what signals might mean. If the parents themselves are very anxious about a particular type of condition, there is a fair chance that the child will present at some time or other symptoms which seem to indicate that kind of condition. It very frequently happens that the parents pick up the slightest indications the child gives that he has this kind of problem and become anxious; the child himself becomes anxious, and it can be extremely difficult for the clinicians to reassure the parents or the child that there is, in fact, nothing wrong.

Bond (Glasgow): In addition to learning about the usually accepted significance of pain, mainly that it indicates organic damage of some kind, children also learn from their parents the other meaning of pain; that pain can be used to manipulate people, that pain can be equated in gaining pleasure and affection and so forth. One should bear this in mind when looking at pain problems in young children.

Mascia (Brooklyn): Dr. Bond, can you comment on the remarkable reactivation or remobilization of patients following psychological interventions?

Bond: I think there is not a simple answer. One can look at the question of the effect of the disease on the individual, the effect of the response of those around him or her to the illness, that is, both the medical personnel and the family; and I think the various factors involved have been mentioned during the course of the day by Chapman, myself, and others. Psychologic intervention usually means reestablishing contact with the patient, it may mean the making of a diagnosis of depressive illness which does occur in such people which, when treated, can produce considerable improvements in mood and motivation. It may mean removing the sense of helplessness, of hopelessness, of loneliness which often afflicts people who feel that doctors have nothing more to offer.

Bistolfi (Genova): Dr. Foley, have you had any experience about the worsening of radiationmyelitis by subsequent BC and U treatment?

Foley (New York): Patients with any neurological illness commonly become much worse when they receive chemotherapy. We do not see it as commonly with BC and U as we see it with vincristine or vinblastine or with high doses of methotrexate, since both drugs are neurotoxic in high doses.

Giugiaro (Torino): Dr. Morpurgo, what is the role of the following components in decoding the pain symptom: physiological cortex representation of the sensitive areas; progressive expansion of the representation of the diseased neoplastic area; drastic reduction of the exogenous stimuli following the patient's isolation? Furthermore, by which means do you define the body image present in cats? How are the registrations made?

Morpurgo (Milano): We had the impression that the progressive expansion of the area is the determining factor, while the reduction of the stimuli is less important because the visual perception associated with the painful stimulus and the large reduction of the training time would show that the pain stimulus itself is capable of occupying areas other than its own, independently of whether other areas are occupied or not. Everybody here knows that when we have a toothache, it is difficult to follow a show. So I would say that the other sensory inputs are considerably reduced by pain. As for the technique, we follow all the other researchers, from Mountcastle to Albe-Fessard and Spinelli. The cortical area which has to be explored is evidenced by means of electrodes that progressively penetrate it. Every time the machine shows a stable activity due to a neuron, then we analyze peripherally the areas from which such activity is generated. This way we can correlate the cortical image to what happens peripherally.

Raineri (Genova): Dr. Bond, do the patients who know of their disease and the ones who do not show any difference as regards pain sensitivity?

Bond: I think the answer lies in levels of anxiety. When people are told unpleasant things and become anxious, their tolerance tends to fall. So any circumstance which reduces the tendency to raise anxiety, and perhaps being treated at home may, in some circumstances, lower anxiety, whereas, in others, for reasons we have heard, may raise anxiety. Any situation which lowers anxiety will tend to keep pain thresholds up.

Martino (Milano): Italian physicians do not give explanations to the patient more than is necessary and are also reluctant in administration of analgesics. We should know that a percentage of patients, larger than we had thought, is capable of knowing the truth and its conditions, and that hiding the truth can give as much anxiety, even more than knowing the truth. As for hospitalization, it does not improve the survival, and it is isolating both in structure and in practice. Such inconvenience is indirectly confirmed by the literature, which shows a higher percentage of pain incidence in hospitalized patients than in those at home. However, also in this regard, there is no rule. Home can also be isolating depending on the social, cultural, and financial conditions of the family. For this reason, to carry out a correct analgesic therapy, we must estimate, in every single case, not only the psychological conditions of the patient, but also the social and cultural conditions of his home environment. In our experience, the pain symptom in the ambulatory patient is often a signal of his social discomfort. In these cases, to carry out a correct analgesic therapy, we should also work with the family, supporting it psychotherapeutically and financially.

Advances in Pain Research and Therapy, Vol. 2,
edited by J. J. Bonica and V. Ventafridda.
Raven Press, New York © 1979.

Introduction to Management of Pain of Advanced Cancer

John J. Bonica

Department of Anesthesiology, University of Washington, Seattle, Washington 98195

In this chapter we begin consideration of the various modalities currently available for the management of pain of advanced cancer. As is well known this revolves around three main methods of approach: (a) use of anticancer modalities intended to decrease or eliminate the neoplasm and consequently eliminate the etiology and mechanism of the pain; (b) control of the pain without affecting the neoplasm; and (c) a combination of these.

Anticancer modalities include the use of: (a) *chemotherapy,* (b) *endocrine therapy,* (c) *radiation therapy,* (d) *radioisotope therapy,* and (e) *palliative surgery,* including excision of the tumor, bypass operation, and destruction or excision of endocrine organs such as hypophysectomy, adrenalectomy, and castration. It is important to emphasize, however, that regardless of which of the major approaches is to be used that physiologic and psychologic support of the patient and his family is an essential, if not the most essential, part of the management of patients with cancer pain. This will require a well-coordinated, concerted effort by the medical team, sociologists, and religious counselors.

When the aforementioned measures prove totally or partially ineffective or not feasible, it is necessary to control pain symptomatically without affecting a neoplasm (2,3,4). The modalities in current use include: (a) *systemic drugs* consisting of nonaddictive analgesics, sedatives, ataractics, psychotropic drugs, and potent (addictive) narcotics; (b) *therapeutic nerve blocks* which can be achieved either temporarily with a local anesthetic or for a prolonged period by injecting neurolytic agents; (c) *neurosurgical operations,* which may either be ablative, intended to interrupt pain pathways, or use stimulation of pain-modulating mechanisms including transcutaneous stimulation, peripheral-nerve stimulation, dorsal-column stimulation, and stimulation of the brain; (d) *psychologic methods* which include traditional psychotherapy, hypnosis, biofeedback, and operant conditioning. Many patients with cancer pain also need rehabilitation programs, which may include physical therapy, occupational therapy, exercise and support by psychologists, nurses, theologians, etc.

In determining which one or combination of therapies is to be used, it is essential to adhere to certain principles basic to the practice of medicine in general and to oncologic therapy in particular. In introducing the proper management of pain of advanced cancer, I wish to emphasize some of these principles and issues in order to provide a background for the following chapters. Although most of these are well known, all too often many of them are neglected by therapists. They will be discussed in greater detail in the chapters that follow.

One of the cardinal principles for health care is that optimal therapy of any pathologic process, including cancer pain, requires a correct diagnosis. In regard to pain, the therapist must know and appreciate its etiology, mechanism, and physiopathology. It is becoming clear that chronic pain is due to prolonged and persistent dysfunction of peripheral or central neural mechanisms, or psychologic or motivational or cognitive substrates of pain, or, most frequently, a combination of these. In Chapter 2, Zimmermann has already discussed the neurophysiology of nociception and acute pain and some of the peripheral mechanisms of chronic pain. Here I wish to supplement the discussion by presenting some speculations on the mechanisms of chronic pain in general which may serve as background for the discussion of the mechanisms of cancer pain. I emphasize that these are speculations, because scientific data from human studies are meager.

MECHANISM OF CHRONIC PAIN

From a therapeutic viewpoint, it may be useful to classify the suggested mechanisms of chronic pain in a simplistic fashion into "peripheral," "peripheral-central," "central," and "psychologic" mechanisms.

Peripheral Mechanisms

In some patients, including those with cancer, chronic pain is a consequence of a persistent pathologic process that causes persistent biochemical, mechanical, and thermal changes that sustain stimulation of nociceptors or afferent nociceptive pathways in the periphery. Persistent mechanical noxious stimulation probably occurs in various lesions such as tumors which irritate nerve endings or fibers. As Zimmermann has emphasized, sensitization may be caused by some of the pain-producing substances liberated from cellular breakdown or through emotional factors which increase sympathetic hyperactivity. Perl (18) has recently shown that, once the high-threshold A-delta and C-fibers have been damaged or heated and are tested after the evoked discharge has died down, they have become sensitized so that light pressure or mild warming now evokes firing. Moreover, as Zimmermann has mentioned, Wall and Gutnick (21) developed an experimental model for neuroma by cutting rat sciatic nerves and allowing the cut end to regenerate into a sealed polyethylene tube, and thus studied the physiology and pharmacology of the fine sprouts in the neuroma. They showed that the partially damaged nerve membrane and the sprouts within a neuroma become very sensitive to light pressure and to norepinephrine, which is liberated in greater amounts as a result of sympathetic hyperactivity provoked by injury. They also showed that some of the modulation produced by electric stimulation of peripheral nerves resulted from the turnoff of abnormal peripheral nerve generators in the neuroma. The clinical implication of peripheral mechanisms is that pain due to prolonged dysfunction of peripheral parts of the nociceptive system, can be eliminated by interrupting the afferent nociceptive pathways (6).

Peripheral-central Mechanisms

In some patients dysfunction of nociceptor systems initiates in the periphery but subsequently involves parts of the neuraxis. Examples of these are reflex sympathetic dystrophy phantom-limb pain, and the late stages of post-thoracotomy and other postoperative-pain syndromes that may develop in cancer patients. Although the exact mechanisms of this persistent dysfunction are not known, the following are among the most important hypotheses proposed.

The "vicious circle" mechanisms. Initial injury produces reflex responses that, in turn, produce abnormal changes in tissues that contribute to the noxious stimulation (13). The reflex skeletal muscle spasm contributes to the afferent barrage; the sympathetic hyperactivity causes vasospasm with a consequent sequence of ischemia, cellular damage, liberation of pain-producing substances, and sensitization of nociceptors to nonnoxious stimuli. The sympathetic hyperactivity also causes increased liberation of norepinephrine in nerve endings that then augment the firing in the small sensory fibers. One or all of these factors cause persistent noxious stimulation that then causes abnormal firing patterns in closed, self-exciting neuron pools in the spinal cord, which in turn produce more intense reflex responses with consequent increased noxious stimulation (13). Thus, a vicious circle of pain, reflex response, and more pain is initiated and sustained. Invariably, psychologic factors contribute to these mechanisms.

Decrease of peripheral inhibition. These mechanisms, based on the Melzack-Wall theory (16), often have been invoked to explain the chronic pain associated with certain peripheral-nerve disorders that reduce the number of active large fibers and cause the loss of their inhibitory influence on synaptic transmission on dorsal horn cells. This mechanism has been suggested for: (a) painful peripheral neuropathies in which there is an actual loss of large fibers, as in diabetes, post-herpetic neuralgia, and certain toxic neuropathies; and (b) painful disorders in which there is mechanical pressure on peripheral nerves. Since large fibers are more vulnerable to pressure than are small fibers, there is consequent loss of large-fiber inhibition. Wall (20) has suggested that this may be the mechanism of pain associated with neoplasm and other diseases that mechanically impinge on axons and peripheral nerves.

Central biasing mechanism. A hypothesis somewhat related to the preceding two is that of Melzack (15), by which he proposed to explain the pain of phantom limb, causalgia, and other peripheral-nerve injuries. It is based on some of the aforementioned recent data pertaining to the neural systems that exert powerful inhibitory influences on various parts of the neuraxis. According to this concept, a portion of the brainstem reticular formation acts as a central biasing mechanism by exerting a tonic inhibitory influence or bias on transmission at all synaptic levels of the somatosensory system, including the "gate" in the dorsal horn and at other levels of the neuraxis. This inhibitory function of the central biasing mechanism is dependent in part on a normal sensory input. Loss of input to the system, as occurs with peripheral-nerve lesions and amputation, weakens the inhibition and thus causes persistent pain. Emotional stress and certain drugs can also impair the efficacy of the biasing mechanism, thus aggravating the spontaneous pain. Contrarily, increased sensory input by mechanical stimulation or by direct electrical stimulation of the skin or nerve would increase the inhibition and decrease the pain.

Melzack has used this concept to explain the therapeutic efficacy of peripheral tactile and electrical stimulation in peripheral-nerve injuries. He has also used the concept to explain the therapeutic efficacy of nerve blocks in the treatment of causalgia and other reflex sympathetic dystrophies. The nerve block permits temporary return to normalcy by breaking up the activity in the self-sustaining neuron pools, and it thus produces relief of pain that may outlast the pharmacologic effect of the block. After the block has worn off, stimulation again triggers sustained activity, but because of the time necessary for it to spread to a sufficiently large number of neurons within the pools, pain-relief outlasts the action of the local anesthetic. Moreover, the relief of pain permits increased use of the limb, which produces patterned, temporarily dispersed inputs, particularly from the muscles that are out of phase with the rhythmically firing neuron pools, and disrupts their activity. This delays resumption of self-sustaining firing.

Denervation hypersensitivity. To explain the pain, dysesthesia, and paresthesia that often accompany peripheral-nerve injuries and complicate surgical interruption of pain pathways such as rhizotomy and cordotomy, Loeser et al. (14), among others, have proposed that loss of normal sensory input produces an abnormal firing pattern in the somatosensory system proximal to the deafferentation (9). In animal models, he found seizure-like abnormal firing patterns in deafferented dorsal-root fibers and lateral caudate nucleus. He also has recorded high-frequency bursts distal to a spinal-cord injury in a patient exhibiting paraplegic pain and flexor spasm. Black et al. (1) have shown similar abnormal firing patterns following trigeminal denervation consequent to tooth-pulp extraction and section of the nerve. Since damage to a peripheral nerve causes chromatolysis of ganglion cells, and since it has been shown that chromatolytic motor neurons become hyperexcitable, Wall (20) has suggested that peripheral-nerve section produces either a partial central deafferentation with consequent hyperexcitability, or a change of the location of central terminals.

Central Pain Mechanisms

Disease of certain parts of the central nervous system (CNS) often produces what is generally referred to as "central pain," characterized by spontaneous burning, aching pain, hyperalgesia, dysesthesia, and other abnormal sensations (8). Central pain often accompanies thalamic lesions (so-called "thalamic pain"), surgical interruption of certain parts of the pain pathway, tabes dorsalis, and other painful diseases of the CNS (2,8). Mechanisms of these disorders are not known, but it has been suggested that there is a loss of descending inhibitory influences, or that interruption of certain parts of the pain pathway disturbs the normal balance between the discriminative and motivational systems.

Psychologic Mechanisms

In addition to the important role psychologic factors play in chronic pain produced by injury or disease, in a significant number of patients, chronic pain primarily due to psychologic factors develops. This group can be arbitrarily subdivided into four categories: (a) psychophysiologic mechanisms; (b) operant mechanisms; (c) psychogenic mechanisms; and (d) psychiatric mechanisms (6).

Psychophysiologic (psychosomatic) mechanisms. In some individuals, severe emotional stress, through psychophysiologic (corticofugal) mechanisms, produces skeletal-muscle spasm, local vasoconstriction, visceral dysfunction, liberation of pain substances, or a combination of these (2,19). One or more of these produces peripheral noxious stimulation, with its consequences of pain, reflex responses, and affective reactions, all of which aggravate the emotional stress. This, in turn, provokes more psychophysiologic impulses, thus sustaining the vicious circle of pain. This is probably the mechanism of tension headache and pain due to spasm of muscles in the shoulder girdle, low back, and chest. Psychophysiologic mechanism has also been invoked to explain migraine headache, in which emotional factors provoke the liberation of substances that produce the characteristic vasoconstriction and vasodilatation. It has long been appreciated that this is the probable mechanism of coronary artery disease, peptic ulcer, and colitis, each of which is often accompanied by chronic pain.

Operant mechanism. This mechanism, first proposed by Fordyce (11,12), is responsible in a significant number of patients in whom chronic pain behavior develops following a disease or injury that often is of a minor nature.

The initial injury provokes operant responses and pain behavior on the part of the patient that are reinforced by favorable consequences or reactions on the part of those important to the patient. Thus, a husband who for years has been inattentive to his wife becomes solicitous and concerned and gives special attention when she sustains an injury—favorable consequences that reinforce her pain behavior. This concept involves well-established principles of operant conditioning that state that behavior is subject to the influence of, or under the control of, learning factors, and to a considerable degree is governed by consequences in the environment.

Chronic pain behavior continues as long as the consequences are favorable, and eventually becomes independent of the underlying pathology and persists even after the original pathogenic factor is gone. Under such conditions, a "pain habit" that is real and is readily accounted for by learning or conditioning has developed. The important therapeutic implications are that, to change the chronic pain behavior, it is necessary to eliminate the favorable consequences that are acting as positive reinforcers to the behavior, rather than to seek out and try to eliminate underlying pathology.

Mechanisms of "psychogenic" pain. A significant number of patients who have chronic pain have what is traditionally referred to as "psychogenic" pain, which really means pain due to psychologic causes. It deserves strong emphasis that these patients are not imagining the pain, but that the pain is as real as and is felt and described in much the same way as "somatogenic" pain. The difference between these two major groups is that psychogenic pain is less adequately explained in physical terms. In view of this, Sternbach (19) suggested the definition that "psychogenic pain" refers to "pain which is better understood in psychologic than in physical language." The psychodynamics of "psychogenic" pain have been detailed by Sternbach. Briefly, in these patients' early lives, pain was associated with anxiety and fear of bodily harm and loss of love. Later, the experience of one evokes the sensation of the other: Pain provokes "unnecessary anxiety," or anxiety can cause "psychogenic pain." Anxiety is the affect associated with the experience of acute pain. When what is feared actually does come to pass, depression replaces anxiety. Psychogenic pain symbolizes conflict among unmet emotional needs, internal prohibition, and external realities.

Psychiatric mechanisms. Chronic pain is occasionally a symptom of depression, hysteria, or other psychiatric disorders. The psychodynamics of these are described by Merskey and Spear (17).

Cancer can cause pain by one or more of the following mechanisms: (a) bone tumor invasion, (b) compression of nerve roots, nerve trunks, or plexuses; (c) infiltration of nerves by tumor cells; (d) obstruction of hollow viscera; (e) occlusion of large blood vessels; (f) infiltration, contraction, and swelling in tissue invested snugly by fascia, periosteum, or other pain-sensitive structures; or (g) necrosis, infection, inflammation, and ulceration of pain-sensitive structures produced by the lesion.

MECHANISM OF CANCER PAIN

As emphasized by Foley (10), the etiology of cancer pain may be classified into one of three major categories: (a) pain caused by the oncologic process; (b) pain that develops as a result of therapy; and (c) pain that develops coincidentally with, but is unrelated to, the cancer. In the average cancer-hospital population, pain is caused by the oncologic process in three-quarters of the patients, posttherapy pain is present in 20% of the patients, and about 5% have coincidental pain (10). Although Foley has described the most important causes of pain in cancer patients, the following brief section is intended to summarize the subject. Those aspects discussed in detail by Foley will only be mentioned here.

Pain Caused by the Oncologic Process

The following classification of cancer-induced pain is a modification of the one first proposed by Bonica (2,3) a quarter-century ago and taking into consideration recently acquired information about basic mechanisms as well as the information provided by Foley.

Bone Tumor Invasion

As Foley has indicated, tumor invasion of bone by either primary or metastatic lesion is the most common cause of pain in patients with cancer. This is discussed in greater detail by Foley (*this volume*).

Compression of Nerve Roots, Nerve Trunks, and Plexuses

Compression of nerve roots, nerve trunks, or plexuses by an enlarging tumor or lymph glands or metastatic fracture of bones adjacent to the nerves results in a radiculopathy or neuropathy which is accompanied by fairly sharp, localized neuralgic pain projected to the distribution of the nerve structure involved. In such instances, it is likely that noxious mechanical stimulation produces dysfunction of the nociceptive system which is limited to the periphery for a time, but then it may activate peripheral-central mechanisms.

Tumor Infiltration of Nervous Structures

Infiltration of a peripheral nerve causes constant, burning pain associated with hyperesthesia and dysesthesia in the area of sensory loss. Tumor infiltration of other plexuses or major nerves will produce burning pain with hyperalgesia, hyperesthesia, and dysesthesia along the distribution of the affected nerve. It is important to note that the quality of the pain is usually burning, resembling that of causalgia and reflex sympathetic dystrophy. In fact, reflex sympathetic dystrophy frequently accompanies perineural infiltration by cancer cells.

Infiltration of Blood Vessels

Infiltration of blood vessels by tumor cells results in vasospasm and a perivascular lymphangitis and consequent irritation of nociceptors or nociceptive afferents. This process produces a diffuse burning or aching pain that does *not* have a peripheral-nerve distribution. In many instances, there develops a reflex sympathetic hyperactivity with a consequent increased liberation of norepinephrine which aggravates the basic physiopathology and sensitizes nociceptors. This type of process probably involves peripheral mechanisms, and the pain can be eliminated effectively by interruption of the affected peripheral nociceptive pathways.

Obstruction of a Hollow Viscus or the Ductal System in a Solid Viscus

It is well known that obstruction of the stomach, intestine, biliary tract, ureters, uterus, or urinary bladder causes intense contraction of the smooth muscles under isometric conditions (i.e., when the exit of the viscus is obstructed) with the production of visceral pain which is characteristically diffuse and poorly localized and referred to dermatomes supplied by the same spinal-cord segments which supply the affected viscus. Recent data show that these structures are supplied by A-delta and C-fibers which are activated by ischemia and chemical agents (7). It is likely that the ischemia causes cellular breakdown with production of "pain-producing substances" and probably lowers the threshold of mechanical nociceptors. A similar mechanism is probably operative in oncologic processes which obstruct the outflow of ductal systems of the pancreas, liver, and other solid viscera. In all of these conditions, persistent obstruction produces progressively greater contractions and finally intense distention with consequent progressively greater pain.

Occlusion of Blood Vessels

Occlusion of blood vessels, either partial or complete, by an adjacent tumor produces venous engorgement or arterial ischemia or both. Venous engorgement will result in a tumor of all the structures that are supplied by the obstructing vessel. The edema, in turn, causes distention of facial compartments and other pain-sensitive structures resulting in progressively more severe, intractable pain. Examples are the progressively more severe headaches consequent to obstruction of the veins draining from the head, and the pain in the upper or lower limb caused by obstruction of the venous outflow from these structures. Ischemia produced by obstruction of a major artery probably causes cellular breakdown with production of "pain-producing substances" which lower the threshold of nociceptors. The pain generated by these mechanisms is usually diffuse and does not follow any particular nerve distribution and usually becomes progressively worse. It is likely that the pain arising from these pathologic processes involves purely peripheral mechanisms and theoretically should be relieved by denervation of the affected part, provided that the interruption is extensive enough.

Tumefaction and Swelling in a Structure Invested Snugly by Fascia, Periosteum, or other Pain-sensitive Structures

This type of process is probably responsible for the pain associated with growing tumors of liver, spleen, and certain types of kidney tumors. Each of these processes produces distention of the investing pain-sensitive structure with consequent stimulation of mechanical nociceptors. If the pain-inducing tumor is a superficial somatic structure, the pain is sharp and relatively well localized; whereas if the tumor is situated in deep somatic structures or the viscera, the pain is dull, poorly localized, and usually referred to dermatomes which receive the same nerve supply as the involved structure.

Necrosis, Infection, Inflammation, and Ulceration of Mucous Membranes and Other Pain-sensitive Structures

These pathologic processes produce pain which is frequently excruciating and most likely to occur with cancer of the lips, mouth, and face, and tumors of the gastrointestinal and genitourinary tracts. It is likely that the inflammatory reaction lowers the threshold of nociceptors so that innocuous stimuli produce excruciating pain usually localized to the region.

Pain Syndromes Associated with Cancer Therapy

Pain that develops as a complication of cancer therapy can be further subdivided into three etiologic subgroups: (a) pain that develops following surgery such as postthoractomy pain, postmastectomy pain, pain after a radical neck dissection and phantom-limb pain; (b) postradiation pain syndromes including radiation fibrosis of the brachial or lumbar plexus, radiation necrosis of bone, and radiation-induced secondary injury; (c) pain that develops following chemotherapy such as the pain associated with peripheral neuropathy from *Vinca* alkaloids, post-herpetic neuralgia that develops as a late effect of immunosuppresive therapy and mucositis in which chemotherapeutic agents produce chemical changes in mucous membranes and other pain-sensitive structures with consequent severe pain particularly in the mouth, throat, and nasal passages.

Postsurgical Pain

Pain following thoracotomy and mastectomy is usually due to damage of the nerves during the surgical operation. The nerves may be partially injured or completely severed. The pain becomes evident 1 to 2 months following the operation and is characterized by constant pain in the area of sensory loss with occasional, intermittent, shock-like pains. Dysesthesia in the scar area and hyperesthesia in the surrounding zone are often prominent symptoms. It is likely that the proximal portion of the severed nerve regenerates and produces small neuromata. Moreover, the surgical trauma usually damages nerve membranes of unsevered nerves. The neuroma and damaged membrane are hypersensitive to pressure and norepinephrine (20,21). Consequently, light touch and movement exacerbate the pain. As a result, some of these patients may develop a concomitant frozen shoulder and consequent limitation of motion and disuse atrophy of the arm, and the patient may develop a true reflex sympathetic dystrophy.

A number of patients who undergo radical neck dissection develop constant burning pain, dysesthesia, and lancinating pain in the region of the neck. The physiopathologic process is similar to that of other postsurgical neuropathies. Following amputation of the limb, the patient may develop two types of pain: pain in the stump and pain in the phantom limb. The stump pain is constant and burning in character, whereas the pain in the phantom limb may be either a burning pain or cramping, proprioceptive pain characterized by abnormal position of the missing distal part of the limb.

In all of these postsurgical pain syndromes, peripheral-central mechanisms are usually operative. Initially, the peripheral nociceptive dysfunction predominates, but eventually the disturbance in the neuraxis plays the most important role. The clinical implication of this is that interruption of pain of peripheral nociceptive pathways is likely to produce little or no pain-relief.

Postchemotherapy Syndromes

Painful dysesthesia and paresthesia following treatment with the *Vinca* alkaloid drugs such as vincristine and vinblastine occurs as part of a symmetrical polyneuropathy which usually develops with the doses of the drug required to achieve an antineoplastic effect (10). Dysesthesias are commonly localized to the hands and feet and are characterized by burning pain exacerbated by noxious stimuli.

Steroid pseudo-rheumatism occurs following withdrawal of steroid medications. Some patients develop diffuse myalgia and arthralgia with muscle and joint tenderness on palpitation but without objective inflammatory signs. These symptoms regress with reinstitution of steroid therapy.

Aseptic necrosis of the head of the femur or the humerus or both with consequent pain in the knee or shoulder joint, respectively, occurs as a complication of cancer therapy, specifically, chronic steroid therapy. This is discussed in detail by Foley.

Post-herpetic neuralgia is a complication of radiation therapy, or it may occur following herpes zoster that develops in the area of tumor pathology. The patient usually experiences continuous, burning pain in the area of sensory loss, painful dysesthesia and intermittent lancinating pain. This condition involves peripheral-central mechanisms and is one of the most difficult pain syndromes to treat.

Mucositis occurs after the administration of certain chemotherapeutic agents which apparently produce biochemical changes in mucous membranes and other pain-sensitive structures with consequent severe pain particularly in the mouth, throat, and nasal passages.

Postradiation Therapy Pain

Following radiation therapy to the region of the brachial plexus or the lumbosacral plexus, *fibrosis* of the surrounding or connective tissue occurs with secondary injury to the nerve structures (2,10). The condition is progressive with consequent increasing pain. The pain is often associated with numbness or paresthesia in the structures supplied by the affected nerves, lymphedema in the arm, and radiation skin changes and induration of the supraclavicular and axillary areas present with brachial plexus fibrosis. Similarly, fibrosis of the lumbosacral plexus produces pain associated with progressive motor and sensory changes and lymphedema in the limb. The fibrosis, which is a slow, progressive process, produces injury to the nerves with consequent abnormal firing that eventually produces abnormal function in the somatosensory system in the neuraxis. Consequently, the peripheral-central mechanism produces the pain, which is not likely to respond to interruption of peripheral pathways.

Radiation myelopathy is an important problem which is discussed in detail by Foley (*this volume*).

SELECTION OF THERAPY

In determining the best therapeutic modality or combination of therapies to effectively relieve the pain, it is essential to consider the characteristics of the pain, the chronology of the disease and of previous therapy, and various other aspects which can only be ascertained by a very detailed history and a comprehensive general physical, neurologic, orthopedic and other appropriate examinations (2,10). Since most patients with cancer pain present a complex array of physical, psychologic, behavioral, and affective manifestations, a total psychologic and social evaluation is mandatory to develop the most appropriate therapeutic strategy. These are essential to define the role that psychologic, social, cultural, motivational, and related factors play in the patient's total pain experience.

History

A careful history of the pain complaint is an essential first step in determining a therapy. It is important to consider the location and distribution of the pain and its possible spread, its quality, severity, and time-characteristics (i.e., whether it is continuous or occurs in bouts), and what factors aggravate and relieve the pain. It is also important to elicit information about associated phenomena including sensory deficits, muscle weakness, and visceral dysfunction. For example, in a patient complaining of severe back pain exacerbated by lying down associated with a complaint of difficulty in urinating suggests a diagnosis of epidural spinal-cord compression.

It is also important to obtain a history of the oncologic process in order to determine which of the major etiologic factors is responsible for the pain. If the pain is directly due to the neoplasm, it is essential to know the type and grade of differentiation and site of spread or metastasis. If the pain is the result of therapy, an attempt should be made to predict its time-course. For example, the pain of postradiation fibrosis of the brachial plexus is progressive in severity and often very difficult to control with drugs. Similarly, post-herpetic neuralgia consequent to immunosuppressive therapy and post-thoracotomy, postmastectomy, and postamputation pain are also progressive and require early application of therapeutic modalities that will eliminate the basic mechanisms which, at this stage, involve only the peripheral nociceptive system. Management of such patients with systemic drugs may relieve the pain temporarily but does not prevent progression of the neural mechanism. These are likely to involve the CNS with a consequent progressive increase in the pain and the associated reflex sympathetic dystrophy which, after a period of months, will not be relieved by anything except very destructive procedures in the higher parts of the neuraxis.

Examination

Careful examination of the painful region and the general physical, neurologic, and orthopedic examinations are also essential to acquire objective data and substantiate the clinical history. A detailed neurologic examination is particularly useful in differentiating local pain from referred pain, and in differentiating pain due to peripheral-nerve involvement from pain due to plexus or cord involvement. For example, in a patient with low-back pain and radicular symptomatology in L5-S1 distribution, together with an absent ankle jerk, nerve root rather than plexus involvement is suggested.

Psychologic and Psychosocial Evaluation

A comprehensive psychologic and social evaluation is essential to develop the most effective therapeutic strategy. This should include a general psychologic and behavioral assessment and the application of appropriate psychometric tests. Psychosocial evaluation should include determination of cultural background, religious beliefs, interaction with spouse and family unit, social activities, and the impact of these on the pain. These will be considered in more detail in later chapters.

Special Diagnostic Tests

Various diagnostic tools may be essential to determine the mechanisms of pain. Since plain X-rays have limitations, it may be necessary to supplement them with bone scan, tomography and, in some special cases, computerized transaxial tomography (CT scan). In addition to the usual laboratory examination, special biochemical procedures may be necessary. Cisternal and lumbar myography and cerebrospinal fluid cytology are sometimes necessary to determine the etiology of the pain. The important role that appropriate nerve blocks can play in ascertaining the mechanisms and pathways of cancer pain will be discussed later. The appropriate use of placebo or hypnosis or both may provide important information about the physiologic and psychologic substrates of pain.

Evaluation of Therapeutic Modalities

Knowledge of therapeutic modalities currently available for the relief of cancer pain is crucial to the selection of the most effective therapy. It is essential to know not only the analgesic efficacy and advantages, but also the limitations and disadvantages of each procedure. Only with such knowledge integrated into the information obtained from the history and physical examination will it be possible to determine which is the best method or methods of relieving cancer pain.

Multidisciplinary Team Management

The importance of a multidisciplinary team effort in managing patients with cancer, especially in the terminal phase, has become well established. For many years, cancer hospitals and cancer units of general hospitals have had oncology groups consisting of oncologic surgeons, radiation therapists, medical oncologists, and pathologists to deal with the pathologic process. More recently, the importance of treating the whole patient (rather than just the lesion) has become appreciated; and consequently oncology teams have added nutritionists, nurses, physical therapists, psychologists, social workers, and various other health professionals and chaplains with special interest and expertise in cancer management. Moreover, much has been written on the physiologic and psychologic needs of cancer patients.

Unfortunately, most of these oncology groups in the United States have ignored or neglected one of the most important aspects of the care of cancer patients—the effective control of pain. This aspect is especially important in patients with advanced and terminal cancer. Except for a few of the comprehensive cancer centers with pain-control teams, the management of pain is relegated to the house staff who, as previously mentioned, have had no formal teaching and consequently treat the pain empirically, usually with narcotics prescribed in totally inadequate doses.

Consideration of the numerous mechanisms of chronic pain in general and cancer pain in particular and of the various modalities currently available for its therapy makes it obvious that no one individual has the knowledge, expertise, and skill to provide optimal relief to each and every patient. I recognized this problem 35 years ago when I was given the responsibility of managing patients with severe intractable pain due to wartime injuries (2). As a result of these experiences, I developed the conviction that the management of complex pain problems is best achieved by well-coordinated, concerted efforts of a team composed of the patient's physician and specialists from different disciplines, each of whom contributes individualized knowledge and skills to the common goal of making a correct diagnosis and developing the most appropriate therapeutic strategy. Following World War II, I proved the usefulness of this concept in a community general hospital, and in 1960, I founded the University of Washington Multidisciplinary Pain Clinic. In the course of 18 years, this group has grown to about 25 health professionals representing some 14 basic science and clinical disciplines (5). Despite the numerous publications and hundreds of lectures given throughout the world, until the early 1970s the concept was ignored by the medical profession. Fortunately, during the past 6 years or so, a number of such multidisciplinary facilities modeled after the University of Washington program have been developed in the United States and several other countries.

A detailed description of the organization and function of the University of Washington facility has been published (5). The unique feature of this facility is that the members of the group have close interaction during the diagnostic workup of the patient. The managing physician and the various consultants continuously communicate during the entire process. Once all of the diagnostic information is collected, it is presented at the conference which is held at frequent intervals. This is followed by vigorous interchange among the members of the group until there is a consensus about the diagnosis and best therapy. Long experience has shown that this type of face-to-face group discussion held during the conferences is much more effective and productive in making a correct diagnosis and formulating the appropriate therapeutic strategy than communication by letter or telephone or through the fragmented, independent efforts inherent in traditional medical practice. In addition to providing highly specialized consultant services to the referring physician and the patient, these conferences serve as an excellent forum for the exchange of ideas and information and thus constitute a highly effective teaching mechanism. Moreover, the frequent interchange among the members of the group enhances the cross-fertilization of new ideas and stimulates independent and collaborative research.

Long experience also suggests that this multidisciplinary team approach is even more effective in managing patients with cancer pain. As far back as 1953, I advocated the team approach to provide a more effective therapy for pain of advanced and terminal cancer (2,4). In the ensuing quarter-century, I have espoused the concept repeatedly in numerous articles and lectures given at regional, national, and international cancer meetings. A multidisciplinary pain diagnostic and therapy team is especially indicated in the larger comprehensive cancer centers. Such a team should be composed of basic scientists and clinicians with special interest and expertise in chronic pain in general and cancer pain in particular who would devote the time and effort to evaluate carefully each patient with severe cancer pain and determine the best method or methods of relieving the pain. Such a team should include medical, surgical, and radiation oncologists, clinical pharmacologists, anesthesiologists, neurosurgeons, psychologists, psychiatrists, social workers, nurses with special knowledge and expertise in pain, theologians and others with special expertise and skills that might be needed in the diagnostic workup and in the development of the most appropriate therapeutic strategy.

REFERENCES

1. Black, R. G., Anderson, L., and Abraham, J. (1971): Neuronal hyperactivity in experimental trigeminal deafferentation. *J. Neurosurg.*, 35:444–452.
2. Bonica, J. J. (1953): *The Management of Pain.* Lea & Febiger, Philadelphia.
3. Bonica, J. J. (1954): The management of pain of malignancies with nerve blocks. *Anesthesiology,* 15:134–142; 280–301.
4. Bonica, J. J. (1954): The management of cancer pain. *GP* (*American Academy of General Practice*), 10:34–43.
5. Bonica, J. J. (1974): Organization and function of a pain clinic: In: *Advances in Neurology, Vol. 4: International Symposium on Pain,* edited by J. J. Bonica, pp. 433–443. Raven Press, New York.
6. Bonica, J. J. (1977): Neurophysiologic and pathologic aspects of acute and chronic pain. *Arch. Surg.*, 112:750–761.
7. Bonica, J. J., and Albe-Fessard, D., editors (1976): *Advances in Pain Research and Therapy, Vol. 1: Proceedings of the First World Congress on Pain.* Raven Press, New York.
8. Cassinari, V., and Pagni, C. A. (1969): *Central Pain: A Neurosurgical Survey.* Harvard University Press, Cambridge, Mass.
9. Denny-Brown, D., Kirk, E. J., and Yanagisawa, N. (1973): The tract of Lissauer in relation to sensory transmission in the dorsal horn of the spinal cord in macaque monkey. *J. Comp. Neurol.*, 151:175–200.
10. Foley, K. (1979): Pain syndromes in patients with cancer. In: *Advances in Pain*

Research and Therapy, Vol. 2, edited by J. J. Bonica and V. Ventafridda. Raven Press, New York.

11. Fordyce, W. (1974): Treating chronic pain by contingency management. In: *Advances in Neurology, Vol. 4: International Symposium on Pain,* edited by J. J. Bonica, pp. 585–587. Raven Press, New York.
12. Fordyce, W. E. (1976): *Behavioral Methods for Chronic Pain and Illness.* C. V. Mosby Co., St. Louis.
13. Livingston, W. K. (1943): *Pain Mechanisms.* Macmillan Co., New York.
14. Loeser, J. D., Ward, A. A., Jr., and White, L. E., Jr. (1968): Chronic deafferentation of the human spinal cord neurons. *J. Neurosurg.,* 29:48–50.
15. Melzack, R. (1973): *The Puzzle of Pain.* Basic Books, Inc., New York.
16. Melzack, R., and Wall, P. D. (1965): Pain mechanisms: A new theory. *Science,* 150:971–979.
17. Merskey, H., and Spear, F. G. (1967): *Pain: Psychological and Psychiatric Aspects.* Bailliere Tindall & Cassell, Ltd., London.
18. Perl, E. R. (1976): Sensitization of nociceptors and its relation to sensation. In: *Advances in Pain Research and Therapy, Vol. 1: Proceedings of the First World Congress on Pain:* edited by J. J. Bonica and D. Albe-Fessard, pp. 19–27. Raven Press, New York.
19. Sternbach, R. A. (1968): *Pain: A Psychophysiological Analysis.* Academic Press, New York.
20. Wall, P. D. (1974): Physiological mechanisms involved in the production and relief of pain: In: *Recent Advances on Pain: Pathophysiology and Clinical Aspects,* edited by J. J. Bonica, P. Procacci, and C. A. Pagni, pp. 36–63. Charles C Thomas, Springfield, Ill.
21. Wall, P. D., and Gutnick, M. (1974): Ongoing activity in peripheral nerves: The physiology and pharmacology of impulses originating from a neuroma. *Exp. Neurol.,* 43:580–593.
22. Wall, P. D., Waxman, S., and Basbaum, A. I. (1974): Ongoing activity in peripheral nerve: Injury discharge. *Exp. Neurol.,* 45:576–589.

Advances in Pain Research and Therapy, Vol. 2,
edited by J. J. Bonica and V. Ventafridda.
Raven Press, New York © 1979.

Role and Limits of Anticancer Drugs in the Treatment of Advanced Cancer Pain

Gianni Bonadonna* and Roberto Molinari**

** Division of Clinical Oncology F, Istituto Nazionale Tumori, Milan, Italy; ** Division of Clinical Oncology C, Istituto Nazionale Tumori, Milan, Italy*

For nonmedical people, the image of cancer has always been associated with the fear of prolonged, severe, and intractable pain. Today, despite significant progress achieved with specific drug regimens as well as sophisticated supportive measures, a considerable number of cancer patients die with poorly controlled pain due to progressive disease in some "trigger zones."

In recent years, the medical treatment for various forms of neoplastic disease has markedly improved in terms of strategy, number of effective drugs, and incidence of favorable response. The medical approach to advanced cancer can now be regarded as an established method of therapy with either curative or palliative purposes depending on the histology and stage of the neoplasm. Furthermore, in a large number of patients treated in the United States of America and in Europe, specific drug therapy is administered by qualified physicians.

The specific impact of medical treatment on pain produced by advanced cancer has not yet been the subject of a detailed report. The main reason is probably that, by tradition, the response to anticancer drugs has been considered significant only when documented by an objective regression of measurable parameters (Table 1). Because of frequent concomitant supportive measures, subjective improvement alone, including pain-relief, was almost never regarded as a meaningful response to anticancer drugs (3).

The aim of this report is to summarize briefly the current status of medical treatment for advanced cancer and to delineate those clinical situations in which various anticancer drugs, alone or in conjunction with specific local modalities, are indicated to control pain produced by progressive tumors.

ANTICANCER DRUGS AND THEIR ACTIVITY IN ADVANCED TUMORS

A relatively small number of drugs of different classes are now available for the treatment of advanced cancer. Table 2 lists the most important com-

TABLE 1. *Current criteria for objective evaluation of drug response in advanced solid tumors*

1. *Complete Remission* (*CR*): Complete disappearance of all known disease including recalcification of all osteolytic metastases for at least 1 month.
2. *Partial Remission* (*PR*): A decrease of 50% or greater in the product of the two largest perpendicular diameters of all measurable lesions including partial recalcification of osteolytic metastases for a minimum of 1 month.
3. *Objective Improvement* (*OI*): A decrease of 25–50% of the product of the two largest perpendicular diameters of all measurable lesions with no change in osseous metastases.
4. *Progression*: An increase of 25% or greater over original measurements in the product of the two largest perpendicular diameters of measurable lesions, irrespective of concomitant regression in other tumor sites and/or occurrence of new lesions.
5. *Recurrence*: Appearance of new lesions or increase in the product of the two largest perpendicular diameters of measurable lesions by 50% over the size recorded at the initiation of therapy following a period of initial response or a period of no change.

pounds utilized in clinical practice. They are currently being administered in numerous combinations and through a wide range of dose schedules.

The medical literature is overloaded with publications from different institutions reporting the therapeutic results of a variety of drug regimens in different forms of advanced solid tumors. An effort to summarize those results and relate them to specific combinations is beyond the scope of this report, and the readers are referred to specific publications (1,2,4). Table 3 simply outlines the average response rate currently being obtained with anticancer drugs.

The table indicates that, irrespective of the drug combination utilized, many forms of solid tumors are now showing objective response to specific medical therapy. Although a satisfactory control of most forms of cancer is still far

TABLE 2. *Main anticancer drugs utilized in clinical practice*

Class	Drugs
Alkylating agents	mechlorethamine, cyclophosphamide, chlorambucil, melphalan, busulfan
Antimetabolites	methotrexate, fluorouracil, mercaptopurine, thioguanine, cytosine arabinoside
Plant alkaloids	vinblastine, vincristine, VP-16, VM-26
Antibiotics	adriamycin, daunomycin, bleomycin, actinomycin D, mitomycin C
Hormones	androgens, estrogens, antiestrogens, progestogens, corticosteroids
Miscellaneous	procarbazine, dacarbazine, hydroxyurea, cis-platinum, hexamethylmelamine, dibromodulcitol, nitrosoureas (BCNU, CCNU, MeCCNU, streptozotocin), asparaginase

TABLE 3. *Average expected response rate with various drug combinations in advanced solid tumors*

Neoplasia	CR (%)	CR + PR (%)
Hodgkin's disease	70–80	85–95
Non-Hodgkin's lymphomas	50–60	60–80
Wilms's tumor	60–70	70–80
Testicular cancer	60–70	85–95
Ovarian cancer	25–30	70–80
Breast cancer	12–20	50–70
Soft-tissue sarcomas		
children	30–40	70–80
adults	< 10	25–35
Lung cancer		
small-cell cancer	30–40	70–90
non-small-cell cancer	20–30	40–60
Bladder cancer	< 20	50–60
Head and neck cancer[a]	20–30	40–60
Ewing's sarcoma	< 20	50–60
Gastric cancer	< 15	20–35
Colorectal cancer	< 10	20–30
Endometrial cancer	10–20	40–60
Epidermoid ca. (cervix, esophagus)	< 20	30–40
Malignant melanoma	< 10	20–30

[a] squamous

from being obtained, it cannot be denied that available drug treatments are currently able to produce good partial remission (PR) and even complete remission (CR) in some neoplastic diseases for which 10 years ago only supportive therapy was available. As a general rule, the achievement of significant response (CR + PR) is almost always translated into an improved survival compared with nonresponders. Furthermore, in a fraction of patients with specific forms of neoplasia (pediatric tumors, lymphomas, testicular cancer, ovarian cancer) complete remission of the neoplastic disease is followed by a prolonged disease-free survival compatible with cure (1,2,4).

Table 4 summarizes the main reasons for the limited efficacy of available anticancer drugs in advanced neoplastic disease. The words "inherent low susceptibility" oversimplify the fact that many solid tumors (e.g., gastrointestinal, bronchogenic, renal, thyroid, and epidermoid carcinomas, as well as many adult sarcomas) show only a moderate to minimal response to agents which are very effective in other forms of cancer (e.g., lymphomas, Wilms's tumor, embryonal carcinoma of testicle). Our ignorance as to why certain types of neoplastic cells do respond to given drugs whereas others do not remain vast. However, few reasons for the success or failure of medical therapy have been, in part, elucidated through a number of studies carried out in experimental animals.

TABLE 4. *Main reasons for the limited efficacy of anticancer drugs in advanced cancer*

1. Inherent low susceptibility to available drugs	
2. High tumor cell burden	
Decreased growth fraction	
Prolonged doubling time	
Increased cell loss	
3. Ineffective concentration of drug to the target site for a long enough time (C × T)	
4. Development of drug resistance	
Decreased:	cellular uptake, activation of drug
Increased:	DNA repair, target enzyme, deactivation of drug
5. Development of drug toxicity	
Acute:	e.g., myelosuppression, mucositis
Cumulative:	cardiomyopathy, nephrotoxicity, lung fibrosis

One important reason is represented by the fact that in clinically overt metastatic disease the tumor cell mass ($> 10^{10}$) is too high to be effectively eradicated or reduced by current drug combinations. In large tumor masses many cells are temporarily nondividing (G_0 or prolonged G_1 phase) and are only partially or completely insensitive to drugs, depending on the class of drug and the disease entity. Another reason is related to the pharmacokinetics of drugs in patients. Even if a tumor is susceptible to a drug, it cannot influence the tumor in a favorable way unless the drug reaches the target site and remains there in tumoricidal concentration (C) for a long enough period of time (T) to bring about the desired effect. The effectiveness of an antitumor agent is directly related to its C × T which is markedly affected by dose and schedule. The optimum C × T should kill the maximum tumor cells with minimum lethality in cells of normal tissue.

To be effective, in most cases chemotherapy must be repeated over long intervals. Under these circumstances, repetitive exposure of tumor cells to chemicals can lead to clinical resistance to drugs. The clinician is faced with a two-fold problem: the regrowth of tumor cells between cycles of therapy (which must be separated by intervals sufficient to allow recovery of normal tissue) and reduced amounts of tumor-cell kill with subsequent cycles of treatment owing to the development of resistant cell lines. Largely on the basis of experimental animal systems, various mechanisms have been proposed for the development of resistance.

In susceptible tumors, the eradication of the last neoplastic cell is theoretically possible with chemotherapy, but the toxic effect of drugs on normal cells represents an important limiting factor. Cyclic chemotherapy currently represents the most effective measure to minimize severe bone-marrow suppression as well as oral and intestinal mucositis. Cumulative toxicity can be prevented in the large majority of patients by discontinuing the administration of a given drug before the total risk dose is reached.

ANTICANCER DRUGS AND PAIN-CONTROL OF ADVANCED TUMORS

Several tumor factors are involved in many clinical situations characterized by pain. Table 5 summarizes some of the more obvious mechanisms by which pain is produced in advanced cancer. While a detailed discussion of pain mechanisms is beyond the scope of this chapter, the reader should remember that usually more than one factor can be present at the same time in a given situation (e.g., obstruction plus infection, pressure plus destruction of tissue).

Table 6 outlines the main factors responsible for the limited efficacy of anticancer drugs alone. First of all, solid tumors which often produce pain symptoms usually do not respond well to current drug regimens. In fact, complete remission occurs in less than one-third of patients, and in the large majority of cases is short-lived. Pain is often produced by large tumor masses and, as previously mentioned, a high tumor burden is inversely related to the incidence of a satisfactory drug response. Furthermore, since pain usually develops in late stages of the disease, second- or third-line drug treatments yield a minimal response rate. Finally, in certain target sites (e.g., head and neck area, pelvis) prior radical surgery and especially prior irradiation negatively affect in almost every patient the vascular supply, thus preventing an effective drug $C \times T$.

Despite the aforementioned limitations, effective first-line drug therapy

TABLE 5. *Principal mechanisms by which pain is produced in advanced cancer*

1. Infection	lowered resistance, poor drainage, ulceration of skin or mucous membranes
2. Obstruction	occlusion of a hollow viscus by a tumor mass; occlusion of large vein or artery
3. Destruction of tissue	destruction of bone, skin, soft tissue, and viscera
4. Pressure	growth of tumor in closed areas and/or compression of nervous structures
5. Visceral pain	direct involvement by tumor, rapid enlargement of a viscus due to cancer

TABLE 6. *Main reasons for the limited efficacy of anticancer drugs on pain of advanced malignancies*

1. Many solid tumors associated with pain symptoms are not sufficiently responsive to current drug regimens.
2. Pain usually develops in late stages when the tumor has become resistant to first-line drug therapy.
3. Pain is often produced by large tumor masses.
4. Prior surgery and especially prior radiotherapy applied to the target site almost always prevent effective drug C × T.

does produce pain-relief along with objective tumor regression. Some practical examples are provided in Table 7. For instance, advanced local breast cancer may be painful when inflammatory reaction distends the breast, when local extensive infiltration of the chest wall occurs, and when the tumor ulcerates. In all these situations, medical therapy (chemotherapy and/or endocrine therapy) produces complete plus partial remission in 50 to 70%, and the objective response is almost always associated with marked regression and even disappearance of pain. In contrast, in the presence of skeletal metastases, tumor response to drugs is usually slow, and pain-control is best

TABLE 7. *Activity of current drug regimens on pain characteristics of certain tumors*

Disease	Pain characteristics	Drug activity on pain[a]
Breast cancer	Tumor ulceration, infiltration of chest wall	+++
	Skeletal metastases	++
	Lymphedema of the arm (supraclavicular recurrence)	+
Prostate cancer	Skeletal metastases	+++
Leukemia, myeloma	Periosteal irritation or invasion, medullary pressure	+++
	Headache (meningeal infiltration)	+++
Lymphomas	Back pain (para-aortic adenopathy)	++++
	Spinal-cord compression	++
Testicular cancer	Back pain (para-aortic adenopathy)	++
Lung cancer	Superior sulcus (Pancoast) tumors	+
Colorectal, cervical, or bladder cancer	Low abdominal, perineal, or back pain due to pelvic recurrence	+
Oral, pharyngeal cancer	Tumor ulceration, invasion of nervous structures (e.g., earache)	++
Intracranial tumors	Headache (increased pressure)	+[b]

[a] ++++ complete relief; +++ very good, but incomplete relief; ++ fair relief; + little relief.
[b] Corticosteroids excluded.

achieved by combining drugs with radiotherapy. On the other hand, in prostate cancer, endocrine therapy (orchiectomy, estrogens) produces a high and prompt response rate. Therefore, palliative radiation therapy is utilized only in the late stages of the disease. However, radiation therapy is always the treatment of first choice when supraclavicular adenopathy in breast cancer produces compression of the brachial plexus and lymphedema of the arm.

Diffuse bone pain often occurs at the onset or during the course of multiple myeloma as well as in leukemia with high peripheral blood count. In acute leukemia a frequent cause of pain is meningeal infiltration. In all these situations, initial chemotherapy is successful in producing a prompt remission. This is particularly true in leukemia whereas in myeloma, radiation therapy is often indicated, especially in the presence of bone fractures.

Large retroperitoneal adenopathies can produce back pain. This is promptly and well controlled by anticancer drugs in all types of malignant lymphomas, less well in testicular cancer. The tumors of the thoracic inlet, sometimes called superior sulcus or Pancoast tumors, involve the nerves of the brachial plexus and the sympathetic chain and are characterized by severe shoulder and arm pain. Although combination chemotherapy can produce a fairly prompt objective remission in about 50% of patients, the degree of tumor regression is usually not sufficient to achieve satisfactory pain-control. Therefore, it is always advisable to combine chemotherapy with irradiation. This strategy should also be applied to intracranial tumors (either primary or metastatic) when not resectable. In fact, available drugs such as nitrosoureas do not induce a satisfactory remission rate which could relieve a severe and persistent headache.

Recurrence of various types of tumors in the low abdomen, in the pelvis as well as in the pharyngeal and cervical regions, often produces pain which is difficult to control by means of anticancer drugs. The large majority of tumors with recurrence in these sites have been previously subjected to extensive surgery and irradiation. For this reason, almost always drug C × T is ineffective. To circumvent this situation, intra-arterial drug infusion has been attempted, mainly in head and neck area. In spite of the above-mentioned modifications of blood supply, the immediate results on pain symptoms are often dramatic, irrespective of the degree of objective response. However, intra-arterial chemotherapy can not be continued for more than 15 to 30 days because of frequent local complications. Therefore, remission is commonly for a short period and requires further systemic chemotherapy to be maintained. In spite of some progress recently achieved in head and neck cancer (5), in clinical situations where severe and protracted pain is caused by infiltration of nervous structures, conventional analgesics, nerve blocks, and/or neurosurgical procedures must be considered as the treatments of choice, rather than waiting for the response of a second or third-line chemotherapy.

CONCLUSION

Medical therapy, and especially cyclical combination chemotherapy, can produce a prompt relief of cancer-induced pain only if the tumor is usually well or fairly well responsive to anticancer drugs. To achieve a prompt and satisfactory pain-relief, anticancer drugs should also be administered as first-line chemotherapy, in patients whose target sites were not previously subjected to extensive surgery and/or radiotherapy and in the absence of very large tumor masses. In the large majority of clinical situations, pain-control is the result of a combined team approach which includes medical oncologists, radiation therapists, neurosurgeons, and anesthesiologists. Although several techniques were recently standardized, optimal management is often the result of an individualized approach.

REFERENCES

1. Carter, S. K., Bakowski, M. T., and Hellmann, K. (1977): *Chemotherapy of Cancer.* John Wiley & Sons, New York.
2. Clarysse, A., Kenis, Y., and Mathé, G. (1976): *Cancer Chemotherapy: Its Role in the Treatment Strategy of Hematologic Malignancies and Solid Tumors. Recent Results in Cancer Research, 53.* Springer-Verlag, Berlin.
3. Karnofsky, D. A. (1961): Meaningful clinical classification of therapeutic responses to anticancer drugs. *Clin. Pharmacol. Ther.,* 2:709–712.
4. Holland, J., and Frei, E., III (1978): *Cancer Medicine,* 2nd ed. Lea & Febiger, Philadelphia.
5. Molinari, R., Mattavelli, F., Cantu', G., et al. (1979): Results of a low-dose, double synchronizing sequence of polychemotherapy (VBM) in the palliative treatment of oral and oropharyngeal squamous cell carcinoma. *Eur. J. Cancer (in press).*

Advances in Pain Research and Therapy, Vol. 2,
edited by J. J. Bonica and V. Ventafridda.
Raven Press, New York © 1979.

Role and Limits of Oncologic Chemotherapy of Advanced Cancer Pain

Georges Brulé

Medical Oncology Unit, Institut Gustave-Roussy, 94800 Villejuif, France

The previous chapter was focused on chemotherapeutics which would delay or inhibit metastatic extension. Unfortunately, despite properly administered medication, a large number of patients do reach the stage of general dissemination, with all the sufferings which accompany this condition. Various mechanisms may be at the origin of oncologic pain including: (a) invasion or compression of the nervous network through the neoplastic process or peritumoral edema; (b) lymphatic or venous stasis; and (c) distant repercussion of a pelvic tumor such as lumbalgia, or renal colic, etc. Therefore, anything which can reduce the size of the tumor will logically lead to relief of pain; chemotherapy manifests its action following this principle but equally by some other processes which still remain obscure.

Antimitotic drugs are far from being harmless and often prove to be highly toxic, particularly in patients in poor general condition either as a result of the disease or previous medication. The whole problem is to find the proper balance between the risk of toxic phenomena and the advantages one may expect from chemotherapy.

It may be recalled that during cancer proliferation, the cells multiply unceasingly and, when the critical mass is reached, their erratic growth leads to the death of the host organism. Moreover, regardless of the mode of cell growth or on the principles of chemotherapy, a given dose of drug will kill a constant proportion and not a constant number of cells, whatever be the number of cells existing during the treatment. Hence, the greater the number of cells existing at the time of medication, the less is the chance of reducing significantly the size of the tumor. It therefore follows that because of this fractional destruction, the proper elimination of the tumor-cell population can only be obtained either by increasing the dose of the drug or drugs within the limit tolerable to the host, or by starting the treatment when the number of cells is still small in the hope of completely destroying the tumor. For patients with advanced cancer, this approach is not possible, because they have already a large number of tumor cells. Therefore, the problem is essentially dosage-oriented. Unlike what very many physicians believe, oncologic chemotherapeutic agents may be more selectively cytotoxic toward cancer cells than normal cells of the host. We will see later that some drugs are more particularly indicated for some anatomic locations or for some types of cancer. Only a fairly small number of cells do proliferate and are chemosensitive, the remainder being quiescent, as they are anoxic or in the process of necrosis.

In order to be effective for most patients, chemotherapy must be repeated at regular intervals so as to allow restoration of normal cell mitosis between each course. Under such conditions, the repeated action of chemical agents or tumor cells may lead to a clinical resistance to the drug. Then, the physician faces a dual problem: (a) the recurrence of tumor growth between courses, which must be sufficiently spaced so as to enable restitution of normal tissues; and (b) reduction of death of tumor cells during later courses because of the occurrence of resistance to drug therapy.

The various mechanisms which may explain the occurrence of this resistance are not known, but it is clear that resistance to anticancer drug makes the problem of advanced cancer treatment even more difficult to solve. The success of any medication depends on the number of resistant lines in the tumor population and the available therapeutic armamentarium as to elaborate effective combination. In addition to the mechanism of cell resistance, other factors inherent in the host may cause an apparent reduction of tumor cells' sensitivity. For example, these factors may interfere with the reduction of the concentration of active ingredient in tumor cells.

The hope of overcoming drug resistance has probably been the most important stimulus for the study of various drug combinations. Similarly, the combination of radiotherapy and chemotherapy has led to target cells in the resting phase which are sensitive to radiotherapy, while they are actually resistant to chemotherapy. Moreover, the toxicity of healthy tissues is different. Normal tissues with a high mitotic index of frequent cell renewal are very sensitive, for example, hematopoietic tissue or digestive epithelium, whereas the conjunctive tissue near the tumor is more sensitive to radiation and allows better penetration of the drug into the tumor. If the combination of radiotherapy and chemotherapy does potentiate the effect of the drug, it also increases the effect of the drug on healthy tissue.

The therapeutic armamentarium of the oncologist has progressed considerably over the last 30 years. Now we have a wide range of drugs having various modes of action, degree of toxicity, and spectrum of effectiveness. Within the framework of this presentation, I cannot describe all of them. Therefore, I shall refer to some drugs used either separately or in combination for some pain syndromes. I will purposefully not discuss dosage because it can vary considerably, depending on the general condition of the patient, the integrity of the core cancer cells, and possible impairment of hepatic and renal functions.

Often patients with advanced cancer have diffuse bone metastases and have in most cases received radiation therapy over a wide target area. Therefore, the initial dosage must be lowered. It must be adapted for each patient. In such circumstances, it is difficult to draw general rules. For most oncologic drugs, administered alone or in combination, it is the destruction of medullar cells which remains the main restriction for the dosage.

A complete hematologic examination just before each chemotherapeutic course is essential. Nevertheless, as these drugs alone or in combination are more effective at full doses, it is preferable to allow more time to elapse between courses than to reduce the doses. In case of severe medullar impairment, adequate precaution may have to be taken, but only a very small number of centers happen to be in a position to cater for such circumstances. Some sensitive tumors may equally, after rapid resorption, cause nephropathy through precipitation of uric acid stones. To prevent this complication, it is therefore essential that the patient takes enough liquid, to keep his urine alkaline and to give him allopurinol during the chemotherapy.

Among 50 drugs currently prescribed by oncologists in specialized hospitals, some are particularly indicated for certain anatomic locations or certain histologic types of tumors which may at times be very specific. The best example is given by hormonodependent carcinomas for which high dose of hormones, often synthetic hormones, will act electively. I will not elaborate on this subject since it will be discussed elsewhere, but it may be recalled that for breast or prostate cancer, it is not a hormonal but a chemical effect which is involved. The best demonstration of this fact is brought by some forms of cancer which apparently have nothing to do with hormones, for example, hypernephroma. In 20% of such cases, the administration of very high doses of progestational agents will give positive results. Such synthetic hormones may equally be indicated not only in endometrial carcinoma but also in some forms of ovarian cancer, even though this mode of action remains debatable.

Streptozotocin, whose mode of action is unknown, is an extremely toxic drug to the kidney, but at the dose of 1 $g/m^2/week$, it manifests specific effectiveness on secretory tumors of the pancreas, that is, tumors of the islets of Langerhans. Similarly, endocrine tumors of the adrenal and their usual pulmonary metastases do not respond to any hormonal treatment, but they are very sensitive to mithotane, a derivative of DTT which manifests a specific necrotic action on normal or pathologic adrenal cortex.

Apart from these two examples of almost specific action on very rarely encountered tumors, many currently administered products show some tropism, either toward some tissues or toward some histologic forms. For example, tumors of the central nervous system, which are protected by the meningeal barrier, are normally resistant to all substances administered by the systemic route because these products do not pool in the nervous tissue. Nitrosourea derivatives offer a striking advantage because they cross the meningeal barrier and enough concentration is obtained in the brain and the spinal cord, so that unlike other products they are effective not only on primarily cerebral tumors, but also in some cases of metastasis. Derivatives of podophyllotoxin, such as VM-26, equally seem to be able to cross the serosa, and that is why the combination VM-26–BCNU may preferably be used in case of cerebrally located secondaries of tumors regardless of the primary location. Finally, it must be mentioned that for meningeal and cerebral localization of acute leukemia, methotrexate may well be injected by the intraspinal route to relieve the terrible headache caused by meningitis during certain forms of leukemia or hematosarcoma, lymphoblastic sarcoma in particular.

5-Fluorouracil is an antipyrimidin extensively used in oncologic chemotherapy. This drug seems to act selectively on the hepatic tissue, particularly on hepatic metastasis of tumors of the colon. Besides this, it also applies to almost all tumors of glandular origin. The more acute the hepatic metastasis with rapid development (whether accompanied by fever or not), the greater are the chances of 5-fluorouracil's being effective. In such cases, the patient is generally very ill, febrile, and suffering dreadfully from the hepatic lesion. Infusions of 15 mg 5-fluorouracil/kg/day during 5 to 6 days will cause dramatic remission in 35% of the patients, and this may extend over several months when courses of 5 days a month are given, even in the absence of corticoids or other products.

When studying the effectiveness of derivatives of doxorubicin, adriamycin, or duborimycin, it occurred to us that duborimycin manifests a particularly specific and unaccountable action on often-unbearable pain of bone metastasis of breast cancer. In a group of 20 patients, pain was relieved in 65% of cases, while radiologically the lesions had remained absolutely unchanged and calcemia had not improved (1). This action of duborimycin is much less marked for adriamycin and seems less obvious for rubidasone, another derivative of this family of drugs.

Mithramycin, which has been abandoned because of its great toxicity at oncologic dose, yields hypocalcemic action at low dose and relieves muscular pain and digestive disorders caused by hypercalcemia, which is so frequent during advanced cancer, particularly in breast cancer.

Very high dose of cyclophosphamide as infusion of 2 g in 30 min often leads to dramatic relief of pain and dyspnea of bronchopulmonary cancer, in particular oat-cell forms which are relatively chemosensitive but grow very rapidly.

Amongst other currently administered drugs, bleomycin seems to show specificity for upper-digestive epidermoid cancer. Described by other authors, this fact has not been confirmed at Gustave-Roussy Institute.

On the other hand, Japanese investigators have reported that mitomycin is particularly effective in large stomach tumors, which do not in general respond to any other chemotherapy. This product is also useful in local or regional spreading which follows such tumors.

It must also be recalled that actinomycin D shows some specificity for embryonary tumors or for some tumors in children, melphalan in ovarian tumors, and decarbazine or DTIC in some melanomas. The effectiveness of the last three products is at times debatable, but it is useful to include them in therapeutic combination which may be used in the treatment of such tumors. For example, in case of melanomas, the combination of decarbazine with vincristine and adriamycin may prove effective.

A wide range of possibilities occurs for the combination of drugs. The same applies for their dosage and schedule of administration. The combination of antimitotic drugs is theoretically based on our knowledge of cell kinetics and biochemical properties of these substances. Actually, clinical results and dogmatic expectations are not always in agreement. Therefore, all these combinations are more essentially based on some empirism and chemotherapeutic experience rather than concrete data. Without going into details, the essential principles are the following:

1. used simultaneously or sequentially, drugs which act at various stages of the cell cycle; for example, an antimetabolite which acts on the synthesis, an alkylating agent which acts on DNA, and a spindle poison which will exert its effect during mitosis. By multiplying the cycles and possibly by changing the substances, one may expect to target a maximum number of cancer cells.
2. all these drugs exert toxic effects on different targets (hematopoietic system, digestive tract, nervous system, kidney, myocardium, etc.) and should therefore be so combined that their respective side effects do not occur concomitantly; hence maximum dosage may be given while avoiding cumulative toxicity.

Table 1 shows a combination which is very often used in the treatment of advanced breast cancer. The first substance used, an alkaloid obtained from the periwinkle, is a poison for the spindle. It acts during mitosis and essentially manifests neurologic toxicity. The second is an alkylating agent and shows mild hematologic toxicity. At times, it causes cystitis. The third one is an antimetabolite. It manifests side effects mainly on the digestive tract and the bone marrow. An interval of 4 weeks between each course causes restoration of normal cells, which occurs more rapidly than for tumor cells.

Examples of such combinations are unlimited in number: For embryonic tumors, actinomycin D is in general combined with cyclophosphamide and methotrexate. In case of resistance to this combination, cis-platinum (CDDP)-bleomycin-vincaleucoblastine sulphate may, in very advanced cases, lead to regression of fairly long duration.

TABLE 1. *Drug combinations used for breast cancer*

Day 1–2	i.v.d. vincristine without exceeding 1 mg
Day 3–4–5–6	i.v.d. Endoxan® without exceeding 400 mg
Day 3–4–5–6	infusion over 1½ hr 5-fluorouracil 500 mg/m^2

Moreover, it may be recalled that the adjunction of heparin to all these chemotherapeutics, either alone or in combination, may, according to some authors, potentiate their therapeutic effects without increasing their toxicity.

Hematosarcomas, leukemias, and other such diseases do respond to several drugs. Unfortunately, they have a tendency to relapse, and it is in this type of disease that some products may serve as substitution to classic medications: for example, L-asparaginase or methyl-glyoxal.

L-Asparaginase in blastic transformation of lymphosarcomas may lead to new remission in patients in apparently desperate condition. The same applies with methyl-glyoxal-bis in blastic transformation of chronic myeloid leukemia having become resistant to Misulban® or other classic therapeutics.

Vindesine, the latest alkaloid of the periwinkle, leads to a high proportion of remission in acute lymphoid leukemia. Some resistant cases of lymphosarcoma and Hodgkin's disease respond to this medication. The most effective daily dosage seems to be 2 mg/m^2 administered as i.v. infusion during 2 days.

As already stated, patients suffering from advanced cancer have, in general, new drugs or original drug combinations. In case of success or transitory improvement, this may lead to the elaboration of an optimal chemotherapy for the treatment of disseminated cancer and finally the integration of local or regional neoplasms. Therefore, this approach shows that, in no circumstance, should the oncologist despair even when the patient appears to be in the ultimate stage. He should always attempt to test new combinations and, in so doing, he may be providing a contribution to the care of other patients. The severity of side effects caused by the treatment should be the only limiting factor to the therapeutic regimen. If there is no hope of recovery and if pain remains unbearable, one must not increase the patient's discomfort through therapeutic insistence. On the other hand, in case of intolerable pain, an effort to find new combinations, even including high-dosage corticosteroids, should delay the use of major analgesics with all the side effects which such drugs may have on the patient's personality. [*Editors' Note:* We vehemently disagree with Dr. Brulé's last statement. The patient's pain *must* be relieved by one of the other modalities, including the use of potent narcotics, while chemotherapy is being tried.]

REFERENCES

1. Brulé, G., Chauvergne, J., Clavel, B., Carton, M., Klein, T., Gary Bobo, J., Guerrin, J., and Pommatau, E. (1975): Essai de chimiothérapie anticancéreuse par la Duborimycine. *Bull. Cancer (Paris)*, 63:41–58.

Advances in Pain Research and Therapy, Vol. 2,
edited by J. J. Bonica and V. Ventafridda.
Raven Press, New York © 1979.

The Role of Endocrine Therapy for Relief of Pain Due to Advanced Cancer

F. Pannuti, A. Martoni, A. P. Rossi, and E. Piana

Division of Oncology, Marcello Malpighi Hospital, 40138 Bologna, Italy

In our experience, pain due to cancer can be basically attributed to: (a) compression and/or infiltration of nerve structures by the neoplastic process; (b) inflammatory process around or within a tumor; and (c) the action of chemical mediators. In the first and second and, more rarely, the third types, pain is located in the region of the tumor or referred to the distribution of the nerves involved and follows the evolution or development of the tumor. In the third type, pain is usually widespread systemically. This report will confine itself to local pain as a direct expression of the presence of neoplastic lesions and in relation to the influence that can be exerted on it by hormonal therapy in the region of so-called "hormone-sensitive tumors."

Of 291 patients with advanced solid tumors treated in our Division of Oncology during the first 4 months of 1977, 186 or 63.9% had moderate to severe pain. The incidence of pain in patients with specific tumors was as follows: 68% with breast cancer (117 of 171 patients); 67% with stomach cancers (14 of 21 patients); 59% with cancer of the prostate (10 of 17 patients); 58% with intestinal tumors (14 of 24 patients); 57% with lung tumors (23 of 40 patients); 55% with kidney tumors (11 of 20 patients); and 47% with head and neck tumors (7 of 15 patients).

Since 1973, we have been carrying out studies on the use of high doses of medroxyprogesterone acetate (MAP) which is capable of having a significant beneficial effect on the pain of these patients (see below). Figure 1 shows the percentage rate of patients who died in pain during the 4-year period 1972 to 1976 (pain evaluation was carried out 15 days before death). Although it is slight, the percentage drop of patients with breast cancer should be noted.

BASIC CONSIDERATIONS

Neoplastic pain is assessed in different ways and with different aims in clinical semiology and pharmacology.

Clinical Considerations

Pain as a symptom can be made use of in diagnosing disease and in the differential diagnosis of several possible disorders. An example is given in

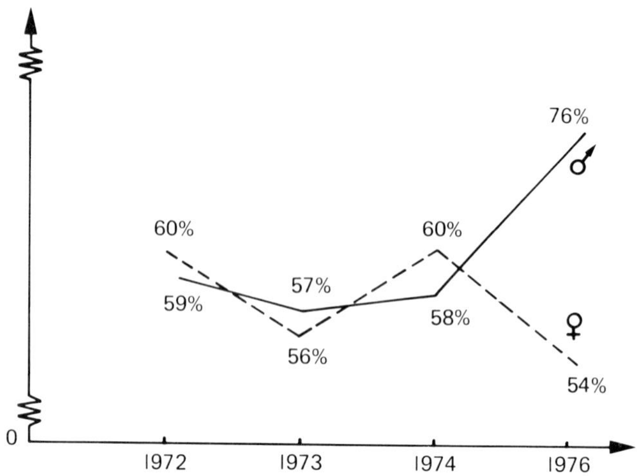

FIG. 1. Percentage rate of patients that die in pain (pain evaluation carried out 15 days before death).

Table 1. The clinical definition of pain is important for a prompt diagnosis of recurrence. The case shown in Fig. 2 refers to a patient who had been subjected to rectal amputation and had intense pain situated in the perineal region. The pain regressed partially only following anticancer therapy. However, clinical evidence for relapse already had existed before the chemotherapy course was effected (location, features, type of pain intensity, lack of sensitivity to anti-inflammatory drugs). Another example is provided by acute colicky pain localized in the liver as an early symptom of hepatic metastases in patients who have had mastectomy for carcinoma of the breast.

Definition of "signal-symptom" includes the clinical, biologic, and hematologic elements capable of characterizing the neoplastic disease in relation

TABLE 1. *Differential diagnosis of painful conditions in the chest*

Characteristics of the pain (location, quality, etc.)	Benign disease of the breast	Cancer of the breast	Angina pectoris	Thoracic neuropathy	Arthrosis
Superficial	+	−	−	+	−
Stable localization	−	+	+	+	+
Diffuse	+	−	−	−	−
Spreading from the breast	−	−	+	+	+
Rapid onset	+	−	+	−	−
Continuous	−	+	−	+	−
Intense	−	−	+	+	+
Upon effort or movement	−	−	+	+	+

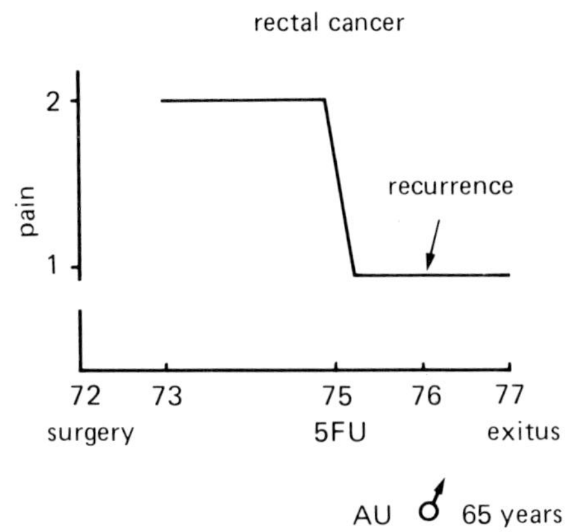

FIG. 2. Patient discussed in text (p. 146) with severe perineal pain partially relieved with 5-fluoro-uracil therapy. Vertical axis pain intensity (2—severe; 1—moderate; 0—none) and horizontal axis time in weeks.

to the treatment adopted. Pain as a signal-symptom in oncology is, by definition, a direct expression of the local presence of the neoplastic lesion and is also capable of indicating with an acceptable degree of clinical approximation the evolution of the disease in relation to the treatment adopted.

Pain as a signal-symptom should be distinguished from non-neoplastic pain and from pain which, even though it is related to the neoplastic process, is not a reliable indication of the evolution of the disease in terms of expansion or regression of the neoplastic mass. An example of the latter is provided by pain due to pathologic fractures of the vertebra. When pain is present as an isolated event during remission of the disease, pain is to be attributed only to fracture rather than to the expansion of the neoplastic process. Even though pain, in this sense, is an index of objective worsening of the patient's conditions (e.g., occurrence of paraplegia in the lower limbs), in itself it is *not* an indication of the failure of the anticancer treatment that may be in progress. It is more probable that the treatment should be integrated into other modalities such as radiotherapy and orthopedic measures.

Pain as a signal-symptom serves to (a) monitor the disease during treatment, and (b) appraise the final results of the treatment. To this end, it should be defined in a qualitative-quantitative fashion. For this purpose, we use the following rating: *grade 0*—absent; *grade 1*—moderate, for which the patient requires not more than one analgesic every 24 hr; *grade 2*—intense, for which the patient requires more than one analgesic every 24 hr. A significant change in pain is referred to only when the change involves the move from one grade to another.

Method of Use of the Pain Rating (43,50)

The patient is told that he can freely avail himself of a certain type of analgesic drug (e.g., acetylsalicylic acid, pentazocine, etc.) in a quantity not exceeding a specified limit in a 24-hr period (e.g., not more than three 0.5-g tablets of acetylsalicylic acid or two 30-mg vials of pentazocine). The physician simply records the quantity of analgesic drug taken during the 24-hr period. These conditions mean that only the *subjective assessment* of the patient is involved.

An advantage of this rating is that only three degrees of intensity of pain are involved. A simple code of this kind is better suited to practical routine clinical evaluations compared with those involving 5 or 6 grades of intensity. Although the latter may be more precise, they are influenced by the fact that both the patient's and the physician's subjective judgments become involved to a greater degree than the simpler rating.

PAIN AND HORMONE THERAPY

From a pharmacologic point of view, pain as a signal-symptom has different meaning and different features in (a) clinical drug tolerance and (b) pharmacodynamics.

Pain and Clinical Drug Tolerance

The administration of hormones for cancer therapy can lead to the production of pain. Obviously, no problems exist in interpreting local pain following intramuscular administration. On the other hand, when the hormone is given intravenously, problems of differential diagnosis can develop. The clinical features that enable a symptom to be categorized as a side effect and not as a symptom of the tumor are the following: (a) continuous pain following administration of the drug; (b) the pain ceases with the end of the metabolic phase responsible for the pain; (c) the site or sites of pain are not subject to change; and (d) the quality of the pain.

An example is provided by pain arising following administration of diethylstilbestrol diphosphate (DES-P). The pain is quite specific, as it arises during intravenous administration and reaches a climax in a few minutes. It then disappears after 5 to 15 min and reappears each time the drug is administered. The pain is usually located in the perineal region (but can also appear at the site of metastases) and is experienced as a burning sensation.

Pain and Pharmacodynamics

Hormone Interference

The concept of hormone dependence is based on Huggins' (24,25) clinical and experimental observation that cancer cells, like the normal cells from which they originate, "depend" on the activity of one hormone or more for their metabolism and proliferation. The term *hormone dependence,* according to Tagnon (23,66), has a tendency to oversimplify the relationship between cancer cells and hormones. The administration of estrogens, for example, can induce breast cancer both in man and in animals, and ovariectomy previous to menopause can induce remission in approximately 40% of patients with advanced breast cancer. However, it is also true that small doses of estrogens stimulate the evolution of the disease, whereas higher doses have an inhibiting effect. This is why Tagnon suggests replacing *"hormone dependence* with the term *hormone sensitivity*. In other words, the breast cancer cells do not necessarily depend on a hormone, but "may" be sensitive to one or more hormones. Some time ago we suggested (51) the use of the term *hormone sensitivity* with the reservation that sensitivity can be "absolute" or "relative" (in relation to one hormone or more, or depending on the different doses of the same hormone).

The tendency to divide clinical hormone therapy into additive and subtractive types may certainly simplify the issue, but also contains the risk of an imprecise and schematic approach to these cancer patients. Ovariectomy, for example, involves on the one hand the removal of hormones synthesized by the ovaries and on the other an excess production of the corresponding pituitary trophic hormones due to the inactivation of the feedback mechanism. It is also known that, in this kind of situation, the adrenal glands are also able to produce greater amounts of sexual hormones in order to effect compensation. It is apparent that, following surgery, we are faced with a situation entailing both addition and subtraction of hormones, which are all capable of interfering with the growth and reproduction of this kind of tumor cell. For example, administration of hormones such as progestins is in itself an "additive hormone therapy" which involves inhibition of the secretion of a series of hormones at different levels (ovaries, pituitary gland, and perhaps adrenal gland) and a "subtractive" effect which occurs concomitant with the "additive" effect brought about by the therapy itself.

The problem is further complicated by the fact that a few hormones are undoubtedly able to carry out pharmacologically autonomous activity in the host organism and also modify the state of the relationship between the tumor and the organism (for example, immunosuppressive activity of MAP), leading finally to important subjective and objective improvements. This situation validates the statement that these hormones are capable of significantly "interfering" with the evolution of the neoplastic disease. The tumor should not simply be considered as a pool of atypical infiltrating and proliferating cells, but a clinical situation which involves a complex relationship between the tumor cells and the organism.

At this point, we believe that the term *hormone interference* as described above can be introduced into oncologic literature alongside the term *hormone sensitivity*. The latter term stresses the possibility of response to hormone treatment, independently of the problems connected with the direction followed by the response, the type of hormone, or the dosage selected. By using *hormone interference* as a term, we are attempting to shift the emphasis from the cancer cells to the hormone employed in pharmacologic terms with the intention of: (a) underlining the complexity of hormone therapy, as it is usually not only "additive" or "subtractive" but both at the same time; (b) underlining the possibility that interference may be effected at the level of tumor-cell kinetics, regardless of the type of effect the hormone will have; and (c) indicating that the hormone also interferes with the evolution of the tumor with the understanding that the neoplastic disease is to be thought of in its widest clinical sense and therefore also in function of the state of the relationship between the tumor and the host organism.

ENDOCRINE THERAPY AND PAIN RELIEF

Most authors reporting results of anticancer treatment in patients with advanced malignant neoplasms have usually been concerned only with measuring the volume-reduction of the tumor masses. Most writers have neglected and often deliberately excluded the assessment of subjective response, including that relative to pain, because this factor was not thought to be a reliable measure of the effectiveness of the treatment. In this chapter we shall indicate the incidence of relief or remission of pain and other general subjective symptoms as assessed and reported by the authors of the papers reviewed. In this regard it is necessary to mention the almost complete lack of rating systems of pain assessment on the part of therapists and this obviously leads to heterogeneous results which cannot be compared precisely.

Advanced Prostate Cancer

Table 2 lists the results (subjective results and pain whenever possible) derived by patients with advanced cancer of the prostate following orchiectomy, adrenalectomy, or hypophysectomy. Table 3 lists results obtained with additive hormone therapy and in particular with diethylstilbestrol diphosphate (DES-P), cyproterone acetate (CP) and high doses of medroxyprogesterone acetate (MAP) in doses of 1,500 mg intramuscularly (i.m.) per day for 30

TABLE 2. *Results with hormonal therapy in advanced prostate cancer*

Treatment	No. of pts.	Object. rem.	Subject. rem.	Pain rem.	Authors
Hypophysectomy					
surgery	34	n.d.	12(35.2%)	n.d.	Murphy et al. (38)
^{90}Y	13	n.d.	n.d.	11(85%)	Straffon et al. (64)
^{90}Y	74	n.d.	n.d.	51(69%)	Fergusson (19)
Adrenalectomy	4	n.d.	n.d.	1(25%)	Huggins et al. (26)
	10	2(20%)	n.d.	7(70%)	West et al. (74)
	7	n.d.	n.d.	7(100%)	Archimbaud et al. (3)
Orchiectomy	21	n.d.	15(71.4%)	n.d.	Huggins et al. (27)

Legend: Object. rem. = objective remission; Subject. rem. = subjective remission; Pain rem. = pain-remission. Percentages are given in round numbers. n.d. = no data.

TABLE 3. *Results with hormonal therapy for advanced prostate cancer*

Treatment	No. of pts.	Object. rem.	Subject. rem.	Pain rem.	Authors
Estrogens					
(DES-P)	23	n.d.	19/25(76%)	21(91%)	Colapinto et al. (11)
	10	4(40%)	n.d.	5(50%)	Band et al. (5)
	9	4(44%)	n.d.	8(89%)	Susan et al. (65)
Cyproterone	25	n.d.	n.d.	12(48%)	Smith (62)
acetate (CP)	10	8(80%)	n.d.	8(80%)	Scott (59)
Medroxyprogesterone acetate (MAP)					
300 mg/day i.m.	12	n.d.	n.d.	9(75%)	Rafla et al. (54)
500 mg/day i.m.	12	n.d.	n.d.	9(75%)	Bouffioux (8)
1,500 mg/day i.m.	10	n.d.	10/10	10(100%)	Pannuti et al. (53)

Legend: See Table 2.

TABLE 4. *Results of hormonal therapy for advanced prostate cancer pain/subjective remission*

Additive			Ablative		
	No. of pts.	Pain rem. (%)		No. of pts.	Pain rem. (%)
Oestrogens	42	80	Adrenalectomy	21	71
Cyproterone	35	57	Hypophysectomy	87	71
Medroxy-progesterone acetate (MAP)	22	68			
Total	99	70	*Total*	108	71

Legend: See Table 2.

days. Table 4 shows that additive and subtractive methods on the average gave the same percentage of pain relief (around 70%). For additive methods, the highest percentage rate was found with MAP and DES-P, while for subtractive methods the percentage rates for adrenalectomy and hypophysectomy were identical. Our experience concerns the use of high doses of MAP. The experience we have is limited and refers to a "pilot study" that preceded the definition of the protocol which is now being followed and which envisages prospective and randomized comparison of MAP versus DES-P in this kind of patient.

Advanced Endometrial Carcinoma

Table 5 shows results obtained with progestins on subjective response in the advanced stage of endometrial carcinoma. The average remission rate

TABLE 5. *Results of hormonal therapy (progestins) for advanced endometrial cancer*

Treatment	No. of pts.	Object. rem.	Subject. rem.	Pain rem.	Authors
Medroxyprogesterone					
acetate (MAP)	42	17 (40%)	30 (71%)	n.d.	Smith et al. (61)
(<500 mg/day)	13	2 (15%)	11 (85%)	n.d.	Serment et al. (60)
17-Hydroxyprogesterone	176	58 (33%)	123 (70%)	n.d.	Kistner et al. (29)

Legend: See Table 2.

was 71%. It should be noted that these authors used low doses of MAP (less than 500 mg/day). No data relating to incidence of pain-relief are available in the reports.

Advanced Thyroid Cancer

Although there is a large body of literature on the use of hormones for advanced thyroid cancer, no reliable data relating to subjective response and, in particular, pain, are available.

Advanced Clear-Cell Kidney Cancer

The appearance of kidney tumors in male hamsters following estrogen treatment and inhibition of these tumors employing testosterone or progestins

TABLE 6. *Results with hormonal therapy for advanced renal clear-cell cancer*

Treatment	No. of pts.	Object. rem.	Subject rem.	Pain rem.	Authors
Progestins					
(other than MAP)	16	2 (12%)	14 (87%)	n.d.	Talley et al. (67)
	33	2 (6%)	12 (36%)	n.d.	Van der Werfmessing et al. (70)
Androgens	11	n.d.	11 (100%)	n.d.	Talley et al. (67)
Corticosteroids	38	n.d.	38 (100%)	n.d.	Talley et al. (67)
Total	98	n.d.	75 (76%)	n.d.	
Medroxyprogesterone					
acetate (MAP)	8	1 (12%)	7 (87%)	n.d.	Talley et al.[a] (67)
	9	1 (11%)	4 (44%)	n.d.	Van der Werfmessing et al.[a] (70)
	20	2 (10%)	6/14 (43%)	5/12 (42%)	Pannuti et al.[b] (43)
Total	37	4 (11%)	17 (46%)	n.d.	

Legend: See Table 2.
[a] Low doses.
[b] High doses.

(7) suggested the concept of hormone therapy for renal adenocarcinoma. On the basis of these indications, Bloom was the first to use testosterone and subsequently MAP for treating human renal carcinoma, especially the advanced clear-cell variety.

Table 6 lists subjective remission rates obtained by administering androgens, cortisone substances, and progestins with special reference to MAP. Our results refer to the treatment of a group of patients with high doses of MAP (1,500 mg. i.m. per day for 30 days) (46). High doses of MAP are capable of significantly reducing or completely eliminating pain in 42% of the patients with advanced renal cancer. In light of this and considering the low percentage of objective remission, the treatment protocol we are currently using envisages the use of MAP associated with a multiple chemotherapeutic regimen.

Advanced Breast Cancer

Due to the high incidence, the strong tendency to develop skeletal metastases, and the not-infrequent high life-expectancy that advanced cancer patients have, breast cancer is one of the neoplastic situations where pain treatment is most important. There are few details in case statistics assessing pain-remission employing adrenalectomy and castration (see Table 7). The best results reported indicate pain-relief is obtained by a maximum of 44% of the patients.

TABLE 7. *Results of hormonal therapy for advanced breast cancer*

Treatment	No. of pts.	Object. rem.	Subject. rem.	Pain rem.	Authors
Hypophysectomy					
^{90}Y	100	32 (32%)	42 (42%)	n.d.	Notter et al. (40)
^{90}Y	300	90 (30%)	n.d.	225 (75%)	Denoix (16)
^{90}Y	56	17 (30%)	n.d.	49 (88%)	Abbes et al. (1)
^{90}Y	n.d.	n.d.	n.d.	85%	Juret et al. (28)
Cryohypophysectomy	42	13 (31%)	n.d.	30 (71%)	Abbes et al. (1)
Transsphenoidal-hypophysectomy	146[a]	n.d.	n.d.	140 (96%)	Hardy et al. (22)
Alcohol-injection into pituitary	10	0	0	10 (100%)	Martino et al. (33)
Adrenalectomy	18	8 (44%)	8 (44%)	8 (44%)	Dao[b] (15)
	500	178 (36%)	202 (40%)	n.d.	Fracchia et al.[c] (20)

Legend: See Table 2.
[a] All patients with osseous metastases.
[b] Controlled clinical trial.
[c] In 255 patients + ovariectomy.

TABLE 8. *Results with hormonal therapy (androgens) for advanced breast cancer*[a]

Drug used for therapy	No. of pts.	Object. rem.	Subject. rem.	Pain rem.	Authors
Testosterone propionate	23	3 (13%)	0	n.d.	Brennan et al. (9)
	20	4 (20%)	8–10 (40–50%)	n.d.	Lewison et al. (31)
	27	4 (15%)	9 (33%)	n.d.	Nevinny et al. (39)
	16	2 (13%)	10 (63%)	n.d.	Volk et al. (73)
3β-17β-Androstanedeol	21	2 (10%)	8 (38%)	n.d.	Brennan et al. (9)
11β-OH-17α-Methyl-testosterone	23	2 (9%)	5 (22%)	n.d.	Volk et al. (71)
Fluoxymesterone	25	2 (8%)	8 (32%)	n.d.	Volk et al. (71)
Testost. prop. + 17β-hydroxy-androsten-3-one	25	3 (12%)	? (40–50%)	n.d.	Lewison et al. (31)
2αγ-Methyldihydro-testost. propionate	23	6 (26%)	14/16 (88%)	n.d.	Volk et al. (72)
6β-Dibromethyl-ene-testost. propionate	23	4 (17%)	9/12 (75%)	n.d.	Volk et al. (72)
6-dehydro-17α-methyl-testosterone	20	0	5 (25%)	n.d.	Nevinny et al. (39)
Norandrolone phenpropionate	26	7 (27%)	9 (35%)	n.d.	Volk et al. (73)
Calusterone	44	4 (9%)	n.d.	16/36 (44%)	Aslam et al. (4)

Legend: See Table 2.
[a] All data from controlled clinical trials.

There are more numerous and consistent indications relating to the effect on pain of operations aiming at removing or destroying the hypophysis (Table 7). This type of treatment provides remission of pain in 82% of the patients on the average (from 71% with cryodestruction to 100% with the Moricca technique of alcohol neuroadenolysis) (36). It should be stressed that the ratio between objective remission and remission of pain was 1:3.

The vast literature relating to the use of androgen refers vaguely to subjective remission obtained in an average of 37% of the patients treated (range: 0 to 87.5%). In almost none of the reports is there specific reference to the anti-pain effect of this hormone (Table 8). The same considerations apply to the use of estrogens. In Table 9 results are shown on the use of anti-estrogens, cortisone substances, L-DOPA and progestins (other than MAP). In the case of tamoxifen, reference is made to the fact that pain may become acute again during the first days of treatment (12,35) but then subsides.

Table 10 shows results obtained using additive hormone therapy excluding

TABLE 9. *Results with hormonal therapy for advanced breast cancer*

Treatment	No. of pts.	Object. rem.	Subject rem.	Pain rem.	Authors
Antiestrogens					
Tamoxifen	96	17 (18%)	41 (43%)	n.d.	Cole et al. (12)
Nafoxidine	48	18 (37%)	n.d.	8/24 (33%)	Bloom et al. (6)
Cortisone	20	0	4 (25%)	3 (15%)	Dao[a] (15)
Prednisone	23	1 (4%)	3 (13%)	2 (9%)	Colsky et al.[a] (13)
L-DOPA	30	10 (33%)	10 (33%)	10 (33%)	Minton (34)
Progestins (other than MAP)					
9α-Bromo-11β-ketoprogesterone	23	0	8 (35%)	5 (22%)	Colsky et al.[a] (13)
norethisterone acetate	55	21 (38%)	31 (56%)	n.d.	Curwen (14)
	31	14 (45%)	n.d.	19 (61%)	Sonkin et al. (63)

Legend: See Table 2.
[a] Controlled clinical trial.

TABLE 10. *Results with hormonal therapy for advanced breast cancer*

Drug	No. of pts.	Object. rem.	Subject rem.	Pain rem.	Authors
L-DOPA	30	33%	33%	33%	Abbes et al. (1)
Cortisone	43	2%	16%	12%	Amadori et al. (2)
Androgens	316	12%	37%	44%	Colsky et al. (13)
Antiestrogens	144	24%	43%	33%	Amadori et al. (2)
Progestins (other than MAP)	118	30%	50%	38%	Archimbaud et al. (3)

Legend: See Table 2.

MAP. Compared with an average objective remission rate of 23.5% (range: 2 to 33%), the average subjective remission rate was 35.8% (range: 16 to 50%), and remission of pain took place in 32% of the patients treated (range: 12 to 44%). These give the ratios for objective to subjective results and for objective results to pain relief of 1:1.5.

Medroxyprogesterone Acetate (MAP) and Pain

MAP, a steroid which was synthesized in 1958, has an intense progestative effect on animals, as well as androgen- or estrogen-type effects and a corticoid activity (21). In oncology it has been used, apart from breast cancer, in endometrial carcinoma, renal carcinoma, and prostate carcinoma.

Mechanism of Action of MAP

The anti-tumor effect of MAP would seem to consist of inhibition of the pituitary gland, the ovary, and the adrenal glands, and also a direct effect on the neoplastic cell. In man MAP has a pronounced inhibitory effect on the pituitary-ovary axis (55) and on the adrenal-hypothalamic axis (41) and, in a secondary fashion, blocks the secretion of ovarian hormones and cortisol (57). These effects are brought out in man both with low doses (< 500 mg/day) and high doses.

Our experience can be summarized as follows: High doses of MAP induce a rapid decrease of plasma levels of GH, FSH, and LH—an effect which persists for a few months after treatment is discontinued. On the other hand, prolactin underwent no significant change. MAP also inhibits adrenal function as reflected by the reduction of the excretion of endogenous cortisol and endogenous 17-keto-steroid metabolites (58).

Recently, new information has been acquired concerning hormone receptors. Progesterone and a few synthetic progestins related to MAP are able, *in vitro,* to reduce the bond formed by 17β-estradiol with specific receptors present in breast cancer, and this effect seems to be in proportion to the hormone's concentration (17). MAP also reduces the cell concentration of estradiol receptors (ER) in human endometrium (69) and exhibits competitive effects at hypothalamic level towards estrogens and reduces their capacity to bind to specific receptors (56). Finally, in the uterus of the rabbit, it has been shown that the affinity of MAP for progesterone receptors is approximately 30 times greater than that displayed by natural progesterone (68).

These data lead us to suppose that progestins and particularly MAP are capable of displaying notable interference to hormone-sensitive neoplastic cells at the level of hormone receptor mechanisms.

The response to therapy with a given hormone administered at high doses may be correlated to a direct nonspecific toxic effect of the hormone itself. In fact, with cultured breast cancer cells, identical results are obtained as regards the inhibition of thymidine-tritiate incorporation using both 17α-estradiol and its nonactive isomer 17β-estradiol if the same high concentrations are employed (32).

Results with Low Doses of MAP

The use of MAP in advanced breast cancer goes back to the beginning of the 1960s. The average dose used was 100 mg/day given orally or intramuscularly. Table 11 shows results obtained using "low doses" of MAP with specific reference to remission of pain or subjective remission. The rates of remission are statistically dispersed (range: 18 to 92%). Results relating to remission of pain are also of little significance, and the relative percentage values are lower than 33%.

TABLE 11. *Results with hormonal therapy (low doses of MAP) for advanced breast cancer*

Doses of map	No. of pts.	Object. rem.	Subject. rem.	Pain rem.	Authors
50 mg/os	30	11/30 (37%)	n.d.	9/27 (33%)	Bucalossi et al. (10)
100–125 mg i.m.	27	15/27 (55%)	25/27 (92%)	n.d.	Dogliotti et al. (18)
100 mg i.m. × 3	34	7/34 (20%)	6/34 (20%)	n.d.	Muggia et al. (37)
20–300 mg/day/os	40	4/40 (10%)	n.d.	5/40 (12%)	Klaassen et al. (30)

Legend: See Table 2.

Results with High Doses of MAP

In 1973, we showed it was possible to use daily doses of MAP that were greater than those previously in use (usually less than 500 mg i.m. per day): the maximum tolerable dose (MTD) of MAP given i.m. was found to be 1,500 mg/day for 30 days (52). Subsequently (48), we treated 54 patients suffering from advanced breast cancer with MAP at the MTD, obtaining 44% of objective remission.

Even before objective remission became apparent, treatment with high doses of MAP was shown to be capable of inducing prompt subjective remission and producing an impressive anti-pain effect. During a study aimed at identifying the maximum therapeutic dose (MTD), it was found that MAP was able to induce pain-remission in 90% of the patients treated (52).

Subsequently, in a group of 54 patients treated with doses of 1,500 mg i.m. per day for 30 days the subjective remission rate was 86% (38 of 44) and partial or complete relief of pain occurred in 95% (35 of 37) of the patients (48). Table 12 shows that the remission of pain became apparent as early as 1 week from commencement of treatment and became propor-

TABLE 12. *Pain-remission in relation to time and total doses of MAP in 37 patients with grade 1 and 2 pain*

	Pain intensity			
	Grade 2 (no. of pts.)	Grade 1 (no. of pts.)	Grade 0 (no. of pts.)	MAP total dose (gm)
Before treatment	26	11	8	0
After 1 week	7	25	13	10.5
After 2 weeks	2	24	19	21
After 3 weeks	1	18	26	31.5
After 4 weeks	1	15	29	42
After 5 weeks	0	11	34	50
After 6 weeks	0	11	34	n.d.

Legend: Grade 2 = severe pain; grade 1 = moderate pain; grade 0 = no pain.

tionally greater during the following weeks and while the treatment was still in progress. By 5 weeks of the therapy all of the 26 patients who had severe pain before treatment had been totally or partially relieved of the pain. The anti-pain effect was especially noticeable in patients with very advanced breast cancer with multiple osseous metastases who were forced to keep completely still and were thought to be no longer susceptible to chemotherapy. Together with the anti-pain effect, we also noted an improvement in the ability to walk in 63% (15 of 24) of the patients. For the purpose of assessing the latter, we considered walking-impairment as a signal-symptom and therefore as being correlated to the presence of probable neoplastic foci capable of inducing motor impairments. We used the following rating scale: grade 0—absent or slight; *grade 1*—the patient spends less than 50% of the day in bed; *grade 2*—the patient is forced to spend more than 50% of the day in bed.

In this group of patients, the incidence of objective remission [complete remission (CR) + partial remission (PR)] was 44% (20 of 45) with an average duration of 7 months (48). Prior to therapy 79% of this group of patients had pain and nearly one-half of these had severe pain. After 1 month of treatment only 15% had pain and none had severe pain. However, this remission lasted about 6 months, when pain recurred in 48% of the patients and of these nearly one-third had severe pain. In 23 patients of this group, upon reappearance of pain, we repeated MAP treatment employing higher doses (2,000 mg i.m. per day for 30 days) with a more-concentrated MAP pharmaceutical preparation.[1] As a result of this repeated therapy, we noted remission once again in 21 patients (91%). In this second group of patients the incidence of objective remission (CR + PR) was 18% (49).

Subsequently, we treated another group of 25 patients with the same type of advanced disease with daily doses of 2,000 mg i.m. per day for 30 days. We noted an objective remission rate of 45% and subjective remission rate of 70% (48).

A new group of 92 patients with the same type of disease was studied as part of a prospective, randomized, multi-institute study with the aim of assessing the effectiveness of two different dose-levels of MAP. Forty-six patients received 500 mg/day for 30 days and 46 patients received 1,500 mg/day for 30 days. The drug was administered intramuscularly (47). Statistical analysis of objective results revealed that a larger percent of the patients who received 1,500 mg doses had complete or partial remission but the differences were not significant. However, the remission rates in all the signal-symptoms considered were consistently higher for MAP at the 1,500-mg dose-level (Table 13). Moreover and very importantly, remission of pain which occurred during the treatment was more rapid and greater for the higher dose-level than the lower dose-level (Table 14).

[1] Farlutal 500–1,500, F.I. 7401, 200 mg/ml vials.

TABLE 13. *Significant reduction or disappearance of the signal-symptoms present before treatment with high and low doses of MAP*

	Patients tested with MAP 1,500 mg			Patients tested with MAP 500 mg		
Symptomatology	Before therapy	After therapy	Remission rate	Before therapy	After therapy	Remission rate
Pain	26	4	85%	28	7	75%
Dyspnea	9	3	67%	6	3	50%
Asthenia	25	7	72%	24	8	67%
Anorexia	10	0	100%	16	3	81%
Walking-impairment	10	3	70%	12	7	42%

TABLE 14. *Behavior of the pain during the treatment (rate of remission)*

Drug dose (mg)	Patients with pain before therapy	Rate of remission during therapy (weeks) (in % of total patients with pain)			
		1	2	3	4
MAP 1,500	20	40%	60%	70%	80%
MAP 500	21	29%	38%	48%	71%

The results we obtained using high doses of MAP were subsequently confirmed by other authors (2,33). On the whole, MAP induced remission of pain in 83% of the patients (Table 15).

Moreover, review of the literature reveals that with MAP doses of 500 mg or less per day pain-relief was obtained by 21% of the patients compared with the 83% rate achieved with high doses. Although we are well aware of the limitations of retrospective comparisons, the difference in the remission of pain induced by high doses and low doses of MAP appears quite clear.

TABLE 15. *Results with hormonal therapy (large doses of MAP) for advanced breast cancer*

Authors	MAP dose (mg/day i.m.)	No. of pts.	Objective remission		Pain before therapy No.	Pain before therapy %	Pain remission No.	Pain remission %
Pannuti et al. (51)	1,500	44	18	41	40	91	37	92
Amadori et al. (2)	1,000–1,500	44	25	57	37	84	21	57
Martino et al. (33)	1,500	20	6	30	20	100	20	100
Pannuti et al. (44)	500– 1,000–2,000	168	76	45	114	70	98	86
Total/Averages		276	125	45	211	76	176	83

TABLE 16. *Effect of MAP orally/2,000 mg on pain of advanced breast cancer*

Effects on pain	Hormone-sensitive tumors (no. of pts. = 9)	Not hormone-sensitive tumors (no. of pts. = 16)	Total of the two groups
Decrease or complete relief	67%	50%	56%
No change	22%	44%	36%
Increase	11%	6%	8%

Administration of 1,500 mg of MAP intramuscularly is associated with a 15% incidence of abscess. Because of this complication, we began a series of studies concerning the oral administration of high doses of MAP (2,000 mg/day for 30 days) aimed at appraising: (a) the effect on the appetite and body-weight of the patient (anabolic effect); (b) the anticancer effect on hormone-sensitive tumors; (c) the effect on pain. At the moment, we have already shown an anabolic effect in 58 patients who experienced a statistically significant increase in body-weight and appetite (45). Studies concerning points b and c are still in progress. Preliminary results regarding pain relief are shown in Table 16.

Table 17 summarizes some of the results obtained with different hormone therapies for advanced breast cancer. It is apparent that of the subtractive measures, those that induced the highest remission of pain involved the destruction of the pituitary gland, whereas among the additive measures were high doses of MAP. In this regard, we should mention an important study made by Martino and Ventafridda (33) who compared the anti-pain effects of pituitary neuroadenolysis (alcohol-injection of the pituitary gland) with those obtained with 1,500 mg/day doses of MAP for 30 days (in the way

TABLE 17. *Results of therapy for advanced breast cancer: hormonotherapy*

Additive therapy			Ablative therapy		
Drug	Pain rem.	Subject. rem.	Organ	Pain rem.	Subject. rem.
L-DOPA	10/30 (33%)	10/30 (33%)	Hypophysis	454/554 (82%)	42/100 (42%)
Cortisonics	5/43 (12%)	7/43 (16%)	Adrenals	8/18 (44%)	8/18 (44%)
Androgens	16/36 (44%)	77/209 (37%)	Adrenals + ovary	n.d.	202/500 (40%)
Progestins (other than MAP)	24/54 (44%)	39/78 (50%)			
MAP low doses	14/67 (21%)	n.d.			
MAP high doses	176/211 (83%)				

Legend: See Table 2.

TABLE 18. *Advanced breast cancer (MAP/500, 1500, 2000 mg/day × 30 days) side effects*

Infiltration	12/166	(7%)
Abscess	31/166	(18%)
Facies lunaris	28/166	(16%)
Fine tremors	27/166	(16%)
Sweating	25/166	(15%)
Vaginal bleeding	18/166	(10%)
Thrombophlebitis	2/166	(1%)
Cramps	15/166	(9%)

we first suggested) and with the two therapies combined for patients with very advanced breast cancer. Their patients were no longer responsive to multiple chemotherapy and had very severe, continuous pain which was no longer controllable with narcotic analgesic drugs. They found a more prolonged anti-pain effect in the two groups treated with MAP, compared with the group treated with pituitary alcoholization. Furthermore, in 6 of the 20 patients who had been given MAP there was objective remission of the disease, but none occurred in the 10 patients who had undergone only pituitary alcoholization.

The relative profile for the toxicology of MAP at high doses is reported in Table 18. All side-effects are reversible within 20 days after the end of treatment and do not delay or interrupt further treatment.

CONCLUSIONS

Our experience concerning the effect of MAP on pain in the treatment of advanced hormone-sensitive tumors and especially in breast cancer leads us to conclude that the analgesic effect is at least in part independent of the pure anticancer effect. This conclusion is based upon two considerations: (a) In breast cancer the incidence of remission of pain is considerably greater than the incidence of objective remission of the tumor; and (b) there is a proportion of patients who, although they exhibit progression of the neoplastic disease, also experience reduction of pain-intensity. One comes to the same conclusion when one considers the results of hypophysectomy. These considerations lead one to the attractive hypothesis that there may be an analogy in the mechanisms of action. This is further suggested by the data of Martino and Ventafridda and also by data which show that MAP is capable of inhibiting pituitary-hormone activity in a less destructive fashion and without the immediate and long-term side effects of hypophysectomy.

Although the mechanism of the anticancer activity (direct or mediated by pituitary blocking) may be the prime factor to explain the anti-pain effect of MAP, one cannot rule out that the analgesic effects of this hormone may also be due to its actions on such factors as prostaglandin inhibition, anti-inflammatory effects, etc. These are worthy of study separately and systematically, not only in man but also in suitable pre-clinical experimental animal systems.

Regardless of the possible mechanism of action, it should be stressed that MAP is certainly an anticancer agent which, when given in high doses (as we first suggested), is able to induce remission of pain in hormone-sensitive tumors to an extent that has never been observed previously. The value of this therapeutic intervention certainly takes on greater importance when one considers that it is associated not only with quite considerable objective remission rates, at least in breast cancer, but also with a strong anabolic effect that is no small contribution to the quality of life of cancer patients.

ACKNOWLEDGMENTS

We are grateful to Dr. Antonia Cricca, to Dr. Fiorenza Fruet, and to Ms. Ida Rubino for help in the preparation of this manuscript.

REFERENCES

1. Abbes, M. M., Bourgeon, G., Paillaud, F., Juillard, G., Kermarec, J., Cambon, P., and Namer, M. (1972): À propose de 111 destruction hypophysaires pér yttrium 90 on cryothérapie pour cancer du sein avancé. *Ann. Chir.*, 26:521–531.
2. Amadori, D., Ravaioli, A., and Barbanti, F. (1976): L'impiego del medrossiprogesterone acetato ad alte dosi nella terapia palliativa del carcinoma mammario in fase avanzata. *Min. Med.*, 67:1–14.
3. Archimbaud, J. P., Dex Roseax, M., and Picq, P. (1973): Le traitement des douleurs des métastases osseuses de l'épithélioma prostatique par la surrénalectomie unilatéralle gauche. *J. Urol. Nefrol.*, 79:415–419.
4. Aslam, J., and Maxwell, J. (1977): Calusterone therapy for advanced breast cancer. *Cancer Treat. Rep.*, 61:371–373.
5. Band, P. R., Banergee, T. K., Patwardhan, V. C., and Eid, T. C. (1973): High-dose diethylstilbestrol diphosphate therapy of prostatic cancer after failure of standard doses of estrogens. *CMA J.*, 109:697–699.
6. Bloom, H. J. G., and Boesen, E. (1974): Antioestrogens in treatment of breast cancer: Value of nafoxidine in 52 advanced cases. *Br. Med. J.*, 2:7–10.
7. Bloom, H. J. G., Dukes, C. E., and Mitchley, B. C. V. (1963): Hormone-dependent tumours on the kidney. 1. The oestrogen-induced renal tumour of the Syrian hamster—hormone treatment and possible relationship to carcinoma of the kidney in men. *Br. J. Cancer*, 17:611–645.
8. Bouffioux, C. (1976): Traitement du cancer de la prostate par les agents progestatifs. *Acta Urol. Bel.*, 44:336–353.
9. Brennan, H. J., Beckett, V. L., Kelley, J. E., and Betanzos, G. (1960): Treatment of advanced mammary cancer with 3-β-17-β-androstanediol. *Cancer*, 13:1195–1200.
10. Bucalossi, P., Di Pietro, S., and Gennari, L. (1963); Trattamento ormonico del carcinoma mammario diffuso con un progestativo sintetico: il 6-α-methil-17-α-acetossiprogesterone. *Min. Chir.*, 9:358–366.
11. Colapinto, V., and Aberhart, C. (1961): Clinical trial of massive stilbestrol diphosphate therapy in advanced carcinoma of the prostate. *Br. J. Urol.*, 33:171–177.
12. Cole, M. P., Jones, C. T. A., and Todd, D. H., (1971): A new anti-oestrogenic agent in late breast cancer in early clinical appraisal of ICI 46474. *Br. J. Cancer*, 25:270–275.
13. Colsky, J., Shnider, B., Jones, R., Jr., Nevinny-Stickel, H. B., Hall, T., Regelson, W., Selawry, D. S., Owens, A., Brindley, C. D., Frei, E., III, and Uzer, Y. (1963): A comparative study of 9α-bromo, 11β-ketoprogesterone and prednisolone

in the treatment of advanced carcinoma of the female breast. *Cancer,* 4:502–505.
14. Curwen, S., (1963): The value of norethisterone acetate in the treatment of advanced carcinoma of the breast. *Clin Rad.,* 14:445–446.
15. Dao, T. L. (1961): In: "Progress report: results of studies by the cooperative breast cancer group 1956–1960." *Cancer Chemother. Rep.,* 11:109–141.
16. Denoix, P. (1970): *Breast Cancer: Treatment of Malignant Breast Tumours.* pp. 1–92. Springer Verlag, Berlin.
17. Di Carlo, F., Pacilio, G., and Conti, G. (1975): Sul meccanismo d'azione dei progestinici nella terapia dei tumori mammari ormono-dipendenti. *Tumori,* 61:501–508.
18. Dogliotti, G. C., Gavosto, F., and Molinatti, G. M. (1968): Trattamento del cancro avanzato della mammella con progestatici di sintesi. *Min. Med.,* 81:42–83.
19. Fergusson, J. D. (1971): *Life Sciences Monographs, 1, International Symposium on the Treatment of Cancer of the Prostate.* Pergamon Press, Vieweg.
20. Fracchia, A. A., Randall, H. J., and Farrow, J. H. (1967): The results of adrenalectomy in advanced breast cancer in 500 consecutive patients. *Surg. Gynecol. Obstet.,* 125:747.
21. Glenn, E. N., Richardson, S. L., and Bowman, B. J. (1959): Biologic activity of 6α-methil compounds corresponding to progesterone, 17-α-hydroxyprogesterone acetate and compounds. *Metabolism,* 8:265–285.
22. Hardy, J., Grisoli, F., Leclercq, T. A., and Somma, M. (1975): Hypophysectomie transphenoidale dans le cancers du sein metastatiques (160 cas). *Nuov. Presse Med.,* 4:2387–2390.
23. Heuson, J. C., Kenis, Y., and Tagnon, H. J. (1969): Hormones et cancer mammaire. Base espérimentale et traitment endocrinien. In: *Traitment médicaux des cancers et des léucemies,* Masson et Cie, Paris.
24. Huggins, C. (1956): Control of cancers of man by endocrinologic methods. A review. *Cancer Res.,* 16:825–830.
25. Huggins, C. (1967): Endocrine-induced regression of cancers. *Cancer Res.,* 27:1925–1930.
26. Huggins, C., and Scott, W. W. (1945): Bilateral adrenalectomy in prostatic cancer. *Ann. Surg.,* 122:1031–1045.
27. Huggins, C., Stevens, R., and Hodges, C. V. (1941): Studies on prostatic cancer. II. The effect of castration on advanced carcinoma of the prostate gland. *Arch. Surg.,* 43:209.
28. Juret, P., and Hayem, M. (1974): Pituitary ablation in the treatment of breast cancer. In: *Mammary Cancer and Neuroendocrine Therapy,* edited by B. A. Stoll, pp. 283–311. Butterworths, London.
29. Kistner, R. W., Griffiths, C. T., and Craig, J. M. (1965): Use of progestational agents in the management of endometrial cancer. *Cancer,* 12:1563–1579.
30. Klaassen, D. J., Rapp, E. F., and Hirte, W. E. (1976): Response to medroxyprogesterone acetate (NSC-26386) as secondary hormone therapy for metastatic breast cancer in postmenopausal women. *Cancer Treat. Rep.,* 60:251–253.
31. Lewison, E. F., Trimble, F. H., Grow, G. L., and Masukawa, T. (1963): Results of combined hormone therapy in advanced breast cancer. *Cancer,* 16:1243–1245.
32. Lippman, M., Bolan, G., and Huff, R. (1976): The effect of estrogen and antiestrogen on hormone-responsive human breast cancer in long-term tissue culture. *Cancer Res.,* 36:4595–4601.
33. Martino, G., and Ventafridda, V. (1976): Effetto antalgico dell'alcolizzazione ipofisaria, del medrossiprogesterone acetato ad alte dosi e della loro associazione nel carcinoma mammario in fase avanzata. *Tumori,* 62:93–98.
34. Minton, J. P. (1974): The response of breast cancer patients with bone pain to L-DOPA. *Cancer,* 33:358–363.
35. Morgan, L. R., Schein, P. S., Hoth, D., McDonald, J., Posey, L. E., Beazley, R. W., and Trench, L. (1976): Therapeutic use of tamoxifen in advanced breast cancer: A correlation with biochemical parameters. *Proc. Am. Assoc. Cancer Res.,* 17:126.
36. Moricca, G. (1974): Chemical hypophysectomy for cancer pain. *Adv. Neurol.,* 4:470–714.

37. Muggia, F. M., Cassileth, M. O., Ochoa, M., Jr., Flatow, F. A., Gellhorn, A., and Hyman, G. A. (1968): Treatment of breast cancer with medroxyprogesterone acetate. *Ann. Intern. Med.*, 68:328–337.
38. Murphy, G. P., Reynoso, G., Schoonees, R., Gailani, S., Bourke, R., Kenny, G. M., Mirand, E. A., and Schalck, D. S. (1971): Hypophysectomy and adrenalectomy for disseminated prostatic carcinoma. *J. Urol.*, 105:817–825.
39. Nevinny-Stickel, H. B., Dederick, M. M., Haines, C. R., and Hall, T. (1964): Comparative study of 6-dehydro-17α-methyltestosterone and testosterone propionate in human breast cancer. *Cancer*, 17:95–99.
40. Notter, G., and Melander, O. (1966): Pituitary implantation with ^{90}yttrium in the treatment of advanced breast cancer. *Coll. Int.* (*Lyons*), pp. 113–121.
41. Novak, E. (1977): Effects of medroxyprogesterone acetate on some endocrine functions of healthy male volunteers. *Curr. Ther. Res.*, 21:320–326.
42. Ortiz, A., Hiroi, M., Stanczyk, F. Z., Goebelsmann, V., and Mishell, D. R., Jr. (1977): Serum medroxyprogesterone acetate (MPA) concentrations and ovarian function following intramuscular injection of Depo-MPA. *J. Clin. Endocrinol. Metab.*, 44:32–38.
43. Pannuti, F., editor (1977): *Il protocollo terapeutico ed i codici di caratterizzazione e di valutazione in clinica oncologica.* Editrice Universitaria Bolognese, Bologna.
44. Pannuti, F., Castellari, S., Camera, P., Di Marco, A. R., Fruet, F., Giusti, H., Lelli, G., Martoni, A., Piana, E., Pollutri, E., Rossi, A. P., and Strocchi, E. (1977): I protocolli oncologici dell'ospedale M. Malpighi. In: *La chemioterapia dei tumori solidi,* edited by F. Pannuti, pp. 517–553. Editrice Universitaria Bolognese, Bologna.
45. Pannuti, F., Fruet, F., Piana, E., Strocchi, E., and Cricca, A. (1978): The anabolic effect induced by high doses of medroxyprogesterone acetate (MAP) orally in cancer patients. *IRCS Med. Sci.*, 6:118.
46. Pannuti, F., Martoni, A., and Cricca, A. (1978): Treatment of renal clear cell carcinoma by high doses of medroxyprogesterone acetate (MAP): Pilot study. *IRCS Med. Sci.*, 6:177.
47. Pannuti, F., Martoni, A., Di Marco, A. R., and Piana, E. (1978): Results of a randomized clinical trial of two different massive dosages of medroxyprogesterone acetate (MAP) in the treatment of metastatic breast cancer (*in press*).
48. Pannuti, F., Martoni, A., Lenaz, G. R., Piana, E., and Nanni, P. (1976): Management of advanced breast cancer with medroxyprogesterone acetate (MAP, F.I. 5837, F.I. 7401, NSC-26386) in high doses. In: *Functional Explorations in Senology,* pp. 253–265. European Press, Ghent, Belgium.
49. Pannuti, F., Martoni, A., Lenaz, G. R., Piana, E., and Nanni, P. (1978): A possible new approach to the treatment of metastatic breast cancer: Massive doses of medroxyprogesterone acetate. *Cancer Treat. Rep.*, 62 (*in press*).
50. Pannuti, F., Martoni, A., Piana, E., and Palenzona, D. (1977): Proposta di un modello di valutazione della tossicità in chemio-ormonoterapia antiblastica. *Min. Med.* (*in press*).
51. Pannuti, F., Martoni, A., Pollutri, E., Camera, P., and Lenaz, G. R. (1974): Ormonointerferenza da medrossiprogesterone acetato: Risultati relativi a 50 pazienti affetti da carcinoma mammario in fase avanzata. Proposta di una nuova metodologia di caratterizzazione e di valutazione. *Bull. Sci. Med.*, 144:1–43.
52. Pannuti, F., Martoni, A., Pollutri, E., Camera, P., Losinno, F., and Giusti, H. (1976): Massive dose progestational therapy in oncology (medroxyprogesterone). Preliminary results. Acts of the IV symposium on the locoregional treatment of tumours, St. Vincent, 1973. *Pan. Min. Med.*, 18:129–136.
53. Pannuti, F., Rossi, A. P., and Piana, E. (1977): Massive doses of medroxyprogesterone acetate (MAP): Pilot study in the treatment of advanced prostate cancer. *IRCS Med. Sci.*, 5:375.
54: Rafla, S., and Johnson, R. (1974): The treatment of advanced prostate carcinoma with medroxyprogesterone. *Curr. Ther. Res.*, 16:261–267.
55. Rifkind, A. B., Kulin, H. E., Cargille, C. M., Rayford, P. C., and Ross, G. T. (1969): Suppression of urinary excretion of luteinizing hormone (LH) and follicle stimulating hormone (FSH) by MAP. *J. Clin. Endocrinol Metab.*, 29:506.

56. Rosner, J. M., Declercq De Perez Bedes, G., and Gomez, E. (1974): Competition entre l'oestradiol et different progestagens au niveau de l'hypotalamus du rat. *Ann. Endocr.,* 35:173–176.
57. Sadoff, L., and Lusk, W. (1974): The effect of large doses of medroxyprogesterone acetate (MPA) on urinary levels and serum levels of cortisol T4 LH and testosterone in patients with advanced cancer. *Obstet. Gynecol.,* 43:262–266.
58. Sala, G., Castegnaro, E., Lenaz, G. R., Martoni, A., Piana, E., and Pannuti, F. (1978): Hormone interference in metastatic breast cancer patients treated with medroxyprogesterone acetate at massive doses: Preliminary results. *IRCS Med. Sci.,* 6:129.
59. Scott, W. W. (1973): Rationale and results of primary endocrine therapy in patients with prostatic cancer. *Cancer,* 32:1119–1125.
60. Serment, H., Spitalier, J. M., Ayme, E., De Giovanni, E., and Bardin, J. P. (1970): Médroxyprogestérone et adénocarcinomes de l'endométre. *Bull. Fed. Gynecol. Obstet.,* 22:93–97.
61. Smith, J. P., Rutledge, F., and Soffar, S. W. (1966): Progestins in the treatment of patients with endometrial adenocarcinoma. *Ann. J. Obstet. Gynecol.,* 94:977–984.
62. Smith, R. B. (1971): Cyproterone therapy in stage IV. In: *Life Science Monographs, 1, International Symposium on the Treatment of Cancer of the Prostate.* Pergamon Press, Vieweg.
63. Sonkin, R., Coudeyras, M., and Thévenet, M. (1969): L'utilisation de la noréthindrone à doses fortes dans le traitement de certains cancers génitaux hormonodépendants. *Obstet. Gynecol.,* 68:355–372.
64. Straffon, R. A., Kiser, W. S., Robitaille, D. F., and Dohn, D. F. (1968): ^{90}yttrium hypophysectomy in the management of metastatic carcinoma of the prostate gland in 13 patients. *J. Urol.,* 99:102–108.
65. Susan, L. P., Roth, B. R., and Adkins, W. C. (1976): Regression of prostatic cancer metastases by high doses of diethylstilbestrol diphosphate. *Urology,* 7:598–601.
66. Tagnon, H. J., Coune, A., Heuson, J. C., and Van Rymenant, M. (1967): Problems in the treatment of disseminated cancer of the breast: Selection of patients for hormone treatment. In: *New Trends in the Treatment of Cancer,* edited by L. Manuila, S. Moles, and P. Rentchnick, pp. 126–133. Springer-Verlag, Berlin, Heidelberg, New York.
67. Talley, R. W., Moorhead, E. L. Tucker, W. G., San Diego, E. L., and Brennan, M. J. (1969): Treatment of metastatic hypernephroma. *JAMA,* 207:322–328.
68. Terenius, L. (1974) Affinities of progestogen and estrogen receptors in rabbit uterus for synthetic progestogens. *Steroids,* 23:909–919.
69. Tseng, L., and Gurpide, E. (1975): Effects of progestins on estradiol receptor levels in human endometrium. *J. Clin. Endocrinol. Metab.,* 41:402–404.
70. Van der Werfmessing, B., and Van Gilse, H. A. (1971): Hormonal treatment of metastases of renal carcinoma. *Br. J. Cancer,* 25:423–427.
71. Volk, H., Ciprut, S., and Escher, G. (1962): Hormonal therapy in advanced breast cancer. II: Effect of oral 11β-hydroxy-17α-methyl-testosterone compared with fluoxymesterone on clinical course and its effects on metabolism of nitrogen and selected electrolytes. *Cancer,* 15:726–732.
72. Volk, H., Foley, C. J., Sanfilippo, L. J., and Escher, G. C. (1964): Hormonal therapy in advanced breast cancer. III: Effect of 6-β-dibromomethylene-testosterone propionate compared with that of 2α-A-methyl-dihydrotestosterone propionate on clinical course and metabolism of selected serum electrolytes. *Cancer,* 17:1073–1078.
73. Volk, H., Wilde, R. C., Carabasi, R., and Bisel, H. (1965): Anti-tumor efficacy of norandrolone propionate compared with testosterone propionate in advanced breast cancer. *Cancer,* 18:651–655.
74. West, C. D., Hollander, V. P., Whithore, W. F., Jr., Randall, H. T., and Pearson, O. H. (1952): The effect of bilateral adrenalectomy upon neoplastic disease in man. *Cancer,* 5:1009–1018.

Advances in Pain Research and Therapy, Vol. 2,
edited by J. J. Bonica and V. Ventafridda.
Raven Press, New York © 1979.

Radiation Therapy

S. Basso Ricci

Department of Radiology, Istituto Nazionale per lo Studio e la Cura dei Tumori, 20133 Milan, Italy

Pain and other discomforts of different types and intensity almost always occur with advanced carcinoma. Usually pain is related to the location and extension of tumor and individual reactivity, and it may be localized to the site of the primary tumor or referred elsewhere. The questions relevant to the possibility of getting partial or total regression of pain and other symptomatology are often very important in the therapy of these patients, even though recovery is no longer possible for most of them. The analgesic effect of ionizing radiation employed in the radiotherapy of tumors has long been well known. Although the precise basic mechanism of analgesic action from radiation therapy is not known generally, the most important beneficial effects result from: (a) decrease or removal of pressure on the nervous structures, (b) reduction of heteroplastic infiltration under the action of radiation, (c) disappearance of ulcerations and pressure on hollow organs with consequent elimination of colicky pain, and (d) resolution of inflammatory reaction in the tumor and its periphery.

It cannot actually be predicted to what extent these factors will respond to the radiation treatment or what degree of analgesia will be produced. It is this uncertainty of results which is the main restraint of radiation therapy.

The subject matter I intend to treat is dealt with on the basis of data from reports on this subject by others and from my own personal experience. It is subdivided according to the sites at which tumors manifest themselves, so I shall consider them successively under the following headings: (a) the head and the neck, (b) the chest, (c) the female genital system, (d) the male genital system, (e) the nervous system, and (f) the skeletal system. In the end I'll mention systemic tumors.

TUMORS OF THE HEAD AND THE NECK

If very extended, all these tumors can cause pain and, if there has been no previous radiation treatment, they can all show definite relief of pain and improvement of other symptomatology because of ionizing radiation.

Of the tumors in the rhinopharynx, the cases that I will consider are the ones concerning the sensory branches of the trigeminal nerve. It is known that in cases of recurrence this often involves mechanical or inflammatory processes of these nerves, and a second radiotherapy cycle is likely to produce relief of pain and related symptomatology (3). With tumors in the paranasal cavities and especially in the maxillary sinus, pain often occurs both in the cases that can't be operated and with tumors that recur after previous radiation and surgical treatments. These often produce pain because of the inflammatory process. Moreover, the pain often involves structures with different innervation so that surgical interruption or nerve blocks directed to one branch will not produce adequate relief [*Editors' note:* In such cases the neurosurgical procedure or nerve block must involve all of the branches of the trigeminal nerves that are likely to become involved with future expansion of the lesion. Therefore it is best to destroy the gasserian ganglion or sensory root of the trigeminal nerve. (See p. 537.)]

For large tumors in the oropharynx and the hypopharynx, which often cause local and referred pain, especially lesions in the floor of the mouth and the base of the tongue, the analgesic and curative effect of ionizing radiation is well known. On the other hand, when there is persistence or recurrence of these tumors, there develops ulceration in the infiltration zones which are poorly radiosensitive. Consequently, radiation therapy does not produce pain-relief and is therefore not indicated for analgesic action. In these cases it is better to use chemotherapy.

Radiation therapy of large tumors in the thyroid, which affect the nerves of the neck, produces effective pain-relief in most patients. Metastatic adenopathies of the neck deserve special mention, particularly those which progressively enlarge after previous radiation and surgical therapy. These metastatic lesions affect the nerves of the neck and those of the base of the skull by pressure and infiltration from the extralymphonodal component with consequent severe pain which has different location in different patients. Therefore, radiation therapy to produce analgesia must also include the base of the skull.

TUMORS IN THE CHEST

Advanced cancers in the chest considered here include primary tumors of the lung, primary and secondary tumors in the chest wall, and carcinoma of the breast. It is well known that Pancoast tumor early on infiltrates the brachial plexus and later becomes involved in pathology of the ribs.

Other peripheral pulmonary tumors in an advanced stage spread into the pleura and chest walls, whereas the central ones tend to affect the parabronchial and mediastinal nervous structures. In most cases, thanks to the experience which is now common to all radiotherapists, it is possible to obtain prompt and dramatic relief of pain and other discomforts as Haas and his associates pointed out in 1937 (5,9).

In our Institute, in the presence of pain after radiation treatment or surgical intervention, often we use bleomycin with radioactive indium in order to localize the probable site of recurrence and then start a new schedule of radiotherapy. Pain caused by metastatic lesions in the pleura and chest wall is often relieved by radiation treatment. I have no direct experience nor could I find any information about the response to radiotherapy when pain is caused by primary tumors in the pleura.

Carcinoma in the breast, with big, metastatic lymph nodes or ulcerations of tissues may cause pain which can be promptly relieved by radiation therapy. When pain develops in the distribution of part or whole of the brachial plexus in a woman who has received radiation therapy, we must exclude postradiation fibrosis pain before further therapy is considered.

TUMORS IN THE ABDOMEN

Here we will discuss tumors of the pancreas and the large bowel. For tumors of the pancreas, radical curative therapy is hardly ever feasible, and therefore the main object of radiation therapy is to provide pain-relief. Green and associates (4) state that pain-relief is almost always obtained, even with low doses, and should be considered even when hepatic metastases have already become evident.

Remarkable regression and even elimination of pain and related symptomatology may be obtained in the cases of endopelvic metastases of carcinoma of the large bowel and especially the rectum. These metastases are often in the hypogastrium and sacral regions. In the last 5 years, in our Institute, we have irradiated about 40 patients with this type of lesion with good results in most of them.

Recently, Smoron (13) has reported good results with radiation therapy of carcinoma of the biliary tract, even those which were not amenable to surgical therapy.

TUMORS OF THE FEMALE GENITAL SYSTEM

In these cases pain and related symptomatology is caused by infiltration of the parametrium and by hypogastric, sacral, aortic, and inguinal lymph-node metastases. The hypogastric and sacral metastases affect the sacral and parasacral nervous structures, although sometimes pain is due to a heteroplastic infiltration in the the bony structures.

In a series of 313 patients suffering from endopelvic recurrences of carcinoma of the uterus, Basso Ricci and Bianchi (1) noticed the presence of pain in about a third of the cases, with partial relief following radiation therapy. However, the best results have been obtained with anterolateral cordotomy (10).

TUMORS OF THE MALE GENITAL SYSTEM

These include malignant tumors in the testicle and the prostate. The voluminous metastatic adenopathies of tumors in the testicle, especially in the aortic and inguinal regions, often cause pain because of the pressure and infiltration of the individual nerves and lumbosacral plexus in the paravertebral region. When they are teratocarcinomas, we use radiotherapy to relieve pain only in the cases where chemotherapy proves inadequate. However, because these neoplasms are poorly radiosensitive, we should not expect dramatic or total pain-relief, but only partial analgesia.

Radiation therapy from the outside of tumors in the prostate in D stage with consequent neoplastic infiltration into the endopelvic tissues and organs produces regression of pain and at times total relief (6,12).

TUMORS OF THE URINARY APPARATUS

Renal tumors which have not been radically removed by surgery may cause pain in the hypochondrium or in the lumbar region by producing pressure and irritation of lower thoracic and lumbar nerves in the paravertebral region and also by to the concomitant presence of retroperitoneal lymph-node metastases.

Tumors in the urinary bladder with infiltration of the vesical wall, or lymph-node metastases, or even endopelvic recurrences after total cystectomy, can be successfully treated with radiation therapy to relieve pain and related symptomatology.

TUMORS INVOLVING THE NERVOUS SYSTEM

The neoplastic involvement of the central nervous system (CNS) must be differentiated from the ones involving the peripheral nervous system. As is well known, primary malignant neoplasms of the CNS which cannot be operated or have not been surgically removed produce progressively severe cephalalgia. In such cases radiation therapy can produce regression of the symptomatology, but we must add that the headache in these patients can be cured in most cases with surgical procedures which lessen the increased intracranial pressure and can be remarkably improved with the use of cortisone.

According to Hendrikson (7) the cerebral metastases were associated with severe headache in 30% of the patients, and of these at least 85% derived almost complete regression of the symptom with radiation therapy. The latter is carried out along with the use of cortisone in order to lessen the cerebral edema. It is also known that chemotherapy is not effective in cerebral metastases. In our Institute in the last 5 years we have treated 40 patients with this type of lesion, and our results have been similar to those reported by Hendrikson (7). As Posner (11) has emphasized, extracerebral, epidural, or arachnoid metastases can also be associated with headache if there is pressure or thrombus in the sagittal sinus. For these intracranial lesions which seldom are associated with edema, cortisone is not effective, and the only possible treatment is often radiation therapy. According to Posner (11) even the latter therapy is not effective when the sagittal sinus is thrombosed.

Pain is often experienced when the spinal cord is pressed upon by bony vertebral or epidural metastatic lesions. This pain, which is often of the radicular type, may precede even by months other neurologic symptomatology, especially motor disturbances. Therefore, after thorough study of the case including neurologic examination of the meninges, myelography, and possibly scintigraphy, radiation therapy is used possibly after laminectomy. Metastatic lesions can involve the roots of spinal nerves as well as spinal cord. Moreover, as previously mentioned, metastatic lesions may also involve nerve plexuses and more peripheral nerves.

The cauda equina may also be involved with a radicular pain which may be preceded by the loss of vesical and intestinal functions. I agree with Posner (11) that in such cases radiation therapy is more effective in lessening pain than other symptoms. When radiation therapy proves ineffective, we use neurosurgical procedures or neurolytic blocks (10,15).

TUMORS OF THE BONES

Primary tumors of bones deserve only a brief mention here because they can often be operated upon. Nevertheless in these cases, radiation therapy can produce good pain-relief. Metastatic tumors to bones are more important, because they are often the site of pain whether the tumor is in the bone itself, or in the subperiostal region, or if the metastases causes bony destruction and collapse with consequent pressure on nerve roots. These metastases respond promptly to radiation therapy and pain usually regresses rapidly and disappears after just a few treatments.

The osteolytic metastases react more effectively than the osteoblastic ones. Besides the radiation therapy from the outside, there is also the use of 32 radioactive phosphorus for the metastases of prostatic carcinoma, especially when we take care to increase the use of these isotopes for the metastases with parathormone. Hypophysectomy with radioactive yttrium can also give good results.

SYSTEMIC TUMORS

In the subject we are dealing with, the important cases are the ones where the lymph-node localizations cause pressure on paravertebral nerve structures and when there are meningeal, intracranial, or bony metastases.

SEQUELAE OF RADIOTHERAPY

Among the sequelae that arise in the peripheral nervous system, lesions of the nerve plexus and especially the sacral and brachial plexus are most important. Lesions of the sacral plexus are rather rare (8); on the other hand, those of the brachial plexus are relatively frequent following repeated cycles of irradiation of the supraclavicular region in patients with metastases from breast cancer or head or neck tumors. Irradiation in these cases can improve the symptomatology caused by the metastases but can also cause lesions of the brachial plexus, which produce very intense pain-symptomatology associated with alterations of muscle function in the arms. These are diagnosed by clinical and electrophysiologic examinations (2).

Finally, irradiation of bones, as is done, for example, in the case of bone metastases of mammary cancer with excellent pain-relief, can also cause permanent inhibition of the bone-marrow activity, with anemia, leucopenia, and thrombocytopenia. These alterations can be serious and can reduce survival time.

Early local reactions to radiation therapy, such as skin rash, inflammation of the mucosa, loss of hair, and decrease in salivation, in addition to general reactions such as the so-called "radiation disease" are all transitory and do not merit further comment. More important, however, are the delayed sequelae, most of which are not found at clinical examination because, in general, patients affected by advanced cancer have a brief survival. On the other hand, these sequelae in cases with longer survivals are particularly important, because we are usually dealing with patients subjected to repeated cycles of irradiation. Among the most important of these sequelae are those involving the skin, subcutaneous tissue and mucosa, bones, mediastinum, lungs, nervous tissue, and bone marrow.

The skin, subcutaneous tissue, and mucosa can have necrotic ulcers after repeated radiation treatments, and those which arise on the mucosa can produce intense pain. Necrotic lesions, sometimes of the rhinopharynx, are not infrequently the cause of serious hemorrhage after repeated treatment. The bones can also develop necrosis and consequent bone sequestra of fractures, especially of the mandible, the clavicle, or the upper part of the femur (8).

Among the sequelae in organs in the mediastinum, pericarditis deserves mention although it is very rare (14). Irradiation can cause inflammatory processes in the lung that evolve in fibrosis.

Among the sequelae of the CNS, transverse myelitis is the most important because it is almost always irreversible.

CONCLUSION

The significant radiosensitivity of certain neoplasms, the existence of probable contraindications for chemotherapy or surgery, and the opportunity of delaying the use of drugs represent important indications for radiation therapy for the relief of pain of advanced cancer. The more radiosensitive the neoplasm, the more promptly is its response to radiation therapy. So we must also expect a more obvious beneficial effect from radiation therapy in the cases where pain is caused by simple pressure rather than by infiltration of nerve structures which may also be irreparably damaged. The difficulty of localizing the nervous structures involved by the neoplasm or the involvement of many nerves make surgical intervention difficult. In contrast, radiation therapy, using relatively wide fields of irradiation, can act on more structures at the same time, as often happens for involvement of the base of the skull.

In order to make more complete data available on the extension of neoplasms to be irradiated, we have often resorted not only to the clinical examination and the common radiographic examination, but also to scintigraphy with labeled bleomycin, especially in the presence of recurrence of pulmonary carcinomas.

Contraindications of radiation therapy include previous radiation treatments when the latter have been made recently and with very high doses. Even if we take into account the different radiosensitivity of neoplasms, we do not think it useful to go further than a certain limit of doses to obtain some relief of pain rather than complete relief.

The maximum dose for an analgesic effect is different from patient to patient, but it is always below the one which must be reached for a radical elimination of the neoplasm. Sometimes we notice a worsening of the pain after the first application; but this effect, which is due to an initial congestion caused by radiation, rapidly resolves with the successive therapies. Sometimes we obtain not only regression of pain but also an improvement of the general condition of the patient, because narcotics with side effects can be decreased or eliminated.

REFERENCES

1. Basso Ricci, S., and Bianchi, F. (1966): Terapia delle recidive pelviche del carcinoma del collo dell'utero. *Minerva Ginecol.,* 18:603–609.
2. Basso Ricci, S., Ventafridda, V., Zanolla, R., Cassani, L., and Spreafico, R. (1976): Presentazione di 25 casi di lesioni postirradiatorie del plesso brachiale e loro trattamento. *Tumori,* 62:365–372.
3. Felci, U. (1964): La radioterapia dei tumori della rinofaringe. In: *Corso Superiore sulla terapia dei tumori della testa e del collo,* Milano, 6–11 April, pp. 181–215. CEA, Milano.
4. Green, N., Beron, E., Melbye, R. W., and George, F. W. (1973): Carcinoma of pancreas palliative radiotherapy. *Am. J. Roentgenol. Radium Ther. Nucl. Med.,* 117:620–622.
5. Haas, L. L. (1957): The place of the betatron in radiotherapy. *Arch. Intern. Med.,* 100:190–195.
6. Hazra, T. A. (1974): The role of radiotherapy in management of carcinoma of the prostate. *Maryland Med. J.,* 23:48–49.
7. Hendrikson, F. R. (1975): Radiation therapy of metastatic tumors in the brain. *Semin. Oncol.,* 2:43–46.
8. Kaplan, S. H. (1972): Complications of radiotherapy. In: *Hodgkin's Disease,* pp. 327–339. Harvard University Press, Cambridge, Mass.

9. Milani, F., and Lattuada, A. (1975): La radioterapia nei tumori dell'apice polmonare. In: *I tumori polmonari,* edited by P. Bucalossi, U. Veronesi, H. Emanuelli, and G. Ravasi, pp. 233–237. CEA, Milano.
10. Natale, P., and Miserocchi, E. (1952): La cordotomia anterolaterale nelle sindromi dolorose dell'utero incurabile. *Minerva Ginecol,* 5:1–6.
11. Posner, J. B. (1971): Neurological complications of systemic cancer. *Med. Clin. North Am.,* 55:625–646.
12. Rodriguez, A., Cook, S. A., Jelden, G. L., Hunter, A. T. W., Sraffon, R. A., and Stewart, B. H. (1973): Management of primary and metastatic carcinoma of the prostate. *Am. J. Roentgenol. Radium Ther. Nucl. Med.,* 118:876–880.
13. Smoron, G. L. (1977): Radiation therapy of carcinoma of Gallbladder and biliary tract. *Cancer,* 40:1422–1424.
14. Stewart, J. R., Cohn, K. E., Faiardo, L. F., Hancock, E. W., and Kaplan, H. S.: Radiation-induced heart disease: A study of twenty-five patients. *Radiology,* 89: 302–310.
15. Wilson, C. B. (1969): Surgical control of pain in the cancer patients. *Oncology,* 23:44–48.

Advances in Pain Research and Therapy, Vol. 2,
edited by J. J. Bonica and V. Ventafridda.
Raven Press, New York © 1979.

Palliative Surgery

Leandro Gennari

Istituto Nazionale per lo Studio e la Cura dei Tumori, 20133 Milan, Italy

What is the meaning of palliation? By palliation we mean the effect of all the procedures (such as inhibiting the progression of the disease or minimizing the dramatic events that are often produced by the neoplastic disease) that are used when it is impossible to cure a patient and that improve the quality of his remaining life. Palliative treatment of tumors almost always involves the use of physical means or chemical agents, such as radiotherapy or chemotherapy, whereas surgery is generally considered a means of attempting to solve contingent and grave situations, such as intestinal obstruction or bleeding. Recently, the improved knowledge in the field of oncology has altered this opinion, and surgery as a palliative measure is now being used more extensively. However, the meaning that is given to the term *palliation* is important.

If it is true that an operation is really curative when no residual tumor cells are left in the body, a large number of operations can be considered as palliative. In fact, from the survival data, we can state, for example, that in about 80% of the stomach carcinomas and in 50% of the carcinomas of the large intestine, the surgical operation employed was theoretically curative but in essence only palliative.

Perhaps this is both a philosophic and semantic matter; however, it suggests complex problems, the hypothetical solutions of which are not free from criticism and polemics where everybody is right and nobody is wrong. If the concept of surgical palliation is to be given a more restrictive meaning, all the situations in which surgery is required with a definite palliative purpose must be identified. Four different surgical situations are therefore distinguishable:

1. direct palliative surgery: (a) urgent, (b) reductive, and (c) necessary,
2. indirect palliative surgery,
3. palliative surgery for pain,
4. mediate palliative surgery.

DIRECT PALLIATIVE SURGERY

Urgent Palliative Surgery

Urgent palliative surgery means the surgical practice necessitated by emergency conditions, such as intestinal perforation or serious bleeding. Tumors of the gastrointestinal tract frequently cause heavy bleeding owing to the neoplastic erosion of a blood vessel. In these cases it is almost impossible to employ a raphe because of weak tissue, and it is thus essential to do a resection that may not always be carried out according to oncologic criteria of radicality. The surgeon, in this situation, is more concerned with resolving the emergency than removing all of the clearly metastatic lymph nodes. In the same way, a colostomy is required for a closed stenosis at the rectal-sigmoid junction or if the neoplasm is not resectable, Hartman's or Mukuliecz's operations are necessary when peritoneal or hepatic metastases are present.

Experience has demonstrated that, regardless of association with chemotherapy and/or radiotherapy, the survival of these patients is improved, both in the duration and quality of life, because the pain-symptom, due to local inflammatory events, is decreased by the absence of fecal passage. This kind of surgery is insensitive towards reductive palliative surgery.

Reductive Palliative Surgery

Reductive palliative surgery is so defined because at the end of the surgical treatment a notable reduction in the tumor mass is obtained. The result of such a treatment is that the radiologist and/or the chemotherapist have the opportunity to devise a therapeutic scheme that, even though it has no curative purpose, allows in many cases a recovery of the patient's general conditions, a restoration of some compromised functional capacities, and thus not only an extended survival but, more importantly, an improvement of the quality of life.

We have re-examined a group of patients affected by rectal cancer and treated in a nonradical way with surgery alone or in association with radiotherapy. Palliative surgery or radiotherapy alone resulted in a 1-year survival in 30% of the cases and 0% within 3 years. Association of the two types of treatment gave a 100% survival at 1 year, and 20% of the cases are still alive at 5 years. Such data corroborate the fact that palliative surgery as the only therapeutic treatment is extremely limited, but it has a wider application when used as part of a multidisciplinary approach.

Experimental studies and cell kinetic information have formed the basis for associated surgery-chemotherapy treatments. In such cases, however, the surgeon should not lose sight of the initial indications, limits, and objectives of the treatment, which in any case is palliative.

Palliative surgery is not intended only as a means for prolonging life. Its main purpose has been stated by Pack: "Palliation is not simply the duration of life, but rather the measure of comfortable living the individual enjoys in the remainder of his life." On the other hand, the surgeon must consider some elements objectively before making any decision, even if he does not contest every man's right to live as long as possible, regardless of the kind of life he might have. The surgeon must therefore consider: the operative mortality, the postoperative morbidity, the extent of the mutilation, and the kind of survival.

Each surgical operation, however simple, involves the risk of surgical mortality. However, this is a calculated risk that takes into account the possibility of complete recovery of the patient. On the contrary, knowing that a palliative treatment is useless risks death during or immediately after surgery. In these cases, the surgeon must avoid operating and must not become committed to a useless and dangerous course for reasons of ostentation or technical pride. Finally, the surgeon must not forget that the patient, because of the diffusion of the disease, often has only a weak resistance to the surgery. In fact, a tumor in such an advanced stage that it can not be removed, has already lowered the patient's organic resources so much that a simple laparotomy can cause an irreversible process that could be fatal. The weak resistance to surgical trauma also is largely responsible for postoperative morbidity, and therefore between two possibilities of palliative surgery, it is a good rule to chose the less dangerous one.

For example, in the case of a patient with a stenosis and bleeding carcinoma of the sigmoid colon with distant metastases, the surgeon must decide whether to perform a colostomy, which would solve the mechanical problems of the obstruction but not the oncologic ones, or to perform an intestinal resection, which would solve the immediate and delayed problems but might be followed by a high percentage of complications. In other words, is it better for the patient to undergo an operation that might be dangerous or to begin immediately after colostomy chemotherapeutic or radiologic treatment to relieve pain? Moreover, the surgeon must not forget the implications of the mutilation and the relative quality of the patient's remaining life.

For example, it is technically possible to perform a resection of almost all of the small intestine. In the literature cases are reported of patients who have survived for up to 2 years after a resection that left only from 6 to 18 inches of the small intestine. This fact is surprising if we consider the functions of the small intestine, also because the caloric contribution necessary for survival has been assured by the total parenteral nutrition (TPN). Although the survival of these patients is a fact of clinical relevance, we should ask ourselves if the high surgical mortality and the serious hardships during residual life are not too heavy a price to pay in comparison with the hypothetical advantages.

Finally, the choice of extensive palliative resections is conditioned, moreover, by the usual criteria: the duration of the possible remaining life and those factors which influence the outcome of the surgery.

Necessary Palliative Surgery

Necessary palliative surgery means all operations directly performed on primary tumors or metastases and required by their sometimes monstrous growth. Since this kind of surgery is often destructive, is the disarticulation of a limb justified? As long as the above-mentioned rules are taken into account, we feel that such surgery is warranted. In our opinion, such surgery is definitely required in the case of very large, necrotic, ulcerated, infected and malodorous, painful and secreting tumors that result in an early cachexia. In fact, after palliative amputation or disarticulation, patients whose grave general conditions were due to large limb tumors rather than to the presence of pulmonary metastases, have recovered. Moreover, with the improvement of the hematologic picture, these patients can undergo chemotherapy with a greater probability of success. In other words, the two-fold purpose of removing a source of infection and often stabbing pains and of dealing with possible metastases by reducing the tumor mass is realized.

Finally, we should not forget that large superficial tumors, because of the

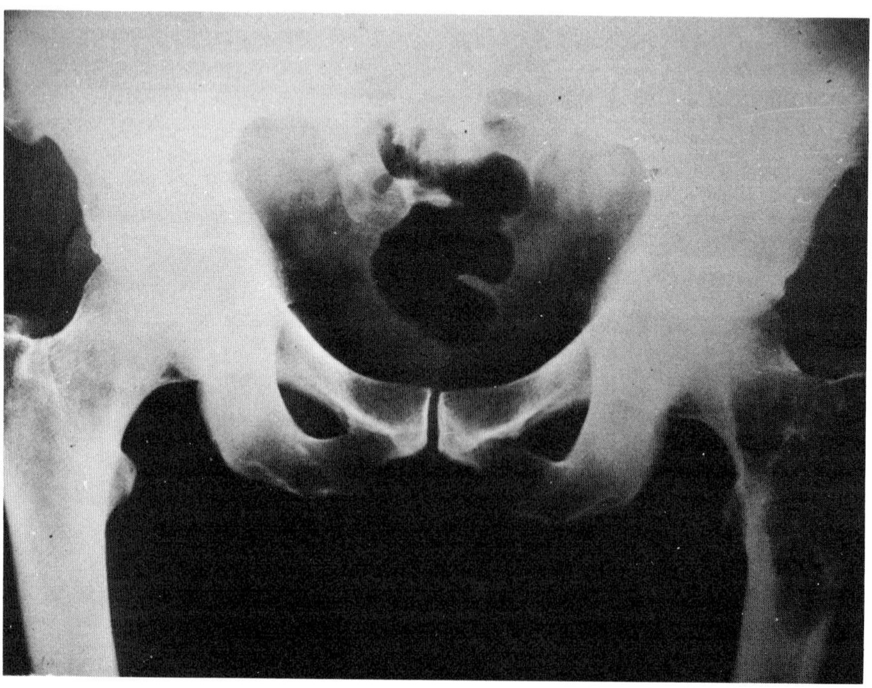

FIG. 1. X-ray of patient with pain in left hip due to metastatic lesion.

obvious discomfort they cause, represent a serious psychologic problem, and their removal gives patients the illusion of a cure that offers, in addition to the physical integrity, a reacquisition of psychologic equilibrium, which is necessary for reinsertion, even if temporary, into society.

Some tumors have a rather restricted activity that is expressed by a late, sometimes single metastasis and by a relatively slow local progression. In these cases, which are represented by bone metastases from thyroid or renal carcinomas, a surgical treatment, aggressive and conservative at the same time, is well justified. We have experimented with such types of surgery and have obtained very good results.

Figure 1 shows the radiogram for a 42-year-old patient who underwent X-ray examination for pain in the hip. The lesion was interpreted as a primary bone tumor, and the tumor was biopsied. The histologic diagnosis

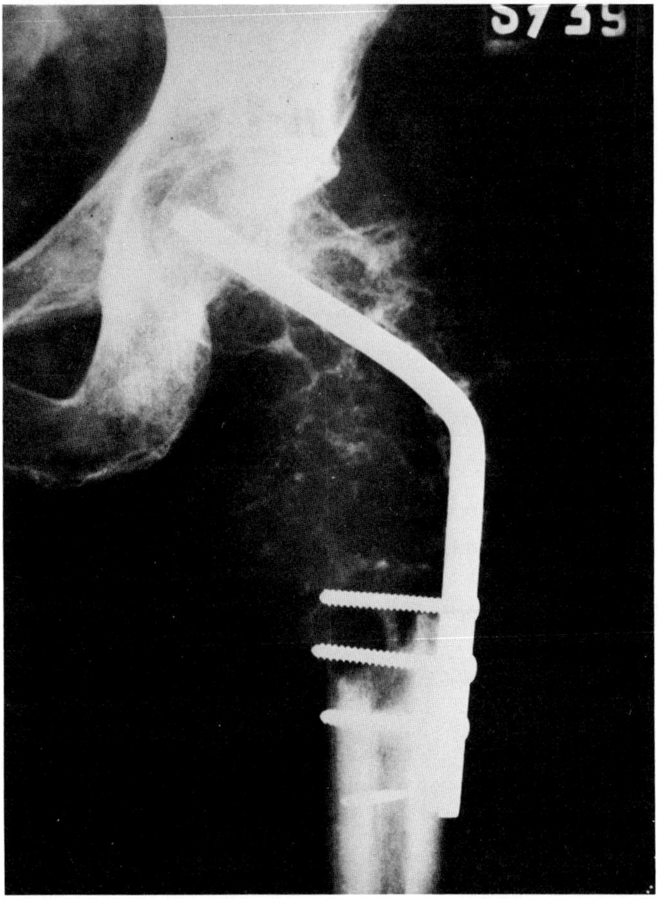

FIG. 2. X-ray showing pin of hip for metastatic fracture of upper femur.

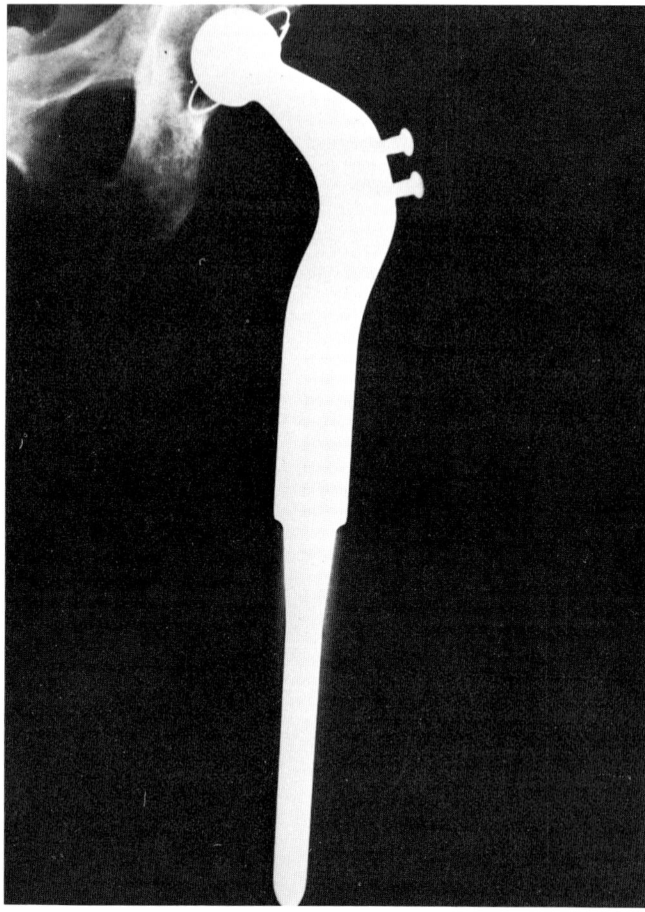

FIG. 3. X-ray showing prosthesis of left hip which resulted in relief of pain.

was "hypernephroma metastasis," and the surgeon performed a nephrectomy. After some time a pathologic fracture was found in the femoral site, and the orthopedist inserted a pin (Fig. 2). The patient remained without additional therapy until December, 1977, when the progressive increase of the femoral metastases caused a complete functional disability. After some time, the metastases were removed, and a prothesis was inserted with good results (Fig. 3).

INDIRECT PALLIATIVE SURGERY

Indirect palliative surgery involves the surgical treatment of organs whose functional activities have an effect on the development of the neoplastic disease. This includes mainly the so-called "ablative surgery" of endocrine organs and is used for patients with metastatic breast or prostatic carcinomas. Of all the forms of palliative surgery, this is the one that has given the best results in terms of response, both subjective (with decrease of pain and recovery of muscle function) and objective (with regression of pathologic parameters). Ablative surgery for ovarian cancer is particularly indicated for younger or premenopausal patients.

The recent finding of the presence of estrogen receptors has been of great assistance in the field of hormone surgery. In other words, on their surfaces, cells of breast cancer may have certain receptors that are able to bind and carry estrogens into the cells. Thus we are able to identify estrogen-receptor–positive (ER^+) and estrogen-receptor–negative (ER^-) tumors. The estrogen-receptor assay could play an important role in the planning of therapy, since it seems that only ER^+ tumors may benefit by an ovariectomy. Castration causes a partial or complete objective remission for an average period of about 6 months in 35% of the cases. Regression of bone and lymph-node lesions is most remarkable and is also accompanied by a complete remission of pain symptomatology.

With the progression of the neoplastic disease, it is possible to perform bilateral adrenalectomy which, however, complicates patient-management because of the necessity of continuous corticosteroid administration. At present, we tend to avoid adrenalectomy, and there is a renewed interest for surgical or radiologic hypophysectomy, not only for the hormonal suppression involved, but also for its analgesic action.

The same theoretical principles are also adopted in the treatment of metastasized prostatic carcinoma. It is generally a neoplasm with a slow evolution, and even after several years important results are obtained with castration or estrogen hormonotherapy. Some important studies, like those of Nesbit and Baum, carried out on 1,818 cases, have led us to conclude that castration is the treatment of choice with respect to estrogen therapy (3). Moreover, surgical treatment, thanks to modern technical devices, is well tolerated by the patient physically and psychologically.

PALLIATIVE SURGERY FOR PAIN

Pain has both a physical and an emotional component; the evaluation of pain-intensity is difficult, chiefly because of the unforeseeable quantification of the subjective component. In this volume, pain has been analyzed in all of its components by renowned specialists. I would like to agree with Pettavel (4) in stating that in a cancer it is the long duration, its increasing severity, and the progressive breakdown of physical and psychologic conditions of the patient that make pain intolerable. Pain is caused by many factors, such as tissue anoxia due to vascular insufficiency, compression, and the deceptive perineural infiltration.

Any palliative surgery, direct or indirect, reductive or mediate, causes a reduction of pain. However, it is sometimes so intense that the analgesic purpose of the surgery can be achieved only by operating on sensitive nerve trunks. It is a good rule to surgically intervene for the alleviation of pain only after all the other therapeutic means, pharmacologic and others, have failed. The main difference between this palliative surgery and the others is represented by the fact that this one tends only to make remaining life more tolerable, whereas the others can also prolong life. There is a wide range of operations for the peripheral nervous system: nerve blocks produced with neurolytic agents such as alcohol or phenol, which have been widely employed, particularly for stabbing pains in the limbs or in the perineal area due to recurrence of rectal carcinoma; and chordotomy, which is the most common operation with the greatest probability of success. Because of complex nervous compromises, blocks for pains in the perineal area must be performed very cautiously, since they can cause unpleasant complications, such as urinary incontinence.

MEDIATE PALLIATIVE SURGERY

Mediate palliative surgery is surgery that acts as an essential tool to carry drugs to the tumor area.

The local administration of antineoplastic drugs is a form of chemotherapy that, if performed on selected cases, gives more advantages than does systemic chemotherapy. Intra-arterial local-regional treatment has been used in various parts of the body and is now considered an important therapeutic tool. Some years ago Dargent (1) obtained good results, of a chiefly analgesic nature, on inoperable or recurrent rectal and uterine carcinomas that were considered beyond the limits of the possibilities of radiotherapy treatment.

For many years hepatic infusion has been performed, according to Watkins and Sullivan (5), via the hepatic artery for patients with metastases from carcinoma of the stomach and, above all, of the large intestine. Results are encouraging, even if not exciting. In a critical review of the treatment of primary and secondary hepatic tumors, Lee (2) reported a mean survival time of 5.6 to 7 months from the moment of diagnosis. Even the best results with chemotherapy, both mono- and polychemotherapy, were only from 17% (with 5-fluorouracil) to 55% (5-fluorouracil + adriamycin + mitomycin), and the duration of remission was also rather brief (about 10 weeks).

Palliative treatment with arterial infusion seems to give more satisfying results. We have treated 44 patients with inoperable primary tumors of the liver or affected by metastases in the gastrointestinal tract, which were responsible in many cases for a pain-symptomatology that was probably due to rupture or involvement of the peritoneal wall because of its proximity. The survival according to the degree of hepatic involvement is very important. For an accurate analysis of the efficacy of infusion treatment, a breakdown by stage is essential. We have adopted the classification of Pettavel (4). The best survival is found for the patients in Stage I and II, with a median survival of more than 1 year. The most impressive fact was the absence of systemic toxicity, even at high doses in a relatively brief time.

The absence of toxicity was apparent mainly when 5-fluorouracil was employed, whereas when adriamycin was used, toxicity was so intense that a patient died following bronchial pneumonia. The lack of systemic toxicity with 5-fluorouracil is probably due to the elimination of the drug partially by the liver and partially by the lungs. Regardless of the extension of survival, infusional treatment has brought about an immediate effect, has diminished severe pain in the hypochondrium, and caused a partial regression of hepatomegaly.

CONCLUSION

In conclusion, even when a radical cure is not feasible, it is possible for the surgeon to carry out an effective therapy, both to improve the quality of the patient's remaining life and to prolong survival. The surgeon must, however, attempt to minimize the physical and psychologic damages that an indiscriminate, aggressive operation can cause in a patient affected by cancer.

REFERENCES

1. Dargent, O. (1977): Lecture given at the National Cancer Institute of Milan, Italy. (Unpublished.)
2. Lee, Y. T. (1977): System and region treatment of primary carcinoma of the liver. *Cancer Treat. Rev.,* 4:195–212.
3. Nesbit, R. M., and Baum, W. C. (1950): Endocrine control of prostatic carcinoma: Clinical and statistical analysis of 1818 cases. *JAMA,* 143:1317–1320.
4. Pettavel, J. (1971): Les limites de la chirurgie palliative du cancer. In: *Oncologie Chirurgical,* edited by F. Saegesser and J. Pettavel. Masson, Paris.
5. Watkins, E., Jr., and Sullivan, R. D. (1964): Cancer chemotherapy by prolonged arterial infusion. *Surg. Gynecol. Obstet.,* 118:2–19.

Advances in Pain Research and Therapy, Vol. 2,
edited by J. J. Bonica and V. Ventafridda.
Raven Press, New York © 1979.

Hyperthermic Perfusion with Sympathectomy for the Treatment of Advanced Painful Limb Tumors

* R. Cavaliere, ** G. Moricca, * G. Stradone, and * F. Di Filippo

**Department of Surgery, **Department of Pain Therapy, Regina Elena Cancer Institute, Rome, Italy*

INTRODUCTION

For many years, after the first report by Busch in 1866 (3), investigators have commented on the destructive effect of heat upon cancer cells (8,12,15,22). In previous papers, we have reported on biochemical and clinical studies which demonstrated that hyperthermia is an effective anti-neoplastic treatment (6,18,19). At the beginning of our clinical attempts, the first problem we were concerned with was the choice of a technique for an effective local heating. Isolation perfusion according to Creech and Krementz (10), but using prewarmed and diluted blood without drugs, seemed to be the right technique for reaching and maintaining a 42.0°C temperature in the perfused area as far as advanced malignant tumors of the limb were concerned.

The first series of hyperthermic perfusions was performed using a sigma-motor heart-lung machine equipped with a digital pump, a disc-oxygenator previously primed with whole, heparinized blood diluted at 50% with an isotonic solution, and a water-circulating heat exchanger unit maintained at about 47 to 48°C. Thermistor needle probes were applied to the arterial line of the circuit, on the skin, in the muscles, and in the tumor. The perfusions were started; no drugs were perfused; pump flows and the perfusion pressure were previously calibrated. Since a long perfusion time has been found to be effective against tumors, the application of a tourniquet was discontinued after the first cases because it caused peripheral nerve dysfunction. Consequently, we have had to standardize flow equilibration and perfusion pressure during the whole time of perfusion in order to control the exchange of blood between the systemic and the perfusing circulations which, when very pronounced, are a considerable handicap to the hyperthermia of the limb and the general condition of the patient.

Many complications occurred in this first series of patients treated with hyperthermic perfusion which was continued until 1967 (6). Nevertheless, the follow-up of this series allowed us to evaluate the long-term results.

These have been encouraging since of all the patients who were alive and well in 1967, only one died of the disease more than 7 years after hyperthermic perfusion; and this patient had a distant metastasis at the time of perfusion.

At that time, we did not have the possibility of dealing with the difficult problem of limb pain, because we were compelled to improve the technique in order to avoid major complications like acute renal failure, amputations, arterial ruptures, and secondary shocks. These trials were successfully accomplished: The heart-lung machine was replaced by a more reliable one; a flowmeter was inserted into the arterial line of the circuit together with a multichannel monitoring system; and, at the heat exchanger, the temperature was supplied by an independent water-circulating thermostat unit. At the beginning of the perfusion, the temperature in the arterial line was about 42.5°C to 43.0°C, and 42.0°C when hyperthermia was achieved. Mannitol was infused slowly but continuously and continued for some days. A beta-blocking agent was injected into the perfusion circuit at the beginning of perfusion with the aim of reducing the reaction to heat at the microcirculatory level, thus limiting arteriovenous shunts and tissue hypoxia due to the exclusion of the capillary bed.

The mortality rate was reduced to about 2% after the modifications were introduced to the technique. The results obtained in 150 patients clinically confirmed that hyperthermic perfusion is able to cause limb tumors to regress, even if the experimental results do not show complete agreement to the clinical experience (5). However, it is noteworthy that a statistical evaluation of our results published in 1977 (19) showed a 5-year survival rate of about 60% of the patients with osteogenic sarcoma and 75% of the patients with melanoma of the limbs. In spite of these excellent results, there remained the problem of the pain which we continually observed.

For a long period of time, we attached no great importance to this problem of "painful limb," allowing ourselves to be convinced that it was a transient problem of the postoperative period, probably due to swelling with venous stasis and blistering, which were frequently observed, sometimes followed by foot drop. The latter was avoided early by routinely performing anterolateral fasciotomy of the leg, but the problem of painful limb remained unchanged and, in the long run, attracted our full attention. These observations or considerations caused us to focus on this problem.

The first observation—truly disappointing—was the answer obtained from a systematic control of the perfused patients, many of whom were found to be suffering from painful limb, although the limb itself was apparently normal. The second observation concerned the discrepancy between the intensity of persistent pain and the gravity of circulatory disturbances following perfusion. The third observation had to do with the definite improvement obtained with sympathetic blocks, whose effectiveness was greater when the blocks were performed as early as possible in the postoperative period. This suggested that the pain was nonmalignant in nature though obscure in its exact mechanisms, and imprecise in its character, which is possibly mediated by the autonomic nervous system. On the basis of descriptions in the literature (1,2,7,25), we think this kind of painful limb may represent a form of reflex sympathetic dystrophy because of the absence of direct nerve damage, the persistent burning pain, the hyperesthesia and, sometimes, the presence of edema or intermittent cyanosis (4). We are in agreement with Gross (13) when he states that the "autonomic irritation syndromes occur either after irritation of the vessel or of the sympathetic trunks." It is a matter of fact that hyperthermic perfusion can reasonably be considered sufficient stimulus to give rise to painful limbs and that it possesses almost all the characteristics of a minor causalgia: the abnormal topography of pain, dyskinesia, dyscrasia, and dystrophy.

On the basis of these considerations, and because we noted complete, but transitory relief of pain following sympathetic blocks, we decided to tackle such a difficult problem at its origin. We therefore tried to find a new surgical approach that could allow us to perform hyperthermic perfusion and sympathectomy at the same time. This report describes the preliminary results obtained with this combined form of therapy.

MATERIAL AND METHODS

Thirteen patients undergoing hyperthermic perfusion for cancer of the limb were included in this clinical trial: 7 had osteosarcoma, 3 had soft-tissue sarcoma, and 3 had recurrent melanoma. Of the 7 patients with osteogenic sarcoma of the lower limbs, 6 had very extensive tumors and had to be amputated some weeks after perfusion in accordance with our protocol regarding the hyperthermic treatment of limb tumors. The 7th patient underwent bone resection followed by endoprosthesis 4 weeks after hyperthermic perfusion.

Of the 3 patients treated for soft-tissue sarcoma, 1 had a rhabdomyosarcoma of the left arm, and the others had large recurrent fibrosarcoma of the thigh and the calf, respectively. The treatment protocol for these tumors is to use hyperthermic perfusion followed by endoarterial antiblastic infusion and, finally, the excision of the tumor.

Of the 3 patients treated for melanoma, 2 underwent hyperthermic perfusion and dissection of involved nodes for recurrent multiple melanomas of the lower limb. The 3rd one underwent perfusion without node dissection for recurrent melanoma with satellitosis of the upper limb.

All the above patients were treated with sympathectomy at the time of hyperthermic perfusion, involving a single surgical approach. The addition of the sympathectomy does not significantly increase the surgical problems: The exposition, insulation, and cannulation of both iliac and axillary vessels are not affected by the modifications to the technique performed in order to remove the sympathetic chain. The surgical procedure is as follows:

For upper limb tumors, the patient is placed in the supine position with the head turned to the opposite side and the arm in abducted position with the palm upward. The incision is made from the midportion of the sterno-cleidomastoid muscle, 4 cm above the clavicle, laterally and downward along the deltopectoral groove. The clavicle could be divided in its midportion, but this can be avoided and we prefer to do so in order to permit the prompt mobilization of the perfused limb. The clavicular head of the sternocleido-mastoid muscle, the omohyoid muscle, and the anterior scalene muscle are divided above the clavicle, obviating retracting the phrenic nerve. The insertion of the major pectoralis muscle over the short head of the biceps muscle is incised, and the tendinous insertion of the pectoralis minor muscle is divided on the coracoid process. At this time, the content of the axilla is bared below the clavicle, while the subclavian artery is exposed in the upper part of the wound. It is easy to divide the thyreocervical arterial trunk, to palpate the stellate ganglion, and to dissect the sympathetic chain in the extrapleural

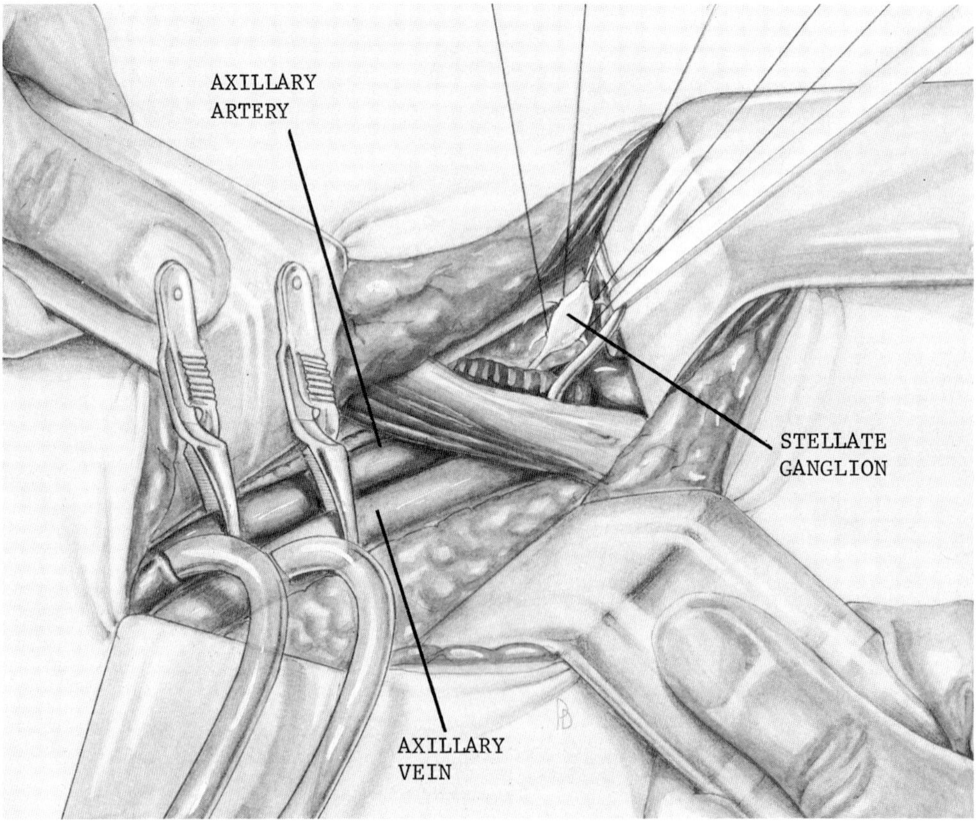

FIG. 1. The stellate ganglion is to be excised above the clavicle (the schematic drawing does not show that the upper part of the ganglion is left *in situ*). Below the clavicle, the axillary artery and vein are cannulated.

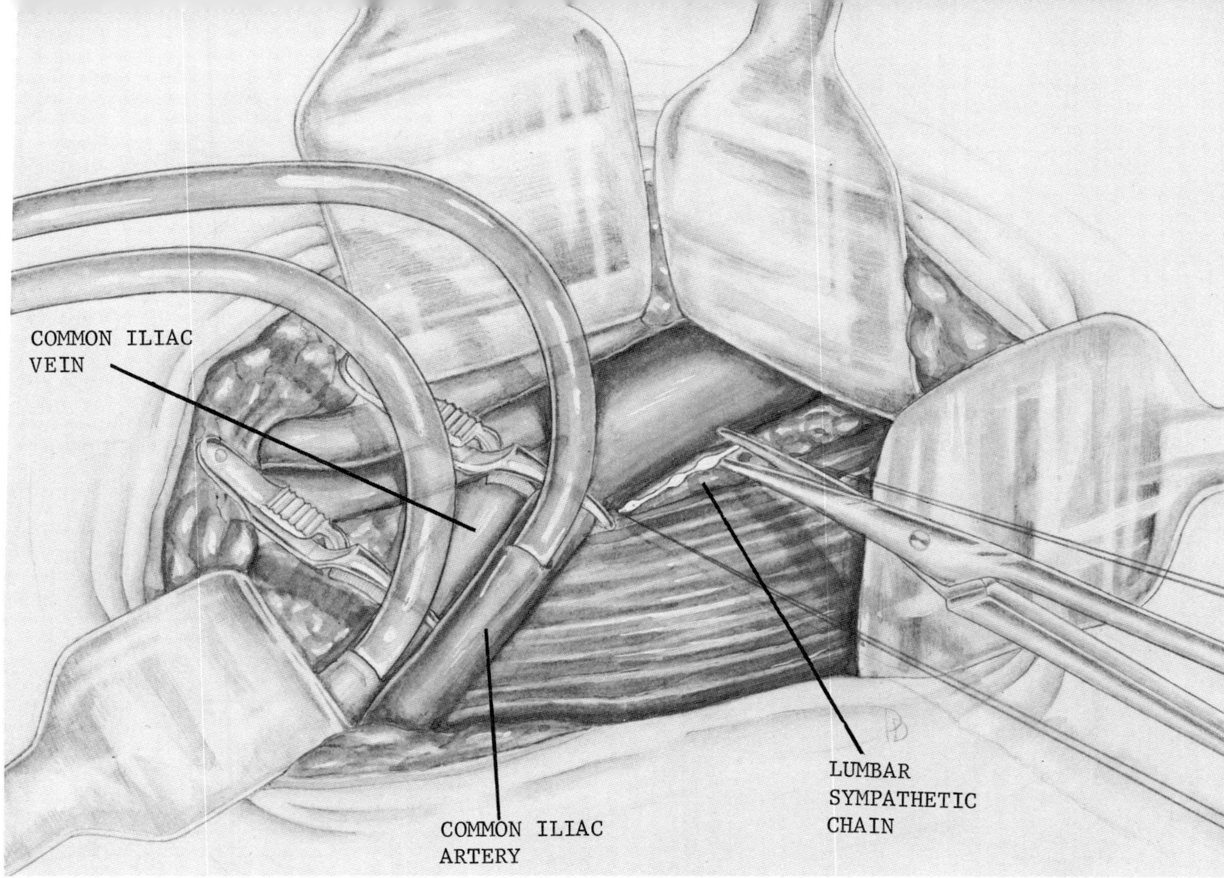

FIG. 2. The bifurcation of the aorta and the first portion of the vena cava are exposed; the lower lumbar sympathetic chain is to be cut between ligatures. The common iliac artery and vein are cannulated.

space. A nerve hook is placed under the sympathetic chain, the various rami are clipped with silver clips, and the chain is divided between the distal part of the stellate ganglion and the 3rd dorsal ganglion (Fig. 1). The cannulation of the axillary vessels and perfusion are performed as described in previous papers (5,19).

For lower limb tumors, the patient is placed in the supine position, and the whole abdomen and the limb to be perfused are included in the operative field. A transverse abdominal incision is made approximately 2 cm below the umbilicus, omolaterally to the limb. The rectus muscle and the external oblique and internal oblique muscles are incised in the direction of the skin incision. The transversus abdominis may usually be incised in the direction of its fibers. The peritoneum is opened; the liver and aortic nodes are exposed. After this maneuver, the peritoneum is sutured, and the peritoneal sac with its contents is bluntly directed medially. The psoas muscle, the distal portion of the abdominal aorta on the left side, or the first portion of the vena cava on the right side, the iliac vessels, and the other structures in the retroperitoneal area come into view. Following Hershey and Calman (14), the sympathetic chain is palpated laterally on the vertebral bodies. By gently lifting the chain with silk threads, the last 3 lumbar ganglions and their rami are identified (Fig. 2). Silver clips are applied between the second lumbar ganglion and the terminal division branches. Other silver clips are applied on the remaining part of the rami, and sympathectomy is performed.

The sympathectomy can be carried out before or after the perfusion; our experience did not show any difference between the two modalities, although it could theoretically be more correct to perform it at the end of the hyperthermic perfusion.

For both upper and lower limbs, a drainage is placed and the incision is closed in layers. No special postoperative care is necessary in relation to adjunctive sympathectomy.

RESULTS

Of the 7 patients treated for osteogenic sarcoma, 6 were suffering from "painful limb," presumably due to the tumor mass's infiltrating the soft tissues around the bone disease. The pain was continuous, markedly increased by palpation and walking, but not well defined in its characters and variable in its intensity. After hyperthermic perfusion and lumbar sympathectomy, the continuous pain was greatly reduced, while the intense and provoked pain disappeared. Neither edema nor venous stasis nor foot drop were observed. These considerations remained until the patient underwent surgery in accordance with the protocol for the treatment of extensive osteogenic sarcoma. The last patient of this group did not present preoperative painful limb; the postoperative period was very comfortable because of the complete absence of pain and of circulatory disturbances. After 4 weeks, he underwent a second operation for bone resection with metallic endoprosthesis; even then, the limb was not painful nor edematous. None of the patients who underwent amputation developed a painful phantom limb.

Of the 3 patients treated for soft-tissue sarcoma, one underwent this combined therapy for a rhabdomyosarcoma of the arm, a very large ulcerated tumor with an important edema of the hand and forearm. The tumor was recurrent and the limb very painful, with a burning, superficial type of discomfort. After the combined treatment, the burning sensation disappeared, although the arm remained heavy; the edema decreased in a few days. These effects cannot, however, be attributed to the therapeutic action of hyperthermic perfusion on the tumor because of their rapidity.

The other 2 patients treated for soft-tissue sarcoma were not suffering from painful limb, although their tumors were large. In these cases, however, the effectiveness of combined therapy was immediately evident in view of the condition of the perfused limb: Swelling, edema, venous stasis, postoperative pain, and foot drop were completely absent, so neither fasciotomy nor debridements were necessary. The patients walked promptly after surgery, and mobility of the limb was also recovered without any trouble.

The same effect of such combined therapy was observed in the 3 patients treated for recurrent melanoma. They did not need fasciotomy or debridements either, and they never complained of painful limb. The only complication encountered was 1 case of Bernard-Horner syndrome, presumably due to a mistake in the identification of the lower portion of the stellate ganglion and first ramus communicans.

DISCUSSION AND CONCLUSION

The first consideration concerns the mechanism of the pain in the limbs. The characteristics of the pain and associated symptomatology suggest that postperfusional circulatory disturbances, such as swelling and edema, can be excluded, because of the persistence of the pain in many patients after their limb had completely recovered. A causative mechanism identified with some direct traumatic action on the vessels appears more likely. A twofold origin can be recognized for such action: at a surgical level, due to the handling of major vessels and/or at a diffuse level, throughout the limb, because of the action of heating on vascular walls. This origin can explain reasonably well why other authors (16,24) who have performed antiblastic hyperthermic perfusion at lower temperatures with shorter durations observed minor incidences of postoperative, long-lasting, painful limb.

The aforementioned preliminary results have convinced us to pursue this clinical trial. The postoperative conditions of the perfused limbs after the association of sympathectomy show such significant differences in comparison with the conditions observed prior to using sympathectomy, that this form of combined therapy should no longer be ignored. Moreover, complications of sympathectomy are few and can be entirely avoided by correct surgical management. At the cervicothoracic level, it is not necessary to accomplish total stellectomy; the goal consists in the excision of the lower part of the stellate ganglion together with the 2nd and 3rd thoracic ganglia. The lower part of the stellate ganglion is identified as the 1st thoracic and may be recognized by its shape and because of the presence of the communicant ramus with the 1st thoracic nerve. The approach we describe permits—without any differences—the perfusion procedure and the excision of the 1st, 2nd, and 3rd thoracic ganglia; and this is sufficient to control the pain even if the innervation of the axilla is avoided (21).

At a lumbar level, surgical implications were emphasized by Simeone (23) and are unchanged in respect to our surgical approach. The only difference concerns the possibility of injuring, on the right side, a large lumbar vein which emerges at approximately the first lumbar vertebra and crosses the sympathetic trunk to enter the vena cava. It can be injured by the retractor because of the reduced direct exposition that our incision permits. On the other hand, such an approach did not present great difficulties if the retractors were correctly applied. Because of the limited extent of sympathetic resection that we have carried out, the first two lumbar ganglia are not affected. This prevents sexual complications (impotence) while allowing us to obtain good physiologic effects, as it prevents the regeneration of preganglionic fibers to the 4th and 5th lumbar ganglia with consequent reactivation of postganglionic neurons whose axons contribute to the femoral and sciatic nerves passing through the lower roots of the lumbosacral plexus. The prevention of regeneration is quite important in our opinion, even in the absence of primary vascular disease, because of the possibility of other kinds of operation such as bone resection or amputation for osteosarcoma, or endoarterial antiblastic infusion for soft-tissue sarcoma, or another perfusion at a different level for melanoma.

The literature indicates it is obvious that postsympathectomy neuralgia is a common complication, occurring to a significant degree in approximately 25% of cases. However, there is great variability between reports, ranging from 2 to 100% (11,17). Fontaine (11) attributes little importance to this complication, observed in 5% of his patients. The nature of the neuralgia is not precisely known, but it is likely due to injury of the somatic lumbar nerves during the operation (1,2). In the opinion of Cooley and Herman (9), the ligature of the sympathetic trunk with nonresorbable thread, as we do, prevents the onset of this kind of postoperative pain. In our limited experience, no complications occurred related to the sympathectomy with the exception of the Bernard-Horner syndrome in 1 patient.

The combined use of sympathectomy with hyperthermic perfusion is to be considered an important achievement, which has encouraged us to continue to use it. As a matter of fact, for the treatment of advanced tumors of the limbs, we are developing a very complex multi-step therapy in which hyperthermic perfusion plays the most important role; but the final goal consists of obtaining limbs definitely free of disease and pain which will be at the same time functional and working. Even if it is too early to draw firmly definite conclusions on this subject, it is our opinion that such a combined approach is an advance toward the solution of the problem and is to be considered a progress because it does not affect the mortality and morbidity in comparison with perfusion alone.

REFERENCES

1. Bonica, J. J. (1959): *Clinical Applications of Diagnostic and Therapeutic Nerve Blocks.* Charles C Thomas, Springfield, Ill.
2. Bonica, J. J. (1953): *The Management of Pain.* Kimpton, London.
3. Busch, W. (1866): Über den Einfluss, welchen heftigere Erypsipeln zuweilen auf organisierte Neubildungen austuben. *Verhandl. Naturh. Preuss. Westphal.,* 23: 28–30.
4. Carron, J., and Weller, H. C. (1974): Treatment of post-traumatic sympathetic dystrophy. In: *Advances in Neurology, Vol. 4: International Symposium on Pain,* edited by J. J. Bonica. Raven Press, New York.
5. Cavaliere, R. (1976): In: *Proceedings of the International Symposium on Cancer Therapy by Hyperthermia and Radiation.* American College Radiology Press, Baltimore, Md.
6. Cavaliere, R., Ciocatto, E. C., Giovanella, B. C., Heidelberger, C., Johnson, R. O., Margattini, M., Modavi, B., Moricca, G., and Rossi-Janelli, A. (1967): Selective heat sensitivity of cancer cells, biochemical and clinical studies. *Cancer,* 20(9): 1351–1381.
7. Challenger, J. H. (1974): Sympathectomy nervous system blocking in pain relief, Monographs in Anaesthesiology. In: *Relief of Intractable Pain,* Vol. 1, edited by M. S. Swerdlow. Excerpta Medica, Amsterdam.
8. Coley, W. B. (1893): The treatment of malignant tumors by repeated inoculations of erypsipelas—With a report of ten original cases. *Am. J. Med. Sci.,* 105:487–511.
9. Cooley, D. A., and Hermann, B. E. (1963): Simple means for prevention of post-sympathectomy neuralgias. *Surgery,* 53:587.
10. Creech, O., Jr., and Krementz, E. T. (1961): Cancer chemotherapy by perfusion. *Adv. Cancer Res.,* 6:111–147.
11. Fontaine, R. (1977): Histoire de la sympathectomic lombaire de sa naissuance à ce jour. *Acta Chir. Belg.,* 1:3–16.
12. Fowler, G. A. (*unpublished report*): Effects of acute concurrent infection on cancer in man (Series A)—Pyrogenic infection in inoperable cancer, 152 cases.
13. Gross, D. (1974): Pain and autonomic nervous system. In: *Advances in Neurology, Vol. 4: International Symposium on Pain,* edited by J. J. Bonica. Raven Press, New York.
14. Hershey, F. B., and Calman, C. H. (1967): *Sympathectomy, Atlas of Vascular Surgery,* C. V. Mosby, St. Louis.
15. Johnson, H. J. (1940): The action of short radio waves on tissues—III. A comparison of the thermal sensitivities of transplantable tumors *in vivo* and *in vitro. Am. J. Cancer,* 38:533–550.
16. Krementz, E. T., and Ryan, F. (1972): Chemotherapy of melanoma of the extremities by perfusion: Fourteen years of clinical experience. *Am. Surg.,* 175:900–917.
17. Litwin, M. S. (1962): Postsympathectomy neuralgia. *Arch. Surg.,* 84:121.
18. Mondovi, B., Strom, R., Ratilio, G., Finazzi-Agro, A., Cavaliere, R., and Fossi-Janelli, A. (1969): The biochemical mechanism of selective heat sensitivity of cancer cells. *Eur. J. Cancer,* 5:129.
19. Moricca, G., Cavaliere, R., Caputo, A., Bigatti, A. and Calistro, F. (1977): Hyper-

thermic treatment of tumors: Experimental and clinical applications. *Recent Results Cancer Res.,* 59:112–152.
20. Pettigrew, R. T., Galt, J. M., Ludgate, C. M., and Smith, A. N. (1974): Clinical effects of whole-body hyperthermia in advanced malignancy. *Br. Med. J.,* 4:679.
21. Robb, C. and Smith, R. (1977): *Operative Surgery—Vascular Surgery.* Butterworth, London.
22. Rohdenburg, G. L. (1918): Fluctuations in the growth of malignant tumors in man, with special reference to spontaneous recession. *J. Cancer Res.,* 3:193–225.
23. Simeone, F. A. (1977): The lumbar sympathetic—anatomy and surgical implications. *Acta Chir. Belg.,* 76:17–26.
24. Stehlin, J. S., Giovanella, B. C., et al. (1975): Results of hyperthermic perfusion for melanoma of the extremities. *Surg. Gynecol. Obstet.,* 140:338.
25. White, J. C. (1974): Sympathectomy for relief of pain. In: *Advances in Neurology, Vol. 4: International Symposium on Pain,* edited by J. J. Bonica, pp. 629–638. Raven Press, New York.

Advances in Pain Research and Therapy, Vol. 2,
edited by J. J. Bonica and V. Ventafridda.
Raven Press, New York © 1979.

Combined Whole-body Hyperthermia and Chemotherapy in the Treatment of Advanced Cancer with Diffuse Pain

* G. Moricca, ** R. Cavaliere, † M. Lopez, and ‡ A. Caputo

**Department of Pain Therapy, **Department of Surgery, †Department of Medicine, ‡Scientific Department, Regina Elena Cancer Institute, Rome, Italy*

INTRODUCTION

The therapeutic effect of high temperatures on neoplastic diseases has been known for several decades. Probably the first clinical report is that of Busch (2), who described a patient who had complete regression of sarcoma of the face after two attacks of erysipelas. Bruns in 1877 (1) reported on a patient with disseminated melanoma who had an attack of erysipelas with a sustained fever of more than 40°C (104°F) for several days. All tumors disappeared, and the patient was alive and free of disease 8 years later. Coley, in 1893 (5) discussed 38 patients with histologically proved advanced cancer who had accidental or deliberate infections of erysipelas with high fever; of these, 12 had complete disappearance of their tumors, and the survival of 2 of the patients with sarcomas was 7 and 27 years, respectively. Subsequently, there were numerous reports on the beneficial effects of high fever or locally applied heat on malignant tumors (17,25,27,28), but much of this information went unnoticed because of the unpredictability of the results related to the methods used to elevate body temperatures.

A renewed interest in the use of heat in the treatment of cancer arose from our demonstration of the selective lethal effect of elevated temperatures on tumor cells, both experimentally and clinically (3). Our successes in tumor control and pain-relief, obtained initially with hyperthermic perfusion and then following Stehlin's experience (23) with hyperthermic-antiblastic perfusion, led us to evaluate the therapeutic possibilities of whole-body hyperthermia alone, and then in combination with antiblastic drugs in the treatment of advanced cancer with diffuse pain.

Table 1 shows the most common methods used to produce total-body hyperthermia. Coley induced hyperpyrexia in cancer patients through the so-called "Coley's toxins" (filtered extracts of *Streptococcus erysipelatis* and *Bacillus prodigious*). Although beneficial effects were recorded for several types of cancer (15), this method fell into disuse because of the great diffi-

TABLE 1. *Methods used to produce whole-body hyperthermia*

Resetting the hypothalamic thermostat using pyrogens:
live organisms (e.g., malaria, erysipelas)
vaccines
bacterial extracts (e.g., Coley's toxins)
nonspecific proteins (e.g., milk)
Introduction of heat into the body:
inflation of the lungs with heated gases
hot-air cabinet
hot baths
irrigation of body cavities with heated fluids
shunt of the blood through a heat exchanger
diathermy
electric blanket
heated wax
hot-water blanket
Inhibition of the evaporative heat loss
sealed polyethylene bag

culty of standardizing the bacterial toxins biologically, and the correspondingly capricious results.

Apart from this technique, the most commonly employed method of obtaining high body temperature was immersion in hot baths. Schmaberg and Tseng (22), in a review of the literature, found that the water temperatures used varied between 35.5 and 53.3°C (96 to 120°F) with a mean temperature commonly used of 40°C (104°F). The duration of immersion also varied widely, but was generally short, ranging between 4 and 5 min. In their experiments, they concluded that the maximum safe water temperature was 43.3 to 45.5°C (110 to 114°F) and that, at a bath temperature of 40°C (104°F) an immersion of 30 min was necessary to achieve a body temperature of 39.4°C (103°F).

Although von Ardenne (26), from his own Institute in East Germany, with his program of "cancer multi-step therapy" based on extreme hyperthermia induced by hot baths, tumor hyperacidity, and changed glucose concentration, has claimed spectacular successes, the considerable problems of control in the application of extreme hyperthermal procedures led him to stop these experiments. He observed "precollapse or collapse states" also, after about 200 or 300 min of hyperthermia at 40°C in the middle-aged patients, and after 120 min in the advanced-age patients.

In fact, the detailed case reports that we have been able to consult are few. Kirsch and Schmidt (12) reported on 5 out of 48 patients with inoperable cancers who were treated with whole-body hyperthermia in a hot-water bath with additional diathermy: 1 of the 5 patients died shortly after the treatment and the other 4 showed minor clinical improvement. Suryanarayan (24), using combined whole-body hyperthermia at 42°C by immersion in hot baths, and chemotherapeutic drugs, treated 9 patients with advanced cancer. He observed pain-relief and regression in tumor size, but the results were not impressive.

In 1968, we started our experiments with a cabinet in which forced-air ventilation at controlled temperature and humidity was maintained. Under general anesthesia, the patient was put into the cabinet with, above him, a cable from a Siemens 608 Ultratherm diathermy machine. The head of the patient was kept outside of the cabinet and enclosed in a helmet in which cold water circulated continuously. Two patients were treated in this manner, and the preliminary results were reported in a previous paper (14). Because of these not-very-satisfactory results, we modified the technique. After a series of various experimental approaches, among which a two-chamber hyperthermia bath with a cooling head-chamber was also used, a final assessment of the technique was possible.

METHOD

At the present time, we are using the following method: After premedication with atropine and promethazine, the patient is anesthetized with an intravenous barbiturate, curarized, and intubated with an endotracheal canula. Anesthesia is maintained with a 60–40% N_2O and O_2 mixture supplemented as needed with intravenous short-acting barbiturates. Leads for the electrocardiograph are applied on the chest, and an intravcnous catheter is inserted to monitor central venous pressure and to replace fluid losses. A nasogastric tube is passed to prevent vomiting due to fluid accumulation, and an indwelling catheter serves to control urine output. Temperature probes are placed in the esophagus, in the rectum, in contact with the tympanic membrane and, whenever possible, in the tumor.

After these procedures, the patient is entirely wrapped in a polyethylene bag to inhibit evaporative heat loss (Fig. 1). (As known, evaporation of 1 liter of sweat from the skin takes 580 kcal from the body.) The major source of heat is a blanket containing water at 50°C that surrounds the polyethylene-enclosed patient (Fig. 2). Endotracheal gases are preheated to 38°C, mainly in order to diminish heat loss in this way.

Core temperature generally rises about 2° to 3°C per hr in relation to body weight, so an average of 2 hr is necessary to obtain the optimal esophageal temperature of 41.8°C. When the esophageal temperature reaches 41°C, the circulation of hot water is stopped. This avoids overshooting of the predetermined temperature, and slows down the rate of heating. By exposing the head and the anterior thorax and adjusting the temperature of the circulating water, it is easy to maintain predetermined esophageal

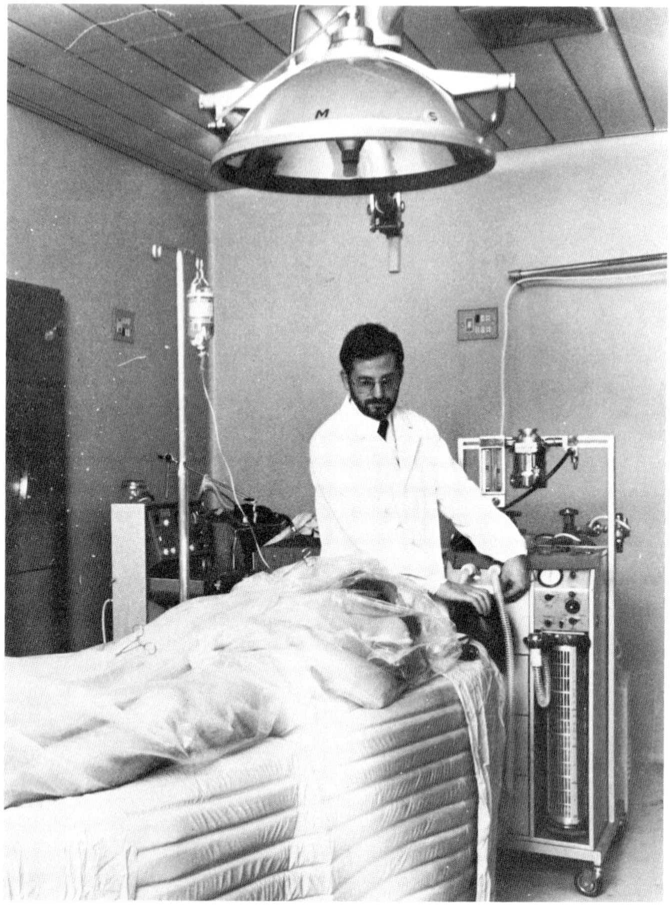

FIG. 1. Patient wrapped in a polyethylene bag.

temperature for the established time (generally 3 hr). If the core temperature rises too rapidly, the procedures designed to diminish the rate of heating are carried out early.

During the treatment, EKG and core temperature are monitored constantly; at intervals, blood pressure, central venous pressure, heart rate, serum electrolytes, urine output, and intratumor temperatures are recorded. Extracellular fluids and serum electrolyte losses are replaced with solutions preheated to 36°C. The monitoring of cerebral function during treatment has proved unnecessary. After treatment, when the water blanket is removed and the patient's body surface is exposed, cooling is rapid, and normal body temperature is reached within 2 hr.

Antiblastic drugs are injected in a single dose when the esophageal temperature of 41°C is achieved. All the drugs used are administered by

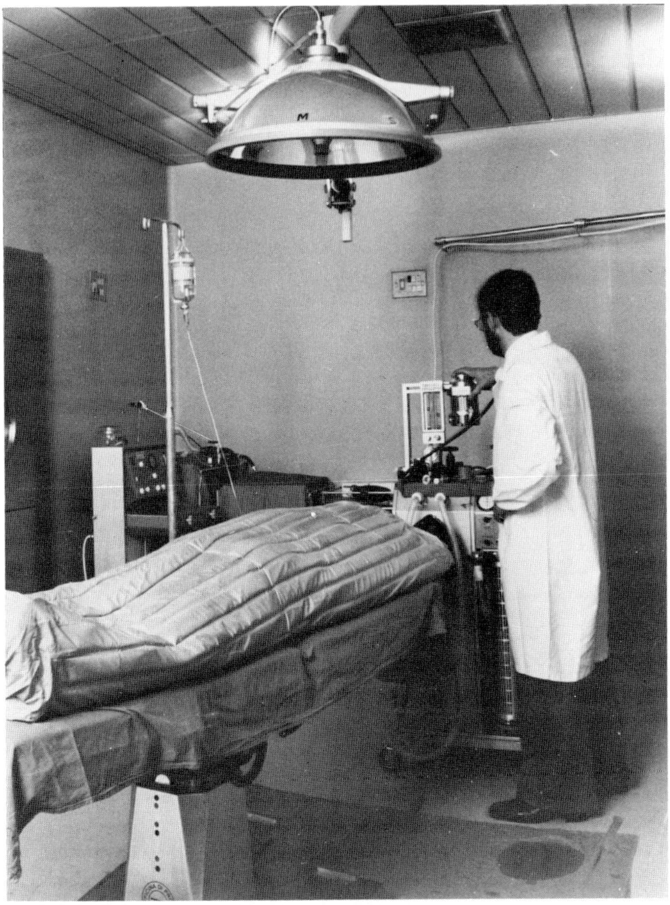

FIG. 2. Hot-water blanket surrounding the polyethylene-enclosed patient.

bolus i.v. injection with the exception of VM-26, a semisynthetic podophyllotoxin derivative, which was given by i.v. infusion over a period of 30 to 40 min in order to obviate the hypotension reported from rapid drug administration (21).

Gastrointestinal and pancreatic carcinomas were treated with 5-flourouracil, 600 mg/m^2, and BCNU, 60 mg/m^2. Breast cancers and soft-tissue sarcomas were treated with vincristine, 1.4 mg/m^2 (maximum dose, 2 mg), and adriamycin (ADR), 60 mg/m^2. The only patient with cerebral neoplasia was treated with VM-26, 100 mg/m^2, and BCNU, 60 mg/m^2, which have a high degree of lipid-solubility and a low molecular weight, i.e., the chemical characteristics required to cross the "blood-brain barrier."

After 4 or 8 weeks depending on the therapeutic schema, bone-marrow toxicity and the patient's clinical response, the thermochemotherapy is repeated. The criteria for response evaluation are both subjective (pain-relief, weight gain, performance status improvement) and objective (tumor regression as seen in serial measurement clinically, or in radiologic changes).

PATHOPHYSIOLOGIC CONSIDERATIONS

The circulatory and biochemical effects of whole-body hyperthermia as seen in our series of patients are the following: The increase in pulse rate was, on the average, 10 beats per min per centigrade degree. In order to avoid undue stress on the heart, we were very careful to avoid overshooting 180 beats per min, both maintaining stable narcosis and administering, if necessary, beta-blocking agents, generally oxprenolol, 2 to 6 mg, intravenously.

Unlike what happened in conscious patients, in whom hypotension and decreased central venous pressure due to peripheral dilatation were observed, there were no significant changes in these parameters in anesthetized subjects. Cardiac dysrhythmias occurred sporadically and generally took the form of ventricular ectopic beats controllable with the usual anti-arrhythmic agents such as lidocaine, initially administered with a bolus i.v. injection of 1 mg/kg body weight, with additional doses every 5 min, either until the arrhythmia was abolished or until 5 mg/kg had been administered.

Out of 6 patients treated with adriamycin, 3 showed ST-T changes returned to normal within 48 hr after treatment. No changes in serum enzymes were observed in adriamycin patients. Fluid losses through sweating were considerable—as much as 500 ml per hour—but serum electrolytes changed remarkably little, and infusions of 700 ml/hour of fluids (we alternated the use of 500 ml of normal saline and 500 ml of 5% dextrose) were generally sufficient to maintain sodium and chloride serum levels within normal limits. Urine output was about 130 ml/hour.

In some cases, a slight fall in the serum calcium and phosphate levels was observed, but normal values were achieved spontaneously within 3 days. Table 2 shows that the average serum activities of lactate dehydrogenase (LDH), alanine aminotransferase (SGPT), aspartate aminotransferase (SGOT), alkaline phosphatase, and gamma-glutamyl-transpeptidase (Gamma-GT) changed little after hyperthermic treatment, and also in patients treated with adriamycin. Significant increases in the serum enzyme activities were observed only when the temperature was held between 42.0°C and 42.3°C for periods of 15 to 20 min. These data agree to a certain extent with those reported by Pettigrew et al. (19).

Renal function tests, serum urea nitrogen and creatinine did not reveal renal dysfunction due to high temperature. Uric acid levels generally rose proportionately to tumor necrosis, so that allopurinol was given (100 mg, 3 times a day, starting 3 days before treatment) to the patients in whom necrosis of large tumor masses was expected.

TABLE 2. *Serum enzyme levels before and after hyperthermia*

Enzyme	Normal level (U/l)	Before heating	After heating	
			24 hr	72 hr
SGOT	< 12	4	6	6
SGPT	< 12	6	9	7
LDH	< 240	163	170	165
Gamma-GT	♂ 6–28	16	22	18
	♀ 4–18	10	15	12
Alk. phosphatase	20–48	31	42	35

Coagulation parameters, prothrombin time (PT), and partial thromboplastin time (PTT) did not change remarkably, whereas platelet counts tended to drop later, mostly in patients treated with BCNU. Nevertheless, neither bleeding diathesis nor disseminated intravascular coagulation (DIC) was observed.

Leukocytosis was observed during hyperthermia, probably related to the letting into the circulation of an amount of white blood cells owing to the hyperthermic stress. Hemoglobin concentration did not change from base-line values, suggesting that hemolysis did not occur at the temperatures involved. This is in accordance with the slight change observed in the serum bilirubin concentration.

RESULTS

Effects on Pain and Neoplasm

As of March 2, 1978, a total number of 15 patients ranging in age from 21 to 77, had been treated with combined whole-body hyperthermia and chemotherapy. The patients were suffering from unbearable diffuse pain due to disseminated cancers and were considered unsuited for further conventional treatments. A total of 39 treatment sessions were carried out and the total number of hours over 40°C was 156. Table 3 shows the data on the malignancies treated, the number of treatment sessions for each patient, the chemotherapeutic agents used, the responses observed, and the survivals as from the start of chemotherapy. The number of treatment sessions to which each patient was subjected was not high, varying from 1 to 4. This reflects our main purpose, which was pain-relief; in the responders, therefore, the interval between courses was prolonged.

The 3 cases of pancreatic carcinoma had a bulky abdominal mass with intractable pain in the epigastrium and in the lower-quadrant areas, radiated to the back. In one patient ascites was present, and another had lung metastases. All 3 patients showed favorable response, with relief of pain and

TABLE 3. *Results of treatment using combined whole-body hyperthermia and chemotherapy*

Type of tumor	No. of patients treated	Previous treatments			No. of treat-ments	Antiblastic drugs	Objec-tive resp.	Subjec-tive resp.	No resp.	Survival as from start of therapy (wks)
		Surg.	Radio-therapy	Chemo-therapy						
Pancreatic cancer	3	0	1	2	4,2,1	5-FU, BCNU	1	3	0	20,10,5
Gastric cancer	3	3	0	2	4,2,3	5-FU, BCNU	2	3	0	26,8,15
Breast cancer	4	4	4	3	3,4,1,4	VCR, ADR	2	2	2	9,17,2.5, 19+
Soft-tissue sarcomas	2	2	2	2	1,4	VCR, ADR	1	1	1	3, 18+
Colon cancer	2	1	0	1	1,3	5-FU, BCNU	1	1	1	3,12
Cerebral neoplasia	1	1	1	0	2	VM-26, BCNU	1	1	0	9

Legend: 5-FU = 5-fluorouracil; BCNU = 1–3 *bis* (2-chloroethyl)-1-nitrosourea; VCR = vincristine; ADR = adriamycin; VM-26 = 4′-demethyl-epipodophyllotoxin-β-D-thenylidene-glucoside.

discontinuance of opiates, but only one showed objective response with considerable regression of lung metastases (Figs. 3 and 4) and a decrease of more than 50% in the 2 perpendicular diameters of measurable abdominal mass.

Out of 3 patients suffering from gastric carcinoma, 2 had unbearable pain in the epigastrium with anorexia, vomiting, and weight loss. After thermochemotherapy, both subjective and objective response was observed with complete pain-relief, decrease in size of measurable abdominal tumor mass and weight gain. The third patient, with diffuse, severe pain from bone metastases, showed only subjective improvement with pain-relief; he died after 2 months.

Of the 2 patients listed with colon carcinoma, only one demonstrated favorable response with complete pain-relief and decrease of metastatic liver involvement. The other died 3 weeks after treatment with acute hemorrhage, and necropsy showed multiple areas of necrosis in the tumor metastases.

Of the 4 patients with carcinoma of the breast, treated with thermochemotherapy, a 28-year-old woman showed no response. At necropsy, involvement of the liver, pancreas, both kidneys, uterus, both lungs, and skeleton was found. Another patient died 18 days after treatment, without pain-relief, and necropsy showed multiple areas of necrosis in the tumor. Two patients who had diffuse, severe pain had pain-relief and objective regression of measurable lesions and were able to lead a relatively normal life.

Of the 2 patients with sarcomas treated, the nonresponder was a 21-year-old man suffering from recurrent fibrosarcoma in the lateral wall of the left hemithorax, and previously treated with chemotherapy for multiple lung metastases. The second patient was a 65-year-old woman, twice operated on in the past for recurrent retroperitoneal fibrosarcoma. She had unbearable pain due to a very large mass occupying the right hemi-abdomen (Fig. 5). Shortly after the first treatment, pain-relief and decrease in tumor size occurred (Fig. 6). The subjective and objective conditions progressively improved with further treatments.

A favorable response was also obtained in the only patient suffering from recurrent malignant glioma. This patient, obtunded and totally hemiplegic prior to therapy, recovered a normal mental status and had an almost complete return of motor function. Improvement was maintained for 2 months until he died from intratumor hemorrhage.

Complications

Six patients developed herpes labialis, generally following first treatment. In 2 cases, a metabolic acidosis developed, with a base excess of −8 and −10 and a fall in serum potassium to 2.4 mEq/l, respectively. Promptly treated, these situations reversed rapidly.

No problems were encountered in controlling ventricular ectopic beats,

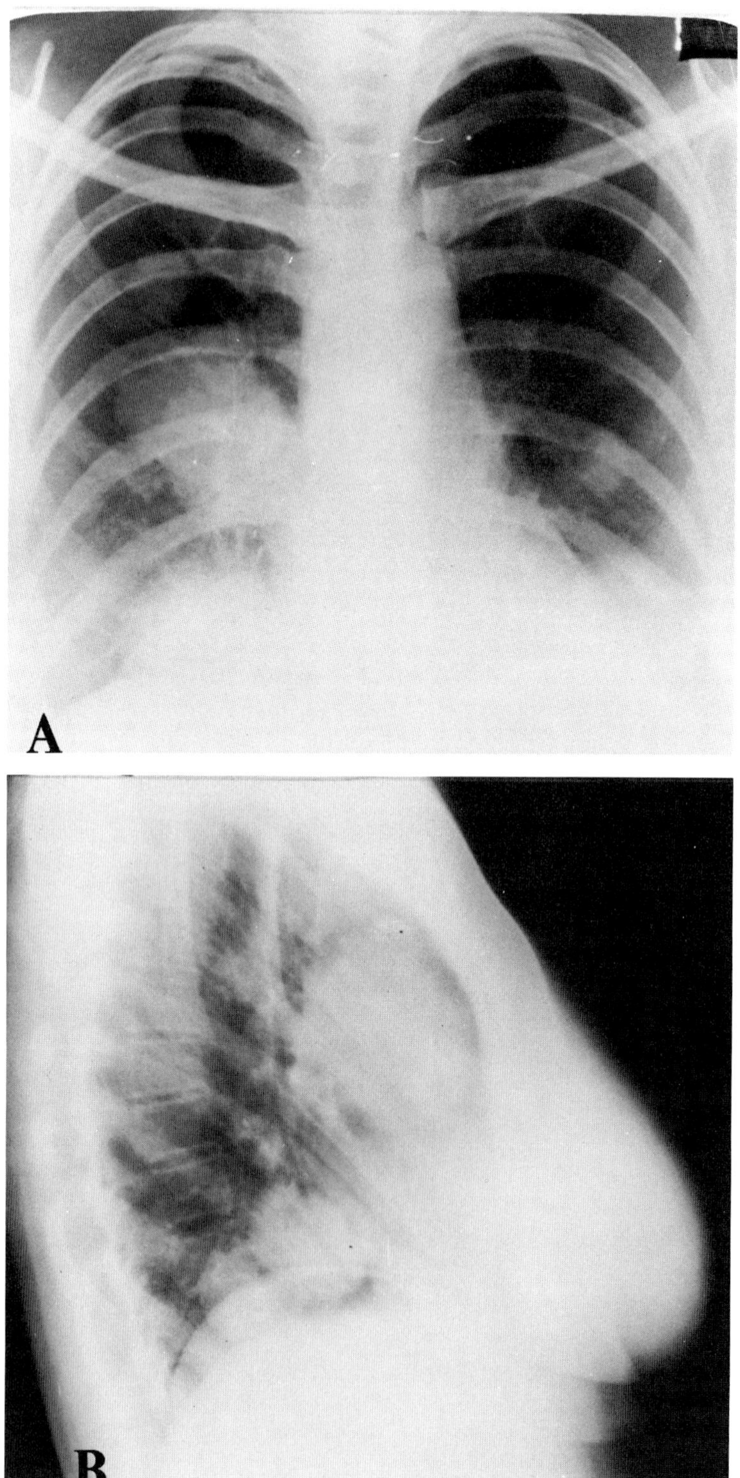
A
B

generally with lidocaine. Sore throats and superficial burns at recognized pressure points occurred in a few patients. During the recovery period some patients showed restlessness and disorientation, but they returned to normal during the subsequent 2 days.

In our series of patients, no deaths were attributable to the treatment. Adriamycin, a potentially cardiotoxic agent, as mentioned above, caused reversible ST-T changes, but not cardiac dysrhythmias or cardiomyopathy. On the other hand, the 550 mg/m^2 dose limit was not exceeded.

Ventricular fibrillation occurred once in Mackenzie's series (13) and once in Pettigrew's series (20); then it was attributable to the temperature level (43°C) or to biochemical disturbances.

Associated heart disease was not encountered in patients receiving adriamycin. It is our opinion that cardiovascular effects of whole-body hyperthermia do not increase the risk of adriamycin cardiotoxicity in comparison with patients not treated in this way if the patient is carefully controlled in order to prevent other myocardial sensitizer factors.

DISCUSSION

Tumor cures have not been achieved so far with whole-body hyperthermia, and complete clinical remissions have generally been few and short-lasting. Nevertheless, pain-relief with discontinuance of opiates and objective responses obtained in some cases of advanced cancer are sufficient to justify this method for the treatment of advanced cancer unsuited to further therapy by conventional methods. Moreover, the relatively easy method, in experienced hands, permits very short hospitalization times.

With present knowledge and technology, it is not very likely that whole-body hyperthermia can produce total neoplastic cell necrosis. Johnson (11) believes that over 20 hr would be needed at 41.8°C in order to obtain this result. On the contrary, Dietzel et al. (6), in their experiments with high frequency heating, showed that the higher thermosensitivity of the tumor cells is not sufficient to achieve cures in a generalized tumor because of the impossibility of separating nonmalignant cells geometrically, even if they are less thermosensitive.

Therefore, it is likely that the best results can be obtained with short and moderate hyperthermia in combination with chemotherapy. Several workers have observed a synergistic effect between high temperatures and certain antiblastic drugs (7,8,9,10,23), but the explanation of such synergism is not

---

←

FIG. 3A. Chest X-ray image before treatment (lung metastases from pancreatic carcinoma): frontal view. **B.** Chest X-ray image before treatment (lung metastases from pancreatic carcinoma): lateral view.

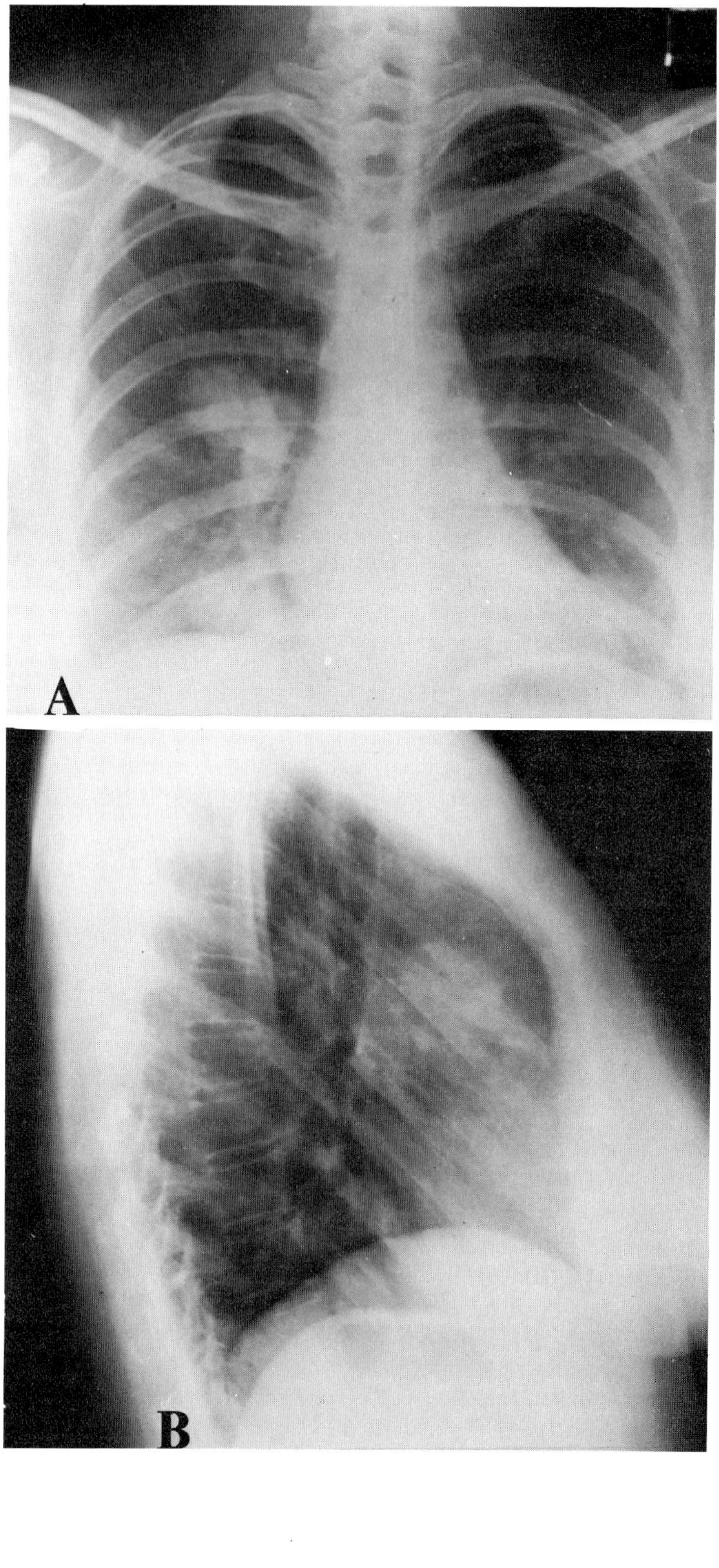
A
B

yet completely known. Hahn et al. (9) showed that *in vitro* and *in vivo* treatment of mouse mammary tumor cells with a combination of elevated temperature (42 to 43°C) and adriamycin increased cell death irrespective of the duration of the combined treatment. Further experiments (10) on Chinese hamster cells exposed to simultaneous hyperthermia (43°C) and adriamycin showed that the cells initially were sensitized to the cytotoxic agent. If the duration of combined treatment exceeded about 30 min, however, the cells became refractory to additional destruction by adriamycin. If heat was applied before exposure to adriamycin, the cells could also be rendered insensitive.

As far as we know, the only trials on man that have been carried out using combined whole-body hyperthermia and adriamycin are our own. It is our impression that, under the experimental clinical conditions described above, the hyperthermia increases the therapeutic effect of adriamycin, because the majority of responders to combined therapy had previously been unsuccessfully treated with adriamycin. We have not observed any increase of toxicity of the drugs used, so this is probably not modified by heating.

A particular problem is that of patients with malignant intracranial neoplasms. To the author's knowledge, the literature contains no case reports on whole-body hyperthermia in combination with chemotherapy. The patient whom we treated received cortisone and mannitol in order to prevent the possible acute elevation of intracranial pressure. It is noteworthy, even though this is only one case, that this patient has not shown particular disturbances, and that he demonstrated favorable response.

Although none of our patients exhibited fatal complications such as disseminated intravascular coagulation (DIC), this problem must be kept in mind (16). Cancer and DIC may be induced by different stimuli. The most important parameters to be evaluated regarding possible fatal complications seem to be the degree of liver involvement, the tumor mass, and the thermosensitivity of the tumor. Liver damage by high temperature is generally slight and reversible under 42.0°C. Over this limit, jaundice may appear. Moreover, some antiblastic drugs have liver toxicity. Therefore, if considerable liver involvement exists and if the tumor is highly thermosensitive, the residual functional parenchyma cannot detoxify the large amount of toxic product brought into the circulation following tumor necrosis.

The results obtained in our series of patients are in agreement with those of Pettigrew (18). He treated 82 patients with hyperthermia using molten paraffin wax as the source of heat. Sixty-four patients had hyperthermia alone, 15 had combined hyperthermia and cytotoxic drugs, and 3 had hyper-

---

←

FIG. 4A. Chest X-ray of the same patient after treatment (6 weeks): frontal view. **B.** Chest X-ray of the same patient after treatment (6 weeks): lateral view.

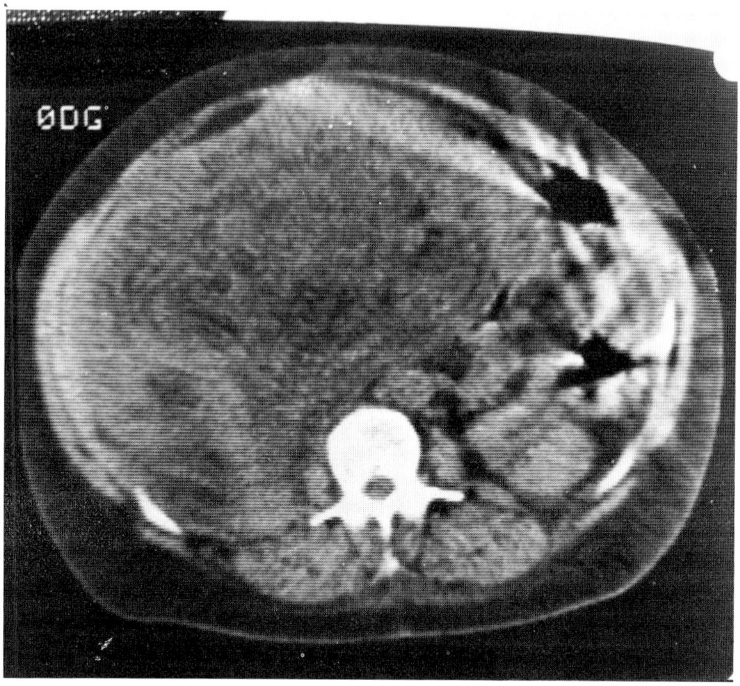

FIG. 5. Abdominal computerized axial tomography (CAT) showing a large mass occupying the right hemi-abdomen (retroperitoneal fibrosarcoma before treatment).

thermia in combination with local radiotherapy. The best results were observed in soft-tissue sarcomas and in tumors of gastrointestinal origin, whereas breast cancers did not respond well to hyperthermia alone but only to thermochemotherapy.

It is of particular interest that pancreatic and gastric carcinomas, which generally have a poor prognosis because of their poor response to the currently available treatments, have shown favorable response. Although the small number of patients treated does not permit the drawing of definite conclusions, further controlled clinical trials are justified.

Another point that should be discussed concerns the possible enhancement of immunologic defenses produced by heating. Since our first clinical experiments with regional hyperthermic perfusion for the treatment of tumors of the limbs (4), the best results have been obtained when amputation or tumor excision was performed some time after hyperthermic perfusion and not immediately afterward. This led us to conclude that the presence of the heated tumor acts as an antigenic source for immunization of the host against metastases even if whole-body hyperthermia can be quite different, from this point of view, from local hyperthermia by perfusion. Experimental work on this subject is underway in our laboratory.

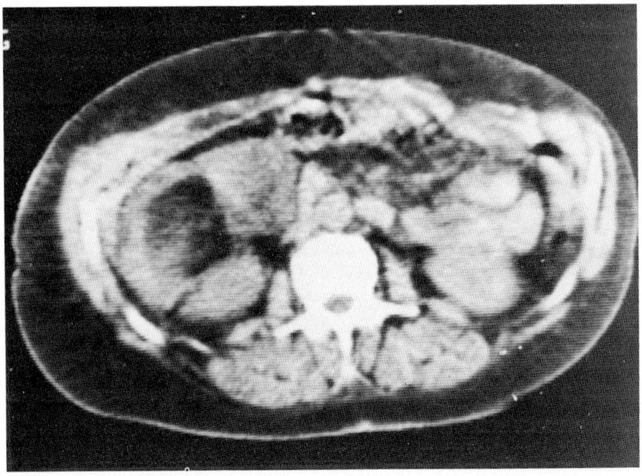

FIG. 6. Abdominal CAT of the same patient after treatment (7 weeks).

The problem of treating tumors using thermochemotherapy has certainly not been resolved. It can, however, be said that the technique is, in any event, valid in view of the success achieved in obtaining pain-relief.

REFERENCES

1. Bruns, P. (1887): Die Heilwirkung des Erpsipels auf Geschwulste. *Beitr. Klin. Chir.,* 3:443–446.
2. Busch, W. (1866): Über den Einfluss, welchen heftigere Erysipelan zuweilen auf organisierte Neubildungen austuben. *Verh. Naturh. Preuss. Rhein. Westphal.,* 23: 28–30.
3. Cavaliere, R., Ciocatto, E. C., Giovannella, B. C., Heindelberger, C., Johnson, R. O., Margottini, M., Mondovi, B., Moricca, G., and Rossi Fanelli, A. (1967): Selective heat sensitivity of cancer cells. *Cancer,* 20:1351–1381.
4. Cavaliere, R., Moricca, G., and Caputo, A. (1975): Regional hyperthermia by perfusion. In: *Proceedings of the International Symposium on Cancer Therapy by Hyperthermia and Radiation.* Washington, April 28–30.
5. Coley, W. R. (1893): The treatment of malignant tumors by repeated inoculations of erysipelas, with a report of ten original cases. *Am. J. Sci.,* 105:487–511.
6. Dietzel, F., Seibert, G., and Klobe, G. (1975): Der Einfluss einer Hochfrequenz-hyper-thermie auf den Verlauf des Ehrlich Ascites Karzinoms der Maus. *Strahlentherapie,* 149:105–107.
7. Giovannella, B. C., Lohman, W. A., and Heidelberger, C. (1970): Effects of elevated temperatures and drugs on the viability of L1210 leukemia cells. *Cancer Res.,* 30:1623–1631.
8. Goss, P., and Parsons, P. G. (1977): The effect of hyperthermia and melphalan on survival of human fibroblast strains and melanoma cell lines. *Cancer Res.,* 37(1): 152–156.
9. Hahn, G. M., Braun, J., and Har-Kedar, I. (1975): Thermochemotherapy: Synergism between hyperthermia (42–43°C) and adriamycin (or bleomycin) in mammalian cell inactivation. *Proc. Natl. Acad. Sci. USA,* 72:937–940.
10. Hahn, G. M., and Strande, D. P. (1976): Cytotoxic effects of hyperthermia and adriamycin on Chinese hamster cells. *J. Natl. Cancer Inst.,* 57(5):1063–1067.

11. Johnson, H. J. (1940): The action of short radio waves on tissues-III. A comparison of the thermal sensitivities of transplantable tumors *in vivo* and *in vitro*. *Am. J. Cancer,* 38:533.
12. Kirsch, R., and Schmidt, D. (1966): Erste Experimentelle und Klinische Erfahrungen mit der Ganzkorper-Extrem-Hyperthermie. In: *Aktuelle Probleme aus dem Gebiet der Cancerologie,* edited by W. Doerr, F. Linder, and G. Wagner, pp. 53–70. Springer-Verlag, Heidelberg.
13. Mackenzie, A., McLeod, K., Cassels-Smith, A. J., and Dickson, J. A. (1975): Total body hyperthermia: Techniques and patient management. In: *Proceedings of the International Symposium on Cancer Therapy by Hyperthermia and Radiation.* Washington, April 28–30.
14. Moricca, G., Cavaliere, R., Caputo, A. Bigotti, A., and Colistro, F. (1977): Hyperthermic treatment of tumors. Experimental and clinical applications. *Recent Results Cancer Res.,* 59:112–152.
15. Nauts, H. L., Fowler, G. A., and Bogatko, F. A. (1953): A review of the influence of bacterial infections and bacterial products (Coley's toxins) on malignant tumors in man. *Acta Med. Scand.,* 145: suppl. 276.
16. Peck, S. D., and Reiquam, C. W. (1973): Disseminated intravascular coagulation in cancer patients: Supportive evidence. *Cancer,* 31:1114–1119.
17. Percy, J. F. (1916): Heat in the treatment of carcinomas of the uterus. *Surg. Gynecol. Obstet.,* 22:77–79.
18. Pettigrew, R. T. (1975): Cancer therapy by whole body heating. In: *Proceedings of the International Symposium on Cancer Therapy by Hyperthermia and Radiation.* Washington, April 28–30.
19. Pettigrew, R. T., Galt, J. M., Ludgate, C. M., Horn, D. B., and Smith, A. W. (1974): Circulatory and biochemical effects of whole body hyperthermia. *Br. J. Surg.,* 61:727–730.
20. Pettigrew, R. T., Galt, J. M., Ludgate, C. M., and Smith, A. N. (1974): Clinical effects of whole body hyperthermia in advanced malignancy. *Br. Med. J.,* 4:679–682.
21. Preclinical Brochure (1967): Sandoz Compound VM-26, Sandoz Pharmaceuticals. Hanover, New Jersey.
22. Schramberg, J. F., and Tseng, H. W. (1927): Experiments on the therapeutic value of hot baths with special reference to the treatment of syphilis: Physiologic observations. *Am. J. Syph.,* 11:337–397.
23. Stehlin, J. S., Jr. (1969): Hyperthermic perfusion with chemotherapy for cancer of the extremities. *Surg. Gynecol. Obstet.,* 129:305–308.
24. Suryanarayan, C. R. (1966): Certain interesting observations during and after hydrohyperthermic chemotherapy in advanced malignancies (preliminary survey). *Indian J. Cancer,* 3:176–181.
25. Vidal, E. (1911): *Travaux de la Deuxieme Conference Internationale pour l'Étude du Cancer,* p. 160. Paris.
26. Von Ardenne, M. (1972): Selective multiphase cancer therapy: Conceptual aspects and experimental basis. *Adv. Pharmacol. Chemother.,* 10:339–380.
27. Warren, S. L. (1935): Preliminary study of the effects of artificial fever upon hopeless tumor cases. *Am. J. Roentgenol.,* 33:75–87.
28. Westermark, F. (1898): Ueber die Behandlung des ulzerierenden Cervix Karzinomes mittels konstanter Warme. *Zentralbl. Gynaekol., pp.* 1336–1339.

Discussion

Part II. Management of Pain of Advanced Cancer: Anticancer Modalities

D. Fink (Moderator)

Questioner: Dr. Bonadonna, do *in vitro* tests of sensitivity to antitumorogens constitute a useful guide to therapy?

Bonadonna (Milano): No.

Questioner: Dr. Pannuti, what are possible side effects associated with MAP treatment given at the high doses discussed in your paper?

Pannuti (Bologna): As I've stated, since 1973, we have used high doses of MAP. The toxic profile of high doses of MAP is known and has also been verified by other authors. Local intolerance is the only limiting factor, because its intramuscular injection leads to 10 to 15% of abscesses. As for the systemic toxicity at the hematochemical level, the only parameter significantly verified is potassium level, which is significantly increased but is still within normal limits. There is an increase of the alpha-2-globuline level, but it also stays within normal limits. Furthermore, one should notice a statistically significant increase of the white cells and platelets, but such effects have already been shown by using MAP even in low doses. As for the other side effects of high doses of MAP, some new findings must be reported as regards low doses:

1. cramps in the legs at night beginning usually after 10 to 15 days and lasting 4 to 5 days.
2. tremors lasting no more than 20 days after the MAP treatment has ended, and
3. night sweats.

Gaining weight has also to be associated with these effects; patients can gain even 10 to 12 kilos. This weight increase is real, and it is due to an anabolic effect. It is not associated with fluid retention or with significant electrolytic alterations. We have also demonstrated this in animals in collaboration with the Pharmacological Institute of our University. In animals, doses such as 4 gr orally or intramuscular produce a significant increase of the anus elevator, which is the best test for deciding whether or not these animals have undergone an anabolic effect. There are no other side effects. We have already begun studies that have also given us the opportunity to use doses higher than the 3 or 4 gr orally for 1 month of treatment with 200 to 280 gr given also as maintenance treatment, showing no significant toxicologic effects.

Questioner: Has MAP been used in other centers?

Pannuti: Dr. Martino's study has compared the administration of 1500 mg MAP for 1 month with the hypophysiolysis achieved by the infusion into the hypophysis of ethanol. Thus, a group of patients has been treated with hypophysiolysis and high doses of MAP. The use of MAP gives pain remission in a larger number of cases than the hypophysiolysis alone. Relief intervenes, as we have already reported, after 3 or 4 weeks and is slower than the hypophysiolysis, but it lasts longer. The average duration of the pain remission is, in our studies, approximately 6 months. It is very important that the administration of high doses of MAP gives not only pain remission in a significantly larger number of patients but also an objective remission of advanced breast carcinoma.

Ricci (Genova): Can a second treatment by radiotherapy for lung cancer be given at the same site as radiotherapy given in the past for control of pain?

Pannuti: For lung cancer, it can be in the same site or in the contiguous site.

Ricci: What is the effect of radiotherapy on pain when given at a dose of 800 to 1000 rads?

Pannuti: This kind of application has been widely used in other institutes but much less in ours, mainly at the level of secondary lesions, of the nervous system, and in or near the bone marrow. Results are not better than the ones achieved with the usual administration of 200 rad instead of 800 rad.

Questioner: Drs. Bonadonna and Basso Ricci, after giving a single, high dose of cyclophosphamide 1,500/2,000 mg or radiation 1,000/1,500 rads to patients with metastasis from Ewing sarcoma or breast cancer, the severe pain is reduced or disappears in a day. How do you explain the mechanism of the relief of pain even though there is not time for reduction in the number of tumor cells?

Bonadonna: If you give treatment with an alkylating agent in susceptible patients, cells are killed within a few hours.

Questioner: Dr. Cavaliere, has hyperthermia been attempted with ultrahigh frequencies?

Cavaliere (Rome): Yes, but mainly at a systemic and not a regional level. We should remember the problems of establishing the temperature we reach, which cannot always be monitored because the thermometers we use are metallic and cannot be kept inside the tumor during the high-frequency heating. Furthermore, the high-frequency heating does not seem really homogeneous, so it is difficult to keep all the tumoral cells exposed at a given temperature and for a given period of time.

Moricca (Rome): Dr. Lopez, does total-body hyperthermia induce intratumoral hemorrhage?

Lopez (Rome): Cases of massive necrosis in various metastatic areas have been reported.

Questioner: What is the relationship of your hyperthermia technique with that described in Germany a few years ago?

Lopez: The technique we used was not substantially different from the Von Norden one.

Questioner: Was the patient with the brain tumor treated with hyperthermia checked with computerized axial tomography before and after the treatment?

Lopez: Computerized axial tomography showed a reduction of the volume of the brain neoplastic growth. But there was also an objective evaluation, because the protrusion of the neoplasm through the residual operative window was not observed anymore after hyperthermia.

Questioner: Is there information about the effect of ovariectomy performed at the time of breast resection in young, still-menstruating women?

Pannuti: The ovariectomy problem in breast cancer is still open. As for us, we do not believe in the use of prophylactic ovariectomy, but only in its therapeutic use. Our present experience is the one also common in the literature, i.e., a remission rate of approximately 40%.

Questioner: Dr. Basso Ricci, in some institutes, multiple bony metastases are submitted to polyirradiation with 850 rad in 2 days. What do you think?

Basso Ricci (Milano): In our opinion, the localized treatment at a lower dose for each metastasis is better.

Questioner: Dr. Pannuti, how useful is calcitonin in bony metastases?

Pannuti: The use of calcitonin in bony metastases, particularly in breast cancer, has not yet been studied in a controlled way. In the terminal stages with hypercalcemia, my personal experience is very disappointing.

Questioner: Why not have a maintenance treatment with MAP after the initial 1-month cycle?

Pannuti: This is a question we have already asked ourselves. As we did not know what side effects could be expected in the future with such high doses, we limited them to the first month. As soon as we verified that there were no dangerous side effects, we used the maintenance treatment that we use now, which is as follows: 1-month treatment, 15 days interruption, and then again high doses, 1 or 2 g for 15 days every month. We have already administered to many patients doses higher than 200 g without their showing any systemic side effects.

Questioner: In your experiments on the MAP analgesic effects, do you consider useful the use of such a general codification of the pain symptom by levels according to the kind of analgesic administered?

Pannuti: This is a very important problem concerning the codification of the pain. When I used the terms *signal tumor* and *signal symptom,* I meant a pain symptom generating from the tumor location. This is the signal symptom definition and its value is established according to the treatment. A pain is defined as being of first degree when a patient is in moderate pain and does not take more than one analgesic. Obviously, if a patient takes only one dose of morphine, he is in a very different position from the one who takes only one aspirin. The patient taking morphine will have more intense pain. The definition of pain is very difficult because different factors have to be investigated: the semantics, the pain quality, and the emotional, psychological, and social connotations of the patient himself.

Advances in Pain Research and Therapy, Vol. 2,
edited by J. J. Bonica and V. Ventafridda.
Raven Press, New York © 1979.

Psychologic and Psychiatric Techniques for the Relief of Advanced Cancer Pain

M. R. Bond

Department of Psychological Medicine, Southern General Hospital, Glasgow, G51 4TF Scotland

At the outset it must be emphasised that pain is a *symptom* of illness and, as such, must be taken as an integral part of that illness. Indeed, in many instances where pain is part of a chronic and potentially fatal illness of the cancer group, success in treatment will not be gained unless this approach is adopted. Consideration of the whole illness also means more than attending solely to physical symptoms, because it means taking account of a patient's emotional problems and the effects of changes caused by his illness in the family in terms of their own emotions and social activities. Thus, management of cancer patients, with or without pain, entails the use of a team of trained individuals—doctors, nurses, social workers, nonmedical therapists of various kinds and, where appropriate, ministers of religion—in such a way that a continuum of care is available at all times between hospital and home.

One of the problems posed by this counsel of perfection is that we know relatively little about the detailed nature of services required for cancer patients in the community other than those of a physical nature, and it is only within recent times that attempts have been made to examine patterns of care needed by patients with chronic, painful diseases who are not in a hospital. In other words there is currently a discrepancy between psychologic and social services needed by cancer patients and their families and the care available (9,10). This is partly due to failure of the medical and social services to recognize and treat emotional and social problems. It is also due to the reluctance of patients to report their needs in this regard, because they see doctors as being concerned with their physical health only and fear being regarded as weak should they complain. This is an unfortunate consequence of the British attitude toward illness and suffering.

In order to comment specifically upon the use of psychiatric and psychologic techniques in pain-relief for cancer patients, it is first necessary to examine the nature of the emotional and social problems raised by various stages of the illness, when pain is present and when it is absent.

THE EMOTIONAL CONSEQUENCES OF CANCER FOR PATIENT AND FAMILY

The diagnosis of cancer is often withheld from patients in Britain, although relatives are told of it at an early stage. The family are quite naturally very distressed by what has been revealed to them, because the illness presents the threat of loss of a loved one, loss of income, and loss of social status. They are often forced by the doctor into a "conspiracy of silence" because of the lack of his or her willingness or inability to tell the patient the true nature of the illness. Moreover, the stress imposed by this knowledge among relatives poses a heavy burden, especially if psychologic support is not offered, as is often the case. Thus, until the chronicity of the disease and the failure of doctors to check its progress becomes evident, or except where fear of cancer appears at the outset as in the case of a woman who develops a breast lump, the level of emotional disturbance may be quite low initially.

In practice, however, patients often become aware through unspoken clues from doctors and relatives or friends that their illness is more serious than they first believed. However, sooner or later overt anxiety develops as a patient faces a series of stresses including uncertainty of the outcome of the illness, threat of loss of identity, self-esteem, and life. Regarding the last point, unspoken awareness of impending death is present in as many as three-quarters of those within 6 months of the end of their lives (5). The chronically ill person, especially when in pain, becomes increasingly withdrawn and introspective, mobility is reduced, social contacts are lost; and preoccupation with physical symptoms, anxiety, and especially depression, are the hallmarks of the mental state. It has been suggested that depression develops out of a sense of helplessness, of being at the mercy of an uncontrollable malignant process; and of hopelessness because others are unable to provide a cure or even satisfactory relief from pain. For some this seems to be a punishment for real or fantasied misdeeds in the past, and to others it is a useless and disturbing experience which produces extreme feelings of loneliness (2).

Pain heightens emotional responses already evoked by illness, and this process increases if the patient feels that doctors have lost control of the disease and have reached the limit of their therapeutic powers. It is a situation with which some doctors cannot cope and causes their withdrawal from close contact with the patient because of personal feelings of inadequacy, or the fact that they see the patient's decline as a failure and a threat to their professional role as a healer. The daily work is then left to others often more junior and less experienced, though perhaps more compassionate. The use of increasingly powerful drugs and surgical treatment bring unpleasant side effects too, including reduced awareness and powers of concentration, anesthesia, dysesthesias, failure of bladder control, dyspnea, nausea, and vomiting, which add yet further to the general level of misery and discomfort.

Cancer patients are said to pass through four stages in their responses to the progress of a fatal illness, and their relatives are said to experience them too, though not necessarily at the same time. In practice all four reactions may occur in the space of hours, may be repeated, and may appear in several different sequences. They are illustrated by the following case history of a 56-year-old housewife who discovered that she had bladder cancer and who survived for a period of 7 months afterward.

Having been told of her cancer after a cystoscopy, performed after two severe episodes of hematuria, the patient appeared to accept the diagnosis with an unusual degree of cheerfulness and apparent lack of concern. At this stage she was reticent to accept major surgery but was persuaded to undergo a course of radiation therapy. It was felt at this time she was coping with the overwhelming anxiety imposed by the nature and the extent of the illness by operating the mental mechanism of denial (Stage 1). Initially the illness was not painful. However, radiation therapy produced severe cystitis and excruciating pain only partially controlled by narcotics. The patient became very depressed (Stage 2), her feelings were mixed with anger, and the comment, "Why should this have happened to me?" was made frequently. Considerable blame was placed on the various doctors for their negligence in not having reached the diagnosis sooner—for which there was some justification (Stage 3). Although the pain was never fully controlled from that time onward the level of depression fell, perhaps because of the use of psychotropic drugs. Although the patient did not mention her impending death, it became obvious about a month beforehand that she had accepted it as inevitable. She became quite composed, cheerful, and reasonably constructive with her remaining weeks of life (Stage 4). About 10 days before she died she asked us if death would be painful, a common fear among cancer patients. After discussing the issue she did not refer to the matter again but became quiet and clearly resigned to her fate. Throughout the illness her husband, with whom she had had a close relationship all their marital life, remained unnaturally cheerful and optimistic in her presence, and yet elsewhere showed extreme agitation, depression with frequent weeping, and expressions of despair. Despite their long and close life together, spoken communication in the final illness was strained. This strained relation clearly would have been improved if an experienced doctor could have become involved in psychotherapy with both the patient and her husband.

The sequence of events described is by no means unique, but it highlights common physical and emotional problems with which doctors and nurses must cope. Examination of studies which have looked at pretreatment and posttreatment levels of emotional disturbance are of interest. A search of the literature did not reveal references referring specifically to cancer patients in pain, but Lee and Maguire (7) who investigated 400 women attending a breast clinic found that anxiety levels were high in all patients and remained so among those admitted for biopsy. It was noted that levels of distress were also high in patients' husbands, and that the surgeons tended to ignore the latter's distress if it were not put into words. Lumps in the breast are greatly feared by virtually all women, and by many they are thought of as malignant until proved otherwise. The findings of Lee and Maguire draw attention to the fact that the patient's need to cope with emotional distress begins, though to a varying degree, at the time of initial consultation with a doctor.

In a more recent paper on breast cancer patients (10), it was reported that many patients have emotional disorders long after surgery at a time when surgeons regard them as having completed treatment. For example, 1 year later a quarter of their patients had anxiety, depression, or both, requiring treatment, and a third had moderate to severe sexual difficulties. However, only a very small proportion (8 of 75) of patients sought help for their emotional problems, and only 2 felt they were given appropriate support. Pain was not a feature of patients in this study, but the point is made that the trials posed by the illness and its treatment are potent causes of psychiatric illness. Undoubtedly if pain had been present, the patient who suffered it would have experienced even more mental distress. Maguire (9) likens the response to mastectomy, as others have done in the case of different mutilating operations, for example surgery for rectal cancer (3), and limb amputation (11), to a bereavement reaction incorporating the following sequence of events: (a) initial shock and disbelief; (b) sadness and weeping; (c) some preoccupation that the individual has become physically unattractive; (d) resentment and hostility revealed in complaints about others, or different aspects of the environment; (e) some loss of self-confidence and self-esteem. It is clear that the reactions described are also those experienced by many patients with a progressive and ultimately fatal disease.

THE TREATMENT OF EMOTIONAL DISTURBANCES AND PAIN

From what has been written it is obvious that an understanding of, and ability to deal with, the emotional consequences of cancer pain are essential if the emotional well-being of patients is to be supported, and relatives' problems are to be resolved. Psychiatrists, psychologists, and social workers are by virtue of their training more able to deal with this aspect of illness than others and have certain methods of special treatment at their disposal including psychotropic drugs, psychotherapies, and social manipulation. However, it should not be thought that this area of work is the sole prerogative of those with a specific training in psychiatry and allied disciplines. Surgeons, radiotherapists, nurses, and others should also acquire and develop some measure of skill.

Kraft (6) recommends that the surgeon should never condemn patients' behavior when it is driven by necessary mental defense mechanisms which he may regard as "neurotic" and that he should produce an empathic response to patients' expressions of anxiety and their need for a sense of control in the face of helplessness. Kraft advocates ready, simple, and direct communications with the patient and the maintenance of compassion at all times, preferably in an environment as free as possible from the complex and perhaps frightening paraphernalia found in certain hospital wards. The surgeon should also remember that the patient's view of him is governed by inner needs for security and safe deliverance rather than by objective facts and that he or she almost always places child-like trust in the surgeon and other doctors directly concerned with treatments, including pain-control. Such dependency demands a warm and comforting approach which will satisfy emotional needs and reduce levels of anxiety and depression.

Psychotropic Drugs

Bearing in mind that the most common disorders of emotion in chronically ill patients with pain are anxiety and depression, it is clear that anxiolytic and antidepressant drugs have their uses. Unfortunately there is surprisingly little reliable information about well-conducted trials of these drugs in the literature. In order to deal with anxiety, and much of this is based in reality and connected with the nature of the illness and apprehensions about treatment, the use of drugs should be carefully controlled. Preferably they should be used in association with counseling designed to remove as much anxiety as possible. This approach has been shown to reduce anticipatory preoperative anxiety substantially and, as a consequence, postoperative pain (4). An alternative, namely the use of benzodiazepines alone, as described by Battelli et al. (1) in the treatment of cancer patients, is less accceptable because they were not combined with counseling.

Patients with cancer may become very depressed (14). Therefore the use of antidepressant drugs is indicated in such instances for those who are deeply depressed, and these are usually easily distinguished from those with lesser degrees of emotional disturbance. It should be remembered that many patients are sad rather than depressed. Consequently, occasionally it is difficult to decide upon the depth of depression because many of the normal biologic features of the malignant disease process simulate organic changes associated with depression in psychiatric patients, e.g., weight loss, anergia, and poor sleep. Thus, care must be taken to avoid unnecessary use of antidepressants, for they have unpleasant side effects. Where the patient is depressed, tense, and anxious, and the medicine preferred is a tricyclic antidepressant, amitriptyline is recommended; and where apathy predominates imipramine is of value as it has an energizing effect.

Psychotropic drugs are commonly and quite properly used as adjuncts to analgesic therapy. Chlorpromazine in doses above 25 mg potentiates analgesics; and some advocate the use of tricyclic antidepressants too, because over and above their ability to reduce depression they also appear to have analgesic properties. The use of chlorpromazine and an antidepressant together has been advocated because chlorpromazine may increase feelings of depression. There are many different tranquilizers and antidepressants available. It is this writer's recommendation that those who wish to use them should select one or two drugs and become familiar with their use, effects, advantages, and disadvantages, for we believe that there is little to choose between different preparations of similar compounds.

Psychotherapy

It has been reported by Maguire (9) that the patients often regard doctors as too busy to listen to them and see them as uninterested in their emotional problems. Many see doctors as individuals who are dealing with their physical symptoms and not people to whom they should take their emotional difficulties (12). However, the mainstay of a psychiatrist's treatment is a psychotherapeutic approach, and although this is not a subject which can be dealt with at length in this paper, several comments about its use are relevant. Firstly, patients with organic illnesses may feel angry and resentful at being interviewed by a psychiatrist. His presence threatens already weakened self-esteem and feelings of self-control, bringing the implications of inability to cope to the bedside. Secondly, patients may feel that doctors engaged in their physical therapy have given up hope and that they have become untreatable. Thirdly, patients may believe they are being troublesome in some way by letting "their nerves get the better of them." These issues must be dealt with at the outset by emphasizing that the physical illness remains a major concern but that inevitably it brings with it both personal and interpersonal difficulties. Most patients recognize and accept this view and come to welcome the psychiatrist's visit.

The main purpose of therapy is to help the patient accept the reality of the threat his or her illness poses in a positive way and to encourage the living of a full emotional life with new and limited but obtainable goals in the remaining weeks or months. Le Shan and Gassmann (8) commented that fear of death, which must be dealt with eventually, is often a reflection of guilt about not having really lived earlier in life and that this may be overcome by engaging the patient in the process of living for the day, for, as Le Shan and Gassmann emphasize (and this can be pointed out with confidence), "no human being has assurances about the future." Thus physical, social, and emotional goals for the day are set and discussed and then adjusted to suit each individual's level of physical and emotional well-being. It should be appreciated that the approach is empathic and that direct expressions of sympathy for the patient are *not* encouraged, for they may be detrimental in causing him or her to focus upon the hopeless aspects of the situation and thus worsen feelings of depression.

The reduction of anxiety associated with psychotherapy and the feeling patients develop that they have not been deserted is often associated with reduction in feelings of futility, hopelessness, and depression. Pain levels often fall too, and the need for analgesic drugs may be reduced or even abolished. Two other major emotional difficulties may be present, and they represent crises in the relationship between the patient and his or her doctor centered upon the failure of the latter to bring expected relief from suffering, or the actual or anticipated rejection of the patient by the physician (13). These conflicts arouse much anxiety, which generally remains unformulated because of the serious threat such feelings pose for the emotional integrity of both doctor and patient. However, they may become manifest in anger and frustration with the doctor, who in turn may react with threats of abandonment or other more subtle forms of punishment—an unpleasant situation which psychiatrists are not infrequently called upon to disentangle.

It should be remembered that psychotherapy is arduous for the therapist as well as the patient. He or she may develop feelings of futility or hopelessness too as a result of working with a dying patient. The therapist must work through this, remembering that the task on hand is helping the patient to achieve a fuller emotional life, which may bring with it relief of physical symptoms and even lengthened life. Nevertheless, the death of the patient when it occurs is a severe blow, and irrational feelings of failure may develop. It is for this reason that the therapist should be protected by being a member of a team caring for the patient. Anxieties are shared and discussed among members of the team with the purpose of resolving feelings of pain and disappointment among colleagues, as well as planning and executing different stages of physical treatment.

Group and Family Therapy

Group therapy may be carried out with patients and has very definite benefits. The function and composition of groups vary from place to place, but in most cases their basic goals are the gaining of emotional support by one patient from another in controlled surroundings and discussion of practical difficulties arising out of pain and disability. The sense of loneliness which tends to afflict patients is removed by sharing difficult experiences with others who have similar problems.

Family therapy is a growing area in psychiatry and also has much to offer in the world of physical disease. All too often physicians, surgeons, and family doctors, confine their interests to the patient, because for many the complexity and taxing nature of the work demanded by relatives is beyond their personal skill and interests (15).

There are three basic steps in family therapy: first, the analysis of emotional interactions between family members with emphasis upon methods they can adopt for coping with stress. Next, the provision of a setting in which previously unspoken fears and feelings can be expressed in a controlled and "safe" fashion. Lastly, the provision of a situation in which correct information about the illness can be delivered to avoid misunderstanding and anxiety in the patient's family. The feeling that the patient's physical and emotional welfare is being controlled is usually a great source of comfort. Eventually members achieve a realistic understanding of the illness and its treatment and improve upon their own ability to cope with personal feelings and therefore those of the stricken family member.

REFERENCES

1. Battelli, T., Bonsignori, M., Manocchi, P., and Rossi, G. (1976): Anxiety therapy in neoplastic patients. *Curr. Med. Res. Opin.*, 4:185–188.
2. Bodley, P. O., Jones, H. V. R., and Mather, M. D. (1974): Pre-operation anxiety: A qualitative analysis. *J. Neurol. Neurosurg. Psychiatry*, 37:230–239.
3. Devlin, H. B., Plant, J. A., and Griffin, M. (1971): Aftermath of surgery for rectal cancer. *Br. Med. J.*, 3:413–418.
4. Egbert, L. D., Battit, G. E., Welch, C. E., and Bartlett, M. K. (1964): Reduction of postoperative pain by encouragement and instruction of patients. *New Engl. J. Med.*, 270:825–827.
5. Hinton, J. M. (1963): The physical and mental distress of the dying. *Quart. J. Med.*, 32:1.
6. Kraft, I. A. (1976): The surgeon's psychological management of his patient. In: *Modern Perspectives in the Psychiatric Aspects of Surgery*, edited by J. G. Howells, pp. 637–658. Brunner Mazel, New York.
7. Lee, E. G., and Maguire, P. (1975): Proceedings: Emotional distress in patients attending a breast clinic. *Br. J. Surg.*, 62:162.
8. Le Shan, L., and Gassmann, M. L. (1958): Some observations on psychotherapy with patients suffering from neoplastic disease. *Am. J. Psychother.*, 12:723–734.
9. Maguire, P. (1976): The psychological and social sequelae of mastectomy. In: *Modern Perspectives in the Psychiatric Aspects of Surgery*, edited by J. G. Howells, pp. 390–422. Brunner Mazel, New York.
10. Maguire, P., Lee, E. G., Bevington, D. J., Küchemann, C. S., Crabtree, R. J., and Cornell, C. E. (1978): Psychiatric problems in the first year after mastectomy. *Br. Med. J.*, 1:963–966.
11. Murray Parkes, C., and Napier, M. M. (1975): Psychiatric sequelae of amputation. In: *Contemporary Psychiatry*, edited by T. Silverstone and B. Barraclough, pp. 429–440. Headley Bros., London.
12. Peck, A., and Boland, J. (1977): Emotional reactions to radiation treatment. *Cancer*, 40:180–184.
13. Pinsky, J. J. (1975): Psychodynamics and psychotherapy in the treatment of patients with chronic intractable pain. In: *Pain Research and Treatment*, edited by B. L. Crue, pp. 383–398. Academic Press, New York.
14. Woodforde, J. M., and Merskey, H. (1972): Personality traits of patients with chronic pain. *J. Psychosom. Res.*, 16:167–172.
15. Worby, C. M., and Babineau, F. (1974): The family interview: Helping patient and family cope with metastatic disease. *Geriatrics*, 29(6):83–90.

Advances in Pain Research and Therapy, Vol. 2,
edited by J. J. Bonica and V. Ventafridda.
Raven Press, New York © 1979.

Hypnotherapy in Pain of Advanced Cancer

Basil Finer

Department of Anaesthesiology, Samariterhemmes, Box 609, S-75125 Uppsala 1, Sweden

This you shall know:
Dull ache wants company
Sharp pain does not want to be alone
So do not go to bed
You may not lie comfortably
even if you can
For then it will be tyrant over your loneliness

No, you shall sit up
You shall rock to and fro
You shall lean in all directions
You shall keep your own company
You shall write letters to someone
if there is someone, otherwise to no one
as I do now
You shall move things and objects
from place to place
You shall do things in the kitchen
if you have one and can walk
You shall think thoughts if you can
or do some handwork, knit a sock
with a foot miles long. You shall keep company
with your ache, you shall entertain it
the whole time until the grey morning.

Gunnar Ekelöf (1907–1968)
Partitur: Posthumous Poems, 1969
(Own translation—by permission)

The Swedish poet wrote this 3 months before his death from larynx cancer.

It was 440 years ago that the far-sighted rulers in the enlightened government of Venice placed Andreas Vesalius in the chair of Surgery with care of Anatomy in their University of Padua. Five years later was published *Fabrica Humani Corporis,* the beginning not only of modern anatomy but of modern physiology, in as much as Vesalius was the distinct forerunner of Harvey. For Harvey's great exposition of the circulation of the blood did for physiology what Vesalius' *Fabrica* did for anatomy: It first rendered true progress possible. And Harvey's great work was the direct outcome of Vesalius' teaching and yet, one reached by successive steps, steps taken by men of the Italian school, of which Vesalius was the founder and father (11). In Uppsala, there is a copy of the anatomy theatre from Padua in the Gustavianum.

We are all involved in trying to alleviate an intolerable situation for our patients, and no one method can as yet suffice. We need to know the best of each other's methods, so that we can administer the most efficient combination.

The method I will discuss, hypnotherapy, is well known and has been used for more than 200 years, but repeated exaggerated claims for its usefulness, followed by the skepticism of repeated disappointment in its failures have cast an unwarranted shadow over the method. I should like to compare hypnotherapy with nitrous oxide–oxygen anesthesia. Both methods alone are rather weak, and it was a long time before scientific research could be used to investigate their physiologic, pharmacologic, and psychologic mechanisms of action. This research is only in its infancy and both nitrous oxide–oxygen anesthesia and hypnotherapy are still best used in combination with other complementary methods, which they can greatly enhance.

As you began to listen to this lecture, you probably went through various procedures. You chose somewhere that was comfortable, warm, and quiet, with suitable lighting. You more or less consciously shook off your previous thoughts and feelings, while your curiosity and interest in the subject motivated a concentrated effort to take in the words of the speaker. As long as the subject matter captures your attention, you forget your surroundings, but as soon as the subject matter becomes boring, or you get tired, or other matters impinge on your consciousness, your concentration wavers. If you can shake off these interruptions, it may be possible to recapture your interest in the lecture, but otherwise you give up and wait to see the lecture in print later on. The brain functions so that it is difficult or impossible to concentrate strongly on more than one thing at a time. If such strong concentration is possible, it usually implies that there is a simultaneous detachment from other stimuli. Concentration and detachment are like two sides of a mirror, which always exist together. Hypnosis is a way of strengthening these qualities.

FEAR OF CANCER

Cancer is usually a frightening condition. Just the word, *cancer,* is often filled with negative associations—in the first place, its literal meaning of "crab." Nowadays, we are very clever at diagnosing cancer early and removing it totally or subtotally. This means that cancer patients often survive much longer these days than they used to and are usually aware of the diagnosis. There is thus plenty of time to develop a state of chronic fear of cancer. It can imply pain, anxiety, stress, suffering, loss of human dignity, hopelessness, total dependency, guilt, ugliness, jealousy, hate, loneliness, and fear of loss of support from family, friends, and hospital staff. There is a possibility of a prolonged, tortured process of dying. Fear of death is usually greatest for the time preceding it; sometimes the fear is for death itself or even for possible suffering after death. All of these factors increase fear, and fear always increases pain. Anything which counteracts the fear-provoking negative associations to cancer has great value in a comprehensive treatment plan for cancer pain. Hypnotherapy is one contribution among several for counteracting these negative associations (5).

HYPNOSIS

Hypnosis is an altered state of consciousness (12), arising during a specific trusting relationship (13) between one or more "teachers" and one or more "pupils." There are various methods of developing this state; mine is by a modified progressive relaxation and training of the imagination (5). In this state, the patient (pupil) is able to develop a selective increase in concentration, e.g., on maximal enjoyment of the life-time that remains, and a selective increase in detachment, e.g., from fear and pain. This ability can be increased to some extent by training. If the teacher is needed to produce this state, it is called *heterohypnosis,* but if the pupil can continue producing the state alone, it is called *autohypnosis*. Both methods can be used on different occasions. The role of teacher in heterohypnosis can be transferred to another member of staff, family, or friend. In addition, the hypnosis-induction program can be recorded on tape, so that the pupil can recapture the heterohypnosis at will, even when no living teacher or stand-in is available. This increases the pupil's independence.

Physiology

Recent work shows that there is a basic normal plasticity of the central nervous system, which can be mobilized under various circumstances, including hypnosis (12). Reflex responses to pain include spinal segmental reflexes with short latency times, slightly susceptible to hypnosis, and suprasegmental (brainstem) reflexes with longer latency times, markedly susceptible to hypnotic influence. Thus, one effect of hypnosis on pain is a conditioned block of reflex, relieving learned pain. Other recent work has shown that in some chronic limb pain, blood-flow changes in skin and muscle can vary with the pain experience. Finer and Graf (7,8) found that the changes were normalized when pain was relieved both by hypnosis and by beta-sympathetic blockade. Furthermore, during an operation for varicose veins with stripping under hypnosis, there was no change in blood pressure, pulse, or catecholamine excretion attributable to the surgical procedure (9). Thus, another effect of hypnosis on pain is a sympathetic block, relieving the autonomic responses and the anxiety component of pain.

Technique

The various factors and mental manipulations of the technique I use are shown schematically in Fig. 1. The pupils are trained in modified progressive relaxation in a permissive manner, preferably in groups. Sometimes it is difficult for a pupil to start in a group, and individual training can be begun until group work is possible. During relaxation, the pupil is encouraged to imagine pleasant scenes or music. This ability is trained, so that the pupil can concentrate on pleasant things at any time. While in this positive state, the pupil is encouraged to tolerate fear and pain in the imagination. This is called *symptomatic desensitization* and results in a greater ability to tolerate fear and pain in reality. Also in this positive state, the pupil can be encouraged to live fully for the moment, no longer comparing the present with the past and not thinking of the future (16,18).

Thus strengthened, the pupil can begin to imagine unpleasant things. Most patients with pain of advanced cancer have many unpleasant emotions bottled up inside, which they readily release while in the hypnotic state. Thus the pupil reduces tension and consequently pain is diminished. The patient can also be encouraged to accept reality as it is, tolerating and enduring the change in attitude to life and death which this entails. While concentrating on these things, the pupil can be trained to detach from anxiety, stress, and pain.

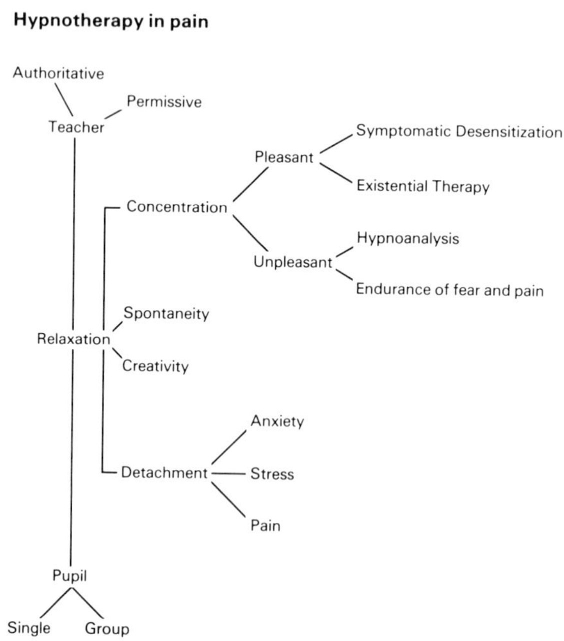

FIG. 1.

The pupil can be encouraged to develop spontaneity and creativity, taking responsibility for himself during the life that remains.

HYPNOTHERAPY FOR THE MANAGEMENT OF CANCER PAIN

The patient with pain of advanced cancer needs: (a) pain reduction with as little mental clouding as possible; (b) emotional support with training in maximal independence. Hypnotherapy is a system of treatment, in which patients and staff interact to produce maximal placebo effects, together with detachment from symptoms (19). My own clinical experience is fairly similar to that of other workers in the field of chronic pain, and especially cancer pain, including Crasilneck and Hall (2), Erickson (4), Kroger (15), LaBaw et al. (17), Sacerdote (21), and particularly Hilgard and Hilgard (14).

Hypnotherapy in the comprehensive management of advanced cancer pain is of value for patient, family, friends, and hospital staff. Patients are easier to work with when they have less pain and are more conscious through less need for narcotics. Where possible, the patients are trained in groups, encouraging and helping each other. The program can be recorded on tape to suit individual patients, so that they can play back at any time night and day and recollect the warm, encouraging atmosphere of the groups. This contact can even be transmitted by telephone when direct contact is delayed and distances are long. Sleep is improved: Patients fall asleep more easily, sleep is calmer and more restful, and they wake more refreshed. Appetite is improved, food and drink better retained. It is easier to perform unpleasant diagnostic and therapeutic procedures and anticipatory fear is reduced. At the same time the patients become more independent, helping themselves and each other in the group to make the remaining life-time more worth-while (20). The efficacy of hypnotherapy in cancer pain can be increased if the patient is trained before the symptoms become severe. Sometimes small operative procedures can be performed under hypnotic analgesia, e.g., on small skin or gland metastases, as shown in my film (6).

Advantages

Hypnotherapy is a comparatively simple method for helping patients with advanced cancer pain. Contrary to popular misconception, it is not particularly time-consuming, especially when compared with other procedures routinely used. In addition, time is greatly reduced by group treatment, the patients helping each other, while the stress and fatigue in the therapist, reported by Butler (1) is eased by the sharing of responsibility. The method is not at all exclusive, being usefully combined with other psychotherapeutic and routine physical and pharmacologic methods. Finally, hypnosis lends itself readily to physiologic and psychologic research analysis in the laboratory and clinic.

Disadvantages

The main disadvantage is the variability in patients' susceptibility to hypnosis, so that it is difficult to know in advance how much the method will help until it is tried. Intelligent use of the method requires adequate training of the whole staff, and this necessitates an educational program to counteract misunderstanding and scepticism.

Deficiencies

The main deficiency is the variability in effectivity, so that an expectant attitude is necessary. While many patients can be helped to some extent and some can be helped very much, the staff must be positive in their attitudes, for skepticism and misunderstanding weaken the method.

RECOMMENDATIONS

The whole staff should be trained in hypnotherapy. They can be trained by the therapist, then train on each other, and finally take part in therapy with patients. Associate therapists are welcome, and the staff will have a much more positive attitude to the therapy.

It is suggested that the therapist should go into therapy too, and particularly go into a supervisory group. Being a therapist to patients close to death arouses much anxiety, and it is important to have help in coping with one's own problems. This will also help to reduce the fatigue and stress described by Butler (1).

The efficacy of hypnosis can be increased by adjuvants. A pilot study by Finer et al. (10) suggested that small concentrations of nitrous oxide–oxygen have this effect. Further research is indicated and indeed necessary. In general, research on hypnosis and hypnotherapy must be expanded, parallel with research in other areas of pain, e.g., acupuncture and endomorphines.

It is increasingly clear that patients with pain of advanced cancer have the right to expect the help that hypnotherapy can give in any effective plan of treatment. It is the duty of the professions involved in the care of patients with pain of advanced cancer to train themselves in this method and to further develop hypnotherapy as an integral part of the comprehensive management of these patients.

ACKNOWLEDGMENTS

I should like to express my sincere thanks to my colleagues, medical, nursing, auxiliary, and secretarial at Samariterhemmes for their support and help. Dr. Elisabet Olander has continuously encouraged me in my work. My debt to her is great.

I should also like to express my appreciation to the Floriani Foundation of Milan and the Scientific Program Committee for organizing this International Symposium on the Management of Pain of Advanced Cancer.

REFERENCES

1. Butler, B. (1954): The use of hypnosis in the care of the cancer patient. *Cancer,* 7:1–14.
2. Crasilneck, H. B., and Hall, J. A. (1975): *Clinical Hypnosis.* Grune & Stratton, New York.
3. Ekelöf, G. (1971): *En självbiografi.* Albert Bonniers Förlag, Stockholm.
4. Erickson, M. H. (1967): An introduction to the study and application of hypnosis for pain control. In: *Hypnosis and Psychosomatic Medicine,* edited by J. Lassner, pp. 83–90. Springer-Verlag, Berlin.
5. Finer, B. L. (1974): Clinical use of hypnosis in pain management. In: *Advances in Neurology, Vol. 4: International Symposium on Pain,* edited by J. J. Bonica, pp. 573–579. Raven Press, New York.
6. Finer, B. L. (1975): Hypnotherapy in cancer pain. Paper read at the International Symposium on Cancer Pain, Florence, Italy.
7. Finer, B. L., and Graf, K. (1968): Circulatory changes accompanying hypnotic imagination of hyperalgesia and hypoalgesia in causalgic limbs. *Z. Ges. Exp. Med.,* 146:97–114.
8. Finer, B. L., and Graf, K. (1968): Mechanisms of circulatory changes accompanying hypnotic imagination of hyperalgesia and hypoalgesia in causalgic limbs. *Z. Ges. Exp. Med.,* 148:1–21.
9. Finer, B. L., Jonzon, A., Sedin, G., and Sjöstrand, U. (1973): Some physiological changes during minor surgery under hypnotic analgesia. *Acta Anaesthesiol. Scand.* [*Suppl.*], 53:94–96.
10. Finer, B. L., Lundberg, M., and Wigh, G. (1975): *Research Report,* Psychological Institute, Uppsala University.
11. Foster, Sir M. (1970): *Lectures on the History of Physiology.* Dover Publications, Inc., New York.
12. Hagbarth, K.-E., and Finer, B. L. (1963): The plasticity of human withdrawal reflexes to noxious skin stimuli in lower limbs. *Prog. Brain Res.,* 1:65–78.
13. Haley, J. (1963): *Strategies of Psychotherapy.* Grune & Stratton, New York.
14. Hilgard, E. R., and Hilgard, J. R. (1975): *Hypnosis in the Relief of Pain.* William Kaufmann, Inc., Los Altos, California.
15. Kroger, W. S. (1963): *Clinical and Experimental Hypnosis.* Lippincott, Philadelphia.
16. Kurosawa, A. (1952): "Ikiru." Film.
17. LaBaw, W., Holton, C., Tewell, K., and Eccles, D. (1975): The use of self-hypnosis by children with cancer. *Am. J. Clin. Hypnosis.* 17:233–238.
18. LeShan, L. (1964): Mobilizing the life-force: An approach to the problem of arousing the sick patient's will to live. In: *Psychosomatic Aspects of Neoplastic Disease,* edited by D. Kissen and L. LeShan, pp. 109–120. Lippincott, New York.
19. Orne, M. T. (1974): Pain suppression by hypnosis and related phenomena. In: *Advances in Neurology, Vol. 4: International Symposium on Pain,* edited by J. J. Bonica, pp. 563–572. Raven Press, New York.
20. Pirsig, R. (1976): *Zen and the Art of Motor Cycle Maintenance.* Corgi Books, London.
21. Sacerdote, P. (1968): Involvement and communication with the terminally ill patient. *Am. J. Clin. Hypnosis,* 10:244–248.
22. Tart, C. (1975): *States of Consciousness.* E. P. Dutton and Co., Inc., New York.

Advances in Pain Research and Therapy, Vol. 2,
edited by J. J. Bonica and V. Ventafridda.
Raven Press, New York © 1979.

Psychophysiologic Control of Cancer Pain

Sophia S. Fotopoulos, Charles Graham, and Mary R. Cook

Midwest Research Institute, Kansas City, Missouri 64110

The etiology and underlying mechanisms of pain associated with carcinoma are complex and difficult to delineate (2,6). Theoretical models of pain generally assume that activation of higher neural substrates, such as integrative functions of the cerebral cortex or the brainstem reticular formation, forms the basis of sensory responding and perception of pain. With pain related to carcinoma, structural and functional physiologic factors combine with psychologic factors to play a crucial role in the pain experienced. In the past, psychologic factors have been classified under the heading of suffering, and were considered merely subjective "feelings" separate from underlying neural mechanisms. Experimental evidence, however, indicates that these reactive components of the pain experience have, to some degree, a conditioned physiologic basis and are related to the neural substrate through complex mechanisms (6). Consequently, traditional stimulus-response models of pain, which assume that pain is a specific sensation reflecting a direct correlation between intensity and extent of tissue damage, are inadequate to characterize chronic pain states. Pain is influenced by cognitive variables, attention, suggestion, motivation, and affective factors, as well as stimulus, organizational, and interpretive functions of the brain and central nervous system.

This model suggests that techniques that alter the decision-making aspects of the pain experience, the affective factors associated with pain, or the conditional responses associated with intense stimulation could be effective in reducing pain without stress, central nervous system (CNS) and autonomic nervous system (ANS) side effects, or danger of diminishing effectiveness. They would leave the individual fully alert and in control of his or her life and death.

Behavioral modification approaches to the reduction of pain attempt to induce change in overt as well as physiologic behavior. Operant conditioning techniques, which entail reinforcement of an emitted response, and its subsequent learning and perpetuation, use strategies for establishing contingencies such as lack of complaining about pain for a specified time and for reinforcement produced by attention by a loved one, going out to dinner, etc. Maladaptive behaviors often tend to intensify pain and frequently lead to affective disturbances, such as depression, which negatively affect the patient's network of family and friends. Behavior-modification techniques can be effective in decreasing secondary gain and in reducing the frequency of behaviors developed as a consequence of the pain syndrome. Operant behavioral techniques are minimally effective in decreasing the pain itself. More appropriate behavioral techniques are classical conditioning, hypnosis, or biofeedback, which are more closely linked to both sensory and affective physiologic sensory processes.

A previous report made at the 1975 International Symposium on Cancer Pain by Fotopoulos et al. (3) described the clinical use of biofeedback in the treatment of 12 cancer-pain patients. Electroencephalographic (EEG) feedback of 8 to 12 Hz activity (alpha) appeared to have little effect on pain. Electromyographic (EMG) feedback had more positive effects, but pain-relief was brief. Significant pain reduction was observed, however, when EMG feedback was presented in combination with EEG feedback of 4 to 8 Hz activity (theta). This type of combined feedback resulted in a state of low physiologic arousal, often accompanied by pain reduction, vivid imagery, and increased feelings of well-being and physical relaxation. While little work has been reported with theta feedback, Beatty (1) has presented evidence suggesting that individuals can learn to suppress theta activity. Stoyva et al. (9) and Graham et al. (5) have reported the enhancement of theta activity with biofeedback techniques and also observed concomitant increases in relaxation and feelings of well-being. The combination of EMG and EEG theta feedback seemed, therefore, to hold great promise for the management of cancer pain.

The findings reported by Fotopoulos et al. (3) were obtained under clinical treatment conditions where psychotherapeutic techniques were employed, in addition to the use of EEG and EMG biofeedback. It was important, therefore, to submit this apparently effective biofeedback procedure to controlled laboratory evaluation. As part of a larger experimental program, the therapeutic effectiveness of a biofeedback technique was evaluated in ambulatory cancer-pain patients. The therapeutic goal was not the total elimination of pain; rather it was to reduce chronic pain to a level which would allow more normal daily function, both psychologically and physiologically. The biofeedback procedure focused on the alleviation of reactive pain components and reduction of physiologic pain concomitants. The hypothesis that providing combined EEG/EMG biofeedback would result in a physiologic state of low autonomic activation, accompanied by a subjective state of well-being and comfort, was tested. The evaluation included: (a) extensive pre- and posttreatment physiologic and psychologic assessments; (b) multiple measures of physiologic activation obtained during biofeedback sessions; (c) assessment of pain parameters and concomitants in the laboratory and at home; and (d) evaluation of the relationship between therapeutic success and the degree of physiologic control achieved.

EXPERIMENTAL METHODS AND PROCEDURES

The overall experimental program called for separate evaluation of the use of biofeedback or self-hypnosis in the treatment of cancer pain. Participation in the program was voluntary. Criteria for participation included: medical diagnosis involving carcinoma; current medical treatment specifically for pain; and ambulatory condition. When subjects completed the pretreatment assessment procedures described below, they were assigned on a pseudo-random basis to receive either biofeedback or self-hypnosis. Material presented here focuses on those subjects who were assigned to the biofeedback treatment condition. Where such information is either not generally available in regard to cancer-pain patients, or may be of interest to other investigators in the area, data from hypnosis subjects are included.

The subject population consisted of 10 females and 7 males between the ages of 31 and 68. The most common diagnoses were carcinoma of the bladder, breast, and lung. Subjects had been in pain an average of 15.7 months and were using both narcotic ($\overline{X} = 10.04$ mg morphine equivalent per day) and nonnarcotic analgesics ($\overline{X} = 1{,}204$ mg aspirin equivalent per day). Of these 17 subjects, 7 were assigned to the experimental biofeedback treatment group.

PRETREATMENT MEASURES

Psychologic and Demographic Measures

The initial interview included a sociodemographic inventory (age, sex, race, ethnic origin, and background) and a detailed pain history. In the second assessment session, a psychologic test battery was administered and consisted of: Eysenck Personality Inventory (EPI), Repression-Sensitization Scale (RS), Ego-Strength (ES), Locus of Control (LOC), and the McGill Pain Questionnaire (MPQ).

Psychophysiologic Battery

A psychophysiologic assessment examines the interaction between a particular individual's physiologic responsivity and a variety of standardized situations varied for physical, cognitive, and affective demands. The dynamic base line allows examination of possible changes in these relationships before and after treatment. This information provides understanding of the effects of biofeedback treatment, as well as information concerning physiologic responsivity over time in individuals in pain. To evaluate individual response patterns, it was necessary to record a variety of autonomic functions continuously during diverse stress and performance situations. The measures and experimental procedures are summarized in Table 1.

TABLE 1. *Procedures for psychophysiologic battery*

I. *Physiologic measures*

Measure	Recording Site	Purpose
Electroencephalograph (EEG)	Left occipital Right occipital Right central	Allow examination of EEG amplitude and percent time at various frequencies
Electromyograph (EMG)	Frontalis area Muscle associated with pain site Stress site	Allow evaluation of patterns of skeletal muscle response to various stressors
Heart rate (HR)	Clavicle vs. 3rd intercostal space	Evaluate base levels and responsivity from a variety of autonomic variables
Skin conductance level (SCL)	2nd and 4th fingers of nondominant hand	
Photoplethysmograph (ppg)	3rd finger of nondominant hand	
Temperature (Temp.)	Oral Skin	Evaluate metabolic and homeostatic lability
Blood pressure (B.P.)	Nondominant arm	Determine suitability for stressors
Respiration (R)	Halfway between umbilicus and xyphoid process	Allow evaluation of relationship between respiratory changes and autonomic changes

II. *Experimental conditions*

Class	Task	Duration
Physiologic base lines	Uninstructed relaxation	2 min
	Instructed "eyes open" (EO)	2 min
	Instructed "eyes closed" (EC)	2 min
Physical stressors	Valsalva's maneuver	varies
	Arm-lift	varies
	Cold-pressor	varies
Cognitive stressors	Serial subtraction of 7's	2 min
	Name nouns beginning with "Y"	2 min
Affective stressors	Word-association to neutral, personally relevant, and disease-relevant stimuli	varies
Instructed relaxation	Zen breathing exercise	5 min
	Pleasant fantasy	5 min

Hypnotic Susceptibility

As a final pretreatment measure, all subjects were individually administered a standardized hypnotic-susceptibility scale [Stanford Scale of Hypnotic Susceptibility, Form C: Weitzenhoffer and Hilgard (10)].

Biofeedback Procedures

The original study protocol called for 20 treatment sessions to be given over a 9-week period. During the first week there were to be daily 2-hr sessions; subsequently, the interval between sessions was to be gradually increased so that the last three sessions were held on a weekly basis. The physical condition of the subjects often made it impossible to adhere to this schedule.

Prior to each biofeedback session, the subject rated his pain, and measures of weight, oral temperature, blood pressure, pulse, and respiration rate were obtained. Electrodes were then attached precisely as for the psychophysiologic battery, and three 2-min physiologic base-line measures obtained: sitting quietly with eyes open, then with eyes closed, followed by a volitional control period during which the subject was asked to relax as deeply as possible without feedback. Each session of biofeedback began with three 5-min periods of EMG training.

Feedback was alternated among the three EMG sites, so that each session began with the muscle showing the highest level of activity, and continued until that muscle group was no longer highest. The highest site was again selected, feedback given from that site, and so forth. An operant shaping procedure was employed to reinforce reduction of muscle activity at each EMG site. Specified levels of EMG activity, relative to base-line EMG activity, were selected. The subject was required to produce EMG activity below this specified microvolt threshold 50% of the time in order to hear the biofeedback tone. Based on this criterion, the threshold was changed at 1-min intervals.

EEG feedback from C_2 followed the EMG biofeedback conditioning procedure. The object of this was to teach subjects to emit EEG activity in the 4 to 8 Hz range (theta). The frequency filter was set initially at 4 to 12 Hz, with the lower amplitude cutoff at 10 μv. When the subject emitted EEG activity within this range, he received the audio biofeedback signal. If EEG activity was in the range selected for a period of time equal to 50% of a 1-min trial, the upper frequency limit was lowered to 11 Hz. This process continued until activity in the theta range was continuously produced as recorded both in polygraphic record and in the digital displays. Once activity was predominantly in the theta range, the lower level of the amplitude cutoff was gradually raised in order to enhance the amplitude of theta bursts.

Combined feedback was then given. During this period the subject had to maintain both EMG and EEG levels within the selected ranges in order to receive feedback. There were three 5-min trials with 30-sec pause periods interspersed, during each session. The three 2-min base-line periods (eyes closed, eyes open, and volitional control) were repeated at the end of each session, followed by oral temperature, blood pressure, and subjective pain ratings. The electrodes were removed, and the day's session discussed with the subject.

Posttreatment and Outcome Measures

After the 20 biofeedback sessions were completed, the protocol called for the psychophysiologic battery and the psychologic test battery to be administered again, and a posttreatment interview conducted. Death or hospitalization of the subjects often made it impossible to adhere to this schedule.

A variety of measures was used to evaluate treatment outcome: subjective pain report, changes in physiologic reactivity to stimuli, changes in use of analgesic medication, and changes in psychologic factors.

PRELIMINARY RESULTS

Pretreatment Characteristics of the Subjects

Because few data on the cancer pain patient are available, pretreatment measures were analyzed for all 17 subjects.

Psychologic Tests

Pretreatment scores were summarized (see Table 2) and compared with appropriate standardization samples or samples of hospitalized patients who did not have a diagnosis of carcinoma. Cancer-pain patients showed significantly lower ego-strength scores ($p < .01$) than either normative or

TABLE 2. *Psychologic test data summary*

		ES	RS	EPI E	EPI N	EPI L	SRI	McGill Sensory	McGill Affective	McGill Evaluative
Males	$\bar{X}$	35.2	65.6	12.9	13.4	2.4	10.6	17.4	5.1	3.1
	S.D.	6.4	17.2	4.8	5.3	1.3	2.4	8.6	3.7	1.1
	N	5	5	7	7	7	7	7	7	7
Females	$\bar{X}$	33.2	51.0	10.9	11.1	4.3	10.6	18.5	4.5	3.3
	S.D.	7.1	22.8	5.1	4.7	1.6	4.3	9.1	3.9	1.5
	N	10	10	10	10	10	10	10	10	10
Total	$\bar{X}$	33.9	55.9	11.7	12.1	3.5	10.6	18.1	4.8	3.2
	S.D.	6.7	21.6	4.9	4.9	1.7	3.6	8.6	3.7	1.3
	N	15	15	17	17	17	17	17	17	17

Legend: EPI = Eysenck Personality Inventory; ES = Ego-Strength; RS = Repression-Sensitization Scale; E = Extraversion; N = Neuroticism; SRI = Social Reaction Inventory (Rotter Internal-External Control Scale).

hospitalized patients with tuberculosis. The neuroticism (N) scale on the EPI resulted in significantly higher N scores for cancer patients compared to normal samplės ($p < .05$). On the Locus of Control Scale, male cancer-pain patients were more "internal" ($p < .05$) than college undergraduate males; no such difference was found for the female patients. Cancer patients did not differ from normative samples on Extraversion or Repression-Sensitization.

Pain Ratings

Multiple measures of pretreatment pain were employed: physicians' ratings of subject pain using a scale of 0 to 100, with 100 indicating intolerable, intractable pain; the subject's mean pretreatment pain rating using the same scale; the rating of present pain intensity from the McGill Pain Questionnaire (MPQ); the Sensory, Affective, and Evaluative scores from the MPQ. These data are summarized in Table 3. An experimental cold-pressor, pain task measure from the psychophysiologic battery was also employed where the subject's physical condition allowed.

Significant agreement was found among the various pain measures as indicated by Kendall's $W = .59$, $p < .001$. A correlation matrix using Spearman's rho was also computed. Of particular interest are the findings that: (a) the sensory, affective, and evaluative scales of the MPQ were highly correlated; (b) the subject's mean pretreatment pain ratings did not correlate significantly with the sensory scale of the MPQ; and (c) the physicians' ratings were highly correlated with all subjects' self-report measures except the evaluative and global MPQ scale scores.

Subjects were divided into high- and low-pain groups using a median split of their pretreatment pain ratings. A correlational analysis showed higher pain levels to be associated with more external control (higher external scores on the LOC) and lower Extraversion scores ($p < .05$). High- and low-pain groups did not differ with regard to age, sex, tumor site, time since diagnosis, or occurrence of metastases. Of particular interest is the observation that the two groups did not differ on the 12 variables assessed during the base-line portion of the pretreatment psychophysiologic battery (see Table 4).

TABLE 3. *Summary of pain data*

Measure	Mean	Standard deviation
Physician rating	55.5	28.7
Subjects' base-line rating	42.9	26.7
MPQ "Now"	33.1	26.0
MPQ Sensory	18.1	8.6
MPQ Affective	4.8	3.7
MPQ Evaluative	3.2	1.3

TABLE 4. *Comparison of base-line physiologic measures for high- and low-pain report groups*[a,b]

Variable	N (H/L)	Group $\bar{X}$ High	Group $\bar{X}$ Low	t	dF	p
EMG: pain site	5/7	3.196	3.219	0.022	10	ns
stress site	3/9	4.892	3.123	1.562	10	ns
frontalis	5/9	5.126	9.33	1.509	12	ns
EEG: amplitude	5/9	12.72	12.217	0.201	12	ns
% time θ	5/9	35.99	40.27	0.658	12	ns
Heart rate	5/8	87.08	88.25	0.134	11	ns
Skin conductance level	4/7	9.35	15.72	0.867	9	ns
Respiration rate	5/8	4.0	4.75	0.941	11	ns
Weight	4/8	154.75	143.12	0.496	10	ns
Systolic blood pressure	5/9	133.80	131.89	0.151	12	ns
Diastolic blood pressure		81.69	81.56	0.006	12	ns
Oral temperature	5/9	98.46	98.49	0.074	12	ns
Pain site rating[c]	4/9	50.0	33.33	0.954	11	ns
Total pain rating[c]	5/8	190.8	48.13	2.82	11	.05

[a] All psychophysiologic measures obtained from first EC period of pre-battery.
[b] High- and low-pain groups defined as above or below the median of base-line period ratings.
[c] Pain site and total pain ratings taken from pain picture data collected at beginning of pre-battery session.

Psychophysiologic Battery

Physiologic data obtained during the eyes-closed (EC) base line of the pretreatment psychophysiologic battery are presented in Table 5. As previously mentioned, the population consisted of men and women who differed as to primary tumor site, chemotherapy, and radiation therapies. Overall the

TABLE 5. *Pretreatment physiologic measures*

Measure	Mean	S.D.
EMG: pain site	3.25 μv	1.59
stress site	3.61 μv	1.74
frontalis	7.71 μv	5.06
EEG: amplitude in range (4–8 Hz)	12.22 μv	4.21
% time in range	42.7%	38.5%
Heart rate	87.8 bpm	14.1
Skin conductance level	14.5 μMho	11.7 μMho
Respiration rate	14.4	2.94
Weight	146.5 lb	35.4
Oral temperature	98.4°F	0.67
Systolic blood pressure	132 mm Hg	21.2
Diastolic blood pressure	81 mm Hg	11.6

patients' physiology did not differ markedly from that observed in a normal adult sample, except that theta amplitude and percent time were elevated.

Results of Experimental Biofeedback Treatment

Subjective Pain

Pain ratings obtained before and after each biofeedback session were compared by separate *t*-tests for each subject. All subjects showed pain-relief after biofeedback sessions, with significance levels ranging from $p < .05$ to $p < .001$. Complete daily home ratings were available for 5 of the 7 subjects and showed mixed results. Four subjects did not show any significant reduction in home pain ratings. However, 1 of these 4 subjects (No. 03) completely ceased use of opiates, and her pain ratings increased minimally. The remaining subject (No. 14) showed significant decrease ($p < .01$) on the daily measures. In summary, the pain-relief obtained in the laboratory appeared to generalize to the home situation for 2 of the 7 subjects.

It was not possible to statistically evaluate changes on the McGill Pain Questionnaire as 4 of the 7 subjects died or were hospitalized before the final test battery. Of the remaining subjects, MPQ scores indicated that pain was greatly alleviated for 1 subject, increased for another, and the final subject's affective pain was better, while the sensory and evaluative pain factors were worse.

Physiologic Changes

It was expected that learned EMG decreases and EEG theta increases would be associated with reduced autonomic responsivity and concomitant pain reduction. Biofeedback-session data were therefore examined to determine whether learning occurred, whether the expected "relaxation response" was observed, and the relationship to pain reduction.

Learning. Three learning criteria were defined: (a) better control of a physiologic variable when feedback was being provided compared to when it was not; (b) better control of EEG/EMG activity during feedback than during EC base line; and (c) a significant rank-order correlation between time in feedback and level of physiologic activity (positive for EEG, negative for EMG). A subject was designated a learner only if two out of three of these criteria were met. Based on this operational definition of learning, two subjects (Nos. 03 and 14) were designated EMG learners; only subject 03 met any of the criteria for learned control of EEG activity.

Autonomic responsivity. Only subjects 03 and 14 met the dual criterion of decreasing autonomic arousal during feedback and lower levels of arousal after feedback. The response was stronger for subject 14, but not significantly so.

Relationship with pain reduction. It was pointed out above that only subjects 03 and 14 showed pain-relief which generalized to the home environment. These two subjects also learned EMG control and showed decreased autonomic responsivity during biofeedback sessions.

Psychophysiologic Battery

Comparisons of pretreatment versus posttreatment changes in the psychophysiology battery focused on two autonomic indicators, heart rate (HR) and skin conductance level (SCL). Because of the great variance among subjects, nonparametric tests were used. Results are shown graphically in Fig. 1. Despite marked increases in SCL during the posttreatment EC base

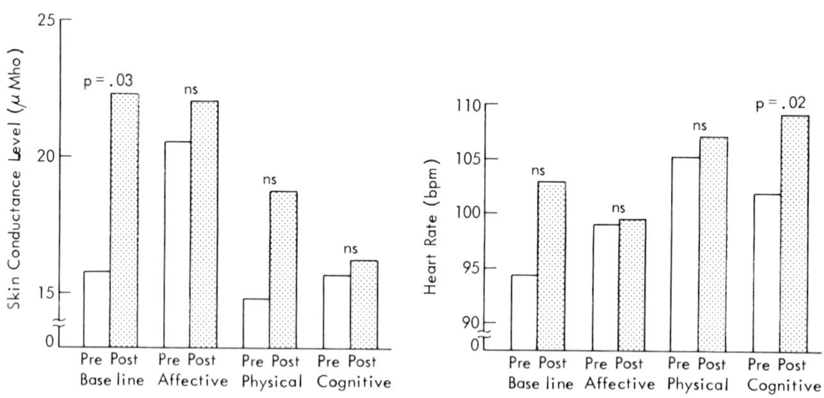

FIG. 1. Skin conductance and heart rate during pre- and posttreatment psychophysiologic batteries for various stress tasks.

line, no significant differences were observed for the affective, physical, or cognitive stress tasks.

DISCUSSION

Significant pain-relief was obtained during biofeedback sessions for all subjects; however, only two of the subjects (29%) were able to generalize this pain-relief to the home environment. These two subjects also were successful in learning EMG control and responded during the biofeedback sessions with decreased autonomic arousal. These results are encouraging in that they partially support the hypothesis being tested, and clearly indicate the importance of further work in the area. Such further work should take into account the complexities of physiologic learning, as well as the difficulties encountered because of the physical state of the subjects.

Conditioning of physiologic parameters is not a simple process. The physiologic variables chosen for conditioning should be closely linked to the disease process(es) itself. In attempting to develop techniques to decrease pain related to cancer, the lack of specific knowledge as to etiology and exacerbation of pain confuses the issue.

From a theoretical standpoint, and on the basis of our previous experience with cancer patients (3) and opiate addicts (4), we expected that simulating the CNS and/or cortical effects of opiates (increased 4 to 10 Hz activity with elevated amplitude) would result in decreased pain. Because of the low levels of physiologic learning observed in the present study, this question remains unanswered. It is possible, however, that the use of lower EEG frequencies as a feedback parameter is not the best choice for pain reduction. Previous research (8) on the production of alpha and theta in normal subjects has frequently reported distortions in time-perception (time-slowing). Such time-distortion associated with low-frequency EEG activity might lead to increased attention to, or perception of, pain because of the perceptual elongation of the sensory and/or reactive components of pain. Alternatively, pain itself might increase the occurrence of cortical responses related to attention or orienting, such as the contingent negative variation (CNV), and increase pain perception. If so, such cortical responses might be subject to deconditioning or extinction. These are speculations, but issues which need to be addressed.

Regardless of the appropriateness of the feedback variables chosen, the low level of learning observed suggests that the biofeedback procedures were not optimal. Because of instrumentation limitations, the feedback procedure was not ideally time-linked to the subject's physiology. Shaping consisted of establishing a set threshold for EEG (decreased by specified degrees) of the immediate dominant frequency emitted during the trial period. Additionally, the most appropriate shaping procedures and reinforcement schedules for the enhancement of theta activity are not known. Progress is being made, however, and systematic controlled experiments are continuing. Appropriate feedback parameters and appropriate conditioning procedures (shaping limits, schedules of reinforcement, etc.), be they operant, classical, or combinations, need to be delineated. Experiments concentrating on the specific sensory or affective components of pain as well as placebo aspects of pain-relief also need to be further examined.

Such experiments are particularly difficult to perform in pain populations suffering from a disease process which is often unpredictable and progressive. Changes in metabolic functioning and other aspects of the disease as well as changes in medical regimens markedly influence pain perception, sensory aspects, ANS and CNS changes, motivation, participation ability, pre-post comparisons, and generalization of treatment effects. Ideally, changes in chemotherapy treatment, other medications, etc., would be controlled experimental variables; however, the patient's health is always foremost, and this degree of control is seldom possible. Such factors should be taken into account in designing future studies of experimental treatment for cancer-related pain.

The work reported here suggested a somewhat different approach to the use of biofeedback techniques for pain reduction. Subjects currently receive biofeedback for both EMG and skin conductance level. Skin conductance level was selected because it is directly related to levels of autonomic arousal. An alternating treatment-base line-treatment design (ABA) with multiple base lines and reduced treatment time is now employed in an attempt to deal with the progressive physical deterioration often associated with cancer. Specific techniques for generalization of pain-relief to the home environment are also included in the protocol.

It is important to note that the cancer-pain patients who entered the current research program had been in continuous pain for 15 months and were in poor psychologic and physiologic health. They had been referred only after other sources of pain management proved unsuccessful. For many of them, biofeedback represented a "treatment of last resort." It is significant that under these circumstances any pain-relief at all was observed. The fact that all patients obtained relief during the sessions and some patients were able to extend this relief to the home environment indicates that biofeedback holds definite promise. Whether the physiologic parameters of choice for conditioning should be cortical, autonomic, or a combination is yet to be determined. The effectiveness of this approach to pain management if applied early in the pain/disease process is also a question of importance. Pain and associated effects such as energy-depletion and suffering are devastating to both the person with cancer and to his or her family. Our efforts are worthwhile so long as there is hope that increasing numbers of patients will experience some freedom from their continuing anguish.

ACKNOWLEDGMENT

This investigation was supported, in part, by Grant No. 5R18 CA17936–03 CCG, awarded by the National Cancer Institute DHEW, and, in part, by Midwest Research Institute. We wish to thank Harvey D. Cohen, Theodore M. Knapp, Susan S. Bond, and Whitney P. Sunderland for their research contributions, and Florence I. Metz for her critical review of the manuscript.

REFERENCES

1. Beatty, J. (1974): Theta feedback, attention, and performance. Paper presented at the Biofeedback Research Society Annual Meeting.
2. Bonica, J. J. (1973): Fundamental considerations of chronic pain therapy. *Postgrad. Med.*, 53:81–85.
3. Fotopoulos, S., Graham, C., and Cook, M. R. (1977): Biofeedback and cancer pain. Unpublished manuscript. Paper presented at the International Symposium on Cancer Pain, Florence, Italy, 1975.
4. Graham, C., Cook, M. R., and Fotopoulos, S. (1976): Studies on the use of bio-

feedback techniques with opiate addicts. Final Report, Contract No. ADM–45–74–139, National Institute on Drug Abuse.

5. Graham, C., Cook, M. R., and Fotopoulos, S. (1976): Studies on the use of biofeedback techniques with opiate addicts. Final Report (Addendum), Contract No. ADM–45–74–139, National Institute on Drug Abuse.
6. Liebeskind, J. C. (1977): Psychological and physiological mechanisms of pain. *Annu. Rev. Psychol.,* 28:41–60.
7. Pos, R. (1974): Psychological assessment of factors affecting pain. *CMA J.,* 111: 1213–1215.
8. Stoyva, J., and Budzynski, T. (1974): Cultivated low arousal—An anti-stress response? In: *Limbic and Autonomic Nervous System Research,* edited by L. DiCara, pp. 265–290. Plenum Press, New York.
9. Stoyva, J., Budzynski, T., Sittenfeld, P., and Yaroush, R. (1974): A two-phase biofeedback approach to sleep onset insomnia. Paper presented at the Biofeedback Research Society Annual Meeting.
10. Weitzenhoffer, A. M., and Hilgard, E. R. (1962): *Stanford Hypnotic Susceptibility Scale, Form C.* Consulting Psychological Press, Palo Alto, California.

Advances in Pain Research and Therapy, Vol. 2,
edited by J. J. Bonica and V. Ventafridda.
Raven Press, New York © 1979.

Psychosocial and Nursing Technique

Ada G. Rogers

Analgesic Studies Section, Sloan-Kettering Institute for Cancer Research, New York, New York 10021

In caring for patients with pain due to advanced cancer, we must consider all the ramifications of the illness. To achieve this goal the most important thing is to communicate with the patient. Developing effective communications will open avenues of good rapport between the patients and those caring for him. Although the physician is primarily responsible for the patient's care, it seems unreasonable to expect him to attend to all aspects of the care of the patient. Part of this responsibility must, by necessity, be transferred to other health-care professionals.

In recent years, it has been recognized that the best care given to the patient has been accomplished through a multidisciplinary team approach. Each discipline has its own specialized techniques that may contribute to the ultimate goal of enabling the patient to function as normally as possible under the circumstances. It should be understood that full cooperation among these specialists is essential to achieve this goal. There are some health-care professionals who may be reluctant to relinquish part of the patient's care to others in fear of losing "control" over the patient. Although not all patients with advanced cancer will require the services of these specialists, these services should always be available to the patients who require them and the patients should be informed of these services.

ROLE OF HEALTH PROFESSIONALS

Although all cancer patients may be depressed and at times may find it difficult to cope with the many aspects of his or her illness, this may not mean he or she will need a psychiatrist. However, there are patients with prior psychiatric problems, patients with suicidal tendencies, patients in an acute psychotic episode due to the aftermath of surgery or medications (e.g., steroids), sudden death of a member of the family, diagnosis of advanced disease, age and pain, who will need crisis intervention. Other situations not so acute may warrant help from the psychiatric service. Unfortunately, in many of these cases, the patient may be reluctant to see a psychiatrist. His reaction may be, "I'm not crazy—why do I *need* a psychiatrist?" In this instance a good rapport with the patient is most essential. An approach, that at times has been successful, has been to indicate to the patient that he or she may need a medication that will help him or her to relax or help his or her depression and the only person who could decide the right kind of medication would be a psychiatrist. The patient may also agree to see a psychiatrist if a member of the staff that he has confidence in will be present at the interviews.

The patient may not be the only one who is having difficulty in communicating and coping with pain of advanced cancer: the family and hospital staff may also be under pressure. In many hospitals, psychiatrists or psychologists have weekly meetings with nurses, social workers, families, and medical staff to enable these members to interact, ventilate their feelings and frustrations, and establish better communication. The feeling should be that all are in this together, and together we can promote better living for the patients, their families, and the health team.

The role of the psychologist parallels that of the psychiatrist except that the psychologist may be interested in gaining more information about the patient, family, and other members of the team through the use of psychologic testing and studies. Some of the tests used are the Rorschach Test (2), the Minnesota Multiphasic Personality Inventory (MMPI) (8), Symptom Check List (SCL-90) (6), Verbal Rating Scale and the Visual Analogue Scale (10) to name a few.

For some time the social service worker's role has been in the area of specific social problems that relate to relationships within the family, parent-child tensions, personal relationships outside the family, household management, health care, use of community resources, and public relief if needed (7). Social service workers have meetings with family members on a one-to-one basis or in groups. Many have teamed up with nurses, physical therapists, and physicians on a weekly basis to discuss various problems. Some social service workers have meetings with patients and families to discuss discharge planning. They have been involved in the education of other social service workers by conducting programs and institutes.

The social service worker is responsible for investigating and planning for financial aid, assistance with employment problems, nursing services outside the hospital, such as nursing homes or terminal care facilities, visiting nurse service, private-duty nursing in the home, transportation, equipment, household help, and self-help groups. The patient should be encouraged to utilize the services of the social worker and contact should be made with them as early as possible during the course of the patient's illness. This may help to eliminate or minimize some of the anxieties that may arise from certain types of problems. One patient tried to commit suicide because she did not want her husband to mortgage their house in order to pay for her many hospitalizations. Another dying patient was concerned about her mentally retarded daughter and who would care for her. In both cases, the social service worker was able to find solutions to these problems.

REHABILITATION PROGRAMS FOR CANCER PATIENTS

Rehabilitation programs involve the physical therapist, occupational therapist, speech therapist, and volunteer, as well as the social service worker, nurse, and physician. The programs available in many comprehensive cancer centers include: (a) *Laryngectomee:* Members of the International Association of Laryngectomees, who teach these patients esophogeal speech and/or use of the electro-larynx. Speech therapists have had an effective role with patients with facial paralysis and/or partial removal of any of the oral articulators. (b) *Mastectomy—Reach to Recovery Programs:* These are intended to aid women who have had surgery for breast cancer to adjust psychologically and physiologically. (c) *Ostomy Program:* This program was designed to assist the colostomy and urinary ostomy patients, but now includes ileostomy. The program includes training of enterostomal therapists (ET), a new category of allied health professionals. Since 1970, 500 ETs have been trained. The training takes 6 weeks, and these therapists are prepared to assist in the total rehabilitation of ostomates (1). In most hospitals ostomy care is provided by registered nurses.

A new program established at Memorial Sloan-Kettering Cancer Center is a preoperative teaching program for the thoracotomy patient. This involves a nurse, a social worker, and a physical therapist. Its purpose is to teach perioperative care regimes and to emphasize the importance of these regimes by explaining the underlying physiologic rationale to the patient and the family.

Physical therapists are involved in the rehabilitation of all types of patients, pre- and post-surgery, in ambulation, which includes the proper way to move and turn, get out of bed into a chair, use a walker, adjust properly to crutches and prosthesis, and in passive and active exercises. These techniques are also useful in patients with muscle-wasting and pain. Some patients may need an overhead trapeze to facilitate moving in bed. Patients have to be taught how to breathe and cough to avoid pulmonary complications at any time during their illness. Today, in many hospitals, this function is conducted by respiratory therapist.

Occupational therapists can help the patient by teaching and aiding in the recovery of patients through interesting occupations and pastimes. The idea behind occupational therapy dates back to Galen (7) who said "Employment is nature's best medicine and essential to human happiness." Many occupational therapists have artistic and creative abilities, and they are able to teach patients how to knit, crochet, sew, paint, and how to do ceramics, wood-carving, metalwork, weaving, etc. The occupational therapist may teach the patient who has lost an upper extremity the use of the other arm and hand in eating, dressing himself, and writing. If a hospital does not have occupational therapists, these activities may fall under the direction of the Recreational Department.

SOCIAL ACTIVITIES

Patients are encouraged to participate in any social activity that is available in the hospital or in their communities. These are techniques that are used to distract the patient, diminish the feeling of isolation and, in general, help him back into a social setting. Many hospitals have hours set for movies, bingo, Las Vegas nights, and live entertainment performed by well-known artists. Women patients always feel better if they can get their hair washed, cut, and set. These services should be provided for both men and women.

In a long hospitalization, a day or weekend pass perhaps will help to decrease the feeling of isolation that so often is a part of depression and hostility. This is especially true during holidays, when all family members will be missed. Patients with small children are particularly affected. If a pass is not feasible, arrangements should be made to allow children under-age to see their parents. Brown (3) has said, "To deprive a mother or father when sick of even a glimpse of what may be most dear and important in life runs counter to the current philosophy of the therapeutic value of meeting patients' psychological needs. To prevent a child from seeing his parents . . . to whom he is psychologically tied, may do him severe damage."

DIETARY ASPECTS

In some cancer patients and their families, eating is synonymous with survival. Unfortunately, many aspects of the patient's illness and treatment may inhibit the patient's ability to eat, as in cases of nausea, vomiting, intestinal obstruction, esophagitis, stomatitis, and loss of appetite. The dieticians, or as they now are called "nutritionists," play an important role. Patients may be on special diets, have food allergies, religious restrictions, and at certain times certain foods may not appeal to them.

Although this may not be the best way, patients usually are given menus to fill out a few days ahead, and the set hours for the delivery of the meals may not be at the time that the patient is hungry. Unfortunately, the routine of most hospitals demands this. However, there are times when the dietician may be able to substitute something more suitable for the patient or the patient's tray may be held for a short period of time. At Memorial Sloan-Kettering Cancer Center, a new computerized system is being considered whereby the patient will be able to select the meals for the day in the same morning. In some hospitals, a dining room facility is provided for patients on each floor, and this allows ambulatory patients to eat and socialize in a more congenial fashion. When a patient's intake decreases, i.v. feedings can be substituted, or in patients with consistent weight loss and/or malabsorption, total parenteral nutrition (TPN) can be started. In some cases, patients may have to be discharged on TPN. Patients are taught how to mix the formula and how to care for the equipment.

ROLE OF THE CLERGY

In recent years, the clergy has been taking a more active role as members of the group of counseling services. Their education has been expanded to include all aspects of the patient's care. Priests, ministers, and rabbis are members of hospital committees, group therapy programs, as well as being involved in educational symposia and workshops. Their input is an important part of the team approach. There are some religious beliefs that are based on superstition rather than doctrine, and these beliefs may be detrimental to the patient who is ill. The clergy may be helpful in changing these misconceptions. The religious patient may feel that his or her church representative is the only person whom he or she can communicate with, who will understand about his or her suffering, or whom he or she will talk to about death and dying. The clergy have had to reexamine their own feelings about death and dying, and as one minister reminded us, even Jesus Christ said as he was dying on the cross, "Oh Father, why have you forsaken me?"

ROLE OF VOLUNTEERS

Volunteers have always been important in time of need and illness. Some volunteers get close to the patients; others prefer to be behind the scenes. In times of disasters such as blackouts, snowstorms, and strikes, it is the volunteers who will replace many of the employees who are unable to get to work. Many volunteers are also former patients and are used in self-help modality in patient-visitors programs.

A "self-help" group can be defined as a group of people sharing common needs and experiences who organize action-oriented programs to help others with the same problems, usually because traditional systems cannot meet their needs. Cancer patients commonly report that almost immediately following their diagnosis a wall of silence begins to grow between them and their families, friends, clergy, and physicians with whom they had shared their anxieties, fears, and concerns. With the progression of the disease and its complications, all communications may stop. Members of the self-help group may be able to break down these barriers by sharing mutual experiences. The visitor—former patient is a vivid demonstration that life goes on in the face of death. The visual impact of the socially active visitor restores the patient's confidence in his or her ability to cope with the continuing trauma of cancer. At some comprehensive cancer centers, this type of volunteer has helped the patient to realize that his pain can be controlled, by informing the patient that there is a group available to deal with pain problems.

VISITORS

Visitors are welcomed by family members. The family can express fears, misunderstandings, or distorted communications, and may ask questions that they would be reluctant to impose on the patient, the nurses, or the physician. Professional resistance to using lay counselors has been a major impediment to the success of self-help programs. Resistance stems from the lack of volunteer accountability and supervision, and the failure to seek direct professional intervention when necessary. Professional health-care givers may fear that this group will either deliberately or unwittingly damage the relationship between the patient and the health-care professionals. Granting lay persons access to patients implies approval, and many professionals may feel that volunteers are not adequately educated or supervised (9).

THE ROLE OF THE NURSE

Traditionally, the nurse has been the liaison between the patient and the physician. She not only spends more time with the patient, but she is administering to many of the patient's basic needs. If the patient has confidence in the nurse, he will likely relate his problems to her. When the problem is understood, then the nurse can be instrumental in applying, obtaining, or suggesting the appropriate means of dealing with the problem. Unfortunately, for many years nursing care has been fragmented because of the team approach. Instead of having a nurse responsible for the patient's total basic care, the care was administered by dividing the responsibility so that there was a medication nurse, a treatment-room nurse, an i.v. nurse, and other specialized nursing duties. This system confused the patient; the patient did not know whom to ask for what and this contributed to delay, duplication of effort, and inefficiency.

Today, the primary care approach is being started in many hospitals, but in one institution in New York, it has been in effect since 1969 (4). Their philosophy of nursing is based upon the thesis that the relationships among the human beings who are members of the health team are, at all times, dynamic and collaborative and not limited by the walls of the hospital temporarily surrounding the patients. The members of the team are the patient, his or her family, nurses, doctors, social workers, and other members of the hospital organization. The end result sought by the members of the team is the attainment of a satisfactory resolution of the patient's health problem. In order to implement this philosophy, it is essential that the primary nursing model be the structure within which the nursing process takes place. Moreover, nurses must be free from involvement with nonnursing functions, which should be the responsibility of Unit Service Management. Human beings have inalienable rights to be respected at all times and to pursue happiness, and the nurse has a major role in assisting the patient in the attainment of these rights.

In this milieu the nursing process is defined simply as the sum of the activities jointly performed by the patient and the nurse. The sum of these activities can be divided into a three-part problem-solving approach: (a) assessment (includes nursing history and nursing diagnosis); (b) intervention (includes nursing orders and nursing care plan); and (c) evaluation (includes nursing prognosis) (5). Moreover, the special sheet for nurses' notes has been eliminated, and instead, along with other members of the health team, the nurses chart their observations in the progress sheets. This chronologic data gathered by all who are caring for the patient can be used by them in assessing the patient's problems and tailoring their care to fulfill the patient's needs.

Nursing History

The nursing history is obtained by the nurse who is admitting the patient, and she greets, orients, and interviews the patient and his family. Certain prerequisite information such as vital signs, dentures, allergies, diet, and medication are specifically elicited. Additional information includes the nurse's observation of the physical status of the patient, his reaction to his illness and the hospital, his social, occupational, and educational history, recreational activities, and additional pertinent information. These data are based on the nurse's knowledge of human behavior in health and sickness. The process of diagnosis is identification of the patient's needs in order to begin a plan of nursing care. The nursing history is included in and becomes a part of the patient's permanent record.

Nurses Order Sheet

The Nurses Order Sheet, also known as the Nursing Care Plan, is inserted in the Doctor's Order Book, and it becomes a part of the patient's chart. Orders are written by the nurse who admitted the patient, and these orders are followed by the nurses on all other shifts. This ensures continuity of care. Orders are written according to the problems identified on a Master Problem List (5). Some orders for a patient with advanced lung cancer and pain may read:

1. *Problem of depression*
   a. Elicit the patient's and family's understanding of the reason for this hospitalization.
   b. Encourage verbalization.
   c. Explain any diagnostic procedures that have been ordered.
   d. Obtain any available information about proposed definitive therapy and review with patient.
2. *Relief of pain*
   a. Assessment of the patient's pain, onset, site, character, what makes it worse or better.
   b. Assessment of analgesics, prior to admission.

c. Explain to patient PRN orders, time interval, route of administration, name of drug.
d. Medicate patient for relief of pain as per M.D. and assess the effectiveness of medication, onset of action, degree of relief, duration of effect, side effects (11).

3. *Discharge planning*
   a. Refer patient to social service worker (this should be done early in patient's care).
   b. Discuss family situation and home environment.
4. *Immediate care*
   a. Demonstrate and encourage the patient to practice techniques for coughing and deep breathing.
   b. Explain machines that may be used for pulmonary problem.
   c. Explain the role of the respiratory therapist.
   d. Check intake and output.
   e. Constipation should be avoided. Make sure orders are written for stool softness, laxatives, and/or enema.
   f. Health teaching about diet and medication other than analgesics.

These orders are transcribed onto the Kardex just as doctors' orders are transcribed by the unit receptionist. The Kardex is kept in pencil and as nursing orders change, the Kardex is changed, but there is always a permanent record of nursing intervention on the patient's nursing order sheet.

Centers with this type of philosophy and services by nurses usually have lists of nurse specialists available for consultation. Unfortunately, in most institutions the list does not include a nurse who can be consulted for pain problems.

The above primary care approach will enable the nurse to become better acquainted with the patient and the patient's needs. It will give the patient a feeling of security, a feeling that someone really cares about all of him, and he will be able to relate to the nurse. These nurses will be reliable and trustworthy, and the genuine interest will inspire confidence.

Regardless of the kind of nursing-care approach used, the nurse must apply psychologic, biologic, and social knowledge to the understanding of the individual as a member of a family and of a specific social group. The nurse must examine her unconscious as well as conscious motivation, prejudices, and objective and subjective reasons for her feelings and behavior toward a particular patient. Every bit of information is important. The nurse has preconceived attitudes and misconceptions learned through education and experience, and she can not assume that her attitude is correct. She should refrain from imposing these judgments on the patient. Accusatory questions or those with hostile implications arouse fear, suspicion, or anger and do not inspire confidence. This is particularly true of the patient who has pain due to cancer. The patient needs to know that the nurse believes he has pain and that she will do something about it. There should be a mutual feeling of confidence, trust, respect, and empathy. The nurse may use gestures to enhance such optimal relationships by holding the patient's hand or stroking the forehead. She should use sympathetic facial expressions, her voice should have a warm tone and quality, and she should use words of encouragement and avoid arguing. Patients often find pep talks to be depressing and patronizing. Schedules of physical activity must be planned with common sense. Patients may be unable to reach goals set by the nursing team, and this causes mutual frustration. The nurse can be most effective when she recognizes that her role and the role of other health-care givers is to help the patient understand his or her life processes so that he or she can better control and cope with the illness (5). Our guidelines should be: Stop, look, and above all, listen.

ACKNOWLEDGMENTS

Supported in part by grants awarded by the National Institute on Drug Abuse (DA 01707–02).

I wish to thank Miss Julie Franchi and Mr. George Heidrich, R.N., B.S.N., for their assistance in the literature search and Miss Natalie M. Rogers for her assistance in the preparation of the manuscript.

REFERENCES

1. American Cancer Society (1978): *Cancer Facts and Figures.* American Cancer Society, New York.
2. Beck, S. J. (1949): *Rorschach Test,* Vols. I, II, and III. Grune & Stratton, New York.
3. Brown, E. L. (1961): *Newer Dimensions of Patient Care,* Part I, pp. 64–84. Russell Sage Foundation, New York.
4. Carlson, S. (1969): An experiment in self-determined patient care. *Nurs. Clin. North Am.,* 4(3):495–506.
5. Carlson, S. (1972): A practical approach to the nursing process. *Am. J. Nurs.,* 72(9):1589–1591.
6. Derogatis, L. R. (1976): The SLC-90 and the MMPI: A step in the validation of a new self-report scale. *Br. J. Psychiatry,* 128:280–289.
7. Hardy, R. E., and Cull, J. G. (1975): *Counseling and Rehabilitating the Cancer Patient, No. 964: American Lecture Series.* Charles C Thomas, Springfield, Ill.
8. Hathaway, S. R., and McKinley, J. C. (1951): *The Minnesota Multiphasic Personality Inventory,* Rev. ed. Psychological Corporation, New York.
9. Mantell, J. E. (1976): Social work and self-help group. *Health and Social Work,* 1(1):86–100.
10. Ohnhaus, E. E., and Adler, R. (1975): Methodological problems in the measurement of pain: A comparison between the Verbal Rating Scale and the Visual Analogue Scale. *Pain,* 1(4):379–384.
11. Rogers, A. (1977): *Drugs for Pain: Proceedings of the Second Nursing Conference on Cancer Nursing,* pp. 39–43. American Cancer Society, New York.

Advances in Pain Research and Therapy, Vol. 2,
edited by J. J. Bonica and V. Ventafridda.
Raven Press, New York © 1979.

Nonnarcotic Analgesics

H. U. Gerbershagen

Institut für Anaesthesiologie, Klinikum, Johannes Gutenberg-Universität Mainz Postfach 3960, Langenbeckstrasse 1, 6500 Mainz, West Germany

This chapter will discuss the role of nonnarcotic analgesics in the management of cancer pain. First, some factors important to drug treatment have to be considered.

BASIC CONSIDERATIONS

In considering the use of drugs for cancer pain it is essential to appreciate the placebo effect. Clinical studies show that a placebo drug will be effective in pain in some 30 to 40% of patients (1,4,5). It is our experience that in cancer pain this effectivity is reduced to some 20% and that the effect is limited to a period of 2 to 3 weeks. Moreover, it is necessary to appreciate that outpatients will take not only the prescribed drugs, but also other medication.

The aim of responsible treatment for physicians and patients alike is the reduction of pain to a tolerable degree. Painlessness or complete freedom from pain is difficult and in some patients impossible to achieve with current therapeutic modalities. Narcotic drugs, including morphine and its derivatives will produce ample pain-relief only in about 75 to 80% of patients, provided that large doses are administered.

Stage of disease. In cancer pain the stage of the neoplastic disease plays an important role. Nevertheless, the psychophysiology of pain is such that the physician cannot adopt the view that terminal cancer pain is more severe than that of the earlier stages. At the same time there is no basis for assuming that a severe pain necessarily demands a narcotic analgesic. The quality, the type, and localization of pain and the attendant circumstances often matter most. Many patients with advanced cancer can be managed by nonnarcotic analgesics.

Mental state of the patient. The psychologic, emotional, and behavioral aspects of pain and the reactions to pain have been reviewed and emphasized by Bond and Chapman (*this volume*). It is important to adopt a qualitative rather than a quantitative viewpoint in such a complex psychophysiologic problem as cancer pain.

PHARMACOLOGIC CONSIDERATIONS

For the rational use of nonnarcotic analgesics an understanding of the basic principles of drug action and a knowledge of the pharmacologic effects are essential. Nonnarcotic analgesics constitute a heterogeneous group of substances with divergent chemical structures and various pharmacologic actions.

Nonnarcotic analgesics most often are derivatives of salicylic acid, ρ-aminophenol, pyrazolone, dioxopyrazolidine, indole, anthranylic acid, phenylpropionic acid, malonic acid, and nicotinic acid.

In addition to their analgesic property, *p*-aminophenol, pyrazolone, and salicylic acid derivates display a central nervous system (CNS)–mediated antipyretic effect. Pyrazolone, indole, anthranylic and phenylpropionic acid derivates, and salicylates are potent anti-inflammatory agents as well (Table 1).

TABLE 1. *The main effects of nonnarcotic analgesics*

	Effects			
	Analgesic[a]	Antipyretic	Anti-inflammatory	Adverse
Acetylsalicylic acid	++	++	++	++
Paracetamol	++	++	0	+
Metamizol	+++	+++	+++	+
Phenylbutazone	+	++	+++	+++
Indomethacin	++	+++	++	+++
Mefenamic acid	++	++	++	++
Ibuprofen	++	++	+	+
Naproxen	+	+++	++	+
Nefopam	+++	0	0	+

Legend: +++ = high; ++ = medium; + = low; 0 = none.
[a] In cancer pain.

Salicylates

Salicylates in particular reduce pain arising from muscles, ligaments, tendons, and bone. Visceral pain is usually said to be poorly influenced (23). In my experience, pain of pancreatic neoplasms is often partially, and in a few instances, completely controlled for weeks and months.

Acetylsalicylic acid is the most frequently used drug of the salicylate group. Numerous alternative compounds have been synthesized in the hope of obtaining a more rapid onset, greater peak analgesic action, prolonged duration of analgesia, and a reduced incidence of side effects. No study has proved the superiority of these compounds.

Soluble, buffered, enteric-coated, and sustained-release acetylsalicylic acid formations have been introduced, but it has not been possible to demonstrate improved analgesic activity or reduced adverse effects. *Injectable* acetylsalicylic acid should be thought of if the patient is already receiving intravenous nutrition or other drugs. *Salicylamide* contained in many analgesic mixtures has no proven analgesic effect.

Para-aminophenol Derivates

Phenacetin and one of its metabolites, paracetamol (N-acetyl-*p*-aminophenol), are equieffective alternatives to aspirin (21). The para-aminophenols can relieve moderate pain arising from integumental and musculoskeletal structures (9).

Many reports have linked chronic consumption of phenacetin-containing drugs with renal papillary necrosis and renal cancer (22). Well-controlled studies are lacking. Nevertheless many countries prohibit the use of phenacetin. Paracetamol does not cause nephropathy and gastrointestinal hemorrhage. It has the advantage of producing less gastric irritation than acetylsalicylic acid and is a good alternative to acetylsalicylic acid in spite of its lacking anti-inflammatory activity.

Pyrazolone and Dioxopyrazolidine Derivates (20)

Aminophenazon (aminopyrine), *noramido-pyrinmethansulfonate-sodium* (metamizol), and *phenylbutazone* are the commonly used drugs of this group (14,15). Aminophenazone can induce fatal agranulocytosis and will form dimethyl-nitrosamine, a very potent cancerogenic, in the stomach and should therefore no longer be administered (3).

Metamizol, a good analgesic and smooth muscle relaxant fell into disrepute because of poorly controlled reports by Discombe (3) and Huguley (11,12) in which they stated that a high incidence (0.5 to 1%) of agranulocytosis is associated with its use. Worldwide surveys show that agranulocytosis may be induced in some 0.001% of cases (10). There is no nitrosamine formation by this drug. Metamizol can be administered orally, intramuscularly, and intravenously.

Phenylbutazone is a drug for muscle and skeletal pain. Because of its frequent and marked side-effects, it should only be used for periods up to 8 days. *Oxyphenbutazone,* a metabolite of phenylbutazone, should also only be used for severe pain states.

Indole, Anthranylic Acid and Phenylpropionic Acid Derivates

The compounds of these groups are about as potent as the groups already mentioned. We feel that they are especially advantageous because they allow a frequent rotation to different analgesic groups. For the past 10 years we have rotated nonnarcotic analgesics every 6 to 8 weeks in order to reduce side effects and abuse liability. In spite of employing larger doses in moderate and severe cancer pain than usually recommended, we have never observed any serious side effects.

Nefopam

Nefopam, a benzoxacine derivate, is a centrally acting, nonnarcotic analgesic and has no antipyretic and anti-inflammatory effects (8). It is approximately one-third as potent as morphine in its parenteral application form. This drug has a mild cardiovascular stimulating action. Respiratory mechanics and pulmonary gas exchange are not influenced (7). This compound, like most nonnarcotic analgesics, does not cause mood alterations or sedation, so that in cancer pain the simultaneous administration of a neuroleptic drug is advisable. Nefopam should not be given with paracetamol because of possible drug interaction causing hepatoxicity.

ADVERSE EFFECTS OF NONNARCOTIC ANALGESICS

The adverse effects, listed in Table 2, are very similar with all groups, differing only in degree and frequency. Provided that the contraindications (Table 3) and drug-rotation scheme are considered, adverse side effects are infrequent and mild with all compounds.

TABLE 2. *Adverse effects of nonnarcotic analgesics*

Derivates of	Adverse side effects
Salicylic acid	Damage to gastrointestinal tract (bleeding, ulceration), allergic reactions (skin rash, angioedema, asthma)
p-Aminophenol	Methemoglobinemia, hemolytic anemia, nephrotoxicity, headache
Pyrazolon	Skin rash, leukopenia, agranulocytosis (0.001%)
Pyrazolidine	Gastrointestinal bleeding and ulcer, leukopenia, agranulocytosis, renal-function disturbances (sodium and water retention), dizziness, headache
Indole	Gastrointestinal bleeding and ulcer, fatigue, mental confusion, depression
Anthranylic acid	Diarrhea, gastrointestinal bleeding, allergy, fatigue
Phenylpropionic acid, phenylformic acid	Gastrointestinal disturbance, ulcer
Malonic acid	Gastrointestinal disturbance, skin rash
Benzoxacine	Sweating

TABLE 3. *Contraindications for nonnarcotic analgesics*

Derivates of	Contraindications
Salicylic acid	History of gastrointestinal ulcers
p-Aminophenol	Anemia, liver disease, severe pulmonary disease
Pyrazol, pyrazolidine	History of gastrointestinal ulcers, myocardial insufficiency, reduced renal function, porphyria, granulocytopenia
Indole	Parkinsonism, epilepsy, psychosis
Anthranylic acid	History of gastrointestinal ulcers
Benzoxacine	Elevated pulmonary-artery pressure

SITE AND MODE OF ACTION OF NONNARCOTIC ANALGESICS

Several hypotheses have been advanced to explain the actions of nonnarcotic and nonsteroid anti-inflammatory agents. These include stabilization of lyosomal membranes (13), inhibition of lyosomal enzymes (13,19), hyperpolarization of neuronal membranes (16), the displacement of an endogenous anti-inflammatory peptide from plasma protein (17,18), interference with the migration of leukocytes (2), and interference with phosphorylation (24). One of several possible modes of action is the inhibition of the biosynthesis of prostaglandins and precursors and similar substances in inflamed and traumatized tissues (6,19). Thus, the prevention of prostaglandin release reduces or prevents the sensitization of pain receptors to nociceptive stimuli. There is also the possibility that acetylsalicylic acid and *p*-aminophenols involve central mechanisms. Nefopam acts on CNS pain mechanisms (26).

EFFICACY OF NONNARCOTIC ANALGESICS

The analgesic efficacy of nonnarcotic analgesics is usually underrated. This may partly be due to the general availability, the general use in mild discomforts, and low susceptibility of experimental pain, and numerous papers published by pharmacologists not involved in patient-care. Unfortunately, the various groups have been defined as weak or minor analgesics for several decades. The nonnarcotic analgesics are potent analgesics if dose-effect relationships are considered. Most often it is ineffective to treat cancer pain, for instance, with single doses of 200 to 500 mg of acetylsalicylic acid.

Nonnarcotic analgesics must be administered in larger doses than usually prescribed. Table 4 gives the dosage required to achieve effective concentrations at their site of action. This brings up the problem of analgesic mixtures. Analgesic mixtures have been compounded in the belief that a synergistic or better-than-additive effect could be obtained, and that adverse effects could be reduced. There is no proven synergistic potency, and the side effects are

TABLE 4. *Effective doses of nonnarcotic analgesics for control of cancer pain*

Generic name	Dose (mg)	Interval of administration during day
Acetylsalicylic acid	750–1250	q. 3 hr
Salicylamide	750–1000	q. 3 hr
Phenacetin	400–600	q. 3 hr
Paracetamol	600–800	q. 3 hr
Acetylaminosalol	400–800	q. 3 hr
Phenazon	500–1000	q. 3 hr
Propyphenazon	450–800	q. 3 hr
4-Aminophenazon	450–800	q. 3 hr
Aminophenazon	450–800	q. 3 hr
Noramidopyrin methansulfonate-sodium (metamizol)	750–1000	q. 3 hr
Mofebutazon		
monophenylbutazon	200–400	q. 4 hr
phenylbutazon	200–400	q. 4 hr
oxyphenbutazone	100–200	q. 4 hr
Mefenamic acid	500	q. 3 hr
Flufenamic acid	200	q. 4 hr
Indomethacin	50–75	q. 4 hr
Benzydamin	100	q. 4 hr
Ibufenac		q. 4 hr
Ibuprofen	200–400	q. 3 hr
Naproxen	250–500	q. 3–4 hr
Niflumic acid	250–500	q. 3–4 hr
Bumadizon	220	q. 4 hr
Alclofenac	500–1000	q. 4 hr
Nefopam	60–120	q. 3 hr

not lessened. They are only different and therefore more dangerous. Owing to drug interactions between nonsteroid anti-inflammatory agents (19) the effectiveness might even be reduced. There are only few analgesic mixtures that contain adequate dosage of analgesics. Therefore, individual drugs should be administered.

Reasonable mixtures of analgesics might contain an analgesic with a chiefly peripheral action and an analgesic with a central site of action, e.g., acetylsalicylic acid plus nefopam or dextropropoxyphene. In most instances the full dose of each drug must be given.

Caffeine, local anesthetics, vitamins, barbiturates, and many other ingredients of compounded analgesic drugs do not increase the analgesic potency (9). Vitamins, in particular, have no potentiating effect and are not analgesics. Perhaps, it may be assumed that the placebo effect of vitamin-containing drugs is slightly greater than with other mixtures. Barbiturates, tranquilizers, and neuroleptics are usually contained in doses which are insufficiently large to produce a clinical effect. However, the dosage is sufficient to induce dependence, and since these compounded drugs are ineffective and also produce side effects, they should *not* be prescribed. If sedative, anxiolytic, or mood-elevating effects are desired, they can be achieved by using an adequate dosage of sedative or psychotropic drug. Drugs containing barbiturates, phenacetin, or ergotamine may induce pain, for instance, headache (25).

In treating cancer pain it is important to differentiate between pain caused by tumor infiltration, by metastatic disease, by complications of cancer therapy, and by problems unrelated to cancer (see Foley, *this volume*). Thus, it is often realized that positive feedback mechanisms, causing motor and sympathetic nervous system hyperactivity, are active. The reflex sympathetic disturbances are often amenable to nonsteroid anti-inflammatory agents and neuroleptic drugs. The painful reflex muscular hypertonicity can be controlled with nonnarcotic analgesics and centrally acting muscle relaxants, such as orphenadrine citrate or chlormezanon.

Antipyretic anti-inflammatory analgesics (with the exception of metamizol) relieve pain of visceral spasm poorly. Therefore, smooth muscle relaxants, e.g., butopromide, should simultaneously be given.

Most nonnarcotic analgesics do not cause subjective effects and do not influence psychoreactive processes of pain. Therefore, it has been our policy for the past decade to simultaneously give nonnarcotic analgesics and neuroleptics. In the treatment of cancer pain only low doses of neuroleptics, far below the so-called "neuroleptic threshold," are required. Some 15 to 20% of our cancer-pain patients, managed with nonnarcotic analgesics and neuroleptics also need small doses of a tricyclic antidepressant. This drug combination often delays the usage of narcotic analgesics.

The timing of drug administration is important. Most nonnarcotic analgesics have an effective duration of some 3 to 5 hr. Therefore, they are regularly given at 3-hr intervals. In cancer patients the pharmacologic considerations are as important as behavioral aspects.

Drug treatment of cancer pain, at any stage of the disease, should begin with nonnarcotic analgesics and neuroleptics. Therapy has to provide ample pain-relief; the patient should be comfortable. If this aim is not achieved by the treatment outlined, narcotic analgesics have to be administered without delay.

REFERENCES

1. Beecher, H. K. (1970): *Research and the Individual Human Studies.* Oxford Press, New York.
2. Di Rosa, M., Papadimitriou, J. M., and Willoughby, D. A. (1971): A histopathological and pharmacological analysis of the mode of action of nonsteroidal anti-inflammatory drugs. *J. Pathol.,* 105:239–256.

3. Discombe, G. (1952): Agranulocytosis caused by aminopyrine. *Br. Med. J.,* 1:1270.
4. Evans, F. J. (1974): The placebo response in pain reduction. *Adv. Neurol.,* 4:289–296.
5. Feather, B. W., Chapman, C. R., and Fisher, S. B. (1972): The effect of a placebo on the perception of painful radiant heat stimuli. *Psychosom. Med.,* 34:290–294.
6. Ferreira, S. H., and Vane, J. R. (1974): New aspects of the mode of action of nonsteroid anti-inflammatory drugs. *Annu. Rev. Pharmacol.,* 14:57–73.
7. Gerbershagen, H. U., and Schaffner, E. (1978): Das Verhalten der Atmung nach intravenöser Verabreichung von Nefopam-HCl und Pentazocin bei Lungengesunden. In: *Nefopam, ein potentes Analgetikum,* edited by H. U. Gerbershagen and G. E. Cronheim. Fischer, Stuttgart, New York.
8. Gerbershagen, H. U., and Cronheim, G. E. (editors) (1978): *Nefopam, ein potentes Analgetikum.* Fischer, Stuttgart, New York.
9. Goodman, L. S., and Gilman, A. (1975): *The Pharmacological Basis of Therapeutics.* Macmillan, New York.
10. Hoechst, Comp. (1977): *Dipyron, eine Übersicht 1977.* Fa. Hoechst AG, Frankfurt (Main).
11. Huguley, C. M. (1964): Agranulocytosis induced by dipyrone, a hazardous antipyretic and analgesic. *JAMA,* 189:938–941.
12. Huguley, C. M. (1964): Drug-induced blood dyscrasias. *JAMA,* 188:817–818.
13. Ignarro, J. L., and Colombo, C. (1972): Enzyme release from guinea-pig polymorphonuclear leucocyte lysosomes inhibited *in vitro* by anti-inflammatory drugs. *Nature New Biol.,* 239:155–157.
14. Krohs, W., Hensel, O. (1961): *Pyrazolone und Dioxopyrazolidine.* Edito Cantor, Aulendorf, Württ.
15. Krohs, W. (1965): Pyrazole derivates. In: *Analgesics,* edited by G. de Stevens. Academic Press, New York.
16. Levitan, H., and Barker, J. L. (1972): Effect of non-narcotic analgesics on membrane permeability of molluscan neurones. *Nature New Biol.,* 239:55–57.
17. McArthur, J. N., Dawkins, P. D., Smith, M. J. H., and Hamilton, E. B. D. (1971): Mode of action of antirheumatic drugs. *Br. Med. J.,* 2:677–679.
18. McArthur, J. N., Dawkins, P. D., and Smith, M. J. H. (1971): The displacement of L-tryptophan and dipeptides from bovine albumin *in vitro* and from human plasma *in vivo* by antirheumatic drugs. *J. Pharm. Pharmacol.,* 23:393–398.
19. Paulus, H. E., and Whitehouse, M. W. (1973): Nonsteroid anti-inflammatory agents. *Annu. Rev. Pharmacol.,* 13:107–125.
20. Roth, H. J. (1978): Pyrazolone und Nitrosamine. *Pharmaz. Z.,* 123:625–633.
21. Shelley, J. H. (1967): Phenacetin, through the looking glass. *Clin. Pharmacol. Ther.,* 8:427–471.
22. Smith, P. K. (1958): *Acetophenetidin: A Critical Bibliographic Review. Interscience Publ., New York.*
23. Smith, M. J. H. (1967): *The Salicylates.* Wyley, London.
24. Whitehouse, M. W., and Haslam, J. M. (1962): Ability of some antirheumatic drugs to uncouple oxidative phosphorylation. *Nature,* 196:1323–1324.
25. Wörz, R., Baar, H., Draf, W., Gerbershagen, H. U., Gross, D., Magin, F., Ritter, K., Scheifele, J., and Scholl, W. (1975): Kopfschmerz in Abhängigkeit von Analgetika-Mischpräparaten. *Münchn. Med. Wschr.* 117:457–462.
26. Zimmermann, M. (1978): Neurophysiologische Untersuchungen über einen spinalen Wirkungsort von Nefopam. In: *Nefopam, ein potentes Analgetikum,* edited by H. U. Gerbershagen and G. E. Cronheim. Fischer, Stuttgart, New York.

Advances in Pain Research and Therapy, Vol. 2,
edited by J. J. Bonica and V. Ventafridda.
Raven Press, New York © 1979.

Systemic Analgesics and Related Drugs: Narcotic Analgesics

Raymond W. Houde

Department of Medicine, Memorial Sloan-Kettering Cancer Center, New York, New York 10021

NARCOTIC ANALGESICS

The narcotic analgesics are, without doubt, the most efficacious of the drugs employed for the relief of intractable pain and suffering due to advanced or terminal cancer. The narcotics have long been recognized to be singularly capable of modifying both the perception of, and reaction to, pain, as well as of inducing a sense of calm indifference to other physical and psychologic stresses not uncommonly experienced by the dying patient and the patient with cancer (12,20). Ironically, the capacity to induce a sense of well-being, or euphoria, is a property of the narcotics which we have been making a great effort to eliminate from the so-called "ideal analgesic" of our aspirations (1). This unfortunate paradox has been the result of an association of euphoria with drug abuse and with the popular misconception that drugs with this capability enslave, demoralize, and lead the unwitting patient down the primrose path to addiction (16).

There has, in fact, been a trend to substitute the term *addictive analgesics* (5) as a more specific designation for what we have traditionally called the *narcotic analgesics*. For the purpose of this presentation, however, we shall adhere to the older term. The drugs about which we shall be speaking are morphine and its surrogates, and their agonist-antagonist congeners, which have been employed for the treatment of pain due to cancer.

INDICATIONS

The major indication for the administration of a narcotic is severe or intractable pain. Customarily, the narcotics are not administered for chronic pain, even in advanced cancer, unless the milder, simple analgesics have been found wanting in being able to relieve the patient of suffering. There are times, however, when we should resort directly to narcotics, for not all pain due to cancer is the same, and it is better to be governed by the demands of the particular clinical situation than by dogma.

Like the mild analgesics, the narcotics are generally readily available and require no special facilities or technical skills to administer them. Because they act centrally to relieve pain, the effects of narcotics are less likely to be influenced by the site or source of pain—which may be an important consideration in a patient with widely disseminated cancer. Not infrequently, the effects of narcotics will also relieve suffering from other causes than pain (8).

Most narcotic analgesics can be given by any of the commonly employed routes of administration, whereas most analgesics of the antipyretic–anti-inflammatory class can only be given by mouth or by rectum. Because the narcotics are much more potent than the simple analgesics, there is a greater risk of acute dose-related toxicity. However, specific antagonists are available (such as naloxone) which can promptly counteract or reverse those effects. Paradoxically, the antipyretic–anti-inflammatory type analgesics are more hazardous, for their more serious acute toxic manifestations, such as gastrointestinal hemorrhage and agranulocytosis, are less predictable but just as formidable as the acute side effects of narcotics. Moreover, the acute hepatic necrosis and "analgesic nephropathy" associated with the overuse of the mild analgesics are far more serious and irreversible than any form of chronic toxicity due to narcotics. There are no specific nonnarcotic drug antagonists (21).

The chronic administration of narcotics can, of course, produce a number of familiar, undesired central nervous system, gastrointestinal, and genitourinary side effects. Tolerance to the analgesic and sedative effects of narcotics appears to develop more rapidly than tolerance to their constipating and sphincteric effects, so that reliance on the use of narcotics for analgesia over long periods of time can complicate the management of the patient with advanced cancer. Unfortunately, many physicians also equate tolerance with drug addiction and believe that the patient will become refractory to all drugs and other methods of relieving pain when in the throes of terminal illness. In keeping with this viewpoint, the caveat that, "The physician should use morphine only as a miser spends his gold," (4) has been the prevailing doctrine of American physicians.

CLINICAL PHARMACOLOGY

The narcotic analgesics are comprised of drugs of several different origins and chemical classes which share, at least in part, the properties of the classic narcotic agonist, morphine. The major groupings are the *opiates* and the *opioids*. The former are comprised of the naturally occurring opium alkaloids and their semisynthetic derivatives; the latter are comprised of a number of purely synthetic classes of drugs of which the most important are the *morphinan* series, the *benzomorphan* series, the *phenylpiperidine* (meperidine) series, and the *diphenylpropylamine* (methadone) series. There are literally hundreds of derivatives of these compounds, as well as a few other purely synthetic narcotics such as the benzimidazoles, thiambutenes, and phenampromide series. Most of the latter have either not been released for clinical use or have not been used to any appreciable extent in the management of pain due to advanced cancer.

For the purpose of our discussion, we shall speak of the individual, clinically important drugs as being of one of three types. The first type would be those drugs which are most similar to morphine in their pharmacologic properties; the second, those which more closely resemble codeine; and the third, those which resemble nalorphine. Codeine, which is simply 3-methyl morphine is very similar to morphine in its pharmacologic actions except that it is less potent and more commonly administered by the oral route, primarily because it is less subject to first-pass effects than morphine. Nalorphine, on the other hand, is both a narcotic agonist and an antagonist, and it differs appreciably in its pharmacologic profile from both morphine and codeine. Although, currently, nalorphine is *not* employed clinically as an analgesic, it is the prototype of the series of which the drug best known as an analgesic is pentazocine (Talwin®). The distinguishing features of the mixed agonist-antagonist analgesics are that they do not produce physical dependence of the morphine type, that tolerance develops more slowly to their repeated administration, and their dominant agonist or antagonist effects are largely determined by whether they are administered before or after a patient has developed physical dependence to narcotics (14).

CHOICE OF ANALGESIC

The choice of an appropriate analgesic and its proper dose should be based on what is known of the nature and the character of the pain and an understanding of the patient and his disease. Virtually all kinds and intensities of pain may be encountered in advanced cancer, and treatment is likely to be most successful if the drug, dose, and route of administration are tailored to fit that individual patient's needs. This requires that we exercise some clinical judgment based on our past experiences with patients in similar circumstances. Reports of pain intensity, in themselves, are not always reliable, particularly if one does not know the patient well. However, it is usually possible to reach a reasonable decision based on physical and laboratory findings and what is known of the extent of the disease and its probable course. The initial goal should be to provide *relief promptly* but not at the expense of inducing adverse side effects. If it were felt that this could be accomplished by the use of a simple analgesic, such as aspirin or acetaminophen, we should surely try that first. After those drugs have been tried in adequate doses, then it is time to take the next step.

Table 1 is a list of relative potencies of analgesics commonly employed for severe pain, expressed in terms of the intramuscular and oral doses approxi-

TABLE 1. *Relative potencies of analgesics commonly employed for severe pain, expressed in terms of the intramuscular (i.m.) and oral (p.o.) doses approximately equivalent in total effect to a 10-mg i.m. dose of morphine*

	i.m. (mg)	p.o. (mg)	Major differences from morphine
Oxymorphone (Numorphan®)	1	6	None
Hydromorphone (Dilaudid®)	1.5	7.5	Shorter-acting.
Levorphanol (Levo-Dromoran®)	2	4	Relatively high p.o. to i.m. potency.
Phenazocine (Prinadol®)	3	15	None
Metopon	3	18	None
Heroin	4		Shorter-acting.
Dextromoramide (Palfium®)	7.5	10	High p.o. to i.m. potency.
Piminodine (Alvodine®)	7.5		None
Methadone (Dolophine®)	10	20	Relatively high p.o. to i.m. potency.
Morphine	*10*	60	
Oxycodone	15	30	Shorter-acting. Relatively high p.o. to i.m. potency.
Dipipanone (Pipadone®)	20		None
Methotrimeprazine (Levoprome®, Nozinan®)	20		Phenothiazine—unlike morphine.
Anileridine (Leritine®)	30	50	Relatively high p.o. to i.m. potency.
Alphaprodine (Nisentil®)	45		Very short-acting.
Pentazocine (Talwin®)	60	180	Narcotic antagonist analgesic.
Meperidine (pethidine, Demerol®)	75	300	None
Codeine	130	200	Relatively high p.o. to i.m. potency. Relatively more toxic in higher doses.
Dextroproxyphene (Darvon®)	240		Similar to codeine but more toxic in high doses.

Relative potencies of analgesics employed orally for less severe pain, expressed in terms of doses approximately equivalent in total effect to 650 mg of aspirin

	p.o. (mg)	Salient features
Pentazocine (Talwin®)	30	Weak narcotic—narcotic antagonist, high analgesic potential,[a] low addiction liability.
Codeine	32	Weak narcotic, high analgesic potential, relatively low addiction liability.
Meperidine (Demerol®)	50	Narcotic, high analgesic potential, high addiction liability.
Propoxyphene (Darvon®)	65	Weak narcotic, low analgesic potential, low addiction liability.
Aminopyrine (Pyramidon®)	600	Nonnarcotic, low analgesic potential, no addiction liability, risk of agranulocytosis.
Aspirin (ASA)	*650*	Nonnarcotic, anti-inflammatory, low analgesic potential, no addiction liability or tolerance.
Phenacetin (acetophenetidin)	650	Similar to aspirin but with limited anti-inflammatory properties.
Acetaminophen (paracetamol)	650	Similar to phenacetin, less potential renal toxicity.
Sodium salicylate	1000	Similar to aspirin.

[a] "Analgesic potential" refers to level of analgesia attainable by increasing dose to point of limiting side effects.

mately equianalgesic in total effect to a 10-mg intramuscular dose of morphine. Where both the intramuscular and the oral equianalgesic doses are stated, that has been based on a double-blind crossover comparison within the same patients of the same drug by two different routes of administration (7). In the lower portion of the table, the relative potencies of analgesics employed orally for less severe pain are expressed in terms of the doses approximately equivalent in total effect to 650 mg of aspirin. It has been our experience (15) that doses in excess of 650 mg of either aspirin or acetaminophen are not as likely to provide the desired increment in analgesia that we could more easily achieve by giving an equianalgesic dose of a weak narcotic analgesic such as codeine or pentazocine along with the aspirin or acetaminophen (10). If this were not sufficient, the dose of the narcotic in the combination should be increased.

There is no single standard dose of any narcotic for all clinical situations. Only after our initially chosen drug and dose have been observed to be ineffective *and* produced adverse effects, should we consider changing to another without titrating either up or down. All too frequently, physicians tend to switch prematurely to another medication simply because they started with the wrong dose of a drug which was otherwise appropriate for the circumstances. Switching from an inappropriate dose of one drug to an equianalgesic but equi-inappropriate dose of another drug really does not help matters. On the basis of our studies, there are no significant differences in side effects at the equianalgesic doses stated (9).

Differences among Analgesics

The terms *potency* and *relative potency* appear to be interpreted in quite different ways by clinicians and pharmacologists. To a clinician, the statement that drug "A" is more potent than drug "B" generally conveys to him the impression that drug "A" is capable of producing a greater effect than drug "B." The pharmacologist would merely conclude that it takes a smaller dose of drug "A" to produce the *same effect* as drug "B," and that it does not follow that either drug is capable of producing a greater effect than the other. The analgesic potencies of narcotic drugs in man differ by as much as several hundred-fold, and yet there is no substantial evidence that even the extremely potent drugs, such as etorphine (an oripavine derivative of thebaine), etonitazine (a substituted benzimidazole), and azidomorphine are any more effective than morphine when all drugs are given in their maximal tolerated doses. Whether or not there are any differences in ceiling effects of the morphine-type analgesics has been the subject of some controversy. When the dose is increased on a logarithmic scale, the increment effect appears to be linear, virtually to the point of loss of consciousness. However, before that level is reached, other undesired pharmacologic effects of the drug become manifest;

and we have observed that the level at which this occurs for different drugs can differ appreciably.

Route of Administration

The narcotic analgesics may differ in other ways. Some (alphaprodine, fentanyl, azidomorphine) have very prompt but short durations of action, whereas others (methadone, buprenorphine) do not act so quickly but have relatively long durations of action. Moreover, some drugs, such as morphine, have a relatively low oral/parenteral potency ratio, whereas others, such as methadone and dextromoramide, have relatively high ones. Thus, if we were to choose an oral narcotic equal in effect to a 10-mg intramuscular dose of morphine, methadone would be a better choice than oral morphine, if only because the patient would probably find swallowing two tablets at a time more acceptable than six.

As patients become tolerant, the dose-effect curves shift to the right, so that one has to give a larger dose to achieve the same effect. In these circumstances, if the patient were receiving a parenteral medication, questions of solubility of the drug and of the concentrations in which it is available may become important considerations. In America, most parenteral narcotics come in fixed concentrations, usually the amount contained in 1 ml of solution being the equianalgesic dose of 10 mg of morphine. The drug with which we are provided the widest latitude is morphine, for it is available in concentrations as high as 30 mg/ml. For that reason, many of us in America tend to reserve morphine for the last, if our patients are expected to need large doses of narcotics by injection. Although morphine sulfate is actually soluble in water to the extent of about 65 mg/ml, it is only about one-eighth as soluble as diamorphine (heroin). Since diamorphine is also 2 to 3 times as potent as morphine by intramuscular injection, diamorphine provides physicians in those countries in which its use is permitted (U.K. and Belgium) even greater dose flexibility in treating terminal cancer patients requiring parenteral analgesics (18).

Insofar as possible, oral medications should be employed rather than injections, for they are usually easier to administer and less likely to cause complications. Tolerance and physical dependence can, of course, develop on the repeated administration of even an orally administered narcotic, and this is a predictable dose-related phenomenon. However, pain due to cancer does not always remain the same or, necessarily, continue to get worse. It is, therefore, incumbent on the physician to monitor the patient closely, and it is just as important to recognize when to titrate downward as when to titrate upward in the course of events. When possible, it is usually advisable to give an antipyretic-type analgesic together with the narcotic, since there is little reason to believe that tolerance develops to that class of drugs, and the added analgesic effect which it provides will help stay the rapid development of tolerance.

Pain Behavior and Drug Dependence

In any consideration of the treatment of pain, we must never lose sight of what might be causing the pain. If there is any chance that some definitive measure—such as radiation therapy, steroids, chemotherapy, or even surgery—is feasible and capable of removing the cause for pain, then, obviously, this is probably the most effective way of preventing or delaying the development of analgesic tolerance and physical dependence.

The prescription governing when the patient can take or receive narcotics may also influence the degree and rate of development of tolerance and physical dependence. Twycross (17) maintains that by administering narcotics *by-the-clock* in amounts sufficient to prevent the patient from having pain, the daily amount of narcotic is less than if the patient were requesting it on-demand. We have little reason to doubt this from our observations, since the more severe that pain is allowed to become, the more difficult it seems to be to control. The conventional way in which analgesics are prescribed is p.r.n. This *on-demand* method of administering drugs has been implicated in the acquisition of what is known as "pain behavior"—which generally means that the patient uses the complaint of pain as a means of manipulating others (2,3). The narcotics are felt to be a prime cause or reinforcer of this behavior and, in addition, the patient is often suspected of being addicted or of getting some vicarious pleasure from the drug. We have not seen any outward signs of elation in our cancer patients receiving on-demand narcotics. However, these patients do frequently develop tolerance to narcotics. Physicians and nurses often speak of such patients as being "clock-watchers" or "addicts" when, in fact, they have simply failed to recognize that one of the cardinal signs of developing tolerance is shortening of the duration of effect. We would assume that Dr. Twycross' patients do not develop pain behavior, for his patients are assured of receiving large enough doses of narcotics regularly to prevent pain from recurring. Whether we should consider those patients addicted will depend on how one wishes to define "addiction." The term *addict* connotes opprobrium. Applying this epithet to a sick and dying patient becomes a matter for one's conscience.

The by-the-clock method of prescribing narcotics with the intention of preventing pain may not always be the wisest course to follow in some cancer patients. When the patient is not being closely monitored, as is the case for most outpatients or home-care patients who are being seen only periodically, potentially serious complications which are commonly heralded by pain could be masked just long enough for there to be disastrous consequences for the patient. By the same token, patients whose pains tend to be intermittent and unpredictable, or are likely to lessen in response to definitive therapy, could be exposed to larger amounts of narcotics than they may actually need and, consequently, experience unwanted dose-related side effects. However, the customarily employed *pro re nata* approach is, itself, not without limitations, some of which have been mentioned above. More importantly, the on-demand prescription forces the patient to re-experience pain before taking or requesting medication, which can be very damaging to the morale of many patients.

NARCOTIC AGONISTS-ANTAGONISTS

In the quarter of a century since the discovery that nalorphine had significant analgesic activity (13), it has been well established that the classic properties of narcotics, their ability to relieve pain, and their capacity for inducing physical dependence, are not inseparable. Since then, a large number and variety of narcotic congeners with mixed agonist-antagonist properties have been developed. Although very few have thus far been introduced into medical practice as analgesics, they have had appreciable impact on how narcotic analgesics are employed.

Pentazocine, the only one of these currently marked for use in the United States, has enjoyed some popularity in the management of severe chronic pain despite its limitations, for the drug is a relatively short-acting analgesic, and it can precipitate some rather disturbing, though transitory, psychotomimetic reactions. Although pentazocine is not free of potential for abuse, it is not listed as a controlled substance in our country. That it is used so much in spite of its shortcomings is, perhaps, an indication of the importance many physicians give to what is construed as addiction liability in their choice of analgesics for the management of chronic pain. The prospects for the future, however, are more promising, for there are now several new drugs of this class under investigation which appear not only to be more potent and to have longer durations of action, but also to produce fewer of the undesired side effects of pentazocine (11).

The narcotic agonist-antagonists vary appreciably in their relative agonist and antagonist properties. Consequently, there are more substantial differences in the pharmacologic profiles of drugs of this type than there are among the typical morphine surrogates. However, they do share in common the property of increased antagonistic potency in the presence of physical dependence. Thus, if pentazocine or any of the newer drugs of this class were to be employed, the best time to do so would be before the patient is first placed on a narcotic analgesic. Drugs of this type act centrally, and they are always used to best advantage when they are given together with the simple analgesics of the antipyretic–anti-inflammatory type. Pentazocine, currently available as an analgesic, is also marketed as a compound mixture with aspirin. Propiram, a phenampromid analog, and tilidine, which has some structural relationship to meperidine, are two agonist-antagonists with very weak antagonist properties. Both of these drugs are marketed in Europe and, at this time, are investigational drugs in the United States. Three agonist-antagonists with more potent antagonist properties are nalbuphine, an analog of naloxone; butorphanol, a morphinan; and buprenorphine, an oripavine. All of these are still investigational drugs that have proven to be very effective analgesics which are felt to have low abuse-potential.

LOW-POTENCY NARCOTICS

The weaker or low-potency narcotic agonists consist of propoxyphene, a methadone analog; meperidine, the prototype of its class; and codeine, a natural opium alkaloid. Both codeine and propoxyphene have good oral/parenteral potency ratios so that, in effect, they are low-potency agonists even when given parenterally. Meperidine, on the other hand, is only about one-quarter as potent by mouth as it is by intramuscular injection (19), so that it is considered with the weaker narcotics when given by mouth and with the potent narcotics when given by injection. When administered by mouth, all of these drugs are best used in combination with other simple analgesics and, in fact, all are marketed in mixtures containing either aspirin, acetaminophen, or APC (aspirin, phenacetin, and caffeine).

HIGH-POTENCY NARCOTICS

Oxycodone, which bears the same chemical structural relationship to oxymorphone as codeine does to morphine, is a potent narcotic agonist which is available to us in America only in fixed-dose combinations with either APC (Percodan®) or acetaminophen (Percocet®). In these formulations, the highest unit dose of oxycodone is 5 mg, which is approximately equivalent to 60 mg of oral codeine.

Other potent narcotics which have relatively high oral/parenteral potency ratios and are not commonly marketed as mixtures include levorphanol, methadone, anileridine, and dextromoramide. The latter drug is not available in the United States but is marketed in Europe. Like oxycodone, all of these drugs are what are considered Schedule II drugs in the United States, a designation applied to drugs with recognized medical uses but high addiction liability. The pharmacologic profiles of virtually all of these drugs are quite similar to morphine, except that morphine has a poor oral/parenteral potency ratio. However, many hospitals and institutions in the United States are now administering morphine orally in some variation of the British Euphoriant Elixir. Diamorphine (heroin), which is more commonly used in the mixture in the U.K., is, of course, illegal in the United States. To my knowledge, the only systematic study of this combination is that reported by Twycross (18), who found that morphine substituted well for diamorphine if added to the solution in a dose 1½ times that of diamorphine.

As usually employed in British hospices, the Brompton Cocktail consists of an orally administered mixture of cocaine, ethyl alcohol, chloroform water, and varying amounts of diamorphine, ranging from 5 to 100 mg, tailored to fit the patients' needs for analgesia. This Elixir is generally administered on a regular 4-hr schedule around-the-clock. Comparable mixtures containing morphine and methadone are generally being administered in the same manner to patients with terminal cancer in the United States and Canada.

SUMMARY

In summary, the use of narcotic analgesics plays an essential role in the effective management of pain due to advanced or terminal cancer. These drugs are the most efficacious of all the systemic analgesics and are capable of relieving virtually all types of pain regardless of site or sites of origin. However, there is no single drug, dose, or route of administration which is appropriate for all patients with advanced cancer. Important to success in controlling pain is titrating the dose within the limits of tolerable side effects before deciding to change to another drug. Pain due to advanced cancer is not static. These patients require continuous monitoring for indicated modifications of their analgesic regimens. The narcotic agonist-antagonists are best employed before the patient has had appreciable exposure to pure narcotic agonists. There are several drugs of this class which appear to have substantial advantages over the presently available pentazocine. An orally administered by-the-clock regimen designed to keep the patient from experiencing pain has many advantages if it can be closely monitored. In the final analysis, successful management of pain in the patient with advanced cancer will, in large measure, depend on understanding the patient, the underlying disease, and the reason for the patient's having pain (6).

ACKNOWLEDGMENT

Supported in part by a grant from the National Institute on Drug Abuse, No. DA-01707.

REFERENCES

1. Eddy, N. B., Halbach, H., and Braenden, O. J. (1957): Synthetic substances with morphine-like effect. Clinical experience: side effects, addiction liability. *Bull. W.H.O.*, 17:569–863.
2. Fordyce, W. E. (1974): Pain viewed as learned behavior. In: *Advances in Neurology, Vol. 4: International Symposium on Pain,* edited by J. J. Bonica, pp. 415–422. Raven Press, New York.
3. Fordyce, W. E. (1974): Treating pain by contingency management. In: *Advances in Neurology, Vol. 4: International Symposium on Pain,* edited by J. J. Bonica, pp. 583–589. Raven Press, New York.

4. Goodman, L. S., and Gilman, A., editors (1941, 1955): *The Pharmacological Basis of Therapeutics,* 1st and 2nd editions, Macmillan, New York.
5. Halpern, L. M., and Bonica, J. J. (1976): Analgesics. In: *Drugs of Choice,* edited by W. Modell, pp. 195–232. C. V. Mosby, St. Louis.
6. Houde, R. W. (1956): Pain and the patient with cancer. In: *The Medical Clinics of North America—Symposium on the Medical Aspects of Cancer,* edited by D. A. Karnofsky and R. W. Rawson, pp. 687–703. W. B. Saunders Co., Philadelphia and London.
7. Houde, R. W. (1974): Medical treatment of oncological pain. In: *Recent Advances on Pain: Pathophysiology and Clinical Aspects,* edited by J. J. Bonica, P. Procacci, C. A. Pagni, pp. 168–188, Charles C. Thomas, Springfield, Ill.
8. Houde, R. W. (1974): The use and misuse of narcotics in the treatment of chronic pain. In: *Advances in Neurology, Vol. 4: International Symposium on Pain,* edited by J. J. Bonica, pp. 527–536. Raven Press, New York.
9. Houde, R. W., Wallenstein, S. L., and Beaver, W. T. (1965): Clinical measurement of pain. In: *Analgetics,* edited by G. de Stevens, pp. 75–122. Academic Press, New York.
10. Houde, R. W., Wallenstein, S. L., and Beaver, W. T. (1966): Evaluation of analgesics in patients with cancer pain. In: *International Encyclopedia of Pharmacology and Therapeutics, Section 6, Volume I: Clinical Pharmacology,* edited by L. Lasagna, pp. 59–97. Pergamon Press Ltd., Oxford.
11. Houde, R. W., Wallenstein, S. L., Rogers, A., and Kaiko, R. F. (1976): Annual report of the Analgesic Studies Section of the Memorial Sloan-Kettering Cancer Center. *Proceedings of the Thirty-eighth Annual Scientific Meeting of the Committee on Problems of Drug Dependence,* National Academy of Sciences, pp. 149–168.
12. Krueger, H., Eddy, N. B., and Sumwalt, M. (1941): *The Pharmacology of Opium Alkaloids, Part 1, Suppl. No. 165 to the Public Health Reports,* pp. 26–29. U.S. Gov't. Printing Office, Washington, D.C.
13. Lasagna, L., and Beecher, H. K. (1954): The analgesic effectiveness of nalorphine and nalorphine-morphine combinations in man. *J. Pharmacol.,* 112:356–363.
14. Martin, W. R. (1967): Opioid antagonists. *Pharmacol. Rev.,* 19:463–521.
15. Modell, W., and Houde, R. W. (1958): Factors influencing clinical evaluation of drugs. *JAMA,* 167:2190–2198.
16. Terry, C. E., and Pellens, M. (1928): *The Opium Problem,* pp. 94–136. Bureau of Social Hygiene, Inc., New York.
17. Twycross, R. G. (1975): Relief of terminal pain. *Br. Med. J.,* 4:212–214.
18. Twycross, R. G. (1977): Choice of strong analgesic in terminal cancer: Diamorphine or morphine? *Pain,* 3:93–104.
19. Wallenstein, S. L., and Houde, R. W. (1959): Relative oral and parenteral potencies of anileridine and meperidine. *Fed. Proc.,* 18:456.
20. Wikler, A. (1950): Sites and mechanisms of action of morphine and related drugs in the central nervous system. *Pharmacol. Rev.,* 2:435–506.
21. Woodbury, D. M., and Fingl, E. (1975): Analgesic-antipyretics, anti-inflammatory agents, and drugs employed in the therapy of gout. In: *The Pharmacological Basis of Therapeutics,* 5th ed., edited by L. S. Goodman and A. Gilman, pp. 325–358. Macmillan, New York.

Advances in Pain Research and Therapy, Vol. 2,
edited by J. J. Bonica and V. Ventafridda.
Raven Press, New York © 1979.

Psychotropics, Ataractics, and Related Drugs

Lawrence M. Halpern

Department of Pharmacology, University of Washington School of Medicine, Seattle, Washington 98195

Recent advances in our understanding of central factors which play roles in the perception of pain and its modulation emphasize the need to parcel out and separately treat various psychologic factors which can intensify or decrease pain experiences in cancer patients. Depression as a temporary mood state, i.e., normal depression or grief states, depression secondary to psychiatric or medical disorders or chronicity of illness, and primary depression or melancholia, may exacerbate pain or make preexisting pain worse. Elation, excitement, or mania may relieve or ameliorate pain. Anxiety may be responsible for *de novo* pain or may make preexisting pain considerably worse. It is now a generally accepted principle that the psychologic circumstances described above may centrally modulate pain arising from nociceptive sources and may even give rise to pain in the absence of nociceptor input.

The last 10 years of progress in the area of chronic pain management have renewed our interest in the actions of psychotropic drugs as "pain medications." Psychotropic agents have been employed to reduce anxiety, provide nighttime sedation, elevate mood, block emesis, or produce analgesia. These alternative uses for psychotropic drugs have emerged empirically as a result of clinical experience with these agents and careful clinical observation by individuals interested in the newly emerging field of chronic pain management. Unfortunately, there are very few studies in the literature which could qualify as good clinical pharmacology. In a recent survey of the cancer-treatment literature this author was able to find few studies of the effects of psychotropic drugs done using reasonable parametric techniques. This is at once surprising and shocking when one considers that the frequency of occurrence of painful malignancy requiring palliative therapy with analgesic and other drugs is reasonably high.

INDICATIONS

Treatment of moderate and severe terminal-cancer pain syndrome is frequently complicated by inappropriate drug selection, inadequate dosage, and in the case of the narcotic analgesics, the development of dependence. Failure

TABLE 1. *Some psychologic ramifications of cancer-pain syndrome and their management with psychotropic drugs*

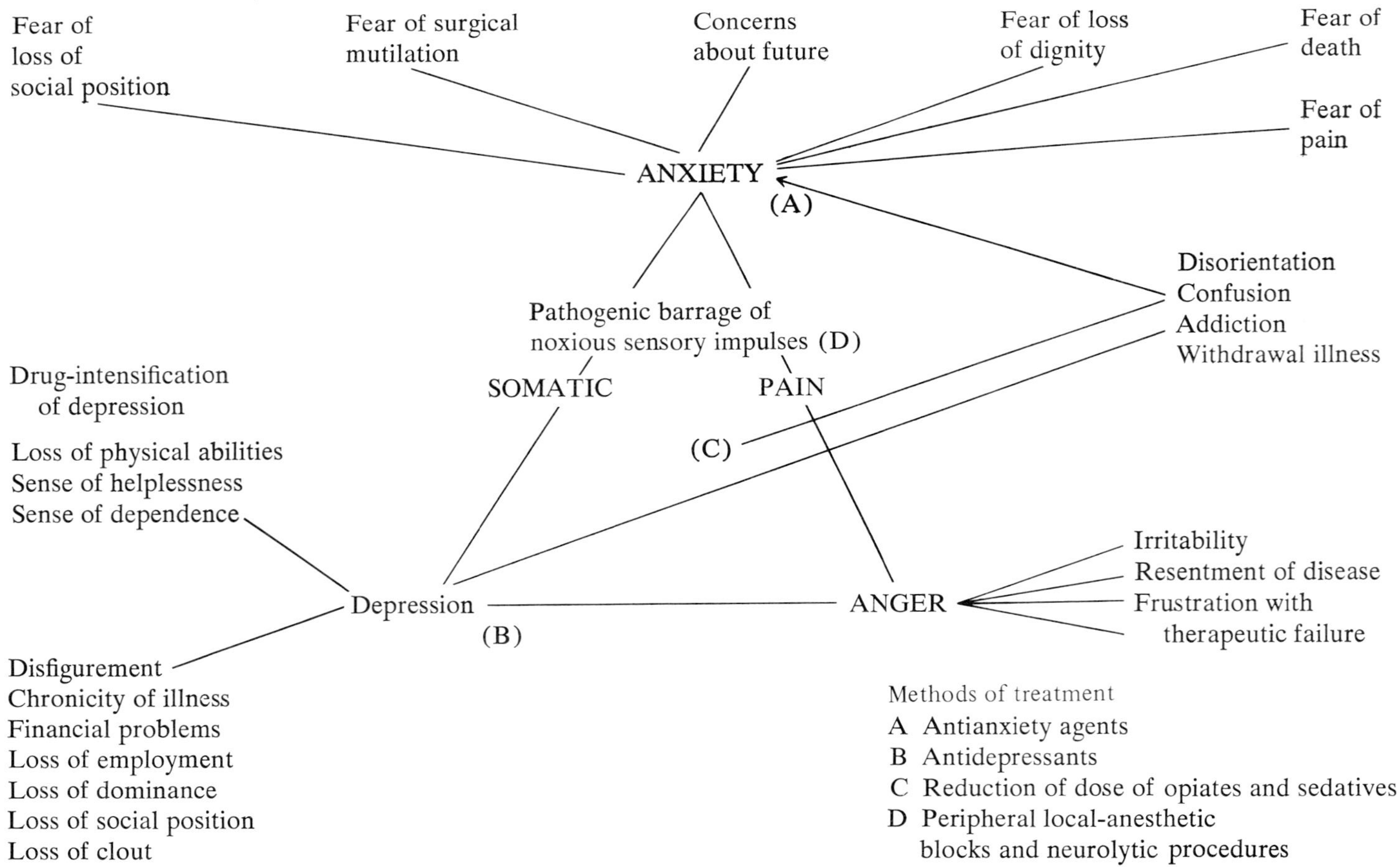

to recognize and appropriately treat the narcotic-analgesic–tolerant individual results in the patient not only receiving inadequate pain-relief, but also having to deal with the unpleasantness of unsupported opiate withdrawal. Narcotics dependence *per se* is not a problem so long as attention to the rising intake levels prevents the patient from discomfort. Once dependence on narcotics is involved, personality change, drug-induced intensification of depression, uncomfortable constipation, and emotional consequences some patients have difficulties dealing with, and reduction in activities outside of maintenance of adequate narcotics dosage severely limit the interactions of the patient with his/her former activities. For these reasons methods of pain control involving psychotropic drugs have begun to appear and are becoming more common as our collective experience with them grows.

Reduction of anxiety with psychotherapy, reassurance, progressive muscular relaxation techniques, transcendental meditation, or drugs; reversal of depression with psychotherapy or drugs; use of selected phenothiazines, sympathomimetic amines, sedative antihistamines, cannabis and its derivatives, and even psychodysleptic agents such as LSD have been used to modify psychologic variables in the management of terminal pain.

Chapman's model for pain associated with advanced cancer (*this volume*) describes many of the psychologic variables which form the rationale for psychotropic drug selection for the management of terminal pain syndrome in advanced cancer (Table 1). While it is true that narcotic analgesic drugs and their potentiators and antianxiety drugs are probably the most frequently used agents for the management of cancer pain, these agents add yet another dimension to the variables in Chapman's model.

As a result of chronic cancer pain and its management with opiates and antianxiety agents, the cancer patient has to deal with the additional burden of chronic drug-induced disorientation, excessive sedation alternating with withdrawal illness, and in some cases uncomfortable feelings of almost a sexual nature which some patients find disquieting. In addition drug-induced intensification of depression may increase fear, anger, and frustration levels and even pain itself. Family members are sensitive to and quick to note progressive personality changes centering around isolation and withdrawal from family members due to drug use. The patient's main preoccupation becomes an involvement with pain medication. Medication is used in anticipation of pain. Inappropriate doses of analgesic drugs are used in attempts to calm anxiety, reduce fear, prevent uncomfortable drug withdrawal symptoms, and to achieve excessive sedation.

TECHNIQUES OF MANAGING PAIN IN THE ADVANCED CANCER PATIENT

Because of the concerns discussed above, our experience has centered around two basic alterations in the usual strategy for providing pain-relief for the terminally ill patient. First, orally active doses of long-acting drugs are used whenever possible, i.e., methadone or levo dromoran, phenobarbital or chlordiazepoxide. Secondly, attempts are made to minimize the dose and duration of usage of narcotics and sedatives by prolonging the time before it becomes necessary to administer them. This is accomplished by use of appropriate psychotropic medications, systematic partial or total detoxification, and the use of local-anesthetic nerve block and peripheral neurolytic procedures where appropriate.

Long-acting drugs prevent euphoria-withdrawal swings, medication in anticipation of pain, and inappropriate use of narcotics for the treatment of anxiety. This allows reduction in opiate and sedative dosage, and as a consequence of lowered dosage, disorientation and withdrawal illness are reduced. In many cases, reversal of chronic drug-induced intensification of depression results in better pain control as a result of lessened depression. Reduction in sedative dosage seems to lessen anger-agitation and emotional lability resulting in a calmer, less-upset patient.

Substitution-withdrawal using long-acting opiates and sedatives (6) allows for reduction of drug-induced effects as described above. Tricyclic antidepressant drugs, usually amitryptiline or doxepine, are started immediately and maintained at 150 mg for the duration of pain treatment. Anxiety and agitation and emotional lability decrease as a consequence of reduction of barbiturate-diazepam dosage. Sedation and an antianxiety effect can be achieved with doses of sedative antihistamines, i.e., diphenhydramine or hydroxyzine, and by taking advantage of the sedative qualities of the antidepressants given H.S. This medication technique permits stable pain-control. As pain reappears during opiate-dosage reduction, the dose of long-acting opiate is held constant at levels which do not completely obliterate pain.

Diagnostic local-anesthetic blocks are done, and if the results show promise, permanent peripheral neurolytic procedures may be employed. Should the peripheral neurolytic procedure provide adequate relief of pain, the dosage of methadone or other long-acting opiates can be reduced even further. In many cases the patient becomes much more active, personalities change toward their former direction, and patients and their families are more comfortable with the dying process.

SYMPATHOMIMETIC AMINES

Amphetamine has recently been shown to potentiate the action of narcotic analgesic drugs (5), 5 mg and 10 mg P.O. produce 1.5 and 2 times the analgesia for a given dose of morphine. Because of the rapid development of tolerance to sympathomimetic amines, this agent should not be used for long periods of time, but is quite useful for short periods where its use can brighten up an excessively sedated patient and provide increased analgesia. This agent antagonizes phenothiazine sedation and is itself antagonized by

TABLE 2. *Psychotropic drugs useful in the management of chronic pain*

Action	Example
Sympathomimetic amines	D-Amphetamine
Elevate mood	Methylphenidate
Potentiate analgesia	
Prevent withdrawal	
Antidepressants	
Elevate mood	Amitryptiline
Increase sedation	Doxepine
Potentiate analgesia	
Analgesic action	
Phenothiazines	
Confusion	Levomepromazine
Delirium	Perphenazine
Psychotic manifestations	Chlorpromazine
Increase sedation	
Analgesic action	
Sedative antihistamines	
Antianxiety	Diphenhydramine
Sedative hypnotic	Hydroxyzine
Analgesic action	
Benzodiazepines	Clonazepam
Cannabis derivatives	
Antianxiety	Marihuana
Antinauseant	Nabilone
Antidepressant	

phenothiazine. Methylphenidate (Ritalin®) has been used for this purpose and reportedly can substitute for meperidine, maintaining good analgesia and preventing opiate withdrawal after discontinuation of meperidine (14).

COCAINE

Cocaine was first used in combination with morphine by Snow (13), who claimed that this substance helped to "sustain vitality." It is a relatively brief, amphetamine-like agent, and its use in fixed-dose combinations with an opiate cannot be recommended. Appropriate dosage of antidepressant drugs, i.e., amitryptiline and doxepine pushed to adequate levels not only serve to brighten the patient but may also have an analgesic action of their own.

TRICYCLIC ANTIDEPRESSANTS

Amitryptiline and doxepine have been used successfully in the management of cancer pain. Prior to the use of narcotic analgesics these agents may be used alone or in combination with the phenothiazines levomepromazine or perphenazine. Levomepromazine is a phenothiazine with analgesic potency (8); when used alone or in combination with an antidepressant, narcotic-like analgesia results without the development of physical-dependence–withdrawal concerns which interfere with narcotic analgesic therapy. One must exert care that excessive sedation does not develop and that the orthostatic hypotension occurring as a result of use of the phenothiazine does not result in falling and further injury to the patient. It is recommended that patients being started on this psychotropic combination be at bed rest until tolerance to these symptoms and appropriate dosages are achieved. Maintenance of patients without narcotic analgesics, or with low doses of narcotic analgesics potentiated with appropriate psychoactive agents, prolongs the patient's ability to interact with family and friends, and may even keep the patient alert and active enough to maintain a job or participate in other outside activities.

Once narcotics have been started, the antidepressants may potentiate narcotic analgesia, have an analgesic action of their own (10), or reduce pain by elevating mood. In any case, the presence of antidepressant drug permits overall reduction in the dosage of narcotics while maintaining adequate analgesia.

The combination of amitryptiline and perphenazine (15) or doxepine and perphenazine is frequently used in the management of post-herpetic neuralgia, which can plague already uncomfortable cancer victims. This is thought to occur as a consequence of supression of immune responses as a result of radiotherapy or chemotherapy. In this situation, the antidepressant is administered at doses of 50 mg H.S. for 3 days, 100 mg H.D. for 3 days and up to 150 mg H.S. thereafter. The perphenazine is started at 1 mg and the dosage increases at 5-day intervals, until doses of 5 to 6 mg/day have been reached.

PHENOTHIAZINES

Methotrimeprazine (Levomepromazine, Levoprome) is a phenothiazine derivative possessing many of the pharmacologic characteristics of the group. Levomepromazine has no antitussive properties, and less respiratory depression occurs as compared with the narcotics. It does not produce psychologic or physical dependence, nor does it suppress the symptoms of morphine withdrawal. It produces narcotic-like analgesia and seems to be half as potent as morphine on a milligram basis (2). Equianalgesic doses for 15 mg of mephotrimeprazine are 10 mg morphine and 75 to 100 mg meperidine. The onset of action of this agent is as rapid as morphine, with a similar duration of analgesic action. As with all phenothiazines, orthostatic hypotension develops, which may outlast the duration of the analgesia produced by this drug. Dizziness, blurred vision, disorientation, and marked sedation are all undesirable side effects which may tend to limit the use of this drug to nonambulatory patients in whom addiction to narcotics is to be avoided. Thus, its major use in the management of cancer patients is to provide full analgesia during the period prior to the introduction of narcotic analgesics. The drug has successfully been combined with amitryptiline and doxepine to provide potentiated analgesia at doses low enough to provide for some careful ambulation while not producing excessive sedation.

Phenergan

Phenergan potentiates the sedation produced by narcotic analgesic drugs while antagonizing the analgesia they produce (4). Thus phenergan is a poor choice of psychotropic agents to be used in the management of cancer pain.

Chlorpromazine

Chlorpromazine is an early member of the group of phenothiazine tranquilizers and is useful for potentiating sedation from narcotic analgesic drugs as well as dealing with confusion, delirium, and psychotic manifestations, should these occur.

SEDATIVE ANTIHISTAMINES

The diphenylmethane antihistaminics diphenhydramine and hydroxyzine have been found to be helpful in the management of chronic pain, and especially cancer pain. An interesting question is raised as to whether the beneficial effect of the agents is due to their antianxiety effect or because these agents have some additional analgesic effect. Beaver (1) has demonstrated an analgesic effect similar to that of morphine, i.e., 100 mg hydroxyzine i.m. is equivalent to 8 mg of morphine sulfate. Kantor (7) was unable to demonstrate analgesic activity for hydroxyzine after doses of 100 mg P.O.

The beneficial effect in cancer patients may be due to a wholly different mechanism. It has been our experience that cancer patients on elevated doses of sedative hypnotic agents, such as diazepam, are likely to have mood-swings which include spontaneous crying for no apparent reason that the patient can describe. Substitution-withdrawal from diazepam or other sedative and the use of diphenhydramine or hydroxyzine eliminates mood-swings and spontaneous crying.

The use of diphenhydramine 100 mg P.O., H.S., or hydroxyzine 100 mg P.O., H.S., often eliminates the need for additional nighttime sedation. When antidepressants are used, the sedative effect of the antihistamines is enhanced, and this combination can be used to good advantage in most patients. Hydroxyzine offers some advantages over diphenhydramine in that maximum daily dosage tolerated without potentially dangerous central side effects is greater.

BENZODIAZEPINES

As a group, the benzodiazepines have not been valuable in the management of cancer pain because of problems associated with physical dependence after chronic use. Barbiturates and meprobamate have been shown to have antianalgesic properties. While there is no clear demonstration as yet, at least after chronic use the benzodiazepines may indeed possess antianalgesic properties. Clonazepam has been recently reported to differ from other members of the benzodiazepine group. This agent has been described to possess valuable intrinsic analgesic activity and has been described as useful in the treatment of neuralgias, atypical facial pain, and other resistant conditions of the head and neck (3).

CANNABIS DERIVATIVES

Studies of delta-9-tetrahydrocannabinol have demonstrated that it possesses euphoriant, analgesic, appetite-stimulant, and antiemetic effects. These effects may have use in the management of the despondency, weight loss, and pain which pose difficult problems, since other psychotropic agents currently in use prove inadequate (12). Studies of these effects in cancer patients suggest that delta-9-THC has value as an antidepressant and can be of value in the management of both inpatient and outpatient cancer patients, provided that somnolence, dizziness, and depersonalization do not result in early discontinuation.

NABILONE

Nabilone is a new THC homologue (9) which has antianxiety properties (11) and is currently being evaluated for use as a substitute. Should this agent prove to be of value, it would simplify problems currently encountered in the administration of marihuana or delta-9-tetrahydrocannibinol, since nabilone is reportedly water-soluble and parenterally injectable.

REFERENCES

1. Beaver, W. T., and Geise, G. (1975): Comparison of the analgesic effects of morphine, hydroxyzine and their combination in patients with post-operative pain. In: *Advances in Pain Research and Therapy, Vol. 1: Proceedings of the First World Congress on Pain,* edited by J. J. Bonica and D. Albe-Fessard. Raven Press, New York.
2. Beaver, W. T. (1976): Comparison of morphine, hydroxyzine and morphine plus hydroxyzine in postoperative pain. *Hosp. Prac.* (Special Edition) p. 19.
3. Budd, K. (1978): Psychotropic drugs in the management of chronic pain. *Anesthesiology,* 33:531–534.
4. Dundee, J. W., Love, W. J., and Moore, J. (1963): Alterations in response to somatic pain associated with analgesia and further studies with phenothiazine derivatives and similar drugs. *Br. J. Anesth.,* 35:597–609.

5. Forrest, W. H., Brown, L. R., Mahler, D. L., Katz, J., Schroff, P., Defalque, R., and Brown, B. (1973): The evaluation of morphine and desamphetamine combination for analgesia. *Clin. Pharmacol. Ther.,* 14:132.
6. Halpern, L. M. (1977): Analgesic drugs in the management of pain. *Arch. Surg.,* 112:861–869.
7. Kantor, T. G., and Steinberg, F. P. (1975): Studies of tranquilizing agents and meperidine in clinical pain. Hydroxyzine and Meprobamate. In: *Advances in Pain Research and Therapy, Vol. 1: Proceedings of the First World Congress on Pain,* edited by J. J. Bonica and D. Albe-Fessard, p. 567. Raven Press, New York.
8. Lasagna, L., and DeKornfeld, T. J. (1961): Mephotrimeprazine: A new phenothiazine derivative with analgesic properties. *JAMA,* 178:827.
9. Lemberger, L., and Rowe, H. (1975): Clinical pharmacology of nabilone, a cannibinol derivative. *Clin. Pharmacol. Ther.,* 18:720–726.
10. Merskey, H., and Hester, R. A. (1972): The treatment of chronic pain with psychoactive drugs. *Postgrad. Med. J.,* 58:594–598.
11. Nakano, S., Gillespie, H. K., and Hollister, L. E. (1978): Nabilone and diazepam. *Clin. Pharmacol. Ther.* 23:51–62.
12. Regelson, W., Butler, J. R., Schulz, J., Kiek, J., Peek, L., Green, M. L., and Zalis, M. O. (1976): Delta-9-tetrahydrocannabinol as an effective antidepressant and appetite-stimulating agent in advanced cancer patients. In: *The Pharmacology of Marihuana,* edited by M. C. Braude and S. Szara. Raven Press, New York.
13. Snow, H. (1897): The opium cocaine treatment of malignant disease. *Br. Med. J.,* 1:1019–1020.
14. Stambaugh, J. E.: Personal communication.
15. Taub, A., and Collins, W. F., Jr. (1974): Observations on treatment of denervation dysesthesia with psychotropic drugs: Post-herpetic neuralgia, anesthesia dolorosa, peripheral neuropathy. In: *Advances in Neurology, Vol. 4: International Symposium on Pain,* edited by J. J. Bonica, pp. 309–315. Raven Press, New York.

Advances in Pain Research and Therapy, Vol. 2,
edited by J. J. Bonica and V. Ventafridda.
Raven Press, New York © 1979.

The Use of Psychotropic Drugs in the Treatment of Cancer Pain

R. Kocher

Psychiatrische Universitätsklinik Basel, Neurologischer Dienst und EEG-Station, 4025 Basel, Switzerland

Since the introduction of psychotropic drugs, especially thymoleptics and neuroleptics, the treatment of all chronic and severe pain including cancer pain has been decisively improved. Shortly after the introduction of neuroleptics (1951 to 1952) and of thymoleptics (1957) in medicine, the first reports of their effective analgesic actions were published. Furthermore, an analgesic potentiating action and a narcotic analgesic-sparing effect were described. These reports suggested to us that we treat the patients of chronic pain including cancer pain with a combination of drugs of both groups. In this report we briefly summarized the results obtained in our clinic and those reported by others.

CLINICAL MATERIAL

Personal Experience

We have been using combinations of drugs of both groups for chronic pain therapy for over a decade. In a previous report (8) we summarized the results of psychotropic drug combinations in patients with a variety of chronic pain syndromes including cancer pain. The results were rated as follows: *very good to excellent* when patients had complete relief of pain and were able to terminate narcotic analgesics; *good to fair* when there was significant (but not total) pain-relief and narcotic analgesic intake could be reduced significantly; and *no improvement* when there was no change in the pain and it was impossible to reduce the dosage of analgesics the patient had been taking. In a group of 91 patients who received the drug combination, 22 (24%) had excellent results; 60 (66%) derived fair to good results; and 9 (10%) had no improvement. The failures occurred in patients with degenerative disk disease and other serious musculoskeletal problems. Among the small group of patients who had moderate to severe cancer pain, all derived good results. During the subsequent 2 years we have continued to use this drug-combination therapy for patients with pain of advanced cancer as well as other chronic pain syndromes with similar results.

Dosage Schedule

As a result of our experience, a clear-cut dosage schedule has been established for inpatients and outpatients. A therapy based on these guidelines has been shown to be without relevant side effects. For outpatients the best combination consists of chlorimipramine 25 mg by mouth 3 times daily and haloperidol beginning with 0.5 mg 2 times daily and then carefully increasing the dosage to 1 mg given 2 or 3 times each day.

For inpatients the best dosage schedule is as follows: chlorimipramine given via an intravenous infusion containing 25 to 50 mg of the drug in 250 ml of 5% glucose solution administered over the course of 2 to 3 hr daily. After 1 week this is changed to 25 mg given by mouth 3 times daily. At the same time, haloperidol is given in initial doses of 0.5 mg 2 times daily and then carefully increasing the dosage to 1 mg 2 to 3 times each day. It is important that in elderly, debilitated persons the daily dosage of haloperidol should not exceed 1.5 mg daily.

Results Reported by Others

Review of the literature reveals that it is difficult to compare the therapeutic results of one group with those of others. This is because there is

TABLE 1. *The analgesic efficacy of psychotropic drugs for cancer pain*

Author	Drug used	No. of pts.	Cause of pain	Improvement of pain
Thymoleptics				
Daxelmüller (5)	Imipramine	40	Neurol. pat. incl. cancer	80%
Gebhardt et al. (7)	Chlorimipramine	52	Cancer	67%
Mönkemeier and Steffen (9)	Imipramine	20	Cancer	75%
Adjan (1)	Imipramine	31	Cancer	80%
Adjan (1)	Chlorimipramine	50	Cancer	90%
Barjou (2)	Imipramine	30	Surg. pat. incl. cancer	70%
Deutschmann (6)	Imipramine	44	Cancer	80%
Neuroleptics				
Bloomfield (4)	Laevomepromazine	18	Cancer and arthritis	>50%
Combinations				
Bernard and Scheurer (3)	Chlorimipramine + laevomepromazine or haloperidol	83	Inoperable cancer (ENT)	87%
Put (10)	Fluanxol and dixeran	17	Visceral cancer	67%

TABLE 2. *Results with use of psychotropic drugs in the treatment of cancer pain*

	No. of pts.	Psychotropic drugs[a]	Improvement in %
Germany			
Duisburg	100	T, N, A	10
Göttingen	250	T, N, A	41
Berlin	300	T, N	30
Austria			
Vienna (2. Med.)	50	A, N	70
Switzerland			
Zürich	134	A, N	30
St. Gallen	1500	A, N	80
Basel	100	T, N, A	30
Neuchâtel	20	T, A	75

[a] T, tranquilizer; N, neuroleptic; A, antidepressant.

usually a lack of uniformity of experimental design of clinical trials and significant variation in the clinical measurement of pain and pain-relief. Despite these reservations of mine, I have listed the results obtained by other clinicians who have used various psychotropic drugs for the management of patients with cancer pain. Review of the data in Table 1 reveals that although the number of patients reported by each writer or group of writers is relatively small, an average of about 80% of the patients had improvement reflected by decrease of the severity of the pain and reduction of narcotic analgesic requirements.

In order to obtain additional data, we carried out a survey of various cancer centers of the German-speaking countries. A questionnaire was sent to the important cancer centers in Austria, Germany and Switzerland. Of 39 questionnaires sent out, 20 were returned consisting of 11 from Germany, 3 from Austria, and 6 from Switzerland. Of these 20 centers, 4 reported no experience with these drugs; in each of 3 other centers, only 1 patient had been treated; and in the reports of 5 centers some of the data were lacking. Table 2 lists the results reported by the remaining 8 centers.

DISCUSSION

The results obtained in the literature, as well as our own personal results, indicated that psychotropic drugs are useful and effective in managing patients with pain of advanced cancer. In general, one can expect improvement in the form of partial or complete pain-relief and reduction or complete elimination of narcotic drugs in about 60 to 80% of the patients, depending on the drug combination used.

In contrast, the results obtained from the survey of some of the cancer centers in the three German-speaking countries strongly suggest that: (a) in general, the use of psychotropic drugs for the treatment of pain of advanced cancer is not well known in these centers. This lack of knowledge should be eliminated by more intense efforts in diffusing information, including all publications on the subject; and (b) the percentage of patients who experience improvement varied greatly among the different centers, which is somewhat in contrast to the publications found in the literature. This suggests that each center should carry out a prospective study in the future in order to ascertain the efficacy of the drug and the best combination of drugs and doses of each agent.

The advantages in using psychotropic drugs for the treatment of cancer pain (as well as other chronic pain syndromes) include: (a) they improve the general emotional condition of patients by their action as antidepressants; (b) they appear to be effective in patients who have developed tolerance to established treatment with narcotic analgesics; (c) properly used, these drugs are associated with few, if any, harmful side effects; and (d) there is evidence that they potentiate the analgesic efficacy of narcotics.

Drug combinations, but particularly the administration of neuroleptics and thymoleptics concomitantly, offer the following additional advantages: (a) a smaller dose of each drug is usually sufficient, and consequently, we can minimize incidence and severity of troublesome side effects; (b) combined thymoleptic and neuroleptic effects are valuable because one of them may be missing or insufficient when a drug of one group alone is given; and (c) the spectrum of pharmacologic action is broadened.

Mode of Action

The generally favorable results for relief obtained with psychotropic drugs, especially when a combination of thymoleptics and neuroleptics is used in the treatment of pain, suggests that these drugs do not have only one but a variety of pharmacologic actions which, as previously mentioned, is greatly broadened when a combined therapy is used. It is now believed that psychotropic drugs have both central and peripheral pharmacologic action. In regard to their *peripheral action,* one thinks immediately of the pain-producing substances. It is possible that psychotropic drugs have their peripheral effect by interfering in some way with these pain-producing substances such as prostaglandins. This is merely a speculation, because evidence to support such a hypothesis is lacking.

Central action. Psychotropic drugs, especially when both thymoleptics and neuroleptics are given, alter pain perception and pain sensation. The drugs effect a "depersonalization of the pain" or a "pain distancing." Many patients have said: "I still have the pain, but it no longer hurts" or "I still have the pain, but it is far away." In addition, thymoleptics and neuroleptics are able to interrupt or prevent the vicious circle: pain→anxiety→depression→pain and so on. In states of anxiety and depression, which often accompany cancer pain, the probability of an interruption or prevention of this vicious circle is greater with a combination therapy than with thymoleptics or neuroleptics alone.

REFERENCES

1. Adjan, M. (1970): Zur therapeutischen Beeinflussung des Schmerzsymptoms bei unheilbaren Tumorkranken. *Ther. Gegenw.*, 109:1620–1627.
2. Barjou, B. (1971): Étude du Tofranil sur les douleurs en chirurgia. *Revue med. Tours,* 6:473–482.
3. Bernard, P., and Scheurer, H. (1972): Action de la Chlorimipramine (Anafranil) sur la douleur des cancers en pathologie cervicofaciale. *ORL,* 21:723–729.
4. Bloomfield, S., Simard-Savoie, S., Bernier, J., and Tetrault, L. (1964): Comparative analgesic activity of leavomepromazine and morphine in patients with chronic pain. *Can. Med. Assoc. J.*, 90:1156–1159.
5. Daxelmüller, L. (1966): Zur Therapie schwerer Schmerzzustande mit Tofranil. *Med. Welt.*, 43:2339–2340.
6. Deutschmann, W. (1971): Tofranil in der Schmerzbehandlung bei Krebskranken. *Med. Welt.*, 22:1346–1347.
7. Gebhardt, K. H., Beller, J., and Nischk, R. (1969): Behandlung des Karzinomschmerzes mit Chlorimipramin (Anafranil). *Med. Klin.*, 64:751–756.
8. Kocher, R. (1976): Use of psychotropic drugs for the treatment of chronic severe pain. In: *Advances in Pain Research and Therapy, Vol. 1: Proceedings of the First World Congress on Pain,* edited by J. J. Bonica and D. Albe-Fessard, pp. 579–582. Raven Press, New York.
9. Mönkemeier, D., and Steffen, U. (1970): Zur Behandlung von Schmerz mit Imipramin bei Krebserkrankungen. *Med. Klin.*, 65:213–215.
10. Put, I. R. (1974): Traitment des douleurs rebelles a l'aide du flupenthixol et du melitracene. *Ars. Medici,* 29:1401–1413.

Advances in Pain Research and Therapy, Vol. 2,
edited by J. J. Bonica and V. Ventafridda.
Raven Press, New York © 1979.

The Brompton Cocktail

Robert G. Twycross

The Churchill Hospital, Headington, Oxford, England

INTRODUCTION

For many centuries opium has held a unique place in the physician's armoury on account of its ability to relieve severe pain without undue sedation. With the extraction and purification of opium alkaloids in the 19th century, morphine was increasingly substituted for opium. In 1896, Snow, a surgeon at the Cancer Hospital (now the Royal Marsden Hospital, London), reported the combined use of morphine and cocaine in advanced cancer, though subsequently he stopped adding cocaine because of the cost (6,7). Some 30 years later, however, it was re-introduced by Roberts, a surgeon at the Brompton Hospital, who used a morphine-cocaine elixir as a post-thoracotomy analgesic (2). At other hospitals, similar elixirs were used in advanced malignant or terminal respiratory disease. These were known by a variety of names, such as *Mistura pro moribundo, Mistura pro euthanasia,* and *Mistura euphoriens*. It was not until 1952, when the Brompton Hospital produced its own supplement to the National Formulary, that the composition of a morphine-cocaine elixir appeared in print; in this supplement it was called *Haustus E* and contained:

Morphine hydrochloride	¼ grain	(15 mg)
Cocaine hydrochloride	⅙ grain	(10 mg)
Alcohol 90%	30 minims	(2 ml)
Syrup	60 minims	(4 ml)
Chloroform water to	½ fl. oz.	(15 ml)

This was a modification of the pre-war Brompton formulation which contained gin and honey instead of alcohol and syrup. It appeared subsequently in Martindale's *Extra Pharmacopoeia* (4) together with three variant formulations. In recent years, diamorphine (diacetylylmorphine, heroin) has commonly been used instead of morphine as the analgesic component in such elixirs, now generally known as the *Brompton Cocktail.* The correct method of use is summarized in Table 1.

There is, however, a tendency to endow the Brompton Cocktail with almost mystical properties and to regard it as the panacea for terminal cancer

TABLE 1. *Use of the Brompton Cocktail in cancer pain compared with the use of injected morphine for acute severe pain*

	Brompton cocktail (cancer pain)	Injected morphine (acute pain)
Aim	Pain-relief	Pain-relief
Sedation	Usually undesirable	Often desirable
Desired duration of effect	As long as possible	2–4 hr
Timing	Every 4 hr regularly (in anticipation)	Every 2–6 hr as required (on demand)
Dose	Individually determined (5–100 mg)	Usually standard (10 mg)
Route	By mouth	Injection
Adjuvant medication	Common	Uncommon

pain. Experience at St. Christopher's Hospice, London, and similar units specializing in symptom control in far-advanced cancer, while testifying to the cocktail's general usefulness, emphasizes that to obtain the best results, the cocktail must be used within a comprehensive pattern of total patient care (5,10).

It does, however, contain four substances all of which have a side-effect potential and which, on occasion, have led to noncompliance by the patient and continued unrelieved pain. In view of this, it is necessary to examine in the light of present knowledge and experience whether such a mixture is a prerequisite of success or whether a simple solution of morphine or diamorphine would be equally effective.

DIAMORPHINE OR MORPHINE

A randomized, controlled trial of orally administered diamorphine and morphine when given every 4 hr in individually optimized doses to advanced cancer patients has recently been completed at St. Christopher's Hospice, London (9). The primary aim was to compare the incidence and severity of the side-effects of the two preparations when prescribed at the effective analgesic dose for each patient (Fig. 1). Patients, stratified for sex, were randomly allocated to receive either diamorphine or morphine by mouth as first treatment. All the patients received a phenothiazine; other medication was prescribed when indicated clinically. There were 699 patients, of median age 67 years, who entered the trial, of whom 146 were well enough to cross over. Of these, 89 remained on an unchanged dose of "diamorphine equivalent" and did not have their adjuvant medication modified during the 5-day period

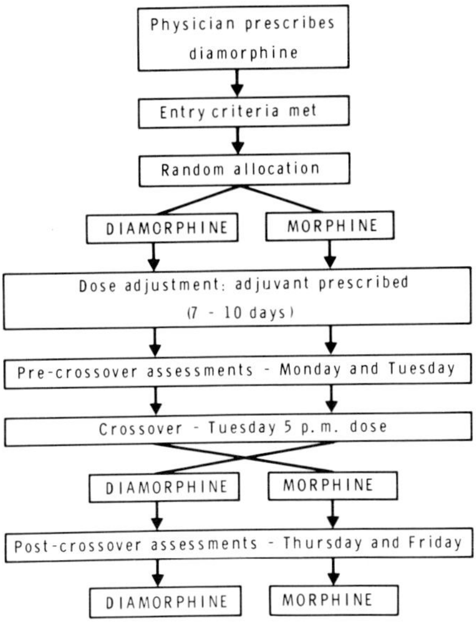

FIG. 1. Flow diagram describing method of diamorphine/morphine trial.

of observation. A potency ratio for orally administered diamorphine and morphine of 1.5:1 was assumed on the basis of a pilot trial.

In the 51 satisfactory female crossover patients, no statistically significant difference was noted in relation either to pain or the other symptoms evaluated. On the other hand, 38 satisfactory male crossover patients experienced significantly more pain and were significantly more depressed, while receiving diamorphine. In these, the potency ratio of diamorphine to morphine appeared to be less than 1.5:1. If this is allowed for, then the difference in mood is probably not significant. The patients who did not cross over appeared to do equally well on either opiate (Fig. 2).

It was concluded that, provided allowance is made for the potency difference between the two opiates, diamorphine and morphine are equally efficacious when given in a solution *by mouth* every 4 hr in individually optimized doses with a fixed dose of cocaine hydrochloride (10 mg) and in association with a phenothiazine such as prochlorperazine or chlorpromazine. (The oral/parenteral potency ratio of morphine when used in *solution* in this way appears to be of the order of 1:3, though this has not been tested formally.)

In a parallel study of urinary excretion of morphine in patients receiving diamorphine or morphine regularly, the results indicated that diamorphine is completely absorbed by the gastrointestinal tract but that morphine is only some two-thirds absorbed (11). This suggests that the potency ratio of orally administered diamorphine and morphine merely reflects the alimentary absorption ratio of the two preparations. This accords with the view of Way and his associates (13,14), based largely on studies using organ homogenates

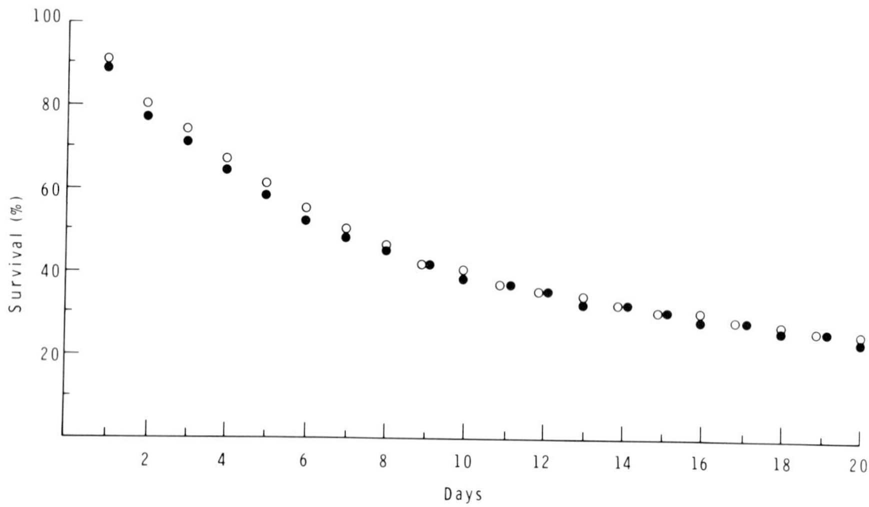

FIG. 2. Survival chart for 350 diamorphine-receiving patients (open circles) and 349 morphine-receiving patients (filled circles).

from both animals and man, that diamorphine is so rapidly deacetylated *in vivo* to O^6-monoacetylmorphine and morphine that it has only a transient pharmacological action of its own even after intravenous injection, its effects being almost entirely mediated via its two biotransformation products.

COCAINE

Cocaine was first used with morphine by Snow at the end of the last century on the grounds that it helped "sustain vitality" (6). More recently it has been claimed that the addition of cocaine enhances the mood of the patient: "The euphoria renders the patient comparatively cheerful, and relieves his mental and physical distress" (3). On the other hand it has been reported that the longer an opiate-cocaine elixir is administered, the greater is the likelihood that the patient will become depressed (12).

In order to clarify matters a randomized, controlled trial of morphine and diamorphine elixirs with and without cocaine was undertaken, again at St. Christopher's Hospice (8). After stabilization on an individually determined 4-hourly regimen only 61 out of 400 patients were well enough to cross over. Surprisingly, it was found that although introducing cocaine (10 mg/dose) resulted in a small, statistically significant increase in alertness, stopping cocaine had no detectable effect. Although debatable, it was considered that these findings could be explained if, in this dose, cocaine was of borderline efficacy and that tolerance to this borderline effect occurred within a few days. That tolerance does not always readily occur, however, is indicated by the occasional phenomenon—not seen in this trial—of the patient who becomes restless, agitated, confused, or hallucinated when prescribed cocaine and whose symptoms abate only when cocaine is withdrawn.

As a result of the trial, cocaine is no longer used routinely at St. Christopher's Hospice or at Sir Michael Sobell House. Cocaine is added only if a patient remains drowsy after 3 or 4 days on a steady dose of morphine. Even then my policy is to give a test dose of dexamphetamine or methylphenidate in order to help determine whether the addition of cocaine is likely to be of benefit. I have, in fact, used cerebral stimulants in only 2 patients out of some 200 during the past year. It is a matter of regret, therefore, that the current British National Formulary includes both morphine- and diamorphine-cocaine elixirs, since inclusion lends official blessing to the efficacy of such combinations. More regrettable is the inclusion of variant mixtures containing chlorpromazine. I would suggest that, given their respective doses, any stimulant action of cocaine will be antagonized by the chlorpromazine.

It should be mentioned that, by and large, it is standard practice in those British hospices where cocaine is still administered with diamorphine or morphine to use a standard 10 mg of cocaine hydrochloride. Occasional prescribers of the Brompton Cocktail not infrequently use a higher dose of cocaine and, moreover, commonly vary the dose of the opiate by varying the volume rather than the strength of the mixture. This means the dose of cocaine is increased in parallel with that of the opiate. This is true of its use in a number of American centers. It is perhaps not surprising that, at one center known to the author, hallucinations are so common a concomitant of the use of the Brompton Cocktail, that patients are warned to expect them and are taught to accept them as the necessary price to pay for pain-relief.

FORMULATION

In 1972, a survey of more than 90 teaching and district general hospitals throughout the United Kingdom confirmed that such elixirs were still in widespread use and also demonstrated considerable variation in composition (Twycross, *unpublished observations*). Differences existed both in the active constituents and in the vehicle in which they were dissolved. In addition to morphine or diamorphine, the majority included cocaine. A number also contained a phenothiazine (chlorpromazine or prochlorperazine) and, in some, morphine and diamorphine were both included. The variation in the vehicle was even greater; for example, the alcohol content ranged from 0 to 40% and was frequently replaced by gin, whisky, or brandy. The syrup content varied from 0 to 50% and honey was often substituted for sucrose. In the light of this, the introduction of standard diamorphine- and morphine-cocaine elixirs is welcome (11). Even with these, however, some patients complain about the "sickliness" of such mixtures, while other dislike the alcoholic "bite." As a result it is now my practice to dispense morphine in water alone, the patient adding blackcurrant juice or other flavoring as desired. If dispensed in combination with prochlorperazine or chlorpromazine, the incorporation of one of the flavored proprietary syrups usually circumvents the need for additional flavoring.

SIDE EFFECTS

Most patients with terminal cancer have more than one symptom. Nausea and vomiting are both common, and the use of a narcotic analgesic tends to precipitate or exacerbate these symptoms, particularly if the patient is ambulant. Patients prescribed the Brompton Cocktail should be questioned about nausea and vomiting and either have an antiemetic prescribed simultaneously or the need for such reviewed 2 or 3 days later. A patient will not continue to take an analgesic if it results in nausea or vomiting. At St. Christopher's Hospice a phenothiazine (generally prochlorperazine) is prescribed routinely. It acts not only as an antiemetic but also supplements the sedative effect of the narcotic analgesic. This is often replaced by chlorpromazine or, occasionally, methotrimeprazine in patients with an appreciable psychological component to their pain—for example, the patient with lung cancer experiencing both pain and dyspnea and who fears death by suffocation, or the woman who feels that her fungating breast cancer is jeopardizing her relationship with her husband. Chlorpromazine or promazine are also used to control confusion, delirium, or psychotic manifestations. Because many patients are both elderly and debilitated, it is wise to prescribe not more than 12.5 mg of chlorpromazine initially, to be administered every 4 hr with the (dia)morphine.

Some patients require an additional antiemetic such as cyclizine or metoclopramide. Constipation often occurs and requires an appropriate regimen of diet, laxatives, suppositories, and/or enemas.

A quarter of the patients at St. Christopher's Hospice are also prescribed either a tricyclic antidepressant or a benzodiazepine tranquilizer. Generally speaking, the latter are used for short periods to help patients at times of severe anxiety, whereas the former are used for longer periods if the patient becomes depressed. This occurs more frequently in patients who have a prolonged terminal phase.

Physicians not used to prescribing oral (dia)morphine are often concerned about the possibility of drowsiness. In fact, no study to determine whether there is a relationship between dose administered and drowsiness has yet been reported. In practice, it is generally found that the initial drowsiness experienced by some patients when prescribed (dia)morphine and a phenothiazine diminishes after a day or two. Persistent drowsiness is unusual and is possibly related more to advanced physical debility than to (dia)morphine itself.

As stated above, persistent drowsiness unrelated to debility is so infrequent that the author has prescribed a cerebral stimulant in only 1% of patients prescribed oral morphine during the past year. Inactivity or boredom drowsiness does persist in the majority of patients, but this does not prevent normal activity. In fact, the ability of many patients to "cat nap" when alone or resting is generally seen as an advantage in that it helps to pass the time during what often seems a long 16 hr between getting up in the morning and retiring to bed at night.

CONCLUSIONS

The Brompton Cocktail is, therefore, merely a traditional way of prescribing oral (dia)morphine. It is not the panacea nor does it possess magical properties. The results are best when the cocktail is used within the context of general emotional support for the patient and his family (5). Attention to the several other symptoms the patient is likely to be suffering from is also important. In practice a combination of drug, nondrug, and common-sense measures are necessary to achieve maximum benefit (10).

Although the median 4-hourly dose of oral diamorphine is 10 mg (Fig. 3) and that of morphine 15 to 20 mg, *the effective analgesic doses of both range from as little as 2.5 mg to more than 100 mg*. It is important not to transfer the concept of a "maximum dose" from acute parenteral use to the relatively long-term *oral* use in patients with advanced cancer. Not only does

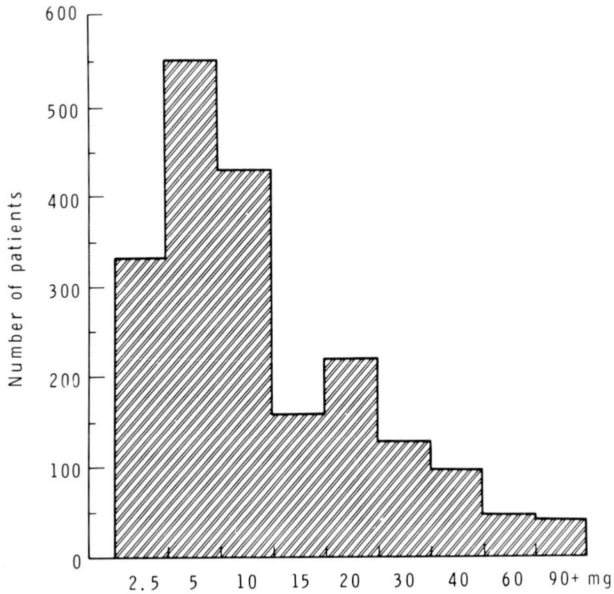

FIG. 3. Histogram of maximum 4-hr doses of diamorphine given to 2,000 patients admitted to St. Christopher's Hospice, 1972–1975 inclusive.

the effective dose vary considerably, but problems associated with continuous parenteral use, such as tolerance, are minimal (12).

Whether or not a physician prescribes the Brompton Cocktail or, simply, morphine in tap water will probably depend on personal inclination. Provided, however, the physician appreciates that each of the four constituents has a side-effect potential and enquires of his patients about untoward effects, including unpleasant taste and a burning sensation in the throat, there is no reason for his not continuing to use the cocktail. On the other hand, he should be aware that it is simpler for the pharmacist, cheaper for the patient, and easier for the physician to manipulate opiate doses if a simple solution of morphine hydrochloride or sulphate is used.

SUMMARY

The use of the Brompton Cocktail, an opiate-cocaine elixir, for the relief of pain in far-advanced cancer is recorded. Results from a comparative trial of diamorphine (diacetylmorphine, heroin) and morphine are summarized. These indicate that, by mouth, both opiates are equally efficacious, though diamorphine is about 1.5 times more potent than morphine. The value of cocaine is questioned, as is the automatic inclusion of alcohol and syrup. The place of antiemetics, laxatives, and other adjuvant medication is discussed. It is emphasized that the Brompton Cocktail is no more than a traditional British way of administering oral morphine to cancer patients in pain. Moreover, if prescribed, it should be used within the context of a comprehensive pattern of patient care, and as one prong of a broad-spectrum approach to the relief of pain.

ACKNOWLEDGMENT

I thank Dr. Cicely Saunders, Medical Director, St. Christopher's Hospice, London, for her continued encouragement and support. The studies reported were carried out at St. Christopher's on patients under her care between 1971 and 1976.

ADDENDUM

Pain-Relief in Advanced Cancer—General Principles

Aim: To keep the patient both free of pain and fully alert.

Assessment

1. *Treatment* varies according to the cause of the pain; use *body chart* to record sites of pain and their probable mechanism.

2. Because a person has cancer, it does not mean that the malignant process is necessarily the cause of the pain.

Choice of Analgesics

1. Establish a simple, practical *analgesic "league table"*
   a. *Non-narcotic*—aspirin (alt. acetominophen)
   b. *Weak narcotic*—codeine (alt. DHC, *d*-propoxyphene)
   c. *Strong narcotic*—morphine (alt. papaveretum, diamorphine)
2. *Avoid* pentazocine, meperidine, and dextromoramide (Palfium®).
3. *Methadone* should be used with caution, particularly in the elderly and debilitated.
4. The use of a narcotic analgesic is dictated by intensity of pain and not by brevity of prognosis.
   "Morphine exists to be given, not merely to be withheld."

Use of Analgesics

1. *Oral medication* is normally possible. When injections are necessary, use freeze-dried ampoules of diamorphine.
2. *Persistent pain requires preventive therapy*. This means that analgesics should be given regularly and prophylactically: "as required" medication is both irrational and inhumane.
3. Doses should be determined on an *individual basis;* the right dose is that which gives relief for at least 3, preferably 4 or more hr.
4. Adjuvant medication is the rule rather than the exception. *Laxatives* are almost always necessary, an *antiemetic* commonly so.
5. If very anxious, an *anxiolytic* such as diazepam should be tried; if depressed, an *antidepressive*.
6. The perception of pain requires both attention and consciousness. *Diversional therapy*—people to talk to, activities to attend, etc.—is of great value.
7. *Tolerance* is not usually a practical problem.
8. Rightly used, *psychological dependence* (addiction) does not occur.
9. *Physical dependence* does not prevent the downward adjustment of the dose of a narcotic analgesic should the pain ameliorate.
10. Neither diamorphine nor morphine is the panacea for terminal pain. Their use does not guarantee automatic success, particularly if the psychological component of pain is ignored.

Reassessment

1. *Relief of pain* should be assessed in relation to comfort achieved
   a. during the night,
   b. in the daytime at rest,
   c. on movement.
2. Reassessment remains a continuing necessity; old pains may get worse and new ones may develop.

REVIEW. REVIEW. REVIEW. REVIEW. REVIEW.

REFERENCES

1. British Pharmaceutical Codex (1973): Pharmaceutical Press, London. p. 669.
2. Kerrane, T. A. (1975): The Brompton Cocktail. *Nursing Mirror,* 140:59.
3. Love, M. (1962): Management of advanced cancer. *Br. Med. J.,* 2, 1192.
4. Martindale (1958): *Extra Pharmacopoeia* (24th ed.), p. 911. Pharmaceutical Press, London.
5. Melzack, R., Ofiesh, J. G., and Mount, B. M. (1976): The Brompton mixture: Effects on pain in cancer patients. *Can. Med. Assoc. J.,* 115:125–129.
6. Snow, H. (1896): Opium and cocaine in the treatment of cancerous disease. *Br. Med. J.,* 2:718–719.
7. Snow, H. (1897): The opium-cocaine treatment of malignant disease. *Br. Med. J.,* 1:1019–1020.
8. Twycross, R. G. (1976): *Studies on the Use of Diamorphine in Advanced Malignant Disease.* D. M. Thesis, University of Oxford.
9. Twycross, R. G. (1977): Choice of strong analgesic in terminal cancer: Diamorphine or morphine? *Pain,* 3:93–104.
10. Twycross, R. G. (1978): Bone pain in advanced cancer. *Topics in Therapeutics 4,* edited by D. W. Vere, pp. 94–110. Pitman Medical, Tunbridge Wells.
11. Twycross, R. G., Fry, D. E., and Wills, P. D. (1974): The alimentary absorption of diamorphine and morphine in man as indicated by urinary excretion studies. *Br. J. Clin. Pharmacol.,* 1:491–494.
12. Twycross, R. G., and Wald, S. J. (1976): Long-term use of diamorphine in advanced cancer. *Advances in Pain Research and Therapy, Vol. 1: Proceedings of the First World Congress on Pain,* edited by J. J. Bonica and D. Albe-Fessard, pp. 653–661. Raven Press, New York.
13. Way, E. L., Kemp, J. W., Young, J. M., and Grassetti, D. R. (1960): The pharmacologic effects of heroin in relationship to its rate of biotransformation. *J. Pharmacol. Exp. Ther.,* 129:144–154.
14. Way, E. L., Young, J. M., and Kemp, J. W. (1965): Metabolism of heroin and its pharmacological implications. *Bull. Narcot.,* 17(1):25–33.

Discussion

Part II. Management of Pain of Advanced Cancer: Systemic Analgesics and Related Drugs

R. Houde and B. R. Fink (Moderators)

Moricca (Rome): Dr. Twycross, can you make a short comment on the use of addictive drugs for the relief of pain in advanced cancer patients for the doctor?

Twycross (Oxford): I don't talk about addictive drugs; it's as alien to me as referring to, let's say, aspirin as a drug which induces deafness.

Hildebrandt (Göttingen): Dr. Kocher, is haloperidol useful as a neuroleptic agent for the treatment of pain?

Kocher (Basel): I think so. At first we began with neuroleptic caevomepromazine (nozinan) and the analgesic effect was better, but we had too many side effects. Now we use haloperidol because you have practically no side effects, and for me, it has the same analgesic effect.

Gerbershagen (Mainz): One should always use these drugs. If you want to have anxiolytics, you would not use that. But if you want to have a sleeping effect, then you would use haloperidol.

Procacci (Florence): Dr. Houde, I have found that atarax has been effective in the treatment of postoperative pain. Has your experience in cancer pain been similar?

Houde (New York): We have not evaluated hydroxyzine in a controlled study, but we do use it clinically, and we have found it to be an effective adjuvant when given along with morphine, generally from 25 to 50 mg.

Iacono (Ragusa): Dr. Twycross, how do you reduce the gastrointestinal effect of analgesics? Which analgesics do you use in patients affected by peptic ulcer?

Twycross: First of all, I tend to give the aspirin with alkali or milk or after food. Most patients seem to be able to tolerate that. In fact, the main reason for stopping aspirin in my ordinary cancer patients has been deafness when I have been using it in doses of 4 g or more a day. But if there is obvious gastric upset, then I may try enteric-coated phenabutizone, which was a favorite; I would tend to use phelebepropane now. What do I do if the patient has a peptic ulcer? So far, I haven't had the combination of a patient with active advanced cancer and active peptic ulcer. Maybe that will happen next week. Until I do, I tend to avoid soluble aspirin if there is a strong history of peptic ulcer, and I tend to use one of these alternatives.

Sapio (Taranto): Dr. Gerbershagen, what is the analgesic effect of cortisone derivatives and the relevant dosage? What is the analgesic effect of local anesthetics by intravenous and relevant dosage?

Gerbershagen: There are many effects of cortisone derivatives. I think the most important effect, besides, of course, the antiproliferative effect, is the antiedema effect. Local anesthetics are mainly used in South America and in some hospitals in Germany, but in South America they are used even for anesthesia in large doses; 1, 2, 3 g of procaine for instance. I think we use it only if there is itching—one type of pain—and then we give i.v. tetracine, about 200 mg in ½ liter of normal saline, and then the itch is usually gone for about a day or two and sometimes it stays away.

Twycross: As regards prednisolone, I agree that we are using it for the antiedema effect and, therefore, perhaps we could list three or four common situations where I find it useful: (a) Headache due to raised intracranial pressure. Often we use dexomethazone, the far more potent corticosteroid, starting at a dosage of 4 mg t.i.d. or q.i.d., and reducing down to about 2 mg t.i.d. subsequently. But sometimes prednisolone is adequate. (b) In patients with head and neck cancer, you get extensive soft-tissue infiltration and secondary edema, and the drug can be remarkable in easing the pain associated with that. (c) For nerve compression pain, it is always worth treating with a combination of morphine and prednisolone initially, perhaps in a dose of 10 mg t.i.d., reducing to 5 mg t.i.d. before you call your anesthetist for a nerve block. (d) The pelvic cancer patient where, again, you have extensive pelvic malignancy with extensive soft-tissue infiltration and secondary edema; and here again, the use of morphine plus prednisolone and often aspirin or other anti-inflammatory drugs together produce very good results when on their own you don't get more than 50/60% relief.

Hildebrandt: Dr. Houde, what do you think of Tiladine®?

Houde: Tiladine is a drug that has narcotic agonist and very weak antagonist properties, like morphine. I realize it is abused quite a bit in Germany. We found it about 1/25 or 1/24 as potent as prophine by injection. It is a little more effective orally, about 1/15 as potent as morphine—not too promising.

Tommasi Morgano (Torino): What do you think of physical and psychological drug dependence from morphine and heroin?

Houde: The question is directed to what the relative physical and psychological dependence potentials are of morphine and heroin. The physical dependence potentials of the drugs are very similar. Whether one has a greater psychological dependence-producing potential than the other is unresolved. The general opinion today is that there is very little to choose between them.

Netti (Conversano): Which measures do you adopt to avoid dependence and tolerance development of narcotic analgesics? How do you evaluate when a patient has developed tolerance when instead there is an insufficient dosage?

Houde: Tolerance development and physical dependence development are dose-related phenomena; we know that. The way of avoiding it is to use drugs in low enough doses or in combinations such that you do not too rapidly escalate the dose. But these are properties of narcotics. They are not important if you adjust your doses. Remember that though patients can gain tolerance and physical dependence, they can also lose it, particularly if you also pay attention to definitive means of treating or removing the cause of pain.

Twycross: When morphine or diamorphine (heroin) is used in an individually determined dosage in association with other treatments, then in those controlled circumstances, associated with attention to other symptoms and emotional support of family and patient, tolerance is not a practical problem. Please get away from all that you have learned from basic pharmacologists and from the addiction center of Lexington. In advanced cancer, tolerance is not a practical problem; physical dependence may occur but doesn't prevent the progressive downward adjustment of dose should the pain ameliorate. A craving for the drug does not occur if the drug is administered prophylactically. (Houde does not agree with all that but will discuss it later.)

Advances in Pain Research and Therapy, Vol. 2,
edited by J. J. Bonica and V. Ventafridda.
Raven Press, New York © 1979.

Introduction to Nerve Blocks

John J. Bonica

Department of Anesthesiology, University of Washington School of Medicine, Seattle, Washington 98195

Nerve blocks, or analgesic block, whereby a local anesthetic or a neurolytic agent is injected near or into a nerve or nerves, have been used to relieve the pain of cancer for over a century (2). Personal experience during the past 35 years and experience reported by many others suggests that, skillfully administered in properly selected patients, nerve blocks are among the most effective methods of relieving cancer pain (1,3,4,5,6,7). On the other hand, improperly applied, these procedures often result in failures and, at times, serious complications. Despite the long use of the procedures, there is still some serious misconception about their role in managing chronic pain in general and cancer pain in particular. The objective of the chapters in this section is to evaluate the efficacy, indications, and advantages, as well as the limitations, disadvantages, and complications of various nerve-block techniques used to relieve cancer pain. I will introduce the discussion by briefly giving a historical perspective, discussing the bases and indications for the application of nerve blocks, emphasizing certain conditions and requisites that must be met in order to obtain optimal results, and giving a brief overview of the various agents and techniques that are used.

HISTORICAL PERSPECTIVE

The first recorded use of analgesic blocks to relieve cancer pain occurred in 1875 when Fauvel (9), Collins, Taglia and others (30) applied cocaine to the larynx in patients with severe cancer pain. This was 9 years before Karl Koller (12) gave the first clinical demonstration of the local anesthetic properties of cocaine for eye surgery, an event considered to be a milestone in the history of anesthesia, because it ushered in the widespread use of local and regional anesthesia for surgery. In 1894, Corning (7), an American neurologist, wrote what was probably the first book devoted to the use of regional analgesia for the relief of pain. In this little-known monograph Corning mentioned the use of cocaine injection into the subarachnoid space and near nerves to relieve neuralgia and other forms of chronic pain including cancer pain. However, the widespread use of nerve blocks for definitive control of cancer pain did not really begin until sometime after 1900, when Schlosser (26) began experimenting with the injection of alcohol near and into nerves for the treatment of neuralgia with particular emphasis on trigeminal neuralgia. The numerous reports of the successful use of alcohol block for trigeminal neuralgia prompted other clinicians to use it for the relief of cancer pain (11,13,20). Similarly, the report of Lewy (14) in 1911, in which he described the successful use of alcohol block of the superior laryngeal nerve to relieve the pain of tuberculosis, led Lukens (16) and, subsequently, Swetlow (29) to apply this technique for the relief of cancer pain.

Another technique which was developed right after the turn of the century was paravertebral block, which entails the injection of spinal nerves as they emerge from the intervertebral foramen (2). Although this technique was first used in surgical anesthesia, it soon became applied as a diagnostic tool to ascertain visceral pain pathways and, subsequently, it was used for the therapy of severe intractable pain. In 1926, Mandl (18) reported the successful use of paravertebral block with procaine to relieve severe pain of cancer of the pancreas. In the same year, Swetlow (29) reported the use of paravertebral alcohol block for a variety of painful conditions including the pain of cancer.

One of the most important events in the history of analgesic block for the relief of cancer pain is the report by Dogliotti (8) in 1931, describing the successful use of the injection of alcohol into the subarachnoid space to achieve chemical rhizotomy. This technique was promptly used widely, and in the ensuing decade, dozens of reports were published attesting to the efficacy of the procedure in relieving cancer pain (10,22,24,25). Five years later, Putnam and Hampton (23) published the first report on the use of aqueous phenol as a neurolytic agent for gasserian ganglion block. About a decade later, phenol was used by Mandl (18a) and others to achieve chemical sympathectomy.

The report by Maher (17) in 1955, in which he described the injection of hyperbaric phenol into the subarachnoid space to produce chemical rhizotomy for the relief of cancer pain must be considered another milestone in the history of the use of nerve block for this purpose. This report had the same type of impact as the report by Dogliotti about alcohol. Consequently, many, many reports have been published attesting to the efficacy of this technique (15,19,21,27,28,31). Since the history of subarachnoid neurolysis will be discussed in detail by Dr. Swerdlow and Professor Papo and others in this volume, I will make no further comments. A detailed discussion of the use of nerve blocks for cancer therapy can be found elsewhere (2,3,6,32).

BASES AND INDICATIONS

The basis for the efficacy and utility of nerve blocks to relieve cancer pain is the interruption of specific sensory, and particularly nociceptive or pain pathways and, in certain circumstances, block of the sympathetic nerves. Sensory block relieves pain and interrupts the afferent limb of any abnormal reflex mechanisms that may be contributing to the physiopathology of the pain and associated phenomena. By using low concentrations of local anesthetics, it is possible to block the small, myelinated A-delta fibers and the unmyelinated C-fibers, some of which are involved in nociception, without significant impairment of motor function. As will be discussed by Professor Gerbershagen, in many instances, block with local anesthetics produces pain-relief which outlasts the pharmacologic action of the drug by hours, days, and sometimes weeks. The exact mechanism for this almost enigmatic phenomenon is not definitely known. It has been suggested that the block of sensory input for several hours brings about a cessation of the self-sustaining activity of the neuron pools in the neuraxis which are considered to be responsible for some chronic pain states (5). Alcohol and phenol produce prolonged pain-relief by destruction of nociceptive pathways. These procedures may be used as diagnostic and prognostic tools, as well as for the definitive therapy of pain.

DIAGNOSTIC BLOCKS

Properly applied and skillfully executed, nerve blocks may be used effectively as diagnostic tools to: (a) help to ascertain the specific nociceptive or pain pathways; (b) help to define the mechanisms of the cancer pain; and (c) aid in differential diagnosis of the site of the pain. For example, nerve blocks help to define the nociceptive pathways in patients with pain in the angle of the jaw, which can be caused by involvement either of the trigeminal nerve or the glossopharyngeal and vagal nerves. Moreover, nerve blocks are useful to differentiate pain due to involvement of viscera from the pain of somatic origin. Examples are patients complaining of chest pain, epigastric pain, or suprapubic pain. Block of those intercostal nerves which supply the area of the chest wall where pain is felt will completely relieve pain due to somatic tissue or chest wall involvement by the cancer, but will have little or no effect on pain from the thoracic viscera. Similarly, pain in the suprapubic region which is relieved by block of the lower two thoracic and first and second lumbar spinal nerves suggests that its cause is in the abdominal wall rather than its being a referred pain from pelvic viscera, which are supplied by the middle three sacral segments.

Prognostic Blocks

Prognostic blocks are useful to predict the effects resulting from prolonged interruption, either by injection of a neurolytic agent or by neurosurgical operation. Moreover, prognostic blocks afford the patient an opportunity to experience the numbness and other side effects that follow surgical section on neurolytic block and thus help the patient decide whether or not to have the procedure.

Therapeutic Blocks

Therapeutic blocks can be achieved with either a local anesthetic or a neurolytic agent. Local anesthetic blocks are very useful in the temporary relief of very severe pain due to cancer in the chest, abdomen, pelvis, and lower limbs. Although various techniques may be used for this purpose, continuous segmental epidural block permits the repeated injection of local anesthetics at intervals to produce continuous pain-relief. In addition to blocking the nociceptive pathways, the local anesthetic eliminates reflex muscle spasm and reflex sympathetic mechanisms which may be acting as positive feedback mechanisms to contribute to the nociceptive input. Thus, for example, in patients with cancer of the pancreas, continuous epidural block limited to the fifth to tenth thoracic segments will provide complete relief of pain which can be continued for several days and as long as a week. As will be emphasized by Professor Gerbershagen, repeated single injection with long-lasting local anesthetics may also prove effective in producing prolonged pain-relief in many patients with cancer.

Neurolytic blocks achieved by the injection of alcohol or phenol involve the intentional destruction of the nerve or nerves for a period of time to produce prolonged pain-relief. If the neurolytic agent is injected into the subarachnoid space, it should, theoretically, destroy the nociceptive fibers in the dorsal root proximal to the spinal ganglion and thus produce permanent interruption of some or all of the affected axons and thus simulate surgical rhizotomy. Similarly, injection of alcohol into the gasserian ganglion should destroy many or all of the nerve cell bodies and, consequently, produce permanent interruption. The efficacy and duration of analgesia are dependent on the completeness of the destruction of the nerve roots or ganglion cells by the neurolytic agent. It deserves reemphasis that neurolytic blocks should be limited to control of pain due to inoperable or recurrent cancer.

GENERAL CONSIDERATIONS

Skillfully administered in properly selected patients, nerve blocks are among the most effective methods of relieving cancer pain. These procedures are especially indicated in patients with moderate to severe pain of advanced cancer whose physical and emotional conditions place them at risk and may contraindicate neurosurgery and whose life-expectancy is less than 6 months. In contrast to narcotics and other systemic drugs, nerve blocks usually produce complete relief of pain without the side effects of systemic drugs. Nerve blocks do not tax the physiologic and emotional resources of the patient to the same extent as neurosurgery. Moreover, since they require short hospitalization, they impose less financial strain on the patient and family. By relieving the pain, they facilitate improved nutrition and enhance the physical and emotional condition of the patient to permit radiation therapy or other oncologic treatments and even neurosurgery. Since the nerves to any part of the body can be blocked, nerve blocks are applicable to relieve the pain of virtually any type of cancer.

REQUISITES FOR OPTIMAL RESULTS

To obtain optimal results for nerve blocks it is essential to adhere to certain basic principles which I originally developed a quarter-century ago and whose importance I have repeatedly emphasized since then (1,4,5). The first is that the physician using this method must be willing to devote the necessary time to evaluate the patient thoroughly. Experience has shown that this is essential even if the patient has already been evaluated by a highly competent colleague. A detailed history and thorough physical examination not only provide additional information but also afford the opportunity for the physician to become acquainted with the patient, to investigate his or her personality, and most important to establish rapport and win the confidence of the patient. A careful neurologic examination not only provides useful information, but will constitute a base line in evaluating the effects of the block. It is also essential to determine the presence of cardiovascular or vesical dysfunctions prior to initiating the procedure.

Another requisite is that the physician must be highly skilled in carrying out the most appropriate nerve block procedure and know thoroughly the immediate and long-term effects. Patients with cancer pain are not good subjects on whom to practice nerve blocks. The skill should be acquired in the application of nerve blocks for surgical anesthesia and in patients with nonmalignant chronic pain. Moreover, nerve blocks must be performed carefully, with meticulous attention to anatomic detail and with utmost gentleness.

In order to select the best nerve block procedure in each particular case it is essential that the physician know well the distribution of the pain, its etiology and mechanisms, the nociceptive pathways involved, the type of neoplasm, its grade of differentiation and possible extension, and the structures it might invade, and all of the other issues I mentioned in my introductory remarks to the management of the problem (pp. 115–130).

An obviously important requisite is to prepare the patient carefully for the procedure. This includes informing the patient and his family of what is going to be done, how it will be done, and what is to be accomplished with the procedure. If the patient and family do not realize beforehand that the diagnostic or prognostic block is only to gain information and will provide only temporary relief, he or she may be disappointed prematurely and become bitter. Moreover, the patient and the family must be made to realize that since the intractable pain of cancer is a difficult problem to manage and complete relief is not always obtained in the first treatment, it may be necessary to do several blocks. If this is explained beforehand, the patient is much less likely to become discouraged before treatment is completed. In addition, it is important to inform the patient and his family, and even the referring physician, of the possible complications because, although these patients often express a desire for relief at almost any price before the procedure, they may become bitter if urinary disturbances or rectal incontinence occur or the extremities become weakened or paralyzed as a result of the block. When the patient is cognizant of the true status of the disease, he or she should be made to understand clearly that the nerve block procedure itself is palliative and not curative. Finally, the patient should receive pharmacologic preparation for the block procedures in the form of sedatives/analgesics.

If the block procedures are to be done for diagnostic or prognostic purposes prior to permanent interruption, it is essential to localize exactly and precisely the involved nerve or nerves. This can be accomplished by eliciting paresthesia, by checking the position of the needle with X-ray with or without prior injection of a contrast medium, or by the use of a nerve stimulator. Moreover, in using diagnostic or prognostic blocks, three essential principles must be adhered to: (a) The injection should entail only small amounts of local anesthetic solution to avoid diffusion to adjacent segments and thus preclude misleading information; (b) no decision should be made until two or three blocks produce consistent responses; and (c) it is best to use local anesthetics of different duration for each of the procedures so that the duration of block can be correlated with the duration of subjective pain-relief.

During and following the block it is essential to assess carefully the results. Observation of the reaction of the patient to the insertion of small needles, the formation of intracutaneous wheals and other parts of the procedure help in evaluating the patient's reactions to noxious stimuli. Following the block, it is essential to ascertain whether the appropriate nociceptive pathways have been interrupted by repeating the neurologic examination.

Once it is established that the procedure has interrupted the intended nociceptive pathways, the effects of the procedure in relieving the pain must be carefully assessed. This usually requires observation for from a few hours to several days or weeks. The amount, type, and duration of relief obtained should be carefully noted and recorded on the patient's chart. In addition to observation by the physician, the results should be evaluated by the patient and his or her family, if they are available, and, most importantly, by the nursing staff.

It is important that all concerned fully appreciate the fact that nerve blocks have certain limitations and should be integrated with other therapeutic measures. It deserves reemphasis that the pain of cancer not only involves nociceptive input, but the emotional, psychologic, and affective responses thereto. While nerve blocks and neurosurgical operation may eliminate the nociceptive input, they do nothing for the other aspects of the cancer pain and, therefore, other therapeutic modalities need to be used.

Finally, it is also essential that the patient and the physicians realize two important disadvantages of these techniques: (a) pain-relief may be incomplete or, if it is complete, may not last until the patient's death. Fortunately, since the block can be extended or repeated several times, these are only minor disadvantages. (b) More importantly, side effects and serious complications can occur during or after the block. The most important of these are orthostatic hypotension from extensive sympathetic interruption, paresthesia and dysesthesia, limb-muscle weakness or dysfunction of vesical or rectal sphincter, or a combination of these. It is the responsibility of the administrator to carry out all prophylactic measures against these undesirable side effects and complications.

REFERENCES

1. Bonica, J. J. (1952): Management of intractable pain with analgesic blocks. *JAMA*, 150:1581–1586.
2. Bonica, J. J. (1953): *The Management of Pain*. Lea & Febiger, Philadelphia.
3. Bonica, J. J. (1954): The management of cancer pain. *GP (American Academy of General Practice)*, 10:34–43.
4. Bonica, J. J. (1955): Teaching residents diagnostic and therapeutic nerve blocks. *Anesth. Analg.*, 34:202–213.
5. Bonica, J. J. (1974): Current role of nerve blocks in diagnosis and therapy of pain. In: *Advances in Neurology, Vol. 4: International Symposium on Pain,* edited by J. J. Bonica, pp. 433–453. Raven Press, New York.
6. Bonica, J. J. (1954): The management of pain of malignant disease with nerve blocks. *Anesthesiology*, 15:(March) 134 and (May) 280–301.
7. Corning, J. L. (1894): *Pain in Its Neuropathologic, Diagnostic and Neurotherapeutic Relations*. J. B. Lippincott, Philadelphia.
8. Dogliotti, A. M. (1931): Traitment des syndromes douloureux de la peripherie par l'alcoholisation sub-arachnoidienne. *Presse Med.*, 67:11.
9. Fauvel, H. (1884): De l'anesthesie produite par le chlorhydrate de cocaine sur la muquese pharyngienne et laryngienne. *Gas des hop., Nr.*, 134, S. 1067.
10. Greenhill, J. P. (1935): Intraspinal (subarachnoid) injection of alcohol for pain associated with malignant conditions of the female genitalia. *JAMA*, 105:406.
11. Hartel, F. (1914): Über die intracranielle injections behandlung der trigeminus neuralgie mit intrakraniellen alkoholeinspritzungen. *Deutsche. Ztschr. f. Chir.*, 126:429.
12. Koller, C. (1884): Vorläufige Mittheilung über local Anästhesirung am Aug. *Klin. Monatsb. f. Augenh.*, 22, Beilagenheft, p. 60.
13. Levy, F., and Baudouin, A. (1906): Les injections profondes dans le traitment de la neuralgia facial rebelle. *Presse Med.*, 13:108.
14. Lewy, A. P. (1911): Analgesia of the larynx by alcohol injection of the internal branch of the superior laryngeal nerve. *Laryngoscope*, 21:9.
15. Lifschitz, S., Debacker, L. J., and Buchsbaum, H. J. (1976): Subarachnoid phenol block for pain relief in gynecologic malignancy. *Obstet. Gynecol.*, 48:316–320.
16. Lukens, R. McD. (1918): Dysphagia in tuberculous laryngitis. *N.Y. State J. Med.*, 107:353.
17. Maher, R. M. (1955): Relief of pain in incurable cancer. *Lancet*, 1:18–20.
18. Mandl, F. (1925): Die anwendungsbreite der paravertebralen injektion. *Klin. Schnschr.*, 4:49.
18a. Mandl, F. (1950): Phenol as a substitute for alcohol in sympathetic block. *J. Int. Coll. Surg.*, 13:566–568.
19. Nathan, P. W. (1972): Pain in cancer: Comparison of results of cordotomy and

chemical rhizotomy. In: *Present Limits of Neurosurgery,* edited by I. Fusek and Z. Kung, pp. 513–516. Excerpta Medica, Amsterdam.
20. Ostwald, F. (1905): Traitment des neuralgies rebelles par les injections profondes d'alcohol. *Presse Med.,* 12:812.
21. Papo, I., and Visca, A. (1974): Phenol rhizotomy in the treatment of cancer pain. *Anesth. Analg.,* 53:993–997.
22. Poppen, J. L. (1936): Subarachnoid alcohol injection: Indication, contraindications, technique and results in 82 patients. *Surg. Clin. North Am.,* 16:1663.
23. Putnam, T. J., and Hampton, A. O. (1936): A technique of injection into the Gasserian ganglion under roentgenographic control. *Arch. Neurol. Psychiatry,* (Chicago), 35:92–98.
24. Russell, W. R. (1937): *Intraspinal Injection of Alcohol for Intractable Pain.* M. J. May, Edinburgh.
25. Saltzstein, H. C. (1934): Intraspinal (subarachnoid) injection of absolute alcohol for the control of pain of advanced malignant growths. *JAMA,* 103:242.
26. Schlosser, H. (1907): Erfahrungen in der neuralgiebehandlung mit alkoholein-spritzungen. *Verhandl. d. Cong. f. innere Med.,* 24:49.
27. Stovner, J., and Enrenen, R. (1972): Intrathecal phenol for cancer pain. *Acta Anaesthesiol. Scand.* 16:17–21.
28. Swerdlow, M. (1973): Intrathecal chlorocresol. A comparison with phenol in the treatment of intractable pain. *Anaesthesia,* 28:297–301.
29. Swetlow, G. I. (1925): Injection of the superior laryngeal nerve with alcohol for the relief of pain in laryngeal tuberculosis. *Am. Rev. Tuberc.,* 12:189.
30. Taglia, S. Cited by Bonica, J. J. (1953): *The Management of Pain.* Lea & Febiger, Philadelphia.
31. Wilkinson, H. A., Mark, V. H., and White, J. C. (1964): Further experiences with intrathecal phenol for the relief of pain. *J. Chron. Dis.,* 17:1055–1059.
32. Wood, K. (1978): The use of phenol as a neurolytic agent: A review. *Pain,* 5:205–229.

Advances in Pain Research and Therapy, Vol. 2,
edited by J. J. Bonica and V. Ventafridda.
Raven Press, New York © 1979.

Blocks with Local Anesthetics in the Treatment of Cancer Pain

H. U. Gerbershagen

Department of Anesthesiology and Interdisciplinary Pain Clinic, Johannes Gutenberg University, Mainz, West Germany

Regional block procedures for the relief of cancer pain are usually performed with neurolytic substances such as alcohol or phenol. There are, however, pain states associated with neoplastic disease which do not require destructive nerve blocks with their inherent side effects and complications. Local anesthetic blocks useful for cancer pain include sympathetic block, somatic nerve block, and extradural block.

SYMPATHETIC NERVE BLOCKADE

Cancer pain amenable to local anesthetic blocks is characterized by symptomatology of so-called carcinomatous (or sarcomatous) neuritis, which is identical to the signs and symptoms of reflex sympathetic dystrophy. These include: (a) pain; (b) hyperpathia (hyperesthesia and/or hyperalgesia); (c) neurovascular instability (vasoconstriction with cyanosis and edema or vasodilatation); (d) sudomotor disturbances (hyper-, hypo-, or anhidrosis); and (e) pilomotor changes.

The quality of pain is burning, throbbing, dull, and in some cases even sharp and stabbing (21). Characteristically, the pattern of distribution of this constant pain and of the hyperpathic area does not correspond to segmental or peripheral nerve innervation. Therefore, physicians who are not familiar with these pain syndromes do not accept the patient's symptom-report and search for neurotic or hysterical traits. Nonrecognition and nontreatment of these conditions almost regularly result in trophic tissue changes which eventually become irreversible. It is therefore essential to initiate treatment with sympathetic blocks promptly after the onset of pain and related symptomatology.

In the initial state of tumor-induced reflex sympathetic dystrophy, which usually occurs 6 to 10 months after radical and effective tumor surgery, objective signs of tumor recurrence are lacking (3). However, in many instances carefully performed *sweat tests* (16,21) are helpful, because tumor infiltration of the cervicothoracic and lumbar sympathetic chains results quite early in hypohidroses or anhidroses in the upper and lower limbs respectively (10,22). These changes, which precede any X-ray evidence of tumor recurrence by months and sometimes years, are particularly likely to occur with lymphogenous spread of Pancoast, breast, urogenital, and rectal tumors (5,6,9).

Another distinct clinical entity frequently observed with cancer pain can be ascribed to reflex sympathetic dystrophy: the quadrant syndrome or vascular zone disturbance described by Gross (12), Laux (14), and Pette (19). These conditions present with burning, dull pain; nonsegmental sensory disturbances; vasomotor, sudomotor, and pilomotor changes; and a special quality of pain which can be detected on careful physical examination. These patients will either indicate a latency between a nociceptive stimulus with a pinprick and pain perception *or* immediately feel a sharp pain on stimulation followed by a dull, severe burning pain.

The distribution of the pain is the typical sympathetic vascular innervation pattern. Thus, the pain distribution can correspond (a) to one or more quadrants of the body in accordance with the sympathetic nervous system

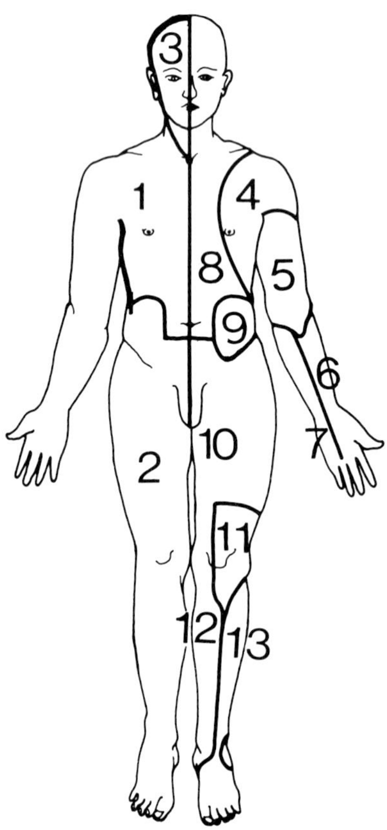

FIG. 1. Arterial supply of the skin (front). The identity of each artery by number is given on page 313.

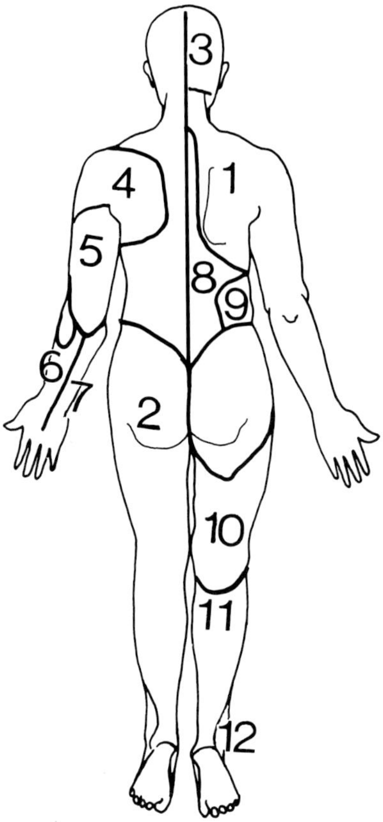

FIG. 2. Arterial supply of the skin (back). See below for identity of each artery.

distribution of subclavian and iliac arteries (Fig. 1) or (b) to the vascular zone of one arterial branch such as the axillary or external carotid arteries (Fig. 2).

Arterial Supply of the Skin

Topographically abnormal sensory disturbances, such as hyper- or hypoalgesia, frequently accompany peripheral nerve and vascular injuries. These nonsegmentally distributed sensory disturbances do not correspond to the innervation of peripheral nerves but can be traced to a typical sympathetic vascular innervation pattern. Gross (12)—and our clinical findings endorse his topographical findings—ascribes the skin areas to the following vascular innervation: (1) subclavian artery = right cervicothoracic trunk outflow = upper quadrant of the body; (2) iliac arteries = right lumbar sympathetic outflow = lower quadrant of the body; and subdivisions of these major trunks; (3) common carotid artery; (4) axillary artery; (5) brachial artery; (6) radial artery; (7) ulnar artery; (8) thoracic aorta; (9) abdominal aorta;

(10) femoral artery; (11) popliteal artery; (12) posterior tibial artery; (13) anterior tibial artery.

About 10 years ago we observed that one diagnostic sympathetic block with a local anesthetic prior to planned neurolytic injections relieved the burning cancer pain and the often-associated muscle-tension pain for days and even weeks. This unexpectedly long effective duration of a local anesthetic block is explained by the following actions of local anesthetics on pain mechanisms. The local anesthetic: (a) blocks pain receptors (nociceptors) and thus prevents transformation and coding of nociceptive impulses in these specialized nerve endings; (b) blocks nociceptive impulse-

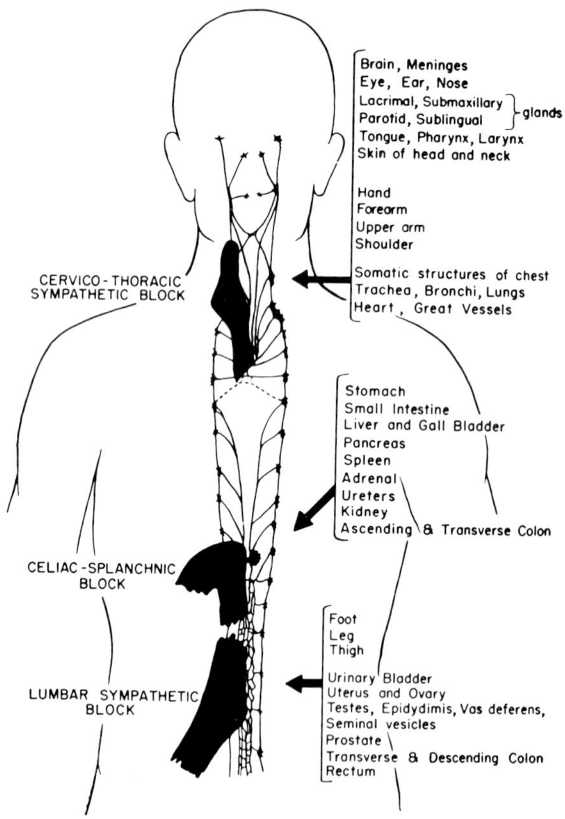

FIG. 3. Diagram illustrating the three "critical sites" which may be employed to interrupt the peripheral sympathetic nervous system. On the reader's left the diagram shows the pattern of diffusion (black) of local anesthetic solutions injected in the vicinity of the cervicothoracic (stellate) ganglion, celiac plexus, and lumbar sympathetic ganglia. On the reader's right are the names of the structures affected with each block. (After F. A. D. Alexander, courtesy of J. J. Bonica, *Clinical Applications of Diagnostic and Therapeutic Nerve Blocks,* Charles C Thomas, Springfield, Ill., 1959).

transmission in those efferent fibers associated with sympathetic fibers and thus prevents such impulses from reaching the central nervous system; (c) blocks sympathetic pathways and thus interrupts sympathetic reflex mechanisms, which act as positive feedback mechanisms and which are usually active in painful conditions (Zimmermann, *this volume*), (d) reduces or eliminates the increased skeletal muscle activity, which contributes to the sustenance of the vicious circle of pain; and (e) regional anesthetic blocks possibly influence higher cortical functions, altering mental constitutional conditions (more directness, spontaneity, integrative tendencies, higher distinctivity, clarity, availability of mental functions) (24).

The pain-relieving effects of regional anesthetic blocks often outlast the pharmacologic impulse-blocking effect of the local anesthetic (11,12). This prolonged analgesic effect, which is obtained even in neoplastic disease, is presumably due to interruption of the aforementioned vicious circle. In treatment of pain, the goal of regional analgesia is interruption of C- and A-delta fibers and of efferent sympathetic fibers (7). This requires only low concentrations of local anesthetics such as 0.5% lidocaine or mepivacaine, or 0.125 to 0.25% bupivacaine. Because of the long duration of action of bupivacaine, an almost-continuous, small-fiber blockade can be achieved with blocks performed once daily (11,17). Our experience clearly has demonstrated that best results with regional analgesic block will be achieved if a series of 6 to 8 blocks are performed at 1- or 2-day intervals. The results achieved with local anesthetics in tumor-induced reflex sympathetic dystrophy are comparable with those attained with neurolytic blocks, i.e., 4 to 6 months of pain relief (11), for interrupting the sympathetic chain and its branches as depicted in the three critical sites (Fig. 3).

Stellate ganglion and cervicothoracic sympathetic blocks are performed for burning cancer pain of the face, head, and neck and celiac plexus blocks, for upper abdominal pain. The following is a brief description of these techniques.

Stellate Ganglion Block

The stellate ganglion, usually a fusion of the inferior cervical and first thoracic ganglia, is located between the anterolateral surface of the seventh cervical vertebral body and the neck of the first rib. Although several methods of blocking the stellate ganglion have been described, the anterior paratracheal technique is the simplest and most widely used (Fig. 4).

The patient lies in the dorsal recumbent position with a pillow under his shoulder and his head slightly hyperextended. A thin, 4- to 5-cm-long needle is inserted 3 cm above the sternoclavicular joint of the side ipsilateral to the block and passed horizontally between trachea and carotid artery to contact the base of the sixth (or seventh) cervical transverse process. (The top of the sixth transverse process (Chassaigniac's tubercle) is easily palpated at the level of the cricoid cartilage.) After the needle is withdrawn 0.5 cm, the needle point lies in the tissue plane anterior to the prevertebral fascia where the stellate ganglion lies. Figure 4 points out that the paravertebral sympathetic chain is enclosed by a fascial sheath. Thus, any solution injected into the correct fascial plane will achieve a *volume-dependent* sympathetic block distribution. Two ml of local anesthetic solution will produce a stellate ganglion block and thus interrupt sympathetic fibers to face and head; 10 ml will interrupt cervicothoracic sympathetic outflow to the upper extremity, intrathoracic organs, and the chest (2,4).

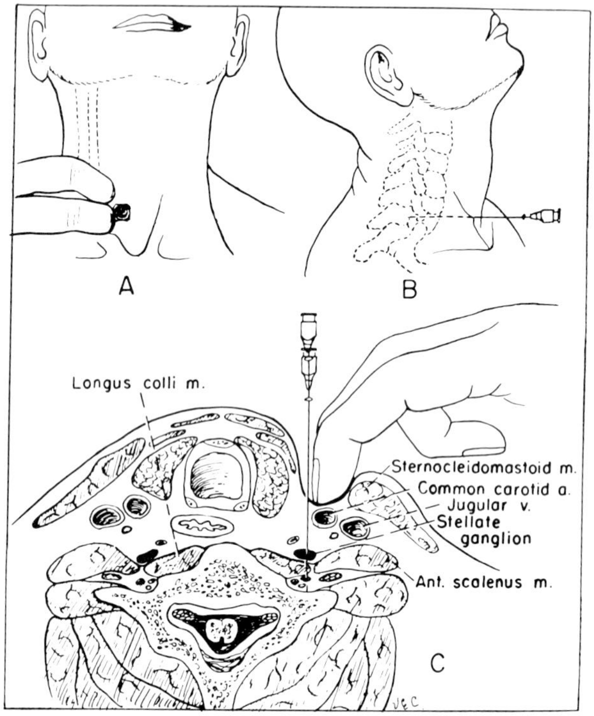

FIG. 4. Technique of stellate ganglion block by the anterior (paratracheal) approach. **A:** Anterior view, showing the maneuver of retracting the large vessels laterally and placing the needle medial to the fingers. **B:** Lateral view showing the needle in place with its tip on the base of the transverse process of the 6th cervical vertebra. **C:** Cross-section depicting the technique. Note the relationship of the fingers to the common carotid and jugular vein and these to the stellate ganglion. After contact with the bone, the needle is withdrawn about 5 mm until its point is anterior to the longus colli muscles and in the same fascial plane as the stellate ganglion. Injection of the solution in this fascial plane permits its diffusion cephalad to involve the lower portion of the cervical sympathetic chain and caudad to affect the upper portion of the upper thoracic chain. Should the needle not be withdrawn and the injection made into the muscle, the diffusion of drug will be limited. (From J. J. Bonica, *Clinical Applications of Diagnostic and Therapeutic Nerve Blocks,* Charles C Thomas, Springfield, Ill., 1959).

Lumbar Sympathetic Block

Technique of lumbar sympathetic block. The lumbar sympathetic ganglia lie along the anterolateral surface of the vertebral bodies and medial to the psoas muscle (Fig. 5). The patient lies in the lateral position on the side opposite the one to be blocked. A 10-cm-long needle is inserted perpendic-

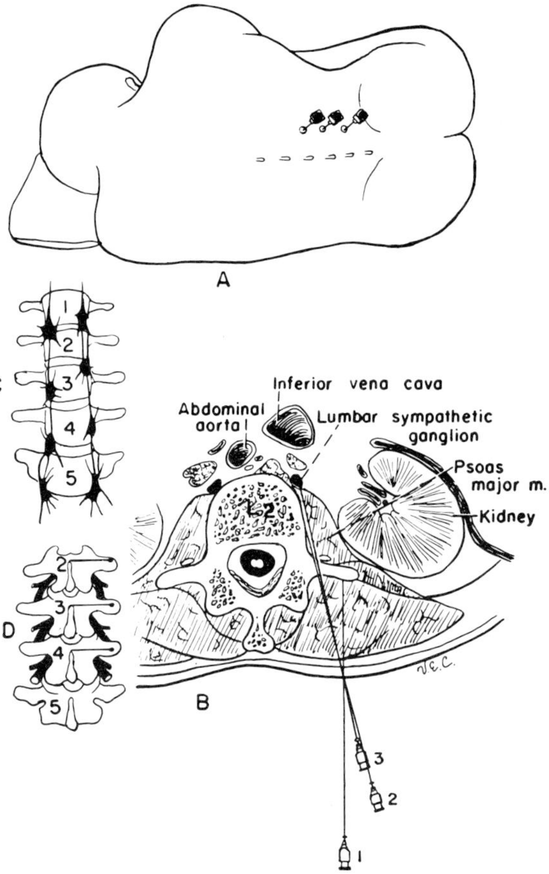

FIG. 5. Anatomy and technique of blocking the lumbar sympathetic ganglia by the paravertebral approach. **A:** Position of the patient for unilateral block. Note the skin wheals are opposite the upper edge of the spinous processes of the 2nd, 3rd, and 4th lumbar vertebra. **C:** Cross-section showing details of technique. The ganglia are on the anterolateral surface of the vertebra anterior to the margin of the psoas major muscle and posterior to the large vessels and abdominal viscera. In the diagram, needle 1, depicting the first step of the procedure, impinges the transverse process; needle 2, the lateral surface of the vertebra; and needle 3, with its point in the proximity of the lumbar sympathetic chain. **C:** Anterior, and **D:** posterior view of the vertebral column showing relation of sympathetic chain. The lines in **D** indicate the landmarks used on the overlying skin. (From J. J. Bonica, *The Management of Pain,* Lea & Febiger, Philadelphia, 1953.)

ularly to the skin surface 4 cm lateral from the middle of the second or third lumbar spinous process. The needle is then advanced until the transverse process is contacted (usually at a depth of 4 cm). The needle point is withdrawn to the subcutaneous tissue, then directed cranially and slightly medially to pass between the transverse process and make contact with the anterolateral aspect of the vertebral body. The correct position of the needle point can fairly well be tested by injection of 2 ml air. If the needle is well placed, there will be no resistance to the air injection; if the needle point is within the psoas muscle or subperiostally a resistance to air-injection will be obvious. After negative aspiration tests, 10 ml of local anesthetic are injected. The lumbar sympathetic block will interrupt sympathetic innervation of the lower ipsilateral extremity and part of the pelvic viscera (1,4,13).

Celiac Plexus Block

Block of the celiac plexus with a local anesthetic can be used as a diagnostic or prognostic aid or for temporary relief of upper abdominal visceral cancer pain. The technique we use is similar to that described by Moore (*this volume*).

Somatic Nerve Block

Since 1972, we have most often interrupted sympathetic and afferent C-fiber impulse-transmission within *somatic plexus* and the *peridural space* instead of performing standard sympathetic-block procedures. Thus, we have used axillary nerve blocks with low concentrations of local anesthetic instead of cervicothoracic sympathetic blocks for the treatment of pain and functional disturbances (such as lymphedema) of the upper extremity and caudal blocks and 3-in-1 blocks instead of lumbar sympathetic blocks for pain states of the pelvis and lower extremities (26). Studies in volunteers (21,23) and pain patients (11) proved that the sympathetic-fiber blockade was comparable and that patient's acceptance of these block types was better than with series of classic sympathetic-block procedures.

Caudal Block

The signs and symptoms of reflex sympathetic dystrophies, especially those of the lower half of the body, often have a bilateral distribution. Therefore, a bilateral sympathetic nerve blockade is necessary to obtain good pain-relief and reduction of functional disturbances. Lymphangiographic studies in our department have shown that bilateral sympathetic blockade produced with caudal block achieved with 30 ml of 0.125 to 0.25% bupivacaine is very effective in reducing edema and in improving lymph drainage from para-aortic and pelvic lymph nodes within a period of 4 to 5 days.

Technique of caudal block. The local anesthetic is injected through the sacral hiatus into the peridural space. The patient is asked to assume the prone position. The posterosuperior iliac spines are palpated, marked, and a connecting line drawn. On this base line an equilateral triangle is drawn, the apex of which usually overlies the sacral cornua. A 3- to 4-cm-long, thin needle inserted in a slightly cranial direction, will palpably pierce the sacrococcygeal ligament. Thirty ml of local anesthetic (low concentration!) is injected. Sympathetic and C-fibers of the lower extremities and the pelvis will be interrupted in some 20 min. (10).

Axillary Block

Burning pain due to tumor infiltration into the supraclavicular fossa can be controlled for several months by performing axillary nerve blocks with 30 ml of 0.25% bupivacaine or cervicothoracic sympathetic blockade achieved by injecting 10 ml of bupivacaine using the standard paratracheal stellate ganglion block technique. In the proximal third of the shaved axilla the axillary artery is palpated and a short, thin needle (23 g) is inserted directly lateral to the artery to a depth of 1.0 to 1.5 cm. After a negative aspiration test, 20 to 25 ml of local anesthetic is injected. With this paravascular technique it is unnecessary to elicit paresthesias, since artery, vein, and nerves are contained in a neurovascular sheath.

Pain and dysfunction in the upper abdomen due to lymphogenous spread of tumors can also be controlled for several weeks with local anesthetic blocks of the celiac ganglion. In these cases, however, we feel that a celiac plexus block with small volumes (15 ml) of 50% alcohol is relatively harmless and a preferable procedure (see Moore, *this volume*).

In comparison of neurolytic nerve blocks, local anesthetic blocks have minimal side effects and no permanent complications if good block techniques are employed (11). The block can be repeated without significantly increasing the risk.

SOMATIC NERVE BLOCKS

Somatic nerve blocks, which include block of A-delta and C afferent and sympathetic fibers, are employed advantageously in patients with acute, severe cancer pain, such as develops with pathologic fractures (rib, femur) or severe pain associated with a radiculopathy caused by tumor compression. These blocks are performed to keep the patient comfortable until more definite therapeutic measures are carried out. For these blocks, it is advisable to use higher-concentration local anesthetics such as 0.5% bupivacaine in order to achieve a more profound and long-lasting nerve block. More often, paravertebral somatic blocks are performed (Fig. 6).

We block paravertebral somatic nerves according to a technique described

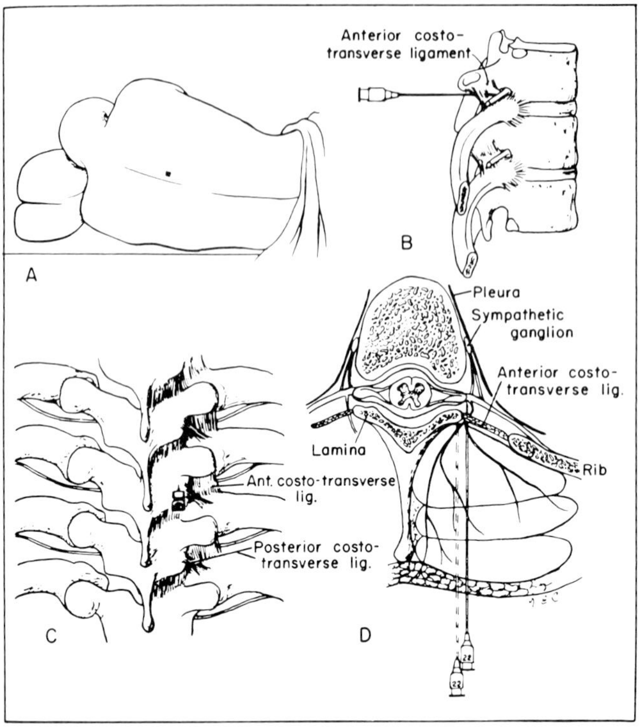

FIG. 6. Technique of paravertebral thoracic somatic nerve block.

by Fervers (8) and reintroduced by Shaw (20) and Bonica (1a) (Fig. 6). It is the only technique described which prevents the needle point from entering the vertebral canal. A 5- to 6-cm-long needle is inserted perpendicular to the skin surface 1 to 1.5 cm lateral of the spinal process and advanced until contact is made with the vertebral lamina. The needle point is withdrawn to subcutaneous tissue and skin moved laterally ½ cm, and the needle point is aimed at the lateral margin of the lamina. After one or two corrections, the needle point will palpably slip off the lamina. The needle is advanced 0.5 cm, an aspiration test performed, and 5 ml of local anesthetic solution injected.

CATHETER TECHNIQUES

In hospitalized patients, *catheter technique* is often preferable. Although the results of this continuous fiber blockade do not differ from the daily, single-injection technique, the catheter technique is advantageous in irritable and aggressive patients and in patients in poor general health.

There is another small group of patients who can benefit from local anesthetic blocks. Patients suffering from cancer pain which cannot be con-

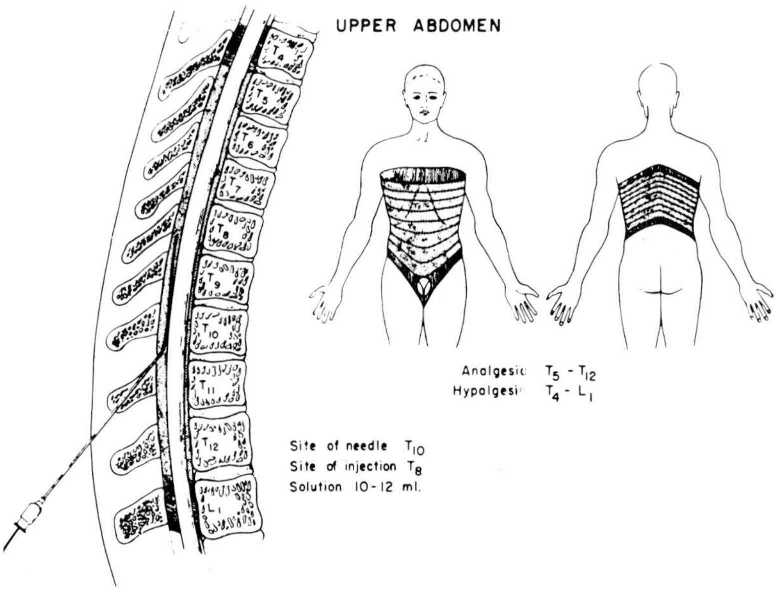

FIG. 7. Pattern of analgesia and hypalgesia produced by means of continuous epidural block to control pain in the upper abdomen, as occurs with acute pancreatitis. (From J. J. Bonica, *Clinical Applications of Diagnostic and Therapeutic Nerve Blocks.* Charles C Thomas, Springfield, Ill., 1959).

trolled by narcotic analgesics and other systemic drugs during their terminal 2 to 3 weeks of life can receive complete pain-relief by continuous nerve blocks via catheters. In most such cases, the catheters are introduced into the epidural space to effect continuous segmental epidural analgesia (2,11) (Fig. 7). These patients are usually dependent on narcotics and should continue to receive these drugs to keep them comfortable. We feel strongly that no dying patient should have to suffer pain, but should spend the last few weeks of life in relative comfort.

Disadvantages

A disadvantage of local anesthetic blockade is the need to repeat the block daily or every other day, which is inconvenient as it subjects the patient to repeated needling. However, taking into consideration that prior to neurolytic block a diagnostic block with local anesthetic should be performed, and that in many patients neurolytic blocks have to be repeated, the aforementioned disadvantage of local anesthetic blocks is not so great. Another significant disadvantage of block with local anesthetic is that in about 10 to 20% the procedure only produces transient relief of pain and the related symptomatology. In these patients neurolytic blocks should then be performed.

REFERENCES

1. Bonica, J. J. (1968): Autonomic innervation of the viscera in relation to nerve block. *Anesthesiology,* 29:793.

1a. Bonica, J. J. (1959): *Clinical Applications of Diagnostic and Therapeutic Blocks.* Charles C Thomas, Springfield, Ill.

2. Bonica, J. J. (1953): *The Management of Pain.* Lea & Febiger, Philadelphia.
3. Bues, E. (1954): Gezielte Grenzstrangresektion. Höhendiagnostik des Sympathikusgrenzstranges und ihre chirurgische Bedeutung. *Chirurg.,* 25:443.
4. Challenger, J. H. (1974): Sympathetic nervous system blocking in pain relief. In: *Relief of Intractable Pain,* edited by M. Swerdlow. Excerpta Medica, Amsterdam.
5. Chiappa, S., Bonadonna, G., Uslenghi, C., and Veronesi, U. (1967): Lymphangiography in the diagnosis of retroperitoneal node metastasis in rectal cancer. *Br. J. Radiol.,* 40:584.
6. Dargent, M. (1948): Role of the sympathetic nerve in cancerous pain; inquiry into 300 cases. *Br. Med. J.,* 1:440.
7. de Jong, R. (1963): Theoretical aspects of pain: Bizarre pain phenomena during low spinal anesthesia. *Anesthesiology,* 24:628.
8. Fervers, C. (1929): Eine vereinfachte Technik der paravertebralen Anästhesie und ihre Anwendung. *Zentrabl. Chir.,* 37:2318.
9. Fuchs, W. A. (1969): *Lymphangiography in Cancer.* Springer, Heidelberg, New York.
10. Gerbershagen, H. U. (1973): Behandlung chronischer Schmerzzustände mit Nervenblockaden. In: *Lokalanästhesie und Lokalanästhetika,* edited by H. Killian. Thieme, Stuttgart.
11. Gerbershagen, H. U., Panhans, C., and Schwarz, R., editors (1978): *Regionalanästhesie in Schmerzdiagnostik und -therapie.* Acron, Berlin.
12. Gross, D. (1972): *Therapeutische Lokalanästhesie.* Hippokrates Verlag, Stuttgart.
13. Haugen, F. P. (1968): The autonomous nervous system and pain. *Anesthesiology,* 29:785.
14. Laux, W. (1958): *Über Quadrantensyndrome. Ein Beitrag zu Klinik und Pathogenese der "Vegetativen Körperviertelstörungen" als Grundlage Chronischer Schmerzzustände.* Karger, Basel, New York.
15. Mandl, F. (1947): *Paravertebral Block in Diagnosis, Prognosis and Therapy.* Grune & Stratton, New York.
16. Moberg, E. (1958): Objective methods for determining the functional value of sensibility in the hand. *J. Bone Jt. Surg.,* 3:454.
17. Nolte, H., Meyer, J., Köpf, B., and Renz, M. (1974): Klinische und elektrophysiologische Parameter zur Differenzierung der Wirkung von Lokalanästhetika. *Anaesthesist,* 23:165.
18. Oeser, H., Taenzer, V., and Behrendt, C. (1971): Das Syndrom nach Rektumamputation (Postproktektomie-Syndrom). *Dtsch. Med. Wochenschr.,* 23:973.
19. Pette, H. (1927): Das Problem der wechselseitigen Beziehungen zwischen Sympathicis und Sensibilität. *Dtsch. Z. Nervenkh.,* 100:143.
20. Shaw, W. M. (1952): Medial approach for paravertebral somatic nerve block. *JAMA,* 148:742.
21. Schenk, C. (1978): *Objektivierung sympathischer Blockaden.* PhD. Thesis, Johannes Gutenberg-Universität, Mainz, West Germany.
22. Schliack, H., and Schiffer, R. (1971): Anhidrose der Fuss-sohle: Symptom retroperitonealer Tumorinvasion. *Dtsch. Med. Wochenschr.,* 96:977.
23. Theiss, D., Robbel, G., Theiss, M., and Gerbershagen, H. U. (1977): Experimentalle Bestimmung einer optimalen Elektrodenanordung zur elektrischen Nervenlokalisation. *Anaesthesist,* 26:411.
24. Türk, H., Frey, R., and Gerbershagen, H. U. (1975): Regional anesthesia as a psychotherapeutic method: A new approach to the psychic system (an experimental study). Paper read at the First World Congress on Pain, Florence, Italy, September 5–8, 1975.

25. White, J. C., and Smithwick, R. H. (1944): *The Autonomic Nervous System.* Kimpton, London.
26. Winnie, A. P., Rammamurthy, S., and Durrani, Z. (1973): The inguinal paravascular technic of lumbar plexus anesthesia: The 3-in-1 block. *Anesth. Analg.,* 52:989.

Advances in Pain Research and Therapy, Vol. 2,
edited by J. J. Bonica and V. Ventafridda.
Raven Press, New York © 1979.

Subarachnoid and Extradural Neurolytic Blocks

M. Swerdlow

Regional Pain Relief Centre, University of Manchester School of Medicine, Salford, M6 8HD, Lancashire, England

It is nearly 50 years since a neurolytic agent (alcohol) was first injected into the theca deliberately to produce pain-relief (7). Strangely enough, although Dogliotti introduced the procedure for noncancer pain, most of the subsequent use has been for relief of cancer pain. The method has seen many changes in frequency of use in the intervening years. In the early decades after Dogliotti's reports, inadequate techniques of asepsis rendered intrathecal injections somewhat hazardous. By the late 1950s this problem had been solved, and the introduction of phenol gave a new impetus to the use of the method (26). During this period, the extradural injection of neurolytic agents to relieve cancer pain was also initiated. Apart from chlorocresol, which Maher (24) introduced in 1963, no important new neurolytic agents have appeared.

During the 1960s neurosurgeons were exploring new surgical techniques of interrupting central nervous system pain transmission and during the present decade percutaneous cordotomy, chemical hypophysectomy, and cytotoxic drugs have been shown to have important roles to play in the treatment of intractable cancer pain. It is the purpose of this report to provide a comprehensive, albeit concise, review of neurolytic subarachnoid and extradural block within the framework of other therapeutic modalities currently used for the control of pain of advanced cancer.

SUBARACHNOID NEUROLYSIS

What is the present position of the intrathecal neurolysis? I believe that it still has an important place in the total spectrum of methods of relieving cancer pain for the following reasons: (a) When properly employed it provides good quality pain-relief in a reasonable proportion of patients; (b) it could easily be made available to all patients with cancer pain; (c) it requires only brief hospitalization; (d) it provides an adequate duration of relief for many of the patients and can be repeated if necessary; (e) it can be applied to the old and very ill; and (f) complications are usually absent or slight.

Pathologic studies have shown that neurolytic solutions injected intrathecally affect large and small fibers indiscriminately (38). The degree of block produced depends on the number rather than the type of fibers destroyed, and this in turn is related to the quantity and concentration of solution employed (41). However, as Papo and Visca (32) point out, the extent of parenchymal damage is not always directly related to the success of the block.

Subarachnoid Phenol and Alcohol

In the early years phenol was often used dissolved in iophendylate. It has been subsequently shown that phenol solutions in iophendylate are less active than those in glycerine, and there is now a consensus that iophendylate is only indicated when it is necessary to have radiological control of the injection (30).

Nathan et al. (31) consider that phenol has a biphasic action—an almost immediate but temporary local anesthetic action and a permanent destructive action on the blocked fibers. According to Gonsette and Andre-Balisaux (9) chlorocresol has only a slight anesthetic action, a fact which is obvious in clinical practice. The destructive effects of alcohol are more intense (41) and less localized (14) than those of phenol.

Technical Considerations

The technique of intrathecal neurolytic injection is now well established. For injections of hyperbaric solutions the patient is positioned with the pain-

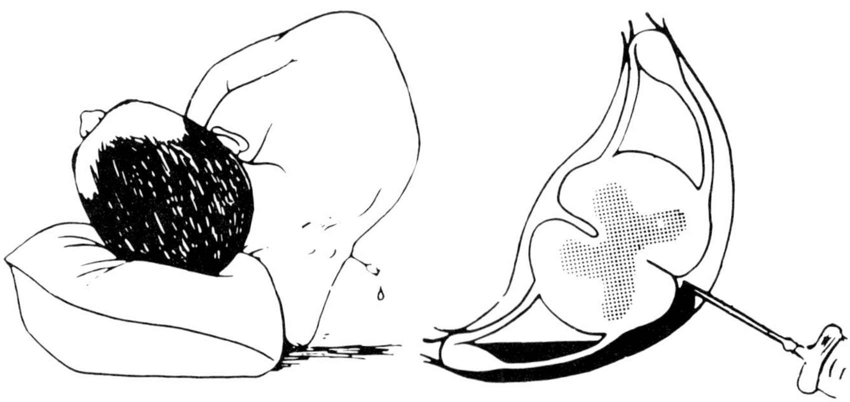

FIG. 1. Subarachnoid injection of hyperbaric neurolytic solution (hyperbaric phenol) to interrupt the posterior rootlets of spinal nerves. The subarachnoid puncture is made with the patient on his side with the affected side underneath. Once subarachnoid fluid emerges from the hub of the needle, the upper part is displaced posteriorly so that the posterior surface of the back makes an angle of 45° with the superior surface of the table. This will place the posterior (sensory core) rootlets of the nerves involved in conducting the pain lowermost. (Courtesy of J. J. Bonica.)

ful side underneath, and the spinal puncture is made at a level such that the neurolytic solution will fall onto the appropriate posterior nerve roots (Fig. 1). When alcohol is being injected, the patient is placed with the painful side upward (Fig. 2). The patient should be retained in the injection position for about 20 min to allow the neurolytic agent to become "fixed" to the nerve roots.

In my opinion, proper siting of the needle is more important than tilting in obtaining good localization of the solution. I also believe that it is important to avoid excessive dosage. Occasionally, with hyperbaric solutions the patient's report of symptoms on the upper side signals that the bevel of the needle is not pointing downward as it ought to be. Judging from published reports (32,45) and personal enquiries, phenol is now the most widely used agent for this purpose; the optimum concentration appears to be 5 to 7%. As will be seen below, I have found that chlorocresol in a concentration of 1:40 or 1:50 is slightly more efficacious than phenol, but side effects are liable

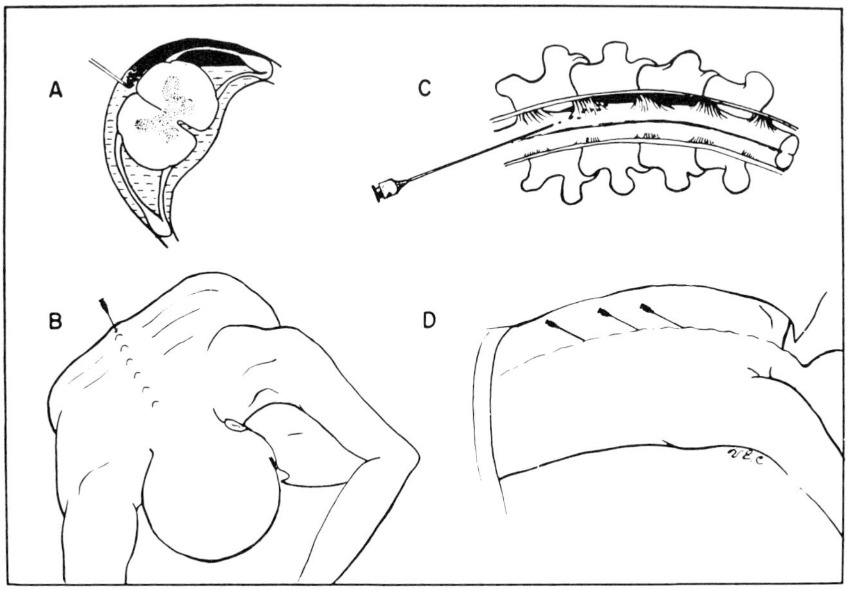

FIG. 2. Diagram showing the position of the patient for subarachnoid alcohol block in the thoracic position. Note that the patient is placed in the lateral-prone position so that the posterior surface of the back makes an angle of 45° with the superior surface of the table. **B:** One or two pillows are placed under the region to be blocked and the table flexed so as to produce a scoliosis of the spine with a maximum curve corresponding to the nerve roots conveying the pain. This will place the posterior (sensory) nerve roots involved in conducting pain uppermost **(A)** with the head and extremities lower than the point of injection. **C:** Longitudinal section showing diffusion of the hypobaric alcohol to involve the uppermost sensory roots. **D:** Note that three needles are used in order to permit the injection of small volumes of solution and thus minimize complications. (Courtesy of J. J. Bonica, *Clinical Applications of Diagnostic and Therapeutic Nerve Blocks,* Charles C Thomas, Springfield, Ill., 1959.)

to be longer-lasting with chlorocresol. Furthermore it has the disadvantage of not causing localizing symptoms at the time of injection, so that it is more difficult to assess exactly which nerve roots are being affected. In order to obtain some of the advantages of chlorocresol whilst avoiding its disadvantages, some workers (27,32) use a mixture of the two agents.

Indications

Subarachnoid neurolysis is particularly appropriate in patients with fairly localized pain. When there is widespread pain and especially in those in whom pain arises early in the course of the disease, a percutaneous cordotomy (or in appropriate cases pituitary adenolysis) would offer a better chance of long-term relief. In patients with bilateral multifocal pain, however, many workers consider that the serious risks of bilateral cordotomy should be avoided by performing cordotomy only on the worse side and applying subarachnoid neurolysis on the other side (47). In patients who are unfit, unwilling, or unable to have a cordotomy, an intrathecal neurolysis is usually the best therapy.

Although techniques of blocking both sides at one injection have been described both with alcohol and phenol, the consensus of opinion favors the two sides' being injected on separate occasions (29).

There is little to choose between the results of alcohol and phenol in expert hands. The choice usually depends on the operator's training and experience, but sometimes the state of the patient, (e.g., marked dyspnea in the Trendelenburg position, inability to lie on the painful side) will dictate whether hypobaric (alcohol) or a hyperbaric (phenol) solution is used. In my opinion the method of choice is to use phenol for blocks in the lumbosacral segments and chlorocresol at higher spinal levels. In view of the superior results reported (15,16) when alcohol rather than phenol was used in the cervicothoracic region, it would seem that alcohol should be given a trial in cases of shoulder and neck pain. At any spinal level it is worthwhile giving a second injection if the first is unsatisfactory; but if two injections fail, there is little chance of a third's being effective and there is an increased risk of complications.

Results

One of the most contentious aspects of intrathecal neurolysis is the nature of the results. This is not surprising when we consider the differences among the patients being treated and the variations in assessment and reporting of results (45). There are a great number of factors involved in the pain of patients with malignant disease: the condition at the time of the injection; the rapidity of growth of tumor; the tissues involved in the production of pain; the type of tumor and part of the cord affected; whether there is sheltering of nerve roots by secondary tumor cells; whether there has been radiotherapy to the cord region or a previous intrathecal injection, both of which can affect results; how long the patient has been suffering pain at the time of the block and how widespread the pain. Moreover, following treatment, growth of the tumor or the advent of new secondary deposits can cause new pain which may make it difficult to assess whether the effects of the block have worn off. Furthermore, in many cases the general condition deteriorates rapidly, or the patient is put on medication which makes pain assessment difficult. Finally, different reports adopt different standards of what is a "good," "moderate," or "poor" result. In general "good" relief implies a high degree of freedom from pain with little curtailment of activity and little need to take analgesic drugs, whereas "moderate" relief implies that the pain level is reduced but that pain may still be causing some curtailment of activities and some analgesic supplementation may be necessary. Tables 1 and 2 are compiled from results reported by different workers with alcohol and phenol respectively.

To date, I have treated over 300 patients with cancer pain with intrathecal neurolysis. The earlier ones were followed up for 3 months (or until death if that occurred earlier), and those results have already been reported (47). Of that group, 44% obtained good relief, 30% had moderate relief, and 26% had little or no relief. It will be seen that further experience has resulted in a rather higher success rate.

The more recently treated patients have, as far as possible, been followed up until death. Analysis of the cases of 130 patients treated shows 69 received phenol and 61 chlorocresol. Of the 130 patients, 79 received one injection, 39 were given two injections, 9 received three, 2 were given four injections and 1 patient received six. Table 3 shows the duration of effectiveness of the block (or time from injection date to death if analgesia was still effective at death) in all single-dose cases or bilateral-dose cases, and also the duration of the first dose in patients who later had more than one therapy.

TABLE 1. *Results with subarachnoid alcohol block for relief of cancer pain*

Author(s)	No. of patients	Efficacy of therapy (% of patients)		
		Good relief	Fair relief	Little or no relief
Kuzucu et al. (16)	322	58	26	16
Hay (11)	252	46	32	22
Dogliotti (7)	150	59	25	16
Greenhill (10)	100	60	10	30
Bonica (2)	182	53	29	18
Perese (35)	95	57	32	11
Stern (40)	50	63	27	10
Total/Average	1151	56	27	17

TABLE 2. *Results with subarachnoid phenol block for relief of cancer pain*

Author(s)	No. of patients	Efficacy of therapy (% of patients) Good relief	Fair relief	Little or no relief
Maher (23)	433	62	6	32
Papo & Visca (32)	282	40	35	25
Ciocatto et al. (5)	207	78	11	11
Swerdlow (46)	200	56	19	25
Stovner & Endreson (42)	151	77%		23
Brown (3)	114	68	5	27
Total/Average	1387	61	15	24

Among this group, 27 patients died within 1 month and 62 within 3 months of the subarachnoid injection.

Pain-relief of more than 1 year's duration is somewhat exceptional, although such cases have been reported by a number of workers. Wilkinson et al. (50) and White and Sweet (49) had patients with analgesia lasting over 2 years and Papo and Visca (32) have reported analgesia lasting 2 to 3 years in several patients. Brown (4) and Lassner (17) have also reported long-lasting relief.

The type of cancer involved is detailed in Table 4. Analysis of the results shows that the type of cancer and the stage at which the patient was presented for treatment play a greater part in determining the duration of relief

TABLE 3. *Analysis of results in 130 patients given subarachnoid neurolysis*

Duration of relief	Agent administered: Phenol — Result of treatment: Good	Phenol: Moderate	Phenol: Poor	Chlorocresol — Result of treatment: Good	Chlorocresol: Moderate	Chlorocresol: Poor
Less than 1 month	11	5	6	14	6	3
1–2 months	6	3	2	7	4	2
2–3 months	7	1	3	3	2	1
3–4 months	3	1	2	2	2	1
4–5 months	8		1	1		1
6–8 months	6	1		8	1	
8–10 months	1			1		
10–12 months	1					
Over 1 year	1					
Over 2 years				1	1	
Total	44	11	14	37	16	8
%	64	16	20	61	26	13

TABLE 4. *Type of cancer in the author's latest 130 patients*

Disease	No. of patients
Ca Rectum	31
Ca Bronchus	30
Ca Cervix	24
Ca Breast	9
Ca Pancreas	7
Ca Colon	5
Ca Stomach	3
Ca Bladder	3
Ca Ovary	2
Ca Kidney	2
Others	14
Total	130

than the nature of the neurolytic solution. Pain-relief lasting 3 to 6 months occurred in the following number of patients with the various lesions: cervix, 7; rectum, 5; breast, 3; colon, 2; bronchus, 1; pancreas, 1; and stomach, 1. Relief lasting 6 months or more was derived by 10 patients with carcinoma of the rectum, 4 with carcinoma of the breast, 3 with lesions of the bronchus, and 3 with lesions of the cervix.

Complications

The easy accessibility of the nerve roots to subarachnoid neurolytic agents sometimes results in complications, some of which are due to involvement of unintended nerves or even vessels, whereas others (such as headache) are unrelated to effect of the neurolytic agent. Furthermore, neurolysis may sometimes aggravate a preexisting deficit such as paresis or dysuria. A comprehensive list of complications of intrathecal neurolysis has been given elsewhere (44). Table 5 lists complications lasting more than 7 days.

The complications are usually transient, but some persist and cause difficulties in patient-management. Headache, paresthesias, and numbness are common, give little trouble, and are unpredictable. Less common and much

TABLE 5. *Complications lasting longer than 7 days in 300 patients.*

Drug(s)	No. of patients	Bladder paresis	Bowel paresis	Muscle paresis	Headache	Paresthesia	Numbness
Phenol	145	7	1	4	—	1	4
Chlorocresol	138	10	1	7	1	1	4
Phenol and chlorocresol	17	3	1	—	1	—	1

TABLE 6. *Duration of complications*

Duration of complications	No. of patients
Lasting more than 3 days	48
Lasting more than 1 week	28
Lasting more than 2 weeks	19
Lasting more than 1 month	10
Total no. of patients	300
Total no. of injections given	453

more serious are muscular pareses and interference with rectal and vesical sphincter action. These complications are to some extent predictable; there is very little risk of interference with rectal or vesical action except when a neurolytic agent is being applied for the first time to the lumbosacral nerves. Likewise, there is a very small risk of significant muscular weakness except when the lumbar or the cervicothoracic outflow are being blocked. Table 6 shows the duration of complications in my series of 300 patients.

It is not generally realized that there are dangers from the effects of neurolytic agents on the blood supply to the cord, although these have been demonstrated by pathologic studies (14,51). There have been few clinical publications of such complications, although anecdotal and medicolegal reports suggest the incidence is not negligible. A recent case report by Superville-Sovak and her colleagues (43) is of interest. These workers report a case in which a subarachnoid injection of 6% phenol in glycerine at the level of T5–6 was followed by temporary respiratory arrest and subsequent weakness and sensory loss in the right upper limb. Respiratory infection led to death 5 weeks after the intrathecal injection, and post-mortem examination showed lesions of many small arteries supplying the posterolateral aspect of the cord.

Intrathecal neurolysis may fail to produce relief. Sometimes this is due to the sheltering action of neoplastic infiltration of the nerve roots (1,25) or of previous radiotherapy. On the other hand, Pellegrini et al. (34) have found gross meylin and axon damage in patients in whom treatment failed altogether. Papo and Visca (32) consider that in chronic cases, failure may be due to development of central summation and that a good result on pain of recent onset is due more to the fact that central changes have not yet developed rather than to absence of sheltering. Nathan (28) found that 32 of 112 patients with cancer pain were not relieved by intrathecal phenol and required anterolateral cordotomy. An adequate explanation is not easy to find.

Conclusion

There is a need to provide the training which will enable subarachnoid neurolysis to be made more widely available. The rapidly increasing spread of worthwhile pain-relief centers should in due course be able to satisfy this need. More should be done to inform doctors providing primary treatment for cancer of the methods which are now available for relief of cancer pain so that more patients are referred earlier for pain-relief therapy. Finally, there is a need to discover a more effective neurolytic agent—an agent with better penetrative and destructive ability, even though such an agent would result in a longer duration of complications. There is also a need to investigate the reasons why intrathecal neurolysis is sometimes totally ineffective.

Intrathecal Saline

Hitchcock (12) and subsequent workers have shown that saline can produce a certain amount of neurolysis that results in pain-relief when injected into the subararchnoid space. The effects appear to be due to the hypertonicity of the saline rather than its temperature (18). However, the injection causes painful twitching, paresthesias, confusion, and a rise in blood pressure and is therefore done under sedation or general anesthesia (47). The method has been used mostly for pain due to malignant disease, but some workers have employed it in such conditions as causalgia and post-herpetic neuralgia (6).

Technique

The patient lies on his side with the painful side underneath, the table being tilted foot down for pain in the lower half of the body and head down for pain in the upper half. After lumbar puncture is performed and some cerebrospinal fluid is removed, 20 ml of 7.5% to 15% saline is injected rapidly, and the needle is then removed. For bilateral pain the patient is now placed supine; for unilateral pain he is kept lying on the painful side.

Results

The results are often disappointing. In Hitchcock's series (13) fewer than half the patients obtained more than 1 month's relief. Furthermore the method is unfortunately not so free from complications as was originally hoped; Lucas et al. (21) reported an 11% incidence of temporary complications with 1% incidence of serious sequelae. Subarachnoid saline is probably better reserved for terminal cases, particularly those with widespread pain from metastases.

More recently barbotage of the cerebrospinal fluid has been experimented with as a method of producing pain-relief (19). The barbotage is performed via a Tuohy needle inserted at the spinal level of the pain. The duration of relief is usually unsatisfactorily brief and it cannot be recommended for clinical use.

EPIDURAL NEUROLYSIS

Now for a few words about epidural neurolysis. Although the epidural route avoids the risks of meningeal irritation and allows good localization of the neurolytic solution, the method is not widely used for relief of intractable pain. Moreover, there does not appear to have been increased usage parallel with the contemporary popularity of epidural block for both surgical and obstetric analgesia. One reason may be that at the time of injection it is not so easy to gauge the response and effectiveness as it is with subarachnoid injection.

Patterson and Marcello (33) and Spaetz and Wagner (39) claimed good results with extradural alcohol, but the injection is often painful and may be followed by postinjection neuropathy with neuralgia. Phenol appears to be a more promising agent for epidural use. A number of workers employ extradural phenol for pain in the cervical and higher thoracic segments to avoid the risks of subarachnoid neurolytics at this level (20).

Results

Lourie and Vanasupa (20) claim pain-relief of more than 9 months with 6% phenol, but Madrid (22) although finding the method successful could only achieve 2 to 4 weeks relief with 7½% phenol in glycerine. Sometimes I use extradural 7 to 10% phenol for neck and shoulder pain of malignancy, especially when subarachnoid injection proves impossible or unsuccessful. Raftery (37) has reported the use of intermittent, small doses of 6% aqueous phenol via an indwelling epidural catheter. The technique was used at all levels of the spinal cord and was often found to give good relief. Extradural phenol has also been used by Doughty (8) to relieve attacks of tenesmus and burning pain which occur with rectal cancer.

Complications

Muscular palsy has been reported by Usubiaga (48) after lumbar epidural injection of both phenol and alcohol for cancer pain; recovery occurred after a period of time. Hypertonic saline has been administered via the epidural route, but it is not yet clear whether this is a worthwhile procedure. Reports suggest that unfortunately it is not without risk (48).

Continuous Epidural Analgesia

Finally, the extradural route can be used to provide useful pain-relief in terminal care. In patients who have widespread pain and are too ill for more major pain-relieving procedures and in whom analgesic drugs are proving unsatisfactory, good relief can be achieved by intermittent injection of a dilute, local anesthetic solution through an appropriately positioned epidural catheter. Such a catheter can be retained for several weeks and can even be used in patients at home. A recent modification of this method is described by Pilon and Baker (36), who connected to the epidural catheter a small reservoir which was then implanted under the skin. Injections of local anesthetic were made percutaneously into the reservoir, pressure on which would "inject" a dose into the catheter. The equipment was maintained *in situ* and gave effective relief for 4½ months.

REFERENCES

1. Berry, K., and Olszewski, J. (1963): Pathology of intrathecal injection in man. *Neurology,* 13:152.
2. Bonica, J. J. (1958): Diagnostic and therapeutic blocks: A reappraisal based on 15 years experience. *Anesth. Analg. Curr. Res.,* 37:58.
3. Brown, A. S. (1976): Pain relief in malignant disease. Symposium on malignant disease. *Roy. Coll. Phys. Edin.,* Publication No. 47.
4. Brown, A. S. (1961): Treatment of intractable pain by nerve block with phenol. *Proc. 2nd Int. Cong. Neurol. Surg. Int. Cong., Series 36.* Excerpta Medica, Amsterdam.
5. Ciocatto, E., Moricca, G., and Cavaliere, R. (1967): L'infiltration sous arachnoidienne antalgique. *Cahiers Anesth.,* 15:747.
6. Collins, J. R., Duras, E. P., Van Housen, R. J., and Spruell, L. (1969): Intrathecal cool saline solution: A new approach to pain evaluation. *Anesth. Analg. Curr. Res.,* 48:816.
7. Dogliotti, A. M. (1931): Traitement des syndromes douloureux de la peripherie par l'alcolisation sub-arachnoidienne. *Presse Med.,* 67:11.
8. Doughty, A. (1972): In: *A Practice of Anaesthesia,* edited by W. D. Wylie and H. Churchill-Davidson. Lloyd Luke, London.
9. Gonsette, R., and Andre-Valisaux, G. (1964): Resultats éloignés dans le traitement neurochirurgical de la spasticité des membres inferieurs dans la sclerose en plaques. *Acta Neurol. Belg.,* 64:481.
10. Greenhill, J. P. (1947): Sympathectomy and intraspinal alcohol injections for relief of pelvic pain. *Br. Med. J.,* 2:859.
11. Hay, R. C. (1962): Subarachnoid alcohol block in the control of intractable pain. *Anesth. Analg. Curr. Res.,* 41:12.
12. Hitchcock, E. (1967): Hypothermic subarachnoid irrigation for intractable pain. *Lancet* 1:965.
13. Hitchcock, E. (1976): The treatment of intractable pain with subarachnoid saline infusion. In: *Current Controversies in Neurosurgery,* edited by T. P. Morley. Saunders, Philadelphia.
14. Hughes, J. T. (1966): Pathological findings following intrathecal injection of ethyl alcohol in man. *Paraplegia,* 4:1671.
15. Katz, J. (1975): Subarachnoid alcohol injections for the management of chronic pain. In: *Recent Progress in Anaesthesiology and Resuscitation.* Excerpta Medica, Amsterdam.
16. Kuzucu, E. Y., Derrick, W. S., and Wilber, S. A. (1966): Control of intractable pain with subarachnoid alcohol block. *JAMA,* 195:133.
17. Lassner, J. (1962): L'analgesie prolongée par l'alcolisation sous-arachnoidienne. *Anesth. Analg.,* 19:5.
18. Lipton, S. (1976): Pain relief. In: *Recent Advances in Anaesthesia and Analgesia,* 12th ed., edited by C. L. Hewer and R. S. Atkinson, p. 239. Churchill Livingstone, Edinburgh.

19. Lloyd, J. W., Hughes, J. T., and Davies-Jones, G. A. B. (1972): Relief of severe intractable pain by barbotage of the C.S.F. *Lancet,* 1:354.
20. Lourie, H., and Vanasupa, P. (1963): Comments on the use of intraspinal phenol-pantopaque for relief of pain and spasticity. *J. Neurosurg.,* 20:60.
21. Lucas, J. T., Ducker, T. B., and Perot, P. L. (1975): Adverse reactions to intrathecal saline for control of pain. *J. Neurosurg.,* 42:557.
22. Madrid, J. (1975): Proceedings of Symposium on Cancer Pain, Florence, Italy.
23. Maher, R. M. (1960): Further experiences with intrathecal and subdural phenol. Observations on two forms of pain. *Lancet,* 1:895.
24. Maher, R. M. (1963): Intrathecal chlorocresol in the treatment of pain in cancer. *Lancet,* 1:965.
25. Maher, R. M. (1957): Neuroma section in relief of pain. Further experience with intrathecal injections. *Lancet,* 1:16.
26. Maher, R. M. (1955): Relief of pain in incurable cancer. *Lancet,* 1:18.
27. Mehta, M. (1973): *Intractable Pain.* Saunders, London.
28. Nathan, P. W. (1963): Results of antero-lateral cordotomy for pain in cancer. *J. Neurol. Neurosurg. Psychiatry,* 26:353.
29. Nathan, P. W. (1970): Treatment of intractable pain by chemical rhizotomy with phenol solution. In: *Gillingham Clinical Surgery. Neurosurgery,* edited by J. F. Gillingham. Butterworths, London.
30. Nathan, P. W., and Sears, T. A. (1961): Some factors concerned in differential nerve block by local anaesthetics. *J. Physiol. (Lond.),* 157:565.
31. Nathan, P. W., Sears, T. A., and Smith, M. (1965): Effects of phenol on the nerve roots of the cat. An electrophysiological and histological study. *J. Neurol. Sci.,* 2:7.
32. Papo, I., and Visca, A. (1976): Intrathecal phenol in the treatment of pain and spasticity. *Prog. Neur. Surg.,* 7:56.
33. Patterson, A., and Marcello, M. (1963): Cited by F. A. D. Alexander and L. W. Lewis (1963): In: *Anesthesiology,* edited by D. E. Hale, p. 801. Blackwell, Oxford.
34. Pellegrini, G., Visca, A., and Papo, I. (1969): Considerazioni sul meccanismo d'azione antalgica delle soluzioni di fenelo intratecali. *Acta Neurol. (Bari),* 24:85.
35. Perese, D. M. (1958): Subarachnoid alcohol block in management of pain of malignant disease. *Arch. Surg.,* 76:347.
36. Pilon, R. N., and Baker, A. R. (1976): Chronic pain control by means of an epidural catheter. *Cancer,* 37:903.
37. Raftery, H. (1977): *Proceedings of the Intractable Pain Society of Great Britain.*
38. Smith, M. C. (1963): Histological findings following intrathecal injections of phenol solutions for relief of pain. *Br. J. Anaesth.,* 36:387.
39. Spaetz, . . and Wagner, . . (1963): Cited by F. A. D. Alexander and L. W. Lewis (1963): In: *Anesthesiology,* edited by D. E. Hale, p. 801. Blackwell, Oxford.
40. Stern, E. L. (1937): Dangers of intraspinal (subarachnoid) injection of alcohol. Their avoidance and contraindications. *Am. J. Surg.,* 35:99.
41. Stewart, W. A., and Lourie, H. (1963): An experimental evaluation of the effects of subarachnoid injections of phenol-pantopaque in cats: A histological study. *J. Neurosurg.,* 20:64.
42. Stovner, J., and Endresen, R. (1972): Intrathecal phenol for cancer pain. *Acta Anaesth. Scand.,* 16:17.
43. Superville-Sovak, B., Rasminsky, M., and Finlayson, M. H. (1975): Complications of phenol neurolysis. *Arch. Neurol. (Chicago),* 32:226.
44. Swerdlow, M. (1979): Complications of neurolytic blocks. In: *Neural Blockade,* edited by M. Cousins and P. Bridenbaugh. Lippincott, New York.
45. Swerdlow, M. (1978): Current views on intrathecal neurolysis. *Anaesth.,* 33:733.
46. Swerdlow, M. (1975): Proceedings of Symposium on Cancer Pain, Florence, Italy.
47. Swerdlow, M. (1978): *Relief of Intractable Pain,* 2nd ed. Excerpta Medica, Amsterdam.
48. Usubiaga, J. E. (1975): *Neurological Complications Following Epidural Anesthesia.* Little, Brown & Co., Boston.

49. White, J. C., and Sweet, W. H. (1969): *Pain and the Neurosurgeon.* Charles C Thomas, Springfield, Ill.
50. Wilkinson, H. A., Mark, V. H., and White, J. C. (1964): Further experiences with intrathecal phenol for the relief of pain. *J. Chron. Dis.,* 17:1055.
51. Wolman, L. (1966): The neuropathological effects resulting from the intrathecal injection of chemical substances. *Paraplegia,* 4:97.

Advances in Pain Research and Therapy, Vol. 2,
edited by J. J. Bonica and V. Ventafridda.
Raven Press, New York © 1979.

Phenol Subarachnoid Rhizotomy for the Treatment of Cancer Pain: A Personal Account on 290 Cases

I. Papo and A. Visca

Neurosurgery Division, Regional General Hospital, 60100 Ancona, Italy

Inasmuch as we have recently surveyed the literature in previous papers (10,11,12), and Dr. Swerdlow has already updated the basic knowledge of subarachnoid and extradural neurolytic techniques, in this brief report we shall deal only with our personal experience with intrathecal phenol in the treatment of cancer pain.

Over the past 18 years we have used phenol rhizotomy on 290 patients. We should distinguish two different phases in our experience. At the beginning we were very impressed with the results reported by Maher (4,5,7) and Brown (1), and we thought that intrathecal phenol would be the most suitable procedure for cancer pain, whereby it would be possible to avoid cordotomy and other conventional surgical procedures in most cancer patients. On these grounds, for about 3 years all patients complaining of painful syndromes from advanced cancer underwent phenol rhizotomy at different levels. During this phase, surgical operations were carried out only in patients in whom chemical rhizotomy had previously failed.

After the clinical experience during this first phase, we realized that the high hopes aroused by previous reports on subarachnoid neurolysis were not entirely justified, because not-negligible failures and complications had been observed. Consequently, we revised our criteria and attempted to outline the specific indications for intrathecal phenol and to establish well-defined guidelines for the future clinical management of these patients. As a consequence of these steps, the overall number of phenol rhizotomies dropped abruptly, but at the same time the rate of good results rose significantly.

RESULTS

Overall we have treated 290 patients with the following major categories of neoplastic lesions: (a) gynecologic tumors, 92; (b) rectal tumors, 44; (c) tumors of abdominal organs, 49; (d) tumors of lung, pleura, and mediastinum, 46; (e) primary and metastatic bone tumors, 52; and (f) kidney and bladder tumors, 7; with a total of 290.

TABLE 1. *Summary of overall therapeutic results*

Neoplastic disease	No. of pts.	Results					
		Good		Fair		Failure	
		No.	%	No.	%	No.	%
Gynecologic cancer	92	37	40.2	30	32.6	25	27.2
Rectal cancer	44	21	47.7	15	34.1	8	18.2
Abdominal cancer	49	23	46.9	17	34.7	9	18.4
Tumors of lung, pleura, mediastinum	46	10	21.8	20	43.4	16	34.8
Primary and secondary bone tumors	52	23	44.2	16	30.8	13	25
Kidney and bladder tumors	7	3	42.8	2	28.6	2	28.6
Total/Average	290	117	40	100	35	73	25

In assessing the results we have accepted the criteria suggested by Mark et al. (8). A result is classed as "good" if the patient is pain-free until death; as "fair" if pain-relief is sufficient to allow a significant decrease in the amount of analgesic medication required to keep the patient comfortable for a prolonged period or if pain is completely relieved for over 3 weeks. The overall results are summarized in Table 1. In Table 2 the results are analyzed in detail according to the localization and type of pain. Complications are listed in Table 3.

DISCUSSION

If we look at the overall results we see that we succeeded in relieving pain satisfactorily in about 40% of patients. In most of these patients the average duration of the analgesia was 2 to 4 months, which was long enough to keep the patient pain-free until death. Moreover, several patients who lived longer than 3 or 4 months died pain-free at 6 to 12 months, and some of these up to 2 or 3 years without recurrence of pain.

The overall rate of *good results* is not very high. However, it must be borne in mind that in this overall series the highest rate of failures occurred in the patients treated in the first phase of our experience when the proper indications of phenol rhizotomy were still not well defined. The *fair results* deserve further explanation. Whereas in patients who lived for a short period they can be considered as very worthwhile (good) because the patient was painfree until death, when survival was longer very often the pain, though relieved for a short period, recurred and further analgesic treatment was required. Recurrence took place mostly in patients with chest and/or upper limb pain from lung and breast cancer that invaded the chest wall and the brachial plexus. Also, pain in lower limb due to nervous compression from

TABLE 2. *Therapeutic results in different types and locations of pain*

Neoplastic disease	No. of pts.	Good No.	Good %	Fair No.	Fair %	Failure No.	Failure %
Gynecologic cancer							
Lower limb pain	45	—	—	22	49	23	51
Groin hemiabdomen, and thigh pain (survival 3 months)	9	4	44	4	44	1	12
Visceral pain (plexalgia pelvica)	8	3	38	3	38	2	24
Abdominal and lumbar pain (somatic)	14	14	100	—	—	—	—
Saddle pain	16	16	100	—	—	—	—
Rectal cancer							
Saddle pain	28	16	57	8	29	4	14
Sciatic pain	7	1	14	2	29	4	57
Sciatic and saddle pain (only saddle pain relieved)	5	—	—	5	100	—	—
Abdominal pain	4	4	100	—	—	—	—
Abdominal cancer (abdominal and lumbar pain)							
Stomach	16	10	63	5	31	1	6
Pancreas (girdle pain)	14	5	36	4	28	5	36
Colon	12	7	58	2	17	3	25
Liver and peritoneal carcinosis	7	1	14	6	86	—	—
Tumors of lungs, pleura, and mediastinum							
Apical and upper chest pain	21	3	14	9	43	9	43
Upper chest pain (above T_6)	8	1	12	6	75	1	13
Lower chest pain (below T_6)	17	6	35	5	30	6	35
Primary and secondary bone tumors							
Bone pain	25	16	64	6	24	3	12
Radicular pain (only the pain from thoracic roots compression was relieved)	27	7	26	10	37	10	37
Kidney and bladder cancer							
Lumbar, abdominal, and hypogastric pain	7	3	42.8	2	28.6	2	28.6

TABLE 3. *Complications*

	Mild and/or transient No.	Mild and/or transient %	Severe No.	Severe %
Lower limb weakness	9	3	11	3.8
Upper limb weakness	4	1.4	1	0.3
Bladder function disturbance	Transient		Permanent	
Urine retention	9	3	5	1.7
Urinary incontinence	2	0.7	—	—

pelvic and vertebral cancer often recurred. Therefore, from a rigid viewpoint, it would seem logical that one should consider only good results in assessing the practical value of phenol rhizotomy and in identifying the proper indications of this procedure. With fair results, though useful to the patients because they reflect good pain-relief for a time, the fact that the pain recurs makes their interpretation less reliable.

The proper range of applications on intrathecal phenol can be derived from the data in Table 2. The efficacy, advantages, limitations, and complications in the therapy of the different types of pain will be briefly discussed.

Saddle Pain

Saddle pain, including superficial and deep sacrococcygeal and perineal pain. Many other authors (2,3,5,6,8,9,13,14) have reported similar results. Small amounts of the neurolytic agent (about 0.5 ml phenol in glycerin) usually relieve saddle pain. Altogether we have treated 49 patients: 16 were suffering from gynecologic cancer (carcinoma of the cervix) and 33 from rectal cancer. Of these, 32 patients obtained good relief of pain and 8 patients improved significantly so that the amounts of systemic analgesics could be reduced until their death.

In 5 patients with rectal cancer, phenol was ineffective. In 5 patients who complained of perineal and sciatic pain, phenol abolished the saddle component; but a spinothalamic cordotomy was necessary to control the sciatic pain, which was not modified by phenol rhizotomy. Four patients underwent sacral surgical rhizotomy, in 3 of whom phenol had failed to relieve the pain at all and in the other pain recurred 3 months after the injection and further introduction of phenol proved ineffective.

Complications consisted of permanent urinary retention in 5 males in whom vesical function was presumably already impaired.

Abdominal, Lumbar, and Inguinal Somatic Pain

A total of 67 patients complaining of these types of pain from different cancers were treated. Pain from pelvic cancer (cervix or rectal carcinoma) was satisfactorily relieved in all 18 patients. In patients with intraperitoneal carcinomas, in whom pain was more protean with a visceral component in several cases, the rate of good results was lower. However, complete relief was achieved in 23 patients out of 49. Fair results were obtained in an additional 17 patients. In 9 patients the treatment was ineffective.

Girdle pain from pancreatic carcinoma was the most refractory (5 failures among 14 patients) so that the highest doses had to be used. Visceral pain seems to be much less affected by subarachnoid phenol neurolysis. The technique may produce good results in some patients with pelvic plexus pain, but is completely ineffective in relieving pain from smooth muscle dyskinesia and subocclusive crisis, as Maher (4) noted long ago.

Bone Pain

Of 25 patients with typical bone pain without root compression, 16 were satisfactorily relieved and in 6 others the pain was significantly reduced. Conversely, radicular pain from bone metastases is seldom abolished. Of 27 patients, only 7 had any significant benefit from chemical rhizotomy. All of them had radicular compression at the thoracic level; therefore high doses could be introduced to produce extensive destruction of sensory fibers with no risk of damaging motor or sphincter fibers. In the remaining patients the results obtained can be considered less than gratifying.

As most of these painful syndromes which are relieved by phenol rhizotomy are bilateral, the advantages of a method that can avoid the well-known disadvantage of bilateral cordotomy become evident. Moreover, although myelotomy has also been advocated for the treatment of bilateral abdominal and saddle pain, these can be managed effectively with the much simpler and less traumatic procedure of chemical rhizotomy. On the other hand, we believe that subarachnoid phenol neurolysis should not be attempted for the relief of lower limb pain except typical bone pain.

Lower Limb Pain

In patients with lower limb pain from root compression and massive edema, the results are usually disappointing and the incidence of complications is high. In fact, in about 25% of our patients treated for lower limb pain, chemical rhizotomy, even using small doses that never exceeded 1 ml of 5% phenol in glycerin, made the ipsilateral lower limb weak. The motor loss was mild and/or transient in 9 patients, but severe and permanent in 11. Muscles innervated by L_2, L_3, and L_4 were selectively involved, with serious functional disability. In contrast, motor disturbances in musculature innervated by the sciatic nerve were seldom observed.

For many years we have not performed chemical rhizotomies for lower limb pain except for bone pain: instead we have been carrying out spinothalamic cordotomy at the outset, especially in all patients expected to survive more than 3 months.

Upper Chest and Upper Limb Pain

The overall results with intrathecal phenol were likewise poor in upper chest and/or upper limb pain from lung and breast cancer. Only lower thoracic pain (below T_6) was permanently relieved in a significant percentage of patients (6 out of 17). In the latter instances we feel that phenol rhizotomy is a valuable procedure which produces beneficial effects similar to surgical rhizotomy provided that high doses are used, so as to produce massive destruction of sensory fibers without impairing motor and sphincter function. For this reason, abdominal, lumbar, and groin pain are usually very well controlled, with no residual neurologic disorders. Oddly enough, thoracic pain from lung cancer is much more refractory even though high amounts of phenol are introduced.

MECHANISM OF THERAPEUTIC ACTION

It is also noteworthy that in nearly all cases no definite cutaneous analgesia is produced. As Maher first pointed out (5), it seems as though the nerve roots were sheltered from the action of the neurolytic agent. The therapeutic effect of phenol on saddle pain is even more difficult to explain. Small doses produce very little, if any, sensory loss, and yet the procedure abolishes even the most severe pain. We speculate that the mechanism of this peripheral somatic pain involves only small branches and terminal arborizations of the lumbosacral nerves and these are effectively interrupted by small doses of neurolytic agent. However, when major nerve roots and plexuses are affected by more invasive neoplasias, the analgesic effects are much less even for sacrococcygeal and perineal pain, and hence more complete surgical procedures should be used.

CONCLUSIONS

We would like to reemphasize that phenol rhizotomy is by no means the last resort for severe pain of terminal cancer in which more effective surgical procedures would not be warranted. The main criteria for the proper selection of patients for subarachnoid neurolysis are the site, type, and extent of the pain. The patient's condition usually plays a minor role in making the decision for this modality. In fact, if intrathecal phenol is likely to be ineffective, as in lower limb pain from major nerve compression and massive edema, it should not be considered whatever the condition of the patient. Although the use of large doses may increase the chance of success, the procedure should be used with caution, if at all, because of the high risk of complications and incomplete relief of pain.

On the other hand, when it is indicated, phenol rhizotomy should be used early. The argument that the effects of chemical rhizotomy are of too short duration to be considered of real clinical value is not valid. In actual fact, the mean duration of the therapeutic action of phenol rhizotomy is 2 to 4 months, and this is enough to keep most patients pain-free until death. Furthermore, on some occasions, particularly when high dosages can be used (e.g., trunk) in patients who survive for a long period, pain-relief may last as long as 8 to 12 months and even longer. In this regard, it is relevant to point out that the problem of long survivals often arises in patients in whom phenol rhizotomy is not indicated, such as in patients with pain from lung tumors or lower limb pain from pelvic malignancies. Moreover, in patients with saddle pain from rectal or cervical carcinoma, phenol rhizotomy usually produces effective relief long enough to keep the patients pain-free until death. Since intraperitoneal cancers which produce abdominal, lumbar, and/or inguinal pain usually run a rather rapid course, surgical procedures are seldom indicated and chemical rhizotomy should be used.

On the basis of our experience we believe that phenol rhizotomy still retains an appreciable range of applications. It is especially indicated in abdominal, lumbar, inguinal, saddle, and bone pains. Properly executed, this technique produces good pain-relief in about 70 to 75% of patients complaining of these painful syndromes. Of course, if doubtful indications are included, the overall results will be less satisfactory. In patients for whom chemical rhizotomy is indicated, we never perform surgical operations before trying subarachnoid neurolysis. In the event two injections fail to modify the pain or if it recurs quickly, within a few hours or days, it is most likely that further injections will prove ineffective, and other forms of treatment must be attempted without wasting time.

In conclusion, although we feel that phenol rhizotomy is not effective in as many patients suffering from cancer pain as was previously believed, nonetheless it remains a valuable weapon in our armamentarium against pain and enables us to avoid more major procedures. If subarachnoid neurolysis has been given up by many workers and neglected in the past few years, it is likely due to failures and complications caused by wrong selection of patients.

REFERENCES

1. Brown, A. S. (1958): Treatment of intractable pain by subarachnoid injections of carbolic acid. *Lancet,* 2:975–978.
2. Kuhner, A. (1976): La valeur des interventions sur les racines sacrées dans le traitement des syndromes douloureux du bassin. *Neuro-Chirurgie,* 22:429–436.
3. Kuhner, A., and Assmus, H. (1975): Intrathecal applications of phenol in the treatment of intractable pain. In: *Advances in Neurosurgery, Vol. 3,* edited by H. Penzholz, M. Brock, J. Hamer, M. Kunger, and O. Spoerri, pp. 256–263. Springer, Berlin.
4. Maher, R. M. (1960): Further experiences with intrathecal and subdural phenol. Observations on two forms of pain. *Lancet,* 1:895–899.
5. Maher, R. M. (1957): Neurone selection in relief of pain. Further experiences with intrathecal injections. *Lancet,* 1:16–19.
6. Maher, R. M. (1966): Phenol for pain and spasticity. Pain. *Henry Ford International Symposium,* pp. 335–343. Little, Brown, Boston.
7. Maher, R. M. (1955): Relief of pain in incurable cancer. *Lancet,* 1:18–20.
8. Mark, V. H., White, J. C., Zervas, N. T., Ervin, F. R., and Richardson, E. P. (1962): Intrathecal use of phenol for the relief of chronic severe pain. *N. Engl. J. Med.,* 267:589–593.
9. Mullan, S. (1971): The surgical relief of pain. *Clin. Neurosurg.,* 18:208–224.

10. Papo, I., and Visca, A. (1973): Intrathecal phenol in the treatment of cancer pain. *J. Neurosurg. Sci.,* 12:146–156.
11. Papo, I., and Visca, A. (1976): Intrathecal phenol in the treatment of pain and spasticity. *Progress in Neurological Surgery, Vol. 7,* pp. 56–130. Karger, Basel.
12. Papo, I., and Visca, A. (1974): Phenol rhizotomy in the treatment of cancer pain. *Anesth. Analg.,* 53:993–997.
13. Robbie, D. S. (1969): General management of intractable pain in advanced carcinoma of the rectum. *Proc. R. Soc. Med.,* 62:1225.
14. Tank, T. M., Dohn, D. F., and Gardner, W. J. (1963): Intrathecal injections of alcohol or phenol for relief of intractable pain. *Cleveland Clin. Q.,* 30:111–117.

Advances in Pain Research and Therapy, Vol. 2,
edited by J. J. Bonica and V. Ventafridda.
Raven Press, New York © 1979.

Cranial Nerve Blocks

Jose L. Madrid and John J. Bonica

*Department of Anesthesiology and Pain Clinic, Ciudad Sanitaria "10 de Octubre," Madrid, Spain; and *Department of Anesthesiology, University of Washington, School of Medicine, Seattle, Washington 98195*

The head and neck frequently are sites of malignant tumors, which in their terminal stages are often accompanied by pain. In many instances the pain is severe, persistent, and continuous, interfering with the patient's nutrition and sleep and thus rapidly sapping the sufferer's strength and morale. Relief of pain in such patients is a matter of urgent necessity and the primary objective of management. In such patients the symptomatic management of pain is influenced to a great extent by the physical and emotional condition and the life-expectancy of the patient. Although many patients can be managed with narcotic analgesics, in many, if not most instances, it is far better to interrupt pain pathways by either chemical or surgical means. If a patient's condition is good, then surgical interruption should be considered. Unfortunately, however, in many instances these patients are not likely to tolerate a major operation and nerve block should be used. The success of nerve block depends in part on how early it is performed. Unfortunately there is a misconception among colleagues about the efficacy of these procedures, for most of them do not refer patients with severe pain for this type of treatment until the patient has had pain not adequately relieved with systemic analgesics and the lesion is so far advanced that it presents technical difficulties in carrying out the nerve block.

Proper provision for nerve blocks requires a thorough study of the course of the lesion and the location and the nature of the pain, a thorough knowledge of the structures supplied by the various cranial nerves and the upper four cervical nerves and, of course, skill in carrying out the various techniques.

ANATOMIC CONSIDERATIONS

It may be recalled that the trigeminal nerves supply sensory fibers to the anterior two-thirds of the head, including the skin of the face, and anterior two-thirds of the scalp, the mucous membranes of the cheek, the upper and lower teeth, gums and hard palate, the anterior two-thirds of the tongue, the anterior pillar of the tonsil, the mucous membranes of the nose, the eyelids and orbit, the maxillary, frontal, ethmoid, and sphenoid sinuses. (See

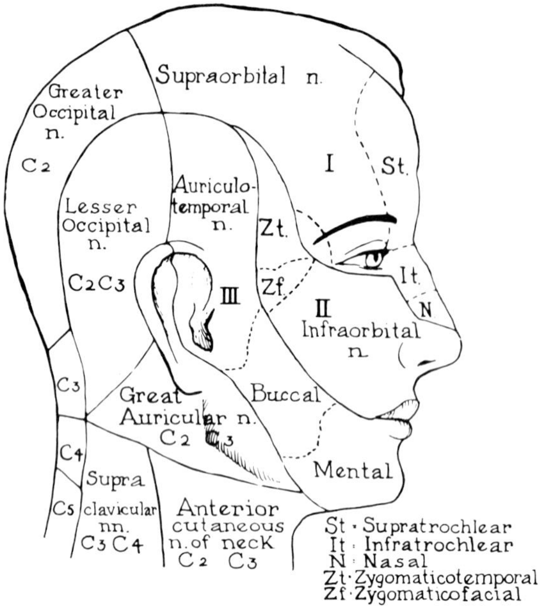

FIG. 1. The cutaneous distribution of the trigeminal nerve and its branches. (Courtesy of J. J. Bonica, *The Management of Pain,* Philadelphia, Lea & Febiger, 1953).

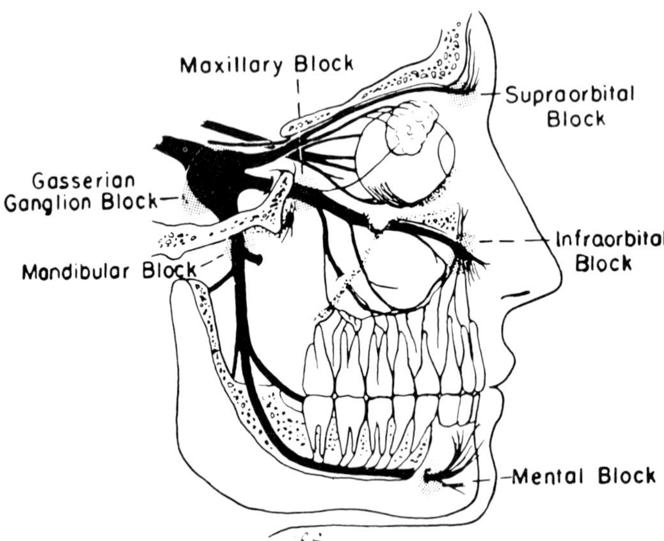

FIG. 2. Diagram showing the anatomy and distribution of the trigeminal nerve and the optimal sites of injecting it (stippled areas). Gasserian ganglion block is accomplished by passing a needle through the foramen ovale and into the gasserian ganglion; maxillary nerve block is accomplished in the pterygopalatine fossa just after the nerve passes through the formen rotundum; mandibular block is accomplished just below the foramen ovale; supraorbital block is accomplished at the supraorbital ridge; infraorbital block is accomplished at the infraorbital foramen or canal, and mental block at the mental foramen. (Courtesy of J. J. Bonica, *Clinical Applications of Diagnostic and Therapeutic Nerve Blocks,* Charles C Thomas, Springfield, Ill., 1959.)

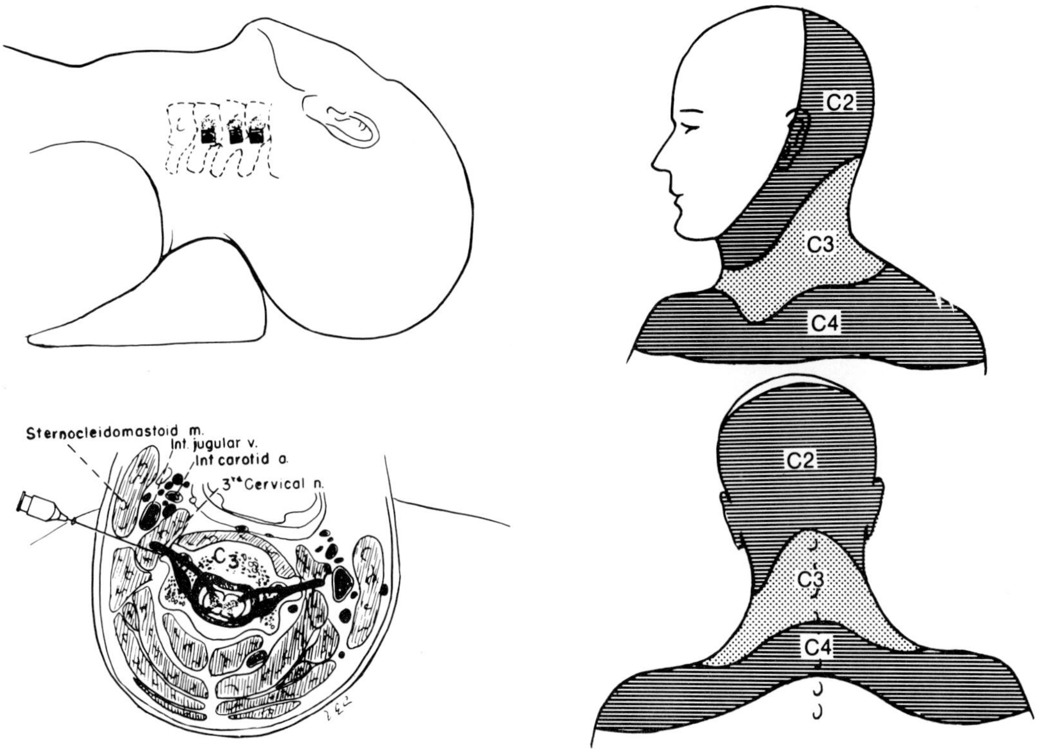

FIG. 3. Anatomy and technique of injecting the superficial cervical plexus. Area of anesthesia resulting from injecting the cervical plexus shown on the right. (Courtesy of J. J. Bonica, *The Management of Pain,* Lea & Febiger, Philadelphia, 1953).

Figs. 1 and 2.) It also contributes sensory fibers to the soft palate, uvula, and tonsils, which also receive fibers from other nerves.

The sensory area of the glossopharyngeal nerve comprises the nasopharynx, the eustachian tube, soft palate, uvula, tonsil, tonsillar pillar base of the tongue, and the pharynx as far as the epiglottis and possibly below it. It contributes fibers to the external auditory canal. The vagus nerve contributes sensory fibers to the ear, the external auditory canal, and the tympanic membrane, and supplies the larynx. The second, third, and fourth cervical nerves supply the neck, the posterior portion of the scalp, the ear, and the skin over the angle and lower portion of the mandible, as shown in Fig. 3. Sympathetic fibers supply the entire region by accompanying somatic nerves and the blood vessels.

CLINICAL CONSIDERATIONS

Chemical section is particularly applicable to cancer pain within the distribution of the trigeminal nerve, and all such cases should be first treated with this method, because experience shows that alcohol injections produce analgesia for 6 to 18 months, sufficiently long to afford relief until death in most patients with cancer pain. Moreover, if pain returns either because the chemical interruption has disappeared or because the tumor has spread beyond the confines of the anesthesia, the injection can be repeated. In some patients block of one of the major divisions of the trigeminal nerve (e.g., maxillary or mandibular) is sufficient but in most instances it is far better to carry out a gasserian ganglion block to produce widespread analgesia because probably the disease will spread if the patient lives sufficiently long. Although gasserian ganglion block is inherent in the risk of keratitis, the problem is quite different than when dealing with patients with tic douloureux in whom life-expectancy is long and where a corneal ulcer would be a serious complication.

Obtaining radiographs prior to the block may be of great importance in some cases. If, for example, a block of the trigeminal nerve at the level of the gasserian ganglion in Meckel's cave is planned, a radiographic plate of the base of the skull is required in order to ascertain the presence of the foramen ovale. In patients with carcinoma of the nasopharynx and the floor of the mouth, the tumor may destroy bone structures of the base of the skull, making it impossible to identify the foramen ovale. In these cases it will be necessary to adopt a different approach for the block or a different procedure. Alcohol diffuses very poorly in tissues so that, if the block is to be effective, exact positioning of the needle in the nerve or nerves is necessary. This is one of the main reasons for the use of radiologic control when these blocks are undertaken (4). Another reason is to obtain objective evidence of the position of the needles at the time of the injection of the neurolytic agent. Moreover, the use of X-ray control allows even the beginner to ensure the exact positioning of the needles in the correct anatomic region so that the solution achieves the desired effect.

TECHNIQUE OF BLOCKING THE GASSERIAN GANGLION

The following brief description of the technique of blocking the gasserian ganglion is included. For a more detailed description, the reader is referred to Bonica's book (1). The most frequently used and best technique of blocking the gasserian ganglion (and also the mandibular nerve) is by the anterolateral (Härtel) approach. The needle is inserted through a skin wheal which is on the skin overlying the 2nd upper molar tooth and advanced in a direction so that when it is viewed from the side its point is directed to the midpoint of the zygomatic arch, and when viewed from the front it is directed to the pupil of the ipsilateral eye. It is advanced until it contacts the infratemporal plate lateral to the base of the pterygoid process just anterior to the foramen ovale. The depth mark is then set 1.5 cm from the skin surface, the needle withdrawn until its point is in the subcutaneous tissue and then reinserted so that its point will eventually go through the foramen.

For the injection, the patient is made to lie in the supine position looking straight ahead. The skin overlying the midpoint of the zygomatic arch and the skin overlying the articular tubercle are marked with a pencil. These points act as a guide to the infratemporal plate and the foramen ovale, respectively. A wheal is made with a local anesthetic in the skin of the cheek 3 cm lateral to the angle of the mouth at the level of the 2nd upper molar tooth. A 10-cm, 22-gauge needle threaded with a depth marker is introduced through this wheal and is advanced in a posteromedial and superior direction, so that when it is viewed from the side, its axis points to the midpoint of the zygomatic arch, and when it is viewed from in front, the axis of the needle points to the pupil (Fig. 4). After piercing the skin, the needle progressively passes through the buccinator muscle, then beneath the mucous membrane between the mandibular ramus and tuberosity of the maxilla, and finally through the external pterygoid muscle before it makes contact with the infratemporal plate lateral to the base of the pterygoid process and just anterior to the foramen. As soon as this contact is made, usually at a depth of about 5 cm, the depth marker is set 1.5 cm from the skin surface, the needle is withdrawn until its point is in the subcutaneous tissue, and it is then reinserted so that its point will eventually go through the foramen. During this second insertion, the axis of the needle, when viewed from the side, points to the articular tubercle, while when viewed from the front, it still points to the pupil. Usually when the needle has been inserted to a depth just 1 cm short of the rubber marker, its point makes contact with the mandibular nerve, causing paresthesia along the course of the latter. These

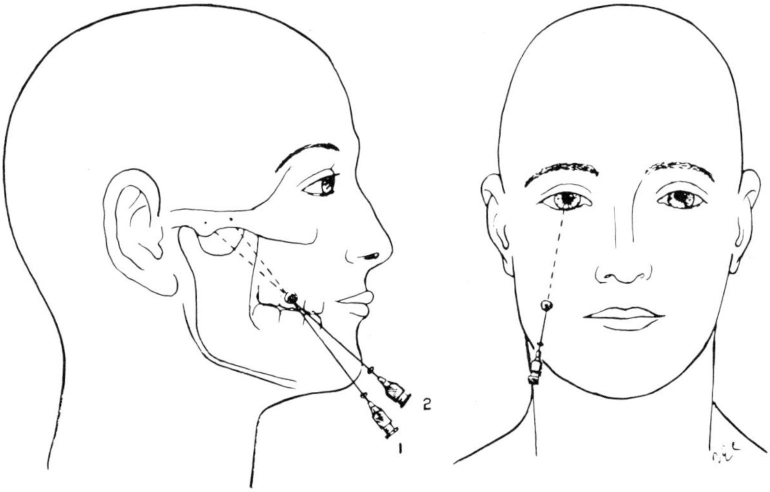

FIG. 4. Gasserian ganglion and mandibular nerve block by the anterolateral technique (Härtel). Note the relationship of the skin wheal to the second upper molar and the direction of the needle in relation to the zygomatic arch (*lateral view*) and to the pupil of the eye (*anterior view*). (Courtesy of J. J. Bonica, *The Management of Pain,* Lea & Febiger, Philadelphia, 1953).

lancinating sensations, usually radiating to the lower jaw and ear, indicate that the point of the needle is in the right position at the inferior entrance of the foramen. The needle is then advanced until the marker is flush with the skin, and presumably its point lies within Meckel's cave or within the ganglion itself. Lack of paresthesia indicates that the needle has been improperly placed, and it should be withdrawn and reinserted correctly. Once the needle is in place, 0.5 ml of local anesthetic is injected to ascertain its correct position. This should produce some analgesia in the region of the Gasserian ganglion. Subsequently, 1 ml of alcohol is injected slowly in increments of 0.2 ml at a time.

The complications of this technique include hematoma of the cheek and herpetic eruptions on the face several days following the injection. Keratitis and corneal ulcers may occur if the eye is not properly cared for. Accidental subarachnoid injection may cause unconsciousness and subsequent involvement of several of the cranial nerves.

TECHNIQUES OF BLOCKING THE MAXILLARY AND MANDIBULAR NERVES

The maxillary and mandibular nerves are best approached by the lateral extra-oral route shown in Fig. 5. The figure on the left indicates the point of entrance into the skin just below the midpoint of the zygomatic arch where a skin wheal is formed for the local anesthetic. For the average patient a 8 cm long 22-gauge security needle is used. The needle is inserted perpendicular to the skin and advanced slowly until the lateral pterygoid plate is contacted. To carry out maxillary nerve block, the needle is withdrawn until its point is in the subcutaneous region; it is then reinserted so that it will pass slightly anteriorly and superiorly and advance until its point enters the pterygopalatine fossa and contacts the maxillary nerve therein (needle 2). In carrying out mandibular nerve block, needle 1 is withdrawn and reinserted in a direction slightly posterior. It is advanced until its point contacts the mandibular nerve just below the foramen ovale (needle 3). It is best to inject 0.5 to 0.75 ml. of alcohol intraneurally to produce complete destruction of the nerves.

TECHNIQUE OF BLOCKING THE GLOSSOPHARYNGEAL AND VAGUS NERVES

Figure 6 depicts the technique of blocking the glossopharyngeal and vagus nerves. The figure on the left shows the site where the skin wheal is formed, approximately midway between the posterior border of the mandible and tip of the mastoid process. The needle is inserted perpendicular to the skin and advanced until its point impinges on the styloid process, as depicted by

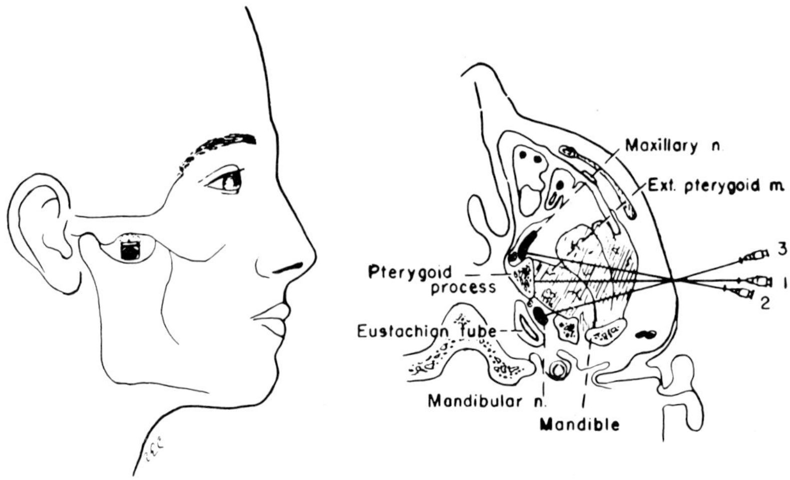

FIG. 5. Diagram depicting the technique of maxillary and mandibular nerve block by the lateral extra-oral route. **Left:** The point of entrance into the skin is just below the midpoint of the zygomatic arch. **Right:** A schematic cross-section. The point of the needle (needle 1) is impinging on the lateral pterygoid plate. To carry out maxillary nerve block, the needle is withdrawn until its point is in the subcutaneous region and then reinserted so that it will pass slightly anteriorly and superiorly, and advance until its point enters the pterygopalatine fossa and contacts the maxillary nerve therein (needle 2). In carrying out mandibular nerve block, needle 1 is withdrawn and reinserted in a direction slightly posterior. It is advanced until its point contacts the mandibular nerve just below the foramen ovale (needle 3). After contacting each nerve and eliciting paresthesia, 1 to 2 ml of solution is injected. (Courtesy of J. J. Bonica, *Clinical Applications of Diagnostic and Therapeutic Nerve Blocks,* Charles C Thomas, Springfield, Ill., 1959.)

needle 1 in the cross-sectional diagram on the right. The needle is then withdrawn and redirected so that it will pass anterior to the styloid process and slightly deeper until its point is in contact with the glossopharyngeal nerve (needle 2). The vagus nerve is blocked by passing the needle posterior to the styloid process and advancing it about 1 cm deeper than the bone (needle 3). Injection of 3 to 5 ml of solution is sufficient.

RESULTS

Table 1 lists the neurolytic cranial nerve blocks performed during the past 11 years by the senior author in patients with malignant tumors localized in the areas innervated by the trigeminal nerve. As may be noted, most of the procedures have involved the gasserian ganglion block, which was carried out in a total of 371 patients representing 41% of all the cranial nerve block procedures done. For blocking the branches of the trigeminal nerve we have used exclusively absolute alcohol. On blocking the gasserian ganglion we used alcohol in 267 cases. Phenol in glycerine 7.5% solution has been in-

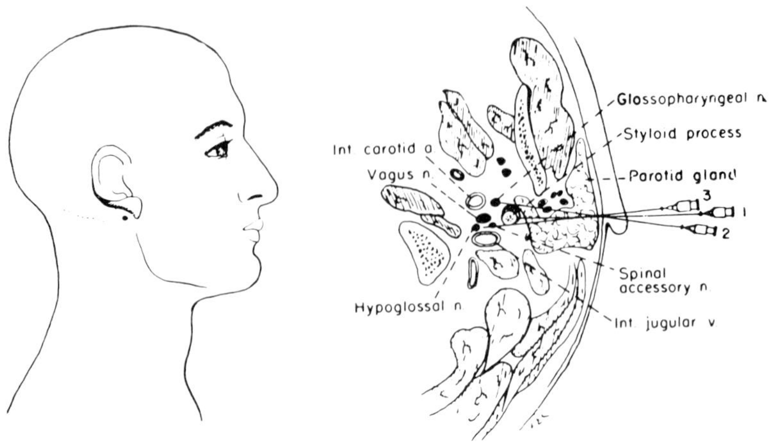

FIG. 6. Technique of blocking the glossopharyngeal and vagus nerves. **Left:** The site where the skin wheal is formed, approximately midway between the posterior border of the mandible and tip of the mastoid process. The needle is inserted perpendicular to the skin and advanced until its point impinges on the styloid process, as depicted by needle 1 in the cross-sectional diagram on the right. The needle is then withdrawn and redirected so that it will pass anterior to the styloid process and slightly deeper until its point is in contact with the glossopharyngeal nerve (needle 2). The vagus nerve is blocked by passing the needle posterior to the styloid process and advancing it about 1 cm deeper than the bone (needle 3). Injection of 3 to 5 ml of solution is sufficient. (Courtesy of J. J. Bonica, *Clinical Applications of Diagnostic and Therapeutic Nerve Blocks,* Charles C Thomas, Springfield, Ill., 1959.)

jected in 82 patients. Early in our series we carried out 22 gasserian ganglion blocks with hypertonic saline, but we have given it up due to poor results. Phenol in glycerine for blocking the gasserian ganglion is well tolerated by the patient, and its injection is painless. The only disadvantage is the need of a larger needle, usually a 20-gauge needle; otherwise, it is difficult to inject the phenol. With a larger needle there is risk of hemorrhage and/or fistula along the path of the needle.

TABLE 1. *Neurolytic cranial nerve blocks (July, 1966 to July, 1977)*

Type of block	Absolute alcohol	Phenol in glycerine	Hypertonic saline	Total
Gasserian ganglion	267	82	22	371 (41%)
Supraorbital	89			89 (9.8%)
Maxillary	57			57 (6.3%)
Infraorbital	198			198 (21.8%)
Mandibular	101			101 (11.2%)
Lingual	12			12 (1.3%)
Mental	74			74 (8.2%)
Glossopharyngeal	4			4 (0.4%)
Total	802			906

As the majority of these patients have been treated with some form of radiotherapy when it becomes necessary to block the cervical nerves, this may represent a difficult task owing to the intense fibrosis in the neck area when the cervical chain has been irradiated.

We feel that the posterior approach to the cervical nerves is not precisely an accurate technique and can be very painful for the patient. We prefer to carry out an extradural cervical block with phenol (3). In our hands this technique has proven to be safe and well tolerated by the patient.

REFERENCES

1. Bonica, J. J. (1953): *The Management of Pain.* Lea & Febiger, Philadelphia.
2. Bonica, J. J. (1959): *Clinical Applications of Diagnostic and Therapeutic Nerve Blocks.* Charles C Thomas, Springfield, Ill.
3. Madrid, J. L. (1975): Experience de 363 cas d'analgesie par alcool et phenol. *Cah. Anesthesiol.,* Fr., 23, no. 7, 825–827.
4. Pender, J. W., and Pugh, D. G. (1951): Diagnostic and therapeutic nerve blocks: Necessity for roetgenograms. JAMA, 146:789–801.

Advances in Pain Research and Therapy, Vol. 2,
edited by J. J. Bonica and V. Ventafridda.
Raven Press, New York © 1979.

Celiac (Splanchnic) Plexus Block with Alcohol for Cancer Pain of the Upper Intra-Abdominal Viscera

Daniel C. Moore

The Mason Clinic, Seattle, Washington 98101

Celiac plexus block is the most effective, least hazardous means of palliative therapy for cancer of the upper intra-abdominal viscera (9,10,14). The celiac plexus can be blocked with 50 ml of 50% alcohol without the alteration of motor, sensory, or visceral function which occurs when most other nerves or plexuses are chemically sectioned. Block of this plexus is definitive treatment for intractable pain from cancer that is limited to one or more of the following upper intra-abdominal organs: (a) stomach and/or duodenum, (b) liver, (c) gallbladder, (d) pancreas, and (e) adrenal glands. Its most frequent use is to alleviate pain from cancer of the pancreas.

RESULTS

In the past 30 years, 168 patients with the established diagnosis of cancer of one or more of the previously noted organs have received 186 alcohol celiac plexus block (18 were reblocked) (Table 1). In these 168 patients, the effectiveness of the alcohol block ranged from 5 days to approximately 1 year. Death from the cancer occurred in 2 days to 14 months following the block. Of the 168 patients, 157 (94%) had good to excellent relief of pain. In addition to pain-relief, other side benefits included: (a) less nausea and vomiting; (b) increased food intake and even occasionally a gain in weight; (c) improved bowel motility, with passing of flatus and stool; and (d) elimination or marked reduction of the need for narcotics. From the time of the block until their death, many patients used only tranquilizers, aspirin with or without codeine, or only small doses of narcotics [first 41 cases document this in a previously published article (3)]. Similar results have been reported by others (2,8,17).

In the patients who had little or no relief, the cancer had metastasized beyond the organs innervated by the celiac plexus. Even though the alcohol blocked the celiac plexus, the patients continued to have pain of a different nature, often in a different area, which was as incapacitating. Therefore, it is advisable to perform a diagnostic block with a long-acting local anesthetic

TABLE 1. *Primary site of cancer of patients treated with alcohol celiac plexus block (1947–1977)*

Site	No.
Pancreas	121
Stomach	11
Liver and bile ducts	7
Gallbladder	2
Liver metastases from:	
Retroperitoneal	2
Rectum	1
Uterus and ovary	5
Lung	11
Kidney	2
Esophagus	6
Total	168

drug—namely, 50 ml of 0.25% bupivacaine (Marcaine®) with 1:200,000 epinephrine—prior to employing alcohol.

TECHNICAL CONSIDERATIONS

Celiac plexus block is not too difficult to master, and complications are minimal provided that the physician performing the procedure: (a) knows the anatomy of the plexus; (b) carries out the technique of the block meticulously; (c) injects the stated amount of alcohol; and (e) employs roentgenography, especially while learning the technique, to determine correct placement of the needles. Because of its high efficacy, it should be used more frequently than it is being used at present. The following detailed discussion of the anatomy and technique of the procedure is included with the hope that it will induce more physicians to learn and use the procedure.

Anatomic Bases

The celiac plexus is situated in the prevertebral region at the level of the body of the first lumbar vertebra. It is composed of right and left celiac superior mesenteric and arteriorenal ganglia and a dense network of nerve fibers that connects them. It surrounds the celiac artery and the base of the superior mesenteric artery. It lies in areolar tissue behind the peritoneum, the stomach, and the omental bursa; in front of the crura of the diaphragm and the commencement of the abdominal aorta; and between the suprarenal glands (Fig. 1).

The celiac plexus contains: (a) the endings of the greater splanchnic nerves, which are made up of branches contributed by the fifth to the ninth or tenth thoracic sympathetic ganglia; (b) the endings of the lesser splanchnic

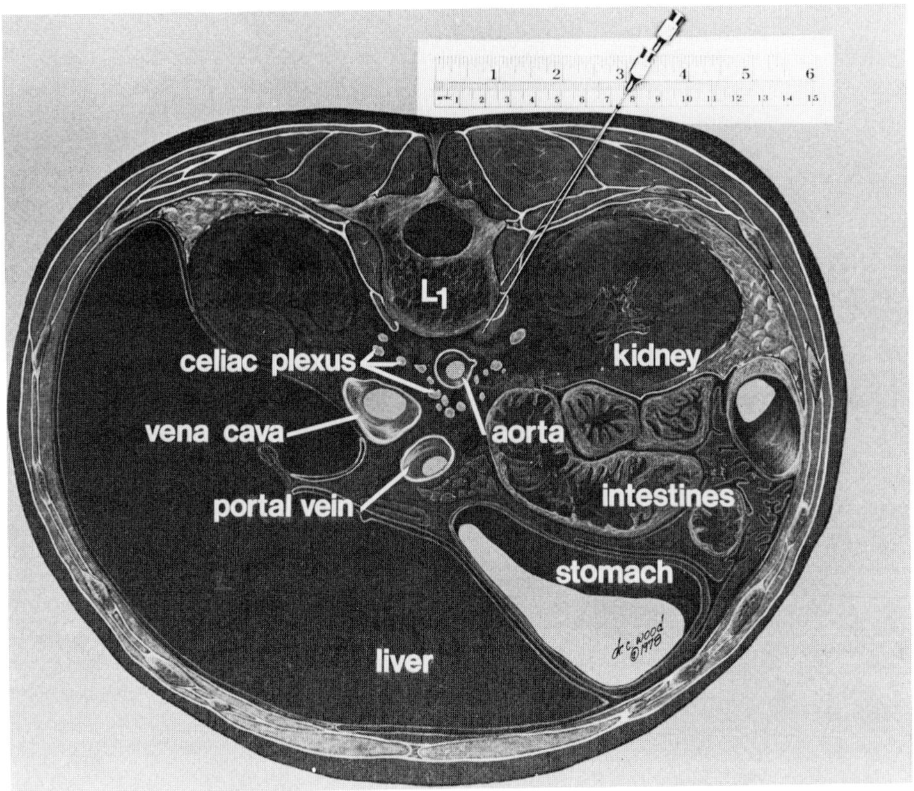

FIG. 1. Schematic cross-section at the level of first lumbar vertebra of a cadaver whose circumference is 36 inches. Size of vertebra, nerves, and organs is scaled accurately. The short-beveled security needles are 20-gauge and 10 cm (4 inches) long.

nerves, composed of branches derived from the ninth, tenth, and sometimes the eleventh thoracic sympathetic ganglia; (c) the endings of the lowest splanchnic nerves, composed of branches contributed by the last thoracic ganglion; and (d) some filaments from the right vagus. The plexus gives off secondary plexuses to the diaphragm, liver, spleen, stomach, adrenal glands, pancreas, ovary and fundus of the uterus, spermatic cord, abdominal aorta, mesentery, small intestine, and colon. While sympathetic and parasympathetic motor fibers themselves do not transmit pain, afferent (sensory) nerve fibers that course with them transmit nociceptive impulses from the viscera.

Technique of Alcohol Block

The posterior approach described by Kappis in 1918, and since advocated in all articles and books describing this block, which were reviewed, is employed (1–17). Prior to performing the block, the anesthetist must explain to the patient its effectiveness in relieving pain, as well as the discomfort experienced during the injection of the alcohol and possible complications. The patient's chart should contain documented evidence of acceptance of the block. As previously mentioned, it is essential to carry out a prognostic block with a local anesthetic before considering alcohol injection. This is done to ascertain that the alcohol block will produce adequate pain relief. For the reasons mentioned below, it is best to carry out the prognostic block at least 12 hr before the alcohol injection is done.

Premedication and/or the Injection of a Local Anesthetic Drug Prior to Injecting Alcohol

The patient is not premedicated or given anesthesia prior to injection of the neurolytic drug, because accurate description of the pain while the alcohol is being injected confirms placement of the needles. Injection of local anesthetic drugs prior to administration of the alcohol is not advised for the same reason, but also because the local anesthetic solution will further dilute the alcohol, resulting in an inadequate block or one of short duration. This does not preclude the use of 3 ml or less of local anesthetic solution while attempts are being made to locate the body of the first lumbar vertebrae.

Position

The patient is placed in the prone position with a pillow between the iliac crests and the rib cage so as to reduce the lumbar curve of the vertebral column to a minimum (Figs. 2 and 3). Any other position increases significantly the likelihood of misplacing the needles.

Landmarks

The landmarks are located by palpation and marked on the skin with a line or an X, using a felt marking pen whose ink when dry will not be washed off by an antiseptic solution (Figs. 2 and 3). The required landmarks are: (a) the spinous processes of the first and second lumbar vertebrae; (b) the cephalad edge of the spinous process of the first lumbar vertebra—the celiac plexus lies at the level of the upper part of the first lumbar vertebra; and (c) a point on the lower borders of the twelfth ribs 5 cm to a *maximum* of 7.5 cm (2 to 3 inches) from the midpoint of the spinous process of either of the marked vertebrae. These distances vary, depending on the size of the patient, and must be measured by a ruler—not estimated (Fig. 1).

The X's marking the cephalad edge of the spinous process of the first lumbar vertebra and those on the twelfth ribs are connected by straight lines. This forms a flat triangle whose apex is seldom more than 2.5 cm (1 inch)

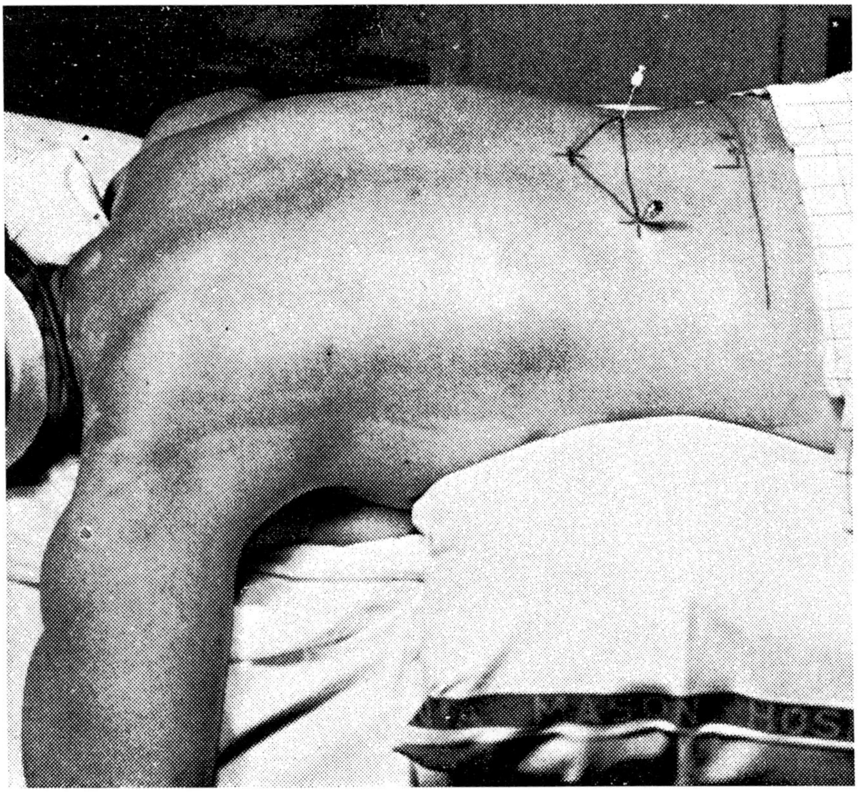

FIG. 2. Lateral view showing the flat triangle formed by joining the three X's which are the landmarks for the celiac plexus block. The straight line between the iliac crests passes through the interspace between the spinous processes of the third and fourth lumbar vertebrae.

above the base (Fig. 2). If the apex of the triangle greatly exceeds 2.5 cm, then either the cephalad edge of the wrong spinous process was marked or the distance from the midline of the spinous process to the 12th rib exceeds 7.5 cm, or both have occurred.

These markings are critical, particularly the maximum of 7.5 cm from the midline to avoid puncture of the kidney or the uteropelvic junction. It is important to remember that the kidneys lie adjacent to the vertebral column and behind the peritoneum, surrounded by loose areolar tissue and a mass of fat (Fig. 4). They are in the same compartment with the celiac plexus, the aorta, and the vena cava (Fig. 1). Moreover, the medial surfaces of the upper and lower poles of the kidney lie approximately 5 cm (2 inches) and 7 cm (3 inches), respectively, from the midline with the right kidney 1 cm lower than the left. Also, the upper poles are at the level of the twelfth thoracic vertebra and the lower poles at the upper border of the body of the

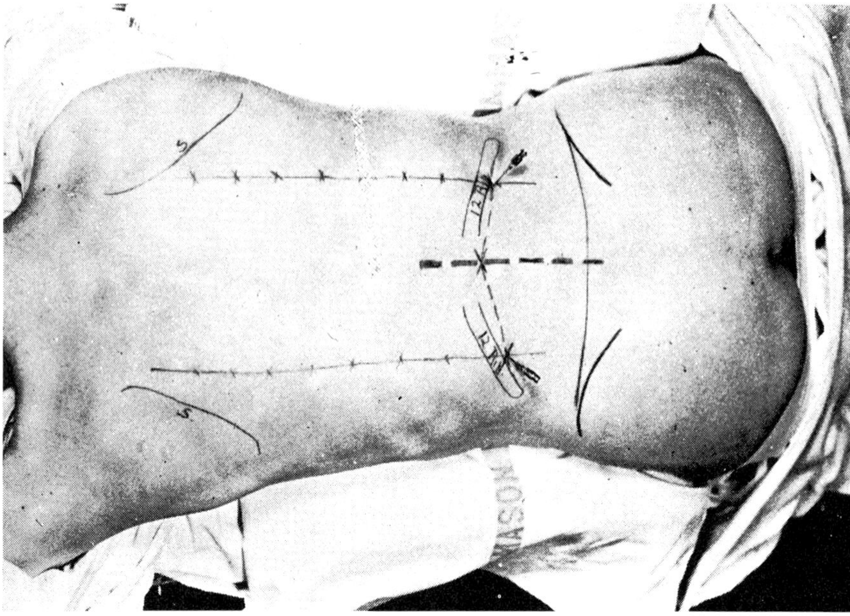

FIG. 3. Posterior view of 4-inch (10.2-cm) needles in place for the execution of the celiac plexus block. Note the direction of the needles as they course along the line from the twelfth rib to the superior edge of the spinous process of the first lumbar vertebra. Also the 55-degree angle formed by the shaft of the needles and the skin.

third lumbar vertebra. Finally, the twelfth ribs lie over the kidneys (Fig. 5).

Therefore, if puncture of the kidneys is to be avoided, the needles must pass medial to them in the 2 to 3 cm (¾ to 1¼ inches) of tissue which lies between the kidneys and the lumbar vertebrae (Figs. 1 and 6). The needle's point may be placed intravascularly or subarachnoidally and withdrawn prior to injecting alcohol with little chance of a complication resulting. Contrarily, if the kidney or the ureteropelvic junction is traumatized when the needle is inserted [and this will occur consistently when the distance for inserting the needle is greater than 7.5 cm (3 inches) from the midline] and if alcohol is injected into or in close proximity to the kidney or the ureteropelvic junction, a serious inflammation may result (17). Sequelae of this may be degeneration of the kidney, extravasation of urine from the ureter, and so forth, requiring nephrectomy.

Neurolytic Solution

A solution of 50 ml of 50% alcohol is preferred. This concentration is prepared immediately prior to its injection by opening ampules of absolute alcohol and mixing their contents with normal saline. Mixing alcohol with a

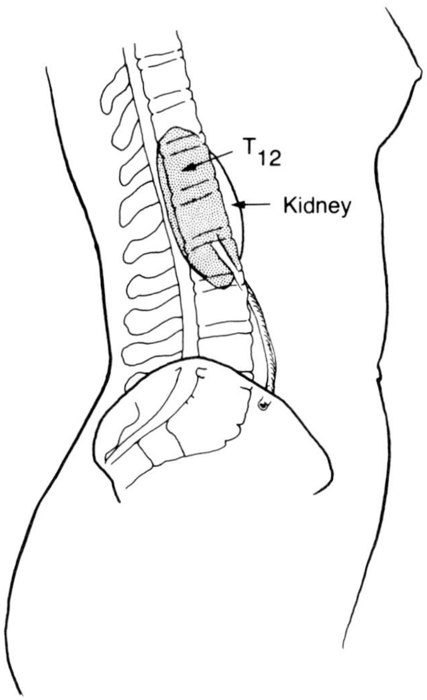

FIG. 4. Schematic drawing showing position of kidneys lateral and opposite to the vertebral column.

local anesthetic solution rather than normal saline will somewhat decrease but not abolish the severe pain from the alcohol, which lasts for 5 to 10 sec. Since the pain from the alcohol is still excruciating and since such a mixture may result in the test dose's giving signs which are difficult to evaluate, I use only normal saline for dilution. Following the injection of the alcohol, the

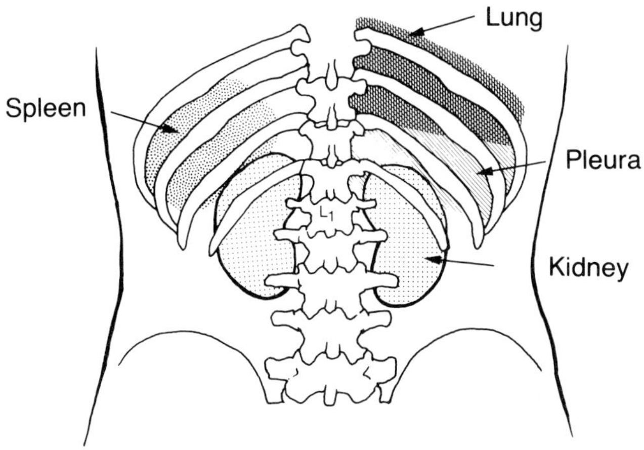

FIG. 5. Schematic drawing of back of the lumbar region, showing position of kidneys in relationship to vertebrae, twelfth rib, pleura, lungs, and spleen.

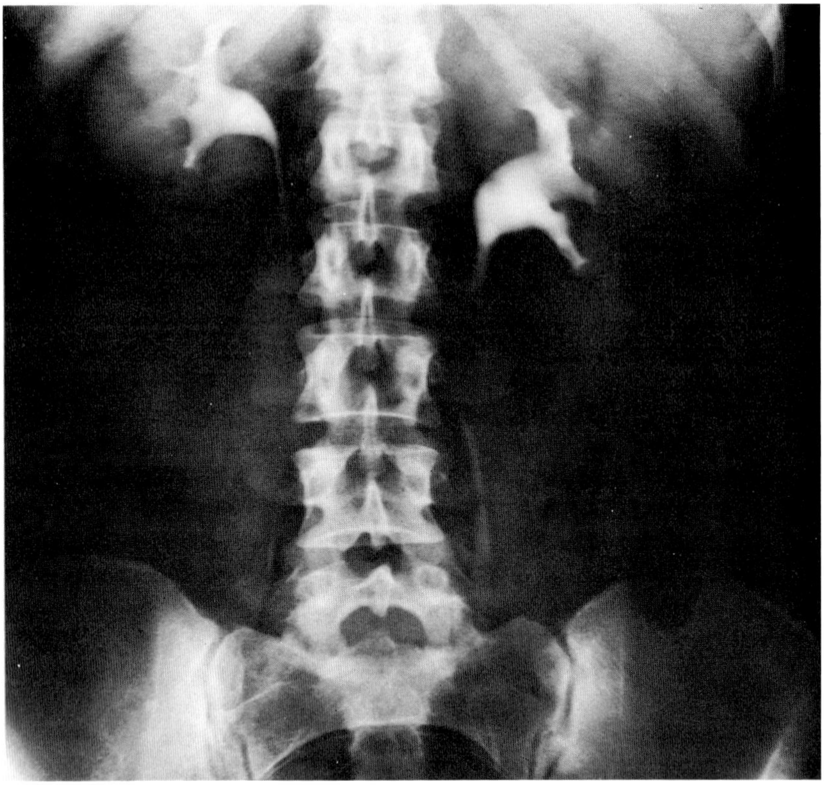

FIG. 6. Intravenous pyelogram showing relationship of kidneys and ureteropelvic junction to vertebrae.

cancer pain is usually markedly reduced or completely abolished in 2 to 10 min, but on occasion 24 hr may be required for maximum effect. The effects of alcohol last 3 weeks to 6 months and on occasion longer. If the block dissipates prior to the patient's death, it is repeated.

Using a smaller amount and stronger concentrations of alcohol is not advocated. The described technique depends on the fact that the solution is injected safely away from the vital organs and diffuses so as to bathe the entire celiac plexus. Pinpoint accuracy of needle placement at the celiac plexus is not necessary. Furthermore, when smaller amounts of absolute alcohol are used, the incidence of unsatisfactory results is higher and the destructive effects greater than required for neurolysis. This increases the possibility of damage to other organs adjacent to the celiac plexus.

Although 50 ml of 6 to 7% aqueous phenol may be used in the same way as alcohol, alcohol is preferred. The onset of analgesia with phenol is somewhat slower, the incidence of satisfactory block less, and the duration shorter. For these reasons, I do not use it.

Placement of the Needles

Although a small-gauge needle may be less painful, two 20-gauge needles are employed, for when they are correctly placed there is no resistance to the injection of the anesthetic solution, and the anesthetist has the feeling that he is injecting intravenously. This feeling indicates correct placement of the needle. If a smaller-gauge needle—for example, a 22-gauge—is used instead, this feeling is decreased, and the physician cannot tell whether the resistance is due to the needle's gauge or whether the needle's point is misplaced under the periosteum of the vertebrae, in an organ's wall, or in other tissue. In the average patient, a 10-cm (4-inch) needle will be sufficient, but on occasion, a 12.5- or 15-cm (5- or 6-inch) needle will be required if the patient is large and/or obese. If in the average-sized patient a needle longer than 10 cm (4 inches) is needed to contact the body of the first lumbar vertebra, the X at the lower border of the twelfth rib is incorrectly placed more than 7.5 cm (3 inches) from the midline of the back.

The following steps are used in blocking the celiac plexus:

The physician stands by the patient at the side into which the needle is to be inserted. A skin wheal is made at the X's on the lower borders of the twelfth ribs using a 26-gauge or smaller needle—if a 30-gauge needle is available, it is used. One of the 20-gauge needles is introduced through the skin wheal at the X at the lower edge of the twelfth rib at a 45-degree angle to the skin. Using the line of the side of the marked triangle as a guide, the needle is slowly advanced as 3 ml or less of local anesthetic solution is injected so as to make its advancement less painful. When the needle contacts the cephalad part of the body of the first lumbar vertebra, the depth of the needle is noted (Fig. 1). The needle should have contacted the lateral side of the body of the vertebra just below the body's midpoint.

To be in the correct position for the celiac plexus block, the needle must be inserted 2 to 2.5 cm (¾ to 1 inch) deeper than the lateral side of the midpoint of the body of the first lumbar vertebra. The needle is then withdrawn 2.5 cm (1 inch), and the angle between its shaft and the skin lateral to the needle is increased by 5 to 10 degrees—that is, from 45 degrees to 50 or 55 degrees—and then the needle is again advanced. This maneuver is repeated, increasing the angle slightly each time, until the needle is felt to slip off the body of the vertebra. At this point, it is advanced another 2 to 2.5 cm (¾ to 1 inch). Now its point should lie in prevertebral areolar tissue which contains the celiac plexus (Figs. 1, 6, and 7). In the average patient, the distance from the skin to the celiac plexus is usually 8.8 to 10 cm (3½ to 4 inches).

So the needle is "walked" slowly anteriorly on the lateral surface of the vertebra; not infrequently contact with the bone is lost, but the needle point is felt to enter into a dense fibrous tissue, which is the periosteum of the vertebra. The periosteum is a valuable landmark because with the next withdrawal of the needle and another slight increase of the angle of the shaft with the skin, the needle will slide anterior to the body of the vertebra. Also, when the needle is inserted *very* slowly on the left side past the body of the vertebra, frequently the pulsation of the aorta may be felt or seen if the needle hub is released. This indicates that the needle is correctly placed. For this reason, placement of the needle first on the left side and then on the right side may be preferable, as the needle's depth on the left side may then be used as a guide for the right side. When the needle's bevel inadvertently is placed in either the aorta or the vena cava, as evidenced by blood appearing at the hub, the needle is withdrawn slowly until blood no longer appears at the hub. Then it is withdrawn another 0.2 to 0.3 cm (⅛ inch) to be certain that it is not in the vessel wall. Puncture of either the aorta or the vena cava is no indication to discontinue the block.

After placing the needle on one side, a second is placed in the opposite side in the same fashion. When the technique is being mastered or in the event of abnormal pathology, posteroanterior and lateral roentgenograms

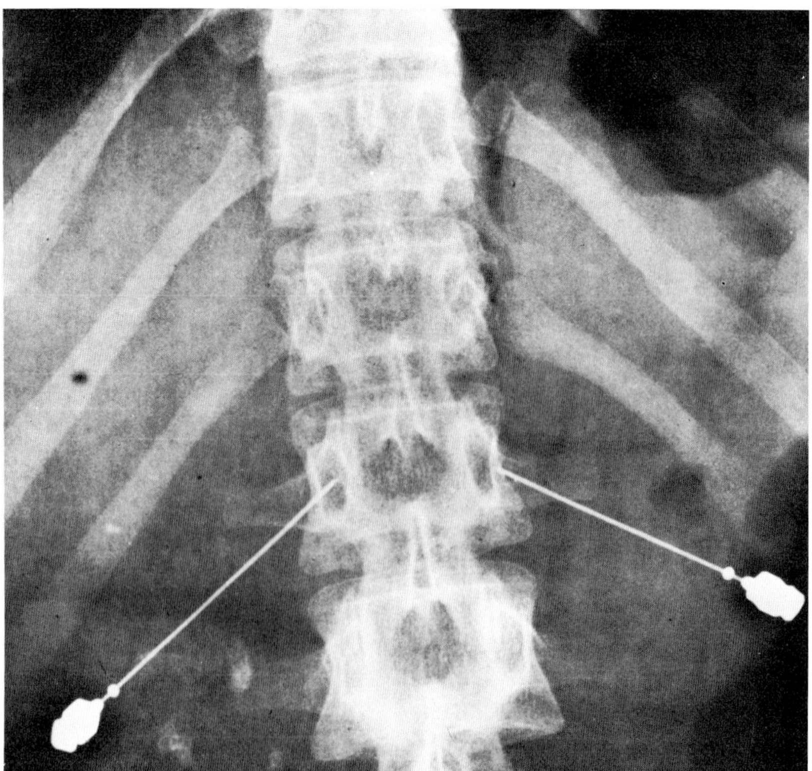

FIG. 7. Posterior-anterior view of needles correctly placed anterior to the body of the first lumbar vertebra.

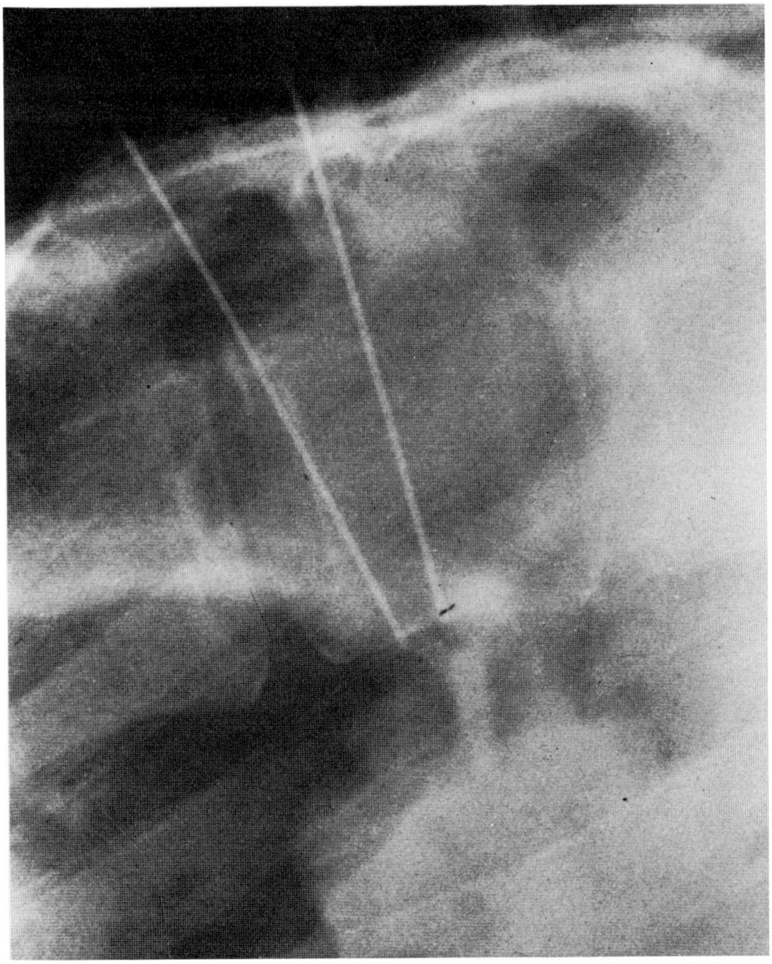

FIG. 8. Lateral view of Fig. 7.

should be taken at this point. These help to rule out epidural or subarachnoid placement of the needle point and confirm its placement anterior to the midpoint of the body of the first lumbar vertebra (Figs. 7 and 8). However, roentgenograms do not rule out intravascular placement. Ideally the needle point should be in this position, but if roentgenograms show the point of the needle to be anterior to the caudad part of the vertebra (rather than at its midpart), nothing further needs to be done because the solution will spread to involve the entire plexus.

After both needles are in place, 2 ml of air is injected through each needle to clear any plugs of tissue which may have entered the needle during its insertion. Then an attempt is made to aspirate for blood or spinal fluid.

When both needles are considered to be properly placed, the syringe filled with dilute alcohol is adapted to the needle and the patient is again warned of the type of pain the alcohol will cause. Aspiration is repeated and if nothing is obtained, 20 to 25 ml of the alcohol are injected at the rate of 2 to 3 ml per sec. As the neurolytic drug is injected, the patient will usually cry out: (a) "It burns like fire," (b) "It is difficult to breathe," or (c) "I cannot stand the pain." Such pain is diagnostic of correct placement of the alcohol, and it subsides in a period of 5 to 10 sec.

Immediately following the injection of one side and even if the patient is still having pain, disconnect the syringe from the needle, *leaving the needle in place,* and refill the syringe. Warn the patient that the pain may increase, and inject another 20 to 25 ml of the alcohol through the second needle. After injection of the first side, the needle is not withdrawn because when the bevels of both needles are correctly placed inside the fascial compartment containing the celiac plexus, injection through the second needle will often force solution to reflux from the first needle. This is another valuable sign that the needles are correctly placed. Subsequently, 2 ml of air are injected through each needle to avoid spilling onto the first lumbar nerve as the needle is withdrawn. Both needles are then removed.

COMPLICATIONS

With the exception of the low blood pressure from block of the celiac plexus and pain in the back from the destructive effects of the neurolytic drug, the complications of celiac plexus block are a result of incorrect landmarks, inaccurately placed needles, or both. If there is any doubt regarding needle placement, posteroanterior and lateral roentgenograms should be taken.

Arterial Hypotension

Following completion of the block, the majority of patients experience hypotension from interruption of the vasoconstrictor fibers to a wide area and the "pooling" of blood in the viscera, particularly in the omentum, the small bowel, and the colon. In the young patient, who can compensate by vasoconstriction in the unaffected vessels, it causes no problem. However, older, arteriosclerotic patients frequently feel faint when they sit up or are ambulated. In 3 days or less, they usually compensate for this splanchnic vascular dilatation.

Oral administration of ephedrine is effective to combat this type of hypotension, but we do not use it. Rather, the patient is warned about fainting or feeling faint when in an upright position or ambulating, and the following orders are written on the patient's chart: (a) wrap both legs to midthigh with a 6-inch elastic bandage or apply elastic stockings; (b) apply a tight abdominal binder before ambulation; (c) when the patient is sitting up for the first time, a nurse should be present and ambulation should be allowed only with an assistant on each side; (d) check blood pressure and pulse every 15 min for 2 hr; and (e) if systolic pressure falls below one-third of the patient's normal, notify Dr. ______, telephone number ______.

Pain

While the cancer pain may be relieved immediately or within a few hours, the patient may experience dull, aching back pain for 24 to 48 hr following the block. Presumably, the tissue irritation from the alcohol causes the pain in the back at the site of the injection. For control, this pain may require small amounts of an analgesic compound—for example, Empirin® #3 which contains phenacetin, 150 mg; acetylsalicylic acid, 200 mg; caffeine, 30 mg; and codeine, 30 mg.

Subarachnoid Injection

When the needles for celiac plexus block are introduced into the skin more than 7.5 cm (3 inches) from the midline and/or at an angle with the skin of less than 45 degrees, the needle may enter the subarachnoid space through an intervertebral foramen or between the lamina of the vertebra.

In more than 3,000 celiac plexus blocks performed with either a local anesthetic solution or alcohol, this has occurred 18 times (0.006%). In all but one case (0.0003%), the spinal fluid dripped from the 20-gauge needle and the needle was withdrawn and placed correctly in the prevertebral space. In the one patient who did receive a subarachnoid injection, the resident physician had not done the prescribed tests prior to injecting the agent. Fortunately, the ensuing total block resulted from a local anesthetic solution and its effects disappeared in a few hours.

Epidural or Lumbar Somatic Nerve Block

Either of these complications may occur if the needle rests in the epidural space, lateral rather than anterior to the body of the vertebra, or in the psoas muscle. In one instance, in an obese, terminally ill woman who had massive ascites, a block was attempted with the patient in a lateral position—a position not used by the author. This compromise in technique coupled with the anatomic distortions of obesity resulted in spread of the alcohol solution to the nerves of the lumbar plexus, and she developed a partial unilateral leg paralysis. Chemical neuropathy with neuralgia (pain) of the first lumbar nerve from slight spillage of the neurolytic drug has been reported, but none of our patients developed such complications.

Puncture of the Lung, Kidney, Blood Vessels, and Other Viscera

Unless a complication occurs, it is difficult to evaluate whether the needles used in celiac plexus block puncture these organs and, if so, how often. Irrespective of the anesthetist's ability, at times they must. However, when a local anesthetic solution is used, complications resulting from this kind of puncture must be minimal and usually go unrecognized. Contrarily, when a neurolytic drug is injected, serious complications (particularly from puncture of the kidney) may result, requiring surgical intervention.

Puncture of the viscera, with peritonitis and hemoperitoneum following a celiac plexus block has not been seen by the author, and none has been noted in the literature. However, grossly bloody urine has been observed once in a patient who also had a pneumothorax from the same block and on whom the landmark for the insertion of the needle was misplaced 12.5 cm (5 inches) from the midline rather than the stated maximum of 7.5 cm (3 inches). Such complications—particularly puncture of the kidney—as previously noted, are more likely to occur when: (a) the needle is inserted more than 3 inches (7.5 cm) from the midline of the spinous process of the first or second lumbar vertebra; (b) the body of the first lumbar vertebra is not contacted by the needle's point prior to advancing it anterior to this vertebra; (c) the needle's point does not lie immediately in front of the body of the lumbar vertebrae but lies 2 cm (¾ inch) or more lateral and/or anterior to the body; and (d) attempts are made to place the needle's point higher than the body of the first lumbar vertebra—that is, at the body of the eleventh thoracic vertebra, as in the supradiaphragmatic technique, which is not advocated by the author.

The following must be emphasized. The major portion of the celiac plexus lies in front of the aorta, but the anesthetist should not attempt to put the needles there because puncture of vital organs is more likely. If the advice of a roentgenologist is sought regarding placement of the needles and if the needles are *correctly* placed 1 cm (⅜ inch) anterior to the body of the vertebra, the roentgenologist may state that the needles are not correctly placed because they are behind rather than in front of the projected location of the aorta (Figs. 7 and 8). *The anesthetist should not move the needles.* The 50 ml of solution will diffuse sufficiently to compensate for the placement of the needle behind rather than in front of the aorta.

Deposit of the neurolytic solution in dilute concentrations in either the aorta or the vena cava can result, but this has not occurred in our series of celiac plexus blocks. Carefully performed aspiration tests and the use of a 20-gauge needle evidently have avoided this complication. Even if 50 ml of 50% alcohol were injected intravascularly, it is doubtful that any untoward effects would result because alcohol infusions are often used for control of pain and other therapy. Whether absolute alcohol or phenol would be equally innocuous is questionable.

Necrosis of Contents in Close Proximity to Celiac Plexus

While necrosis of tissue in the retroperitoneal space from 50 ml to 50% alcohol might be anticipated, repeat autopsy observations have shown no grossly discernable changes.

Blood Levels of Alcohol

Alcohol is readily absorbed following the block as shown by the rapid rise of the drug over the first 20 min. The maximum level measured was 0.021 g/100 ml which is about one-fifth of the common legal standard for intoxication (16).

CONCLUSION

To reiterate, celiac plexus block using a bilateral approach and 50 ml of 50% alcohol relieved safely intractable pain of cancer of the upper intra-abdominal viscera in 94% of patients. Therefore, every physician who treats cancer pain should learn this block.

REFERENCES

1. Adriani, J. (1954): *Nerve Block.* Charles C Thomas, Springfield, Ill.
2. Bonica, J. J. (1953): *The Management of Pain.* Lea & Febiger, Philadelphia.
3. Bridenbaugh, L. D., Moore, D. C., and Campbell, D. D. (1964): Management of upper abdominal cancer pain. *JAMA,* 190:877.
4. Brown, E. M., and Kunjappan, V. (1975): Single-needle lateral approach for lumbar sympathetic block. *Anesth. Analg.,* 54:567.
5. Collins, V. J. (1976): *Principles of Anesthesiology,* 2nd ed. Lea & Febiger, Philadelphia.
6. Dale, W. A. (1952): Splanchnic block in treatment of acute pancreatitis. *Surgery,* 32:605.
7. Hale, D. E. (1963): *Anesthesiology,* 2nd ed. F. A. Davis, Philadelphia.
8. Jones, J. J., and Gough, D. (1977): Coeliac plexus block with alcohol for relief of upper intra-abdominal pain due to cancer. *Ann. R. Coll. Surg. Engl.,* 59:46.
9. Kappis, M. (1919): Sensibilität und lokale anästhesia im chirurgischen gebiet der bauchhöhle mit besonderer berücksichtigung der splanchnicus-anästhesie. *Bruns' Beiträge Zur Klin. Cher.,* 15:161.
10. Labat, G. (1922): *Regional Anesthesia,* 1st ed. Saunders, Philadelphia.
11. Lundy, J. (1945): *Clinical Anesthesia.* Saunders, Philadelphia.
12. Macintosh, R. R., and Bryce-Smith, R. (1953): *Local Anesthesia: Abdominal Surgery.* E. & S. Livingstone, Edinburgh.
13. Moore, D. C. (1965): *Regional Block,* 4th ed. Charles C Thomas, Springfield, Ill.
14. Pauchet, V., Sourdat, P., Labat, G., and D'ormont, R. D. B. (1927): *L'Anesthesie Regionale.* Gaston Dion et Cie, Paris.
15. Southworth, J. L., and Hingson, R. A. (1946): *Conduction Anesthesia.* Lippincott, Philadelphia.
16. Thompson, G. E., Moore, D. C., Bridenbaugh, L. D., et al. (1977): Abdominal pain and alcohol celiac plexus nerve block. *Anesth. Analg.,* 56:1.
17. Walton, F. A. (1952): Coeliac ganglion block. *Can. Med. Assoc. J.,* 67:342.

Advances in Pain Research and Therapy, Vol. 2,
edited by J. J. Bonica and V. Ventafridda.
Raven Press, New York © 1979.

Chemical Hypophysectomy

John Miles

Centre for Pain Relief, Department of Neurosurgery, Walton Hospital, Liverpool, England

For the last 5 years, in the Centre for Pain Relief in Liverpool, we have been using Moricca's technique of alcohol injection into the pituitary gland for the relief of pain in patients with advanced cancer (1,2). We prefer to call it just that, *alcohol injection into the pituitary gland,* rather than "chemical hypophysectomy" or Moricca's term of "neuroadenolysis" because we would rather *not* imply that the undoubted pain-relieving effect that results, is due necessarily to destruction of the pituitary gland. As you will note, many other exciting explanations are possible.

The technique has been used only when the pain syndrome seemed unlikely to respond to conventional methods such as regional nerve blocks or cordotomy. It has been used particularly for widespread bilateral pain, pain in the head and neck, or midline body pain.

We originally considered that it could be used as an alternative to cordotomy in patients with cancer so advanced as to render the patient unfit for cordotomy. This we no longer believe. Patients being considered for pituitary alcohol injection require as much or more biologic resilience if they are to benefit from it, than do those undergoing cordotomy.

TECHNICAL ASPECTS

To date we have performed 179 injections in 122 patients (Table 1). In 75 instances a single injection was made, but frequently more than one needle was introduced to obtain more complete injection into the gland. Regardless of whether one or more needles were used, a maximum of 1.25 ml of absolute alcohol was injected in increments of 0.1 to 0.2 ml. In all cases 0.5 ml of contrast medium, either water- or oil-soluble, was injected prior to the alcohol. Only one injection was made if a good result had been obtained, or when the patient did not survive long enough to require subsequent injection. Occasionally, although no relief was obtained by the first injection, some other form of treatment was considered more appropriate than repeating it. Otherwise multiple injections were expected.

Thirty-seven patients had a second injection when the pain returned, or if the relief was not sufficient, or when dealing with carcinoma from the breast

TABLE 1. *Pituitary alcohol injection (total experience, 1973–1978)*

Total:	179 Injections in 122 patients
	75 Single
	37 Twice
	10 Three times

when it was considered ethically advisable to achieve pituitary destruction as well as pain-relief. Ten patients underwent a third injection. One to two weeks was the usual interval for elective repeating of the injections.

RESULTS

The quality of pain-relief has been classified as: *excellent* in patients who after the procedure required no analgesics except for perhaps an occasional dose of a nonnarcotic drug; *some relief* was considered to have been achieved when the patient obtained partial relief and would still require nonnarcotic analgesics (but not narcotics) on a regular basis; and *no relief* was considered to occur if the patient still required narcotic analgesics (Table 2).

Seventy-six injections were followed by excellent relief of pain; 59 patients derived some relief of pain, and 26 derived no relief. Eight patients died within the first week and before an assessment was possible. The data on 10 patients are too incomplete to allow accurate assessment.

The duration of pain-relief varied greatly, and so far we have not been able to correlate it with the type of cancer, the sex of the patient, the radiologic evidence of diffusion of contrast within or outside the gland, or even the particular physician who carried out the technique. There have been more than six different doctors administering the procedure.

In the majority of patients the pain-relief has lasted weeks or months (Table 3). The more complete it was, the longer it lasted. The longest relief was most impressive, there being two patients with total suppression of pain for more than 1 year. We cannot guarantee that other medical therapy has not contributed to this relief, but they have certainly had excellent and immediate response without recurrence.

TABLE 2. *Pain-relief after pituitary alcohol injection*

Excellent	76 (42.5%)
Some	59 (33.0%)
None	26 (14.5%)
Died before assessment	8
Untraceable	10
Total	179

TABLE 3. *Duration of pain-relief after pituitary alcohol injection*

Quality	1/52	1/12	3/12	>3/12	Total	Longest
Excellent	17	17	26	16	76	14 months
Some	24	30	5	0	59	6 weeks

TABLE 4. *Types of cancer pain treated by pituitary alcohol injection*

Carcinoma breast	41%
Carcinoma prostate	15%
Carcinoma lung/bronchus	13%
Uterus	10%
Gut (rectum especially)	10%

Pain from almost all forms of cancer has been treated (Table 4). The commonest has been associated with metastases from carcinoma of the breast. The next most frequent has been from carcinoma of the prostate. Usually this has been a picture of slowly progressive infiltration in the pelvic bones or plexus or from distant bony metastases. Usually the sufferer was in good general physical condition. Patients with more fulminating carcinomatoses rarely survive long enough to require surgical treatment specifically for their pain.

SIDE EFFECTS AND COMPLICATIONS

There is a definite morbidity associated with the injection of alcohol into the pituitary gland. There is what one might term an obligatory hormonal morbidity, and this most commonly takes the form of diabetes insipidus. This is common, occurring in over 60% of the patients when their fluid intake and output charts are compared. However, this side effect required treatment in only 20 to 30%. Pitressin® nasal spray is usually sufficient, though Pitressin® injection has been used occasionally. In only 2 cases has the diabetes insipidus continued beyond 6 weeks. Because many of our patients already had had courses of steroids and to prevent corticosteroid deficiency, a dose of 2 mg prednisolone 3 times a day was usually prescribed. It is well to remember that long-surviving patients may require thyroxin.

Morbidity as a result of technical problems occurred, with the most common being cerebrospinal fluid (CSF) rhinorrhea. This occurred to some extent in between 10 and 20% of the patients but usually stopped within a day or so. We have had only 1 patient who took more than 6 weeks to stop leaking. Meningitis must always remain a threat, particularly in the presence of CSF rhinorrhea, and it is our practice to give prophylactive sulfonamide.

Among our patients there have been 2 cases of presumed meningitis successfully treated by antibiotics.

Neurologic complications are of major concern. The most commonly seen complication involves the second and third cranial nerves and is presumably due to the alcohol's diffusing up from the pituitary gland to these structures. In an attempt to minimize this risk, a close observation is kept on the pupils and their ability to react in response to light during the alcohol injection. Five patients have apparently had some deficiency in function of either the second or third cranial nerve following injection. Two of these developed optic nerve impairment with visual-field defects which were marked in the first few days and gradually diminished over succeeding weeks. It is probable that in each of these incidents some permanent deficiency resulted.

Two patients have appeared to show definite evidence of hypothalamic injury. In each there was impairment of conscious level that progressively developed in the days following injection, and in one this was associated with hemiparesis. In each case autopsy confirmed extensive infarction of the pituitary stalk and suggested infarction of the hypothalamus with separation of the ependyma.

We have had 8 deaths within the first week following injections. Two appeared to result from technical failures associated with the transphenoidal puncture. In one of these patients the needle passed through an unsuspected empyema of the sphenoidal sinus which resulted in fatal meningitis. The other patient had a bleeding diathesis associated with her cancer and had a fatal hemorrhage following the puncture. Prior to the injection, the majority of patients were in very poor physical condition due to the advanced state of their cancer. It is this fairly recent experience with some serious complications that has caused us to call into question our previous attitude regarding the fitness of the patient to undertake this procedure. We now feel that the patient must be at least as fit as we consider necessary before undertaking cordotomy.

MECHANISM OF PAIN-RELIEF

As there is usually no alteration in the patient's neurologic and psychologic functions when he is relieved from his pain by this method, we have been very interested to discover an explanation for the analgesic effects. As previously mentioned, in our clinical practice we routinely inject a contrast medium, prior to the injection of alcohol. Consequent, we have observed spread of the contrast out of the gland up the stalk into the hypothalamus and even into the ventricular system in some 20% of patients (Fig. 1). This spread is easily observed during the monitoring of the injection and occurs without excessive pressure. After the route has been opened up, either immediately or late in the injection, all subsequent increments are seen to follow briskly the same track, unless the needle is moved.

We performed a study on cadavers using the same technique but injecting

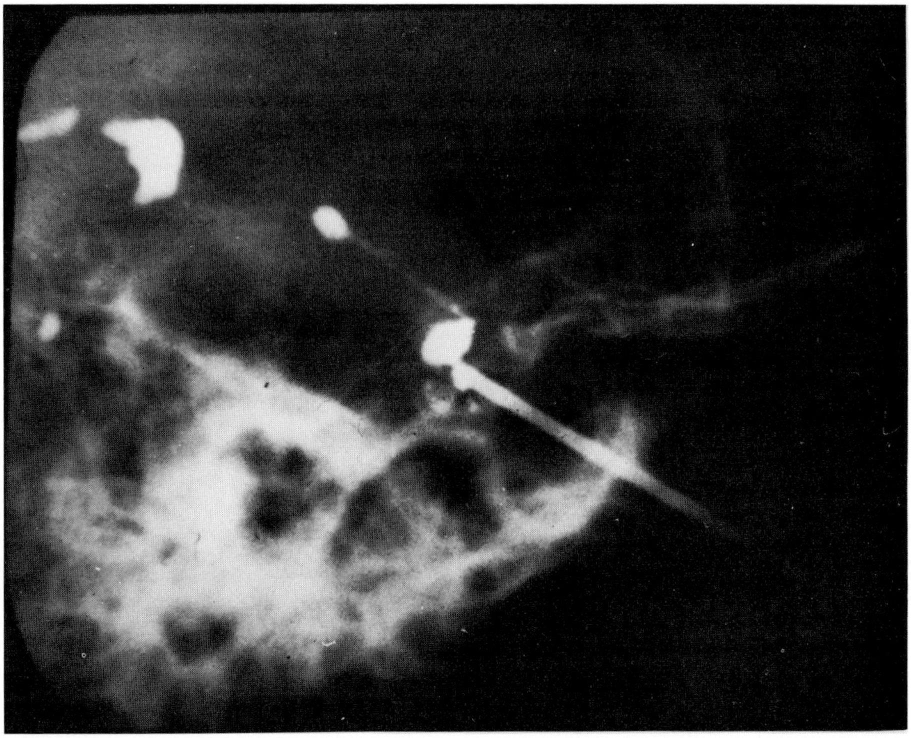

FIG. 1. Lateral radiography of skull, showing spread of iophendylate from the pituitary gland, up the stalk, into the hypothalamus, and into the third ventricle.

a mixture of contrast medium and India ink and observed the same radiologic spread upward to the hypothalamus. However, we also noticed a free movement out of the pituitary gland via the hypophyseal veins to the systemic blood circulation (Fig. 2).

Serial sections of the pituitary, its stalk, and the hypothalamus showed the India ink particles in the portal venous system of the stalk and hypothalamus (Fig. 3). Rupture of the upper ends of the system appeared to have occurred with India ink in the parenchyma of the hypothalamus and within the ependyma of the ventricles.

This suggested the possibility of injury to the hypothalamus, to the hypothalamic-thalamic pathways, and perhaps even the forebrain bundle. Autopsy evidence supported this hypothesis and perhaps explains the very rapid (within minutes or hours) pain-relief that occurs in 10 to 15% of patients. However, since the majority of patients achieve their pain-relief gradually and progressively over the second, third and fourth days, we wondered about the possibility of a chemical explanation.

With the help of Professor H. W. Kosterlitz of Aberdeen University, we

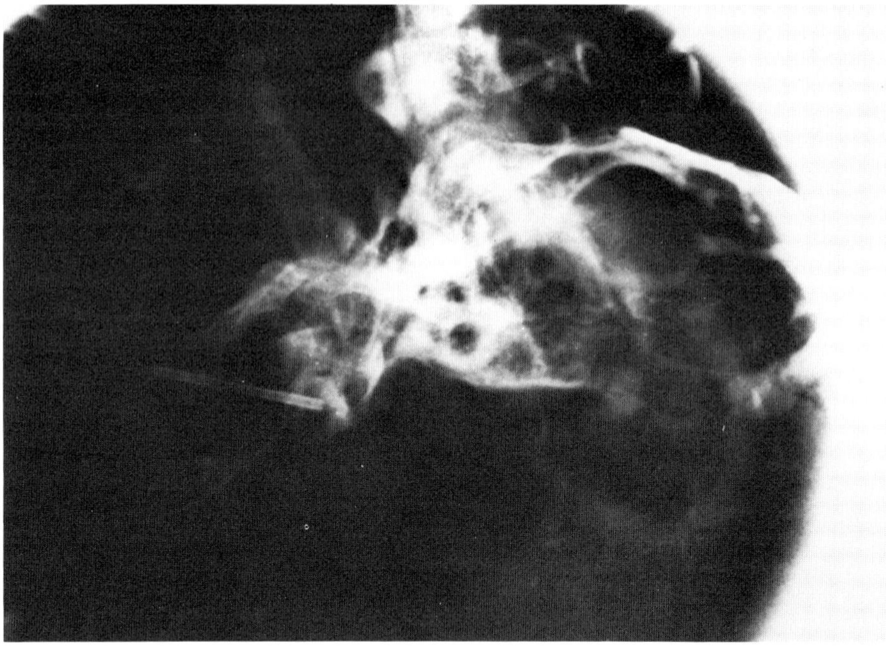

FIG. 2. Lateral radiograph of skull of cadaver during injection of Meglumine Iocarmate showing spread of the contrast medium out into the intracranial veins and sinuses.

sampled lumbar CSF, before, immediately after, and 5 hr after pituitary injection but have failed to show an elevation in either metencephalin or beta endorphin. Nevertheless, we are still wondering about the possibility of this effect's being associated with the currently exciting pituitary/hypothalamic peptide system. Dr. David Bowsher of the Neurobiology Unit at Liverpool University has been challenging patients, whose pain has been relieved by pituitary alcohol injection, with an injection of naloxone. In his initial series of 12 patients, 4 have experienced definite evidence of return of their original pain. This return occurs slowly after 15 to 20 min and lasts for 1 hr and then resolves. Several patients have developed forms of narcotic-withdrawal syndrome that might be associated with their previous medication.

With the help of Dr. Derek Smyth of the Medical Institute for Research, Mill Hill, London, we have just begun to search for the presence and possible elevation of beta endorphin in the blood of patients undergoing pituitary injection. The cadaver study suggests the possibility that there might be a flushing out from the pituitary via the hypophyseal veins of some analgesic peptide, and we await these results.

Naturally we have been interested to know how much pituitary or hypothalamic hormonal suppression results from alcohol injection. It is extremely difficult to subject these patients who are suffering severely from

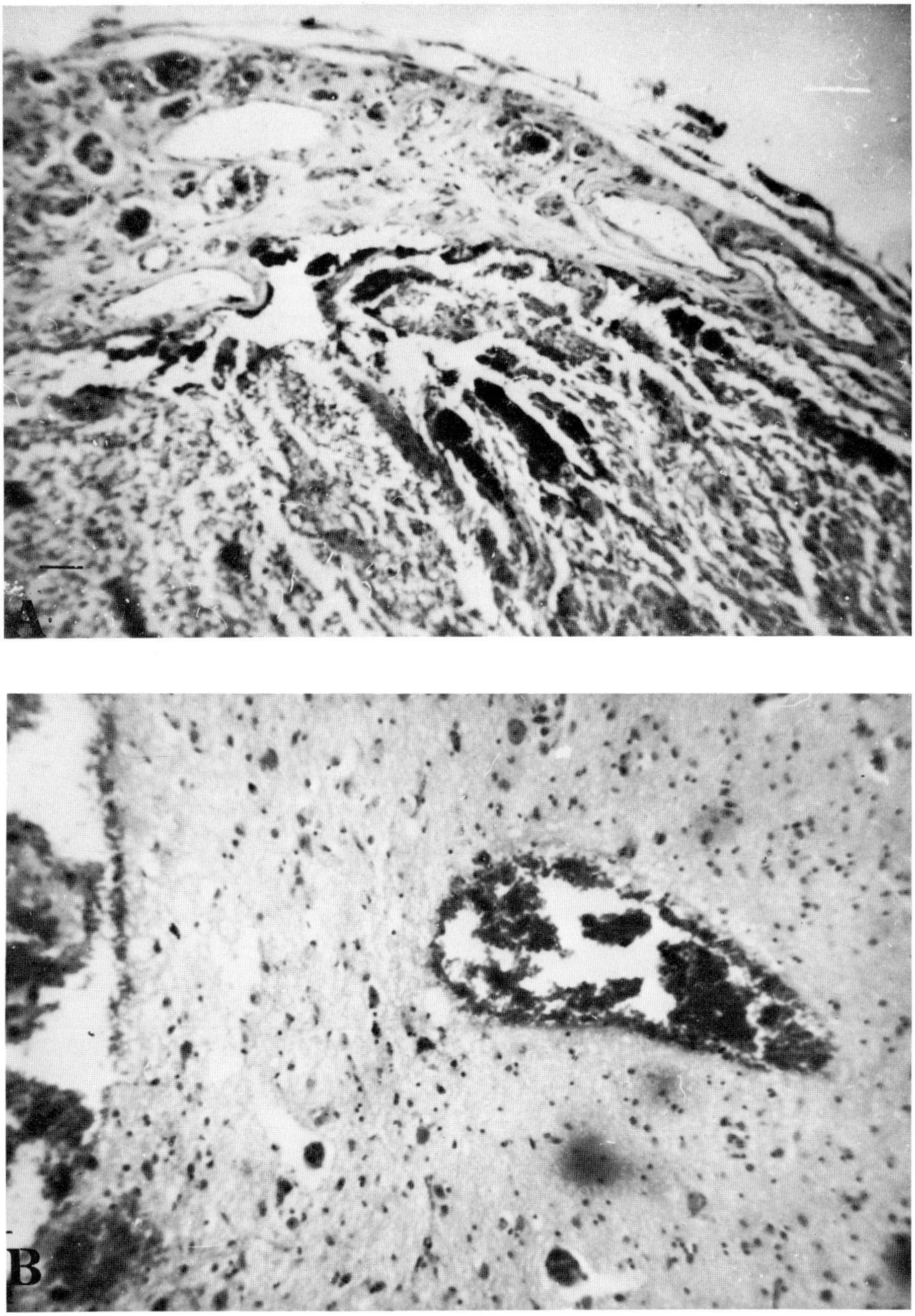

FIG. 3. Photomicrographs showing India ink particles in **(A)** the portal veins of the pituitary stalk; and **(B)** in the upper terminations of the portal veins in the hypothalamus.

very advanced cancer to sophisticated and tedious studies, especially when repetition is necessary. However, we have now developed an endocrinologic protocol condensed into a 4-hr period by which the main pituitary and hypothalamic functions can be assessed, before and 1 month after injection. Dr. Norton Williams, another member of our group, has found that the effects of injection are rather surprising. There is a massive suppression of the growth hormone and prolactin secretion in response to a glucose load; there is a regular and major depression of gonadotrophin activity; there is a rather variable depression of thyroxin output; and there is little or no suppression of ACTH release or of the adrenocortical hormones. Further studies should help in the interpretation of these results.

We obviously do not have a complete explanation for the relief of pain by pituitary alcohol injection and further research needs to be done. The elucidation of the therapeutic effects might result in a considerable advance in our basic knowledge of methods of pain relief and indeed of pain itself.

Despite our lack of understanding of the mechanism of pain-relief, injection of alcohol into the pituitary gland is a simple and very effective procedure for many patients with widespread pain of advanced cancer.

REFERENCES

1. Lipton, S., Miles, J. B., Williams, N., and Bark-Jones, N. (1978): Pituitary alcohol injection for the relief of pain. *Pain,* 5:73–82.
2. Moricca, G. (1974): Chemical hypophysectomy for cancer pain. In: *Advances in Neurology, Vol. 4, International Symposium on Pain,* edited by J. J. Bonica, pp. 707–714. Raven Press, New York.

Advances in Pain Research and Therapy, Vol. 2,
edited by J. J. Bonica and V. Ventafridda.
Raven Press, New York © 1979.

Chemical Hypophysectomy

Jose L. Madrid

Department of Anesthesiology and Pain Clinic, Ciudad Sanitaria "10 de Octubre," Madrid, Spain

The endocrine ablation for cancer of the breast was advocated more than 80 years ago, and the role played by the different hormones in breast cancer and its dissemination has been extensively documented. However, it was not until 1953 that Luft and Olivecrona (4) published the results of the first surgical hypophysectomies by way of a frontal craniotomy. This method became a standard procedure for the treatment of advanced cancer of the breast. Since then, the inactivation of the pituitary gland through surgical or nonsurgical methods has been accepted as a therapeutic procedure in the management of cancer of the breast with bone metastases. It has also been observed (10) when total pituitary ablation was accomplished in patients with hormone-dependent tumors, regression of the carcinoma was possible as evidenced by radiologic examination by post-necropsy studies. Moreover, an effective and lasting pain-relief in the majority of these patients was observed which could not be accounted for by tumor regression, because pain-relief developed promptly after the procedure was done.

Surgical ablation of the pituitary gland represents an extensive and risky procedure in many patients. In an effort to develop safer and simpler techniques, extracranial approaches for hypophysectomy have been carried out via the transsphenoidal approach. These include coagulation by radiofrequency, cryohypophysectomy, and implantation of radioactive elements, ^{90}Y, ^{198}Au or ^{32}P (1,2,3,6,11). All these methods have some limitations, as they are associated with severe and important complications or require very expensive apparatus.

In 1963, chemical hypophysectomy was introduced by Moricca (7) at the Regina Elena Cancer Institute in Rome. Essentially, this technique consists of introducing a special needle via transnasal and transphenoidal route into the sella turcica and subsequently injecting absolute alcohol into the pituitary gland (9). In 1976, Moricca (8) reported 2,775 neuroadenolyses, as he came to call the procedure, in a total of 1,139 patients with very impressive results: 86.5% of the patients had excellent pain-relief. Besides, he reported evidence of improvement in the neoplastic disease after neuroadenolysis in the case of hormone-dependent tumors.

Our experience with this technique is related to those patients with diffuse metastatic cancer in whom it was not possible to perform the usual neurosurgical procedures or any appropriate neurolytic nerve block owing to the multiple location of pain. It is important to emphasize that the purpose of the chemical injection of the pituitary was mainly as an analgesic measure rather than as a therapy for the tumor.

MATERIAL AND METHODS

Up to January 1978, we have treated 329 patients with this technique. All patients but one were suffering of intractable pain due to diffuse bone and/or visceral metastases from malignant tumors. The only exception in these series was a case of diabetic retinopathy.

TABLE 1. *Age of 329 patients subjected to chemical hypophysectomy*

Age group (yrs)	Patients	
	No.	% of total
11–20	1	0.3
31–40	47	14.2
41–50	110	33.4
51–60	86	26.2
61–70	70	21.3
71–80	15	4.6
Total	329	100.0

Our cases consisted of 189 patients with breast carcinoma; 67 patients had prostate carcinoma; 32 patients had some forms of carcinoma of the endometrium; in 24 cases the patients were suffering from lung carcinoma; 11 patients had carcinoma of the pancreas; and 5 cases underwent a chemical hypophysectomy for hypernephroma.

The ages of our patients are represented in Table 1. Our youngest patient was an 11-year-old boy with primary lung carcinoma with diffuse bone metastases, and the oldest patient was an 80-year-old man with carcinoma of the prostate. The largest group of patients treated with chemical hypophysectomy fell into the 41 to 50-years-old group.

A single procedure was performed in 233 patients; 84 patients underwent a second injection 15 days to 4 months after the first one; and 12 patients had a third injection 6 months to 1 year after the second injection, bringing the total number of neuroadenolyses performed to 437.

Technique

The technique we use at the Ciudad Sanitaria "1° de Octubre" General Hospital in Madrid is as follows. Under light, general anesthesia we insert

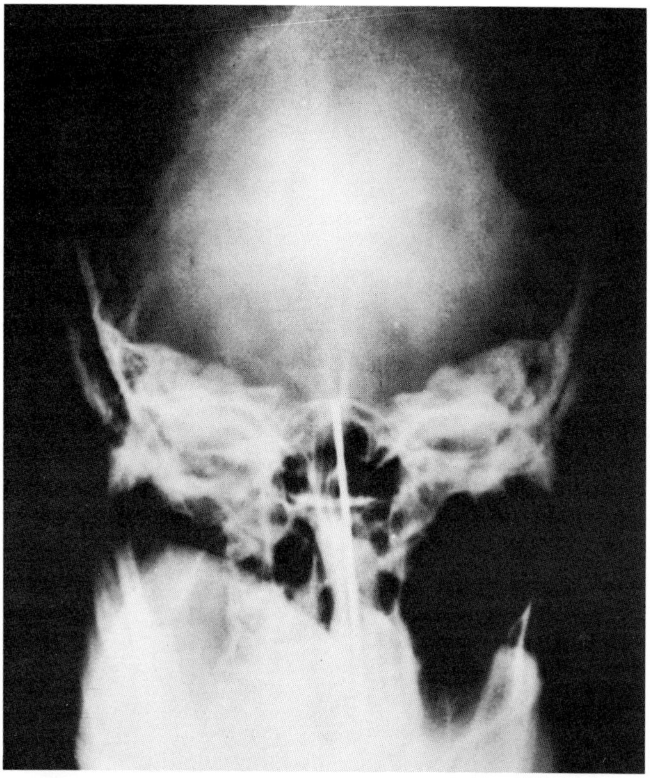

FIG. 1. An anteroposterior roentgenogram taken with Towne's projection permits accurate identification of the sella turcica and the clinoid process, confirming the midline position of the needle.

the Moricca's needle via the right nostril under constant monitoring with an image-intensifier until its tip is just past the floor of the sella turcica. An A-P film taken with Towne's projection enables us to confirm the midline position of the needle into the pituitary fossa (Fig. 1).

Once the correct position of the needle has been achieved, we introduce through the first-placed needle a 20-gauge needle (with stilet) which is 1 inch longer than the first-inserted needle. This second needle has a rubber marker to control the depth into the sella turcica. We feel that with this modification of the original technique the risk of contamination is reduced, and most of the time we are able to feel when the gland has been pierced and the tip of the needle is inside the gland.

After the needle has been properly positioned, we carry out a Queckenstedt test, and if this is negative we confirm the intraglandular position of the needle point by injecting 0.2 ml of Myodil® through the 20-gauge needle. We have observed the spread of the contrast medium moving up the pituitary stalk (Fig. 2A). Once these preliminary steps have been completed, we begin to inject absolute alcohol very slowly, while at the same time we check for

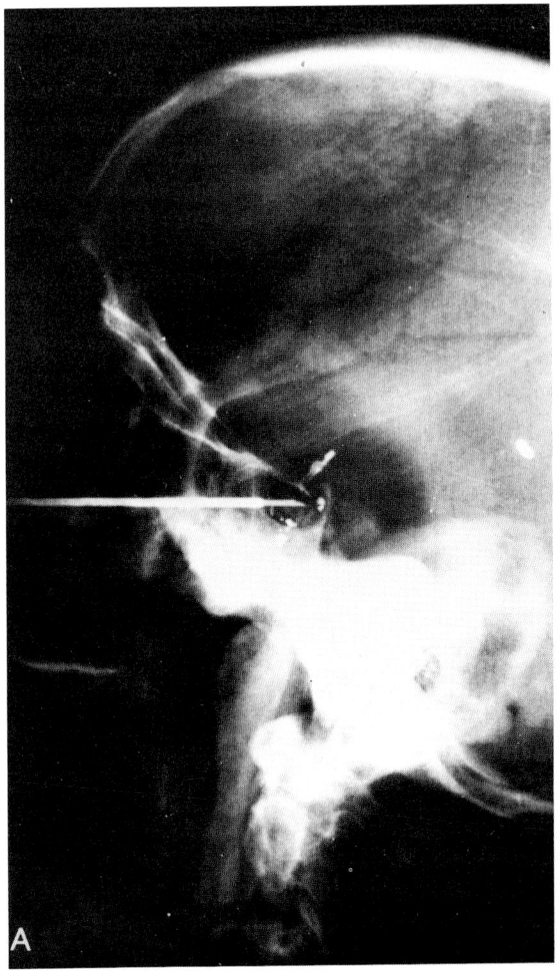

FIG. 2. Lateral roentgenogram showing the position of the needles and diffusion of the Myodil. **A:** After injection of 0.2 ml of Myodil the contrast medium is moving up the pituitary stalk. **B:** After injection of 0.4 ml of alcohol the Myodil® has diffused upward into the third ventricle.

any abnormalities of the pupil or dysfunction of other cranial nerves. After injection of 0.4 to 0.6 ml of alcohol, we are able to observe diffusion of the dye into the third ventricle. Our experiences confirm previous reports by Miles and Lipton (5) about the possibility of the alcohol's using this path (Fig. 2B).

Provided that there are no abnormalities in pupil size, we continue to inject alcohol up to a total of 2 ml. Should dilatation of the pupil appear during injection, we stop the procedure and proceed to inject into the cisterna magna 40 mg of methylprednisolone with the patient still under general anesthesia.

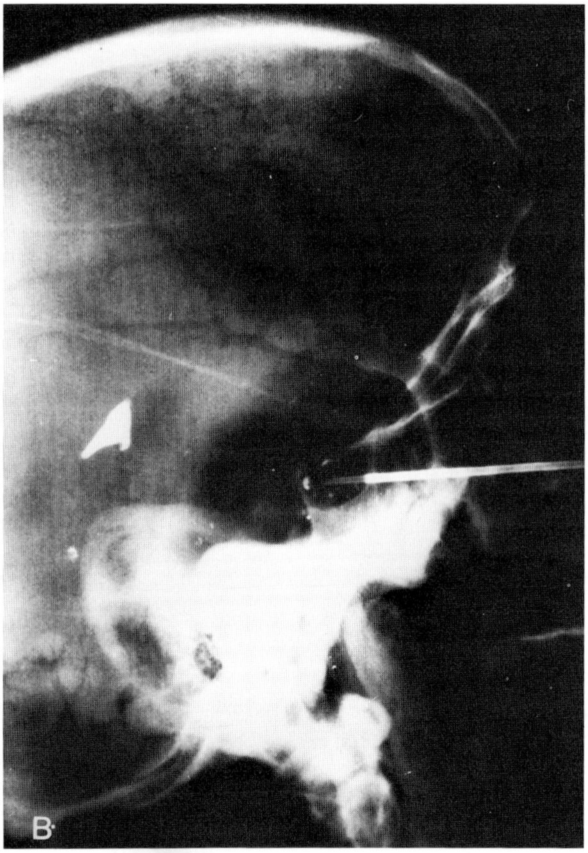

With this procedure the mydriasis has subsided by the time the patient is transferred to the recovery room.

Once the injection has been completed, we insert a nasal tube with two cuffs instead of packing the nostril with gauze as practiced by Moricca. This modification permits a posterior and anterior packing and allows the patient to breathe freely through that nostril.

RESULTS

The immediate results are listed in Table 2. There were no deaths during the procedure, and in general it was well tolerated by the patients in spite of their poor physical condition.

Pain-Relief

Complete pain-relief has been obtained in 221 patients, which represents 67% of the total. We were unable to follow up many of the patients after

TABLE 2. *Immediate results from chemical hypophysectory in 329 patients*

Results	Patients No.	Patients % of total
A. *Pain Relief*		
Complete	221	67.2
Partial	88	26.8
None	20	6.0
B. *Side Effects*		
Anisocoria during injection	32	9.7
Cephalalgia 24–48 hr duration	311	94.5
Cephalalgia 48–72 hr duration	64	19.4
Hyperthermia	28	8.5
Normal diuresis	49	15.0
Diuresis of 3 to 6 L/24 hr	210	63.8
Diuresis of 6 to 8 L/24 hr	62	18.8
Diuresis of more than 8 L/24 hr	8	2.4

leaving the hospital, so we cannot present data on the duration of the pain-relief and correlate it to patient survival. However, we were able to follow some of the patients at regular intervals, and virtually all of them were taking only nonnarcotic analgesics and tranquilizers. Apparently, the combination of hypophysectomy and minor drug therapy provided good relief of pain until the patient's death.

Our longest survival following this procedure was a woman with carcinoma of the breast and multiple bone metastases who died 4 years after she underwent the first treatment. At the time of the first chemical hypophysectomy, this patient was in such agonizing pain that it was necessary to move her on a sheet to the operating table because she would not permit anyone to touch her. On the second day after the hypophysectomy she was able to move around, and after her discharge from the hospital she went to work. She continued to do well for almost a year, when she came back to the hospital complaining of the same type of pain as she did on her first admission. A second chemical hypophysectomy was carried out which made her free of pain for almost another year. A third injection of alcohol into the pituitary gland (assuming there was some left) was performed, giving her partial relief. This together with administration of nonnarcotic analgesics kept her comfortable until her death.

Side Effects and Complications

The most common complication by far in our cases is diabetes insipidus which is transient and usually subsides spontaneously, probably because there is an incomplete destruction of the hypothalamic nuclei by the neurolytic

TABLE 3. *Complications of chemical hypophysectomy in 329 patients*

Complications	Patients No.	Patients % of total
Rhinorrhea	8	2.4
Diplopia	7	2.2
Hemianopsia	2	0.6
CSF leak	2	0.6
Meningitis	1	0.3
Myxedema	1	0.3
Total	21	6.4

agent. These cases of diabetes insipidus were transitory, and the patients were able to compensate by drinking fluids. Eight patients had diabetes insipidus with production of more than 8 liters of urine in 24 hr. They were treated with Pitressin.® (Table 2, B.)

Eight patients in whom the nasal cavity was packed with a gauze soaked with povidone-iodine developed rhinorrhea. We have not seen rhinorrhea in patients with pneumatic packing of the nasal cavity (Table 3).

Diplopia occurred in 7 patients, 5 of whom recovered and 2 had the complications permanently. Two patients developed right hemianopsia, which persisted during the time we were able to follow them.

Two patients had leak of cerebrospinal fluid (CSF), which persisted for several days and cleared up with bedrest in supine position avoiding any maneuvering tending to increase CSF pressure. One patient developed pneumococcic meningitis, which was treated with high doses of penicillin, and the patient recovered completely. Another patient had a myxedema 30 days after the chemical hypophysectomy and required supportive treatment.

We were able to perform postmortem studies in 5 patients who died after chemical hypophysectomy. All of them presented a complete necrosis of the anterior pituitary lobe, while the posterior lobe was apparently intact (Figs. 3 and 4). None of these cases had evidence of pathologic damage of the hypothalamic nuclei. However, in one case we found leptomeningeal edema and some hemorrhagic changes in the lower part of the infundibulum which could be attributable to the effect of alcohol (Fig. 5).

DISCUSSION

Although not exempt from controversy, the important feature of this technique is its simplicity and efficacy, which permit it to be used in those hospitals lacking the facilities to carry out more complicated and expensive techniques to relieve intractable painful syndromes due to neoplastic diseases. The dramatic pain-relief obtained in the majority of these patients *cannot* be

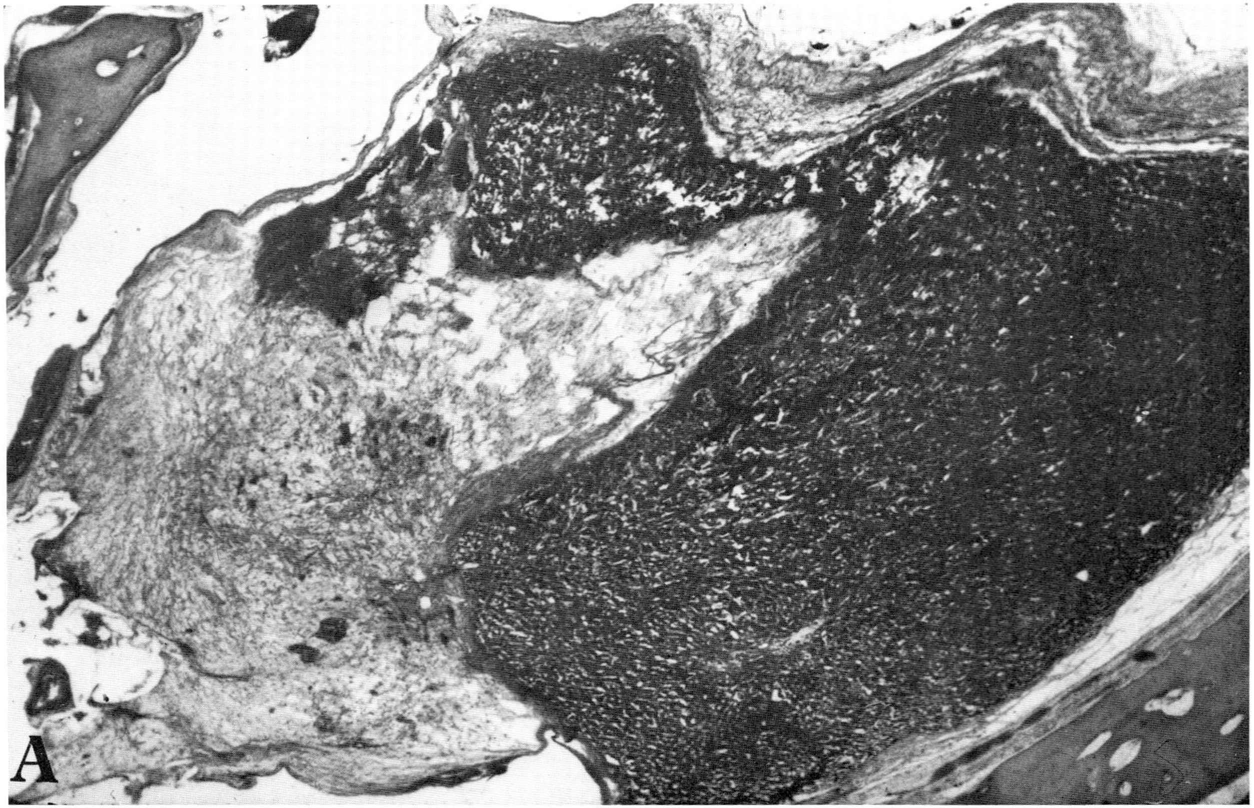

A

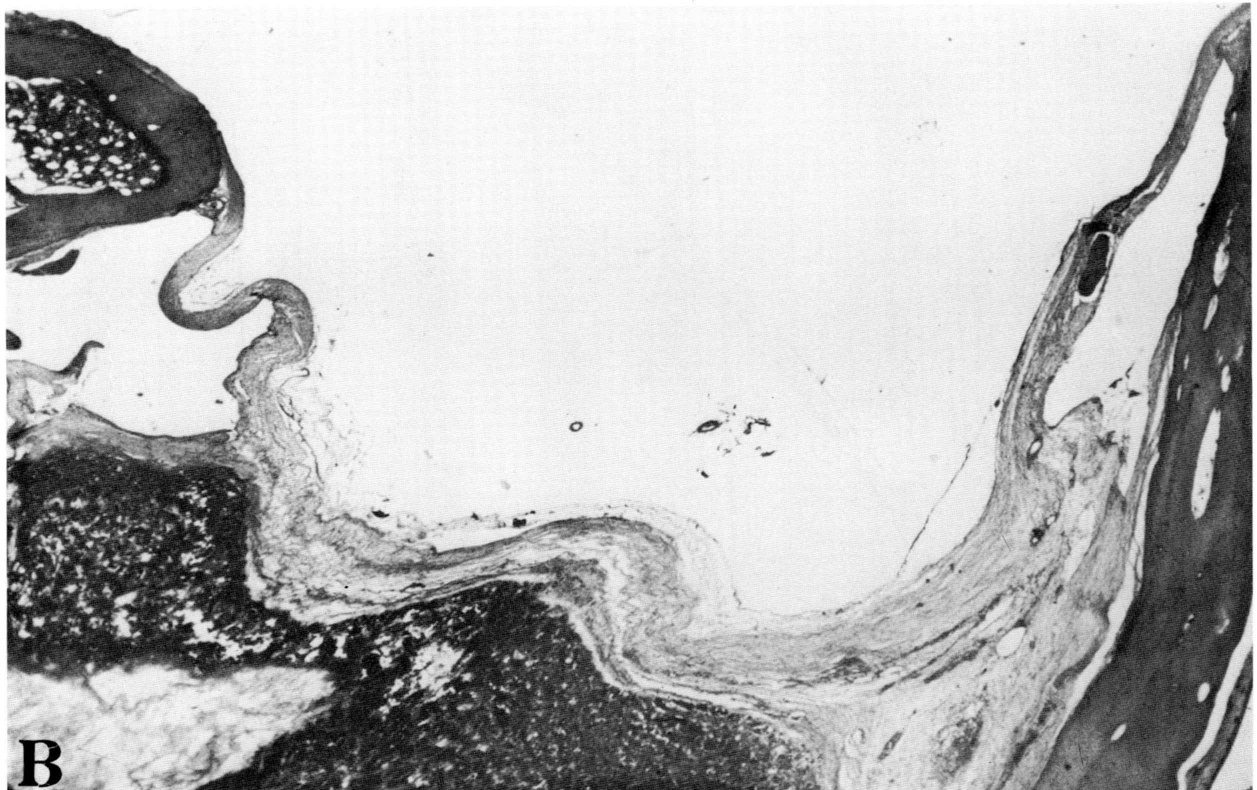

FIG. 3. Autopsy specimens taken from a patient who had had chemical hypophysectomy. **A:** shows the sella turcica with the pituitary gland *in situ*. On the left upper corner the anterior clinoid process can be seen. The anterior part of the pituitary gland shows a total necrosis, whereas the posterior part seems to be intact. **B:** View of the superior aspect of the pituitary gland. Note that the otherwise intact tentorium remains attached to the bone, but its surface is sunken due to a volume decrease of the sella turcica content.

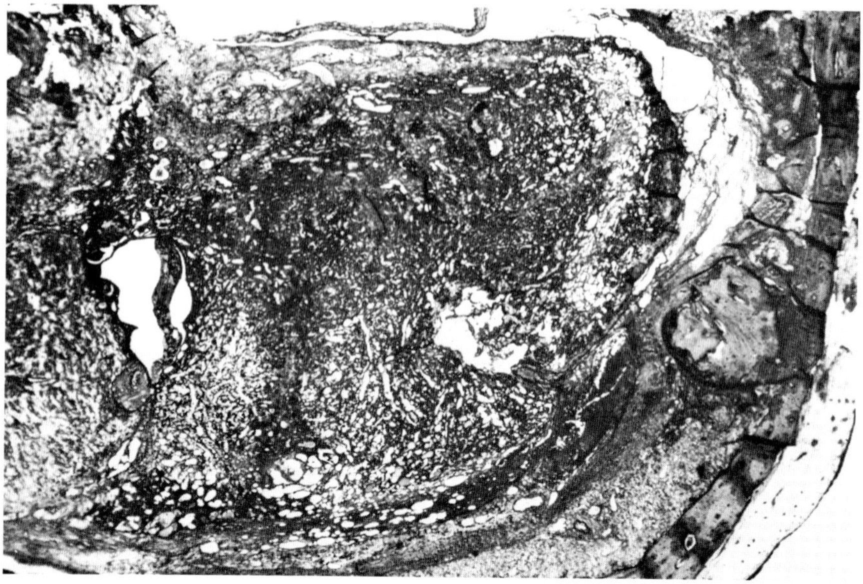

FIG. 4. Autopsy specimen of another patient showing the changes following an injection of alcohol in the anterior pituitary gland. The pituitary lobe has been replaced by necrotic material and extensive fibrosis.

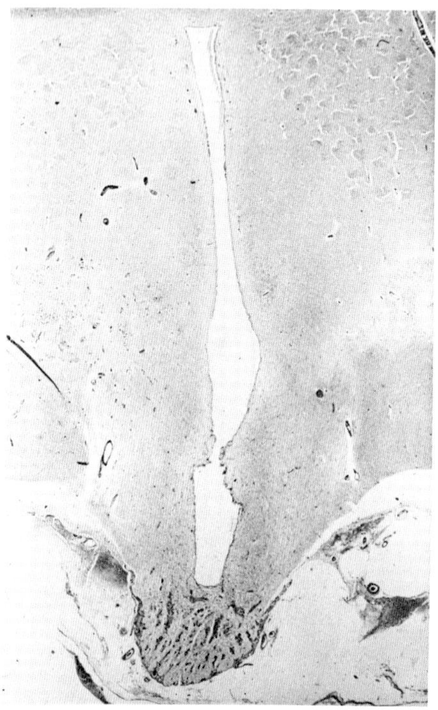

FIG. 5. Coronal section of the hypothalamus and third ventricle. In the upper part of the interthalamic commissure, while in the lower part of the infundibulum can be seen a leptomeningeal edema and some hemorrhagic changes in the neurovascular zone attributable to the effects of alcohol.

attributed solely to removal of some hormones, because similar results can also be seen in patients with non-hormone-dependent tumors.

Moricca's hypothesis regarding progressive involvement of the hypothalamohypophysis connections by direct action of the alcohol is a plausible explanation of the mechanism of action of chemical hypophysectomy. However, there are probably other mechanisms operative with this procedure. These are discussed by Miles (*this volume*).

While there are still many questions that need to be answered to explain the exact mechanisms of pain-relief with this technique, there is no doubt that it is an extremely useful procedure in patients with widespread pain of advanced cancer. Our favorable experience is especially impressive in view of the fact that most of the patients sent to us could not be relieved of pain with any other method and were in poor physical condition. As a result of our experience, our staff considers chemical hypophysectomy as a unique method to relieve advanced cancer pain.

REFERENCES

1. Adams, J. E., Seymour, R. J., Earll, J. M., Tuck, M., Sparks, L. L., and Forsham, P. H. (1968): Transsphenoidal cryohypophysectomy in acromegaly. Clinical and endocrinological investigation. *J. Neurosurg.,* 28:100–104.
2. Hartog, M., Doyle, F., Fraser, R., and Joplin, G. F. (1965): Partial pituitary ablation with implants of gold-198 and yttrium-90 for acromegaly. *Br. Med. J.,* 2:396–398.
3. Joplin, G. F., Fraser, R., Steiner, R., Laws, J., and Jones, E. (1961): Partial pituitary ablation by needle implantation of gold-198 seeds for acromegaly and Cushing's disease. *Lancet,* 2:1277–1280.
4. Luft, R., and Olivecrona, H. (1953): Experiences with hypophysectomy in man. *J. Neurosurg.,* 10:301–316.
5. Miles, J., and Lipton, S. (1976): Mode of action by which pituitary alcohol injection relieves pain. In: *Advances in Pain Research and Therapy, Vol. 1: Proceedings of the First World Congress on Pain,* edited by J. J. Bonica and D. Albe-Fessard, pp. 867–869. Raven Press, New York.
6. Molinatti, G. M., Camanni, F., Massara, F., Olivetti, M., Pizzini, A., and Giuliani, G. (1962): Implantation of yttrium 90 in the sella turcica in 16 cases of acromegaly. *J. Clin. Endocrinol. Metab.,* 22:599–611.
7. Moricca, G. (1974): Chemical hypophysectomy for cancer pain. In: *Advances in Neurology, Vol. 4: International Symposium on Pain,* edited by J. J. Bonica, pp. 707–714. Raven Press, New York.
8. Moricca, G. (1977): Neuroadenolysis (alcoholization of the pituitary) for intractable cancer pain. In: *Anaesthesiology. Proceedings of the VI World Congress on Anaesthesiology.* Excerpta Medica, Amsterdam.
9. Moricca, G. (1968): The management of cancer pain. In: *Progress in Anaesthesiology. Proceedings of the IV World Congress of Anaesthesiology,* pp. 266–270. Excerpta Medica, Amsterdam.
10. Pearson, O. H., Ray, B. S., Harrold, C. C., West, D. C., Li, M. C., Maclean, J. P., and Lipsett, M. B. (1956): Hypophysectomy in treatment of advanced cancer. *JAMA,* 161:17–21.
11. Rand, R. W. (1966): Cryosurgery of the pituitary in acromegaly: Reduced growth hormone levels following hypophysectomy in 13 cases. *Ann. Surg.,* 164:587–592.

Advances in Pain Research and Therapy, Vol. 2,
edited by J. J. Bonica and V. Ventafridda.
Raven Press, New York © 1979.

Hypophysectomy for Relief of Pain of Disseminated Carcinoma of the Prostate

Charles R. West, Anthony M. Avellanosa, Alfonso M. Bremer, and Kazuo Yamada

Roswell Park Memorial Institute, Buffalo, New York 14263

The first hypophysectomy for disseminated prostatic carcinoma was performed some 30 years ago (17). At that time, craniotomy was the only practical technique available for carrying out the hypophysectomy. Since this intracranial procedure was usually considered when orchiectomy and estrogen therapy had failed, and since the medical condition of these patients was frequently somewhat deteriorated after relapse, the risks of craniotomy were often regarded as unacceptable. Thus, a number of techniques of less extensive surgery for accomplishing hypophysectomy were eventually worked out (2,14). One of these was the transsphenoidal stereotaxic cryohypophysectomy, a technique considered safe and one which did not require general anesthesia and the usual preparation for major surgery (1,8,10,11, 14,20). After the transsphenoidal stereotaxic cryohypophysectomy was performed in a number of patients, it was found that the procedure did not effect a complete ablation of the adenohypophysis. In fact, Norrell et al. (11) found total cryodestruction of the anterior lobe in only 4 of 18 cases. It is of interest that they found little correlation between the quality and duration of response and the anatomical completeness of the adenohypophysectomy in patients with disseminated prostatic carcinoma.

The present report provides data on the direct correlation between functional ablation of the growth hormone (GH) response to insulin-induced hypoglycemia following hypophysectomy and overall remission in patients with disseminated prostatic carcinoma. Our findings support previous findings that total functional adenohypophyseal destruction is not necessary to achieve satisfactory remission of signs and symptoms of widespread carcinoma of the prostate.

RATIONALE FOR HYPOPHYSECTOMY

The underlying theoretic basis for the palliation of symptoms and signs achieved by hypophysectomy in patients with disseminated carcinoma of the prostate is that it removes the source of trophic hormones which support the metabolic activity of the tumor. Huggins and Hodges (6) proposed that androgens under influence of gonadotropins stimulate growth of prostatic carcinoma and concluded that by removing the testes as the main source or by inhibiting its effects with estrogen therapy, growth of the cancer would often be retarded. Extragonadal androgens may be effectively eliminated from circulation by hypophysectomy and or adrenalectomy, and thus these procedures may be regarded as a rational extension of the orchiectomy.

The mechanism by which pain of osseous metastases is relieved following hypophysectomy, especially when tumor regression cannot be demonstrated, is not clear. However, elucidation of this may be provided soon by the accumulation of information on the highly specific opiate receptors and opioid peptides (α-endorphins, β-endorphins, and enkephalins) recently described in the pituitary and in the hypothalamus (4,7,12,19) and implicated in the regulation of pain (5,7). Indeed, Moricca (9) has presented clinical data which indicate that relief of pain of cancer following hypophysectomy is not limited to patients with endocrine-sensitive tumors (breast and prostate). Thus, since radioimmunoassay techniques have already been developed (15), it would be of great interest to determine the role of endorphins and enkephalins in modulating pain, especially that associated with cancer. Furthermore, it would also be useful to determine whether the hypophysectomy procedure is in some way related to release of endogenous, opioid-like compounds into the general circulation.

INDICATIONS FOR CRYOHYPOPHYSECTOMY

In the sequence of the hormonal regimen for treatment of disseminated carcinoma of the prostate, hypophysectomy may be considered after orchiectomy and estrogen therapy have been proved ineffective. Under these conditions, the main indication for cryohypophysectomy is pain of widespread metastases, usually in the bones of the spinal column, of the pelvis, and of the lower extremities. Metastases in the liver or in other viscera are not contraindications to cryohypophysectomy, nor is advanced age (1,2). Many of these patients will obtain gratifying relief of subjective and objective signs and symptoms in what are often the final weeks or months of their lives (2,10,11,14,17).

PATIENTS AND METHODS

All of these patients treated at Roswell Park Memorial Institute had histologically proved prostatic carcinoma and demonstrated dissemination of disease, despite previously beneficial orchiectomy and estrogen hormonal therapy. They also had substantial bone pain as the main indication for cryohypophysectomy. Adenohypophysectomy was achieved either under direct vision following open craniotomy (8 patients) or following stereotaxic cryoablation (19 patients) under topical anesthesia and sedation. Retrospective review of the records of these patients revealed that those who had general medical conditions judged to be extremely poor were usually treated by cryohypophysectomy. Furthermore, only those patients who underwent GH assay during insulin-induced hypoglycemia once during the preoperative (control) and twice during the postoperative (experimental) period were included for analysis in this report.

Initial workup included detailed history and general physical examination. Laboratory studies included: roentgenological skeletal survey, determination of body weight, concentrations of serum acid and alkaline phosphatase, blood glucose (fasting), urea nitrogen, electrolytes, urinalysis, and peripheral vein hematocrit. All these studies were repeated postoperatively. None of the patients suffered from preexisting diabetes mellitus.

Growth Hormone Assay

In the present study, the GH assay was used to determine an index of adenohypophyseal ablation. Plasma levels were determined in all patients during insulin-induced hypoglycemia following overnight fast as described by Garcia et al. (3). Human GH assay so performed was an accurate measure of adenohypophyseal function (16) and thus was a means of comparing indices of subjective and objective remission. All patients included here underwent GH assay once within 10 days prior to surgery and twice during the postoperative period. The initial postoperative GH assay was performed 2 weeks to 1 month following surgery and repeated between the third and ninth month. The period of hypoglycemia was always carried out with continuous monitoring of blood pressure, pulse, and level of consciousness and a physician in constant attendance. There were no untoward occurrences during the GH assay procedure.

Clinical Criterions for Response

These were as previously described by Scott and his associates (17). Subjective responses were: (a) pain-relief, (b) sense of well-being and (c) improved appetite. Objective responses were: (a) decreases in serum acid phosphatase level, (b) sustained decreases in serum alkaline phosphatase levels (c) weight gain (d) improved radiological appearance of osseous metastases, and (e) improvement in anemia designated by increase in relative hematocrit or stability of hematocrit values at 30% or greater. A persistent deterioration of any of these criterions, when evaluated at monthly intervals, indicated progression of the disease.

Surgical Technique

The techniques used to perform adenohypophysectomy following craniotomy were as previously described by Poppen (13). Those for the stereo-

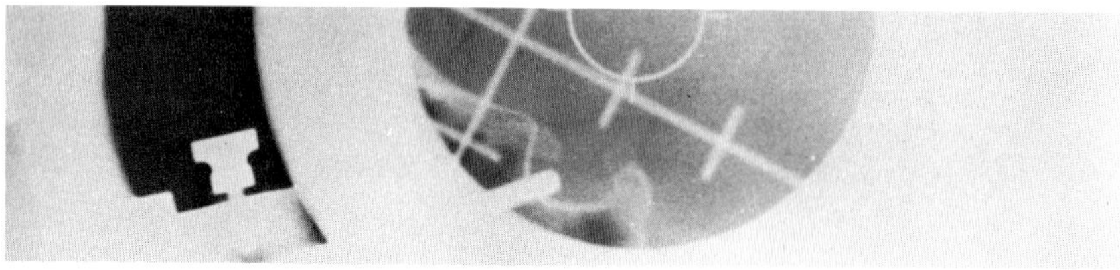

FIG. 1. Transsphenoidal insertion of cryoprobe into the antero-inferior quadrant of the sella turcica.

taxic transsphenoidal cryoablations were as described by Rand et al. (14) with modifications of Norrell et al. (11). Biplane fluoroscopy facilitated placement of a 2.7 mm cryoprobe through the sphenoid sinus and through the floor of the sella turcica. With the cryoprobe properly placed at the target point as shown in Fig. 1, a single midline lesion was created with the probe temperature at − 180 ° to − 190 ° C for 20 min. Routine operative and postoperative hormonal management is described elsewhere (10).

Calculations and Expressions of Data

It has already been shown that insulin-induced hypoglycemia is associated with hypophyseal release of GH (16). Data which we obtained from hormonal assay were plotted as a response curve (Fig. 2). As presented here,

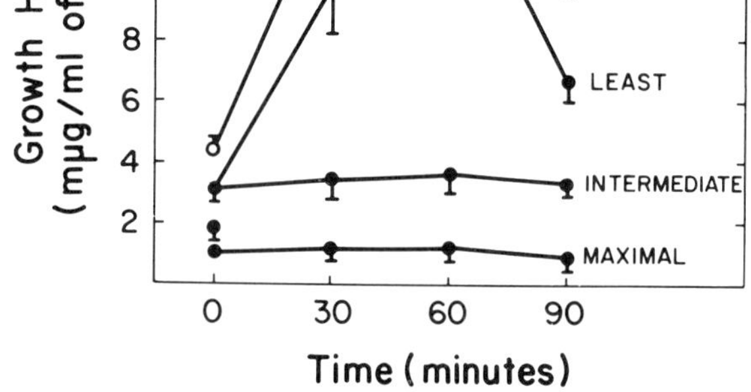

FIG 2. Concentrations of plasma growth hormone and of blood glucose plotted as functions of time following start of intravenous infusion of insulin. Each plotted point represents mean values with standard error of mean (vertical half bars) for 8 to 16 determinations from 8 patients.

numerical integration (18) of data points that describe the curve over the 90-min assay period yielded a single value that reflected the data determined for the entire assay period and permitted direct statistical comparison of groups of data. The survival period of patients was calculated from the time of hypophysectomy to the time of death.

RESULTS

When the plasma levels of glucose fell to less than 50% of the corresponding fasting level after start of intravenous infusion of insulin (0.1 units/kg, regular insulin), the absence of a characteristic increase in plasma GH (Fig. 2) was an indication of suppression of adenohypophyseal function (15). It should be emphasized that valid assessment of anterior pituitary function by GH provocation during the postoperative period is best delayed for at least 2 to 4 weeks, since transient injury by surgical insult might yield an erroneous index of anterior pituitary functional integrity if considered as permanent (10). Thus, in order to avoid this possible error in our study, GH response to insulin-induced hypoglycemia was repeated twice in all cases.

Profound suppression of plasma GH levels secondary to insulin provocation was detected after the pituitary gland was removed under direct vision (Fig. 3). However, the responses following cryohypophysectomy were variable, reflecting varying degrees of adenohypophyseal destruction (Table 1). In fact, as shown in Table 1, three patterns of suppression indicated average

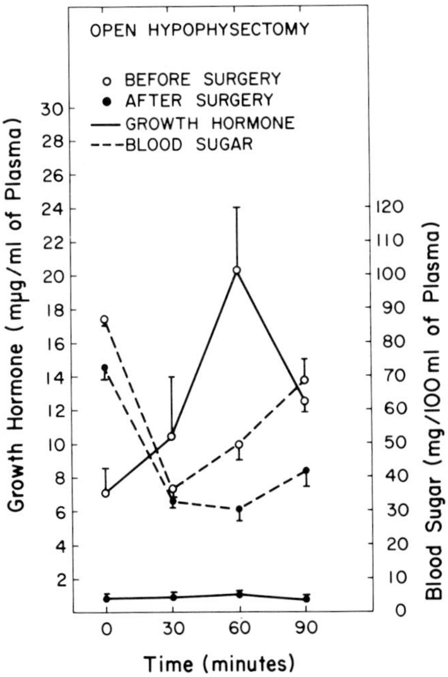

FIG. 3. Concentration of plasma growth hormone plotted as a function of time after start of insulin infusion. Each plotted point represents mean values with standard error of mean (vertical half bars) for 10 or more determinations from 5 or more patients in each group designated.

TABLE 1. *Human growth hormone (GH) responses to insulin-induced hypoglycemia*[a]

Procedure	Integrated average GH level, over 90-min period (mμg/ml of plasma)			Index of adenohypophyseal ablation[b] (%)
	Preoperative		Postoperative	
Craniotomy with hypophysectomy	**8/8** 15.6(±0.9)		**8/16** 0.94(±0.03)	93.9
Stereotaxic cryohypophysectomy		Maximal reduction	**7/14** 1.3(±0.12)[c]	90.3
	19/19 13.5(±1.8)	Intermediate reduction	**5/10** 3.6(±0.6)[c]	73.3
		Least reduction	**7/14** 10.5(±0.8)[c]	22.2

[a] Data tabulated represent mean values (±SEM) for the number of determinations indicated in boldface (no. of patients/no. determinations). All patients underwent GH assay once preoperatively and twice in the postoperative period.

[b] Based on GH suppression; mean differences between respective preoperative and postoperative values are significant at the level of $p < .001$ and are expressed as percent decrease from preoperative values.

[c] Significance of mean difference between adjacent postoperative values at the level of $p < .001$.

reductions of insulin-induced GH levels of 22.2% (least), 73.3% (intermediate) and 90.3% (maximal).

Correlation of the test results with corresponding criterions for clinical remission in the respective groups indicated that the operative procedure was either clinically effective or not effective (Table 2). When adenohypophyseal function was reduced by 73% (intermediate, Tables 1 and 2), it was as effective in extending the postsurgical time of survival and duration of clinical remission as the more totally ablative cryosurgical procedure (maximal, Tables 1 and 2). Furthermore, distinction between the clinical efficacy of open hypophysectomy versus cryohypophysectomy in prolongation of re-

TABLE 2. *Remission and survival periods*[a] *for two operative procedures*

	Stereotaxic cryosurgical adenohypophysectomy			Craniotomy with adenohypophysectomy
	Least[b]	Intermediate[b]	Maximal[b]	
No. of patients	7	5	7	8
Age, year	70.40, (+1.76)	65.0, (+1.78)	67.14, (+2.40)	58.09, (+1.30)
Duration of remission, mo.				
Subjective	0.87, (±0.52)	10.25, (±3.84)	7.54, (±2.22)	5.11, (±1.48)
Objective	0.12, (+0.05)	7.60, (+3.04)	6.25, (+2.55)	6.78, (+2.62)
Survival following adenohypophysectomy, mo.	4.80, (+1.3)	13.58 (+3.0)	13.57, (+2.83)	10.88, (+2.36)

[a] Following adenohypophysectomy for disseminated prostatic carcinoma; values tabulated represent means (±SEM).

[b] Categories of least, intermediate, and maximal effectiveness of GH suppression refer to similar categories designated in Table 1 and Fig. 2; GH indicates growth hormone.

mission and survival times disappeared when at least 73% of anterior pituitary function was destroyed by the cryogenic lesion. Although effective hypophysectomy achieved by either direct or indirect techniques was associated with some improvement of survival time and of subjective and objective remission ($p < 0.05$), dramatic relief of pain was often the most gratifying. In all of the patients reported here who had 73% or more suppression of GH, pain-relief occurred within 4 days or less of the surgical procedure.

COMMENT

More than 50% of the patients with disseminated carcinoma of the prostate who have relapses following previous castration and estrogen therapy will benefit from hypophysectomy (2,8,10,11,17). We found that cryohypophysectomy was the better choice of the two procedures used when the medical condition of the patients precluded extensive surgery. It was clear that total anterior pituitary ablation was not necessary to achieve effective remissions from prostatic carcinoma (11). Furthermore, a specific laboratory criterion which permits a determination of the technical adequacy of the hypophysectomy procedure has been provided by the data presented in this report.

REFERENCES

1. Conway, L. W., and Collins, W. F. (1969): Results of transsphenoidal cryohypophysectomy for carcinoma of the breast. *N. Engl. J. Med.*, 281:1–7.
2. Fergusson, J. D., and Phillips, D. E. H. (1962): A clinical evaluation of radioactive pituitary implantation in the treatment of advanced carcinoma of the prostate. *Br. J. Urol.*, 34:485–492.
3. Garcia, J. F., Linfoot, J. A., Manougian, E., Born, J. L. and Lawrence, J. H. (1967): Plasma growth hormone studies in normal individuals and acromegalic patients. *J. Clin. Endocrinol. Metab.*, 27:1395–1402.
4. Goldstein, A., Lowney, L. T. and Pal, B. K. (1971): Stereospecific and nonspecific interactions of the morphine congener levorphanol in subcellular fractions of the mouse brain. *Proc. Natl. Acad. Sci. USA*, 68:1742–1747.
5. Guillemin, R., Ling, N., and Burgus, R. (1976): Endorphines, peptides, d'origine hypothalamique et neurohypophysaire à activité morphinomimetique. Isolement et structure moleculaire de l'alpha-endorphine. *C.R. Acad. Sci. (Paris)*, 282:783–785.
6. Huggins, C., and Hodges, C. V. (1941): Studies on prostatic cancer: I. Effects of castration, of estrogen and of androgen on serum phosphatase in metastatic carcinoma of prostate. *Cancer Res.*, 1:293–297.
7. Hughes, J. T. (1975): Isolation of an endogenous compound from the brain with and pharmacological properties similar to morphine. *Brain Res.*, 88:295–298.
8. Maddy, J. A., Winternitz, W. W., and Norrell, H. (1971): Cryohypophysectomy in management of advanced prostatic cancer. *Cancer*, 28:322–328.
9. Moricca, G. (1974): Chemical hypophysectomy for cancer pain. In: *Advances in Neurology, Vol. 4: International Symposium on Pain,* edited by J. J. Bonica, pp. 707–714. Raven Press, New York.
10. Murphy, G. P., Reynoso, G., Schoonees, R., Gailani, S., Bourke, R., Kenny, G. M., Mirand, E. A. and Schlach, D. S. (1971): Hypophysectomy and adrenalectomy for disseminated prostatic carcinoma. *J. Urol.*, 105:817–825.

11. Norrell, H., Alves, A. M., Winternitz, W. W. and Maddy, J. (1970): A clinicopathological analysis of cryohypophysectomy in patients with advanced cancer. *Cancer,* 25:1050–1060.
12. Pert, C. B., and Snyder, S. H. (1973): Opiate receptor: Demonstration in nervous tissue. *Science,* 179:1011–1014.
13. Poppen, J. L. (1960): *An Atlas of Neurosurgical Techniques.* W. B. Saunders Co., Philadelphia.
14. Rand, R. W., Dashe, A. M., Paglia, D. E., Conway, L. W. and Solomon, D. E. (1964): Stereotactic cryohypophysectomy. *JAMA,* 189:255–259.
15. Rossier, J., Bayon, A., Vargo, T. M., Ling, N., Guillemin, R., and Bloom, F. (1977): Radioimmunoassay of brain peptides: Evaluation of a methodology for the assay of β-endorphin and enkephalin. *Life Sci.,* 21:847–852.
16. Roth, J., Glick, S. M., Yalow, R. S. and Berson, S. A. (1963): Hypoglycemia: A potent stimulus to secretion of growth hormone. *Science,* 140:987–988.
17. Scott, W. W. and Schirmer, H. K. A. (1962): Hypophysectomy for disseminated prostatic cancer. In: *On Cancer and Hormones: Essays in Experimental Biology,* pp. 175–204. University of Chicago Press, Chicago.
18. Sokolnikoff, I. S. and Redheffer, R. M. (1958): *Mathematics of Physics and Modern Engineering,* p. 717. McGraw-Hill, New York.
19. Terenius, L. (1973): Characteristics of the "receptor" for narcotic analgesics in synaptic plasma membrane fractions from rat brain. *Acta Pharmacol. Toxicol.,* 33:377–384.
20. Tytus, J. S., and Ries, L. (1961): Further observation on rapid freezing and its possible applications to neurosurgical techniques. *Bull. Mason Clin.,* 15:51–61.

Discussion

Part II. Management of Pain of Advanced Cancer: Nerve Blocks

D. C. Moore and G. Moricca (Moderators)

Moricca (Rome): I listened with great satisfaction and interest to the discussions of Madrid, Miles, and Lipton.

But I would like to underline the fact that their results on pain treatment must and can be even better. Our results are better. In Italy also, Acampora in Napoli, Casini in Cagliari, Francesconi in Merano, and Pasqualucci in Perugia often obtain better results. Why? Because I have always been aggressive against pain and my friends feel the same way.

Well, in this case, to repeat the treatment with two or more needles and with greater quantities of neurolytic permits one to obtain far better results. Results that are not obtainable, it must be underlined, with any other medical, surgical method or with any other kind of method.

And this is due not only to the more or less total destruction of hypophyseal tissue but also and mainly to the hypothalamic effect obtainable with the neuroadenolytic treatment in a totally atraumatic way. Neuroadenolysis, a delicate technique but very sure in expert hands, permits one to dominate pain considered intractable generally with only one block. Being atraumatic, it can be done on poor-risk patients.

Why remove the ovaries and testicles when you can strike at a higher level with better results? Why use chemotherapy for pain treatment? Why not recur to neuroadenolysis in hormone-conditioned tumors; neuroadenolysis not only cures the pain but also fights the evolution of the neoplasia; later one can recur to polychemotherapy.

Bond (Glasgow): Dr. Miles, how often are changes in mental functions observed after hypophysectomy? What form do these changes take? How long do they last?

Miles (Liverpool): In our series we have seen recognizable mental changes in fewer than 10 patients. In the patients in whom I suspected hypothalamic injury this took the form of obtunded behaviour. The patient was withdrawn, and in one of them she also had a hemiparesis. One of these two died and we saw evidence of specific hypothalamic injury. In the rest of the cases, euphoria and some degree of lack of insight has been the usual; and in these instances it has lasted only a few weeks.

Meissner (Stuttgart): Dr. Bonica, what kind of written consent of the patient do you have that the patient is informed about the method to be used and about possible complications?

Bonica (Seattle): As I indicated, an essential requisite for carrying out nerve block procedures and for carrying out any management of pain in patients with chronic pain, including cancer pain, is to thoroughly inform the patient of exactly what is going to be done, why it is being done, what is to be expected, and what are the possible complications. Now, in discussing complications, one has to be very sensitive and supportive, indicating that one has had much experience and most patients do not get complications. It is important for them to realize that complications may occur, that failure may occur. And it is up to the patient and to the family to decide whether or not they wish to undertake the risk. In the U.S.A. we must obtain written consent and the patients must be informed in ordinary language so that they understand what they are undergoing.

Swerdlow (Manchester): How is it possible to avoid complications with intrathecal block?

Bonica: You can predict that with a block in the thoracic dermatomes there is almost no chance whatsoever of paralyzing the bladder or the rectum. Muscular paresis is going to occur when a chemical is applied to the cervicothoracic region or in the lumbosacral region and when you are injecting in the middle and lower thoracic dermatomes. You also avoid complications by keeping the dose down. One should not normally inject more than 1 ml of solution, possibly with the exception of the thoracic region, which we are going to be talking about tomorrow. By injecting 2 and 3 cc as I have seen and heard done, you are inviting complications.

In other words, you really have to have great skill and experience, and this must be obtained during a period of training in a setting where individuals who have wide experience can teach you how to do it. You said that it can't happen that injection in the trunk will produce complications in the low limbs, but I know it has been produced. It was very obviously a serious technical error that can be avoided by proper technique.

Questioner: Dr. Gerbershagen, will you comment on the use of intrathecal-water publication by King and Jewett for treatment of intractable cancer pain?

Gerbershagen (Mainz): It has been tried for several years now to inject either water or hypertonic cold or warm saline into the subarachnoid space. We have done it only 3 times with water and about 5 or 6 times with hypertonic saline. It was very painful to the patient in spite of premedication with meperidine, and the effect lasted about 3 days. It is a damaging procedure, because there are histopathological changes that are quite widespread in comparison to the change you see with phenol or alcohol. Regarding intrathecal phenol, we recommend to do a diagnostic block first for practice, and you can get one nerve with 0.5 ml of tetracaine.

Houde (New York): Dr. Miles, regarding the challenge of naloxone to patients whose pain had been relieved by pituitary alcohol injection; were they on narcotics?

Miles: No, they had not been on narcotics for at least 2 weeks.

Schulkes (Amsterdam): Dr. Swerdlow, what were the types of complications encountered in your series?

Swerdlow: Headache, paresthesia, numbness, hyperesthesia, and the two major complications—muscular paresis, weakness of an arm or of a leg, and bladder and bowel weakness.

Questioner: Dr. Swerdlow, how did you define good and fair pain-relief?

Swerdlow: Good relief after the block means that the patient doesn't require any analgesics at all or nothing more than the mild ones. Fair relief means that he has a lot less pain than he used to have, but he still requires a certain amount of medication and maybe some limitation in his activities. As far as I am concerned, poor relief is no relief.

I was very interested in Moore's presentation and would like to make one point. I firmly believe that it is not necessary to inject 25 cc on each side. I think that it is too much. I think that 15 cc on each side is quite enough, and I have made this point to several colleagues in this business; having tried 15 cc, they absolutely agree.

Moore (Seattle): I disagree. Our failures have been with less than 50 ml.

Hildebrandt (Göttingen): Dr. Miles, is thermocoagulation of the pituitary gland an alternative to alcohol injection?

Miles: I don't know that anyone has tried pituitary ablative surgery for the range of cancers that are being treated by alcohol injection. Certainly hypophysectomy by any route has been known to be associated with an amazingly rapid relief of pain in some patients. And the implication, as I see it, is that surgery by whatever means might damage the area of the hypothalamus, as Madrid showed.

Bonica: Regarding nerve blocks and narcotics, and this applies also to neurosurgery, I must assume that people who do these procedures have the skill and experience that we stressed this morning. First of all, it is best to refer the patients early. Often people will prescribe narcotics for months before they think about sending the patient for nerve block. I think that this does several disservices to the patient. First, the degree of analgesia with successful blocks is greater than with narcotics, without some of the side effects. Second, it is important to remember that the pain of the cancer stimulates respiration and counteracts the depressive effects of the narcotics. If the patient has had large doses of narcotics and we then produce either a block or a neurosurgical relief of pain, there is a danger that the patient will have trouble with respiratory depression. I have seen patients develop apnea following a nerve block. Thirdly, the fact that the patient requires narcotics after the block or after hypophysectomy or neurosurgery does not really mean that the procedure has failed to produce analgesia. It may well be that the patient has developed physiologic and psychologic dependence; and although his nociceptive input has been eliminated, either partially or totally, his body still requires narcotics in order to feel well. Finally, I want to dispel the misconception that the continuous use of narcotics is contraindicated in patients with block. One of the serious mistakes one can make is when a patient has been on narcotics for a long period of time and one gets a very good block or successful neurosurgery procedure; if one suddenly stops the narcotics, the patient is likely to develop a withdrawal syndrome and will feel very uncomfortable from the absence of the narcotic drugs. It is a misconception that narcotics are bad to give to patients with chronic pain, including patients with cancer. I think we should forget about the problem of addiction in patients with cancer.

Advances in Pain Research and Therapy, Vol. 2,
edited by J. J. Bonica and V. Ventafridda.
Raven Press, New York © 1979.

General Comments on Ablative Neurosurgical Procedures

Carlo A. Pagni

2nd Chair of Neurosurgery, University of Torino, Torino, Italy

In the past, ablative neurosurgical procedures for pain-relief have been based on the hypothesis that pain is due to activation of specific fibers, tracts, and centers whose destruction would block nociceptive impulses. However, if pain were simply a sensory modality conducted along such specific systems, we should be able to permanently relieve patients by appropriate destruction of these pathways somewhere in their course. As is now well known, such is not the case. What is worse, activity in sensory relays does not disappear following interruption of afferent systems. On the contrary, following such procedures activity can be triggered by nonnoxious stimulation and exaggerated by deafferentation (70).

In the last decade or so, evidence has been adduced that pain is *not* simply due to activation of specific fibers in peripheral nerves or tracts in the central nervous system consisting of long, ascending fibers with the same origin, function, and termination and collected in discrete regions of the neuraxis; or centers located in specific thalamic nuclei or cortical areas where sensory impulses are brought to consciousness to produce pain (1,27, 30,63,70). Sensory mechanisms for localization of the source of painful excitations are only part of the many systems which subserve pain and its affective components. Nociceptive transmission involves not only the long afferents but also short neurons which extend from the spinal cord to the hypothalamus and terminate not only in pain "centers" but also activate a large number of subcortical and cortical structures. Moreover, neuronal systems subserving pain are open to many excitatory and inhibitory influences coming from many sources (nociceptive and other neural systems) which can enhance or block nociceptive impulses at every level of the central nervous system (1). Thus, it seems that pain is due to the activation of many diffuse paths and of many gating mechanisms which allow patterns of activity to develop in widespread subcortical and cortical structures (8).

In less than 70 years about 15 different neurosurgical operations have been devised to treat intractable pain. Certain procedures have been temporarily abandoned in favor of a new one, and then resumed to avoid the drawbacks of the latest procedure (100,101). Moreover, the good results reported with a new operation often keep eluding surgeons who try to duplicate them. The obvious conclusion is that surgical procedures for pain do not produce as satisfactory relief as claimed by their proponents. In this report, I will attempt to give a brief overview and evaluation of the most widely employed ablative procedures for cancer pain based both on personal experience and data found in the literature.

SYMPATHECTOMY

Sympathectomy is of limited usefulness for cancer pain. As White and Sweet (102) state, "pain from carcinoma generally does not arise as long as the disease is confined to a viscus." Nevertheless, pain due to visceral infection, distention, ulceration, or other pathophysiology can be relieved by sympathectomy which interrupts not only the sympathetic motor fibers, but also the afferent (sensory) fibers which supply the viscus. An example of this is the surgical (or chemical) splanchnicectomy to relieve the pain of carcinoma of the pancreas. However, the pain caused by cancer of the abdominal or thoracic viscera usually becomes severe and intractable when the tumor involves somatic spinal nerves or nerve trunks. At this point, only extensive denervation by rhizotomy or interruption of central pain pathways will produce adequate relief.

SPINAL DORSAL RHIZOTOMY

Dorsal rhizotomy of spinal nerves was the first operation successfully employed in the surgery of pain (Fig. 1). However, accurate analyses of long-term results was not attempted until recently. These have shown that the results are not as good as might be expected after complete denervation of a painful area produced by cutting an adequate number of nerve roots. Usually, the operation has been an immediate, complete success, but in a few months patients start anew to complain of pain (46).

In analysis of the results in a group of patients, Loeser (46) found no technical factors accounting for the lack of long-term success of rhizotomy: therefore, he suggested that abnormal physiologic phenomena are at work. Coggeshall et al. (12) suggests that some unmyelinated nociceptive fibers arising from cells of the dorsal ganglion but running in the anterior roots might be responsible for the recurrence of pain. Consequently, Osgood et al. (65) introduced the technique of posterior root "ganglionectomy," which should interrupt even these sensory fibers which pass through the anterior root. However, evidence to support this hypothesis is still lacking. Failures from dorsal rhizotomy are also accounted for by the fact that cancer is a progressive disease which spreads and involves adjacent nerves which have not been surgically interrupted. Although this is undoubtedly true in certain

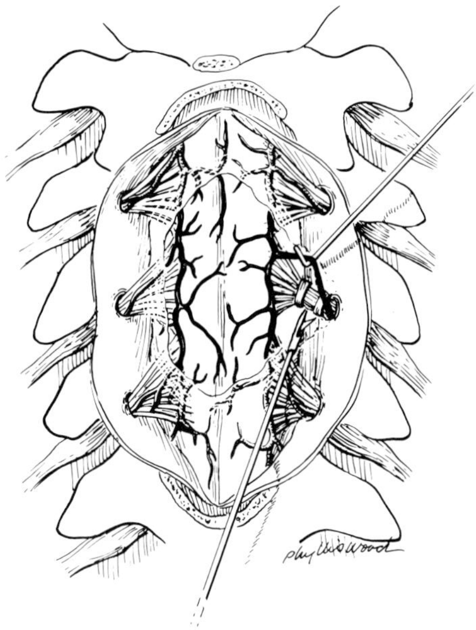

FIG. 1. Spinal dorsal rhizotomy. (Courtesy of Loeser, J. D., in: Bonica, J. J.: *The Management of Pain,* 2nd edition, *in preparation*).

cases, failures have been observed even if the denervation was adequate: Pain "recurs" even in permanently denervated and analgesic areas. In such cases, there is not recurrence of the original pain; an entirely new, strange, annoying, burning or aching, unbearable sensation develops which patients never had before. The abnormal sensation is referred to the anesthetic area or deep under the anesthetic skin: Sometimes denervated limbs feel like a painful phantom (70). In other words, recurrence of "pain" really represents the development of "anesthesia dolorosa": the source of pain does not lie in the peripheral nerves or roots, but in the central nervous system. Initially, deafferentation is followed by decrease of activity in the deafferented central sensory pathways but later spontaneous, persistent, abnormal firing patterns develop which give rise to the sensations patients call pain (see literature in ref. 70). Furthermore, cancer may damage nerve trunks with consequent loss of large, myelinated axons followed by disinhibition of small fibers, resulting in excessive neuronal firing in central pain pathways which contributes to the pain. Further deafferentation by rhizotomy could exaggerate the abnormal firing.

In contrast, nearly four decades ago, Ray (75) and recently Barrash and Leavens (2) reported good results following extensive dorsal rhizotomy. However, Ray (75) did not mention long-term results. The opinions of Barrash and Leavens (2) are based on 72 cases of cancer pain: 40 patients were completely relieved and 10 were satisfactorily relieved. They believe that rhizotomy is a safe and effective procedure for severe intractable pain including that due to cancer.

I obtained favorable results with extensive rhizotomy used to relieve cancer pain in the trunk, upper limb, and shoulder but only in patients who survived less than 4 months. If survival was longer, there was either recurrence or painful anesthesia. In patients with cancer pain in the face, head, and neck, rhizotomy of cranial nerves and cervical spinal roots sometimes gives longer relief (Fig. 2). Moreover, denervation of the neck is well tolerated and suppression of shooting pains is sufficient to make patients more comfortable (71,72). Rhizotomy can successfully be employed even in pain limited to the perineum and sacrococcygeal region due to rectal and anal carcinoma in patients submitted to colostomy (7,20,37). Bilateral rhizotomy from S_5 to S_2 (some of which are to be spared on one side if there are no bladder disturbances) can afford complete relief: The area of perineal and perianal anesthesia is small and well tolerated without anesthesia dolorosa (7,20,37). Unfortunately, if carcinoma spreads to invade lumbar spinal nerves or roots, the operation proves inadequate.

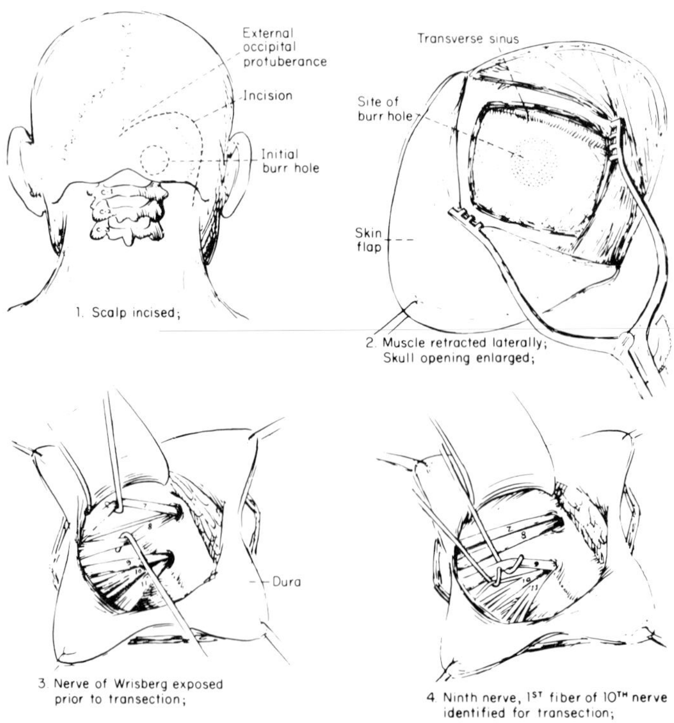

FIG. 2. Section of the VII and IX nerves. (Courtesy of Loeser, J. D., in: Bonica, J. J.: *The Management of Pain,* 2nd edition, *in preparation*).

A significant disadvantage of dorsal rhizotomy is massive denervation of an arm or leg which makes the limb virtually useless. To avoid this, Sindou et al. (87) introduced the "selective spinal posterior rhizotomy" or "radicletomy" or "rhizidiotomy." With the aid of the operative microscope only small-caliber fibers which, as the rootlets enter the cord are collected in a small lateral bundle, are cut; the large, myelinated fibers bound for the posterior funiculi, collected medially, are spared. Only pain sensation should be abolished, leaving intact other sensory modalities. The purposes of the operation are: (a) to spare inhibitory input on nociceptive afferents thus preventing failures due to deafferentation; and (6) to avoid functional impairment of limbs due to massive denervation. Sindou et al. (87,88) reported that among the 20 patients subjected to this procedure, 13 obtained complete relief and 3 partial relief of pain and that, "the best indication would seem to be painful disease of upper limb . . . and cervical roots (mainly Pancoast-Tobias syndrome) where high cervical cordotomy is often inefficient and extensive posterior rhizotomy too severe." (88) Vlahovitch and Fuentes (97) share this opinion, although in their patients they combined "radicletomy" and total rhizotomy. Experience with the procedure is, however, limited.

Percutaneous thermocoagulation of cranial and spinal nerves is a new technique with less risk and is thus worthwhile in patients in very poor condition (38). However, the experience with this procedure is limited.

ANTEROLATERAL CORDOTOMY

Anterolateral cordotomy or spinothalamic tractotomy aims at sectioning the spinothalamic tract in the anterolateral quadrant of the cord, wherein are located the ascending pathways which primarily transmit nociceptive information coming from the opposite side of the body. I will *not* discuss the indications, technique, and complications of the procedure but will limit my comments to the efficacy of open cordotomy and percutaneous cordotomy in relieving pain in the lower half of the body. This will include comments on the problem of recurrence on long-term followup.

Open Cordotomy

Complete unilateral transection of the anterolateral quadrant (Fig. 3) at upper thoracic or cervical levels produces, in nearly every patient, analgesia in the contralateral half of the body, and bilateral section produces bilateral analgesia. Immediate relief of pain is achieved in nearly 60 to 80% of patients (74,102). However, the number of failures rises at long-term followup: Broadly speaking, the incidence of recurrence of pain is about 30 to 50%. Unfortunately, details are often lacking in the published reports. Criteria for evaluation of the results and the length of survival are quite different in the various published series, thus precluding comparison of different series found

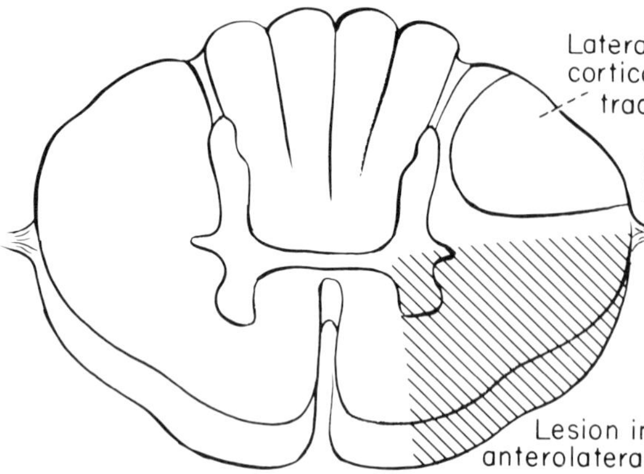

FIG. 3. Cordotomy lesion. (Courtesy of Loeser, J. D., in: Bonica, J. J.: *The Management of Pain,* 2nd edition, *in preparation*).

in the literature. My own personal experience is based on 24 patients I have been able to personally follow up. Among this group, more than 75% of the patients had recurrence of pain 3 months after the procedure was done. This figure is higher than currently estimated in the literature. However, it compares quite well with Bohm's report (6) which, oddly enough, is never quoted even in the most complete reviews on the subject. He reported that out of 29 patients who had bilateral thoracic cordotomy, 20 had recurrence of pain at 3½-months follow-up and only 9 patients who survived only 2 months died free from pain. In other words, there was a recurrence of pain in all surviving patients at 3½ months. No better were the results noted by Siegfried and Krayenbühl (86), who reported that after a few weeks 50% of the patients had recurrence of pain.

The obvious question is, "why the disappearance of analgesia?" Incomplete section of the spinothalamic tract with only temporary damage to ascending fibers has been blamed for the recurrence. Although this may be true in some cases, neuroanatomic studies have shown that fading of analgesia occurs even with complete bilateral sections of the anterolateral quadrant (11,28,63,70,102). Moreover, usually there is not simple recurrence of the pain for which the patient was operated on; patients complain of a new kind of pain, of disagreeable, unbearable sensations (dysesthesia). Peripheral stimuli can give rise to hyperpathia. These symptoms are identical to those of "central pain" and are often more annoying and sometimes more excruciating to the patients than the original cancer pain (11,68,70). Recovery of sensibility and the related symptomatology are not simply due to recovery of function of injured long ascending fibers, but in part due to transmission of impulses by other multisynaptic or alternative spinal pathways which can and often do display abnormal spontaneous activity (11,34,

63,70). These pathways are diffuse and intermingled with other cord tracts. Total interruption of them will never be possible without severe impairment of other functions.

Reliable information is scanty about the effectiveness of cordotomy at C_1-C_2 for the relief of pain in the shoulder and upper arm. The number of patients reported is usually small (6,9,24,25,48,64,66,100), or the problem is not thoroughly discussed (53,57). White and Sweet (102) state that "cervical cordotomy has a very poor chance of producing lasting analgesia of the arm," and Schürmann (82) states that, "with cervical cordotomy at level of C_1-C_2 permanent analgesia very rarely extends higher than C_8-D_1," being ineffective for relief of pain in the shoulder and upper limb. None of the 6 patients I was able to personally follow up for more than 3 months obtained permanent analgesia of, and good relief of pain in the shoulder and arm. In the opinion of White (100) shoulder and upper limb pain is better treated by some form of leucotomy or thalamotomy; others prefer selective posterior rhizotomy (44,88,97) or mesencephalic tractotomy (53). The mechanisms of fading of analgesia, recurrence of pain, and occurrence of central pain are probably the same as in thoracic cordotomy.

Percutaneous Cordotomy

In 1963, Mullan et al. (59) introduced the technique of percutaneous cordotomy. The procedure, refined by others (15,26,41,45,79) entails the interruption of the anterolateral quadrant of the cord by percutaneous insertion of a coagulating probe in the spinal cord at upper or lower cervical level. It is a relatively minor surgical procedure: Operative mortality seems very low (1 to 3%) even following bilateral procedures, and complications are less than those occurring with open cordotomy (78). Percutaneous cordotomy seems to offer the patients the same pain-relief as open cordotomy (26,78) with a rate of immediate success up to 96% (94). However, long-term follow-up studies do not always detail precise results.

Impressively large series of cases are only of moderate interest, because pain-relief seems to have been assessed only at discharge (26,56,60,94) and correlations between survival and pain-relief are sometimes lacking (26,41, 56,60,94). Only Rosomoff (78) made an accurate study of 100 cases of bilateral cordotomy at long-term follow-up. Cancer pain and noncancer pain were grouped together, with results not given separately for pain in the upper or lower half of the body. Rosomoff (78) obtained "complete relief" postoperatively in 80 out of 100 cases (80%); at 6-weeks follow-up, 42 out of 63 (67%) patients were still free from pain; at 3 months the rate was 31 out of 49 (63%); at 6 months, 18 out of 36 (50%) of the patients remained pain-free; at 1 year 9 out of 30 (less than 27%) were still relieved. It seems, therefore, that results of percutaneous cordotomy are neither better nor worse than those of open cordotomy. There is no report in the literature containing a detailed analysis of long-term results and failures in patients with pain of the upper limb and shoulder (56). Lorenz et al. (47) state ". . . failures and bad results were mainly due to difficulties in achieving complete abolition of pain arising from the brachial plexus and not sufficient level of anaesthesia."

Perhaps the most relevant point in Rosomoff's report (78) is that percutaneous cordotomy was given to 34 patients who died in 6 weeks, and to another 13 who died between 6 weeks and 3 months, i.e., high-risk patients in very poor condition, "the majority (of which) had died pain-free." It seems to me the best definition of the role of percutaneous cordotomy in surgery for pain was given by Mullan (58): "Percutaneous cordotomy . . . extends the indication for cordotomy to those patients who are too ill for the open surgical procedure. It does not, however, extend it to types of pain that do not respond to the classical surgical method." Another important advantage is that the procedure may be repeated if necessary. This led to the extension of indications to many patients with advanced cancer who had only a few days or weeks of life-expectancy. That could explain why percutaneous cordotomy "seems" to afford higher success rate than open cordotomy even in upper-half body pain. Clearly, an operation which abolishes pain for 2 to 3 weeks in a patient who will survive for such a short time may not be as successful in relieving pain and suffering if the patient had lived 4 to 6 weeks or longer.

In summary, success of cordotomy—by open or percutaneous method—is strictly tied to the duration of survival of the patient. As to when either open or percutaneous cordotomy is indicated, if the patient is in fair condition with several months of life-expectancy, the open technique done with the aid of the operative microscope which allows better visualization of anatomic landmarks and more complete transection of anterolateral quadrant is to be preferred. In patients with very short life-expectancy, when limited damage to the anterolateral quadrant is sufficient to relieve pain during the last few days or weeks of life, percutaneous cordotomy is to be preferred.

MEDULLARY TRACTOTOMY

Spinothalamic tractotomy at medullary level was undertaken with the hope of attaining better results in pain of upper limb than those given by spinal cordotomy (Fig. 4). No more than 68 cases have been reported, many of which involved pain caused by nonmalignant disease (5,102). It appears that no fewer than 43 out of 56 cases were permanently relieved of upper limb pain at some years follow-up. Maybe the good results are due to the fact that lesions impinged on the extralemniscal pain pathways at bulbar level.

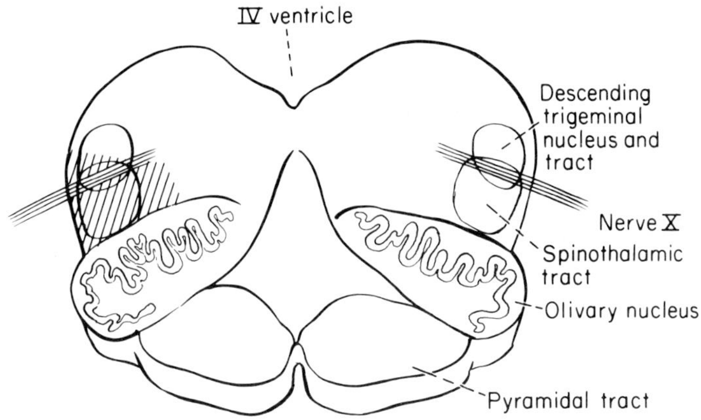

FIG. 4. Medullary tractotomy. (Courtesy of Loeser, J. D., in: Bonica, J. J.: *The Management of Pain,* 2nd edition, *in preparation*).

MESENCEPHALIC TRACTOTOMY

Spinothalamic tractotomy at mesencephalic level was introduced by Dogliotti (17) and Walker (98). The operation entails high operative mortality, complications, and frequent occurrence of central pain and dysesthesia (70,72). Thus, it was given up in spite of the fact that it seemed indicated for pain in face, neck, and upper limb.

The introduction of stereotactic technique by Speigel and Wycis et al. (91) renewed interest in mesencephalotomy. In fact, stereotactic midbrain tractotomy is an operation with low mortality and rare complications (70,72). Furthermore, the stereotactic lesion can be extended beyond the spinothalamic tract to impinge on the reticular formation where polysynaptic pain pathways are supposed to exist (62,77,103). The hope was it would be possible to obtain longer relief of pain and to avoid risk of central pain. The method was employed only in small series of patients with cancer pain (27,31,61,95,103). Opinions about the efficacy of the operation differ: Some writers reported only poor results (103); others believe mesencephalotomy is the technique of choice for the treatment of pain in the head, neck, and arm (61); still others believe that for relief of pain due to cancer it is necessary to combine mesencephalotomy with bilateral cingulotomy (96).

In 1976, Mazars et al. (53) reported they performed 224 stereotactic mesencephalotomies of which 8 were done bilaterally. Of this group, 152 patients had cancer pain. They state the, ". . . effect on pain was immediate and excellent." This is worth noting for patients with cervical and cephalic pain, ". . . which is not relieved by other less valuable procedures." Relief was permanent and complete even in the upper thoracic region and the incidence of complications was very low, but statistical analysis of the results was not reported. Mazars et al. believe that for pain in the lower half of the body cordotomy is still more effective than mesencephalotomy (53). The results reported by Mazars and his colleagues are impressive and suggest further trial of the method.

COMMISSURAL MYELOTOMY

Commissural myelotomy consists of section of the pain fibers at the midline of the cord where they cross to ascend in the contralateral anterior quadrant. It was intended to give large bands of bilateral analgesia in the torso and/or limbs, depending on the cord-splitting level. It would then seem possible to obtain bilateral pain-relief with a single operation, without damage to other spinal tracts and major complications. Successes of the procedure have been rather elusive. Only Wertheimer and Lecuire (99) reported satisfactory results in a large series of cases submitted to lumbar myelotomy for bilateral pain of the legs, pelvis, and perineum. The incidence of complications consisting in operative death, radicular pain, leg dysesthesia, paresis, and/or bladder and/or bowel dysfunction were high. Of 80 patients followed up, 27 (33%) were completely relieved, 25 (32%) were improved, and in 28 (35%) the procedure failed. In 1963, Dargent et al. (16) reviewed the same series and reached the conclusion that commissural myelotomy is effective only for vaginal and visceral pain, and that for rectal and leg pain, cordotomy is preferred.

This operation seemed a matter of only historical interest rather than of practical value, when in 1964, Lembcke (40) reported impressive results in 12 patients submitted to cervical myelotomy. All the patients were relieved and analgesia persisted up to 10 years in 6 long-term survivors; no serious complication occurred. This prompted new interest in the procedure which was employed both for pain in the lower half of the body (10,13,36,44,53, 89,90) and for cervical, upper limb, and thoracic pain (32,73,83). Wertheimer and Lecuire's standard incision was 2 to 3 cm long and a few mm deep (99). Currently most surgeons try to produce a deeper incision with complete splitting of the cord in two halves for several centimeters (10,13, 36,73,90).

As is always the case in surgery for pain, some are happy with the results while others are not. The former group includes Lembcke (40) and Broager (10), who state they gave up bilateral cordotomy in favor of commissural myelotomy. In contrast, Papo and Luongo (73) reported that while pain was completely relieved in all patients, it remained absent for only several weeks: Severe pain recurred within 2 months.

Everyone who has performed commissural myelotomy agrees that, in spite of extensive splitting of the cord, defects in pain and temperature appreciation are relatively mild, that no permanent extensive analgesia ensues and that hypalgesia, when present, fades away in a few weeks. On the contrary, disturbances due to dorsal column injury (loss of positional sense, tactile hypoesthesia, dysesthesia, tingling, ataxia) are frequent and may be marked (44,73). The mechanism by which myelotomy abolishes pain, even if temporarily, is far from clear. Schwarcz (83) suggested pain-relief was due to interruption of extralemniscal polysynaptic pathways close to the central gray matter of the spinal cord: Myelotomy acts like an intralaminar thalamotomy. Sourek (89) and Papo and Luongo (73) report that a close correlation exists between signs of posterior column damage and pain-relief: When these fade away, pain usually recurs, suggesting a role of injury or irritation of dorsal column system responsible for the relief of pain. It seems to me myelotomy is a rather mysterious operation whose mechanisms, indications, and results are far from clear.

STEREOTACTIC THALAMOTOMY

Stereotactic thalamotomy aroused the hope that combined destruction of both the spinothalamic system (VPL-VPM nuclei) and the polysynaptic pathways (CM, Pf, intralaminar, limitans nuclei) might afford longer analgesia and pain-relief than other operations, without occurrence of central pain. Regrettably, experience has shown that it is nearly impossible to achieve persistent analgesia and pain-relief by this technique: In about 70 to 80% of cases pain recurs in a few weeks or months (69). Moreover, destruction of the VPL-VPM nuclei frequently gives rise to central pain (11,51,52,67,69).

Mark et al. (49,50) suggested that the suppression of pain by thalamotomy is not due to lesion of the VPL-VPM nuclei, but to involvement of nonspecific pathways in the CM-Pf-intralaminar complex whose destruction might afford relief of pain without sensory loss and risk of central pain. In my experience unilateral lesions limited to the CM-Pf-intralaminar complex yield only transient results (67,69). Furthermore, clinical-anatomic studies of both personal and published case reports of patients relieved of pain (49,50,93) demonstrate that the lesion actually destroys a variable part of the dorsomedial nucleus with a leucotomic effect which might play a critical role in securing relief of pain in absence of any sensory loss.

An attempt to improve the results was made with bilateral lesions of the basal thalamus including VPL-VPM, CM-Pf-intralaminar complexes: Sometimes results reached the expectation (4,14,35,92). Pulvinarectomy, introduced by Richardson (76) affords no better results for some (22,69), while others are satisfied with this procedure (104).

Stereotactic thalamotomy seems a method of limited practical value. Because of its very low mortality and complication rate, it can be employed in patients in very poor condition with pain of the head, face, neck, and upper limb when other procedures are not indicated or might not be tolerated (72). Therefore, I have read with interest the reports by Fairman (18) and Sano (80) that unilateral or bilateral lesions of the internal medullary lamina including the CM, Pf, and limitans ("thalamolaminotomy") and of the posteromedial hypothalamus ("posteromedial hypothalamotomy") give excellent and persistent relief even in diffuse cancer pain. These data suggest the method merits further trial.

Tractotomy of the descending root of the trigeminal nerve, known as Sjöqvist's operation, is employed for head and face cancer pain. This topic is discussed elsewhere in this volume.

PSYCHOSURGERY

Since the Freeman and Watts statement, "The results of lobotomy . . . have been so gratifying that further efforts in the earlier control of intractable pain are unwarranted" (23), the procedure has been considered for patients with intractable cancer pain. Lobotomy seems to work in that it changes the attitude of the patient toward his pain (23), removes the anticipation and memory of the pain (85), and alters affective and emotional response to it (55); but it does not alter the perception of pain.

Unfortunately, bilateral lobotomy invariably produces apathy and severe psychologic deterioration. Because of this serious complication, less destructive procedures were introduced: unilateral lobotomy (81), undercutting of the frontal cortex (54,84), progressive radiofrequency frontal lobotomy (29), bilateral frontal topectomy (39), and dorsomedial stereotactic thalamotomy (92) (Fig. 5). However, even with those procedures, pain-relief invariably seems to be associated with, and depend on, severe emotional and mental defects. Pain is relieved only so long as changes of personality persist; should they subside, there is recurrence of complaints.

To avoid psychic disturbances, White and Sweet (102) introduced graduated bilateral coagulation of medial frontal white matter. With this procedure small areas of frontothalamic projection fibers are destroyed in successive steps, at intervals of several days. In this way it seems possible to

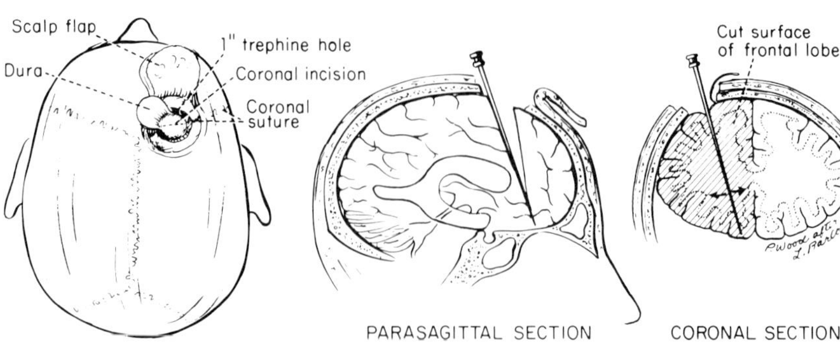

FIG. 5. Prefrontal lobotomy. (Courtesy of Loeser, J. D., in: Bonica, J. J.: *The Management of Pain,* 2nd edition, *in preparation*).

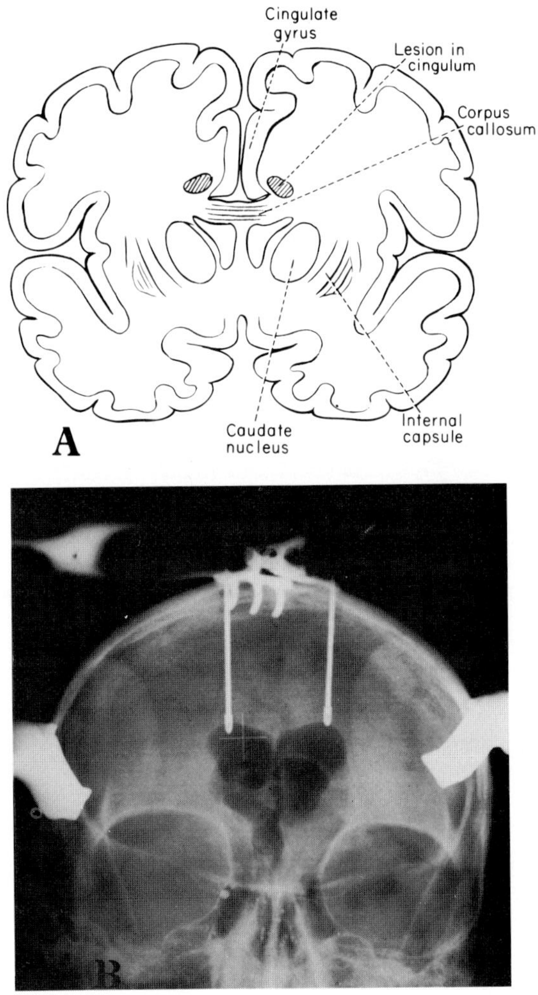

FIG. 6. A and B: Cingulotomy. (Courtesy of Loeser, J. D., in: Bonica, J. J.: *The Management of Pain,* 2nd edition, *in preparation*).

afford pain-relief without severe mental deterioration. Bertrand et al. (3) attempted to obtain the same result by means of stereotactic section of the frontothalamic pathways. Lindstrom et al. (42,43) performed frontal lobotomy by means of ultrasonic beam; "considerable relief from pain" was obtained in 45 of 48 patients thus treated without the mental defects of frontal lobe surgery.

In 1962, Folz and White introduced "cingulotomy" (21). In the cingulum run pathways mediating activities of the limbic system to the entire forebrain; these pathways play a major role in emotional behavior. The hope was to succeed in modifying emotional reaction to pain, relieving suffering with minimal psychic impairment. Foltz and White (21) reported excellent relief at 6 months to 1 year follow-up in a group of patients who showed marked emotional reaction to pain. Recently, Hurt and Ballantine (33) in reporting the results of bilateral cingulotomy in 32 patients with cancer pain, stated they "were unable to document unwanted changes in intellect, memory, personality or other psychological functions in these patients." Marked to complete relief was achieved in 37% of patients, slight to moderate in 28%: but there was "a tendency to progressive decrease in the initial degree of pain relief" (33). It seems, therefore, that cingulotomy has, at least partially, fulfilled expectations (Figs. 6A and B). Duration of relief, however, is briefer than following more-mutilating frontal operations with the attendant persistent mental impairment.

My experience is limited to 4 cases of frontothalamic section (3), 4 cases of cingulotomy (21), 4 of graudated frontal coagulation, and 2 of dorsomedial thalamotomy (92). As far as I can judge by this limited experience, relief of suffering was achieved only with concomitant personality changes and mental deterioration. Thus, I am rather inclined to agree with Falconer (19), who considers frontal surgery a procedure of therapeutic desperation. The less-mutilating procedures in more experienced hands might afford satisfactory relief with only minor personality changes.

CONCLUSIONS

It seems to me that neurosurgical ablative procedures are not always the final answer for relief of pain in cancer. Experience has taught us that if persistent and massive noxious stimuli, as those provoked by cancer, impinge on the central nervous system, not even the largest interruption of the so-called 'pain pathways' might permanently abolish pain and suffering. Owing to vicarious pathways, at least a part of those impulses surface consciousness as pain. Furthermore, sensory deprivation, due both to peripheral or central nervous system lesions, triggers spontaneous discharges in central pain which contribute to the patient's suffering.

However, in cancer pain, surgery has still a definite place. Owing to the fact that patients with malignant disease have a short period of survival, appropriate peripheral or central pain pathways interruption can afford dramatic relief for some months. I think we cannot obtain complete relief for much more than 3–4 months.

Somebody could ask himself whether such a formidable procedure as a surgical operation is reasonable in patients with very short life expectancy. We must recall that in very advanced cancer, for patients who will not survive more than a few weeks, less destructive procedures have been introduced, such as percutaneous cordotomy and stereotactic surgery. They can be employed without major complications. The appropriate procedure must be chosen on the basis of localization of pain, general conditions, and life expectancy. Appropriate selection of operation in selected cases will give the most gratifying results.

REFERENCES

1. Albe-Fessard, D. (1972): Central pathways for noxious stimuli. In: *Cervical Pain,* edited by C. Hirsch and Y. Zotterman, pp. 179–193. Pergamon Press, Oxford.
2. Barrash, J. M., and Leavens, M. E. (1973): Dorsal rhizotomy for the relief of intractable pain of malignant tumor origin. *J. Neurosurg.,* 38:755–757.
3. Bertrand, C., Martinez, N., and Hardy, J. (1966): Frontothalamic section for intractable pain. In: *Pain,* edited by R. S. Knighton and P. R. Dumke, pp. 531–535. Little, Brown, Boston.
4. Bettag, W. (1966): Results of treatment of pain by interruption of the medial pain tract of the brain stem. *Excerpta Medica Int. Cong. Series,* 110:771–775.
5. Birkenfeld, R., and Fisher, R. G. (1963): Successful treatment of causalgia of upper extremity with medullary spinothalamic tractotomy. *J. Neurosurg.,* 20:303–311.
6. Bohm, E. (1960): Chordotomy for intractable pain due to malignant disease. *Acta Psychiatr. Scand.,* 35:145–155.
7. Bohm, E., and Franksson, C. (1958–1959): Coccigodynia and sacral rhizotomy. *Acta Chir. Scand.,* 116:268–274.
8. Bowsher, D. (1974): Thalamic convergence and divergence of information generated by noxious stimulation. In: *Advances in Neurology, Vol. 4: International Symposium on Pain,* edited by J. J. Bonica, pp. 223–232. Raven Press, New York.
9. Brihaye, J., and Rétif, J. (1961): Comparison des résultats obtenuse par la cordotomie anterolaterale au niveau dorsal et auniveau cervical. (À propos de 109 observations personnelles). *Neurochirurgie,* 7:258–277.
10. Broager, B. (1974): Commissural myeolotomy. *Surg. Neurol.,* 2:71–74.
11. Cassinari, V., and Pagni, C. A. (1969): *Central Pain. A Neurosurgical Survey.* Harvard University Press, Cambridge.
12. Coggeshall, R. E., Appelbaum, M. L., Facem, M., Stubbs, T. B., III, and Sykes, M. T. (1975): Unmyelinated axons in human ventral roots, a possible explanation for the failure of dorsal rhizotomy to relieve pain. *Brain,* 98:157–166.
13. Cook, A. W., and Kawakamy, Y. (1977): Commissural myelotomy. *J. Neurosurg.,* 47:1–6.
14. Cooper, I. S. (1965): Clinical and physiologic implications of thalamic surgery for disorders of sensory communication. Part 1. Thalamic surgery for intractable pain. *J. Neurol. Sci.,* 2:493–519.
15. Crue, B. L., Todd, E. M., Carregal, E. J. A., Wright, W. H., and Maline, D. B. (1970): Posterior approach for high cervical percutaneous radiofrequency stereotaxic cordotomy. In: *Pain and Suffering. Selected Aspects,* edited by B. L. Crue, pp. 35–41. Charles C Thomas, Springfield, Ill.
16. Dargent, M., Mansuy, L., Colon, J., and De Rougemont, J. (1963): Les problèmes posé par la douleur dans l'evolution des cancer gynécologiques. *Lyon Chir.,* 59: 62–83.
17. Dogliotti, A. M. (1938): First surgical sections in man, of the lemniscus lateralis (pain-temperature paths) at the brainstem, for the treatment of diffused rebellious pain. *Anesth. Analg.,* 17:143–145.
18. Fairman, D. (1976): Neurophysiological basis for the hypothalamic lesion and stimulation by chronic implanted electrodes for the relief of intractable pain in cancer. In: *Advances in Pain Research and Therapy, Vol. 1: Proceedings of the First World Congress on Pain,* edited by J. J. Bonica and D. Albe-Fessard, pp. 843–847. Raven Press, New York.
19. Falconer, M. A. (1948): Relief of intractable pain of organic origin by frontal lobotomy. *Res. Publ. Assoc. Nerv. Ment. Dis.,* 27:707–714.
20. Felsööry, A., and Crue, B. L. (1976): Results of 19 years experience with sacral rhizotomy for perineal and perianal cancer pain. *Pain,* 2:431–433.

21. Foltz, E. L., and White, L. E. (1966): Rostral cingulotomy and pain "relief." In: *Pain,* edited by R. S. Knighton and P. R. Dumke, pp. 469–491. Little, Brown, Boston.
22. Farioli, B., and Guidetti, B. (1975): Effects of stereotactic lesions of the pulvinar and lateralis posterior nucleus on intractable pain and dyskinetic syndromes in man. *Appl. Neurophysiol.,* 38:23–70.
23. Freeman, W., and Watts, J. W. (1950): *Psychosurgery in the Treatment of Mental Disorders and Intractable Pain.* Charles C Thomas, Springfield, Ill.
24. French, L. A. (1974): High cervical tractotomy: Technique and results. *Clin. Neurosurg.,* 21:239–245.
25. French, L. A., Chou, S. N., and Story, J. L. (1966): Cervical tractotomy: Technique and clinical usefulness. In: *Pain,* edited by R. S. Knighton and P. R. Dumke, pp. 311–320. Little, Brown, Boston.
26. Gildenberg, P. L. (1974): Percutaneous cordotomy cervical. *Clin. Neurosurg.,* 21:246–256.
27. Glees, P. (1953): The central pain tract. *Acta Neuroveg.,* 7:160–174.
28. Graf, C. I. (1960): Consideration in loss of sensory level after bilateral cervical cordotomy. *Arch. Neurol.,* 3:410–415.
29. Grantham, E. G. (1951): Prefrontal lobotomy for relief of pain, with a report of a new operative technique. *J. Neurosurg.,* 8:405–410.
30. Hassler, R. (1960): Die zentrale Systeme des Schmerzes. *Acta Neurochir.,* 8:423–535.
31. Helfant, M. H., Leksell, L., and Strang, R. R. (1965): Experiences with intractable pain treated by stereotaxic mesencephalotomy. *Acta Chir. Scand.,* 129:573–580.
32. Hitchcock, E. (1974): Stereotactic myelotomy. *Proc. R. Soc. Med.,* 67:771–772.
33. Hurt, R. W., and Ballantine, H. T. (1974): Stereotactic anterior cingulate lesions for persistent pain: A report on 68 cases. *Clin. Neurosurg.,* 21:334–351.
34. Kerr, F. W. L. (1975): Neuroanatomical substrates of nociception in the spinal cord. *Pain,* 1:325–356.
35. Kim, Y. K., and Umbach, W. (1972): Comparative evaluation of different psychosurgical methods. In: *Present Limits of Neurosurgery,* edited by I. Fusek and Z. Kunc, pp. 465–469. Avicenum, Praha.
36. King, R. B. (1977): Anterior commissurotomy for intractable pain. *J. Neurosurg.,* 47:7–11.
37. Kühner, A. (1976): La valeur des interventions sur les racines sacrées dans le traitement des syndromes douloureux du bassin. *Neurochirurgie,* 22:429–436.
38. Lazorthes, Y., Verdie, J. C., and Lagarrigue, J. (1976): Thermocoagulation percutanée des nerfs rachidiens à visée analgésique. *Neurochirurgie,* 22:445–453.
39. Le Beau, J., Bouvet, M., and Rosier, M. (1950): Traitement des douleurs irréductibles par la topectomie. *Sem. Hop.,* 24:1946–1952.
40. Lembcke, W. (1964): Über die mediolongitudinale Chordotomie im Halsmarkbereich. *Zentrabl. Chir.,* 89:439–443.
41. Lin, P. M., Gildenberg, P. L., and Polakoff, P. P. (1966): An anterior approach to percutaneous lower cervical cordotomy. *J. Neurosurg.,* 25:553–560.
42. Lindstrom, P. A. (1972): Prefrontal sonic treatment—sixteen years' experience. In: *Psychosurgery, Proc. 2nd Int. Congr. Psychosurg.,* edited by L. Laitinen and K. Vaernet, pp. 357–376. Charles C Thomas, Springfield, Ill.
43. Lindstrom, P. A., Moench, L. G., and Rovnanek, A. (1964): Prefrontal sonic treatment. *Curr. Psychiat. Ther.,* 4:143–149.
44. Lippert, R. G., Hosobuchi, Y., and Nielsen, S. L. (1974): Spinal commissurotomy. *Surg. Neurol.,* 2:373–377.
45. Lipton, S., Dervin, E., and Heywood, O. B. (1974): A stereotactic approach to the anterior percutaneous electrical cordotomy. In: *Advances in Neurology, Vol. 4: International Symposium on Pain,* edited by J. J. Bonica, pp. 689–694. Raven Press, New York.
46. Loeser, J. D. (1972): Dorsal rhizotomy for the relief of chronic pain. *J. Neurosurg.,* 36:745–750.
47. Lorenz, R., Grumme, T., Herrmann, D., Palleske, H., Kühner, A., Stende, U., and

Zierski, J. (1975): Percutaneous cordotomy. In: *Advances in Neurosurgery Vol. 3,* edited by H. Penzholz, M. Brock, J. Hamer, M. Klinger, and O. Spoerri, pp. 178–185. Springer, Berlin.
48. Mansuy, L., Sindou, M., Fischer, G., and Brunon, J. (1976): La cordotomie spinothalamique dans les douleurs cancéreuses. *Neurochirurgie,* 22:437–444.
49. Mark, V. H., Ervin, F. R., and Hackett, T. P. (1960): Clinical aspects of stereotactic thalamotomy in the human. I. The treatment of chronic severe pain. *Arch. Neurol.,* 3:351–367.
50. Mark, V. H., Ervin, F. R., and Yakovlev, P. I. (1963): Stereotactic thalamotomy III. Verification of anatomical lesion site in the human thalamus. *Arch. Neurol.,* 8:528–538.
51. Maspes, P. E., and Pagni, C. A. (1965): Studio critico degli interventi stereotassici eseguiti a livello talamico per il trattamento dei dolori incoercibili. *Riv. Pat. Nerv. Ment.* Atti Congr. Naz. Soc. Ital. Neurol., pp. 1–154.
52. Maspes, P. E., and Pagni, C. A. (1974): A critical appraisal of pain surgery and suggestions for improving treatment. In: *Recent Advances on Pain: Pathophysiology and Clinical Aspects,* edited by J. J. Bonica, P. Procacci, and C. A. Pagni, pp. 201–255. Charles C Thomas, Springfield, Ill.
53. Mazars, G., Merienne, L., and Cioloca, C. (1976): État actuel de la chirurgie de la douleur. *Neurochirurgie* [*Suppl.*], 1:1–164.
54. McKissock, W. (1951): Rostral leucotomy. *Lancet,* 2:91–94.
55. Merskey, H., and Spear, F. G. (1967): *Pain: Psychological and Psychiatric Aspects.* Baillière, Tindall and Cassell, London.
56. Müke, R., and Correia, A. (1975): Potentials and limits of percutaneous cervical cordotomy. In: *Advances in Neurosurgery, Vol. 3,* edited by H. Penzholz, M. Brock, J. Hamer, M. Klinger, and O. Spoerri, pp. 195–198. Springer, Berlin.
57. Mullan, S. (1971): The surgical relief of pain. *Clin. Neurosurg.,* 18:208–224.
58. Mullan, S. (1974): Percutaneous cordotomy. In: *Advances in Neurology, Vol. 4: International Symposium on Pain,* edited by J. J. Bonica, pp. 677–682. Raven Press, New York.
59. Mullan, S., Harper, P., Hekmatpanah, J., Torres, H., and Dobbin, G. (1963): Percutaneous interruption of spinal pain tracts by means of a strontium 90 needle. *J. Neurosurg.,* 20:931–939.
60. Mullan, S., Hekmatpanah, J., Dobbin, G., and Beckman, F. (1965): Percutaneous intramedullary cordotomy utilizing the unipolar anodal electrolytic lesion. *J. Neurosurg.,* 22:548–553.
61. Nashold, B. S. (1972): Extensive cephalic and oral pain relieved by midbrain tractotomy. *Confin. Neurol.,* 34:382.
62. Nashold, B. S., Wilson, W. P., and Slaughter, D. G. (1969): Stereotactic midbrain lesions for central dysaesthesia and phantom pain. *J. Neurosurg.,* 30:116–126.
63. Noordenbos, W. (1959): *Pain: Problems Pertaining to the Transmission of Nerve Impulses Which Give Rise to Pain.* Elsevier, Amsterdam.
64. Ogle, W. S., French, L. A., and Peyton, W. T. (1956): Experiences with high cervical cordotomy. *J. Neurosurg.,* 13:81–87.
65. Osgood, C. P., Dujovni, M., and Faille, R. (1976): Microsurgical lumbosacral ganglionectomy technique, anatomic rationale, and surgical results. In: *Advances In Pain Research and Therapy, Vol. 1: Proceedings of the First World Congress on Pain,* edited by J. J. Bonica and D. Albe-Fessard, pp. 855–862. Raven Press, New York.
66. Owens, G. (1966): Panel discussion. Unsolved problems. In: *Pain,* edited by R. S. Knighton and P. R. Dumke, pp. 540–545. Little, Brown, Boston.
67. Pagni, C. A. (1966): Discussion by Erwin, F. R., Brown, C. E., and Mark, V. H., Striatal influences on facial pain. *Confin. Neurol.,* 27:88–89.
68. Pagni, C. A. (1969): Fisiopatologia del dolore. *Atti. VI Congr. Naz. Soc. Ital. Med. Fis. Riabil.,* pp. 77–116. Mattioli, Fidenza.
69. Pagni, C. A. (1974): Place of stereotactic technique in surgery for pain. In: *Advances in Neurology, Vol. 4: International Symposium on Pain,* edited by J. J. Bonica, pp. 699–706. Raven Press, New York.

70. Pagni, C. A. (1977): Central pain and painful anesthesia. In: *Pain—Its Neurosurgical Management. Part II: Central Procedures,* edited by H. Krayenbühl, P. E. Maspes, and W. H. Sweet, pp. 132–257. Karger, Basel.
71. Pagni, C. A. (1979): Therapy of cancer pain in the head and neck. Role of neurosurgery. In: *Advances in Pain Research and Therapy, Vol. 2,* International Symposium on Pain of Advanced Cancer, edited by J. J. Bonica and V. Ventafridda. Raven Press, New York.
72. Pagni, C. A., and Maspes, P. E. (1970): Problems in the surgical treatment of pain in malignancies of the head and neck. In: *Current Research in Neurosciences, Vol. 10,* edited by H. T. Wycis, pp. 138–153. Karger, Basel.
73. Papo, I., and Luongo, A. (1976): High cervical commissural myelotomy in the treatment of pain. *J. Neurol. Neurosurg. Psychiatry,* 39:705–710.
74. Piscol, K. (1975): Open spinal surgery for intractable pain. In: *Advances in Neurosurgery, Vol. 3,* edited by H. Penzholz, M. Brock, J. Hamer, M. Klinger, and O. Spoerri, pp. 157–169. Springer, Berlin.
75. Ray, B. S. (1943): The management of intractable pain by posterior rhizotomy. *Res. Publ. Ass. Res. Nerv. Ment. Dis.,* 23:391–407.
76. Richardson, D. E. (1967): Thalamotomy for intractable pain. *Confin. Neurol.,* 29:139–145.
77. Roeder, F., and Orthner, H. (1961): Erfahrungen mit stereotaktischen Eingriffen. III Mitteilung. Über zerebrale Schmerzoperationen, insbesondere mediale Mesencephalotomie bei thalamischer Hyperpatie und bei Anaesthesia dolorosa. *Confin. Neurol.,* 21:51–97.
78. Rosomoff, H. L. (1969): Bilateral percutaneous cervical radiofrequency cordotomy. *J. Neurosurg.,* 31:41–46.
79. Rosomoff, H. L., Carroll, F., Brown, J., and Sheptak, P. (1965): Percutaneous radiofrequency cervical cordotomy: Technique. *J. Neurosurg.,* 23:639–644.
80. Sano, K. (1977): Intralaminar thalamotomy (thalamolaminotomy) and posteromedial hypothalamotomy in the treatment of intractable pain. In: *Pain—Its Neurosurgical Management. Part II: Central Procedures,* edited by H. Krayenbühl, P. E. Maspes, and W. H. Sweet, pp. 50–103. Karger, Basel.
81. Scarff, J. E. (1950): Unilateral prefrontal lobotomy for the relief of intractable pain. Report of 58 cases with special consideration of failures. *J. Neurosurg.,* 7:330–336.
82. Schürmann, K. (1972): Fundamental principles of the surgical treatment of pain. In: *Pain—Basic Principles—Pharmacology—Therapy,* edited by R. Janzen, W. D. Keidel, A. Herz, and C. Steichele, pp. 181–193. Thieme, Stuttgart.
83. Schvarcz, J. R. (1976): Stereotactic extralemniscal myelotomy. *J. Neurol. Neurosurg. Psychiat.,* 39:53–57.
84. Scoville, W. B. (1949): Selective cortical undercutting as a means of modifying and studying frontal lobe function in man. *J. Neurosurg.,* 6:65–73.
85. Scoville, W. B. (1972): Psychosurgery and other lesions of the brain affecting human behavior. In: *Psychosurgery, Proceedings of the 2nd International Congress on Psychosurgery,* edited by E. Hitchcock, L. Laitinen, and K. Vaernet, pp. 5–21. Charles C Thomas, Springfield, Ill.
86. Siegfried, J., and Krayenbühl, H. (1972): Clinical experience in the treatment of intractable pain. In: *Pain—Basic Principles—Pharmacology—Therapy,* edited by R. Janzen, W. D. Keidel, A. Herz, and C. Steichele, pp. 202–204. Thieme, Stuttgart.
87. Sindou, M., Fischer, G., Goutelle, A., and Mansuy, L. (1974): La radicellotomie postérieure sélective. Premiers résultats dans la chirurgie de la douleur. *Neurochirurgie,* 20:391–408.
88. Sindou, M., Fischer, G., and Mansuy, L. (1976): Posterior spinal rhizotomy and selective posterior rhizidiotomy. In: *Pain—Its Neurosurgical Management. Part I: Procedures on Primary Afferent Neurons,* edited by H. Krayenbühl, P. E. Maspes, and W. H. Sweet, pp. 201–250. Karger, Basel.
89. Sourek, K. (1969): Commissural myelotomy. *J. Neurosurg.,* 31:524–527.
90. Sourek, K. (1977): Mediolongitudinal myelotomy. In: *Pain—Its Neurosurgical*

Management. Part II: Central Procedures, edited by H. Krayenbühl, P. E. Maspes, W. H. Sweet, pp. 15–34. Karger, Basel.

91. Spiegel, E. A., Wycis, H. T., Marks, M., and Lee, A. J. (1947): Stereotaxic apparatus for operations on the human brain. *Science,* 106:349–350.
92. Spiegel, E. A., Wycis, H. T., Szekely, E. G., and Gildenberg, P. L. (1966): Medial and basal thalamotomy in so-called intractable pain. In: *Pain,* edited by R. S. Knighton and P. R. Dumke, pp. 503–517. Little, Brown, Boston.
93. Sugita, K., Mutsuga, N., Takaoka, Y., and Doi, T. (1972): Results of stereotactic thalamotomy for pain. *Confin. Neurol.,* 34:265–274.
94. Tasker, R. R. (1977): Open cordotomy. In: *Pain—Its Neurosurgical Management. Part II: Central Procedures*, edited by H. Krayenbühl, P. E. Maspes and W. H. Sweet, pp. 1–14. Karger, Basel.
95. Torvik, A. (1959): Sensory motor and reflex changes in two cases of intractable pain after stereotactic mesencephalic tractotomy. *J. Neurol. Neurosurg. Psychiatry,* 22:299–305.
96. Turnbull, I. M. (1972): Bilateral cingulotomy combined with thalamotomy or mesencephalic tractotomy for pain. *Surg. Gynecol. Obstet.,* 134:958–962.
97. Vlahovitch, B., and Fuentes, J. M. (1975): Résultats de la radicellotomie sélective postérieure à l'étage lombaire et cervical. *Neurochirurgie,* 21:29–42.
98. Walker, E. A. (1942): Mesencephalic tractotomy. A method for the relief of unilateral intractable pain. *Arch. Surg.,* 44:953–962.
99. Wertheimer, P., and Lecuire, J. (1953): La myélotomie commissurale postèrieure. À propos de 107 observations. *Acta Chir. Belg.,* 52:568–574.
100. White, J. C. (1966): Cordotomy: Assessment of its effectiveness and suggestions for its improvement. *Clin. Neurosurg.,* 13:1–19.
101. White, J. C., and Kjellberg, R. N. (1973): Posterior spinal rhizotomy. A substitute for cordotomy in the relief of localized pain in patients with normal life expectancy. *Neurochirurgia,* 16:141–170.
102. White, J. C., and Sweet, W. H. (1969): *Pain and the Neurosurgeon. A Forty Years Experience.* Charles C Thomas, Springfield, Ill.
103. Wycis, H. T., and Spiegel, E. A. (1962): Long-range results in the treatment of intractable pain by stereotaxic midbrain surgery. *J. Neurosurg.,* 19:101–107.
104. Yoshimasu, N. (1972): Functional anatomy of the internal medullary lamina based on the results of stereotaxic surgery. *Brain and Nerve,* 24:1277–1292. (In Japanese.)

Advances in Pain Research and Therapy, Vol. 2,
edited by J. J. Bonica and V. Ventafridda.
Raven Press, New York © 1979.

Percutaneous Cervical Cordotomy

Sampson Lipton

Associated Department of Neurological Sciences, Liverpool University, Walton Hospital, Liverpool L9 1AE England

In 1905, Spiller (16) showed that pain and temperature sensation are transmitted through the anterolateral spinal tract. Seven years later, Spiller and Martin (17) reported a patient in whom section of the anterior quadrant of the spinal cord abolished intractable pain. Since then, sectioning of the anterolateral quadrant (ALQ), commonly known as cordotomy, or anterolateral tractotomy, has been used widely to relieve severe, intractable pain located below the cervical spinal segments. Until 15 years ago, the procedure was carried out through a laminectomy and a subsequent section of the tracts at the upper thoracic levels.

In 1963, Mullan (11) first described the technique of percutaneous cordotomy at $C_{1\text{-}2}$. Destruction of the ALQ was achieved through a needle inserted via a posterolateral approach and a radioactive strontium–tipped probe placed in ALQ. Subsequently, techniques entailing lateral, anterior, and posterior approaches were developed (1,6).

Because the percutaneous technique is a minor surgical procedure, it has been largely used for the relief of severe pain of advanced cancer. In this presentation, I will discuss: (a) the anatomic bases of cervical percutaneous cordotomy; (b) techniques of lateral, anterior, posterior, and bilateral percutaneous cervical cordotomy; and (c) the results obtained by our group for patients with cancer.

ANATOMIC CONSIDERATIONS

The anterolateral quadrant of the spinal cord contains crossed sensory fibers which transmit sensations interpreted as pain, heat, and cold. Also in this region are the spinocerebellar tracts, and ataxia may result when these are destroyed. Moreover, in the C_1-C_2 region of the spinal cord are located the respiratory reticular fibers lying close to the anterior horn cells, and these may be destroyed by cordotomy at this level.

The posterior quadrant of the spinal cord contains the cerebrospinal or motor tract, and this is contiguous anterolaterally with the sensory tracts. The dentate ligament at the C_1-C_2 level tends to separate the anterior sen-

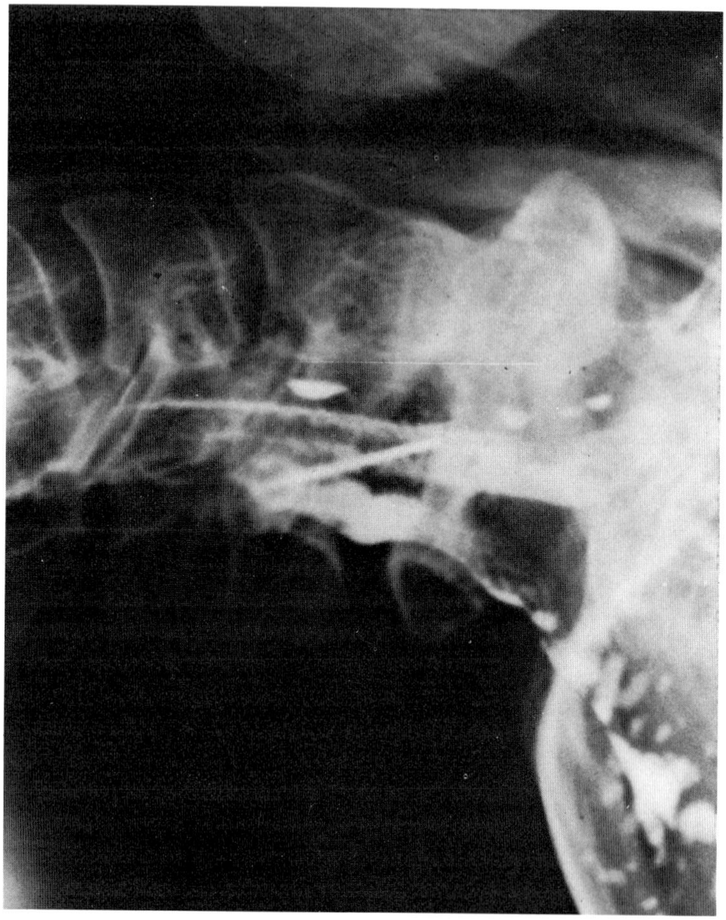

FIG. 1. Lateral roentgenograms of the cervical spine taken in the course of a lateral percutaneous cervical cordotomy. The needle is in place after being inserted through the interspace between C_1 and C_2 vertebra. Injection of the radio-opaque emulsion outlines the anterior border of the spinal cord, the dentate ligament, and the posterior dura. Note that the point of the spinal needle is anterior to the dentate ligament.

sory quadrant from the posterior motor nerve fibers. The position of the ALQ is between the anterior border of the spinal cord anteriorly and the dentate ligament posteriorly.

The cervicomedullary junction is a portion of the spinal cord where rapid rearrangements of nerve fibers are made. Above this level the motor fibers are anteriorly situated while below, the sensory fibers are anterior. Thus, over a short distance, motor fibers move posteriorly, while sensory fibers move anteriorly. This takes place over a definite section of the spinal cord, whose length varies in different patients. Occasionally at the C_1-C_2 level, the motor decussation has not been completed and the motor fibers have not moved completely posteriorly, while the sensory fibers remain partially posteriorly (18).

Another important anatomic fact is that when pain fibers enter the posterior root of the spinal cord, they ascend for a few segments and then cross to the opposite ALQ. However, this crossover is not 100%, and occasionally little, if any, crossover takes place. There are authenticated cases where sectioning of one ALQ has produced analgesia on the same side of the body instead of the contralateral side (20).

The pain fibers in the anterolateral quadrant are segmented in that the sacral fibers are close to the dentate ligament, and those from lumbar, dorsal, and cervical regions lie successively anteriorly The upper cervical pain fibers lie close to the anterior horn cells and the respiratory fibers. A cordotomy, which produces a high level of analgesia by destruction of the cervical fibers, tends to destroy the respiratory fibers also (5,13).

Nerve fibers which control micturition lie close to the lateral horn and may be destroyed in any cordotomy. Bilateral cordotomies at any level of the spinal cord may interfere with micturition. Bilateral cordotomies at the C_1-C_2 level may also interfere with respiration. Loss of reticular respiratory fibers bilaterally produces a peculiar form of apnea in which the patient can breathe voluntarily but does not breathe automatically (4). These patients, therefore, tend to develop a form of sleep apnea ("Ondine's Curse"). This respiratory problem can be avoided by carrying out cordotomy on one side, using the lateral approach, and on the other side, using the anterior approach at the C_5-C_6 level; i.e., below the respiratory reticular fibers and below the outflow of the phrenic nerve. Alternatively, a bilateral C_1-C_2 cordotomy can avoid respiratory problems if the level of analgesia is kept below C_7 on one side. If a patient has reduced lung-function, then a unilateral cordotomy will increase the disability by reducing ventilatory power (8).

TECHNICAL CONSIDERATIONS

The anterior approach can be used at any cervical level but usually is done at C_5-C_6. The lateral approach can be carried out only at the C_1-C_2 space, as the anatomic configuration of the cervical facet joints (zygoapophyseal joints) closes the other spaces. The posterior approach can be made at the C_1-C_2 space or between the base of skull and C_1 if a cervicomedullary lesion is to be made. The technique of the lateral approach will be discussed first.

As previously mentioned, the first technique of percutaneous cervical cordotomy described by Mullan in 1963 (11) entailed the use of ionizing radiation to destroy the ALQ. A spinal needle was inserted from a posterolateral approach, and the tip of the spinal needle was placed against the vertebral body anteriorly. Through this needle was inserted a probe tipped with radioactive strontium which was forced against the bone. The spinal needle was then withdrawn to uncover the radioactive-tipped probe, and a mathematical calculation was used to estimate the irradiation time. This technique led to pain-relief in the lower limb in 1 to 2 weeks. Relief of pain in the arm required a higher dose of radioactivity and took longer to develop. Further, the radiation destruction of nerve fibers was progressive. If the patient lived long enough, damage spread to the contralateral side of the spinal cord and even posteriorly; paresis and even paraparesis could develop.

In 1965, Mullan (12) described a modification entailing the use of a direct electrical current to achieve destruction of the ALQ. This worked well, but a period of at least 20 min was required for adequate analgesia to develop. In the same year, Rosomoff and his co-workers (14) used a radiofrequency current which produced thermocoagulation of the nerve fibers in the ALQ. This method produces a very rapid destruction of the nerve tissues; much more care had to be taken to position the needle correctly. Our center has employed a technique for percutaneous cordotomy based upon the work of Mullan and Rosomoff.

LATERAL PERCUTANEOUS CERVICAL CORDOTOMY

Instrumentation. For the lateral percutaneous cervical cordotomy, the patient lies supine with the head fixed in a special head-holder. A spinal needle of sufficient size to allow the electrode to pass through it is used. The electrode has a stop on it so that only 4 mm of its tip protrudes through the spinal needle. Moreover, the terminal 2 mm of the electrode is free of insulation, and the tip is sharpened. A lesion generator is used to produce the radiofrequency current; and the complete apparatus, which includes the head-holder, micromanipulator to raise or lower the spinal needle, the electrode kit and lesion generator, is sold commercially.[1] Commercial lesion generators usually contain facilities for impedance measurements and a range of stimulation frequencies from 2 to 100 Hz.

Technique of puncture. Under local anesthesia, the spinal needle is inserted approximately 1 cm below and behind the mastoid process and advanced into the subarachnoid space anterior to the dentate ligament. Ten ml of air or 1 to 2 ml of myodil emulsion[2] is injected. Air outlines the anterior border of the spinal cord, whereas myodil outlines the dentate ligament (3,4,10,14) (Figs. 1 and 2). Which of these is used depends upon the patient's life-expectancy; if the patient has a long life-expectancy, air is used, because this avoids the risk of arachnoiditis in those patients sensitive to myodil. The majority of my patients have a short life-expectancy due to inoperable cancer; usually, I employ myodil.

[1] The apparatus the author uses is that of Owl Instruments Limited, 61 Alness Street, Downs View, Ontario, Canada, M3J 2H2.

[2] The myodil emulsion is made up by shaking 3 ml of iophendylate with 6 ml of saline or CSF in a 20-ml syringe with air.

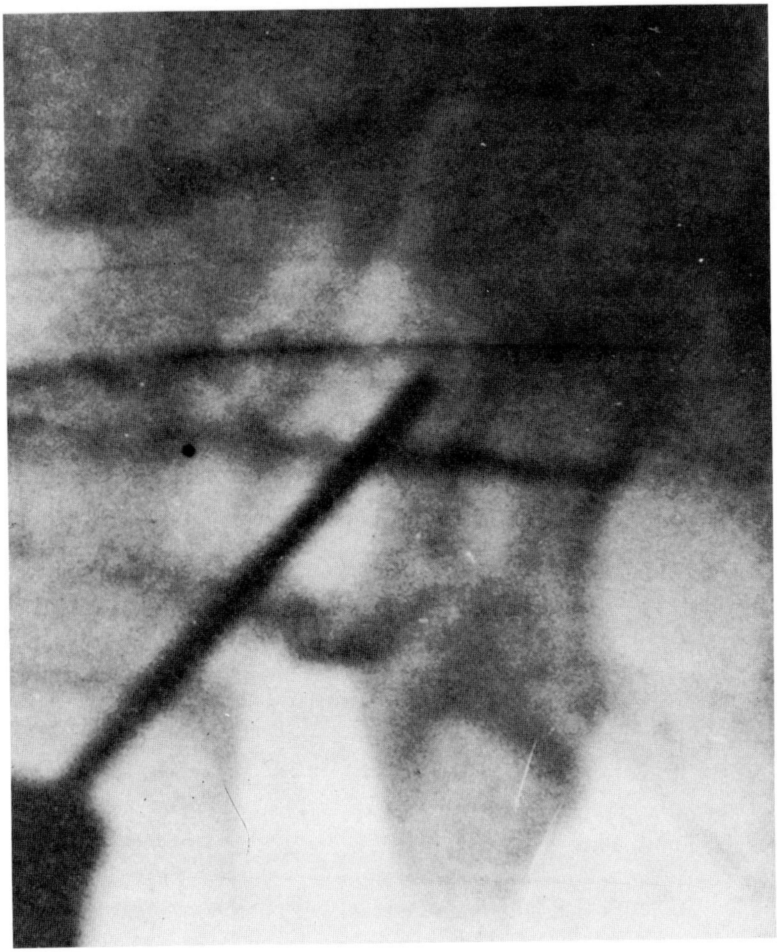

FIG. 2. Close-up of normal appearance after injection of radio-opaque emulsion.

After the injection of air or myodil, the position of the spinal needle is checked by lateral and anteroposterior X-rays using an image-intensifier. The lateral film helps to place the tip of the needle in relation to the dentate ligament or anterior border of the spinal cord (Fig. 3). The anteroposterior film taken through the open mouth allows visualization of the tip of the spinal needle in relation to the pedicles laterally and the odontoid process medially. If penetration is deeper than the lateral border of the odontoid process, the spinal needle has been inserted too deeply (8,10,14,15) (Fig. 4).

The spinal needle is then aimed 1 to 2 mm anterior to the dentate ligament or 3 mm posterior to the anterior border of the spinal cord. Impedance measurements are then used to insert the electrode. When the tip of the electrode is in the cerebrospinal fluid, resistance is about 200 ohms. When the electrode tip is half in the spinal cord and half in the cerebrospinal fluid, the

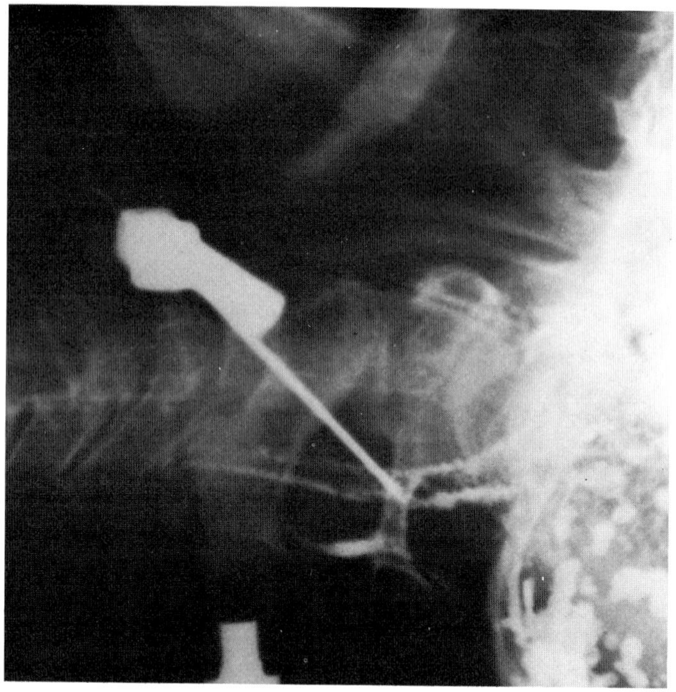

FIG. 3. The hub of the spinal needle is elevated and its tip depressed. Also note that the dentate ligament is depressed.

resistance is slightly higher, approximately 300 ohms. When the tip is entirely in the spinal cord, the resistance rises rapidly to 800 ohms or more.

Stimulation technique. Initial stimulation is at 2 Hz; and at 2 V, stimulation of motor fibers and anterior horn cells may occur. This is shown by rhythmic contractions of the small muscles of the ipsilateral neck causing a turning movement of the head and of the ipsilateral trapezius as well, causing elevation of the shoulder. At this voltage, there should be no activation of arm, body, or leg muscles. If there is, the electrode is too close to the corticospinal tract, and its position must be altered. If the voltage is increased to 4 or 5 V, contractions of the ipsilateral limb or trunk muscles may occur.

Stimulation is then carried out at 100 Hz and 0.2 V; the patient may describe sensation on the contralateral side. These sensory hallucinations may take any form, such as pain, tingling, pins and needles, or sensations of hot or cold wind on the skin. Occasionally, these sensations are ipsilateral, and occasionally bilateral. If consistent ipsilateral sensory hallucinations are produced, the only method of determining whether the patient has an uncrossed sensory tract is by carrying out a small coagulation and observing the development of analgesia. In the author's experience, this has invariably been on the contralateral side; but it must be recognized that sooner or later

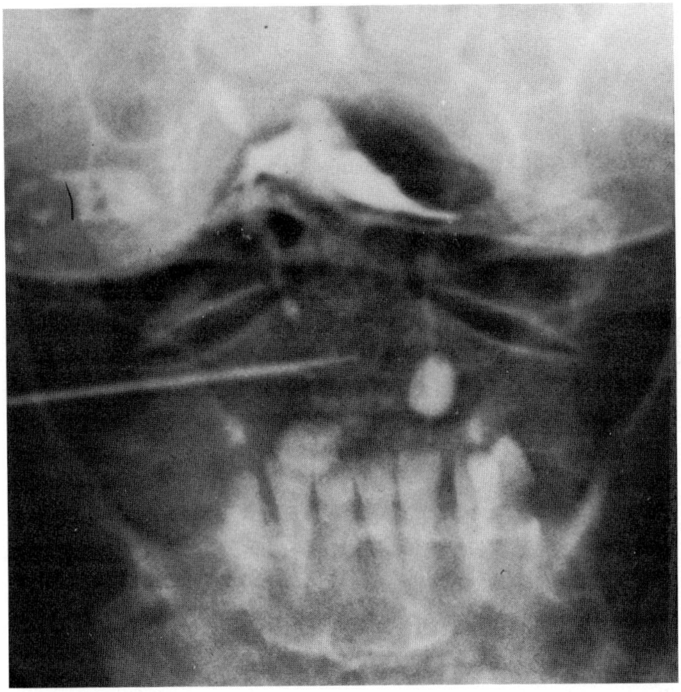

FIG. 4. Anteroposterior view through the open mouth showing the relationship of the tip of the spinal needle and the electrode protruding through it to the odontoid process.

a patient with one of the rare uncrossed sensory tracts will appear, so care must be taken (8,12,19).

Coagulation. Before carrying out coagulation, sensation to pinprick on both sides of the body should be checked; the mere presence of the electrode can produce alterations of sensation in the contralateral side. On rare occasions, the insulated portion of the electrode or even the spinal needle could have been inserted into cord tissue, and this may show itself by a Brown-Sequard syndrome. If penetration of the cord in this fashion occurs, the needle should be withdrawn, the cordotomy postponed and the patient observed for 24 hr. Recovery of normal sensation and power begins in about 15 min and improves rapidly. The following day, the percutaneous cordotomy can be carried out in the usual fashion.

There are two methods of coagulating the ALQ. One is by using a current of about 50 milliamperes (mA) for short periods of time, beginning with 2½ sec and rising to 30 sec in small increments. Testing of analgesia is always carried out between each increment. The second method is to use a time of 30 sec and vary the current beginning with 20 mA, rising to 50 mA and again testing contralateral sensation between each increment. The actual current and time used will depend on the lesion generator; if a commercial instrument is used, these parameters will be indicated by the manufacturer. It is best to err on the cautious side, as a larger lesion can always be made; but damage cannot be eradicated once it has occurred. The series of coagulations continues until analgesia covers the painful area with a few segments to spare. The final coagulation used is repeated 3 times to make sure all fibers in the coagulated region are destroyed.

During coagulation, the ipsilateral arm and leg are carefully observed for the development of weakness: a sign of spread of the lesion to the corticospinal tract. This is quite easily carried out by asking the patient to flex the ipsilateral knee or hold the ipsilateral arm in the air while coagulating. After each coagulation, the grip can be tested as can dorsiflexion of the foot (7).

RESULTS

Analgesia. It is difficult to obtain an accurate figure for this, as many authorities have not published full details (3,8,10). In the author's series, 75% of patients with intractable cancer pain were free of pain until they died. A further 8% had exceedingly good relief of pain, which was not complete but was controlled by simple analgesics, such as aspirin or paracetamol. A further 8% had partial relief of pain which wore off in a variable period, while 9% obtained ineffectual relief of pain or were failures. Of the last two groups, totaling 17%, more than one-third (7%) had successful repeat cordotomies. This brings the total success rate to 90% (8).

Mortality. Mortality depends primarily on selection of patients. In our institution, if the patient is expected to live at least 2 weeks, a cordotomy will be carried out. Over the years, increasingly ill patients have been accepted for the lateral percutaneous cervical cordotomy, and the mortality has increased also. It is now 6.2% in the first postoperative week. The majority of these deaths occurred in patients who had respiratory problems before the cordotomy. The number of percutaneous cervical cordotomies carried out at the Centre for Pain Relief, Walton Hospital, Liverpool, is approaching 700. Fewer than 50 cordotomies have been carried out on patients with long life-expectancies. It is these patients who, in the main, develop dysesthesiae beginning some 6 months postoperatively.

Side effects and complications. Horner's syndrome after a lateral C_1-C_2 percutaneous cervical cordotomy is invariably present in successful cordotomies. It is usually marked in the first few weeks and gradually decreases over a period of months. No cardiovascular disturbances have developed in any of our patients subjected to percutaneous cervical cordotomy. Ataxia is rare but may be masked by weakness and therefore not noted. A few cases have been seen to involve the lower limb and usually improve within 3 weeks. Hemiparesis was present to some extent in 90% of the patients postoperatively. However, 40% of the patients did not have any practical disability; 40% recognized that they had weakness; and 20% were unsteady when they turned around or went up or down stairs due to a weak lower limb. About 10% of the patients had enough weakness to require a walking aid, but the majority of these did not require this walking aid after 1 month. Two percent of patients had a permanent hemiparesis sufficient to prevent them from walking without help. Normally, the leg is affected to a greater degree than the arm; this probably being a reflection of the closeness of the motor fibers to the leg of the ALQ.

Abnormalities of micturition are rare after unilateral cordotomy (1.5%). However, after bilateral cordotomy, urinary problems are much more frequent.

Significant respiratory complications occurred in 8.7%, and approximately half these (4.6%) were fatal. They are very rare after unilateral cordotomy, but more common after a bilateral lesion. These figures are higher than those of most other authorities.

Bilateral Percutaneous Cervical Cordotomy

The two possible complications of bilateral percutaneous cervical cordotomy at the upper cervical level have already been mentioned (14). These are sleep apnea, which has a 50% mortality rate, and problems with micturition, which occur in almost all cases. It is wise, therefore, to consider procedures which can avoid a high bilateral percutaneous cervical cordotomy. Often, a high cordotomy can be combined with an intrathecal phenol block for the pain on the other side. As both these lesions will be made on the same side of the spinal cord, both respiratory and bladder problems can be avoided. Alternatively, a high lateral percutaneous cervical cordotomy can be combined with an anterior percutaneous cervical cordotomy at the C_5-C_6 level.

If a bilateral cordotomy has to be carried out, it is best to have an interval of a week between the two sides, and to aim the electrode on one side cephalad, and on the second side, caudad to try to ensure that the two lesions are not made at exactly the same spinal level. If the analgesic level of one of these lesions can be kept below C_7, there should be no respiratory problems. Great care must be taken when a cordotomy is performed on a patient with pulmonary deficiencies contralateral to the cordotomy (3).

Anterior Percutaneous Cervical Cordotomy

In 1966, Lin (6) reported an anterior approach to the anterolateral quadrant using a lower disk space. The technique consists of inserting the spinal needle through the disk space between C_5 and C_6, entering the subarachnoid space and placing an electrode into the anterolateral tract from

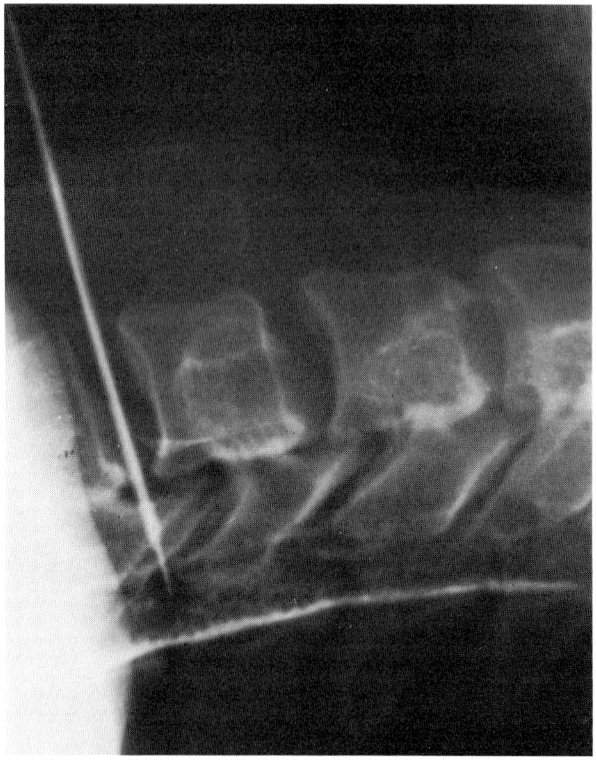

FIG. 5. Anterior-approach percutaneous cordotomy. Note that the spinal needle is in position through the disk space with the electrode protruding. An injection of radio-opaque emulsion has outlined the subarachnoid space with the posterior dura showing up well.

an anterior position. The target is exactly the same as that in the lateral approach, namely 2 mm anterior to the dentate ligament. A series of calculations have to be made from X-ray films to ensure that the direction of the spinal needle is correct. If cervical or thoracic sensory fibers are to be destroyed, the target is 3 to 4 mm from the midline on the contralateral side, whereas for sacral or lumbar pain, the target is 8 mm from the midline. In the anteroposterior direction, the target is 8 mm behind the posterior edge of the vertebral body (Fig. 5).

This technique is difficult because the spinal needle is gripped by the disk material and, once the tip of the needle has entered the disk, its direction cannot be altered. Therefore, this needle must be aimed directly at the target from the very beginning.

The technique is much safer than C_1-C_2 lateral cordotomy because respiratory abnormalities do not occur, as the lesion is made below the outflow of the phrenic nerve. The patient's normal diaphragmatic activity is preserved on the side of the lesion. However, the electrode approaches the sensory fibers by passing through the anterior horn cells, and there is a high risk of damage to the motoneurons. Depending on the level used, there may be weakness of muscles in the upper or lower arm; and, if a lower cervical space is used, in the hand itself. This weakness recovers usually within a week.

Because of the difficulty of approach, a number of stereotactic methods have been designed to help in placing the spinal needle on the correct line (2,9).

Posterior Percutaneous Cervical Cordotomy

Crue et al. (1) reported the technique of using the posterior approach to the anterolateral quadrant of the spinal cord. A bipolar needle is used for recordings, and then the same electrode is used as a monopolar lesion electrode. With the patient lying prone, the electrode is inserted through the skin and muscles of the posterior part of the neck through the C_1-C_2 interspace and thence through the epidural and subarachnoid spaces and into the substance of the spinal cord. A stereotactic frame is used to line up the spinal needle and electrode on the target. The target, of course, is exactly the same as that used in the lateral or anterior approach cordotomy. At the C_1-C_2 level, the target is 3 to 4 mm lateral from the midline; it is assumed that the midline of the odontoid process corresponds to the midline of the spinal cord. The electrode is inserted until it is 1 to 2 mm from the anterior border of the spinal cord.

Stimulation studies are carried out as in the previous techniques with both 2-Hz and 100-Hz stimulation. The position is also checked by X-ray films or through an image-intensifier, and a lesion is made in similar fashion to that previously described for the lateral percutaneous cordotomy. The lesion begins close to the anterior horn and cervical fibers so the initial analgesia tends to develop in the upper part of the body and spreads downward. Lesions closer to the dentate ligament tend to cause analgesia in the lower limb, which spread upward. Posterior percutaneous cervical cordotomy is, therefore, of more value when a high level of analgesia is required.

This technique is more complicated than the other two; and, as the electrode traverses the corticospinal tract, there is more danger of hemiparesis. It requires sophisticated apparatus and highly skilled operators.

CONCLUSION

It is obvious that the techniques of percutaneous cervical cordotomy described in this presentation offer a range of procedures which provide analgesia in the spinal dermatomes. We have found the lateral percutaneous cervical cordotomy the simplest to carry out, although the correct technique must be meticulously followed to prevent complications. Anterior percutaneous cervical cordotomy is technically difficult because the needle is gripped by the intervertebral disk. It does, however, provide a method of avoiding sleep apnea.

The posterior approach has limited application because of its technical difficulty. It has advantages when a very high level of analgesia is required and will produce a higher level of analgesia than the lateral approach. A very small number of patients who have had this procedure have been reported.

The lateral percutaneous cervical cordotomy and the surgical (open) cordotomy provide the most satisfactory and the most profound relief of pain for the intractable pain of inoperable cancer that can be obtained at the present time. The mortality depends on selection of patients; but, because surgical trauma is avoided with the percutaneous technique, its mortality in very ill patients is much lower than that of open (surgical) cordotomy. The lateral percutaneous cervical cordotomy is best for unilateral pain below the C_5 dermatome; but because it has to be performed at the C_1-C_2 space, analgesia may well arise unexpectedly up to the C_5 dermatome; and there is the remote possibility of paresis of the upper limb. For these reasons, when pain is present bilaterally at lumbar and sacral levels, a surgical bilateral, upper-dorsal cordotomy may have advantages in controlling the level of analgesia in patients able to withstand a major operation.

REFERENCES

1. Crue, B. L., Todd, E. M., Carregal, E. J. A., Wright, W. H., and Maline, D. B. (1970): Posterior approach for high cervical percutaneous radiofrequency stereotactic cordotomy. In: *Pain and Suffering—Selected Aspects,* edited by B. L. Crue, Ch. 5. Charles C Thomas, Springfield, Ill.
2. Fox, J. L., and Green, R. C. (1968): Percutaneous stereotaxic cordotomy. II. A guidance technique for the anterior approach. *Acta Neurochir. (Wien)*, 18:318–326.
3. Ganz, E., and Mullan, S. (1977): Chapter 2. In: *Persistent Pain—Modern Methods of Treatment,* edited by S. Lipton, pp. 21–33. Academic Press, London and New York.
4. Hitchcock, E., and Leece, B. (1967): Somatotopic representation of the respiratory pathways in the cervical cord of man. *J. Neurosurg.* 27:320–329.
5. Krieger, A. J., and Rosomoff, H. L. (1974): Sleep-induced apnoes. I. A respiratory and autonomic dysfunction syndrome following bilateral percutaneous cervical cordotomy. *J. Neurosurg.,* 39:168–180.
6. Lin, P. M., Gildenberg, P. L., and Polakoff, P. P. (1966): An anterior approach to percutaneous lower cervical cordotomy. *J. Neurosurg.*, 25:535–560.
7. Lipton, S. (1968): Percutaneous electrical cordotomy in relief of intractable pain. *Br. Med. J.,* 2:210.
8. Lipton, S. (1973): Percutaneous cervical cordotomy. *Proc. R. Soc. Med.,* 66:607–609.
9. Lipton, S., Dervin, E., and Heywood, C. B. (1974): A stereotactic approach to the anterior percutaneous electrical cordotomy. In: *Advances in Neurology, Vol. 4: International Symposium on Pain,* edited by J. J. Bonica, pp. 689–694. Raven Press, New York.
10. Mullan, S. (1971): Percutaneous cordotomy. *J. Neurosurg.,* 35:360–366.
11. Mullan, S., Harper, P. V., Hekmatapanah, J., Torres, H., and Dobbin, G. (1963):

Percutaneous interruption of spinal pain tracts by means of a strontium 90 needle. *J. Neurosurg.*, 20:931.
12. Mullan, S., Mallis, M., Karasick, J., Vailati, G., and Beckman, F. (1965): A re-appraisal of the unipolar anodal electrolytic lesion. *J. Neurosurg.*, 22:531.
13. Nathan, P. (1963): The descending respiratory pathway in man. *J. Neurol. Neurosurg. Psychiatry*, 26:487–499.
14. Rosomoff, H. L. (1969): Bilateral percutaneous cervical radio-frequency cordotomy. *J. Neurosurg.*, 31:41–46.
15. Rosomoff, H. L., Carroll, F., Brown, J., and Sheptak, P. (1965): Percutaneous radiofrequency cervical cordotomy technique. *J. Neurosurg.*, 23:639.
16. Spiller, W. G. (1905): The occasional clinical resemblance between caries of the vertebra and lumbothoracic syringomyelia, and the location within the spinal cord of the fibers of the sensation of pain and temperature. *Univ. Pa. Med. Bull.*, 18: 147–154.
17. Spiller, W. G., and Martin, E. (1912): The treatment of persistent pain of organic origin in the lower part of the body by division of the anterolateral column of the spinal cord. *JAMA*, 58:1489–1490.
18. Taren, J. A., Davis, R., and Crosby, E. C. (1969): Target physiologic corroboration in stereotaxic cervical cordotomy. *J. Neurosurg.*, 30:569–584.
19. Tasker, R. R., and Organ, L. W. (1973): Percutaneous cordotomy. Physiological identification of target site. *Confin. Neurol. (Basel)*, 35:110–117.
20. Voris, H. C. (1951): Ipsilateral sensory loss following cordotomy. Report of a case *Arch. Neurol. (Chicago)*, 65:95.

Advances in Pain Research and Therapy, Vol. 2,
edited by J. J. Bonica and V. Ventafridda.
Raven Press, New York © 1979.

Spinal Posterior Rhizotomy and Commissural Myelotomy in the Treatment of Cancer Pain

I. Papo

Neurosurgery Division, Regional General Hospital, 60100 Ancona, Italy

Unlike open cordotomy, which has been widely used for the treatment of cancer pain, spinal rhizotomy and commissural myelotomy have been erratically used and the subjects of controversies. It is beyond the scope of this brief report to deal exhaustively with pathophysiologic and practical aspects concerning these two procedures. Therefore, I shall confine my remarks to data that will help ascertain the proper role of rhizotomy and myelotomy in the treatment of cancer pain.

SPINAL RHIZOTOMY

Spinal posterior rhizotomy has been infrequently used in the treatment of cancer pain for two reasons. First, cancer is a progressive disease which tends to spread and involve the adjacent areas innervated by nerve roots not severed by the rhizotomy. Consequently, the area denervated surgically often becomes too limited to ensure permanent or at least long-lasting relief. Second, the overlap in spinal dermatomes requires that a significant number of nerve roots must be sectioned to produce a band of analgesia broad enough to secure permanent analgesia in the entire area to which pain is referred. This requires an extensive laminectomy which may not be tolerated by debilitated patients with advanced cancer. Moreover, despite the large laminectomy and extensive rhizotomy, there is no guarantee of good results both in terms of quality and duration of pain-relief. In addition, extensive sensory denervation of limbs gives rise to severe disability. For these reasons, even in the past when ablative surgery was much more popular and used more frequently than at present, spinal rhizotomy was used infrequently for the treatment of cancer pain.

Spinal rhizotomy still may be of practical value in two circumstances: When pain is limited to only a few spinal segments, and when the tumor is localized with no tendency to spread into the surrounding regions.

The largest series of patients subjected to dorsal rhizotomy for cancer pain was reported by Barrash and Leavens (2), who operated on 72 patients. In this group the rhizotomy was done in the following regions: cervical, 17; cervicothoracic, 8; thoracic, 25; thoracolumbar, 2; lumbar, 3; lumbosacral, 3; sacral, 13; and thoracolumbosacral, 1. Altogether, 18 additional operations were needed. The results were as follows: complete relief in 40 patients (57%); good relief in 10 (14%); moderate relief in 8 (12%); minimal relief in 5 (7%); and no relief in 5 (7%). In 2 (3%) patients the results could not be evaluated. According to Barrash and Leavens, dorsal rhizotomy is a valuable procedure in the management of cancer pain.

These very favorable results, however, are not borne out by other reports in the literature in which the percentage of early and, more importantly, late failure is significantly higher. White and Sweet (34) treated a total of 34 patients: Early relief was achieved in 19, but pain recurred subsequently due to extension of disease in 4 patients. In 12 patients rhizotomy was ineffective, and finally 2 patients with advanced cancer died. In Loeser's series (18) only 43% of 13 patients operated for cancer pain benefited permanently from rhizotomy. This procedure was effective in only 5 out of 18 patients treated by Onofrio and Campa (20). Loeser and Onofrio and Campa state that preoperative regional anesthetic blocks are not reliable in predicting the later therapeutic efficacy of posterior rhizotomy. However, to make a more precise assessment of the practical value of this operation, the site, type, and extent of pain must be taken into account.

Cervical Rhizotomy

Painful syndromes in the neck are often successfully managed, as White and Sweet (34) pointed out, by sectioning 3 to 6 roots. I have also satisfactorily treated 3 patients by sectioning 3 or 4 roots. In most of these patients, good results are achieved without residual neurologic disorders. However, pain strictly limited to the neck is rather uncommon.

Cervicobrachial Rhizotomy

Posterior rhizotomy has also been used for the treatment of pain in the apex of the chest and/or in the upper arm due to breast (10,20,34) and lung cancer (23). In such cases, often as many as 8 or 9 roots must be divided to relieve pain in the entire area. Such extensive denervation requires a very large laminectomy which cannot be withstood by patients in poor physical condition.

Except for Ray's favorable report (23), in which no details are given, the results reported in the literature are, on the whole, not very gratifying (10,20,34). Even with extensive denervations, failures and early recurrences occur not infrequently. Moreover, as was previously emphasized, extensive rhizotomies lead to severe disability of the upper limb.

In spite of these considerations, Sindou et al. (27) believe that because other procedures attempted for the relief of cervicobrachial pain are often dangerous or ineffective or both, spinal rhizotomy has a definite role in cancer patients with this type of pain. It is especially indicated in patients with not very advanced Pancoast-Tobias tumors and in patients in whom the function of the upper limb is already lost.

Thoracic Rhizotomy

Dorsal rhizotomy of several thoracic segments may be indicated in patients in good physical condition who have severe segmental neuralgic pain caused by metastasis or collapse of a thoracic vertebra. It is also indicated in patients with thoracic segmental pain caused by a localized tumor which is not likely to spread extensively. On the other hand, in patients with thoracic pain caused by advanced cancer and who are predicted to have a short life-expectancy, chemical rhizotomy is preferable.

Sacral Rhizotomy

For the management of sacrococcygeal and perineal pain from pelvic malignancies (rectal or cervix carcinoma), sacral rhizotomy has also been reported by several writers (3,6,7,9,11,20). Guillaume and Sigwald (11) recommend rhizotomy only in cases of pudendal neuralgia and for pain strictly located in the anal and coccygeal region. They believe this operation should not be done for patients with deep pain. Bohm and Franksson (3) reported on 7 patients complaining of superficial coccygeal pain treated by bilateral rhizotomy of the lowermost 2 or 3 sacral roots. In 3 patients, one of whom lived more than 3 years, relief was complete until death, while the remainder developed subsequent pain caused by recurrence of abdominopelvic tumor. Onofrio and Campa (20) reported long-term relief of perineal pain caused by rectal cancer in only 2 of 7 patients subjected to this procedure.

Kuhner (15) treated 4 patients suffering from rectal cancer pain and 1 from prostatic carcinoma pain. In one patient the S_4 and S_5 roots were sectioned, in the remainder, the rhizotomy included S_3 as well. Coccygodinia was permanently abolished in all the patients. Of 4 patients who also had associated pain, complete relief was obtained in 2 and significant relief in the other two.

Crue et al. (6,7,9) advocate the complete section of the dural sheath together with all spinal roots below S_1 using a simplified technique. The whole dural sheath is divided between two ligatures through a small opening in the bone. In patients having good bladder control, S_2 is spared at least on the less painful side. Crue and his associates believe sacral rhizotomy is effective for treatment of perineal, sacral, and coccygeal pain either superficial or deep. The operation should be performed only in patients with pain of at least 3 months' duration, life-expectancy should be at least 3 months, and all the patients should have a previous colostomy. They reported on 29 patients treated with this technique. Of these, 1 died and the results could not be assessed, while the results obtained in the other 28 patients were as follows: satisfactory in 20; fair in 5; poor in 2; and total failure in 1. Sciatic pain associated with perineal pain caused the poor results, both observed in patients with carcinoma of the cervix.

Personally, I have used Crue's technique in 4 patients suffering from superficial and deep perineal and sacrococcygeal pain from rectal carcinoma. All of them had previous colostomies. In 3 patients, phenol rhizotomy had failed to relieve the pain, and in 1 pain recurred 3 months after an effective subarachnoid neurolysis but subsequent neurolytic injections proved ineffective. In all patients but one who had severe drug addiction, pain was satisfactorily relieved. They remained pain-free until death 3 to 8 months after sacral rhizotomy. I should add, however, that despite sparing of S_2 roots bilaterally, vesical function which was already impaired, was permanently lost.

Sacral rhizotomy is of value in the treatment of pain strictly limited to sacrococcygeal and perineal region whether it is deep or superficial. Because of the very limited denervation produced by this procedure, recurrence of pain due to the spread of pelvic cancer beyond the boundaries of the analgesic area is relatively frequent. The procedure fails to relieve sciatic pain even if S_1 is divided and also fails to relieve abdominopelvic visceral pain. Since phenol rhizotomy produces excellent results in most patients with saddle pain, surgical rhizotomy should be reserved only for patients in whom phenol rhizotomy has failed.

POSTERIOR RHIZIDIOTOMY

In recent years, Sindou and his associates (26,27) have suggested a modified technique to achieve selective section of those rootlets considered primarily responsible for nociceptive transmission. They call this procedure *selective posterior rhizidiotomy*. This is achieved by making an incision 1 mm deep into the spinal cord to interrupt the ventrolateral portion of each rootlet supplying the painful area. In this way the pain-conducting fibers are interrupted in Lissauer's tract. Theoretically, rhizidiotomy should obviate the most disabling complication of total posterior rhizotomy. For the treatment of cancer pain Sindou et al. (26,27) performed rhizidiotomy at the cervical and lumbosacral levels, with results which can be considered very worthwhile. Of 16 patients with different pain syndromes subjected to this procedure, 13

(81%) were relieved satisfactorily. Valuable results were also reported by Vlahovitch and Fuentes (31).

Of course rhizidiotomy should be considered only for the treatment of pain involving roots whose section would entail functional disability (e.g., roots subserving the upper and lower limbs). I have done rhizidiotomy on 2 patients with Pancoast's tumors with pain in the upper chest and the upper limb limited to C_8 and T_1 spinal segments. Total rhizotomy of T_2-T_5 was combined with rhizidiotomy of C_8 and T_1. Pain was abolished with no major disability, but the interval for follow-up is still too brief to make a reliable assessment of the results achieved.

Although rhizidiotomy is certainly a more selective and less dangerous technique than total posterior rhizotomy, it is nonetheless a major surgical operation which requires extensive laminectomy. Therefore, its indications are limited and not substantially different from those of conventional dorsal rhizotomy.

COMMISSURAL MYELOTOMY

Commissural myelotomy at different levels and with different techniques is a recurrent topic in neurosurgery. Since this operation was devised for the management of pain by Armour (1) over a half a century ago, its popularity has waxed and waned. Its very attractive theoretical basis may account for such an undulating history. It would seem quite logical that neurosurgeons should aim at producing bilateral pain-relief with a single harmless procedure, which does not damage the corticospinal, respiratory, micturitory, or other main spinal tracts. Unfortunately, the results produced by commissural myelotomy have been far from what one would have expected. Consequently, neurosurgeons have become disenchanted and myelotomy has been abandoned for a period of time. In a paper published in 1976, Lungo and I (21) reviewed the literature, and since then several other reports have been published (5,14,25,29,30).

To begin with, we must distinguish between two kinds of commissurotomies, according to the technique used to divide the anterior commissure: open commissurotomy, which can be done at different levels required by the location of the painful area; and stereotactic myelotomy, as suggested by Hitchcock (12,13), which is performed in the upper cervical spinal cord.

Conventional Myelotomy

Conventional myelotomy aims at dividing the spinal commissures through a perfectly midline incision. Review of the literature reveals that the depth and the extent of the incision have become increasingly greater. In fact, the French authors who first performed myelotomy on a large scale (19,32,33) during the 'forties and early 'fifties, used to make a small incision 3 mm deep and 2.5 to 3 cm long into the spinal cord. Later, Sourek (28) advocated a complete division of the spinal cord in two halves over the length of 2.5 to 4 cm. More recently, Cook and Kawakami (5) and King (14) carried out complete myelotomies of up to 100- to 110-mm long in an attempt to interrupt all the decussating fibers subserving the painful area.

Despite these very long commissurotomies, clear-cut bands and levels of well-defined thermoanalgesia are very seldom observed. In some patients no analgesia at all can be demonstrated. Moreover, the published results achieved by myelotomy are somewhat contradictory. Mansuy and associates (19) and Wertheimer and his associates (32,33) of Lyon in the initial report stated that myelotomy provided satisfactory results in most patients with bilateral pain. However, subsequently they reanalyzed the same material (8) and concluded that myelotomy was effective only for the treatment of vaginal and visceral pain, whereas rectal and lower limb pain were not significantly influenced. Cordotomy, therefore, should be preferred in most patients.

Sourek (29) believes myelotomy is an effective technique for the management of pain located in lower half of the body, whereas pain located in the apex of the chest and in the upper limbs would recur in most cases after cervical commissurotomy. In contrast, Lembcke (16) reported favorable results in all the 12 patients treated with cervical myelotomy. Still different, were the results reported by Cook and Kawakami (5), who succeeded in relieving pain in the upper part of the body with myelotomy but the procedure was unsatisfactory for lower limb pain due to pelvic cancer. Lippert, Hosobuchi and Nielsen (17) pointed out that the results after myelotomy are gratifying in patients with pain located in the midline or in bilaterally innervated structures, but they are much less favorable in patients with spinal or lower limb pain. In Sunder, Plassmann and Grunert's (30) series of 56 patients, 50 of them with cancer pain, permanent relief was obtained in about one-third of the cases.

Stereotactic Myelotomy

Our results (21) with stereotactic myelotomy have been much less favorable than those reported by Hitchcock (12,13) and Schvarcz (24,25). Although immediate relief is obtained in nearly all patients, it very seldom lasts long enough to keep patients pain-free until death among those who survive for more than 2 or 3 months.

General Evaluation

An overall assessment of commissural myelotomy is very difficult for many reasons. First of all, the surgical technique is not yet standardized: There are no reliable, widely accepted criteria for how long the incision should be in order to interrupt all the fibers subserving a given painful area, though it is generally agreed that the depth of the incision should extend to the anterior sulcus of the spinal cord. Secondly, the sensory changes are too unreliable to allow any physiologic appraisal of the effects of myelotomy. Moreover, the mechanism of therapeutic action of commissurotomy is still hypothetical: none of the explanations suggested is substantiated by definite anatomic or physiologic evidence. Although ascending systems are likely to be involved, the reduced transmission of nociceptive impulses brought about by myelotomy is often insufficient to ensure permanent or even long-lasting relief. In a significant percentage of patients when the effects of the surgical trauma wear off and some fibers not divided anatomically recover their previous function, pain recurs.

In establishing criteria for the use of myelotomy in the treatment of cancer pain, the practical drawbacks of this operation must also be borne in mind. Myelotomy is a major surgical procedure that should be considered with great caution and reservation in the treatment of patients in poor condition and with short life-expectancy. Moreover, even with the largest myelotomies there is no reasonable guarantee of long-lasting results. Therefore, this operation should not be considered as a routine procedure in patients with long life-expectancy. Complications must also be considered. Postoperative dysesthesia may be very distressing and sometimes last several weeks. Temporary disorders of propioception or somatic motor disturbances occur in a significant percentage (4).

Considering the location of pain, we have concluded that commissurotomy for upper chest and upper limb cancer pain may be of some value in selected patients, although there are differences of opinion regarding its efficacy for these conditions. As I have already stressed in the discussion of posterior rhizotomy, virtually all techniques suggested for the treatment of cancer pain in these sites fail to produce adequate relief in a substantial percentage of patients. Since there is no standard effective treatment for these unfortunate patients, myelotomy may be indicated in patients with lung cancer in whom respiratory function is already impaired and life-expectancy rather short. In contrast, commissurotomy will not be very effective for the treatment of bilateral lower limb pain from pelvic or spinal cancer. Moreover, abdominal and saddle pain, which may be relieved by myelotomy, is also satisfactorily controlled in most patients with the much less traumatic phenol rhizotomy.

Survey of the literature does not provide useful criteria for selecting patients for commissural myelotomy. Consequently the indications for this procedure still remain a matter of controversy and personal opinions of various writers. Piscol (22) in assessing open spinal operations for cancer pain, recommends myelotomy only for lower trunk pain, but even in these cases bilateral open cordotomy is a much more reliable and no more traumatic operation.

To conclude, I believe that one should be very cautious about recommending commissural myelotomy as the initial therapeutic modality for the relief of pain of advanced cancer. Less traumatic and better-established procedures should be considered before myelotomy. I believe that on the whole, specific indications for myelotomy seem to be exceedingly rare.

REFERENCES

1. Armour, D. (1927): Lettsorian lecture on the surgery of the spinal cord and its membranes. *Lancet,* 1:691–697.
2. Barrash, J. M., and Leavens, M. E. (1973): Dorsal rhizotomy for the relief of intractable pain of malignant tumor origin. *J. Neurosurg.,* 38:755–757.
3. Bohm, E., and Franksson, C. (1959): Coccygodinia and sacral rhizotomy. *Acta Chir. Scand.,* 116:278–284.
4. Broager, B. (1974): Commissural myelotomy. *Surg. Neurol.,* 2:71–74.
5. Cook, A. W., and Kawakami, Y. (1977): Commissural myelotomy. *J. Neurosurg.,* 47:1–6.
6. Crue, B. L., and Todd, E. M. (1964): A simplified technique of sacral rhizotomy for pelvic pain. *J. Neurosurg.,* 21:835–837.
7. Crue, B. L., Todd, E. M., Wright, W. H., and Maline, D. B. (1970): Sacral rhizotomy for pelvic pain. In: *Pain and Suffering,* edited by B. L. Crue, pp. 24–30. Charles C Thomas, Springfield, Ill.
8. Dargent, M., Mansuy, L., Colon, J., and De Rougemont, J. (1963): Les problèmes posés par la douleur dans l'évolution des cancer gynécologiques. *Lyon Chirurgical,* 59:62–83.
9. Felsoory, A., and Crue, B. L. (1976): Results of 19 year experience with sacral rhizotomy for perineal and perianal cancer pain. *Pain,* 2:431–433.
10. Grant, F. C. (1941): Surgical methods for relief of pain. *JAMA,* 116:567–571.
11. Guillaume, J. Sigwald (1947): Coccygodinie rebelle traitée par radicotomie bilatérale de S5. *Guérison. Rev. Neurol.,* 54:60.
12. Hitchcock, E. (1970): Stereotactic cervical myelotomy. *J. Neurol. Neurosurg. Psychiatry,* 33:224–230.
13. Hitchcock, E. (1974): Stereotactic myelotomy. *Proc. R. Soc. Med.,* 67:771–772.
14. King, R. B. (1977): Anterior commissurotomy for intractable pain. *J. Neurosurg.,* 47:7–11.
15. Kuhner, A. (1976): La valeur des interventions sur les racines sacrées dans le traitement des syndromes douloureux du bassin. *Neurochirurgie,* 22:429–436.
16. Lembcke, W. (1964): Ueber die mediolongitudinale Chordotomie im Halsmarkbereich, *Zbl. Chir.,* 89:439–443.
17. Lippert, R. G., Hosobuchi, Y., and Nielsen, S. L. (1974): Spinal comissurotomy. *Surg. Neurol.,* 2:373–377.
18. Loeser, J. D. (1972): Dorsal rhizotomy for the relief of chronic pain. *J. Neurosurg.,* 36:745–750.
19. Mansuy, L., Lecuire, J., and Acassat, L. (1944): Technique de la myelotomie commissural posterieure. *J. Chirurgie,* 60:206–213.
20. Onofrio, B. M., and Campa, H. K. (1972): Evaluation of rhizotomy: Review of 12 year experience. *J. Neurosurg.,* 36:751–755.
21. Papo, I., and Luongo, A. (1976): High cervical commissural myelotomy in the treatment of pain. *J. Neurol. Neurosurg. Psychiatry,* 39:705–710.
22. Piscol, K. (1975): Open spinal surgery for (intractable) pain. In: *Advances in Neurosurgery, Vol. 3,* edited by H. Penzholz, M. Brock, J. Hamer, M. Klinger, and O. Spoerri, pp. 157–169. Springer, Berlin.
23. Ray, B. S. (1943): The management of intractable pain by posterior rhizotomy. *Res. Publ. Ass. Res. Nerv. Ment. Dis.,* 23:391–407.
24. Schvarcz, J. R. (1974): Spinal stereotactic surgery. In: *Recent Progress in Neuro-*

logical Surgery, edited by K. Sano and S. Ishii, pp. 234–245. Excerpta Medica, Amsterdam.
25. Schvarcz, J. R. (1976): Stereotactic extralemniscal myelotomy. *J. Neurol. Neurosurg. Psychiatry,* 39:53–57.
26. Sindou, M., Fischer, G., Goutelle, A., and Mansuy, L. (1974): La radiacellectomie sélective postérieure. Premiers résultats dans la chirurgie de la douleur. *Neuro-Chirurgie,* 20:391–408.
27. Sindou, M., Fischer, G., and Mansuy, L. (1976): Posterior spinal rhizotomy and selective posterior rhizidiotomy. *Prog. Neurol. Surg.,* 7:201–250. Karger, Basel.
28. Şourek, K. (1969): Commissural myelotomy. *J. Neurosurg.,* 31:524–527.
29. Šourek, K. (1977): Commissural myelotomy. *Prog. Neurol. Surg.,* 8:15. Karger, Basel.
30. Sunder-Plassmann, M., and Grunert, V. (1976): Commissural myelotomy for drug-resistant pain. In: *Clinical Microneurosurgery,* edited by W. Th. Koos, F. W. Boeck, and R. F. Spetzler, pp. 165–170. Thieme, Stuttgart.
31. Vlahovitch, B., and Fuentes, J. M. (1975): Résultats de la radicellectomie sélective postérieure à l'étage lombaire et cervical. *Neuro-Chirurgie,* 21:29–42.
32. Wertheimer, P., and Lecuire, J. (1953): La myélotomie commissurale postérieure. À propos de 107 observations. *Acta Chir. Belg.,* 52:568–574.
33. Wertheimer, P., and Sautot, J. (1949): Les résultats de la myélotomie commissurale postérieure (à propos de 69 observations). *Con. Méd.,* 74:413–414.
34. White, J. C., and Sweet, W. H. (1969): *Pain and the Neurosurgeon: A Forty-year Experience.* Charles C Thomas, Springfield, Ill.

Advances in Pain Research and Therapy, Vol. 2,
edited by J. J. Bonica and V. Ventafridda.
Raven Press, New York © 1979.

Open Cordotomy in the Treatment of Cancer Pain

I. Papo

Neurosurgery Division, Regional General Hospital, 60100 Ancona, Italy

Open cordotomy, either at the cervical or thoracic level, has been one of the most debated topics in neurosurgery for more than 50 years. All technical, pathophysiologic and clinical problems concerning this operation have been exhaustively dealt with in innumerable reports, monographs, and meetings, so that a further appraisal of them appears to be unnecessary. Since the introduction of percutaneous cervical cordotomy 15 years ago and its subsequent widespread use, open cordotomy has been rather neglected and has been the subject of only a few reports. Hence, at present the question arises as to whether it is still rational to perform open cordotomy for the treatment of cancer pain.

Differences of opinion exist regarding the usefulness and indication for open cordotomy for this purpose. Tasker (6), who performs percutaneous cordotomies routinely, believes this procedure can be applied in nearly all patients, even if they are suffering from terminal cancer and in very poor condition. According to him, open cordotomy should be carried out only in the following instances: (a) in uncooperative patients in whom motor and sensory tracts cannot be localized safely by electrical stimulation; (b) in patients with craniospinal malformations in whom no reliable anatomic landmarks are available; and (c) in the unusual cases in which the neurosurgeon is unable to localize sensory and motor pathways. According to Tasker the mandatory indications for open cordotomy would be exceedingly rare.

These opinions, however, are not shared by everyone. For instance, Kuhner (1), who also has ample experience with percutaneous cordotomy, is of the opinion that open and percutaneous cordotomies have the same indications. Percutaneous tractotomy is of course a much less traumatic procedure. However, it has some drawbacks, particularly when a bilateral operation is required. Piscol (5) suggests that open thoracic cordotomy is preferred for the treatment of unilateral or bilateral pain located in the lower half of the body.

In comparing the two procedures, we acknowledge that percutaneous cordotomy is a simple, safe, and effective technique with minimal discomfort for the patients, provided that it is done by experienced surgeons who perform this operation routinely in a large number of patients. If percutaneous cordotomy is done only occasionally, it is likely to take longer to perform and may also be distressing to the patient. On the other hand, open cordotomy done with an operative microscope for magnification is also a safe operation which produces excellent results. Magnification makes anatomic landmarks perfectly clear, and the section of the anterolateral column can be achieved precisely without impinging upon the corticospinal tract. The complication rate of microsurgical cordotomy is negligible, and the level of analgesia is usually satisfactory and long-lasting. Finally, the whole procedure can be completed in 25 to 30 min under general anesthesia.

RESULTS

Analgesia

In the past 2 years I have performed open thoracic cordotomy on 24 patients. In 3 of them a two-stage operation was done at 3- to 6-month intervals. All patients operated on were complaining of excruciating pain in one lower limb mostly from rectal and cervix carcinoma. In all of the patients except 2, extensive analgesia and excellent pain-relief was achieved and persisted until death, which occurred 4 to 12 months later. In 2 patients, despite a very broad section of the anterolateral column, the level of analgesia dropped from T_6 to L_4 in a few weeks, leaving a band of hypalgesia from T_{11} to L_4. Fortunately, both patients had previously been complaining of sciatic pain which was completely eliminated and did not recur.

Complications

No permanent complications were observed with the unilateral operation. However, in the patients in whom pain developed in the contralateral side after the first operation, a second cordotomy on the opposite side resulted in mild weakness of one lower limb and transient urinary retention.

DISCUSSION

On the basis of personal experience, I emphasize that magnification has significantly improved the results of open cordotomy both in terms of quality and safety. In the past, a certain rate of unpredictable short-term failures were observed even with massive open sections of the anterolateral columns (7). Many explanations have been suggested, but none of them is entirely satisfactory. The degree of drop of the level of analgesia remains unpredictable.

In order to establish guidelines for the use of open cordotomy, especially in view of the favorable results produced by percutaneous cordotomy during the past decade, it is necessary to consider the different circumstances in which both techniques are done. If a neurosurgeon performs open cordotomy extensively, the results will be good and the procedure can be used. However, since the vast majority of neurosurgeons do only a few cordotomies a year, the results are likely to be less favorable.

If a percutaneous cordotomy is the routine procedure, I would share Tasker's point of view but on different grounds. First of all, even though open cordotomy under magnification is a safe and effective procedure, it still entails significant surgical trauma and, consequently, there is much more postoperative pain and morbidity, which require a longer hospital stay. Secondly, psychologic factors must also be taken into account: most patients with severe pain of advanced cancer have already been subjected to previous therapy which includes surgical operations with long hospital stays. Consequently, they dislike hospitals and are reluctant to undergo further operations. In contrast, most physicians do not consider percutaneous cordotomy as a major operation and, therefore, this procedure is accepted more readily. Thirdly, percutaneous cordotomy can be carried out in patients in poor physical condition who do not tolerate major surgical operations. Finally, there is no definite evidence that open cordotomy produces better or more lasting analgesia than percutaneous cordotomy (1,2,4).

Some indications for open cordotomy still exist. I believe that for the treatment of bilateral lower limb pain, open thoracic cordotomy should be preferred unless anterior percutaneous tractotomy is performed at a lower cervical level. Moreover, open and percutaneous cordotomies can be properly combined for the treatment of bilateral pain. Open cordotomy is also indicated when neurosurgeons do not perform percutaneous cordotomy. Apart from its specific indications for bilateral lower limb pain, unilateral pain in the lower limb in patients in relatively good condition seems to be the most valuable indication for open thoracic cordotomy. A two-stage procedure is done when pain develops in the contralateral side weeks and months after the first operation.

High or low open cervical cordotomy, as suggested by Mansuy et al. (3), does not seem to provide substantial advantages to warrant its routine use. Finally, for some types of cancer pain, the rationale for open cordotomy, whether unilateral or bilateral, is doubtful when other simpler therapeutic modalities to relieve the pain are available.

REFERENCES

1. Kuhner, A. (1976): La cordotomie cervicale percutanée. *Neuro-Chirurgie,* 22:261–280.
2. Lorenz, R., Grumme, Th., Hermann, H. D., Palleske, H., Khuner, A., Steude, U., and Zierski, J. (1975): Percutaneous cordotomy. In: *Advances in Neurosurgery, Vol. 3,* edited by H. Penzholz, M. Brock, J. Hamer, M. Klinger, and O. Spoerri, pp. 178–185. Springer, Berlin.
3. Mansuy, L., Sindou, M., Fischer, G., and Brunon, J. (1976): La cordotomie spino-

thalamique dans les douleurs cancéreuses. Résultats d'une série de 124 malades opérés par abord direct postérieur. *Neuro-Chirurgie,* 22:437–444.
4. Muke, R., and Correia, A. (1975): Potentials and limits of percutaneous cervical cordotomy. In: *Advances in Neurosurgery, Vol. 3,* edited by H. Penzholz, M. Brock, J. Hamer, M. Klinger, and O. Spoerri, pp. 195–198. Springer, Berlin.
5. Piscol, K. (1975): Open spinal surgery for (intractable) pain. In: *Advances in Neurosurgery, Vol. 3,* edited by H. Penzholz, M. Brock, J. Hamer, M. Klinger, and O. Spoerri, pp. 157–169. Springer, Berlin.
6. Tasker, R. R. (1976): Open cordotomy. *Prog. Neurol. Surg.,* 7:14. Karger Basel.
7. White, J. C., and Sweet, W. H. (1969): *Pain and the Neurosurgeon: A Forty-year Experience.* Charles C Thomas, Springfield, Ill.

Advances in Pain Research and Therapy, Vol. 2,
edited by J. J. Bonica and V. Ventafridda.
Raven Press, New York © 1979.

Medullary Tractotomy for Cephalic Pain of Malignant Disease

Albino Bricolo

Department of Neurosurgery, Ospedale Civile, 37100 Verona, Italy

In spite of varying reports of its efficacy, it is time to reconsider Sjöqvist's (26) brilliant idea of medullary tractotomy as a neurosurgical procedure for the relief of cancer pain in the face and head. However, we still do not have a method which is always applicable and effective in relieving serious cancer pain in this region. This is due to the fact that nociceptive (pain) impulses from these areas are transmitted by several sensory cranial nerves and possibly by the upper cervical dorsal roots. In addition to the major nerve supply to the face by the trigeminal nerve, some somatic sensory fibers of the facial, glossopharyngeal, and vagal nerves transmit pain from the auricle, external auditory meatus, tympanic membrane, posterior third of the tongue, tonsils, tonsillar pillars, uvula, part of the soft palate, and pharynx (1,2,4,7,9, 13,25,27,29). The relief of severe cancer pain in this region remains a challenging problem (3).

Operations including mesencephalic spinothalamic tractotomy, trigeminal tractotomy, multiple rhizotomy, stereotactic mesencephalotomy, and thalamotomy have been proposed for the treatment of this type of pain (20,22,32). The most widely used operation is the section of multiple sensory roots done through a posterior fossa craniectomy and cervical laminectomy and section of the trigeminal nerve, the nervus intermedius, the glossopharyngeal nerve, the upper vagal rootlets, and the upper dorsal roots of the cervical nerves. Apart from the not infrequent failure to produce complete and persistent denervation of the painful area, this procedure subjects the patient to a significant risk of paralytic keratitis, dyspnea, dysphagia, facial and recurrent laryngeal nerve palsy (23,24,30,32).

An alternative operation could be bulbar tractotomy, which is derived from Sjöqvist's (26) trigeminal tractotomy. This technique is based upon the fact that the pain and temperature fibers of the seventh, ninth, and tenth cranial nerves are located in the medulla and upper cervical cord in close proximity to the descending trigeminal tract (13). This procedure, which Kunc (13,14,15,16) has continued to improve, theoretically is the most physiologic one: A small incision relieves pain in the face and anterior two-thirds of the head with preservation of touch sensation and the corneal reflex. Nevertheless, it has never achieved widespread use and has been abandoned by many neurosurgeons because of unpredictable results. Moreover, there has been a high incidence of complications including ipsilateral ataxia and loss of proprioception, paralysis of recurrent laryngeal nerve, lateropulsion, and contralateral analgesia (4,6,17,31). The failures and complications have been due primarily to errors of identification of the descending trigeminal tract in the medulla.

We believe that many of these problems can be obviated as described by Hosobuchi and Rutkin by localizing the anatomic structures with the aid of a surgical microscope, by using a physiologic means of identifying the descending trigeminal tract (8), and producing a precise lesion of the tract with radiofrequency. Recently, we have introduced two new technical aids which should and have improved the results: monitoring of evoked potentials from peripheral stimulation and using a more refined apparatus for producing the radiofrequency lesion. This is a preliminary report of our experience.

OPERATIVE TECHNIQUE

The operation is done under general anesthesia, with the patient in the prone position and head flexed. We prefer this to the sitting position because it prevents loss of large amounts of cerebral spinal fluid and allows the use of controlled respiration with a negative pressure phase, which serves to decrease the risk of air embolism.

After endotracheal anesthesia is established and before the operation is started, a pin electrode is inserted respectively into the supraorbital, infraorbital and mental foramina, coupled with a second pin electrode inserted into the overlying skin to provide intraoperative stimulation of each branch of the trigeminal nerve. Two other electrodes are applied percutaneously for stimulation of the median nerve at the wrist and the peroneal nerve at the neck of the fibula.

A midline incision is made beginning at the inion and extending caudad to the spinous process of C_5. This provides very ample exposure of the suboccipital region and the posterior arch of the atlas and facilitates the performance of tractotomy and, if necessary, rhizotomy of C_2. If section of the lower cervical sensory roots is also required, this incision can be extended caudad so that the laminectomy can be enlarged. The posterior arch of the atlas is first removed, and then 1 cm or more of the posterior rim of the foramen magnum is removed by approaching it from the bottom with a Cloward-Harper laminectomy rongeur.

Once this is accomplished, a longitudinal dural incision is made starting about 5 mm lateral to the midline, ipsilateral to the patient's pain at the level of C_2 and extending the incision cephalad. As the incision approaches the marginal sinus, it is carried slightly more lateral and any bleeding is promptly controlled. Initially, the dura is incised without opening the arachnoid and is then reflected laterally. Only after achieving effective hemostasis is the arachnoid opened to expose the medulla and the upper cervical cord. A Zeiss surgical microscope is used for the remainder of the procedure to facilitate precise identification of nervous structures. Only minimal traction with a spatula inserted below and slightly medial to the cerebellar tonsils is required to identify the obex.

Anatomic Considerations

A clear understanding of the anatomy of the dorsal surface of the medulla and upper cervical cord is essential for optimum results. Lateral to the important anatomic landmark of the obex, the clava and cuneate tubercle are seen; more laterally and ventrally are the bulbar and spinal rootlets of the accessory nerve as they leave the lateral surface of the medulla. Between the point from which the accessory nerve rootlets emerge and the dorsolateral sulcus that limits laterally the fasciculus cuneatus, lies the tuberculum cinereum, which is the bulge made by the fibers of the descending spinal tract of V overlying the caudal nucleus of the trigeminal nuclear complex. These fibers, which conduct pain and temperature, are the proximal branches of neurons whose cell bodies are in the gasserian ganglion. They enter the pons and then turn caudally at the trigeminal spinal tract terminating below the obex. These fibers become most accessible in the lower medulla near the surface within the tuberculum cinereum.

These descending fibers are arranged in a segmental fashion with the ophthalmic fibers lying ventrally and laterally, the mandibular fibers dorsomedially, and the maxillary fibers between them (4,5,15,21,26,27). Tactile fibers, for the most part, turn cephalad after entering the pons. The sensory fibers of the seventh, eighth, and tenth cranial nerves which transmit pain cross the trigeminal spinal tract at their respective levels and descend with it into the cervical spinal cord (1,4,5,17,27). Kunc's contributions (15) are fundamental to the accurate definition of the topographic relationship between the two tracts. The extratrigeminal facial pain fibers, named by Kunc (15) "tractus spinalis, nervi facialis, glossopharyngii and vagi communis," form a narrow bundle that descends between the fasciculus cuneatus and the adjacent trigeminal spinal tract.

Neurophysiologic Consideration

Since the boundaries of the tuberculum cinereum as well as the posterior sulci of the spinal cord are frequently not easily distinguishable, there has always been a need to localize the descending trigeminal tract by means other than anatomic landmarks (4,11,12). In Kunc's (15) procedure, a more precise position of the tract is determined by a delicate local stimulation with a thin needle with the patient under local anesthesia. This direct mechanical stimulation produces a subjective painful response referred to the area of the face supplied by those fibers being stimulated. This technique, especially when carried out by Kunc himself, permits the operator to perform precise and successful tractotomies (16). Furthermore, with the patient awake it is possible to check immediately the results of the section done and to extend it as necessary. To obtain optimal results, it is necessary to use local anesthesia and to have an awake and intelligent patient who responds promptly and correctly to the stimulation. However, because the fibers of the trigeminal tract are primary neurons (33) and their stimulation is often very painful, the stimulation may impair the patient's cooperation (17) and his responses can be misleading (15–32). Moreover, many patients are so stressed by the operation that they are unable to indicate precisely the area in which they feel the stimulation-induced pain.

In view of this, the recording of evoked potentials from the dorsal surfaces of the medulla and upper cervical cord produced by the stimulation of the peripheral trigeminal, median, and popliteal nerves, as suggested by Mullan (19) and carried out by Hosobuchi and Rutkin (8), seems to be a more practical and accurate neurophysiologic method to delineate the descending trigeminal tract and the adjacent funiculi and to preclude the dis-

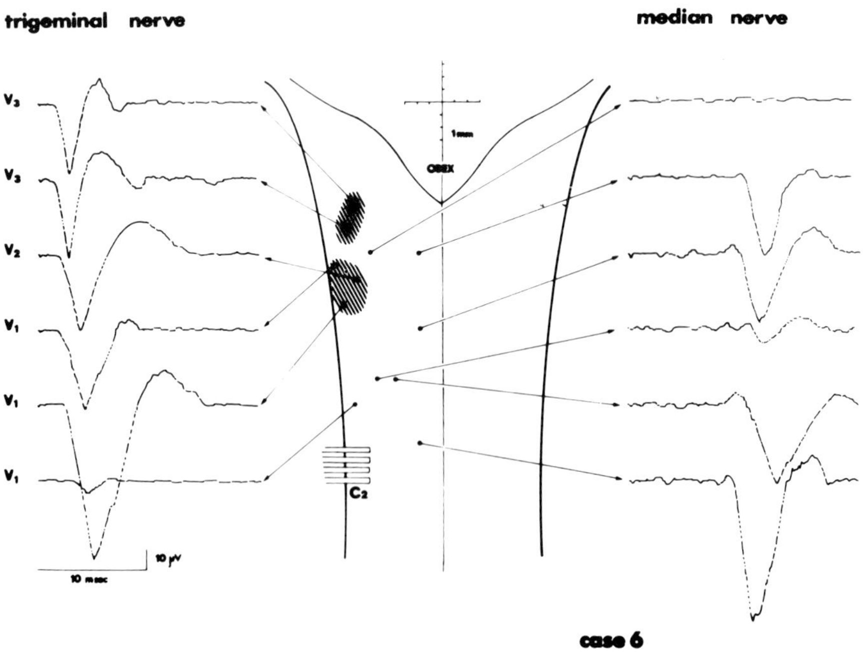

FIG. 1. Case 6 (O.P., 47 yrs). Evoked potentials from the dorsal surface of the medulla and upper cervical cord elicited by ipsilateral trigeminal and median nerve stimulation (monophasic square-wave, 3 Hz, 10 mA, 0.1 msec). Hatching areas indicate radiofrequency lesions.

comfort often experienced with local anesthesia. We have adopted the technique of Hosobuchi and Rutkin (8) which proved very satisfactory, using the O.T.E. Biomedica Neuroaverage 1239 for stimulation and for recording the data.

By monitoring the evoked potentials recorded from the dorsolateral surface of the medulla and upper cervical cord through bipolar concentric electrodes (0.45-mm diameter, 0.07-sq-mm recording area; DISA 9013 K, 0512) it is easy to make a neurophysiologic map that outlines exactly the position of the tract (Fig. 1). The ipsilateral median and/or popliteal nerve is first stimulated, and the dorsal surface of the medulla is systematically explored from the midline in a lateral and caudad-cephalad directions at the emergence of the C_2 posterior rootlets. In this way, we can outline precisely the lateral boundary of the fasciculus cuneatus, which consists of a line beyond which no evoked responses are elicited. After this important boundary is determined, each of the three peripheral branches of the trigeminal nerve is separately stimulated and evoked response recorded from the space between the lateral boundary of the fasciculus cuneatus and the origin of bulbar and spinal accessory rootlets. In this way, it is possible to trace the limits of the descending trigeminal tract and the position within it of the three trigeminal divisions.

Producing the Lesion

Formerly, we made the incision with a scalpel blade prepared so that 5 mm of the cutting edge was exposed. However, now we prefer to produce the lesion with radiofrequency by inserting a stainless-steel electrode insulated with Teflon® which is 0.7 mm in diameter with a 3-mm uninsulated tip into the descending tract to a depth of 1 to 2 mm. Using the Owl Cordotomy System (Model OCS1) and placing the ground electrode subcutaneously in the shoulder region, we make a lesion with a current of 30 mA at 22 to 30 V for 30 sec. This technique permits us to make a precise lesion in the trigeminal tract. If superficial blood vessels are in the way, they are carefully displaced before the electrode is inserted into the medulla.

The majority of authors consider the obex as the most important anatomic landmark in determining the level of tractotomy. However, since the position of the obex is not constant in relation to the inner bulbar structures (17, 32), others prefer to measure the distance from above the uppermost C_2 rootlet rather than below the obex (15). But even these landmarks are far from being reliable, because the distance between them is not constant, varying from 16 to 20 mm.

For these anatomic reasons and other considerations the sites of the incisions used by neurosurgeons have not been uniform. The original incision employed by Sjöqvist (26) in his first procedure in 1938 was much higher, at a level between the middle and the lower third of inferior olive. However, because of certain disadvantages, the level of incision was lowered progressively as far as 5, 6 or 8 mm or more below the obex and extended from the accessory rootlets to the emergence of the C_2 posterior root (5,10,18,28).

The electrophysiologic mapping obtained by evoked responses, which indicates the somatotopic localization of the trigeminal spinal tract, permits us to make the radiofrequency lesions more precisely than do the anatomic landmarks. The point from which the widest potential is evoked by stimulation of the peripheral trigeminal branch is the target zone to be destroyed. Thus, with one or more well-placed lesions, a complete analgesia is achieved of all three divisions of the trigeminal nerve. Moreover, since the pain tracts of the seventh, ninth, and tenth cranial nerves lie between the trigeminal spinal tract and the fasciculus cuneatus, these are also interrupted by extending the lesion dorsomedially to reach the neurophysiologic boundary of fasciculus cuneatus. In addition, the posterior rootlets of the upper two or three cervical nerves can be divided if necessary.

Our previous failures in eliminating pain deep in the ear and posterior oral cavity were probably due to the fact that the incision did not extend dorsally as far as it should have been because of our fear of endangering the fasciculus cuneatus and thereby producing an ipsilateral ataxia.

RESULTS

Ten patients have been treated with the technique described above. These included 7 males and 3 females whose ages ranged from 44 to 71 years. The data are summarized in Table 1. We have had no deaths due to this operation. Despite the poor physical status of some patients due to pain and malnutrition, we were able to discharge all of them from our services. Of these, 8 returned home and 2 were returned to the referral hospital. None had postoperative complications, and those who were able to be out of bed before the operation resumed activities and were able to swallow again. A mild and transitory ataxia in the ipsilateral upper extremity appeared in 2 patients, but none complained of unpleasant dysesthesias or hyperpathia, and those who had no eye neoplastic involvement retained the corneal reflex.

All of the patients experienced immediate complete relief of cancer pain. At their discharge, 1 to 2 weeks later, the results on pain were still very good; 8 patients were pain-free, and 2 developed pain which was less than the original pain. One of the latter, the first operated in this series, developed a pain in the jaw which had been spared by analgesia, and this was due to the fact that the C_2 posterior root had not been sectioned. The second patient (Case 8) in whom pain in the neck persisted, probably would have had complete relief if the C_3 posterior root had been sectioned.

A careful postoperative examination revealed that 9 patients had complete ipsilateral analgesia in all of the three divisions of the trigeminal, as well as analgesia in the distribution of the seventh, ninth and tenth cranial

TABLE 1. *Etiology, site of pain, and results of medullary tractotomy (MT) in 10 patients.*

Case		Age	Sex	Site of pain	Cause	Operation	Pain-relief
1	B.F.	44	M	R. face, ear, throat, jaw	Pharyngeal cancer	MT	Partial
2	C.T.	57	F	L. face, ear, throat	Pharyngeal cancer	MT	Complete
3	C.A.	42	M	R. face, fronto-temp. scalp	Ethmoidal cancer	MT C_1-C_2	Complete
4	B.F.	68	M	L. face, jaw, tongue, throat	Tongue cancer	MT	Complete
5	P.L.	71	M	L. face, tongue, jaw	Lip cancer	MT	Complete
6	O.P.	47	F	L. face, ear, jaw, neck	Pharyngeal ca. cervical metastasis	MT C_2-C_3	Complete
7	B.A.	56	M	L. face, ear, throat	Laryngeal cancer	MT	Complete
8	P.A.	62	F	L. face, ear, neck	Osteogenic sarcoma	MT C_2	Partial
9	M.L.	70	M	R. face, ear, tongue	Maxillary cancer	MT	Complete
10	S.U.	46	M	R. face, neck	Laryngeal cancer	MT C_2-C_3	Complete

nerves (Fig. 2). Tactile sensation was generally spared, even in those patients who had hypoalgesia and analgesia on the face prior to operation as a result of cobalt or surgical therapy. As expected, the neck was also anesthetic in patients who had section of the posterior root of C_3. Our longest follow-up examination has been 6 months, at which time the results were the same as at discharge.

CONCLUSIONS

Our case material is not large enough and the follow-up periods not sufficiently long to allow definite conclusions. However, we feel the following comments are warranted.

The procedure is essentially an extracranial operation. Therefore, it is simpler and less traumatic than any of the other procedures that have been proposed and used for the surgical treatment of pain of cancer of the face and neck. The results of the procedures are quite satisfactory: Pain-relief is achieved while touch sensation and the corneal reflex are preserved, and there are minimal operative risks and complications. In view of this, we wonder why most neurosurgeons prefer a more radical procedure, e.g., multiple rhizotomy, which sacrifices all of the facial sensations in order to relieve

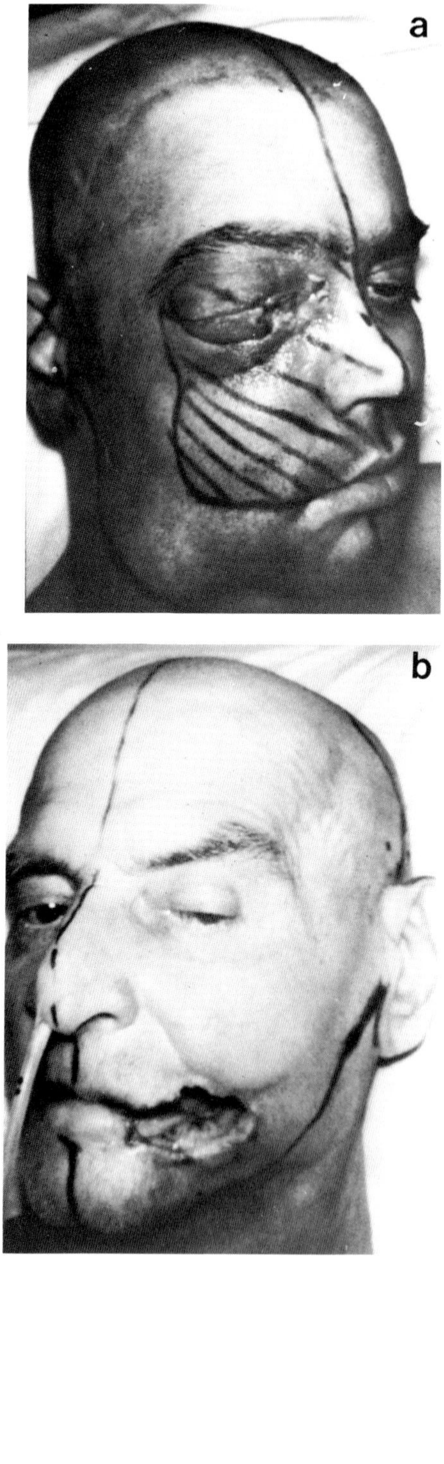

FIG. 2. A: Case 3 (C.A., 42 yrs). Complete relief of pain following right-sided medullary tractotomy and section of C_1 and C_2 posterior roots. **B:** Case 5 (P.L., 71 yrs). Complete relief of pain following left-sided medullary tractotomy. Black line delineates area of complete analgesia; hatching that of anesthesia.

pain and why they consider this more physiologic bulbar tractotomy as only of mere historical interest. These attitudes are probably due to inconsistent results obtained because of the difficulty in localizing precisely the trigeminal tract. We believe that now the neurophysiologic monitoring and precise localization of the tract can be achieved, descending trigeminal tractotomy will become the procedure of choice.

ACKNOWLEDGMENTS

The collaboration of Dr. Galeazzo Sciarretta, of the Bioengineering Research Group of Verona, is gratefully acknowledged for arrangement of electrophysiological instrumentation.

I am also indebted to Mrs. Francesca Pistorelli for her help in translation and typing of the manuscript.

The work is supported in part by the N. H. Marastoni Foundation of Verona.

REFERENCES

1. Brodal, A. (1969): *Neurological Anatomy in Relation to Clinical Medicine.* Oxford University Press, Oxford.
2. Crosby, E. C., Humphrey, I., and Lauer, E. W. (1962): *Correlative Anatomy of the Nervous System.* Macmillan, New York.
3. D'Errico, A. (1973): Mesencephalic and medullary tractotomies. In: *Neurological Surgery,* edited by R. Youmans, pp. 1758–1763. Saunders, Philadelphia.
4. Falconer, M. A. (1949): Intramedullary trigeminal tractotomy and its place in the treatment of facial pain. *J. Neurol. Neurosurg. Psychiatry,* 12:297–311.
5. Grant, F., and Weinberger, L. (1941): Experiences with intramedullary tractotomy. *Surg. Gynecol. Obstet.,* 72:747–751.
6. Guidetti, B. (1950): Tractotomy for the relief of trigeminal neuralgia. *J. Neurosurg.,* 7:499–502.
7. Hamby, W., Shinners, B., and Marsh, I. (1948): Trigeminal tractotomy: Observations on forty-eight cases. *Arch. Surg.,* 57:171–174.
8. Hosobuchi, Y., and Rutkin, B. (1971): Descending trigeminal tractotomy. Neurophysiological approach. *Arch. Neurol.,* 25:115–125.
9. Humphrey, T. (1955): Pattern formed at upper cervical spinal cord levels by sensory fibers of spinal and cranial nerves. *Arch. Neurol. Psychiatry,* 73:36–49.
10. Kempe, L. G. (1970): *Operative Neurosurgery, Vol. 2.* Springer, Berlin.
11. Kerr, F. W. L. (1963): The divisional organization of afferent fibres of the trigeminal nerve. *Brain,* 86:721–732.
12. King, R. B., and Meagher, J. N. (1955): Studies of trigeminal nerve potentials. *J. Neurosurg.,* 12:393–402.
13. Kunc, Z. (1960): La localisation des trajets de la douleur des nerfs IX, X et VII dans la moelle allongée et la possibilité de leur tractotomie séléctive. *Acta Neurochir.,* 8:327–334.
14. Kunc, Z. (1965): Treatment of essential neuralgia of the 9th nerve by selective tractotomy. *J. Neurosurg.,* 23:494–500.
15. Kunc, Z. (1966): Significance of fresh anatomic data on spinal trigeminal tract for possibility of selective tractotomies. In: *Pain,* edited by R. Knighton and P. Dumke, pp. 351–363. Churchill Ltd., London.
16. Kunc, Z. (1977): Data obtained by means of trigeminal tractotomy. *J. Neurosurg. Sci.,* 21:115–120.

17. McKenzie, K. G. (1955): Trigeminal tractotomy. *Clin. Neurosurg.*, 2:50–69.
18. Mracek, Z. (1977): Surgical management of intractable pain due to malignant tumours in the face and neck. *J. Neurosurg. Sci.*, 21:123–125.
19. Mullan, J. F. (1971): Personal communication.
20. Nashold, B. S., Jr., Slaughter, D. G., Wilson, W. P., and Zorub, D. (1977): Stereotactic mesencephalotomy. *Prog. Neurol. Surg.*, 8:35–49.
21. Olivecrona, H. (1942): Tractotomy for relief of trigeminal neuralgia. *Arch. Neurol. Psychiatry,* 47:544–552.
22. Pagni, C. A., and Maspes, P. E. (1970): Problems in the surgical treatment of pain in malignancies of the head and neck. *Topical Probl. Psychiat. Neurol.*, 10:138–153.
23. Pagni, C. A., and Maspes, P. E. (1972): The relief of intractable pain in malignant disease of the head and neck by stereotactic thalamotomy or sensory root section. In: *Pain,* edited by J. P. Payne and R. A. P. Burt, pp. 204–207. Livingstone, London.
24. Pagni, C. A., Maspes, P. E., Visca, A., and Bollati, A. (1969): Riflessioni sul problema del trattamento chirurgico delle algie cranio-cervico-facciali da neoplasia maligna. *Min. Neurochir.*, 13:29–33.
25. Reney, R., Reney, A., and Hunter, C. (1950): Treatment of major trigeminal neuralgia through section of the trigemino-spinal tract in the medulla. *Am. J. Surg.*, 80:11–30.
26. Sjöqvist, O. (1938): Studies on pain conduction in the trigeminal nerve. A contribution to surgical treatment of facial pain. *Acta Psychiat. Neurol.*, Suppl. 17.
27. Taren, J. A. (1964): The position of the cutaneous components of facial, glossopharyngeal and vagal nerves in the spinal tract of V. *J. Comp. Neurol.*, 122:389–398.
28. Taren, J. A., Kahn, E., and Humphrey, T. (1969): The surgery of pain. In: *Correlative Neurosurgery,* edited by E. Kahn et al., pp. 464–508. Charles C Thomas, Springfield, Ill.
29. Walker, A. E. (1966): Neuralgias of the glossopharyngeal, vagus, and intermedius nerves. In: *Pain,* edited by R. Knighton and P. Dumke, pp. 421–429. Churchill Ltd., London.
30. Wetzel, N. (1966): The relief of pain of malignant disease in the head and neck by sensory root section. In: *Pain,* edited by R. Knighton and P. Dumke, pp. 431–437. Churchill Ltd., London.
31. White, J. C. (1962): Evaluation of operations for relief of pain. *Neurol. Méd-chir.*, 4:1–28.
32. White, J. C., and Sweet, W. H. (1969): *Pain and the Neurosurgeon.* Charles C Thomas, Springfield, Ill.
33. Zverina, E. (1977): Location of trigeminal neuralgia development. Preoperative stimulation of descending trigeminal tract. *J. Neurosurg. Sci.*, 21:109–110.

Advances in Pain Research and Therapy, Vol. 2,
edited by J. J. Bonica and V. Ventafridda.
Raven Press, New York © 1979.

Percutaneous Thermocoagulation of the Gasserian Ganglion in the Treatment of Pain in Advanced Cancer

*Jean Siegfried and **Giovanni Broggi

**Neurochirurgische Klinik, Universitätsspital Zürich, CH-8091 Zürich, Switzerland; and*
***Division of Neurosurgery, Istituto Neurologico "C. Besta," via Celoria, 11, 20133 Milano, Italy*

Percutaneous controlled thermocoagulation of the gasserian ganglion permits a clinically complete or partial selective destruction of pain fibers with preservation of some touch sensitivity, carries little stress or danger, has a low complication rate, and can be performed on old patients and/or those in poor general condition with the patient practically ambulatory throughout. After being established as one of the operations of choice in the neurosurgical treatment of classic idiopathic trigeminal neuralgia, its use in symptomatic facial pain appears promising. In our first 6 patients with metastatic or direct invasion of the middle fossa and/or of the face by carcinoma, we obtained good relief of pain (11). Now we have had more experience in patients with pain in one or more trigeminal divisions caused by advanced cancer and managed in two different hospital centers. This report contains a summary of our results.

METHODS AND MATERIALS

In the 6-year period extending from February 1972, to February 1978, 1,106 patients have been operated on in Zürich (742) and Milan (364) for trigeminal pain. In these rather large series, only 20 patients (12 in Zürich, 8 in Milan) were suffering from symptomatic trigeminal pain of advanced cancer. The youngest patient was 37 years old and the oldest 80 years old. The age distribution shows that the majority of patients were between 60 and 70 years old.

The sites of the cancer producing pain in one or more trigeminal divisions are listed in Table 1, and the diagnosis of cancer is listed in Table 2. The general condition of all patients was poor to very poor. They were suffering

TABLE 1. *Site of the cancer producing pain in one or more trigeminal divisions*

Site	No. of pts.
Mandible	5
Epipharynx-mandible	4
Tongue	3
Base of the skull	3
Cerebellar angle	2
Middle fossa	2
Ear-mandible	1

from intractable pain, and most of them were taking narcotics. Carbamazepine was tried in all cases without success. Preoperatively, a diminution of sensitivity (hypesthesia and hypalgesia) was found in 9 patients and hyperpathia noted in 5 patients.

In each patient the technique of percutaneous controlled thermocoagulation of the gasserian ganglion described by Sweet (15) and subsequently by us (12) was used. The anterior approach of Härtel (6) to the foramen ovale with local anesthesia or in some cases with a short-lasting intravenous general anesthetic was used. The needle is introduced into the skin usually 3.0 cm lateral to the labial commissure. The visual landmarks for direction of the electrode are derived from the intersection of a plane 3 cm in front of the ear canal with that passing through the middle of the pupil. Lateral and submento-vertex X-ray views confirm the position of the electrode in the gasserian ganglion through the foramen ovale. For localization of the electrode within the ganglion, low-voltage stimulation (100 to 300 mV, 60-cycle square-wave pulse of 1-msec duration) was performed; nonpainful sensation of itching or tingling in the field of projection of one, two, or sometimes three divisions of the trigeminal nerve permits correct adjustment of the position of the electrode tip. Under an ultra-short-acting barbiturate, one or more radiofrequency coagulations with a temperature of 60°C to 70°C for 1 min are carried out until a dense hypalgesia or analgesia to pinprick in the division mediating the pain is obtained.

TABLE 2

Diagnosis	No. of pts.
Carcinoma	9
Metastasis	5
Fibrosarcoma	4
Cylindroma	2

RESULTS

In patients with cancer pain, a long follow-up is not possible. Moreover, 5 patients could not be evaluated for more than a few weeks after the operation and did not answer the questionnaire we sent them after discharge. Dramatic pain-relief was observed immediately after the operation in all patients, but this relief lasted only a few days in 5 patients. In 6 patients the pain recurred slowly after 1 month, when it was still much less intense than before the operation; but subsequently it gradually became worse and eventually was as intense as before the operation.

Table 3 summarizes the follow-up and shows that about one-half of the patients operated on got very good benefit from the operation with long-lasting effect. The diagnosis of the cancer pain does not play any role, but the site of the cancer producing pain is decisive. As long as the pain is localized in one or more trigeminal divisions, one can expect a favorable result. In two cases, further improvement was obtained with an additional thermorhizotomy of glossopharyngeal nerve. Three cases with bone destruction and deep, burning pain were not improved.

TABLE 3. *Follow-up time and results*

Follow-up	No. of pts.	Pain-free	Less pain	No effect
1 month	20	9	6	5
3 months	15 (2)[a]	9	0	6
12 months	10 (3)[a]	7	0	3
18 months	5 (1)[a]	2	0	3
24 months	2	1	0	1

[a] In bracket: up to death.

Analgesia with hypesthesia was noted in all the patients, and total anesthesia developed in 3 patients. No complications occurred, except itching which was reported by 5 patients.

DISCUSSION

Face and throat pain in advanced cancer pain are common, and the incidence of severe and intractable pain is higher than with malignancy at other sites. Rather surprisingly, the number of patients operated on by us is very small in view of our large experience with the surgical management of facial pain. Cancer pain in the trigeminal region represents only 1.8% of our operations for trigeminal pain. The diagnosis of the cause of pain usually is seen as manifestly clear in patients with demonstrated tissue damage due to the neoplastic disease, and complaints have often a major emotional component.

However, the patients generally state or imply that the emotional effects are necessarily secondary to the pain rather than a primary cause of pain (16). We are thus involved with a chain of morbid processes in which a primary disorder (cancer pain) leads to a second component (emotional pain), which in turn aggravates the first one. In this vicious circle, neurosurgery has a role to play, and pain produced by cancer is certainly one of the best indications for pain surgery.

Combined multiple rhizotomies of cranial nerves and upper cervical nerves are old methods (2,3) and are still indicated in control of pain from malignant tumors involving the face, head, and neck (8,9). A review of several important series made by Sindou et al. (13), included a total of 254 patients of deep and/or extensive cervical and cervicofacial cancers treated by different cranial nerve operations often combined with upper cervical rhizotomy. Of the total, 53% of the patients derived good results (generally short survival), and there was an 18% mortality. The high mortality rate could be explained by the almost invariably precarious state of the patient operated on and the extensive trauma produced by the surgery. The same interpretation can be given for other techniques. Gros et al. (4) reported 24 cases of cervicofacial pain due to cancer, for which they combined an upper cervical rhizotomy and a medullary trigeminal tractotomy complemented by section of the ninth cranial nerve in all the cases and by section of the tenth nerve in 5 cases. They obtained good initial results in 70% of the patients; but this decreased 44% until death, which occurred, on an average, around the sixth month after the operation. Their mortality rate was about 20% (4).

Destruction of only one or two cranial nerves for face and throat pain are rarely mentioned. In his personal experience of 1,433 patients with facial pain treated with alcohol injection of trigeminal nerve, Harris (5) had very few patients with symptomatic pain caused by disseminated sclerosis, antral abscess, sinusitis, etc., but none had advanced cancer. In a series of 637 patients subjected to extradural preganglionic neurotomy (Spiller-Frazier operation), Ruge (10) mentions only one case of carcinoma.

The introduction of the percutaneous coagulation technique by Sweet has led to a resurgence of interest in the neurosurgical treatment of trigeminal pain and its use in cases of advanced cancer. Sweet (14) himself reported on a series of 20 patients of whom 4 were completely relieved until death from 3 weeks to 3 months later. The remainder, after varying short periods of partial or total relief, had recurrence of pain on the same or the opposite side as the lesion spread. Single cases have been reported with success by others (1,7,11).

Our personal experience with this technique in patients with cancer pain suggests the following indications and guidelines:

1. The pain caused by cancer must be localized and tissues supplied by one or more trigeminal branches.

2. If the glossopharyngeus nerve is involved in the pain process, percutaneous thermocoagulation of this nerve can be combined with that of the gasserian ganglion.
3. The preexistence of anesthesia and/or analgesia in the pain area due to destruction of trigeminal roots by the cancer itself is a contraindication to the operation, because the goal of the procedure (analgesia) is already present. An anesthesia or analgesia dolorosa cannot be cured by surgical interruption of pain pathways.
4. Patients with deep, burning pain involving nerve fibers other than those in the trigeminal nerve will derive little or no relief from thermocoagulation of the gasserian ganglion.

SUMMARY

Under strict indications, good to very-good relief of facial cancer pain can be achieved by the percutaneous, controlled thermocoagulation of the gasserian ganglion. This is a procedure devoid of stress, suitable for old patients as well as patients in poor general condition, and has a low complication rate. A series of 20 cases is reported and the indications discussed.

REFERENCES

1. Broggi, G. (1975): Thermorhizotomy in trigeminal neuralgia: Preliminary considerations in 46 cases. *Adv. Neurosurg.*, 3:297–300.
2. Dandy, W. E. (1929): Operative relief from pain in lesions of the mouth, tongue and throat. *Arch. Surg. (Chicago)*, 19:143–148.
3. Fay, T. (1926): Intracranial division of glossopharyngeal nerve combined with cervical rhizotomy for pain in inoperable carcinoma of the throat. *Ann. Surg.*, 84:456–459.
4. Gros, C., Cordier, M., Vlahovitch, B. and Roilgen, A. (1963): Neurotomie combinée et traitement des algies cervico-cranio-faciales d'origine néoplasique. *Ann. Chir.*, 17:533–539.
5. Harris, W. (1940): An analysis of 1433 cases of paroxysmal trigeminal neuralgia (trigeminal-tic) and the end-results of Gasserian alcohol injection. *Brain*, 63:209–224.
6. Härtel, F. (1914): Die Behandlung der Trigeminusneuralgie mit intrakraniellen Alkoholeinspritzungen. *Deutsch. Z. Chir.*, 126:429–552.
7. Onofrio, B. M. (1975): Radiofrequency percutaneous Gasserian ganglion lesions. Results in 140 patients with trigeminal pain. *J. Neurosurg.*, 42:132–139.
8. Pagni, C. A., and Maspes, P. E. (1970): Problems in the surgical treatment of pain in malignancies of the head and neck. *Topical Prob. Psychiat. Neurol.*, 10: 138–153.
9. Pagni, C. A., and Maspes, P. E. (1972): The relief of intractable pain in malignant disease of the head and neck by stereotactic thalamotomy or sensory root section. In: *Pain*, edited by R. Janzen, W. D. Keidel, A. Herz, and C. Steichele. Georg Thieme Verlag, Stuttgart.
10. Ruge, D., Brochner, R., and Davis, L. (1958): A study of the treatment of 637 patients with trigeminal neuralgia. *J. Neurosurg.*, 15:528–536.
11. Siegfried, J. (1977): 500 percutaneous thermocoagulations of the Gasserian ganglion for trigeminal pain. *Surg. Neurol.*, 8:126–131.
12. Siegfried, J., and Vosmansky, M. (1975): Technique of the controlled thermoco-

agulation of trigeminal ganglion and spinal roots. *Adv. Tech. Standards Neurosurg.*, 2:199–209.
13. Sindou, M., Fischer, G., and Mansuy, L. (1976): Posterior spinal rhizotomy and selective posterior rhizidiotomy. *Prog. Neurol. Surg.*, 7:201–250.
14. Sweet, W. H. (1976): Controlled thermocoagulation of trigeminal ganglion and rootlets for differential destruction of pain fibers: Facial pain other than trigeminal neuralgia. *Clin. Neurosurg.*, 23:96–102.
15. Sweet, W. H., and Wepsic, J. G. (1974): Controlled thermocoagulation of trigeminal ganglion and rootlets for differential destruction of pain fibers. Part 1: Trigeminal neuralgia. *J. Neurosurg.*, 40:143–156.
16. Woodforde, J., and Fielding, J. R. (1975): Pain and cancer. In: *Pain,* edited by M. Weisenberg, pp. 326–331. C. V. Mosby Co., St. Louis.

Advances in Pain Research and Therapy, Vol. 2,
edited by J. J. Bonica and V. Ventafridda.
Raven Press, New York © 1979.

Percutaneous Differential Radiofrequency Rhizotomy of Glossopharyngeal Nerve in Facial Pain Due to Cancer

*Giovanni Broggi and **Jean Siegfried

**Division of Neurosurgery, Istituto Neurologico "C. Besta," via Celoria 11, 20133 Milan, Italy; and **Neurochirurgische Universitätklinik, Kantonsspital Zurich, 100 Ramistrasse, Zürich, 8022, Switzerland*

Pain sensitivity of the face and the anterior part of the tongue depends on the trigeminal nerve, while the external ear, oropharynx, larynx, epipharynx, and posterior part of the tongue are innervated by the glossopharyngeal and vagal nerves. The surgical treatment of pain in all these regions may include the partial or total section of these three nerves (7).

After the introduction of percutaneous radiofrequency (RF) differential trigeminal rhizotomy (5) for treatment of trigeminal neuralgia, pain due to cancer in the territory of the trigeminal nerve innervation also has been successfully treated by this technique (Siegfried and Broggi, *this volume*). However, facial pain due to cancer is seldom confined to the trigeminal territory, especially when the base of the skull has been invaded by metastases or there is diffusion of the primary tumor.

Until recently, the surgical treatment of 9th and 10th nerve neuralgia entailed opening of the posterior fossa or extracranial section of the nerve at the posterior foramen lacerum. However, this second surgical approach is not easy in the presence of a tumor or when tissues are modified by previous radiation therapy.

Moreover, the approach to the 9th and 10th nerves through the posterior fossa is not free of operative risk, even when a microsurgical technique is used (4). This operative risk is increased in the cancer patient, who is usually debilitated by the disease and by chemotherapy. Selective bulbar tractotomy (3), indicated when both trigeminal and glossopharyngeal neuralgia are present, poses a similar surgical risk.

Recently (1,6) a percutaneous approach like the one successfully used for trigeminal neuralgia has been proposed for treatment of glossopharyngeal neuralgia. We now suggest the use of this technique for treatment of facial and rhinopharyngeal pain due to cancer.

METHODS AND MATERIAL

In our departments during the past year we have treated 4 patients with glossopharyngeal neuralgic pain with percutaneous RF differential rhizotomy of the 9th nerve at the extracranial side of the posterior foramen lacerum. Two of these patients had cancer of the face.

Case 1 (INM). Male, 50 years old; had a carcinoma of the larynx treated by direct surgery and by two courses of radiation therapy. The pain was located in the right face, in the territory of the 2nd and 3rd trigeminal root, in the ear, in the external auditory canal, and in the tonsillar pillar. The trigeminal pain was continuous, unbearable, burning. The 9th nerve pain was paroxysmal and of the lightning type, triggered by swallowing.

On April 4, 1977, percutaneous RF differential rhizotomy of the trigeminal nerve was done, and 10 days later this same technique was used to produce a rhizotomy of the glossopharyngeal nerve. The pain in the face completely disappeared with analgesia in the territory of the trigeminal nerve. The glossopharyngeal neuralgia also disappeared, but 6 months later the patient had a recurrence of this pain, and on October 3, 1977, a second percutaneous RF rhizotomy of the glossopharyngeal nerve was performed. To date, the patient has remained pain-free. No neurological deficit followed the surgery except for the sensory deficit in the territory of the 5th and 9th nerves. No cardiac problems were present either during or after the surgery.

Case 2 (KSZ). A 68-year-old female had carcinoma of the epipharynx with

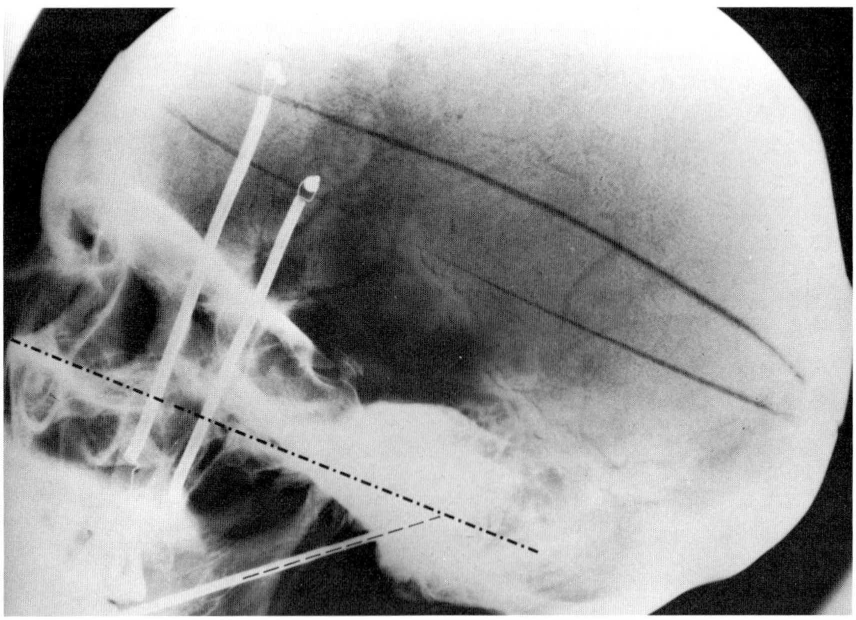

FIG. 1. Lateral X-ray of the dry skull, with the needle inserted in the pars nervosa of the posterior foramen lacerum. Note the angle to the plane passing through the internal auditory meatus and the inferior margin of the orbit.

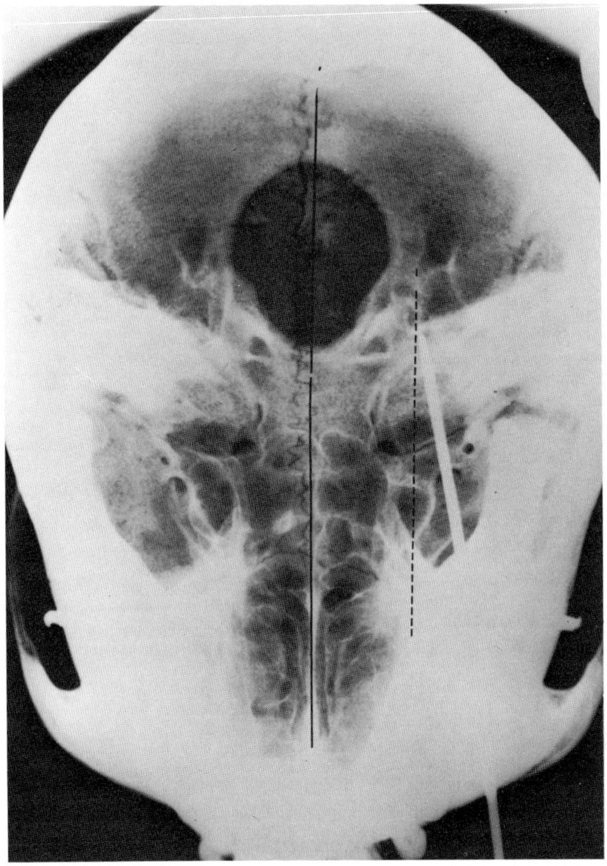

FIG. 2. A-P view of the X-ray of the dry skull. The needle is inserted in the pars nervosa of the posterior foramen lacerum. Note the angle to the plane parallel to the mid-sagittal plane.

pain referred to the mandibular region accompanied by typical glossopharyngeal neuralgia on the left. On January 31, 1978, she underwent in a single session trigeminal and glossopharyngeal percutaneous RF differential rhizotomies. Promptly after the procedure, she had pain-relief associated with analgesia in the mandibular and lower lip regions. She also had difficulty in swallowing, which lasted for 3 weeks and a permanent deficit of the left 12th cranial nerve. No other neurologic deficits followed this percutaneous surgery. She has remained pain-free to the present time.

TECHNIQUE

The technique of 9th nerve percutaneous rhizotomy is similar to the percutaneous approach to the trigeminal ganglion (1). The needle is inserted into the skin of the cheek 2.5 mm lateral to the labial commissure, and is directed under fluoroscopic control along two planes: one of a 12° angle to

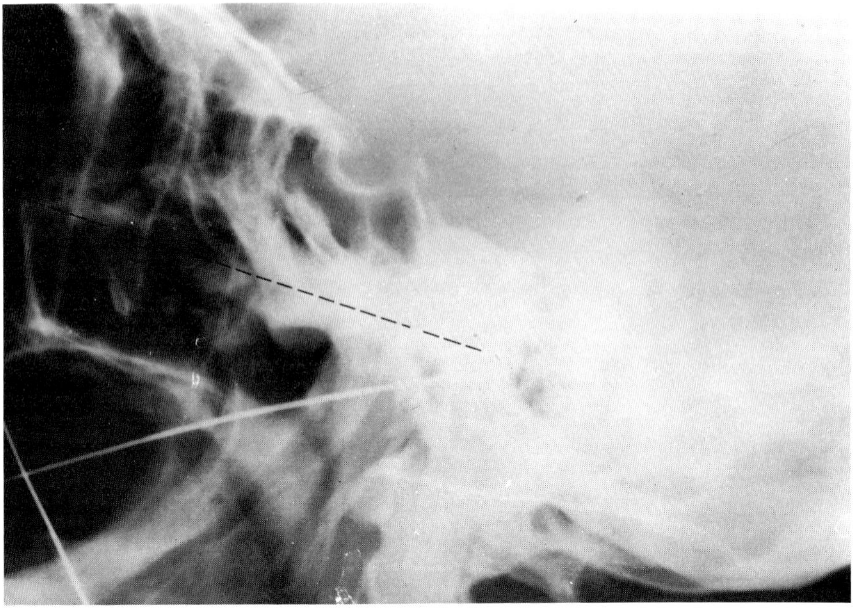

FIG. 3. Case no. 1: Lateral view of the X-ray taken with the image fluoroscopic intensifier. Note that the needle inserted in the position where RF coagulation was performed after electrophysiological control makes an angle to the plane passing through the internal auditory meatus and the inferior margin of the orbit equal to that in the model in Fig. 1.

the vertical plane passing through the pupil of the eye, the second at a 40° angle to the plane passing through the internal auditory meatus and the inferior margin of the orbit.

The needle is advanced to a point lateral to the internal carotid artery where its tip should be at the medial portion of the posterior lacerum. This position is checked with X-ray, then electrophysiologic control is carried out by checking the impedance and evoking 9th, 10th, and 12th nerve responses to confirm the exact position of the needle. EKG monitoring is also recommended. Thiopental sodium (Pentothal®) is administered as a single bolus before the RF coagulation in order to produce amnesia and partial analgesia. The temperature of the probe should be kept between 65°C and 75°C. The lesion is repeated if intraoperative evaluation indicates this is necessary.

Despite the necessity to pass through the tumor or through a tissue hardened by radiation therapy, no difficulties greater than those encountered in noncancer patients have been experienced.

DISCUSSION

A tumor that causes glossopharyngeal neuralgia is rare, but Dandy (2) has also reported a similar case in 1927. In our series, glossopharyngeal nerve involvement in facial pain due to cancer is not infrequent. On the basis of our very limited experience with these 2 patients, we speculate that graded RF percutaneous rhizotomy is a safe and successful technique for the treatment of glossopharyngeal pain due to cancer. It produces minimal trauma, and it can be easily applied to debilitated patients. Since facial pain due to cancer often is not limited to single cranial-nerve involvement, the surgeon can perform the two rhizotomies within a few days or even in the same session as in our second case. Moreover, the hospitalization period is very short, and there is no postoperative pain or morbidity which often follows general anesthesia in the sitting position. Also, the procedure is more readily accepted by patients who believe that it entails no more than a needle puncture. Finally, the operative risk is almost nil, with no mortality and a very selective morbidity.

REFERENCES

1. Broggi, G. (submitted): Percutaneous differential radiofrequency rhizotomy of the glossopharyngeal nerve. *Surg. Neurol.*
2. Dandy, W. E. (1927): Glossopharyngeal neuralgia (tic douloureux): Its diagnosis and treatment. *Arch. Surg.,* 15:198–214.
3. Kunc, Z. (1965): Treatment of essential neuralgia of the ninth nerve by selective tractotomy. *J. Neurosurg.,* 23:494–500.
4. Laha, R. K., and Jannetta, P. J. (1977): Glossopharyngeal neuralgia. *J. Neurosurg.,* 47:313–320.
5. Sweet, H. W. (1976): Treatment of facial pain by percutaneous differential thermal trigeminal rhizotomy. *Prog. Neurol. Surg.,* 7:153–179.
6. Tew, J., Jr. (1977): Percutaneous rhizotomy in the treatment of intractable facial pain (trigeminal, glossopharyngeal and vagal nerves). In: *Current Techniques in Operative Neurosurgery,* edited by H. H. Schimedek and W. H. Sweet, pp. 409–426. Grune & Stratton, New York.
7. White, J. C., and Sweet, W. H. (1970): *Pain and the Neurosurgeon: A Forty Year Experience,* pp. 265–302. Charles C Thomas, Springfield, Ill.

Advances in Pain Research and Therapy, Vol. 2,
edited by J. J. Bonica and V. Ventafridda.
Raven Press, New York © 1979.

Stereotaxic Thalamolaminotomy and Posteromedial Hypothalamotomy for the Relief of Intractable Pain

Keiji Sano

Department of Neurosurgery, University of Tokyo, Tokyo, Japan

The word *pain* has two meanings, one is the pain sensation and the other the suffering. Or one can say that the pain has two aspects, the sensory-discriminative and the emotional-motivational. This is also true with *il dolore, la douleur,* or *der Schmerz*. Moreover, pain sensation can be classified into the truly discriminative "epicritic" pain and the diffuse, or poorly localized "protopathic" pain.

Intractable pain is mainly concerned with this protopathic pain and the associated suffering. The ideal treatment of pain is to cure or minimize the protopathic pain and the suffering without impairing epicritic, discriminative pain sensation. With thalamolaminotomy and posteromedial hypothalamotomy, we are able to achieve such desired results.

THALAMOLAMINOTOMY (INTRALAMINAR THALAMOTOMY)

Since stereotaxic procedures were introduced, but especially during the last three decades, most of our surgical efforts to relieve pain have been concentrated in various parts of the thalamus. In our clinic, one operative procedure on the internal medullary lamina for the relief of intractable pain, which we call intralaminar thalamotomy, or thalamolaminotomy, has been carried out since 1963 (12). The internal medullary lamina comprises the intralaminar nuclei [n. centralis lateralis (CL), centre médian (CM), n. limitans (Lim), etc.] and their adjacent fibers. Standard stereotaxic techniques were used for stimulation and recording at the time of thalamotomy. The technique of the procedure has been reported in detail elsewhere (9,10, 12,13) and is illustrated in Fig. 1.

Clinical Investigations

Neuronal Unit Discharge

In recent cases, before inserting stimulating or lesion-making needles, we have inserted tungsten microelectrodes, 5–10 Megohms, with the tip 1 to 2

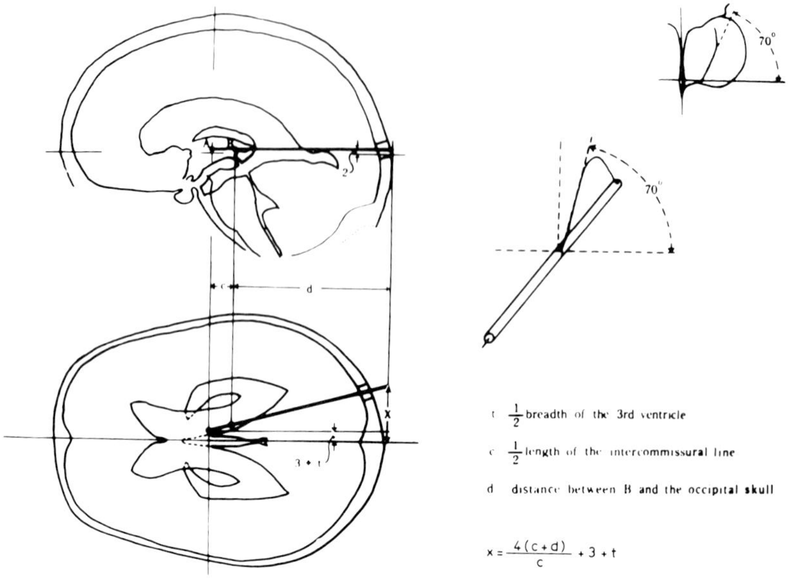

FIG. 1. Technique of thalamolaminotomy. A = point 2–4 mm above the midpoint of the intercommissural line and 3 mm lateral to the wall of the third ventricle. B = point 2–4 mm above the posterior commissure and 7 mm lateral to the wall of the third ventricle. (Courtesy of Sano, K. (1977): In: *Progress in Neurological Surgery,* edited by H. Krayenbühl et al. 8:50–103. Karger Basel.)

μm in diameter, into the brain, in order to investigate spontaneous and evoked neuronal unit discharges from various areas near the target area. With pin pricks of the skin over the wide areas of the body and extremities, both contra- and ipsilateral increase of unit discharge was observed in the nucleus parafascicularis and the center median. Some units also responded to the application of heat to the skin, but did not respond to tactile stimulation.

We have found two types of units, fast-responding and slow-responding. The former units responded with a latency of about 30 to 40 msec and showed a shorter duration of discharge. The latter units responded with a long latency (several hundred msec) and had a longer duration.

In addition, electrical stimulation (1,3,6 Hz and 60,100 Hz, 5–20v̄) of the internal medullary lamina and the adjacent structures was carried out in every 2 mm of the needle (0.8 mm in diameter) track with the parameters mentioned above in order to obtain an accurate localization of the target. Figure 2 (left figure) summarizes the results of high-frequency (60,100 Hz) stimulation in patients under local anesthesia. The stimulated points are projected on the horizontal (+4) plane of the Schaltenbrand and Bailey Atlas (14). Black circles mean that the points showed sensory effects induced by stimulation, whereas white circles mean that the stimulation of the points did not elicit somatic sensation, but produced "unpleasant" sensation which

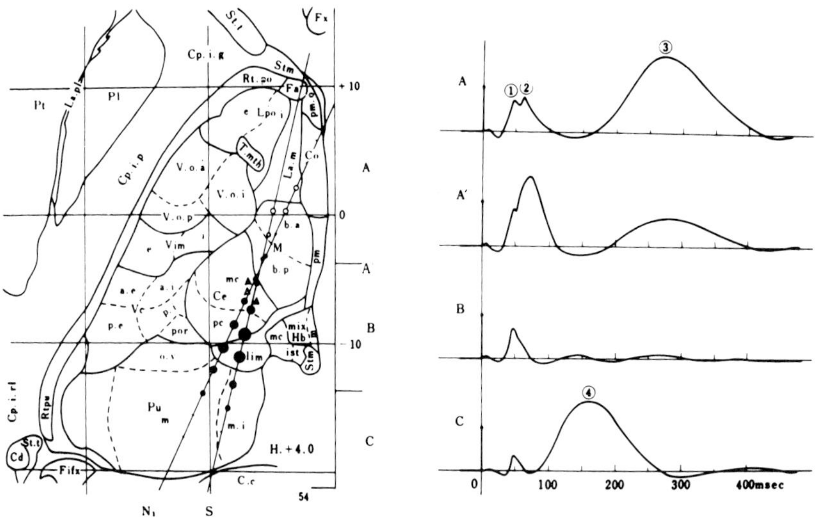

FIG. 2. Left = needle tracks. Right = evoked potentials. *Black circles* = pain effect, the size of the circle being proportional to the effect. *White circles* = unpleasant sensation. *Triangles* = motor effect. (Courtesy of Sano, K. (1977): In *Progress in Neurological Surgery,* edited by H. Krayenbühl et al. 8:50–103. Karger Basel.)

was poorly localized anywhere in the body. The sizes of the circles are proportional to the sensitivity to the stimulation.

As seen in Fig. 2, the white circles are seen in the medial and anterior part of the thalamus (A, left). The black circles are distributed in a wide area of the posterior half of the internal medullary lamina (B, left) which ranges from about 4 mm to 14 mm posterior to the midpoint of the intercommissural line in the anteroposterior direction. The nucleus parafascicularis, the parvocellular portion of the centre médian and the n. limitans are especially sensitive to stimulation. The more forward or upward the stimulating point moves, the weaker the response.

The general character of the sensory responses to the high-frequency stimulation of this area was a diffuse, burning pain in the contralateral half of the body or the whole body. Not infrequently, the spontaneous pain of the patient was exaggerated at a lower intensity than the threshold to produce diffuse, burning pain, irrespective of the side of stimulation.

Among the intralaminar nuclei, the centre médian (CM) occupies the largest area. Although it certainly plays an important role in the perception of pain, it is unlikely that all its parts are related to pain. Only the posterior part which corresponds to the parvocellular portion of the nucleus, is closely related to pain. Several writers have reported the effects of stimulation of the centre médian, but these have differed from author to author. This variety of effects might be partly due to the difference of stimulating points and partly to the difference of parameters. In our experience, the parvocellular portion of the centre médian, the n. parafascicularis (pf) and the n. limitans (Lim) form a most essential area for pain.

High-frequency stimulation of the middle portion of the internal medullary lamina, from the midpoint of the intercommissural line to the point 8 mm behind the midpoint (i.e., the part medial to the Vop and Vim nuclei of Hassler (14) and probably corresponding to the magnocellular portion of the CM), produced, in some patients, tremor and rigidity and in other patients, trembling in the contralateral extremities. These points are represented by triangles in Fig. 2 (A′, left). In cases with extrapyramidal disorders, stimulation of this portion markedly increased tremor and rigidity. Cortical evoked potentials produced by low-frequency (1,3,6 Hz) stimulation showed a good correlation with the sensory-motor effects and were characteristic of each zone (Fig. 2, right).

Conclusions

These data and experimental studies on cats (5,10) led to the following conclusions: (a) The faster-conducting fibers of the spinothalamic tract (fast A-delta) course in the lateral side of the medulla and then turn inside, joining in the lemniscal system, and terminate finally in the specific sensory nucleus of the thalamus contralateral to the side of stimulation. A part of them may terminate in the PO (6,7). (b) The slower-conducting fibers (slow A-delta) course in the more medial part of the medulla; some of them terminate in the lateral part of the central gray, others to the ventral part of the internal medullary lamina of the thalamus, and finally, the rest of the fibers reach the posterior hypothalamus. Some of the slower fibers project also to the side ipsilateral to the side of stimulation. (c) The role of the hypothalamus in pain perception should be emphasized not only because of its effects upon the autonomic and emotional responses to stress, but also because the slow A-delta fibers end here. (d) Unitary discharges could be recorded from various parts in the thalamus which reacted to selective C-fiber stimulation. The results obtained indicate that unitary elements reactive to the C-fiber impulses are widely scattered in the medial structures in the thalamus. But at the same time, they show that the C-fibers terminate most densely in the intralaminar nuclei such as the CM and the CL. We could not find cells in the n. ventralis posterolateralis (VPL) which were activated by the C-fiber stimulation. However, this does not exclude the existence of C-fiber terminals in this nucleus, because the number of cells tested were relatively few.

The latencies of reactions varied very much, ranging from 400 msec to, in most cases, several hundred msec. The longest one was about 2,000 msec, but, in this case, evaluation of the response was very difficult. These results are compatible with those of Albe-Fessard and Kruger (1), as well as those of Collins and Randt (2) who described that the mean latency of the midbrain responses to C-fiber stimulation was 560 msec. The cells in the ventral part of the CM probably receive both slow A-delta and C-fibers. Experimental studies suggest that the intralaminar nuclei exert facilitatory effects upon the specific sensory system and the latter exerts inhibitory effects on the former.

Thus, the specific sensory system and the intralaminar structures constitute a "diencephalic control system" of sensation.

Therapeutic Application

For the relief of intractable pain, the B zone of the lamina where stimulation produces increase of spontaneous pain and burning sensation, namely the zone including the intralaminar nuclei, the parvocellular portion of the centre médian, the n. parafascicularis, the n. limitans with the adjacent fibers, was sterotaxically destroyed.

Patients with thalamic pain; pain due to malignancy; atypical facial pain due to trauma, herpes zoster, carotid basilar anastomosis, etc., causalgia, tabes dorsalis, and other types of central pain in which long-term medication had not been effective, have been subjected to this standard procedure. In some cases stereotaxic destruction of the centre médian–parafascicular complex (usually from the frontal burr hole) was performed.

Results

Table 1 summarizes the results of operations on 41 patients at the time of discharge and 3 months later. Although not shown in the table, the results at 1-year follow-up were the same as those at 3-months follow-up. The numbers in parentheses are cases of stereotaxic destruction of the centre médian–parafascicular complex, while all of the others are cases of thalamolaminotomy. As expected, some patients had less pain-relief at 3 months than at the time of discharge.

The data in Table 1 make it obvious that standard thalamolaminotomy is more effective than the centre médian–parafasciculotomy. The longest follow-up is more than 10 years in a patient with thalamic syndrome who still is pain-free. Except in four instances, the procedure was done bilaterally with an interval of 7 to 10 days. The thalamolaminotomy was especially effective for thalamic pain and other types of central pain. However, pain due to cancer recurred several months later, although when it recurred the pain was still of a tolerable degree as compared with the preoperative state.

No severe complications were observed. Very slight disturbance of consciousness, confusion, or hallucinations were seen in several patients on the second or third postoperative day mostly after the second-stage operation, but they recovered within a week.

In all patients, normal sensations remained intact after the operations.

TABLE 1. *Results with thalamolaminotomy (in 41 patients)*

Cause or type of pain	No. of patients	Degree of pain-relief							
		At discharge				3 Months			
		Complete	Good	Fair	Little or none	Complete	Good	Fair	Little or none
Thalamic pain	9	3	4(1)[a]	—	(1)	3	3(1)	1	(1)
Cancer pain	13	3(1)	(1)	5(3)	—	4(1)	—	4(4)	—
Trigeminal neuralgia	4	1	3	—	—	1	2	1	—
Causalgia	4	3	—	—	1	3	—	—	1
Tabes dorsalis	1	—	—	—	1	—	—	—	1
Other central pain	10	2	2(3)	1	2	2	1(2)	1	3
Total	41	13	14	9	5	14	9	11	6
% of Total		33%	34%	22%	11%	34%	22%	27%	17%

[a] Numbers in parentheses indicate results with the stereotaxic destruction of the centrum medianum–n. parafascicularis complex.

Sensory testing for touch, pressure, temperature and even pain (by pin prick) revealed that these sensations were not impaired compared with the preoperative state.

Autopsy was obtained in 4 cases, 3 of patients with cancer and 1 with thalamic pain. In these cases, the sites of stereotaxic lesions were examined, and with the aid of Nauta Gygax method, the degenerated fibers from the lesion sites were tracked (16). The terminal degeneration was found in the n. ventrocaudalis parvocellularis (Vcpc) and in the second somatosensory cortex on the ipsilateral side. No degenerated axons were found in the medial thalamic nuclei. From these findings, it may be concluded that the posterior portion of the internal medullary lamina has definite connections at least with Vcpc and the second somatosensory cortex, but no connection with the dorsomedial nucleus.

POSTEROMEDIAL HYPOTHALAMOTOMY

This procedure entails making a small stereotaxic lesion in the posterior (ergotropic) hypothalamus which is actually the continuation of the periaqueductal gray. I introduced the procedure in 1962 (8,11), in order to normalize the ergotropic and trophotropic balance for the treatment of violent, very aggressive, and restless behaviors mostly in cases with epilepsy and mental retardation.

Based on the experimental data in animals and on the fact that painful stimuli always cause signs of sympathetic discharges, we started to perform the posteromedial hypothalamotomy for intractable pain in 1971. In the same year, Fairman (4) reported the effects of the posteromedial hypothalamotomy in 12 patients with intractable pain due to metastatic malignant tumor.

Studies of neuronal unit discharges at the time of operation showed the existence of neurons responding to C fiber impulses and A delta fiber impulses in the postero-medial hypothalamus. Electrical stimulation of the area elicited signs of sympathetic discharge (11) and EEG changes similar to those produced by intravenous injection of epinephrine as reported by Venes et al. (15).

There was no operative mortality. As indicated, this procedure was more effective in the treatment of intractable pain due to malignant tumors than that due to other causes (Table 2).

The operation was done bilaterally in 6 patients and unilaterally in 14. It seems that for pain due to lesions below the neck, the operation on the contralateral side was most effective, whereas for pain due to lesions in the face and the head, the operation on the ipsilateral side was more effective.

There was no impairment of sensation noticed after the operation. In our series, regression of metastases of malignant tumors has rarely been ob-

TABLE 2. *Results with posteromedial hypothalamotomy for pain-relief (in 20 patients)*

Cause or type of pain	No. of patients	Degree of pain-relief: At discharge				Degree of pain-relief: 3 Months			
		Complete	Good	Fair	Little or none	Complete	Good	Fair	Little or none
Cancer pain	13	9	3	1	—	9	—	2	2
Causalgia	2	1	1	—	—	—	—	1	1
Neuralgia	4	—	2	2	—	—	—	2	2
Thalamic pain	1	—	—	1	—	—	—	—	1
Total	20	10	6	4	—	9	—	5	6
% of Total		50%	30%	20%	—	45%	—	25%	30%

served, although patients' lives may have been prolonged because of increased appetite and discontinuance of narcotic analgesics.

Five patients with intractable pain due to malignant tumors who lived pain-free for 1 to 3 months following the procedure, after death were submitted to autopsy. The degenerated axons from the lesion site were searched for with the aid of the Nauta-Gygax method. Degenerated fibers were found in the ipsilateral nucleus ventrocaudalis parvocellularis (Vcpc), the second somatosensory cortex, the rolandic sensory cortex, the n. parafascicularis (pf), the pallidum, and downward in the reticular formation. Many of the axons probably terminated in the Vcpc. Moreover, it is noteworthy that no degenerated axons were found in the medial nuclei. It may be concluded that the posteromedial portion of the hypothalamus has connections at least with the Vcpc and probably with the n. parafascicularis and the somatosensory cortices, but no connection with the dorsomedial nucleus.

DISCUSSION

The data suggest that neurons throughout the length of the brain stem, particularly those of the nuclei of the medial two-thirds of the reticular formation, contribute axons to the ascending reticular pathway. This pathway divides at the mesencephalo-diencephalic junction, one portion running a ventral

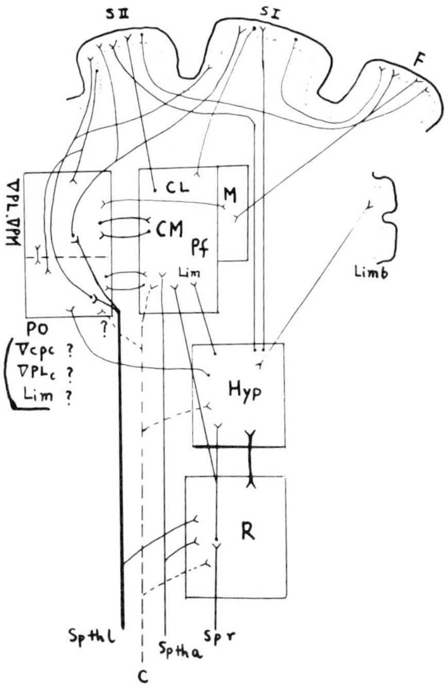

FIG. 3. Diagram of pathways related to pain. C = C fibers; CL = n. centralis lateralis; CM = centrum medianum; F = frontal lobe; Hyp = hypothalamus; Lim = n. limitans; Limb = limbic cortex; M = medial nuclei; Pf = n. parafascicularis; PO = posterior nuclear group; R = brain stem reticular formation; SI = rolandic sensory cortex; SII = second sensory cortex; Spr = spino-reticulo-thalamic pathways; Sptha = anterior spinothalamic tract; Spthl = lateral spinothalamic tract; Vcpc = n. ventro-caudalis parvocellularis; VPL = n. ventralis postero-lateralis; VPM = n. ventralis postero-medialis; VPLc = VPL caudalis. (Courtesy of Sano, K. (1977): In: *Progress in Neurological Surgery,* edited by H. Krayenbühl et al. 8:50–103. Karger Basel.)

course to the hypothalamus, the other ascending and terminating within the intralaminar nuclei of the thalamus (Fig. 3).

According to Dafny and his associates (3), in the posterior hypothalamus of cats there are neurons which respond to somatosensory, visual, and acoustic stimuli respectively; that is to say, there is convergence of impulses of various modalities at the single-cell level. Our data suggest that the posterior hypothalamus in man as well as in the cat contains neurons responding to A-delta as well as C-fiber impulses.

Thus, it is apparent that the hypothalamus is playing a role in sensory functions. Stimulation of the posteromedial hypothalamus in man, however, does not produce any definite sensation but a very unpleasant feeling or great fear. Probably the hypothalamus is important in coloring the emotional aspect of sensations and in provoking autonomic-endocrine responses. This suggests that the posterior hypothalamus is related to unpleasant, fearful, or horrible feelings and sympathetic discharges and endocrine changes which often accompany pain.

SUMMARY

The internal medullary lamina of the thalamus with its nuclei is a composite structure with functional topographic differences: Namely, the anterior, middle, and posterior portions are concerned with emotional, motor, and sensory activities respectively.

The posterior portion of the internal medullary lamina, including the center median (parvocellular portion), n. parafascicularis, n. centralis lateralis, n. limitans, has neurons which respond to slower A-delta-fiber impulses and C-fiber impulses. This portion of the medullary lamina exerts facilitatory influences on the specific sensory system and the latter, in turn, exerts inhibitory influences upon the former, thus both constituting the diencephalic control system of sensation. This posterior portion of the internal medullary lamina has connections, proved by means of the Nauta-Gygax method, with the n. ventrocaudalis parvocellularis and the second sensory cortex. Stereotaxic lesion of the posterior portion of the internal medullary lamina—the intralaminar thalamotomy or the thalamolaminotomy—produces effective relief of intractable pain, especially of central pain, somehow producing no sensory deficits.

The posteromedial hypothalamus has neurons which respond to slower A-delta fiber and C-fiber impulses. Stimulation of this area produces signs of sympathetic discharge (such as rise in blood pressure, tachycardia, pupillary dilation), neck movement, ocular movements, endocrine changes and EEG changes (desynchronization or slow waves of high voltage in the cortical leads) and an unpleasant feeling or fear or horror, but no pain. The posteromedial hypothalamus has connections, proved by means of Nauta-Gygax method, with the n. ventrocaudalis parvocellularis and the n. parafascicularis and probably with the somatosensory cortices.

Stereotaxic lesions of the posteromedial hypothalamus, called posteromedial hypothalamotomy, produce relief of intractable pain due to malignancy, but are not so effective for central pain. No sensory deficits are noted after the operation.

The rationale of the thalamolaminotomy and the posteromedial hypothalamotomy may be that both procedures make lesions not only in one of the main end-stations of the C-fibers and the slow A-delta fibers, but also in the portions that exert influences on the specific sensory system, and thus decrease the intensity of volleys of impulses and change the pattern of impulses which can be interpreted as pain.

REFERENCES

1. Albe-Fessard, D., and Kruger, L. (1962): Duality of unit discharge from cat centrum medianum in response to natural and electrical stimulation. *J. Neurophysiol.,* 25: 1–20.
2. Collins, W. F., and Randt, C. T. (1960): Midbrain evoked responses relating to peripheral unmyelinated or "C" fibers in cat. *J. Neurophysiol.,* 23:47–53.
3. Dafny, N., Bental, E., and Feldman, S. (1965): Effect of sensory stimuli on single unit activity in the posterior hypothalamus. *Electroenceph. Clin. Neurophysiol.,* 19:256–263.
4. Fairman, D. (1972): Hypothalamotomy as a new perspective for alleviation of intractable pain and regression of metastatic malignant tumors. In: *Present Limits of Neurosurgery,* edited by I. Fusek and Z. Kunc, pp. 525–528. Avicenum, Prague.
5. Ishijima, B., and Sano, K. (1971): Responses of specific and non-specific thalamic nuclei to the selective A-δ and C-fiber stimulation, and their interactions in cat's brain. *Neurol. Med. Chir. (Tokyo),* 11:84–100.
6. Mountcastle, V. B., and Henneman, E. (1952): The representation of tactile sensibility in the thalamus of the monkey. *J. Comp. Neurol.,* 97:409–439.
7. Poggio, G. F., and Mountcastle, V. B. (1960): A study of the functional contributions of the lemniscal and spinothalamic systems to somatic sensibility. *Johns Hopkins Hosp. Bull.,* 106:266–316.
8. Sano, K. (1962): Sedative neurosurgery with special reference to posteromedial hypothalamotomy. *Neurol. Med. Chir. (Tokyo),* 4:112–142.
9. Sano, K. (1967): The role of the internal medullary lamina in pain. *Anales del XII Congreso Latinoamericano de Neurocirugia,* pp. 937–952.
10. Sano, K. (1977): Intralaminar thalamotomy (thalamolaminotomy) and posteromedial hypothalamotomy in the treatment of intractable pain. In: *Prog. Neurol. Surg. Vol. 8,* edited by H. Krayenbühl et al. pp. 50–103. Karger, Basel.
11. Sano, K., Mayanagi, Y., Sekino, H., Ogashiwa, M., and Ishijima, B. (1970): Results of stimulation and destruction of the posterior hypothalamus in man. *J. Neurosurg.,* 33:689–707.
12. Sano, K., Yoshioka, M., Ogashiwa, M., Ishijima, B., and Ohye, C. (1966): Thalamolaminotomy. A new operation of relief of intractable pain. *Confin. Neurol.,* 27:63–66.
13. Sano, K., Yoshioka, M., Sekino, H., Mayanagi, Y., Yoshimasu, N., and Tsukamoto, Y. (1970): Functional organization of the internal medullary lamina in man. *Confin. Neurol.,* 32:374–380.
14. Schaltenbrand, G., and Bailey, P. (1959): Einfürung in die Stereotaktischen Operationen mit einem Atlas des menschlichen Gehirns. Thieme, Stuttgart.
15. Venes, J. L., Collins, W. F., and Taub, A. (1972): Evoked cerebral cortical activity from small peripheral nerve fibers in cat. *Electroenceph. Clin. Neurophysiol.,* 33: 207–214.
16. Yoshimasu, N. (1972): Functional anatomy of the internal medullary lamina based on the results of stereotaxic surgery. *Brain & Nerve,* 24:1277–1292 (in Japanese).

Advances in Pain Research and Therapy, Vol. 2,
edited by J. J. Bonica and V. Ventafridda.
Raven Press, New York © 1979.

Central Gray Stimulation for Control of Cancer Pain

Donald E. Richardson

Department of Neurological Surgery, Louisiana State University School of Medicine, and Hotel Dieu Hospital Pain Rehabilitation Unit, New Orleans, Louisiana 70119

This presentation includes a discussion of a new technique for pain-relief that has been applied to only a few patients suffering from cancer pain. A detailed analysis of indications, contraindications, complications, successes, and failures is not available. However, experience to date suggests that this technique has advantages over many others for the control of cancer pain. The potential for control of bilateral pain involving any area of the body from the scalp to the perineum with one operative procedure that can be done under local anesthesia seems to make the procedure ideal for many cancer patients.

Brain stimulation for pain-relief was first done by Heath in 1960 (5). Stimulation of the medial septal area in a woman with carcinoma of the cervix with pelvic pain resulted in pain-relief that was associated with euphoria and a feeling of being intoxicated. Gol (4) did stimulation of this area in several patients with mixed results but, in general, poor pain-relief. Adams and Hosobuchi have stimulated the main sensory nucleus of the thalamus, a procedure comparable to dorsal column stimulation with pain-relief in the area of produced paresthesias (6).

Interest in periaqueductal gray stimulation for pain-relief developed after the report published in 1969 by Reynolds that stimulation of small areas of the central gray produced marked behavioral analgesia in animals (8). This lead was vigorously pursued by Mayer, Liebeskind, Akil, and associates (7) who have been able to produce analgesia consistently by stimulating the area of the dorsal raphe nucleus in the rat. Analgesia was sufficient to allow surgical procedures on the animal without apparent pain and was not associated with motor paralysis or impairment of other sensory modalities. Akil has demonstrated that brain-stimulation analgesia is dependent upon an intact serotonin system, is reduced by dopamine depletion, and is inhibited by norepinephrine (1,2).

Dr. Akil and I carried out a series of experiments in cats and found that stimulation produced analgesia and changes in the evoked response in the medial thalamus comparable to those produced by morphine (9). In addition, naloxone, a morphine antagonist, inhibits these changes in animals (8).

Naloxone given to patients prior to stimulation of the periaqueductal gray also blocks the effect of stimulation with reduction of analgesia (11). In addition, we have measured endogenous opiates in the ventricular fluid of patients undergoing stimulation for pain control and have been able to demonstrate a rise in enkephalin-like compounds in the fluid following stimulation (3). These findings would indicate that the endogenous opiate system, as well as the serotonin system, is involved in the effect of stimulation of the periventricular gray for pain control.

A trial of acute stimulation in 5 patients undergoing thalamotomy was then carried out, with demonstration of excellent bilateral analgesia in 1 and hypalgesia in another 3 patients (10). We found that periaqueductal stimulation produced nystagmus and vertigo, whereas stimulation of the periventricular gray matter in the very medial thalamus produced excellent analgesia with minimal side effects. We have now operated on a large number of patients utilizing a chronic depth-electrode system with an induction receiver and external transmitter that allows chronic self-stimulation for pain control (11). In our published series of 30 patients, 4 patients with cancer pain have been operated on (12). These and 2 additional patients are reported here in detail.

TECHNIQUE

Our present approach is to insert a single, 4-contact, pull-down, platinum-electrode (1) in each patient even if the pain is bilateral. Insertion is done through a coronal burr hole on the side opposite the more intense pain.

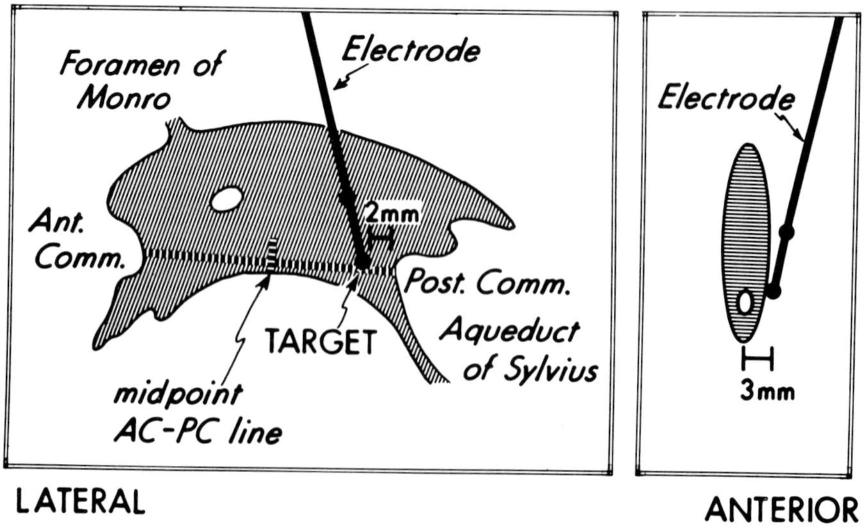

FIG. 1. Placement of electrode for stimulation of periventricular grey.

The procedure is done with a Trent Wells stereotaxic instrument under local anesthesia. Stimulation testing is then carried out for optimum placement based on adequacy of pain-relief and minimal side effects. After the final positioning of the electrode, fine percutaneous leads are brought out through a needle-puncture site some distance from the burr hole, and the electrode is locked in place at the burr hole site by a spherical plug (Fig. 1).

Following surgery, a period of testing of stimulation for effectiveness and side effects is carried out usually lasting approximately 2 weeks. A second procedure for internalization of the system is then done under general anesthesia. The receiver is implanted in the pectoral area and connected to the two most effective electrode contacts through a mating connector in the parietal area, and the percutaneous wiring is removed. A period of parameter-selection, frequency of stimulation, and patient-instruction for proper use of the system is usually necessary. Internal settings on the transmitter allow variations of pulse width, frequency, and maximum voltage which are selected during the period of testing to minimize side effects and maximize pain-relief. The patient is instructed to slowly increase the variable voltage control until side effects are noted and then to reduce the voltage until no side effects are felt, following which a period of stimulation is carried out, typically 10 to 30 min in duration.

RESULTS

The results in 6 cancer patients will be presented in detail with a brief history, since the series is too limited for statistical analysis.

Patient #1. W. S. was a 63-year-old male with recurrent carcinoma of the colon following abdominoperineal resection. His pain was perineal, spreading to the back and legs, increased by lying on his back or standing. Dihydrocodeinone (Percodan®) and morphine 15 mg intramuscularly were insufficient for complete pain-relief prior to surgery, and he was confined in bed lying on his left side most of the time. The electrode was implanted in early September of 1973, on the right side. Following surgery, stimulation at 1 V, 20 Hz, for 20 min every 4 to 5 hr allowed the patient to ambulate and to lie on his back for the first time in months. He described the pain as "floating away." At high current levels, he reported a startled reaction and some dizziness, felt frightened and apprehensive, and demonstrated mild nystagmus. Sensory side effects consisting in a warm sensation down his back were noted at effective pain-relieving levels of stimulation. He remained free of pain on stimulation until he died 2 months following surgery from uremia.

Patient #2. B. M. was a 60-year-old male with a Pancoast tumor of the lung with brachial plexus and spine invasion. He had severe bilateral pain in the neck, shoulders, arm, and chest. Prior to surgery, meperidine (Demerol®), 100 mg every 3 hr, was interspaced with phenothiazines, resulting in partial pain-relief. He was operated on in June of 1974, with implantation in the right periventricular area. Following surgery, he could be maintained almost free of pain with stimulation for 20 min every 2 to 4 hr and amitriptyline (Elavil®), 100 mg daily. Side effects during stimulation consisted of paresthesias of heat in the left face and arm. His disease progressed rapidly, and he expired 2 months following surgery (Fig. 1).

Patient #3. C. G. was a 55-year-old female with carcinoma of the breast with generalized bone metastasis which produced pain in the right shoulder, back, right leg, and both knees. She also had burning in the left leg secondary to previous high thoracic chordotomy. Dihydromorphinone (Dilaudid®), 2 mg every 4 hr, was ineffective in relieving pain, as well as was a previous hypophysectomy. She was implanted April of 1976, on the left side and obtained good relief with stimulation 3 times a day for 30 min. Side effects were heat paresthesias in the left leg and a "locking of her eyes." She did well for 6 months, and then back and right flank pain increased secondary to metastasis to the L_3 vertebra. Increase in stimulation to 10 min every 2 hr controlled pain for 2 more months. She then had a pathologic fracture of the spine which caused severe pain that required resumption of narcotic medication by mouth.

Patient #4. G. S. was a 52-year-old male with carcinoma of the bladder and local recurrence causing low back, pelvic, perineal, and right leg pain. Bed rest and oral codeine, 90 mg every 4 hr, did not relieve his pain, which was markedly increased by ambulation. An electrode was implanted on the left in September, 1976. Following surgery, stimulation for 15 min every 2 to 4 hours and oral amitriptyline, 100 mg daily, gave 80 to 90% relief of his pain while ambulating. Side effects during stimulation were either absent or consisted of slight warmth in the trunk. Pain-relief remained excellent for 5 months until he died from uremia.

Patient #5. J. M. was a 48-year-old female with recurrence of pelvic cancer and consequent perineal and pelvic pain bilaterally. In addition, she had a feeling of pressure described as "sitting on a lump" that was disturbing. In March of 1977, a right periventricular electrode was inserted, and pain-relief was dramatic. However, following surgery, she had persistent complaints of the pressure or lump sensation that disturbed her and had anxiety and depression that was exacerbated by the constant reminder of the pressure of the pelvic mass and perineal drainage. Other physicians placed her on narcotics again, and she discontinued stimulation.

Patient #6. H. L. is a 54-year-old male with generalized peritoneal recurrence of carcinoma of the colon. He developed deep midline and bilateral upper-lumbar and lower-thoracic back pain and upper-abdominal midline pain of constant, aching character. Prior to surgery, he was using meperidine, 100 mg intramuscularly every 2 to 3 hr. A right PVG electrode was inserted in April of 1978, and stimulation every 4 hr produced 80% pain-relief. The addition of amitriptyline, 100 mg at bedtime, gave complete pain-relief with use of the stimulator on a 2-time per day basis. There are no side effects during stimulation, but if stimulation is increased to near maximum for the transmitter, he has blurring of vision.

DISCUSSION

We have demonstrated in this small number of patients that periventricular gray stimulation is effective in relieving severe and widespread pain from recurrent cancer, and that the side effects are mild and easily tolerated. Three obvious problems are demonstrated by these patients. First, on the basis of the fact that 2 patients died only a few months after the electrode implantation, I would advocate not using this procedure unless life-expectancy is predicted to be 4 or more months. Of course it is difficult to predict life-expectancy in these patients, but if the condition of the patient suggests a very short life, I would use percutaneous brain stimulation so as to avoid general anesthesia and the added expense of internalization of the system.

The second problem that has emerged from our experience is that central stimulation may prove insufficient in patients whose disease progresses and whose pain intensity increases. Our experience is not extensive enough to solve this problem, but in the patients with nonmalignant, chronic pain we have operated on, we also have had failures when the pain problem was static or increased. Obviously, the procedure is not perfect and an unknown failure rate will have to be anticipated.

Another limitation of the technique is that associated symptoms, such as pressure or mass effect produced by the tumor growth, are not affected by stimulation. It appears that stimulation affects only pain caused by noxious sensory input. A careful questioning of patients regarding specific type of discomfort and "pain" will help avoid this problem. Anxiety and depression are not controlled by stimulation and should be treated by additional means. The addition of amitriptyline, a tricyclic antidepressant, has improved stimulation results in a number of patients who, prior to surgery, had no effect from the drug. We think this is due to the increased effectiveness of dopamine and serotonin produced by this drug and predicted by Akil's work in animals (2). At present, we routinely place all patients on amitriptyline or a similar tricyclic following surgery. Narcotic addiction also is not controlled by stimulation, nor are withdrawal symptoms modified by stimulation.

Tolerance from excessive stimulation has been observed in rats and also in some patients with chronic, benign pain not included in this report. However, tolerance can be controlled by using the least-effective duration of frequency of stimulation. It can be reversed by discontinuing stimulation for a few days, the addition of tricyclics, norepinephrine (disulfiram), or, more recently, tryptophan.

SUMMARY

The number of patients is too small for a significant analysis of complications and failures. However, our limited experience suggests that brain stimulation in the area of the periventricular gray substance has the promise of being an effective method of relieving severe cancer pain. The procedure can control widespread and bilateral pain with minimal side effects and minimal surgery.

REFERENCES

1. Akil, H., and Liebeskind, J. C. (1975): Monaminergic mechanisms of stimulation-produced analgesia. *Brain Res.,* 94:279–296.
2. Akil, H., and Mayer, D. J. (1972): Antagonism of stimulation produced analgesia by PCPA, a serotonin synthesis inhibitor. *Brain Res.,* 44:692–697.
3. Akil, H., Richardson, D. E., Hughes, J., and Barchas, J. D. (1979): Elevation in levels of enkephalin-like material in the ventricular CSF of pain patients upon analgetic focal stimulation. *Science,* 201 (4354): 463–465.

4. Gol, A. (1967): Relief of pain by electrical stimulation of the septal area. *J. Neurol. Surg.*, 5:115–120.
5. Heath, R. G., and Mickle, W. A. (1960): Evaluation of seven years of experience with depth electrode studies in human patients. In: *Electrical Studies on the Unanesthetized Brain,* edited by E. R. Ramey and D. S. O'Doherty. Haber, New York.
6. Hosobuchi, Y., Adams, J. E., and Rutkin, B. (1973): Chronic thalamic stimulation for the relief of facial anesthesia dolorosa. *Arch. Neurol.,* 29:158–161.
7. Mayer, D. J., Wolfle, T. L., Akil, H., Carder, B., and Liebeskind, J. C. (1971): Analgesia resulting from electrical stimulation in the brain stem of the rat. *Science,* 174:1351–1354.
8. Reynolds, D. V. (1969): Surgery in the rat during electrical analgesia induced by local brain stimulation. *Science,* 164:444–445.
9. Richardson, D. E., and Akil, H. (1975): Comparison of analgesic brain stimulation, peripheral nerve and dorsal column stimulation to morphine sulfate: Effects on evoked responses to noxious input. In: *Abstracts of the First World Congress on Pain (Florence, Italy, 1975)*, p. 262. International Association for the Study of Pain, Seattle.
10. Richardson, D. E., and Akil, H. (1977): Pain reduction by electrical brain stimulation in man, Part I: Acute administration in periaqueductal and periventricular sites. *J. Neurosurg.,* 47:178–183.
11. Richardson, D. E., and Akil, H. (1977): Pain reduction by electrical brain stimulation in man, Part II: Chronic self-administration in periventricular gray matter. *J. Neurosurg.,* 47:184–194.
12. Richardson, D. E., and Akil, H. (1977): Long-term results of periventricular gray self-stimulation. *Neurosurgery,* 1:199–202.

Advances in Pain Research and Therapy, Vol. 2,
edited by J. J. Bonica and V. Ventafridda.
Raven Press, New York © 1979.

Thalamic and Hypothalamic Stimulation

David Fairman

Av. Quintana 49, 8C, Buenos Aires, Argentina

This paper will describe the results of thalamic and hypothalamic stimulation for pain-relief in a series of 750 consecutive patients with intractable pain caused by a malignant neoplasm. My patients can be divided into two groups on the basis of the target selected: intralaminar nucleus of the thalamus (630 patients) or hypothalamic periventricular nucleus (120 patients). The results are contained in Tables 1 and 2.

In 1972, we first performed repetitive stimulation through implanted electrodes in the hypothalamic periventricular nucleus and observed that pain-relief was obtained which outlasted the stimulus for varying periods. We did not need to make a lesion in this region to obtain pain-relief. Effective results were obtained when the stimulation varied between 3 and 4 msec, and total remission of pain was obtained not in stages but instantaneously. These satisfactory results of repetitive stimulation lasted from 1 hr to several days. Repetitive stimulation can be performed as often as necessary (Fig. 1).

Table 2 shows the tabulation corresponding to the hypothalamic procedure for the relief of intractable pain in our series of 120 neoplastic patients in pain.

An essential objective has been to select the optimal target point for electrical stimulation to alleviate pain. Gybels (4) reported interesting studies on electrical stimulation of the thalamic nucleus VPL for the relief of intractable pain. Mazars (7) stated that the integrity of VPL is essential for effective relief of pain by thalamic electrical stimulation. Richardson (8) showed that electrical stimulation of the periaqueductal gray area can be a satisfactory treatment for intractable pain. Most of the reports include patients with various chronic pain syndromes including cancer pain, postherpetic neuralgia, atypical facial neuralgia, phantom limb, and thalamic syndrome. We believe that confusion arises because there is no distinction made between different types of pain. The preoccupation with correct target selection has overlooked the important fact that a prerequisite for success is the proper selection of patients. Target selection should be based upon a careful diagnosis of the type of pain experienced by the patient. In our experience, the essential prerequisite for effective pain-relief by hypothalamic stimulation is the selection of patients based upon the type of pain. This

TABLE 1. *Stereotactic thalamic tractotomy*

Number of cases	Site of carcinoma	Percent
294	Lung	46
122	Head—Neck	19
99	Uterus	15
81	Breast	12
34	G.I. Tract	5
Total 630		100

selection is easier in patients with benign diseases, but in patients with neoplasms the problem is much more complex. The evaluation of the genesis of pain in patients with cancer must establish whether the intractable pain is due to excessive nociception by nerve-fiber compression or due to reduced nervous impulses or deafferentation.

Although deafferentation has been known to affect the central nervous system, it has only recently been incorporated in interpretations of the mechanisms of pain. Therapeutic implications are, of course, derived from understanding of mechanisms. The concept of deafferentation is supported by experimental studies such as those performed by Eccles and McIntyre (2). These investigators severed the dorsal roots of the seventh and first sacral nerves just distal to the dorsal ganglion; i.e., they interrupted the sensory impulses along the root. They found that in a period of time varying between 21 and 40 days there was reduced synaptic efficacy which could be largely restored by brief bursts of repetitive stimulation. Loeser and Ward (6) demonstrated that experimental chronic deafferentation produced by dorsal rhizotomy or hemicordotomy resulted in alterations in both spontaneous and evoked activity. The pathological process that leads to hyperactivity seems to be secondary to chronic deafferentation. Although proof of this concept will require further studies, it can be stated that reduction of the input to the central neurons may produce an increased output in response to a standard stimulus.

TABLE 2. *Hypothalamotomy repetitive stimulation and/or lesion.*

Number of cases	Site of carcinoma	Percent
54	Lung	45
21	Head—Neck	18
19	Uterus	16
14	Breast	11
12	G.I. Tract	10
Total 120		100

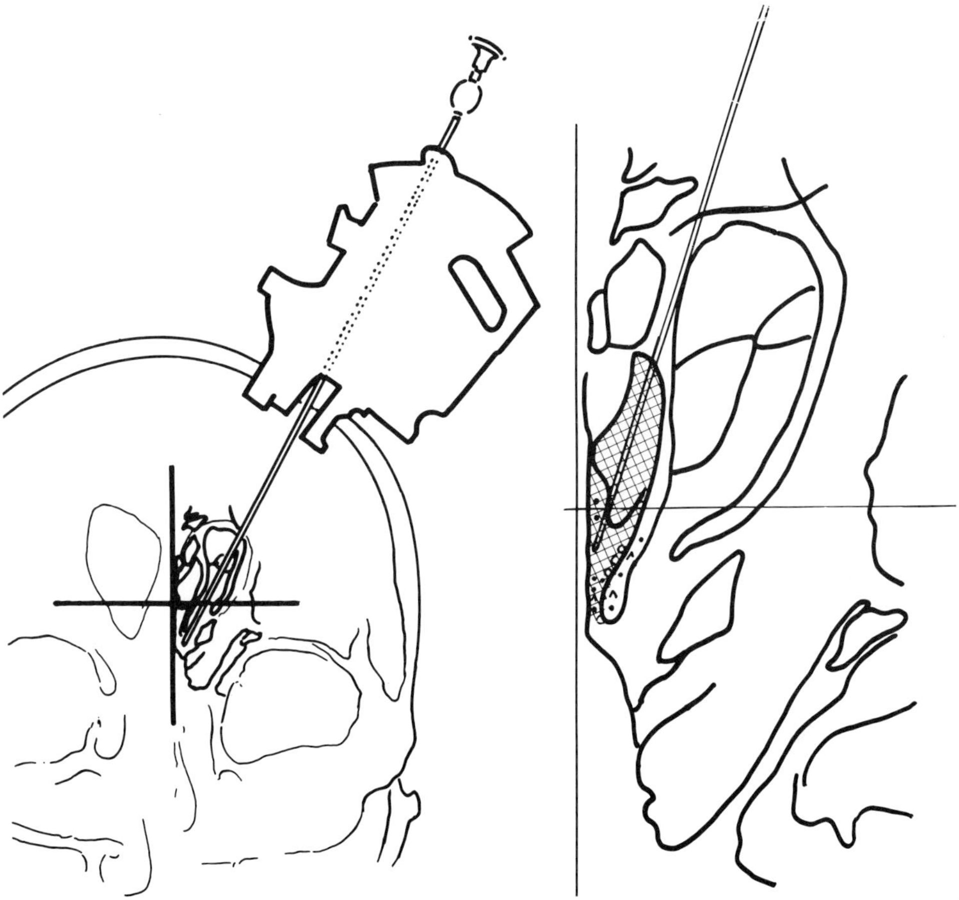

FIG. 1. A. Schema of stereotaxic approach to the hypothalamus. B. Enlargement showing points subjected to stimulation and the different effects mapped on frontal section of the Schaltenbrand-Bailey Atlas.

The concept of deafferentation is pivotal, because it constitutes the indication for repetitive stimulation. The first human experimental studies of deafferentation were performed in 1905 by Head (5) who, after sectioning the superficial radial nerve of his own forearm, described observations made over a 2-year period on the recovery sensation after neurorrhaphy. He observed that the first fibers to regenerate were unmyelinated and of very small diameter. Stimulation of these unmyelinated, free nerve endings produced only unpleasant sensations: a crude, poorly localized sensation of pain. He designated this type of painful sensation "protopathic."

The gradual return of the myelinated, larger fibers was associated with the reappearance of light touch, appreciation of intermediate grades of warmth and cold, and two-point discrimination. He designated this type of sensibility "epicritic." Head postulated that in a normal nerve, these two systems of fibers complemented each other and that the epicritic fibers not only suppressed the unpleasant and diffuse type of protopathic pain but also added the finer modalities of sensation.

We suggest that there is a similarity between these experimental works and the process of deafferentation observed in pain due to neoplastic involvement of peripheral nerves.

As Denny-Brown (1) pointed out, the paraneoplastic neuropathy is a degenerative lesion characterized by demyelinization as well as alterations in the diameter of the nerve fiber. Impulse transmission is probably altered. This process constitutes a process similar to deafferentation. There normally exists an equilibrium between the inhibitory and excitatory impulses transmitted respectively by the myelinated and unmyelinated fibers. Impulses transmitted by the myelinic fibers control the impulses transmitted by the unmyelinated fibers. In the paraneoplastic neuropathy, the process of deafferentation produces a disequilibrium resulting in the protopathic type of severe and diffuse pain due to the lack of inhibition of the epicritic myelinated fibers upon the protopathic unmyelinated ones. In our experience, the optimal procedure for the relief of intractable pain produced by a paraneoplastic neuropathy is electrical stimulation through implanted hypothalamic electrodes and not the surgical interruption of the pain pathways at any level.

In other cases of pain produced by the primary tumor itself or by metastasis, we suggest the presence of a dual mechanism. When compression of the nerve fibers or plexuses is obvious, the excess of nociceptive stimuli is responsible for the production of pain. But, at the same time, there can also be an infiltration process of the neoplastic cells along the perivascular spaces of the nerve fibers. This infiltration can cause a gradual process of demyelinization and partial destruction of the nerves, especially affecting the larger, rapidly conducting fibers which are more susceptible to this. These anatomic changes produce a reduction of nervous impulses so that the pain may be considered to be due to deafferentation. The diminution of the myelinated fibers causes a lack of inhibition of the unmyelinated C pain-conducting fibers. Because of this dual mechanism, we perform repetitive hypothalamic stimulation followed, when necessary, by a lesion at the intralaminar thalamic nucleus.

In 1969 (3), we developed the hypothesis that the hypothalamic periventricular system modulates both inhibitory and excitatory influences of synaptic transmission of pain impulses by blocking the pathways connecting the brainstem reticular formation to the different areas of the paleo- and neocortex which underlie the conscious experience of pain. In Fig. 2, we can see the diagram of the modulating periventricular hypothalamic system (MPHS) that constitutes an area of convergence for the different volleys of sensory, motor, and autonomic fibers which share adjacent neuronal circuits. This hypothesis includes the concept that a dynamic competition for the use

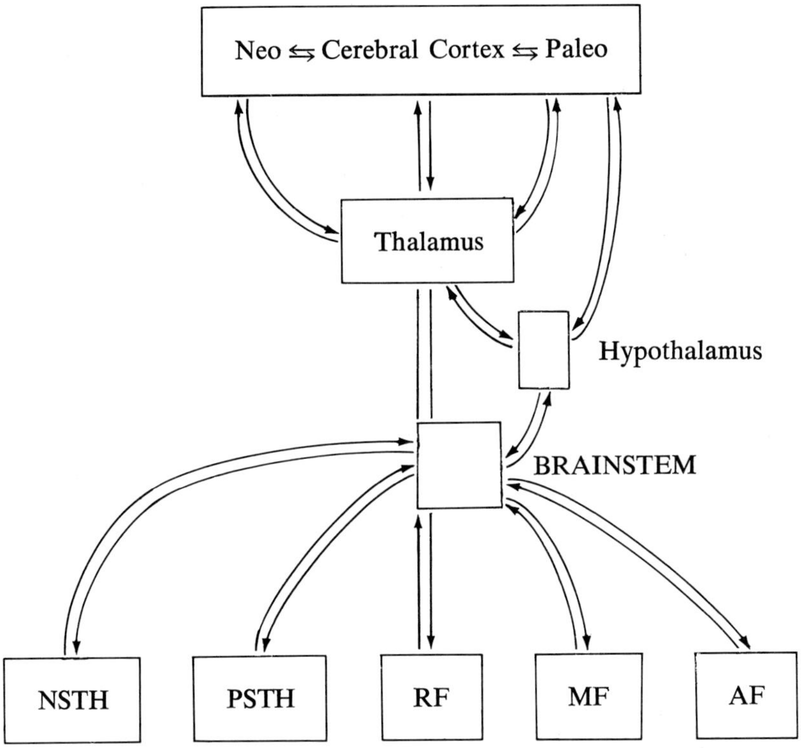

FIG. 2. Theory of the Modulating Periventricular Hypothalamic System (MPHS). NSTH, neospinothalamic; PSTH, paleospinothalamic; RF, reticular formation; MF, motor fibers; and AF, autonomic fibers.

of the same neuronal circuits between the pattern of pain impulses and the pattern of impulses elicited by adequate stimulation results in the effective blocking of the pain impulses.

Our thalamic target is the intralaminar nuclei and our hypothalamic target is the hypothalamic periventricular nuclei whether we perform a surgical lesion or stimulation. We are, therefore, attacking the same neuronal circuits at different levels. We are influencing the phylogenetically old pathways which mediate protopathic pain through the paleospinothalamic tract which relays to the second sensory area.

From the anatomical standpoint, this is the most circumscribed area where repetitive stimulation produces effective and long-lasting results. We are aware, however, that not only at the subcortical level but also at all levels of the nervous system, including the peripheral receptors and the transmission pathways, there exists a process of interrelation. This interaction between the sensory, motor, and autonomic systems is established continuously through the excitatory and inhibitory impulses.

Our theory of the MPHS is based on the fact that the hypothalamus is the highest correlation center of the autonomic nervous system. It integrates at all levels the sensory-motor and motor-sensory systems playing an essential role in the mechanism of pain. Moreover, our model is consistent with the studies suggesting that the hypothalamus could be the coordinating center of the whole brainstem reticular system and, therefore, the primary regulator of cortical activity and consciousness.

At the present stage of our knowledge, many questions can be asked concerning the effects of the mechanism by means of which hypothalamic repetitive stimulation may produce the relief of pain. Therefore, further studies are needed before the exact relationship between electrophysiological alterations of the neural metabolism and repetitive stimulation is established.

REFERENCES

1. Denny-Brown, D. (1948): Primary sensory neuropathy with muscular changes associated with carcinoma. *J. Neurol. Neurosurg. Psychiat.,* 11,1:73–78.
2. Eccles, J. C., and McIntyre, A. K. (1953): The effects of disuse and activity on mammalian spinal reflexes. *J. Physiol.,* 121:492–516.
3. Fairman, D. (1976): Neurophysiological basis for the hypothalamic lesion and stimulation by chronic implanted electrodes for the relief of intractable pain in cancer. In: *Advances in Pain Research and Therapy,* edited by J. J. Bonica and D. Albe-Fessard, pp. 843–847. Raven Press, New York.
4. Gybels, J. (1972): Supraspinal control of experimental pain sensation in man. In: *Pain,* pp. 128–131. Thieme, Stuttgart.
5. Head, H., Rivers, W. H. R., and Sherren, J. (1905): The afferent nervous system from a new aspect. *Brain,* 28:99–115.
6. Loeser, J. D., and Ward, A. A. (1967): Some effects of deafferentation of neurons of the cat spinal cord. *Arch. Neurol.,* 17:629–636.
7. Mazars, G., Merienne, L., and Cioloca, C. (1976): Etat actuel de la chirurgie de la douleur. *Neurochirurgie,* 22,1:1–164. Masson, Paris.
8. Richardson, D. E., and Akil, H. (1973): Pain relief by electrical stimulation of the brain in human patients. *Excerpta Medica,* 219:79.

Advances in Pain Research and Therapy, Vol. 2,
edited by J. J. Bonica and V. Ventafridda.
Raven Press, New York © 1979.

Dorsal Column and Peripheral Nerve Stimulation for Relief of Cancer Pain

John D. Loeser

Department of Neurological Surgery, University of Washington School of Medicine, Seattle, Washington 98195

Electrical stimulation of the peripheral nerves and spinal cord has not yet received an adequate trial in the management of chronic pain due to cancer. It is difficult at this time to present meaningful data on the results obtained; any predictions which I make for the future are based as much upon hope as knowledge. Neurosurgeons have not reported many of their cases; thorough evaluations are often lacking and data are fragmentary. Impediments to clinical research are myriad; my inability to provide an answer to the questions of the efficacy of peripheral nerve stimulation (PNS) or spinal cord stimulation (DCS or PISCES) is based upon both the paucity of reported cases and the methods of evaluation.

We should be cognizant of some of the factors which have led to this unhappy state of affairs. In the United States, governmental regulations have made clinical research and the development of new technologies far too cumbersome. Manufacturers of equipment cannot control the applications of their inventions by well-intentioned but often misguided surgeons. Patient-selection criteria are frequently ignored for reasons of convenience or financial gain. The victim of all this is, of course, the hapless patient.

Practical implanted electrical stimulators have been available for approximately 10 years. These have been manufactured in the United States by Medtronic, Inc, and Avery Laboratories; I am not aware of other commercial suppliers. Many research groups have designed their own equipment for experimental purposes, but the clinical literature seems to report exclusively on Medtronic and Avery stimulators.

These implanted stimulators are inductance-coupled to an antenna driven by a cigarette-pack-sized, battery-operated transmitter; the electronic components have been highly reliable and are certainly safe. There have been no reports of electrical malfunctions resulting in patient problems such as seizures, myocardial dysrhythmia, or other phenomena unrelated to stimulation of the desired neural structures. Batteries do wear out, antenna lead wires break, patients destroy their transmitters by immersing them in bathtubs or dropping them out of windows; the stimulator systems are, in fact, quite durable. The major difficulties have occurred in the electrode system and its interface with the neural tissues. Lead wires break from metal fatigue, electrodes shift in position and become encased in fibrous tissue and this reduces or eliminates their effectiveness. Of course, there are some surgical complications such as infection, rejection of foreign bodies, CSF leaks, and damage to neural tissues. By far the most common long-term problem is related to electrode migration or loss of stimulation efficacy thought to be due to fibrosis about the sites of stimulation.

MECHANISM OF ACTION

Our abilities to cope with failures to achieve pain-relief with electrical stimulation would be enhanced by some comprehension of why electrical stimulation does relieve pain. Review of the more extensive data on patients with pain due to benign diseases suggests that there are few, if any, predictors of long-term efficacy of PNS, DCS, or PISCES systems. All investigators have commented upon the importance of excluding patients whose emotional states preclude meaningful interpretation of the effects of stimulation, but few other generalities emerge. It does seem to be generally true that stimulation must elicit paresthesias in the region of pain to lead to relief of that pain. There is a much higher incidence of immediate pain-relief than long-term amelioration of symptoms. Some of this is undoubtedly placebo effect, but stimulation may also lose its efficacy over time because of mechanisms less related to psychologic factors and related supratentorial functions and more readily ascribed to synaptic or axonal changes. We should, therefore, be cognizant of the fact that long-term stimulation of the spinal cord or peripheral nerves in man has never been shown to be either safe or hazardous. Patients with pain due to cancer are obviously not a suitable group to study for data on long-term hazards of stimulation, but the short and variable life-spans of patients with pain due to cancer make analyses of the efficacy of this mode of therapy quite complicated. I know of not one carefully planned and well-executed study on the efficacy of peripheral nerve or spinal cord stimulation for the relief of pain secondary to cancer. The situation is scarcely better for chronic pain due to benign diseases.

PERIPHERAL NERVE STIMULATION

Peripheral nerve stimulation (PNS) requires the application of an electrode directly upon the nerve to be stimulated via an open surgical procedure. Electrodes have been placed upon such nerves as the sciatic, femoral, ulnar, or median and about the brachialplexus (Fig. 1). The radio receiver is usually implanted subcutaneously in the thigh, abdomen, or supraclavicular fossa. There are very few patients with pain due to cancer who have had a peripheral nerve stimulator implanted (2,12). This is probably due to the

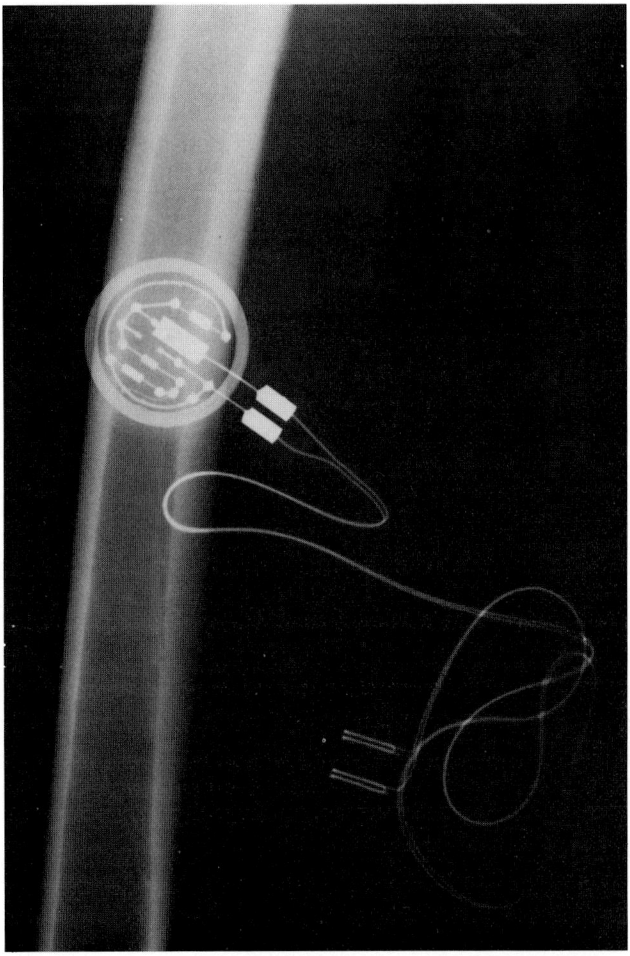

FIG. 1. Lateral X-ray of a sciatic-nerve stimulator and implanted radio receiver in a patient with chronic leg and buttock pain. The receiver is activated by placing an antenna on the skin directly over the receiver.

relative rarity of cancer pain originating from an extremity as well as the limited dissemination of this technique for pain-relief amongst the medical community.

The advantages of peripheral nerve stimulation should not be overlooked; it is a simple, nondestructive procedure for pain-relief. Patients do not have to tolerate a neurologic deficit to be relieved of their pain. The surgery required to insert the electrode and radio receiver can be performed under local anesthesia with minimal surgical risk to the patient. Paresthesias are restricted to the distribution of the nerve being stimulated; one must be certain that all of the noxious sensory inputs are via this nerve. It is desirable to carry out carefully performed local anesthetic block of the nerve before peripheral nerve stimulation is attempted. This procedure should eliminate sensation from the painful region and help predict the effects of PNS.

There is still ambiguity as to whether the locus of noxious sensation must be distal to the site of stimulation for pain-relief to occur. I have one patient whose sciatic-nerve stimulator relieves her pain due to arachnoiditis and epidural adhesions. Peripheral nerve stimulation could relieve pain due to neoplastic invasion of plexuses or epidural space. I believe that the small number of patients with chronic, severe pain in an extremity secondary to cancer can be considered for peripheral nerve stimulation before subjecting them to ablative neurosurgical procedures.

SPINAL CORD STIMULATION

Electrical stimulation of the spinal cord has been utilized since the pioneering work of Shealy approximately 10 years ago (14). The most commonly used commercially available components are manufactured by Avery Laboratories and Medtronic, Inc. In addition, there are parochial experimental devices.

The original concept was that electrical stimulation delivered to the dorsal columns of the spinal cord was responsible for the relief of pain. For this reason, electrodes were designed for implantation via a laminectomy directly upon or within the dura covering the midline dorsum of the spinal cord (Fig. 2). Several varieties of electrode sizes and configurations were evaluated; none were totally satisfactory. Bipolar stimulation proved superior to monopolar; flexible lead wires resistant to fracture by repeated movement were developed.

Surgical complications have been all too common, and morbidity ensued for a significant number of the patients (10,13,16). Among the complications described have been: wound infection, CSF fistula, subdural or epidural hematoma, spinal cord compression, and migration of the radio receiver within its subcutaneous pocket. Some patients have complained of a new pain associated with the implanted equipment. A significant number of patients have described a change in the effects of DCS so that what was a pain-relieving electrical stimulation becomes not only ineffective in alleviating the spontaneous pain but itself becomes unpleasant.

Although the initial concept involved stimulation of the dorsal columns, it became obvious from animal experimentation, human trials, and, later, planned ventral electrode placements, that the actual neural tissues stimulated by the electrodes were uncertain and that stimulation applied to the ventral surface or from dorsal to ventral surfaces could also be effective in relieving pain. The actual current pathways are difficult to determine and the physiologic basis of pain-relief from DCS is uncertain. Whether the effect of electrical stimulation is to activate certain axons which inhibit pain

TABLE 1. *DCS and PNS for cancer pain*

Author	Year	Type[a]	No. of pts.	% Success
Burton (1)	1975	DCS	1	?
Campbell (2)	1976	PNS	3	0
Clark (3)	1975	DCS	3	67
Freidberg (5)	1975	DCS	1	100
Hunt (6)	1975	DCS	1	0
Long (7)	1975	DCS	6	50
Medtronic (4)	1976	PISCES	9	44
Miles (8)	1974	DCS	2	100
Nashold (9)	1972	DCS	1	0
Nielson (10)	1975	DCS	18	61
North (11)	1977	PISCES	2	50
Picaza (12)	1975	PNS[b]	5	60
Pineda (13)	1975	DCS	4	50
Shealy (14)	1969	DCS	2	100
Shelden (15)	1975	DCS	17	47
Sweet (16)	1974	DCS	3	67

[a] PNS = peripheral nerve stimulation; DCS = dorsal column stimulation; PISCES = percutaneously inserted spinal-cord electrode system.
[b] Acute stimulation only.

or to block transmission in axons subserving pain sensations is uncertain. Many patients have reported pain-relief outlasting stimulation by minutes or hours; the neural substrates for such prolonged effects are unknown. Recent studies have suggested that a central neurohumoral system (enkephalins) may be activated by electrical stimulation.

Problems in patient-selection have plagued the assay of the clinical efficacy of dorsal column stimulation. As we might predict, patients whose pain behavior is largely under the control of environmental or emotional factors do not often get relief from DCS. Patients with pain due to cancer do not usually fall into that category and should, therefore, be reasonable candidates for DCS. Table 1 includes all the published cases I can find of DCS for the treatment of cancer pain. Fifty-one patients is not an impressively large group upon which to base an analysis of the efficacy of this treatment modality (1,3,5–10,13–16). Why has not dorsal column stimulation received a wider trial?

The first answer must be that it has, but the patients have not been carefully followed and reported. It is said that over 3,000 DCS units have been employed; roughly 10% of these patients appear in the literature. Data is therefore lost for scientific analysis, although surgeons received fees and manufacturers sold equipment. The development of new technologies cannot be facilitated by this style of slipshod data-collection. Since impressively good results often get reported, my suspicion is that a large proportion of the

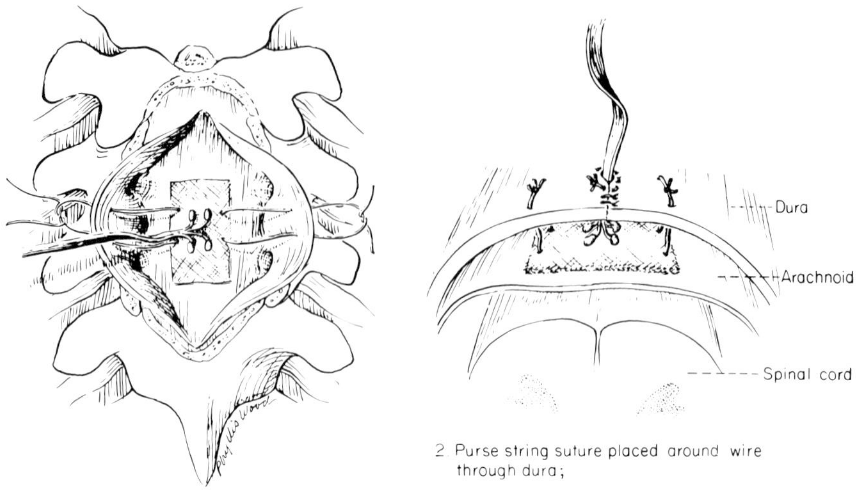

FIG. 2. The insertion of a dorsal column stimulator in the subdural space over the thoracic spinal cord. The lead wires are connected to an implanted radio receiver.

unreported patients did not benefit from DCS. Available case reports suggest that roughly one-half of the patients with pain due to cancer have reported significant relief of their pain when implanted with a dorsal column stimulator (7). Review of the reported cases does not generate any predictors of long-term efficacy. It does seem to be true that paresthesias must be perceived by the patient in the region of the pain if symptomatic relief is to occur.

The insertion of a dorsal column stimulator requires a laminectomy and is usually done with general anesthesia. It is, therefore, a major operation which may not be well tolerated by a terminally ill patient. On the other hand, DCS offers the promise of pain-relief without destruction of any portion of the nervous system and without new neurologic deficits. Almost all of the reported cases have utilized midline dorsal placement of the stimulating electrodes, although some investigators have tried other stimulation sites. Optimal localization of the electrodes has not yet been established (Fig. 2).

The initial enthusiasm for DCS has waned as its modest long-term efficacy and significant complication rate have become apparent. The development of a much simpler electrode system has re-kindled an interest in spinal cord stimulation for pain-relief (4). The PISCES® equipment (Percutaneous Insertion of Spinal Cord Electrode System) eliminates the surgical hazards of DCS but has added new problems with electrode stability. Two flexible electrodes are inserted into the epidural space via standard needles and then threaded into the desired position under fluoroscopic observation. The elec-

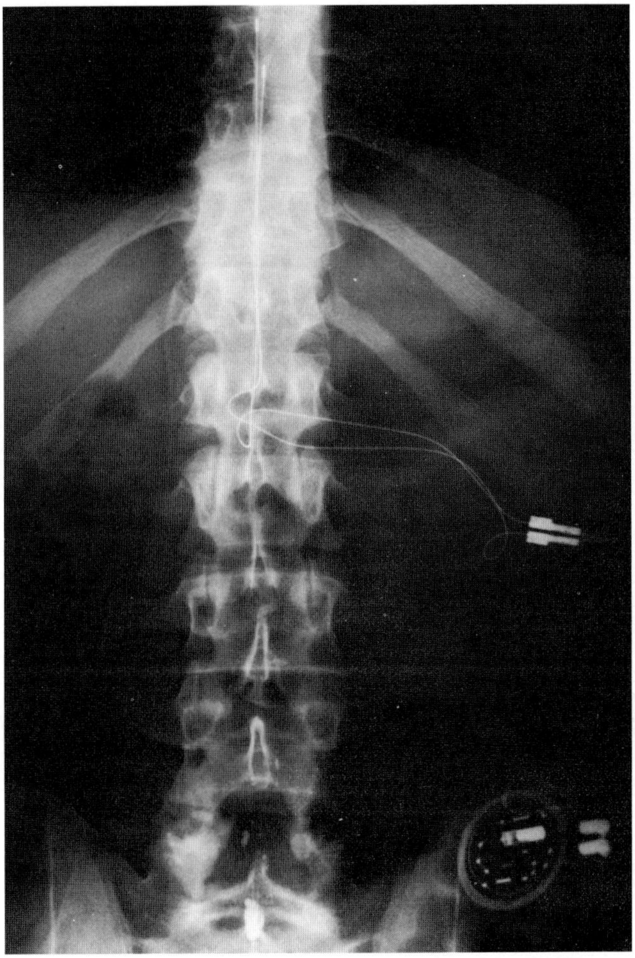

FIG. 3. X-ray of a PISCES system on a patient with chronic back pain. The electrodes were inserted percutaneously at L_1–L_2 and connected to an implanted radio receiver, which can be seen in the left lower quadrant.

trode lead wires are then passed through the skin and connected to an external stimulator (Figs. 3 and 4). The patient then undergoes a trial period; if stimulation is effective, the lead wires are removed and the electrodes connected to an implanted receiver identical to that used for DCS or PNS. This system has eliminated the need for a major surgical procedure and has proven to have a very low rate of complication. The major drawback has been migration of the epidural electrodes hours, days, or months after insertion, with subsequent loss of stimulation efficacy. New electrodes will be required with some type of anchoring devices if this technique is to gain widespread clinical evaluation.

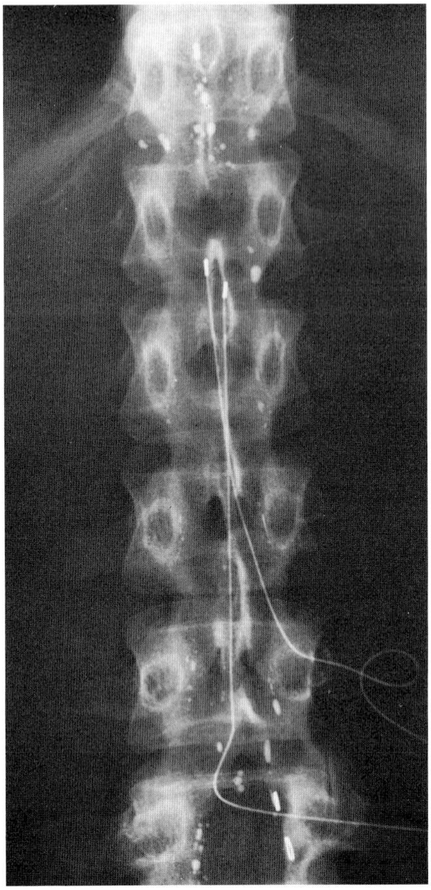

FIG. 4. X-ray of PISCES electrodes in the lumbar epidural space. During the evaluation period, these electrodes are connected to an external stimulator. If stimulation relieves the patient's pain, they are connected to a permanent, implanted radio receiver.

A limited number of patients with pain due to cancer have been reported to have received a PISCES trial; approximately 50% appear to have significant long-term relief (4,11). Experience is too limited to permit a meaningful evaluation.

CONCLUSIONS

In conclusion, I believe that electrical stimulation of the peripheral nerves or spinal cord has the potential for providing pain-relief to patients with cancer. The major problems seem to be related to the perfection of stimulation electrodes and the trial of this technique in a large enough group of patients to generate valid data on the likelihood of pain-relief for other patients with cancer. Clinical efficacy should be demonstrated in well-controlled studies before electrical stimulation of nerve or spinal cord becomes a readily available therapeutic modality.

REFERENCES

1. Burton, C. (1975): Dorsal column stimulation: Optimization of application. *Surg. Neurol.*, 4:171–176.
2. Campbell, J. N., and Long, D. M. (1976): Peripheral nerve stimulation in the treatment of intractable pain. *J. Neurosurg.*, 45:692–699.
3. Clark, K. (1975): Electrical stimulation of the nervous system for control of pain: University of Texas Southwestern Medical School experience. *Surg. Neurol.*, 4:164–166.
4. *Clinical Status Report Medtronic PISCES System Model 3401.* Medtronic, Inc., Minneapolis. 1976.
5. Freidberg, S. R. (1975): Neurosurgical treatment of pain caused by cancer. *Med. Clin. North Am.*, 59:481–485.
6. Hunt, W. E., Goodman, J. H., and Bingham, W. G., Jr. (1975): Stimulation of the dorsal spinal cord for treatment of intractable pain: A preliminary report. *Surg. Neurol.*, 4:153–156.
7. Long, D. M., and Erickson, D. E. (1975): Stimulation of the posterior columns of the spinal cord for relief of intractable pain. *Surg. Neurol.*, 4:134–141.
8. Miles, J., Miles, J., Hayward, M., Bowsher, D., Mumford, J., and Molony, V. (1974): Pain relief by implanted electrical stimulators. *Lancet*, 1:777–779.
9. Nashold, B. S., and Friedman, H. (1972): Dorsal column stimulation for control of pain. Preliminary report on 30 patients. *J. Neurosurg.*, 36:590–597.
10. Nielson, K. D., Adams, J. E., and Hosobuchi, Y. (1975): Experience with dorsal column stimulation for relief of chronic intractable pain. *Surg. Neurol.*, 4:148–152.
11. North, R. B., Fischell, T. A., and Long, D. M. (1977): Chronic stimulation via percutaneously inserted epidural electrodes. *Neurosurg.*, 1:215–218.
12. Picaza, J. A., Cannon, B. W., Hunter, S. E., Boyd, A. S., Guma, J., and Maurer, D. (1975): Pain suppression by peripheral nerve stimulation. *Surg. Neurol.*, 4:105–114.
13. Pineda, A. (1974): Dorsal column stimulation and its prospects. *Surg. Neurol.*, 4:157–163.
14. Shealy, C. N. (1969): Dorsal column electrohypalgesia. *Headache*, 9:99–102.
15. Shelden, C. H., Paul, F., Jacques, D. B., and Pudenz, R. H. (1975): Electrical stimulation of the nervous system. *Surg. Neurol.*, 4:127–132.
16. Sweet, W. H., and Wepsic, J. G. (1974): Stimulation of the posterior columns of the spinal cord for pain control: Indications, technique and results. *Clin. Neurosurg.*, 21:278–310.

Advances in Pain Research and Therapy, Vol. 2,
edited by J. J. Bonica and V. Ventafridda.
Raven Press, New York © 1979.

Transcutaneous Nerve Stimulation in Cancer Pain

V. Ventafridda, E. P. Sganzerla, C. Fochi, G. Pozzi, and G. Cordini

Department of Pain Therapy and Rehabilitation, National Cancer Institute, Milan, Italy; Department of Anesthesiology, Universita degli Studi, Milan, Italy

In the past 10 years there has been a renewed interest in transcutaneous electrical nerve stimulation (TENS) as a means of controlling pain. This simple method of pain modulation was known to the Romans, who used electric eels as current generators. In the 19th century, electrical stimulation was used widely for the treatment of various pain syndromes, and the first electrostatic portable stimulators known as "magneto-electric machines" were built. Because of variable and unpredictable results, electroanalgesia was eventually abandoned by most workers. Although Martini et al. (5) in 1943 demonstrated the analgesic effect of the application of electrical currents to the cat's spinal cord, it was not until after the publication of the gate control theory of pain by Melzack and Wall in 1965 (6) that interest in this method of analgesia was resumed. Of the various techniques developed, transcutaneous electrical nerve stimulation has been the most widely used because it is simple, can be applied on the skin, and produces no important side effects.

Published clinical data reveal that TENS may be acutely beneficial in a large number of patients treated for various pain syndromes, but its efficacy usually declines over a long-term period (7). Results obtained in the management of cancer pain vary among different authors reporting data. In a previous paper (12) we reported good to excellent results in about 43% of the patients with cancer pain managed with this modality. Best results were obtained in patients with moderate initial pain, especially when the pain was located in the head and neck regions and when evident trigger points or hyperalgesic areas were found. Good results were also achieved in patients with post-herpetic neuralgia and with early phantom-limb pain that followed cancer therapy. Using the time that the stimulator was employed by the patient as a criterion, long-term results were less favorable. In 159 patients who obtained an initial benefit from TENS, only 56 (35%) were still using it after 1 month. After 10 days, 92 (58%) had already returned the device, as they did not feel it could help their pain anymore.

In order to obtain a more careful clinical assessment and to better identify the role of TENS in controlling cancer pain, we studied a group of 37 patients who, according to our past experience, were expected to obtain an effective control of their pain with this method. We used a detailed pain-profile questionnaire to assess the efficacy of the technique.

MATERIAL AND METHODS

We evaluated 37 patients with intractable cancer pain or other painful conditions in which cancer was a primary cause. All of them were evaluated with a simplified pain-profile questionnaire according to the model developed

TABLE 1. *Pain profile scoring matrix*

Grade	Daily duration of pain	Intensity of pain	Activity level	Drugs
0	No pain	None	Normal	None
1	Having pain up to 25% of time	Mild	Slightly restricted activity	Antiinflammatory agents
2	Up to 50% of time	Discomforting	Moderately restricted	Psychotropic drugs
3	Up to 75% of time	Distressing	Severely restricted	Hypnotics pentazocine
4	Up to 100% of time	Horrible or excruciating	Incapacitated	Narcotics

by Piccaza, Ray, and Shealy (10). Four major criteria for assessing pain and pain relief were used: (a) severity of pain; (b) the percentage of time each day the pain was present; (c) the effect of pain on physical activity; and (d) the use of drugs (Table 1). In all of the patients, TENS was achieved with a commercially available stimulator and electrodes.[1] Optimal setting of electrical output for pain-relief was empirically determined on an individual basis, by testing the whole range of tolerable outputs in various combinations of pulse width, intensity, and frequency. In every patient, we tried to induce a tolerable tingling sensation, carefully avoiding painful levels of stimulation. Rubber electrodes were usually applied over pain trigger areas, over nerve trunks supplying the painful areas, or over an area of the painful region which, according to the patients, gave the best analgesia. All the patients continued to use the device as long as they obtained some definite benefit from it.

Before entering the study group, all patients were instructed in the use of the stimulating device and used it for a first trial period of 48 hr. All patients who after this first trial obtained a satisfactory pain-relief from the

[1] EPC-Mini—STIM-TECH, Minneapolis, Minnesota.

stimulator were invited to use it as long as they derived benefit from it. At the beginning of the control period and at 10, 20, and 30 days, they were invited to return to the pain clinic where they filled out the pain-profile questionnaire and were clinically evaluated.

For every category of the pain profile and for the total score, the differences observed between the beginning of the treatment and the 10-, 20-, and 30-day evaluations have been calculated. Wilcoxon's *t*-test has been applied to the differences of total scores.

RESULTS

As in our previous experience, this group of patients' TENS had a very high rate of success in the first days of use which rapidly declined during subsequent evaluations. Although the intensity of pain was markedly reduced in 35 (96%) patients during the first 10 days of treatment, only 4 (11%) of the patients experienced reduction of their pain intensity after 30 days. Physical activity initially increased in 28 (76%) patients. This declined to 19% (7 patients) at 30 days. A similar pattern was noted in the total time each day the pain was present or absent: The presence of pain was reduced in 32 (86%) patients at the time of the first evaluation, and 4 (11%) at the last evaluation. In contrast, drug intake was reduced initially in only 13 (35%) patients; but after 1 month, it was reduced in 20 (54%) patients.

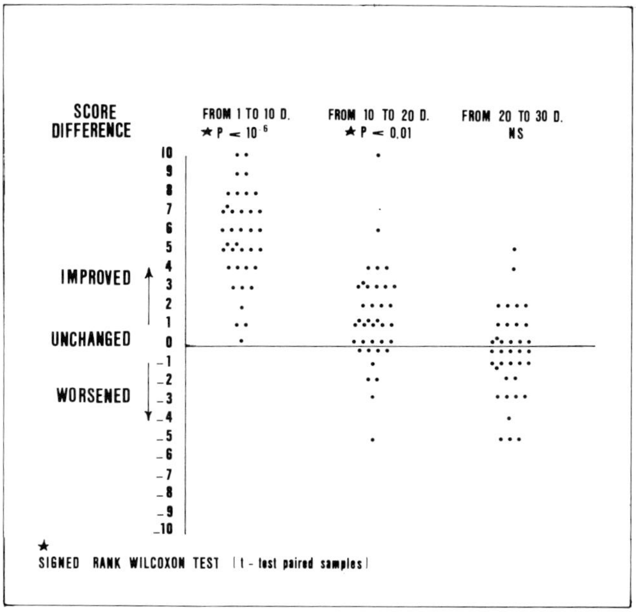

FIG. 1. Total score: differences at 10, 20, and 30 days.

TABLE 2. *Results at 30th. day in 37 oncological patients treated with T.E.N.S.*

Pain character	Pain site	No. patients	Score differences Major +5 +2	Medium +1 −0	Minor −1 −5
Somatic pain	Head and neck	13	3	6	4
with overt	Chest wall	5	—	—	5
trigger points	Abdominal	1	—	1	—
20 patients	Limbs	1	—	—	1
Dysesthesic pain	Phantom (limb)	6	3	1	2
17 patients	Postherpetic neuralgia (chest wall)	8	—	6	2
	Post. surg. neuralgia (chest wall)	3	—	1	2

The differences between the total scores are shown in Fig. 1, which demonstrates that while in the first 10 days, 36 patients (96%) had an overall improvement, follow-up showed significant declines in the effect of the stimulator; and at 30 days, only 27% of the patients still enjoyed an improvement in their pain problem. This was not statistically significant.

Considering the type of pain (Table 2), the best results at 30 days were observed in 3 patients with head and neck pain and in 3 patients with initial phantom-limb pain and to a lesser degree in 6 patients with postherpetic

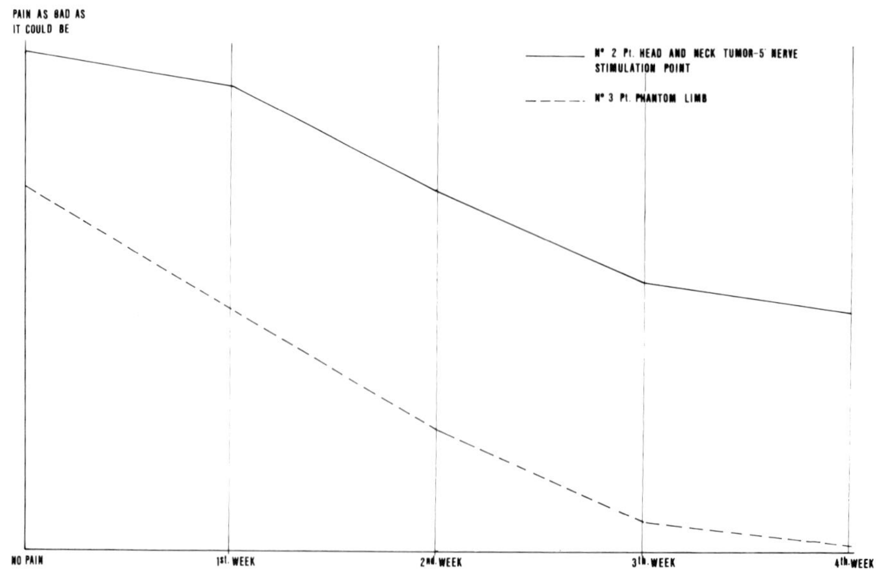

FIG. 2. Worst pain experienced during the week recorded by visual analogue on 5 patients under TENS study.

neuralgia. In the patients who benefited from TENS, there was a constant decrease of pain-appreciation evaluated with the visual analogue technique (2) (Fig. 2).

None of the subjects suffered a complication due to the use of the stimulating device. Skin irritation was avoided by instructing the patients about the frequent cleaning of the electrodes and changing of the conductive paste.

DISCUSSION

Our results with TENS show that in treating patients with chronic pain syndromes of oncologic origin, the long-term usefulness of the stimulating device is quite limited. Even if a high percentage of patients initially respond well to this method of pain modulation, the success rate declines rapidly. After a month or so, it continues to be effective in only a small percentage of patients.

One of the most important factors in the successful use of TENS is the correct positioning of the electrodes and the optimal adjustment of the electrical output. This has to be done with the patient's collaboration, and it is a time-consuming procedure. The patient must be aware of the pain-reducing mechanism of TENS. Pulse width, intensity, and rate combinations have different results for each subject. In order to avoid unpleasant overstimulation and still provide effective levels, these must be carefully determined. Once the analgesic effect is obtained, it is important to test the device for at least 48 hr. Only with such a trial can we determine the correct use and efficacy of the device. Thereafter, the patient must be encouraged to use the stimulator as long as he likes, which may extend from 2 to 3 hr to the entire day.

The presence of a trigger point in an area related to a peripheral nerve fiber is a positive indication for TENS treatment. Richly innervated skin areas are more suitable to pain modulation. Patients suffering from compression by large masses over the cervical nerve trunks or neoplastic involvement on the maxillofacial tissues may get immediate relief. Electrodes must avoid areas of skin erosion or hypesthetic areas. Even if there are no differences between placebo and TENS (11), the placebo effect offered by the use of the stimulating device and its autoregulation by the patient may be useful in diverting the subject's attention from his illness.

Our observations on personality profiles obtained by submitting patients to the MMPI test before treatment indicate that those who had benefit for more than 10 days by the use of TENS revealed significant alterations on their clinical scales compared with the subjects who refused the device at the outset (Fig. 3).

The benefits derived from TENS may be increased by combined therapy with psychotropic drugs and anti-inflammatory agents (13). In fact, antidepressant compounds, such as aminotriptyline with electric stimulation, are

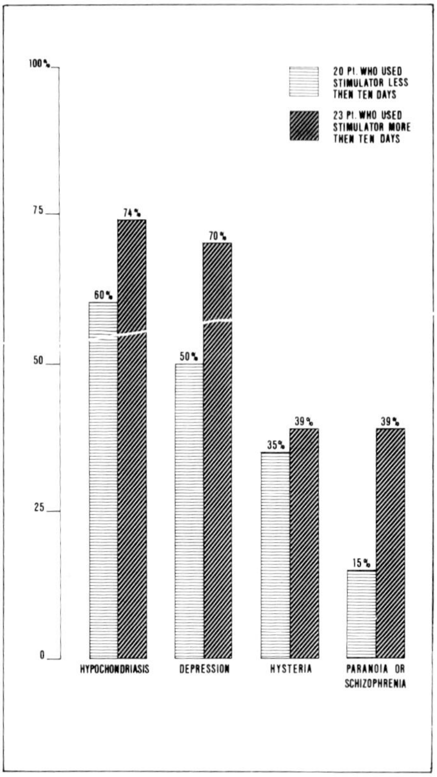

FIG. 3. MMPI significant percent scales with T > 70 on 43 patients who underwent TENS study.

effective in controlling pain from postherpetic neuralgia occurring during chemotherapy for systemic tumors. Electrodes must be placed around the herpetic area until the patient feels a tingling sensation. The tricyclic compound (75 mg daily) not only counteracts the depression, but also restores normal sleep-wakefulness cycling.

Although only a few patients with cancer pain derive long-lasting benefits from TENS, we feel that this simple and innocuous method is worthy of clinical application. Drug-use reduction is a clear index that TENS is worth a trial in oncologic pain control before utilizing more destructive or toxic methods.

REFERENCES

1. Ebersold, M. J., Laws, E. R., Stonnington, H. H., and Stillwell, G. K. (1975): Transcutaneous electrical stimulation for treatment of chronic pain: A preliminary report. *Surg. Neurol.,* 4:96–98.
2. Huskisson, E. C. (1974): Measurement of pain. *Lancet,* 9:1127–1131.
3. Loeser, J. D., Black, R. G., and Christman, A. (1975): Relief of pain by transcutaneous stimulation. *J. Neurosurg.,* 42:308–314.

4. Long, D. M. (1974): External electrical stimulation as a treatment of chronic pain. *Minn. Med.*, 57:195–198.
5. Martini, E., Gualtierotti, T., and Marzorati, A. (1943): Die Rükkenmarkelektronarkose. *Pflügers Arch. Ges. Physiol.*, 246:585.
6. Melzack, R., and Wall, P. D. (1965): Pain mechanism: A new theory. *Science,* 150:971–979.
7. Ray, C. A. (1975): Control of pain by electrical stimulation. A clinical follow-up review. In: *Brain Hypoxia, Pain,* edited by H. Penzholz, M. Brock, J. Hamer, M. Klinger, and O. Spoerri, pp. 216–224. Springer-Verlag, Berlin.
8. Shealy, C. N., and Maurer, D. (1974): Transcutaneous nerve stimulation for control of pain: Preliminary technical note. *Surg. Neurol.*, 2:45.
9. Shealy, C. N. (1974): Transcutaneous electrical stimulation for control of pain. *Clin. Neurosurg.*, 21:269.
10. Shealy, C. N., and Shealy, M. C. (1975): Behavioural techniques in the control of pain: A case for health maintenance vs. disease treatment. In: *Pain: New Perspectives in Therapy and Research,* edited by M. Weisenberg and B. Tursky, pp. 21–33. Plenum Press, New York.
11. Thornsteinsson, G., Stonnington, H. H., Stillwell, G. K., and Elveback, L. R. (1977): Transcutaneous electrical stimulation: A double-blind trial of its efficacy for pain. *Arch. Phys. Med. Rehabil.*, 58:8–13.
12. Ventafridda, V., Fochi, C., and Sganzerla, E. P. (1977): L'Elettrostimolazione transcutanea nel trattamento del dolore oncologico. *Anest. Rianim.*, 18:87–97.
13. Ventafridda, V., Sganzerla, E. P., and Fochi, C. (1979): Considerazioni sull'uso di sostanze psicotrope ad azione antidepressiva in terapia antalgica. *Minerva Med.*, 70 (*in press*).

Discussion

Part II. Management of Pain of Advanced Cancer: Ablative Neurosurgical Procedures and Augmentative (Stimulating) Neurosurgical Procedures

Siegfried (Zürich): I would like to reply to what Pagni said about the utility of percutaneous combined rhizotomy of the trigeminal nerve and glossopharyngeal nerves. I would like to emphasize again that we are talking about cancer patients who are in very poor condition, and I think that open surgery on a posterior fossa carries with it a very high operative risk. I agree that many times pain is outside the trigeminal and glossopharyngeal domain, but we are proposing the percutaneous rhizotomy just for pain of the face. And once you achieve a good relief of pain in the face, you can also perform cervical root rhizotomy if pain is spreading beyond the face.

Broggi (Milano): Dr. Lipton, in my experience, out of 142 cordotomies at the C_1-C_2 level, I had only one paralysis and 6 cases of leg weakness, but 15 of walking ataxia that faded away in 7 to 10 days. Does your experience agree with mine?

Lipton (Liverpool): Our figures vary slightly, I had a paralysis also, a few unexpected cases of leg weakness, and two ataxias, one in the arm, one in the leg. Rosomoff mentions about a 20% incidence of ataxia.

Questioner: Dr. Loeser, have you observed worsening of pain during or after dorsal column stimulation?

Loeser (Seattle): Yes. There is a significant number of patients who usually 6 months to a year after dorsal column stimulation complain that they develop a new sensation when the stimulator is turned on and that that sensation is in itself painful. There is no remedy for that other than not using the stimulator.

Bonica (Seattle): I think it is most appropriate to make a comment about the use of acupuncture for pain management in cancer because it is related to electrical stimulation. I have just reviewed the American literature for some review article and could not find that anyone was using it, and there are, therefore, no statistics. In my 3-week visit to the People's Republic of China, I was very surprised to learn that this is one of the few areas in which the Chinese do not use acupuncture. So, apparently they have tried it and it is no longer used.

Questioner: Dr. Richardson, do you see tolerance with brain stimulation or with central nervous system stimulation for pain-relief?

Richardson (New Orleans): Yes, you do see tolerance to stimulation, Yoshio Hosobuchi has been working with tolerance for some time. We have seen it in a few of our patients. It can be held down to a minimum by using the least amount of stimulation that is effective for pain-relief. And it also can be obviated by the use of drugs.

I have some questions regarding the use of conjoint drug therapy. Almost all of our patients are on tricyclic antidepressives that increase the amount of serotonin in the central nervous system and also obviate sleep problems. These drugs will decrease the amount of stimulation necessary. We have also used anti-norepinephrine agents, such as disulphone, which in the U.S.A. is called Antabuse® and is used for alcoholism. It inhibits norepinephrine and will increase the effectiveness of stimulation by blocking an antagonist modulation system. It will also produce serotonin mania if you use it in conjunction with tricyclics in large doses, and we have had one patient who had serotonin mania and required 2 weeks of hospitalization and treatment with phenothiazenes. We also have a trial going with the FDA on the use of tryptophan as an antitolerance drug. We have little data, but it seems to be more effective than anything else we have.

Questioner: Dr. Richardson, have you measured endogenous opiate levels in relation to stimulation?

Richardson: Yes, we have measured endogenous opiates in ventricular fluid but not in peripheral blood. John Adams has done that and found that there is an increase in opiate-like substances in peripheral blood during central gray stimulation. We have found a marked rise in opiate-like substances in the third ventricular fluid during stimulation, reaching a maximum peak at about 50 min and then gradually decreasing.

Questioner: Dr. Richardson, what is the scientific basis for the assumption that the opiates and paraventricular gray stimulation are mediated through the same system?

Richardson: (a) They are both blocked by nalaxone, a specific morphine antagonist. (b) They are both dependent on serotonin. (c) Dorsal lateral cordotomies in the rat and the cat block the effect of central gray stimulation below the level of the cordotomy in the rat. An animal who has had section of the dorsal lateral column on one side, if given morphine, will show analgesia in the other three extremities and no analgesia in the extremity below the dorsal lateral section. It has also been shown in rats that spinal cord reflexes are released from the effect of morphine by sectioning the cord at the C_1 level.

Questioner: Dr. Richardson, have you noted any behavioral changes?

Richardson: Yes, we have noted very mild but easily observable behavioral changes. Some patients become less depressed. Other patients have had a fright reaction during stimulation. Now, we think this is probably related to having the electrode placed a little too deeply in the hypothalamus, but many patients have excellent pain inhibition with no other side effects. They also will have an obvious elevation of mood apparently unrelated to the pain-relief.

Questioner: Dr. Richardson, is the procedure effective for deafferentation pain, that is, pain in an area of numbness?

Richardson: In some patients, yes; in other patients, we have to use either VLP or internal capsule stimulation. And we have some patients with mixed pain in whom central gray stimulation relieves their chronic mechanical back pain but does not relieve the area of burning pain in their leg caused by nerve injury.

So in some patients you have to choose which pain you are going to attack because you don't want to do two procedures on the same patient at the same time.

Questioner: What is the mortality rate in cordotomy and myelotomy operations, Dr. Papo?

Papo (Ancona): In the past when these operations were performed with broad indications, the mortality rate was about 2 to 4%. Today these operations are reserved for special cases, and mortality rate should be practically negligible. Regarding myelotomy, it is difficult to say. It certainly is very low.

Questioner: Dr. Papo, what is the incidence and mechanism of painful dysesthesia in the lower unilateral limb after cervical cordotomy?

Papo: The current hypothesis is that these are mainly deafferentation pains. The incidence depends mostly on how long the patients survive. In some studies by Guillot, several years ago, all patients operated on for coxalgia and coxarthosis had painful dysesthesias of this kind.

Questioner: Dr. Papo, what do you recommend for cordotomy, local or general anesthesia?

Papo: I believe that general anesthesia is best, because data obtained with local anesthesia have no value since one may be misled by contused fibers that temporarily don't transmit anymore.

Pagni (Torino): Dr. Papo, what about cingulumotomy?

Papo: I performed it some years ago on two groups of patients: some psychiatric patients and some patients in pain; and I noticed that the main difference was in the intensity of psychic deterioration that I could see in the two groups.

While the psychiatric patients tolerated the operation well and the therapeutic results were sometimes useful, in the patients with pain, especially when due to neoplasia, the psychic deterioration was terrible, so I completely abandoned this type of operation.

I recently met Eldon Folz, who introduced this type of operation, and he, too, doesn't perform it anymore.

Loeser: In some of our stimulation procedures for pain-relief, our approach has been to try to reduce the magnitude of the surgical procedures for pain-relief, especially in terminal cancer patients. The selection of the specific procedure should be based on the location of the pain, the prognosis for the particular patient involved, and the extent of the procedure that will be selected.

Advances in Pain Research and Therapy, Vol. 2,
edited by J. J. Bonica and V. Ventafridda.
Raven Press, New York © 1979.

Problems of Cancer Pain in the Head and Neck

Roberto Molinari

Oncology Department, Istituto Nazionale Tumori Milano, 20133 Milan, Italy

Only 35% of head and neck malignant tumors (with the exception of cancer of the lips and larynx) can be successfully treated and cured of the disease. The rest will develop recurrences or metastases or both. Of these 50 to 60% will develop pain. Head and neck cancers usually recur locally and spread to the regional lymph nodes. Distant metastases occur in only 5 to 15%, and only cancer of the nasopharynx and tonsil show general metastases in about 30 to 35%. Pain due to cancer growth tends to be localized in the head and neck, and its pathogenesis depends on the site more than on the histology of the tumor. Epidermoid cancer tends to ulcerate and deeply infiltrate surrounding structures, whereas glandular tumors and lymphomas generally grow by enlargement, so that pain is less frequently encountered in the latter type of tumors. On the whole, histological types of malignant tumors in decreasing order of their importance in causing pain are:

1. Epidermoid squamous carcinoma
2. Undifferentiated carcinoma
3. Adenoid cystic carcinoma
4. Bone sarcoma
5. Fibrosarcoma
6. Condrosarcoma
7. Lymphoma
8. Melanoma

PATHOGENESIS OF THE PAIN

The mechanisms by which head and neck cancer can cause pain include: (a) stimulation of mucosal and submucosal nerve endings, (b) ulceration and superinfection, (c) compression and involvement of sensitive nerve branches, and (d) bone invasion.

Stimulation of Mucosal and Submucosal Nerve Endings

This mechanism is specific for the initial phases of cancer growth. It can be considered to be mainly responsible for local burning sensations, superficial pain, and reflex neuralgic pain, such as otalgia in exophitic or erosive lesions.

Ulceration and Infection

Most of the cancers that arise from mucosal membranes (squamous cancer) of the mouth and pharynx tend to ulcerate, because of both central necrosis and microtraumatisms. Ulceration is not always painful per se, at least in the absence of local irritant agents, such as alcohol or acids, but the ulcer paves the way for infection by the microorganisms that are abundantly present in these cavities. Necrotic tissue and alimentary deposits are excellent culture grounds for bacteria, which can develop and cause subsequent inflammation and edema. Pain due to ulceration is markedly increased by movement of the involved part, and it therefore varies from site to site. Exacerbation by function is minimal in static regions such as cheek, floor of mouth, hard palate, nasal and paranasal cavities, and nasopharynx and is severe in the dynamic structures such as the tongue, soft palate, and faucial arch.

Involvement of Nerve Branches

The deeply infiltrating component of head and neck cancer frequently involves important nerve branches and trunks whose location is constant. Because of this, painful symptoms generally correspond to the anatomic site of the tumor. The most frequently involved nerves are: the lingual nerve by cancer of the mobile part of the tongue and floor of the mouth; the mandibular branch of the fifth nerve by cancer of the inferior gum and of the retromolar space and glossopalatine arch; the glossopharyngeal nerve by cancer of the tonsil and the lateral part of the base of the tongue.

Important sensitive nerve branches are not present in the laryngeal and hypopharyngeal regions, so that problems of pain are unusual in these regions. On the contrary, malignant tumors of nasal and paranasal cavities with particular locations can involve branches of the maxillary nerve, such as the infraorbital or, more often, the superior alveolar nerves. Advanced nasopharyngeal cancers cause mainly palsy of motor nerves, but also serious trigeminal neuralgias when the bone barrier is crossed. Lymph node metastasis causing marked enlargement with the mechanism of direct involvement of nervous branches is practically the only one that can induce severe pain in the neck.

Bone Invasion

Direct involvement of the bone is not painful per se. Pain arises when tumor progression involves nerve branches (as occurs in cancer of the alveolus) or when the path of neoplastic infiltration is followed from the surface by bacterial infection, with consequent osteomyelitis as occurs in alveolar tumors and in cancer of the maxillary antrum, where a superimposed obstructive sinusitis feeds the bone infection.

Adjuvant Factors

The above-mentioned mechanisms can obviously combine themselves in various ways and be all concomitant. Their effects, and consequently the importance of the problems of pain, can be made worse by other factors that are independent of the tumor but that are connected with often unavoidable consequences of the treatment or with functional and psychologic problems.

Post-radiation Damage

These range from simple mucositis to radionecrosis, by many intermediate degrees. When associated with persistence or recurrence of cancer (and consequently with the above-described mechanisms) they give rise to the most distressing situations. More frequent than spontaneous necrosis of a tumor mass is necrosis induced by radiation, which constitutes a rich ground for superimposed infection. Furthermore, it involves healthy tissues that contain sensitive nerve structures that have not been previously destroyed by the cancer. Apart from this extreme complication, radiation induces reactive fibrosis, which can cause more or less painful muscular contractions (trismus). On the whole, the combination of neoplastic recurrence with radionecrosis represents about 70% of the major problems of pain in cancer of the head and neck.

Functional Problems

Functions such as phonetics, breathing, and deglutition are frequently affected in cancer of the larynx and hypopharynx, where, on the contrary, problems of pain are rarely present. In cancer of the nasal and paranasal cavities, pain is mainly due to involvement of bony structures and branches of the fifth nerve; in cancer of the nasopharynx it is very frequently associated with palsy of one or more cranial motor nerves (and functional disorders make persistent pain less tolerable). However, the worst combination of pain and functional trouble is seen in cancer of the mouth and oropharynx, where bouts of hyperalgesia and neuralgia during chewing and swallowing can severely compromise the eating process.

Psychological Problems

All the above-mentioned mechanisms are often intensified by particular psychologic reactions, both basic and progressively acquired.

1. The great majority of the patients with cancer of the mouth and pharynx are heavy drinkers and smokers, with their basic psychologic problems.
2. Combination of pain and functional disorders make the psychologic conditions worse; all these symptoms influence one another in a sort of vicious cycle.

...on the psychologic effects of cancer of the ...ct that these tumors can be seen, so that the ..., day by day, the progress of his illness.

...PECIFIC PAIN SYNDROMES

...dromes associated with head and neck tumors can be listed; ...st frequent and serious are:

... and Type of Lesion	Mechanism of Pain
...r of the floor of the mouth, with bone involvement, with or without radionecrosis	Lingual or mandibular neuralgia complicated by pain caused by the superimposed infection
Cancer of the glossopalatine arch, with involvement of the tongue and the tonsil with or without trismus	Glossopharyngeal neuralgia, with mandibular nerve involvement
Cancer of the maxillary antrum	Maxillary neuralgia
Cancer of the nasopharynx, with invasion of the base of the skull	Dull painful syndrome in the nape of the neck and occipital region
Cancer of the nasopharynx, with invasion of the ethmoidal structure	Trigeminal pain
Advanced neck node metastases or recurrences	Cervical plexus and/or Arnold's nerve neuralgia
Postirradiation "wooden neck"	

Advances in Pain Research and Therapy, Vol. 2,
edited by J. J. Bonica and V. Ventafridda.
Raven Press, New York © 1979.

Oncologic Therapy of Pain in Cancer of the Head and Neck

Roberto Molinari

Head and Neck Oncology Department, Istituto Nazionale Tumori Milano, 20133 Milan, Italy

More than half of the patients with cancer of the head and neck will sooner or later experience pain due to local or regional progress of their illness or, less frequently, to distant metastases. Apart from the latter, which are not specific to these tumors, the present report deals with the etiologic treatment of pain that is strictly localized in the head and neck region.

The weapons at our disposal are traditional: radiotherapy, surgery, and chemotherapy, alone or combined. Since the greatest majority of the problems of pain arise from recurrences after previous treatments, these are to be carefully taken into account for oncologic therapy. It is therefore necessary to consider every treatment not only as an isolated symptomatic measure for palliation, but also as a part of a general therapeutic plan in which we must always remember that progress of the tumor and severity of pain are related. In other words, pain can be frequently expected and avoided in many cases.

Pain can obviously occur in every phase of the illness, but the more advanced the tumor is, the more serious the problems of pain. At the beginning of the illness, every oncologic treatment can and must aspire to cure cancer and prevent pain. In advanced cases, a cure is not the main goal, although it is not to be renounced. However, an active antineoplastic therapy can often represent a valid alternative to a merely passive management of the pain.

RADIOTHERAPY

Radiotherapy is generally the first treatment used in cancer of the head and neck. In very advanced cases that are not suitable for other therapy, radiation therapy alone can often resolve problems of pain, especially when the tumor is highly radiosensitive. These include undifferentiated carcinoma of the nasopharynx and tonsil, ulcerating carcinoma of the tongue and floor of the mouth, and undifferentiated tumors of the nasal and paranasal cavities. In the great majority of cases, however, persistent pain is the consequence of recurrent cancer previously treated with surgery or radiotherapy (2,5). In the latter case, a new course of radiotherapy can hardly achieve consistent results from both an oncologic and a symptomatic viewpoint. On the contrary, the unavoidable overdosage can more often induce radionecrosis and finally increase the pain. Therefore, repetition of radiation therapy must be carefully thought over and performed only if very poor results can be expected from alternative treatments or when there is still some possibility for a cure. This is the case in nasopharyngeal cancer, where intraosseous recurrences are quite frequent and painful and where therapeutic alternatives are not possible. Great caution is needed in order to avoid damage to the spinal cord and to not make the condition of the patient worse by causing mandibular necrosis or trismus. With these precautions and by using different fields, the results are often satisfactory.

Recurrence with consequent pain after surgery represents the larger field of application of radiotherapy. This often happens in cancer of the paranasal cavities, mouth, and oropharynx, where surgery is frequently used as first treatment. On the other hand, in cancer of the larynx and hypopharynx, which is mostly treated with surgery, problems of pain are very rare, both at the initial stage of the disease and after recurrences.

Nevertheless, radiotherapy is a useful means in these cases. The task of the radiotherapist sometimes can be complicated by problems of dosimetry due to modifications resulting from surgery, such as removal of the jaw or other bony structures or removal of muscles such as the sternomastoid. On the other hand, these same changes sometimes facilitate the treatment by making possible and safer the choice of particular techniques not previously usable, such as interstitial radiotherapy or moulded radium apparatus.

It is extremely difficult to quantify the results on the pain of this kind of treatment separately from the oncologic ones. Remission of pain actually comes from the objective neoplastic regression, but the former is not a compulsory consequence of the latter. Radiotherapy pursues certain aims, but these are not always attained; furthermore, it can sometimes cause undesirable side effects, which can undo or even make worse the results achieved.

SURGERY

Symptomatic and Palliative Surgery

Surgical removal of lesions that were previously treated with radiotherapy and have recurred forms part of a combined treatment, even if not planned. This type of recurrence can actually give rise to pain or not, but, apart from oncologic results, remission of pain is a goal that is more frequently and consistently achieved by surgery than by radiotherapy (4).

Recurrence with bone invasion, especially when combined with radionecrosis, is one of the most frequent causes of pain. In this case the removal of bone involved by cancer is the most rapid and direct means of resolving this otherwise difficult problem. When feasible, surgery is repeated if necessary; our duty is only to carefully weigh the pros and cons of this treatment. Postoperative complications due to previous radiotherapy are to be considered in order to avoid life-threatening situations or too-protracted postoperative periods. The evaluation of these risks depends on the personal experience of the surgeon, who must sometimes reject a radical treatment in favor of a shorter and uneventful course with an acceptable expectancy of life with no problem of pain.

Surgery after radiotherapy is applicable and useful in many clinical situations, but mainly in case of:

1. recurrence of cancer of the oral cavity with radionecrosis;
2. osteoradionecrosis of the jaws, with or without neoplastic recurrence;
3. recurrence of oropharyngeal cancer (tonsil, base of the tongue, retromolar space, or anterior pillar);
4. recurrence of tumors of the nasal and paranasal cavities; and
5. recurrence of neck node metastases, after both radiotherapy and surgery.

In case of tumors initially advanced (T_3, T_4) and not previously treated, destructive surgery can be chosen as the first therapy when alternative treatments offer poor chances of resolving pain, independently of purposes of a cure.

Prevention of Problems of Pain

Major problems of pain in cancer of the head and neck can also be prevented by a careful choice of the initial treatment, not only by taking into account the anticipated results of the treatment but also by bearing in mind the future of the patient. When the expected cure-rate is statistically poor, the probabilities that progress of the tumor will cause pain are to be evaluated. As a consequence, we can be induced to modify our therapeutic plan and to choose different approaches, such as surgery instead of radiotherapy. In fact, surgery brings about section of nerve branches and trunks, which is tantamount to a real denervation. Consequences of surgery, such as cosmetic and functional damages, are often more willingly accepted than is the persistence of severe pain; and also an operation is an active therapeutic procedure that provides at least a psychologic relief to the patient, who is aware of his illness. It is often thought that these patients prefer less aggressive treatments, but this is not always true.

In my experience there are three main clinical situations in which the occurrence of severe pain syndromes is strongly affected by the choice of the first treatment:

1. Extended cancer of the mobile tongue and floor of the mouth. If interstitial radiotherapy is not feasible, external conventional irradiation has little chance of success in curing the patient. On the contrary, it

can result in many problems of pain, through radiomucositis or radionecrosis.

2. Cancer of the gums and retromolar space or adjacent structures involving the bone. In these cases, external radiotherapy can only rarely cure the patient but, on the other hand, is able to frequently induce trismus and very painful radionecrosis.
3. Very-large neck node metastases. Except for the more radiosensitive histotypes, such as undifferentiated carcinoma of the nasopharynx or tonsil, lymph node metastases are generally resistant to radiation therapy. Their progress can involve cervical nerve roots and cause severe pain. Very high doses of radiotherapy are to be given to these nodes; if radiotherapy does not succeed in curing them, the so-called "wooden-neck syndrome" often takes place, and in this case any form of curative or palliative surgery is no longer feasible. In all these cases, the initial treatment should be surgery whenever possible, because whatever the oncologic result may be, it is the same as prevention of pain (1).

CHEMOTHERAPY

The rationale of anticancer chemotherapy in patients with severe pain is the assumption that a correlation does exist between regression of the tumor and reduction of the pain. In head and neck cancer this correlation has been clearly demonstrated and is probably due to the fact that the tumor mass is generally smaller than it is in other regions of the body.

Chemotherapy with a palliative purpose has been used for many years in head and neck cancer. Many drugs have been tested including methotrexate, bleomycin, adriamycin, and hydroxyurea. Unfortunately, results have been inconsistent and quite poor. Better results, on the tumor and on the pain, can be achieved by combining different drugs (polychemotherapy) or by increasing the dose of single drugs. The latter was also pursued by using intra-arterial administration to reach the maximum concentration of the drug in a reduced area with no need for a general administration in too high a dose. In this method a catheter is placed in the external carotid artery via its superficial temporal branch; the drug is introduced by slow infusion in 8 to 20 hr daily in 10 to 15 days. Immediate results are very satisfactory: Remission of pain is generally prompt even when the objective regression of the tumor is partial or absent. Tumor regression is achieved less frequently and depends on the type of schedule used (Table 1).

However, intra-arterial chemotherapy cannot be employed in all of the patients because of anatomical or surgical reasons. Moreover, generally it can not be used for more than 15 to 25 days and requires hospitalization. As a consequence, this type of administration is not very suitable for palliative purposes; in addition, it requires further treatment by general administration in order to delay the unavoidable rapid relapse.

TABLE 1. *Immediate results of intra-arterial chemotherapy using different single drugs at the Instituto Nazionale Tumori, Milano (INTM)*

Drug dosage (per day for 10–15 days)	Total cases	% Tumor regression						Overall > 50%	
		< 50%		50%–> 90%		Complete			
		No.	%	No.	%	No.	%	No.	%
MTX[a] 5 mg	26	20	77	5	19.2	1	3.8	6	23
ADM 0.3/kg	9	5	55.5	4	44.5	0	0	4	44.5
MTX 50 mg + CF	11	4	36.4	7	63.6	0	0	7	63.6
BLM 15 mg	30	12	40	14	46.7	4	13.3	18	60
VCR + BLM	27	8	29.6	12	44.4	7	26	19	70.4

[a] MTX = methotrexate; ADM = adriamycin; BLM = bleomycin; CF = citrovorum factor; VCR = vincristine.

General or systemic chemotherapy is more simple and has less risk, at least when drugs are not administered at very high doses. Results on both tumor and pain are not satisfactory when single drugs are used, and only methotrexate causes regression in many cases when it is administered at high doses with Leucovorin® rescue; regressions achieved, however, are rarely very significant (Table 2). Combinations of various drugs have been used by many investigators with better results, but also in this case a strict correlation was observed between clinical response and the number and amount of the drugs used. Severe toxicity is often encountered and is the main limitation of these palliative treatments, which cannot be employed for a long period of time and generally require hospitalization.

In order to overcome this obstacle, we have recently tested a new schedule of low-dose chemotherapy that was expressly set up for palliative, protracted treatments. This schedule is based on some concepts of synchronization of the cell cycle and uses vincristine, bleomycin, and methotrexate (VBM) in a particular sequence (3). In our experience, toxicity was almost negligible and not so different as was expected; oncologic results were very satisfactory in terms of frequency and importance of the regressions achieved (62% of tumors regressed more than 50%, and 32% of the tumors almost completely regressed (Table 3). Patients not previously treated with radiotherapy showed the best results, with 88% of regression greater than 50% of the initial size and 41% of complete regression (Table 4).

The most impressive finding was a clear correlation between clinical objective response and remission of pain; this was almost constant in responsive patients but was also observed in the absence of a significant objective regression (Table 5). The length of the remission was correlated with the importance of the initial response: The mean duration was 2.2 months in the group of less-responsive patients; 4 months in good responders (from 50 to 90% of regression); and 6.6 months among total responders. In 4 of 60 cases the regression achieved lasted 12 to 13 months. When there was a relapse, in 20% of the patients the pain did not occur again, and in 50% it required only simple, conventional treatment. In a certain number of cases we were able to profit from the regression achieved, since it was then possible to employ analgesic procedures (surgery, radiotherapy, or other oncologic treatments), with a palliative purpose.

In conclusion, by applying these principles of oncologic therapy to impending or expected problems of pain, we have noticed during the past 8 years a progressive reduction in the number of patients who require specific major analgesic treatment: 27% of those with head and neck cancer in 1970, 18% in 1973, 13% in 1975, and 10% in 1977. These results can be achieved only by means of a strict cooperation among the surgeon, radiotherapist, and chemotherapist; each must be aware of the limits of his own treatment and of the possibilities of the others.

TABLE 2. *Immediate results of general chemotherapy using different single drug schedules in palliative treatment of head and neck cancer (INTM experience)*

Drugs and schedules		Total cases	% Tumor regression						Overall > 50%	
			< 50%		50%–> 90%		Complete			
			No.	%	No.	%	No.	%	No.	%
CCNU[a]	130 mg/sq m/6 weeks p.o.	11	10	90.9	1	9.1	0	0	1	9.1
MTX	25 mg ×2/week p.o.	14	12	85.7	1	7.1	1	7.1	2	14.3
ADM	60–75 mg/sq m/3 weeks i.v.	35	30	85.7	1	2.9	4	11.4	5	14.3
BLM	10 mg/sq m/×2/week i.v.	14	12	85.7	1	7.1	1	7.1	2	14.3
BLM	15–30 mg/sq m/week i.v.	29	20	68	7	24.1	2	6.9	9	31
MTX	40–60 mg/sq m/week i.v.	23	15	65.2	8	34.8	0	0	8	34.8
BLM	10 mg/sq m ×2/week i.v.	16	14	87.5	2	12.5	0	0	2	12.5
+										
MTX	40 mg/sq m/week i.v.									
VCR	1 mg/week									
+										
BLM	30 mg/week (sequential)	60	23	38.3	18	30	19	31.7	37	61.6
+										
MTX	20 mg/sq m/week									

[a] CCNU = chloroethyl-cyclohexyl-nitrosourea; MTX = methotrexate; ADM = adriamycin; BLM = bleomycin; VCR = vincristine.

TABLE 3. *Results of general chemotherapy with VBM: regression achieved in cancer of the head and neck, by site of the tumor*

		% Tumor regression								Overall	
	Total	0%–< 25%		25%–< 50%		50%–< 90%		90%–< 100%		> 50%	
Site	cases	No.	%	No.	%	No.	%	No.	%	No.	%
Oral cavity (post.)	12	0	0	2	17	5	41.5	5	41.5	10	83.3
Oral cavity (ant.)	22	6	27	3	14	4	18	9	41	13	59
Oropharynx	11	2	18	3	27	4	37	2	18	6	54.5
Larynx-hypopharynx	12	5	41	1	8	4	34	2	17	6	50
Lips, skin	3	1	33	0	0	1	33	1	33	1	33.3
Totals	60	14	23	9	15	18	30	19	32	37	62

TABLE 4. *Results of general chemotherapy with VBM: regression according to previous treatment*

	Responses			
	<50%		>50%	
Previous treatment	No.	%	No.	%
Radiotherapy Surgery + radiotherapy	21	48.8	22	51.2
No treatment Surgery alone	2	12	15	88
Totals	23	38	37	62

TABLE 5. *Relationships between objective regression and remission of pain in 27 patients with problems of pain, using VBM*

	Objective regression							
Remission	0–25%		25%–50%		50%–90%		Complete	
of pain	No.	%	No.	%	No.	%	No.	%
No remission	2/6	33	1/4	25	1/9	11	0/8	0
Slight	2/6	33	1/4	25	0/9	0	0/8	0
Important	1/6	17	2/4	50	5/9	55	0/8	0
Complete	1/6	17	0/4	0	3/9	33	8/8	100

REFERENCES

1. Badellino, F. (1977): Terapia palliativa delle metastasi linfonodali nei carcinomi della testa e del collo. *Nuovo Arch. Ital. Otol.,* 5:561.
2. Hayward, M. (1977): Headache and pain in the head and neck. In: S. Lipton: *Persistent Pain: Modern Methods of Treatment, Vol. I.* Academic Press, London.
3. Molinari, R., Mattavelli, F., Chiesa, F., Cantu', G., Costa, L., and Tancini G. (1978): Results of palliative treatment of advanced or recurred head and neck squamous carcinoma using a sequential low dose combination chemotherapy (V B M), (*in press*).
4. Richard, J., Vandebrouck, C., Lefur, R., and Cachin, Y. (1971): Que faut-il penser de la bucco-pharyngectomie transmaxillaire de rattra-page? *Ann. Otolaryngol.* (*Paris*), 88:663.
5. Wolff, H. G. (1963): *Headache and Other Head Pain.* Oxford University Press, London and New York.

Advances in Pain Research and Therapy, Vol. 2,
edited by J. J. Bonica and V. Ventafridda.
Raven Press, New York © 1979.

Cancer Pain in the Head and Neck: Role of Analgesics and Related Drugs

Raymond W. Houde

Department of Medicine, Memorial Sloan-Kettering Cancer Center, New York, New York 10021

Systemic analgesics of some type are virtually always employed at some stage in the management of pain due to head and neck cancer. The choice of a particular drug, of a particular class of drugs, or of additional adjuvant symptomatic drugs will rest on a number of considerations relating to the patient's present status and past medical history. Head and neck cancer is comprised on a wide diversity of neoplasms which, to name but a few, include the various intracranial and cranial neoplasms, cancers of the mouth, tongue, nasopharynx, oropharynx, larynx, cervical esophagus, salivary glands, thyroid glands, lymph nodes, and skin and underlying soft tissues. The extent to which these cancers produce pain, disability, disfigurement, and suffering is also subject to considerable differences in the clinical evolution of each of these neoplasms, what medical intervention has been undertaken or is being done, and a number of complications which can occur, such as necrosis, ulceration, infection, occlusion of blood vessels or lymphatics, and fractures occurring as a consequence of either the disease or its treatment.

To be considered in decisions of management, particularly as they relate to the use of systemic drugs, are factors relating to the patient's age, social habits, and the social consequences of a disease which may be so visible to one's family, friends, and associates. Some types of cancer, such as those of the brain, eye, thyroid, and blood and lymphatic systems are not uncommonly encountered in the young, but most head and neck cancers, particularly that of the skin and mucous membranes of the upper respiratory system and the upper digestive tract, are chiefly diseases of the middle-aged and the elderly. Patients with cancer of the oral cavity, pharynx, larynx, and esophagus also often give a history of heavy smoking or drinking, or both, and the consequences of these in terms of respiratory or metabolic impairment can be important determinants in the choice of drugs for the management of pain. Finally, the emotional impact of cancer, which may be disfiguring, give rise to offensive odors, or interfere with one's power of speech or ability to communicate cannot be underestimated. Many of these patients present formidable challenges in medical management.

In its varied forms, head and neck cancer can give rise to virtually any type of pain, or none at all. The extent to which pain gives rise to suffering will be influenced, to a great extent, by the presence or absence of other signs or symptoms, such as intractable cough, respiratory distress, nausea and vomiting, profuse or foul-smelling secretions, profound weakness, or even severe anxiety and fear of further disfigurement, invalidism, or death. Depending upon how the patient views these as threats to his being and to his self-esteem, they may take precedence over pain or conversely, and more commonly, they may make any pain worse.

The choice of analgesic medications or adjuvant drugs to control pain, anxiety, insomnia, or any of the other symptoms contributing to suffering must, of necessity, be individualized. Some routes of drug administration will be found to be either impossible or inadvisable, and some drugs and drug combinations contraindicated. The nonnarcotic analgesics of the antipyretic-antiinflammatory type are most frequently employed, primarily because they are less apt to suppress cough and respiration, to cause secretions to become thickened and more troublesome, or to cause an increase in intracranial pressure. Although cancers of the head and neck can be extremely painful, the majority of patients generally respond to the administration of aspirin or acetaminophen, administered either by mouth or crushed and given by nasogastric tube. Mixtures containing other simple analgesics, such as APC tablets and aspirin with antacids, have also been employed, although there is no reason for using them in preference to the simple analgesics. On the other hand, mixtures of simple analgesics with propoxyphene or phenobarbital have been effective when the antipyretic-antiinflammatory drug was not. Consideration must be given to the fact that many of these patients have ulcerations of the mouth or pharynx, severe dysphagia or obstruction, or lesions which are apt to bleed easily and would, accordingly contraindicate aspirin either because of its local effects or antithrombotic effects.

If the pain cannot be controlled with these agents, more potent drugs such as indoprofen appear to be more effective and may make possible the postponement of narcotics. However, if pain is not otherwise controlled, there is no reason to withhold narcotics. Customarily, the milder, orally administered narcotics such as codeine, propoxyphene, or pentazocine are given along with aspirin or acetaminophen. In some patients, codeine's antitussive effects are also a desired attribute of that drug.

With persisting pain and repeated administration of even mild narcotics, some tolerance may develop and require appropriate adjustments in the dose of the narcotic. In some patients with more severe pain, particularly deep in the ear or in the head, it may, in fact, be necessary to use the more potent orally effective narcotics and, if possible, in combination with a simple analgesic.

Many patients with head and neck cancer are quite depressed and can benefit from an antidepressant such as imipramine, amitriptyline, or clomipramine. Tranquilizers, primarily of the phenothiazine type, are occasionally advisable, although some caution should be taken with patients with a history of alcoholism or liver disease. Some head and neck pains are neuralgic in type or lancinating, and in these patients, the use of carbamazapine and/or phenytoin may be indicated. Care should be taken not to administer carbamazapine to patients receiving monoamine-oxidase inhibitors. Both carbamazapine and phenytoin are capable of precipitating a number of hypersensitivity reactions, so that patients should be monitored for the possibility of hematopoietic reactions. In patients with intracranial lesions, steroids primarily in the form of dexamethasone may prove of some benefit.

In summary, the problems of pain in head and neck cancer are extremely complex and generally require some form of combined management directed not only at relieving pain but also at other causes of suffering so commonly encountered in these patients.

ACKNOWLEDGMENT

Supported in part by a Grant from the National Institute on Drug Abuse #DA 01707.

Advances in Pain Research and Therapy, Vol. 2,
edited by J. J. Bonica and V. Ventafridda.
Raven Press, New York © 1979.

Cancer Pain in the Head and Neck: Role of Nerve Blocks

John J. Bonica and Jose L. Madrid*

*Department of Anesthesiology, University of Washington School of Medicine, Seattle, Washington 98195, and *Department of Anesthesiology and Pain Clinic, Ciudad Sanitaria "10 de Octobre," Madrid, Spain*

In patients with moderate to severe pain due to cancer of the head and neck, nerve blocks can be used as diagnostic or prognostic tools or to control the pain for a prolonged period of time. Diagnostic blocks are used to determine the mechanism and pathways of the pain, whereas prognostic blocks are used to predict the effects of neurolytic block or neurosurgical section. The basic principles, advantages, and disadvantages of therapeutic blocks for pain in this region are similar to those mentioned in the panel on nerve blocks.

Pain in the face is often caused by tumors which commonly arise from structures about the mouth, nose, and paranasal sinuses. The physician should not hesitate to inject the gasserian ganglion, because relief of pain must be obtained for the patient even at the price of producing keratitis from block of the ophthalmic branches of the trigeminal nerve. The problem here is quite different from that in patients who have tic douloureux or other benign, chronic pain in whom the life-expectancy is long and a corneal ulcer is a serious complication. Gasserian ganglion block is particularly useful if the lesion involves structures which are supplied by more than one of the major divisions of the fifth cranial nerve. In such cases, it is preferable to carry out a gasserian ganglion block at the onset to produce a widespread field of analgesia into which the cancer can spread without producing more pain subsequently.

Severe pain which often accompanies cancer of the posterior mouth and throat is most effectively relieved by neurosurgical section of the sensory roots of the glossopharyngeal and part of the vagus nerves, a procedure best achieved by the posterior intracranial root (Dandy technique). Blocks of these nerves with local anesthetics may be used as diagnostic and prognostic tools; but, since such blocks also involve motor nerves, neurolytic blocks are contraindicated because they produce prolonged paralysis of pharyngeal and laryngeal muscles, resulting in the loss of the patient's ability to swallow and phonate. This is an especially serious complication if the block is done bilaterally. Unilateral neurolytic block of the glossopharyngeal nerve of the most painful side may be considered in patients with excruciating pain not adequately relieved by narcotics and whose physical condition is too poor to permit neurosurgical section. Pain in the back of the head and upper neck may require block of C_2 and C_3, first with a local anesthetic to ascertain the pain pathways and subsequently with a neurolytic agent. In many instances, cancer of the mouth, tongue, or lower jaw spreads laterally and posteriorly to produce moderate to severe pain and sometimes trismus, which can be effectively relieved by block of the mandibular nerve combined with paravertebral block of the upper two cervical nerves.

Occasionally, tumors of the face and head cause a burning discomfort in addition to the severe neuralgia and deep, aching pain. The burning pain is usually located over one side of the head, the eye, and teeth, and lower and sometimes the upper jaw, the temporal region, and the nape of the neck which is not relieved by block of the somatic nerves. In such cases, cervical sympathetic block should be carried out, first with a local anesthetic; and if it relieves the burning pain, the procedure is repeated with phenol or alcohol as a supplement to somatic block.

Figures 1 through 7 show nerve block procedures used for various types of cancers that produce pain in the face and neck. Figure 1 shows a patient with fibrosarcoma of the left orbit with invasion of the maxilla which produced severe pain in the left eye and ipsilateral side of the face, especially the cheek, which could not be relieved with large doses of morphine. Injec-

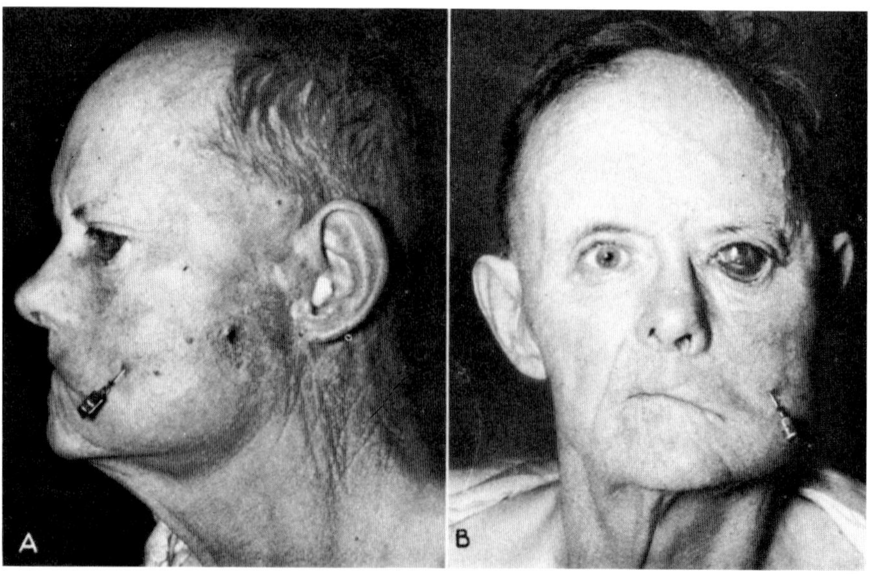

FIG. 1. Fibrosarcoma of the left orbit with invasion of the maxilla. Pain relieved with alcohol block of gasserian ganglion.

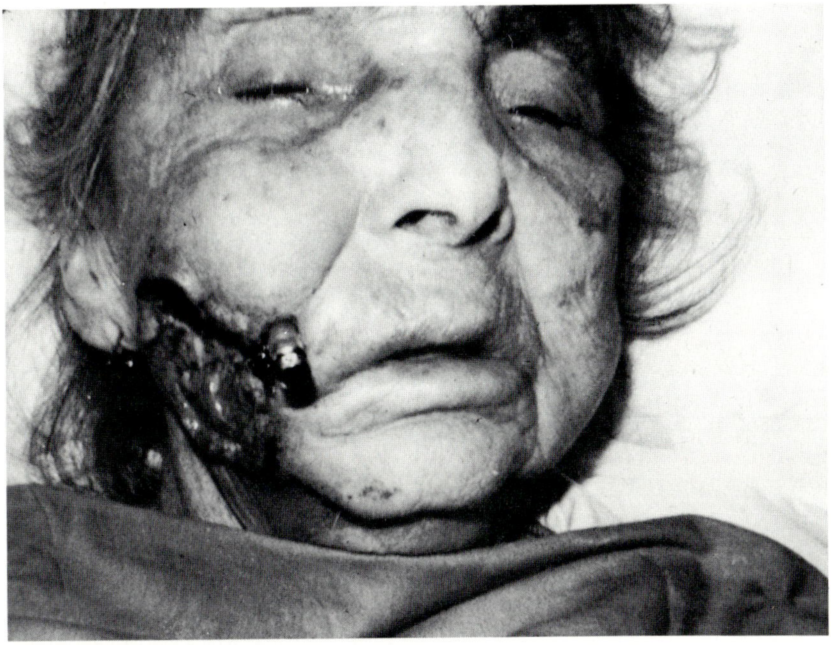

FIG. 2. Invasive epidermoid carcinoma on the skin of the cheek which required an extensive block at the gasserian ganglion level to provide complete analgesia.

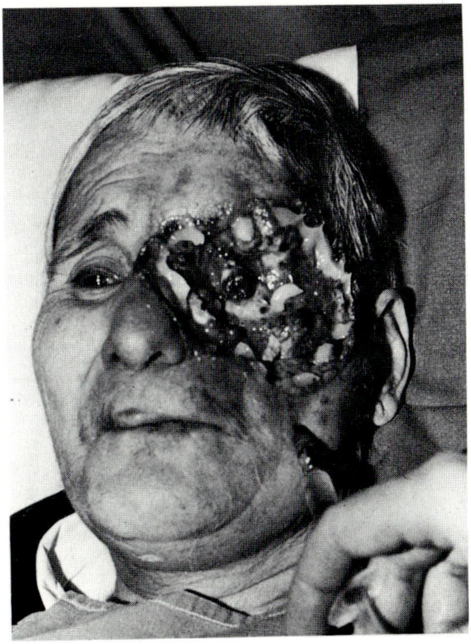

FIG. 3. Advanced carcinoma of the orbit which could not be blocked at the trigeminal division affected by the tumor and also required a gasserian ganglion block.

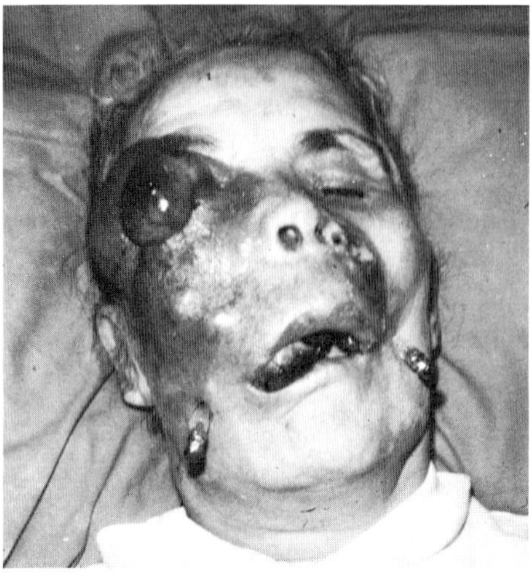

FIG. 4. Advanced cancer which originated in the upper half of the maxillary antrum involving malar, ethmoidal, and orbital structures, and expanding past the midline. In this case it was necessary to block the gasserian ganglion on both sides.

tion of 1 ml of absolute alcohol into the gasserian ganglion produced complete relief. Three months after the block, the patient began to experience diffuse, burning pain over the ipsilateral side of the face. Examination at this time revealed that he still had anesthesia in the distribution of the trigeminal nerve. After three separate cervical sympathetic blocks produced adequate, though not complete, relief of the burning pain, the procedure was repeated with alcohol. By supplementing the blocks with relatively small doses of narcotics several times daily, the patient remained virtually pain-free until he died 5 months later.

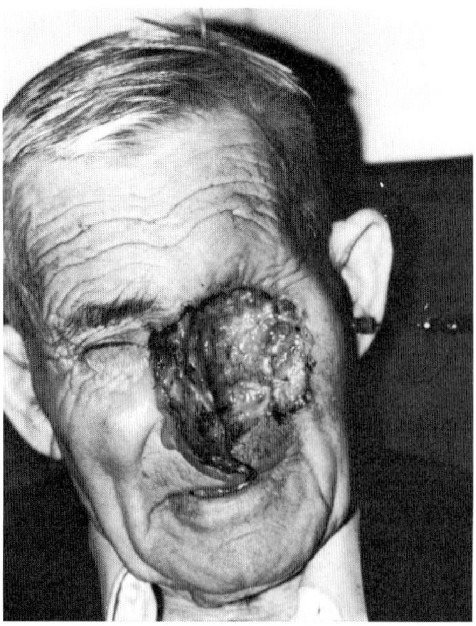

FIG. 5. Invasive and destructive carcinoma treated with alcohol maxillary nerve block by the lateral extra-oral route. Curiously this patient developed a phantom pain at the tip of the nose.

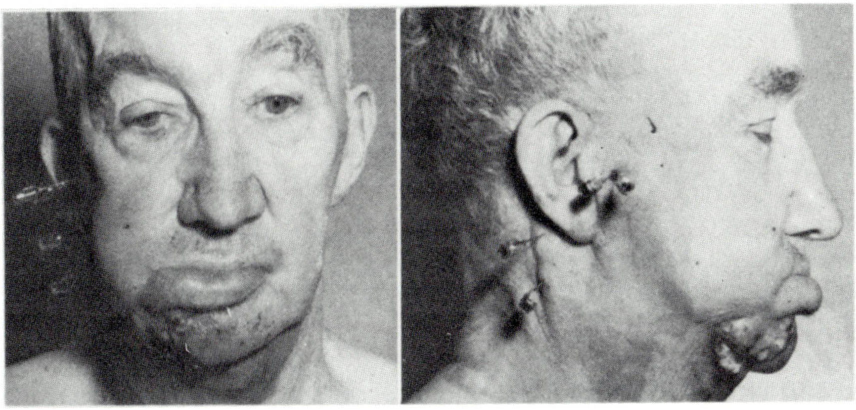

FIG. 6. Patient with cancer of the tongue with invasion of the cheek, lower jaw and chin. Severe pain not relieved by intensive radium and roentgen therapy and large doses of narcotic analgesics, but relieved with alcohol block of the right maxillary, mandibular, and second and third cervical nerves.

When the tumor is localized in the skin of the face, usually it is painless until there is extensive ulceration. Epidermoid carcinoma in the skin of the cheek usually is accompanied by local and referred pain (Fig. 2).

Advanced cancer of the orbit usually spreads to the entire area supplied by the ophthalmic and maxillary divisions of the trigeminal nerve. When the division affected can not be blocked, it is necessary to perform a block at the gasserian ganglion level (Fig. 3).

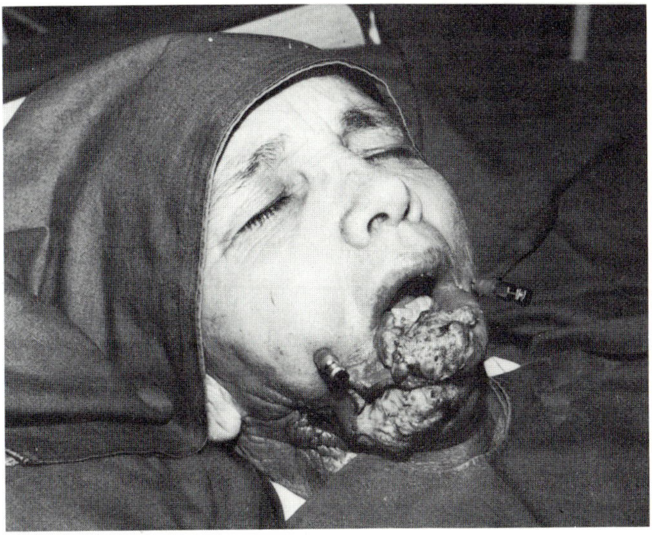

FIG. 7. Epidermoid carcinoma of the lower jaw which invaded both sides of the face. Bilateral gasserian ganglion block.

Advanced cancers originating in the upper half of the maxillary antrum can expand laterally to involve the malar bone, expanding medially to invade the ethmoidal and orbital structures. Moreover they can pass the midline, affecting practically the entire face and requiring a bilateral gasserian ganglion block (Fig. 4).

Block of the branches of the trigeminal nerve can be done in advanced cancer pain of the face. The patient can be blocked by the lateral extra-oral route if the anatomical landmarks are not distorted (Fig. 5).

Figure 6 shows a patient with cancer of the tongue with invasion of the cheek, lower jaw, and chin. Severe pain never relieved by radiation therapy and large doses of narcotic analgesics was effectively relieved with alcohol block of the right maxillary and mandibular nerves and of the second and third cervical nerves.

Epidermoid carcinoma of the lower jaw involves structures supplied by the mandibular nerve and not infrequently invades other areas, requiring block of the cervical nerves to afford relief of pain (Fig. 7).

REFERENCES

1. Bonica, J. J. (1953): *The Management of Pain,* pp. 1445–1466. Lea & Febiger, Philadelphia.
2. Madrid, J. L. (1975): Exferience de 363 cas d'analgesie par alcool et phenol. *Cah. Anesthesiol.,* 23:825–827.

Advances in Pain Research and Therapy, Vol. 2,
edited by J. J. Bonica and V. Ventafridda.
Raven Press, New York © 1979.

Cancer Pain in the Head and Neck: Role of Neurosurgery

Carlo A. Pagni

2nd Chair of Neurosurgery, University of Torino, Torino, Italy

Patients with malignancies of the face, head, and neck often suffer severe pain. Commonly, at the beginning, pain is associated with enlargement of the tumor; and surgery, chemotherapy, and radiotherapy usually afford relief of pain. Intense intractable pain, as a rule, arises only in advanced stages of the disease. When tumor growth can no longer be controlled by anticancer modalities, pain becomes one of the main problems for the patient. Pain is due to various mechanisms: peripheral stimulation of nociceptors due to ulcerative and inflammatory processes; pressure on nerve trunks engulfed by the tumor and fibrosis consequent to surgery and repeated radiation of neoplastic infiltration of nerve trunks and of the base of the skull; and radiodermitis (10,44,60).

At this advanced stage, pain usually is referred to large areas in the peripheral fields of multiple cranial or cervical nerves, bearing no relation to the original tumor site. Sometimes pain is bilateral. Patients usually complain of persistent, progressively increasing pain. A rather common feature is paroxysmal bouts of pain in the face, throat, and ear, which is provoked by talking, mouth movements, or swallowing (preventing food-intake, which worsens the condition of the patient). These agonizing outbursts recall the paroxysmal pain of trigeminal and glossopharyngeal neuralgias. Burning sensations are frequent. Deep-seated pain in the ear is one of the most serious complaints. Other distressing symptoms include difficulty in swallowing, breathing, and talking; loss of taste; dread of repeated bleedings, suffocation, and imminent death. These cause the patient to be depressed and anxious. In spite of these miserable conditions survival is often protracted.

The progressive loss of efficacy of analgesic drugs and the impracticability of peripheral nerve blocks due to the lack of diffusion of drugs in the scleroneoplastic tissues are the causes for referral to the neurosurgeon. Many procedures have been attempted to relieve cancer pain in the head and neck.

TRIGEMINAL OPERATIONS

In pain confined to the trigeminal area, alcohol or phenol blocks of trigeminal branches or ganglion and trigeminal rhizotomy have been attempted (4,18,28,44,54,63). About 50% of patients have satisfactory relief, but detailed information on duration of follow-up and results usually are not reported by the authors. White and Sweet (63) obtained satisfactory relief to time of death or to long follow-up in 17 out of 36 cases. However, partial trigeminal denervation has been shown to have limited efficacy in this kind of cancer pain. In fact, except for very selected cases, patients after trigeminal operation keep complaining of pain in the spared trigeminal areas or in extratrigeminal territories.

MULTIPLE RHIZOTOMIES

Dandy, in 1929 (9), proposed combined rhizotomy of the 5th and 9th root, and if necessary of the upper cervical ones. This method has been used quite extensively with fair results (4,18,30,42,43,44,59,60,63). Advances in anesthesiology and postoperative care permit good results with this operation, which formerly carried a very high operative mortality. Nonetheless, mortality shortly after operation is still high, especially if patients are elderly and in a poor condition. In my series of 12 patients, 1 patient died in the immediate postoperative period, and 4 patients died 15 to 32 days after surgery.

Complete section of the trigeminal and glossopharyngeal nerves is usually successful in affording relief of pain in the face, tongue, jaw, and throat, so that, as White (61) states, this seems not to be the major problem. The rapid disappearance of dysphagia makes swallowing easier and patients quickly gain weight. High cervical and occipital pain is easily controlled by section, bilateral if possible, of the upper cervical roots. Careful search for the second cervical rootlets (which can emerge from the cord above the arch of the atlas) and for a fairly common C_1 root must be made, because both may be easily missed by the unaware surgeon (59,60). Their section is essential for high occipital and submandibular pain-relief.

Deep ear pain is difficult to control. Section of the 5th and 9th nerves is insufficient since the middle ear, tympanic membrane, and external auditory canal are also supplied by the nervus intermedius and by the upper vagal rootlets (45), which must be cut. The use of the operative microscope makes easier identification and section of these rootlets.

Everybody who has used combined rhizotomy agrees that section which includes the 5th, 7th, 9th, upper rootlets of the 10th and upper cervical roots is essential for ample and persistent pain-relief. Unsatisfactory results are usually inadequate denervation of the algogenic areas. Sometimes patients with very long survival, and free from paroxysmal pain, still complain of some discomfort produced by unpleasant sensations in the denervated areas and dryness of the mouth. These and dread of bleeding, suffocation, and death cause the patient to remain anxious and depressed. Therefore, combined therapy with psychotropic drugs may be necessary after rhizotomy.

TRIGEMINAL TRACTOTOMY

Section of the descending root of the trigeminal according to Sjöqvist (51) should block all the pain afferents from the face, because the pain fibers of the 7th, 9th, and 10th enter the descending trigeminal tract collected behind the fibers of the mandibular division of the 5th (29). A few case series have been reported in the literature (18,19,23,29,31,35,38,52,56,62). Usually tractotomy was combined with section of the upper cervical roots to control neck and occipital pain (20,21,56). Gros et al. (20,21) added glossopharyngeal rhizotomy to tractotomy in 27 out of 29 cases, division of the upper rootlets of the 10th in another 7 cases, and cervical rhizotomies in every case.

The reported mortality ranges from 46% (23) to 0% (38). Low mortality is due to better selection of patients, advances in anesthesiology and intensive care, and more frequent use of tracheostomy before operation. Results regarding pain-relief seem to be quite different in the different series. The differences could be due to the different levels of incision, which makes comparison of results difficult; incisions a few mm rostral to the obex could be more effective in producing persistent relief and analgesia than the lower ones, because some fibers of the 5th, 7th, 9th, and 10th might terminate rostral to the obex (62).

In a series of 19 cases, White and Sweet (62), made the incisions above, below, or at the obex level. There were 5 operative deaths, and among the 12 survivors, 7 had recurrence of pain which persisted until death. Subsequent trigeminal rhizotomy did not improve results in some cases. Thus in the opinion of White (61), "medullary tractotomy . . . has not proved to be a successful solution for relief of pain from cancer in the oro-pharynx even if combined with division of the upper cervical sensory roots."

Mracek (38), on the other hand, "successfully performed" medullary tractotomy combined with upper-cervical root section in 12 patients; no other information is given in his short report. Gros et al. (20) reported satisfactory results in a group of 21 patients: 8 of 18 survivors had recurrence of pain or painful dysesthesia, but good relief was obtained by the other 10 patients. In 1969, Gros et al. added 16 new cases of trigeminal tractotomy with satisfactory results (21). It seems to me, however, the good results reported by Gros et al. (20,21) might be due to the fact that in most of the patients they added section of glossopharyngeal nerve, upper rootlets of the vagus, and cervical nerve roots. This emphasizes the need for multiple rhizotomy in order to do ample and sustained pain-relief.

Recently Crue et al. (8) and Hitchcock (26) attempted stereotaxic percutaneous lesion of the trigeminal tract in a few cases. Localization of the tract was based on radiological coordinates, recording of evoked potentials, and clinical effects of stimulations. The procedure produced good results, and it seems indicated in patients in very poor condition.

MESENCEPHALIC TRACTOTOMY

In 1936, Serra and Neri (49) made the first section of quintothalamic fibers at the level of the pons for cancer pain of the face. Then Dogliotti (11,12) introduced spino- and quintothalamic tractotomy at the mesencephalic level. However, the procedure was employed only in a few cases (1,5,13,58). Open mesencephalic tractotomy, in spite of the fact it seemed appropriate to control face and head pain, was abandoned because of the high operative mortality and complications.

The operation was attempted again after the introduction of stereotaxic technique by Spiegel and Wycis (53). Stereotactic mesencephalic tractotomy seems devoid of high operative risks and complications. Only series of a few cases, however, have been reported (25,35,64). Furthermore, results seemed generally very poor (25,64). In 1976, Mazars et al. (37) reported excellent results in an impressive series of 76 cases of head cancer pain. There were neither major complications, nor operative mortality; the risk of occurrence of central pain was minimal (37). Suppression of pain was achieved in 68 out of 76 patients (89%). Unfortunately, detailed results of long-term follow-up are not available. Mazars et al. (37) state categorically that stereotaxic mesencephalotomy is the procedure of choice for pain of the head and neck, and only the lack of experience with it led to the introduction of other less-valuable procedures. Nashold (39) and Voris and Whisler (57) share this opinion and say they prefer mesencephalotomy to multiple rhizotomy.

STEREOTACTIC THALAMOTOMY

Stereotaxic lesions were produced simultaneously at thalamic level in the VPM and CM-Pf-intralaminar nuclei by many surgeons (24,32,40,41,42). The purpose was to block nociceptive impulses bound for the VPM and for so-called "polysynaptic pathways" with the hope of obtaining more-lasting analgesia and relief of pain. Everybody reported "inadequate pain-relief" or "some subjective relief from pain;" every surgeon, however, treated usually only a few cases.

According to Mark et al. (33,34) lesions of the CM-Pf-intralaminar complex which did not produce sensory defects or central pain were sufficient to suppress pain in 12 out of 13 patients. Fairman (14) obtained similar results in 9 cases. In my experience (40,41,42) unilateral lesions exactly targeted on the CM-Pf-intralaminar complex, with minimal involvement of the VPM or other thalamic nuclei, yield only very transient results with recurrence of pain usually in a few days. Voris and Whisler (57) reported similar experience. Careful review of the case reports of Mark et al. (33) reveals that psychic disturbances (confusion, disorientation, memory loss) were recorded. Furthermore their anatomic studies (34) indicated lesions involved the CM nucleus. I wonder whether pain-relief in their patients might have been due to minor leukotomy effects.

I achieved somewhat better results (40,41,42) with combined destruction of the VPM, VPL, CM-Pf-intralaminar and limitans nuclei; the lesions included the thalamo-midbrain junction impinging on the midbrain, the PO region, and the pulvinar. Only patients who died within 2 months of the operation obtained permanent relief; otherwise, there was recurrence of pain (40,41). Lesions including the VPM-VPL nuclei of course entailed the risk of occurrence of central pain (6,40). Tasker (55) obtained permanent relief in 14 out of 19 patients, whose average survival was 4 months, with combined lesions of the VPL, VPM, CM-Pf-intralaminar complex; in 5 cases there was recurrence in a few weeks or months. Thus it seems thalamotomy can afford relief of pain in patients with short life-expectancy, usually for no longer than a few weeks.

Therefore I read with the highest interest the papers of Fairman (15) and Sano (48). Fairman (15) submitted 104 patients to (apparently unilateral) CM-Pf-intralaminar thalamotomy. Sano (48) performed bilateral destruction of the CM-Pf-intralaminar complex ("thalamolaminotomy"). In both series incidence of complications was very low and there was no operative mortality. Mild psychic disturbances cleared up in a few days. "Satisfactory relief of pain—without sensory disturbances—i.e., no pain at all or some tolerable pain no longer requiring narcotic analgesics was obtained in 70% of all the patients. The pain-relief lasted for the entire period of survival, which ranged between 2 and 12 months. . . ." (15); pain was liable to recur only "several months later" (48). In spite of these extraordinarily valuable results, not yet duplicated by others, both Fairman (15) and Sano (48) introduced unilateral or bilateral destruction of the posterior hypothalamus, which is believed to play an important role in the emotional-motivational aspects of pain. This "posteromedial hypothalamotomy" produced results which were better than those achieved with "thalamolaminotomy."

Richardson (47) and Cooper et al. (7) reported excellent pain-relief could be achieved by means of pulvinar lesions. Since then, some cases of head cancer pain were submitted to unilateral or bilateral pulvinectomy (41,50). Experience is limited, but so far it seems pulvinectomy does not improve upon the results of thalamic surgery for pain (17,41,50).

PSYCHOSURGERY

Leukotomy was employed in small series of cases, especially for bilateral pain (63). Pain-relief was very satisfactory, both with large, bilateral transection of the frontal white matter, or with transection limited to the lower frontal quadrants. Sadly, "although these subjects were relieved of pain and suffering . . . apathy and psychologic deterioration were severe" (63). In unilateral extensive leukotomy, too, pain-relief was accompanied by some degree of mental confusion and apathy (63). Large frontal lesions made in a one-stage procedure, make the patient disoriented and apathetic. If lesions of the same size are made in increments over a period of days, or if small lesions are made at short intervals, it is possible to obtain relief of pain without sensibly handicapping the patient's mentation (22). Thus White and Sweet (63) introduced graduated bilateral coagulation of medial frontal white matter. By means of implanted unipolar electrodes an area of fronto-thalamic projection fibers, a centimeter in diameter, is destroyed on both sides. Another two or three such lesions are made at intervals of several days. The patient may be made free from concern about pain, dread of strangulation, death, etc. Destruction of the frontal white matter can be stopped before severe mental deterioration ensues.

Cingulotomy was introduced by Folz and White (16). In the cingulum run pathways mediating activities of the limbic system to the anterior thalamus and the forebrain, which play a major role in emotional behavior. The hope was to modify the patient's emotional response to pain, thus relieving suffering, with only minor psychic impairment. The changes effected by cingulotomy seem identical to those effected by leukotomy; however, these effects appear less damaging to the intellectual faculties (2,27). Folz and White (16) obtained excellent relief, at 6- to 18-months follow-up, with unilateral or bilateral lesions of the cingulum in a group of patients who showed marked emotional reaction to pain with enhancement of their complaints of pain. Rétif et al. (46) obtained poor results in 1 patient.

Bertrand et al. (3) introduced the stereotaxic section of the frontothalamic pathways, on one or both sides, as they lie in the anterior limb of the internal capsule. The operation was performed on 5 patients; all were free from pain and "well oriented" some weeks or months after the operation.

The conservative methods of modern psychosurgery seem to allow good control of pain with moderate psychic impairment. In my own limited experience, however, pain-relief has always been associated with psychic disturbances.

FINAL REMARKS

In head and neck cancer pain, extension of painful areas to territories of multiple cranial and cervical nerves, bilaterality of pain, and psychologic distress due to a devastating disease making patients anxious and depressed make treatment one of the most arduous problems that the neurosurgeon has to cope with. Many surgical procedures have been attempted. There is no consensus about the efficacy and limitations of various methods.

In my opinion two factors should guide the surgeon in the choice of operation: the patient's condition and life-expectancy. If the patient's condition is good and life-expectancy long, multiple rhizotomy is the most useful operation because it assures long-lasting relief. In spite of advances in anesthesiology and intensive care, multiple rhizotomy always carries a certain operative risk. Therefore in the patient in a poor condition with short life-expectancy (limited to 2 or 3 months) stereotaxic surgery is to be preferred, as operative risks are minimal and patients can expect relief as long as they will survive.

Thalamic lesions should be large enough to affect a major part of the VPM-VPL, CM, Pf, intralaminar and limitans nuclei contralateral to the painful side. Such large lesions usually involve the lower part of the dorsomedial nucleus, adding a minor leukotomic effect which may play an important role in producing relief of pain and suffering. Bilateral "thalamolaminotomy" or "hypothalamotomy" (15,48), as well as mesencephalotomy (37) might be more rewarding, but I have no experience with them.

Trigeminal tractotomy either by open or stereotaxic technique in my opinion can be abandoned; the best results are achieved only in association with rhizotomy of the cervical, glossopharyngeal, and vagal rootlets (20, 21,56).

In bilateral pain, psychosurgery, by means of graduated bilateral coagulation of medial frontal white matter (63) or of cingulotomy (16,27) seems to allow good control of pain with moderate psychic impairment.

REFERENCES

1. Bailey, R. A., Glees, P., and Oppenheimer, D. R. (1954): Midbrain tractotomy: A surgical and clinical report with observations on ascending and descending tract degeneration. *Mschr. Psychiat. Neurol.,* 127:316–335.
2. Ballantine, H. T., Cassidy, W. L., Flanagan, N. B., and Marino, R. (1967): Stereotaxic anterior cingulotomy for neuropsychiatric illness and intractable pain. *J. Neurosurg.,* 26:488–495.
3. Bertrand, C., Martinez, N., and Hardy, J. (1966): Frontothalamic section for intractable pain. In: *Pain,* edited by R. S. Knighton and P. R. Dumke, pp. 531–535. Little, Brown, Boston.
4. Botterell, E. H. (1961): Discussion to Parsons H., Opérations sur les nerfs craniens et les racines cervicales postérieures pour d'autres formes de névralgie et de douleur dans des affections malignes. *Excerpta Med. Intern. Congr. Series,* 36:31.
5. Brihaye, J., Thiry, S., LeClercq, R., Rétif, J., and Grégoire, A. (1962): Le traitement chirurgical de la douleur. *Acta Chir. Belg.* [*Suppl.*], 2:255–457.
6. Cassinari, V., and Pagni, C. A. (1969): *Central Pain. A Neurosurgical Survey.* Harvard University Press, Cambridge, Mass.
7. Cooper, I. S., Amin, I., Chandra, R., and Waltz, J. M. (1973): A surgical investigation of the clinical physiology of the LP-Pulvinar complex in man. *J. Neurol. Sci.,* 18:89–110.
8. Crue, B. L., Todd, E. M., and Carregal, E. J. A. (1970): Percutaneous radiofrequency stereotaxic trigeminal tractotomy. In: *Pain and Suffering: Selected Aspects,* edited by B. L. Crue, pp. 69–80. Charles C Thomas, Springfield, Ill.
9. Dandy, W. E. (1929): Operative relief from pain in lesions of the mouth, tongue, and throat. *Arch. Surg.,* 19:143–148.
10. Dodd, G. D., Dolan, P. A., Ballantyne, A. J., Ibanez, M. L., and Chau, P. (1970): The dissemination of tumors of the head and neck via the cranial nerves. *Radiol. Clinics North Am.,* 8:445–461.

11. Dogliotti, A. M. (1937): Trattamento del dolore nei tumori. *Min. Med.*, 28:455–461.
12. Dogliotti, A. M. (1938): First surgical sections in man, of the lemniscus lateralis (pain-temperature path) at the brain stem, for treatment of diffused rebellious pain. *Anesth. Analg.*, 17:143–145
13. Drake, C. G., and McKenzie, K. G. (1953): Mesencephalic tractotomy for pain. Experience with six cases. *J. Neurosurg.*, 10:457–462.
14. Fairman, D. (1966): Evaluation of results in stereotactic thalamotomy for the treatment of intractable pain. *Confin. Neurol.*, 27:67–70.
15. Fairman, D. (1976): Neurophysiological basis for hypothalamic lesion and stimulation by chronic implanted electrodes for the relief of intractable pain in cancer. In: *Advances in Pain Research and Therapy. Vol. 1: Proceedings of the First World Congress on Pain,* edited by J. J. Bonica and D. Albe-Fessard, pp. 843–847. Raven Press, New York.
16. Folz, E. L., and White, L. E. (1966): Rostral cingulotomy and pain "relief." In: *Pain,* edited by R. S. Knighton and P. R. Dumke, pp. 469–491. Little, Brown, Boston.
17. Fraioli, B., and Guidetti, B. (1975): Effects of stereotactic lesions of the pulvinar and lateralis posterior nucleus on intractable pain and dyskinetic syndromes of man. *Applied Neurophysiol.*, 38:23–30.
18. Grant, F. C. (1943): Surgical methods for relief of pain. *Bull. N.Y. Acad. Med.*, 19:373–385.
19. Gros, Cl., Vlahovitch, B., Jourdan, D., and Solassol, A. (1954): Traitement neurochirurgical des algies cranio-faciales d'origine cancereuses. *Sem. Hôp.*, 30:1947–1949.
20. Gros, Cl., Cordier, M., Vlahovitch, B., and Roilgen, A. (1963): Neurotomie combinée et traitement des algies cervico-cranio-faciales d'origine neoplasique., *Ann. Chir.*, 17:533–539.
21. Gros, Cl. (1969): *Montpellier Chir.*, 15:53
22. Hackett, T. P., White, J. C., and Sweet, W. H. (1966): Leukotomy for the relief of pain: The selection of cases and psychological hazards. In: *Pain,* edited by R. S. Knighton and P. R. Dumke, pp. 461–467. Little, Brown, Boston.
23. Hamby, W. B., Shinners, B. M., and Marsh, I. A. (1948): Trigeminal tractotomy. Observations on forty-eight cases. *Arch. Surg.*, 57:171–177.
24. Hassler, R., and Riechert, T. (1959): Klinische und anatomische Befunde bei stereotaktischen Schmerzoperationen im Thalamus. *Arch. Psychiat. Nervenkr.*, 200: 93–122.
25. Helfant, M. H., Leksell, L., and Strang, R. R. (1965): Experiences with intractable pain treated by stereotaxic mesencephalotomy. *Acta Chir. Scand.*, 129:573–580.
26. Hitchcock, E. (1970): Stereotactic trigeminal tractotomy. *Ann. Clin. Res.*, 2:131–135.
27. Hurt, R. W., and Ballantine, H. I. (1974): Stereotactic anterior cingulate lesions for persistent pain: A report on 68 cases. *Clin. Neurosurg.*, 21:334–351.
28. Jefferson, A. (1963): Trigeminal root and ganglion injections using phenol in glycerine for the relief of trigeminal neuralgia. *J. Neurol. Neurosurg. Psychiatry*, 26:345–352.
29. Kunc, Z. (1964): *Tractus spinalis nervi trigemini. Fresh anatomic data and their significance for surgery.* Nakladatelstvì Ceskoslovenské Akadamie. Vêd, Praha.
30. Lapras, C., Fisher, G., and Trouillias, P. (1968): Radicotomie combinée dans le traitement des douleurs cervico-faciales d'origine neoplasique. *Lyon Chir.*, 64:548–556.
31. Le Beau, J., and Billet, R. (1953): Tractotomie bulbare trigeminale et nevralgie du glossopharyngien. *Rev. Neurol.*, 88:265–271.
32. Le Beau, J., Lecasble, R., Choppy, M., and Dondey, M. (1966): Stéréo-thalamotomies localisées pour le traitement des douleurs irréductibles. *Confin. Neurol.*, 27:56–62.
33. Mark, V. H., Ervin, F. R., and Hackett, T. P. (1960): Clinical aspects of stereotactic thalamotomy in the human. I. The treatment of chronic severe pain. *Arch. Neurol.*, 3:351–367.
34. Mark, V. H., Ervin, F. R., and Yakovlev, P. I. (1963): Stereotactic thalamotomy.

III. Verification of anatomical lesion site in the human thalamus. *Arch. Neurol.,* 8:528–538.
35. McKenzie, K. G. (1955): Trigeminal tractotomy. *Clin. Neurosurg.,* 2:50–69.
36. Mazars, G., Rogé, R., and Pansini, A. (1960): Stereotactic coagulation of the spinothalamic tract for intractable trigeminal pain. *J. Neurol. Neurosurg. Psychiatry,* 23:352.
37. Mazars, G., Merienne, L., and Cioloca, C. (1976): État actuel de la chirurgie de la douleur. *Neuro-Chir.* 22, *Suppl.* 1:1–164.
38. Mracek, Z. (1977): Surgical management of intractable pain due to malignant tumors in the face and neck. *J. Neurosurg. Sci.,* 21:123–125.
39. Nashold, B. S. (1972): Extensive cephalic and oral pain relieved by midbrain tractotomy. *Confin. Neurol.,* 34:382.
40. Pagni, C. A. (1966): Discussion to Ervin, F. R., Brown, C. E., and Mark, V. H. Striatal influence on facial pain. *Confin. Neurol.,* 27:88–89.
41. Pagni, C. A. (1974): Place of stereotactic technique in surgery for pain. In: *Advances in Neurology, Vol. 4: International Symposium on Pain,* edited by J. J. Bonica, pp. 699–706. Raven Press, New York.
42. Pagni, C. A., and Maspes, P. E. (1970): Problems in the surgical treatment of pain in malignancies of the head and neck. In: *Current Problems in Neurosciences,* edited by H. T. Wycis, pp. 138–153. Karger, Basel.
43. Pagni, C. A., Maspes, P. E., Visca, A., and Bollati, A. (1969): Riflessioni sul problema del trattamento chirurgico delle algie cranio-cervico-faciali da neoplasia maligna mediante radicotomie multiple. *Min. Neurochir.,* 13:29–33.
44. Parsons, H. (1961): Opérations sur les nerves crâniens et les racines cervicales postérieures pour d'autres formes de nevralgie et de douleur dans les affections malignes. *Excerpta Med. Int. Congr. Ser.,* 36:30–31.
45. Peele, T. L. (1954): *The Neuroanatomical Basis for Clinical Neurology.* McGraw-Hill Book Co., New York.
46. Rétif, J., Crahay, S., and Brihaye, J. (1966): Leucotomie frontale a minima avec interruption sélective du faisceau cingulaire, uni o bilatérale, dans le traitement chirurgical de la douleur. *Acta Neurol. Psych. Belg.,* 66:499–513.
47. Richardson, D. E. (1967): Thalamotomy for intractable pain. *Confin. Neurol.,* 29:139–145.
48. Sano, K. (1977): Intralaminar thalamotomy (Thalamolaminotomy) and posterior medial hypothalamotomy in the treatment of intractable pain. In: *Pain—Its Neurosurgical Management. Part II: Central Procedures,* edited by H. Krayenbühl, P. E. Maspes, and W. H. Sweet, pp. 50–103. Karger, Basel.
49. Serra, A., and Neri, V. (1936): Die elektro-chirurgische Unterbrechung der Zentralbahnen des V Paares am lateralen ventrale Rand des Pons Varoli als erster Behandlungsversuch von hartnätigen Neuralgien des Trigeminus durch Tumoren des Schadelbasis. *Zbl. Chir.,* 63:2248–2251.
50. Siegfried, J. (1977): Stereotactic pulvinarotomy in the treatment of intractable pain. In: *Pain—Its Neurosurgical Management. Part II: Central Procedures,* edited by H. Krayenbühl, P. E. Maspes, and W. H. Sweet, pp. 104–113. Karger, Basel.
51. Sjöqvist, O. (1938): Studies on pain conduction in the trigeminal nerve. A contribution to the surgical treatment of facial pain. *Acta Psychiatr. Scand.* [*Suppl.*], 17:1–139.
52. Sjöqvist, O. (1950): La section chirurgicale des cordons et des voies de la douleur dans la moelle et le tronc cerebral. *Rev. Neurol.,* 83:38–40.
53. Spiegel, E. A., Wycis, H. T., Marks, M., and Lee, A. J. (1947): Stereotaxic apparatus for operations on the human brain. *Science,* 106:349–350.
54. Sweet, W. H. (1976): Controlled thermocoagulation of trigeminal ganglion rootlets for differential destruction of pain fibers: Facial pain other than trigeminal neuralgia. *Clin. Neurosurg.,* 23:96–102.
55. Tasker, R. R. (1975): Neurological concepts of pain management in head and neck cancer. *Can. J. Otolaryngol.,* 4:480–484.
56. Vlahovitch, B., Fuentes, J. M., Choncair, Y., Moreau, P., and Pascal, M. (1976):

Gestes complementaires à l'operation de Sjöqvist dans les algies cancéreuses cervico-faciales. *Neuro-chir.*, 22:503–515.
57. Voris, H. C., and Whisler, W. W. (1975): Results of stereotaxic surgery for intractable pain. *Confin. Neurol.*, 37:86–96.
58. Walker, E. A. (1942): Relief of pain by mesencephalic tractotomy. *Arch. Neurol. Psychiatry*, 48:865–883.
59. Wetzel, N. (1959): Neurosurgical procedures for the control of intractable pain in malignancies of the head and neck. *Am. J. Surg.*, 98:800–804.
60. Wetzel, N. (1966): The relief of pain in malignant disease in the head and neck by sensory root section. In: *Pain*, edited by R. S. Knighton and P. R. Dumke, pp. 431–437. Little, Brown, Boston.
61. White, J. C. (1962): Evaluation of operation for relief of pain. *Neurol. Med-Chir.*, 4:1–28.
62. White, J. C., and Sweet, W. H. (1955): *Pain. Its Mechanisms and Neurosurgical Control.* Charles C Thomas, Springfield, Ill.
63. White, J. C., and Sweet, W. H. (1969): *Pain and the Neurosurgeon. A Forty Years Experience.* Charles C Thomas, Springfield, Ill.
64. Wycis, H. T., and Spiegel, E. A. (1962): Long-range results in the treatment of intractable pain by stereotaxic midbrain surgery. *J. Neurosurg.*, 19:101–106.

Discussion

Part II. Management of Pain of Advanced Cancer: Therapy of Cancer Pain in the Head and Neck

R. Molinari and M. Tiengo (Moderators)

Questioner: Dr. Molinari, what are the complications of intra-arterial administration in chemotherapy of tumors of the head and neck?

Molinari (Milano): The main risk is of pushing the catheter too low, causing the passage of the dose into the internal common carotid and cerebral complications that are, nevertheless, reversible. The most frequent complication is local arteritis. In about 15% of cases, one cannot cannulate the artery for anatomic reasons.

Questioner: Dr. Pagni, what is your experience with the technique of cisternal infusion with cold hypertonic salt solution?

Pagni (Torino): I have used cold salt solution and hypertonic salt solution for pain of the lower limbs, not for this type of pain, with relief never lasting longer than 3 weeks. Many people perform instead a phenolic block with intracisternal phenol. Personally, I have never done a phenolic block of the nerves of the posterior fossa.

Questioner: Dr. Houde, what is your experience in using corticosteroids, notably solumedrol, to control pain?

Houde (New York): We use the corticosteroids as an adjuvant in patients who have special forms and types of problems, primarily associated with increased intracranial pressure or massive edema; and, in these circumstances, you have to recognize the dangers of using steroids, particularly in patients in whom there may be a risk of producing or precipitating a gastric hemorrhage. The drug we use is dexamethazone in fairly high doses, going up to about 16 mg a day and tapering off during the course of a few weeks.

Advances in Pain Research and Therapy, Vol. 2,
edited by J. J. Bonica and V. Ventafridda.
Raven Press, New York © 1979.

Role of Oncologic Therapy in Pain Involving the Chest and Brachial Plexus

Georges Brulé

Medical Oncology Unit, Institut Gustave-Roussy, 94800 Villejuif, France

Pain in the chest may become manifest by major functional signs, e.g., cough, dyspnea, dysphagia, pain either localized in the precordial or in the pleural region. Bone metastasis or infiltration of the brachial plexus by the tissue may cause cervicobrachial or intercostal neuralgia or pain spread over the ribs, the shoulder blade, or the upper limb. Compression of large veins occurs, leading to edema of the face or arms. All these manifestations appear either as an initial sign of the disease or more often at the terminal phase when the patient has already received numerous courses of treatment.

At this stage, the three main therapeutic weapons available in the oncologic armamentorium may still be used: surgery, radiation, or various medical disciplines such as chemotherapy, hormone therapy, or adjuvant medication. The contribution of each of these approaches is discussed briefly.

SURGERY

In case of recurrent and ulcerated breast tumor with involvement of radionecrosis, instead of attempting a radical extensive surgical excision, it seems preferable to proceed with an epiploplasty. The procedure implies stemming the epiploon under the skin and filling up the loss of tissue (following excision of the tumor and radionecrosis) and covering the flap with a dermoepidermal graft. Over the last few years, at Institut Gustave-Roussy, some 50 patients (11) have undergone this type of surgery followed by extremely satisfactory results occurring either immediately or after a period of time. Most patients who died some months after the procedure remained comfortable, and death was not due to local or regional recurrence, but a result of distant complications.

The chest surgeon may also have to interfere in case of isolated pulmonary metastases, particularly if the latter occurs distally near the pleura causing either unceasing bouts of cough or pain. Surgery may extend from partial resection of an isolated metastasis to pneumonectomy or lobectomy.

The neurosurgeon may also become involved in patients manifesting signs of intraspinal neoplastic lesion by performing a laminectomy, which at times prevents paraplegia and relieves the patient's pain.

For carcinoma of the esophagus which despite radiation therapy progresses to the final stage of dysphagia, two techniques may be used. One is the simple Fontan-type gastrostomy which involves opening of a cone of gastric wall sutured to the skin. Special attention must be paid to make sure that reflux through the slit of anastomosis does not occur. Such a direct gastrostomy makes frequent and easy change of the sound possible. With endoscopy, an attempt may be made to insert a cannula through the tumor.

Finally, mention must be made of the value of emergency low tracheotomy for patients showing a high compression of the trachea. The ideal incision is made between the 2nd and 3rd tracheal cartilage under the cricoid cartilage at one finger's breadth above the upper edge of the sternum with the patient's head extended. In case of tracheal tumor, the incision must be made lower, after sternotomy is done and a long cannula is inserted.

Major surgical interventions for tumors of the posterior mediastinum, such as neurinomas, which are usually cured by the operation done before intense pain occurs have not been included. Finally, it may be mentioned that some clinicians still use pleural talc-dusting in recurring metastatic pleural discharge. After drainage of the pleural fluid, the pleura is sealed by the injection of talcum via a trocar. The success of this technique depends on the flexibility of the pleura. Previous radiation therapy of the thoracic wall is a contraindication to the technique.

RADIATION

In regard to the use of radiation therapy, I will discuss exclusively cases involving recurrent or metastatic cancers. Two questions usually arise:

1. Is it possible to resume radiotherapy for a previously irradiated zone?
2. What are the various methods and procedures for palliative irradiation of antalgic interest?

The protocols of irradiation which have been used in the past for treating patients showing recurrence were often crude, and the pattern of dose distribution could be considerably improved by more sophisticated techniques (12). These include individualized beam-shaping by especially tailored lead blocks, by combination of various types of radiation (for instance, photons and electrons), or association of beam therapy and interstitial therapy, a combination that has been made more reliable through the help of computer dosimetry.

The use of a large number of fields (of various sizes, shapes, weight, etc.) considerably improves the dose distribution, but there is an increased risk of errors during the set-up of the patient.

In our institute, radiotherapists have worked out a particular type of palliative irradiation composed of 2 sessions of 8.50 greys (or 850 rads or

650 rads) or 6.50 greys delivered at 48-hr interval. This concentrated irradiation is well tolerated and is most useful for palliative radiotherapy (7). Without considering the radiobiologic problem, it may be said that 3,000 centigreys (15 × 200) in 3 weeks is equivalent to 2 × 850 centigreys in 2 days or 3 × 635 centigreys or 4 × 500 centigreys. Clinical experience shows good tolerance of the normal tissues. Skin and mucosal reactions appear 1 week earlier than for fractionated irradiation, but their maximum is the same and their repair takes no longer. This technique is very handy for carcinoma of the esophagus with very poor prognosis. Over a group of 44 patients, dysphagia was definitely improved in 65% of cases and gastrotomy could be delayed.

Mediastinal Compression

Mediastinal compression due to tumor is managed differently by different radiotherapists. Because of fear of edematous reactions, it is often advised to carry out irradiation with small doses over a long period of time. However, severe compression with vascular and respiratory obstruction requires very prompt relief even at the risk of the use of concentrated radiation therapy. Clinical experience with 14 patients with severe mediastinal compression has shown that these risks are actually limited when doses of 2 × 6.50 centigreys (equivalent to 22.50 greys in 3 weeks) are used.

Of the 14 patients, 13 improved rapidly. Improvement was evident during the first week and in 50% of cases it was evident on the third day. Moderate reactions (nausea in 2 patients, thoracic pain in 4 cases, and marked dyspnea in 2) appeared within a few hours after the first session and lasted about 3 hr. They were less frequent after the second session. The most interesting results concern 7 patients with alarming symptoms of severe respiratory obstruction. In 6, concentrated irradiation caused an immediate relief. Mean survival time was 4 months, extending to a maximum of 12 months.

Bone Metastasis

Concentrated irradiation was used for patients with multiple, painful metastasis of the spine, the ribs, or other sites in order to obtain rapid relief of pain and avoid long-term treatment. The doses used were 2 × 6.50 greys or 2 × 8.50 greys, depending on the extent of the treated volume, the site, and the general condition of the patient. No major side effects were noticed even upon treatment of 3 sites simultaneously. Pain was completely relieved in 35% of patients and significantly 1 week after irradiation. The average duration of the remission lasted 2 months. A second irradiation for recurring pain was usually less effective than the first.

CHEMOTHERAPY

Intra-arterial chemotherapy, a technique which has been widely used, may be employed for lesions of the upper limb, including osteosarcoma, melanoma, or any conjunctive tumor. It may also be injected via the external mammary route when the neoplasm is located in the thoracic wall or the breast (1).

Our own experience at Institut Gustave-Roussy, which dates back 10 years, and the published report on the use of the regional chemotherapy reveal that this has no advantage over the systemic route. Moreover, this procedure is difficult and requires complex equipment. It keeps the patient in bed and leads to complications which are not only systemic but also local, vascular, or cutaneous disorders. For all these reasons, this method was definitely given up.

On the other hand, local or regional chemotherapy is still being successfully used for the treatment of pleural discharge. In this case, local therapy is easier to apply than talc-dusting. I will not consider intrapleural injection of colloidal gold, which has been used for some 10 years. Because of the high cost and special care required for the life-duration of this isotope, therapy with colloidal gold has been abandoned, except maybe in some centers in Switzerland. Intrapleural injections of drugs may be highly effective, provided the proper agent is chosen. Alkylating agents are among the most active drugs, and two of them appear much better than average. The first is Thiotepa® and the second Mannomustine® or Degranol® (1). Easy to handle, these products cause local necrosis at injection-site less frequently than pure nitrogen mustard and unlike cyclophosphamide do not need to be metabolized hepatically to be active.

New liposoluble derivates of podophyllotoxin have been recently introduced. Vehem 26 and VP16 offer the advantage of crossing the seromeningeal or pleural barrier and seem to be as active by the systemic route as by the local route (2). Local intrapleural chemotherapy has considerable advantages; it is not toxic because the product does not diffuse through the pleura and therefore does not cause general hematologic or digestive toxic manifestations as alkylating agents do.

Amongst the increasing number of antimitotic agents available to the oncologist, for therapy of recurrent cancer it is essential to choose the substance which shows the least crossed resistance with previously used drugs. Subcutaneous injection of methotrexate, 6 mg/m^2/day × 4 injections at exactly 6-hr intervals gives satisfactory results in intradermal or cutaneous local or regional recurrence of breast cancer, by reducing the lesion and producing relief of local pain (3). In extended forms of breast cancer, with bone and lymph node involvement, adriamycin-vincristine-methotrexate seems to be the most effective therapeutic combination. It is also used as the initial treatment in breast cancer in preparation for irradiation and possibly surgery. In over 35% of the patients, the primary tumor and nodes are considerably reduced by decreasing the inflammatory reactions of these very rapidly growing tumors (6).

Unfortunately, no chemotherapeutic combination with marked activity in bronchial cancer is available. This also holds true for the resultant compression phenomena, which are usually better controlled by radiotherapy. Nonetheless cyclophosphamide seems to be the most frequent treatment for bronchial oat-cell carcinoma and the local phenomena which they cause. Cyclophosphamide may be used either alone or in combination with nitrourea derivatives.

Mediastinal compression linked with hematosarcoma, particularly immunoblastic lymphosarcomas at times react dramatically with vincristine, a derivative of periwinkle. This response is so consistent that some writers have used it as a therapeutic test if histologic examination proves doubtful. Unfortunately, this dramatic action does not last long and relapse occurs rapidly. The same applies for the effectiveness of bleomycin, mithramycin, and possibly *Cis*-platinum (diamine dichloride) in very rapidly growing pulmonary metastasis of embryonic carcinomas. Often these three products give dramatic results, but unfortunately the benefit is of short duration. Mithramycin has been given up by most clinicians because of its toxicity when administered in effective doses. The combination of bleomycin-*Cis*-platinum and vinblastine seems to give somewhat longer and more frequent remission than when each product is used separately (8).

Combined treatment with radiation and drugs is often used in the treatment of breast cancer, in severe forms of Hodgkin's disease, and in embryonic malignant tumors of the mediastinum in both children and adults. Without going into very complex radiobiological explanations, it is known that cells under formation are radioresistant and yet very sensitive to antimitotic drugs, whereas cells in phase G 1 and not under multiplication are chemoresistant but may be destroyed by radiation. Unfortunately, while this combination is highly effective in damaging tumoral tissues, it also increases normal tissue reaction leading to intense skin or pulmonary manifestations.

Finally, it must be pointed out that addition of heparin to antimitotic drugs, particularly in case of bronchopulmonary cancer seems to potentiate significantly the action of chemotherapy without aggravating the toxicity of these substances.

HORMONE THERAPY

Most forms of pain in the chest and cervicobrachial region in the female result from terminal stages of breast cancer. Therefore reference to hormonal treatment must be made when discussing this subject.

Without discussing the physiology of hormone therapy, hormones may be classified into three groups, each apparently acting specifically on a certain type of lesion. In the elderly female, estrogens, diethylstilbestrol in particular, often exert a striking effect on large, ulcerated and painful lesions. Within 6 to 8 weeks this medication causes disappearance or marked regression of ulcerative and painful lesions extending over a large surface.

Androgens, particularly synthetic androgens, are indicated for younger females. At Institut Gustave-Roussy, we use drostalonone propionate which has the least-virilizing side effects. These synthetic androgens are remarkably effective, especially on bone metastatic lesions of ribs, vertebrae, etc. (4).

High doses of progestational agents, particularly medroxyprogesterone acetate, which is the best tolerated of all such agents and which may be given at high dose by the oral route, often cause complete disappearance of intrapulmonary parenchymatous nodules (10).

Anti-estrogen agents form the latest introduction in hormone therapy. Tamoxifene is by far the easiest to handle. An extensive study of this product during the last few years has revealed that it is somewhat less effective in bone metastasis than are androgens. On the other hand, it is most effective for all metastatic skin nodes and bone lesions of breast cancer. In particular, in the female with primary tumor containing progesterone and estrogen receptors, dramatic results are frequently obtained by combining drostalonone propionate and tamoxifene in case of chemoresistant metastatic dissemination (5).

Major endocrine surgery (i.e., adrenalectomy or hypophysectomy) may yield dramatic relief of bone pain, especially in patients in whom metastasis occurs long after the primary lesion and who have become resistant to hormone therapy.

Finally, as a last resort in the terminal stage, high-dose corticoid medication may improve the patient's general condition. Amongst corticoids prescribed by us, methylprednisolone is particularly well tolerated with hardly any side effects (9). The product is given as a single intravenous injection in the morning, the dose varying between 40 and 300 mg. As reported by other writers, methylprednisolone exerts palliative effects not only on pain but also on dyspnea and cough. This may last several weeks, so that some bed-ridden patients do get up and resume normal life for some time. No satisfactory physiologic explanation seems obvious to justify this beneficial action which other corticoids, being more toxic in equivalent doses, fail to manifest. It seems that in addition to the anti-inflammatory action common to all corticoids, methylprednisolone exerts an effect on the hypothalamus. Several other writers, particularly in France, have noted this effect.

CONCLUSION

In conclusion, pain involving the chest and brachial plexus is a major problem. The oncologist often has to treat a patient who has received several other therapies and who knowingly will not be cured. But there still exist tools which in many cases will give long periods of remission. These tools will delay the terminal stage and the use of major narcotic agents and substances which modify the patient's behavior.

REFERENCES

1. Brule, G., Eckhardt, S. J., Hall, T. C., and Winkler, A. (1973): *Drug Therapy of Cancer,* edited by World Health Organization, Geneve.
2. Brule, G., Chauvergne, J., Guerrin, J., and Klein, T. (1974): Clinical study of new derivatives of podophyllotoxin. *Proceedings of the XI International Cancer Congress,* Florence, Vol. 5. Excerpta Medica, Amsterdam.
3. Brule, G. (1970): Le traitement des tumeurs solides par le Methotrexate Estratto da: *Corso Superiore sulla Chemioterapia dei Tumori,* Milano, 23–27 Marzo, 1970.
4. Brule, G. (1970): Chimiotherapie et hormonotherapie. *Revue du Praticien,* XX, 27:4259–4270.
5. Brule, G. (1976): Cooperative clinical study of 178 patients treated with Tamoxifene. *Symposium on the Hormonal Control of Breast Cancer,* Manchester.
6. Chauvergne, J., Gary-Bobo, J., Pommatau, E., Carton, M., Brule, G., Clavel, B., Guerrin, J., and Berlie, J. (1977): Polychimiotherapie des cancers mammaries en phase avancée. Association ternaire avec doxorubicine. Analyse de 209 observations. *Bulletin du Cancer,* 64,4:667–680.
7. Dutreix, J., Schlienger, M., Chauvel, C., and Daguin, R. (1971): Concentrated irradiation: Concentrated palliative radiotherapy for tumours affecting the oesophagus, brain, bones and mediastinum. *Ann. Clin. Res.,* 3:9–15.
8. Einhorn, L. H., and Donohue, J. (1977): Cis-diamminedichloroplatinum, Vinblastine, and Bleomycin combination chemotherapy in disseminated testicular cancer. *Ann. Intern. Med.,* 87:293–298.
9. Happert, J. L., Catel, P., Allin, O., Bouslama, A., and Engel, J. C. (1973): L'action antalgique du 6 alpha méthyl-prednisolone hémisuccinate de sodium en carcérologie pratique. *Médecin de Paris,* 45–50.
10. Londner, J. (1973): Etude de l'utilisation de la Medroxyprogesterone per os en carcinologie: A propos de 40 observations. *Thêse Paris.*
11. Petit, J. Y., Lasser, P., and Fontaine, F. (1977): Indications de l'épiplooplastie au cours de l'évolution du cancer du sein traité. A propos de 20 épiplooplasties faites à l'Institut Gustave-Roussy. *Bulletin du Cancer,* 64,4:659–665.
12. Tubiana, M. (1974): Achievements to be expected from new developments in tumour radiotherapy. *Europ. J. Cancer,* 10:373–380.

Advances in Pain Research and Therapy, Vol. 2,
edited by J. J. Bonica and V. Ventafridda.
Raven Press, New York © 1979.

Role of Analgesics and Related Drugs in Pain Involving the Chest and Brachial Plexus

H. U. Gerbershagen

Institut für Anaesthesiologie, Univ-kliniken, Langenbeckstrasse 1, Mainz, West Germany

In many countries cancer patients are not informed of the etiology and prognosis of their disease process. The psychologic, emotional, and behavioral aspects of cancer pain are frequently discussed among physicians. With cancer patients, however, this discussion is avoided. Thus, many physicians misjudge the despair and the anxiety of cancer pain patients even if the clinical picture is impressive, e.g., with difficulty in swallowing, dyspnea, lymphedema, postradiation paralysis, etc.

The psychologic and psychotherapeutic guidance of these patients is often wanting. These patients should at least benefit from the selective action of psychotropic drugs. Even in the absence of detectable psychic distress or alteration we do start patients with painful tumor growth of the chest and upper extremities on low dose *phenothiazines* (e.g., thioridazine), *thioxanthenes* (e.g., chlorprothixene), or *butyrophenones* (e.g., haloperidol). The mode and site of action have been aptly described by Halpern and Kocher.

Some patients require *tricyclic antidepressants with anxiolytic properties* (amitriptyline) in addition to neuroleptics. Tumor infiltration of blood and lymph vessels often induces the symptomatology of reflex sympathetic dystrophy. Its typical signs and symptoms are: severe, constant, burning pain; neurovascular instability (e.g., vasoconstriction with cyanosis, edema, cold extremity or vasodilatation); and sudo- and pilomotor alterations. A general hyperactivity of the autonomic nervous system is usually present. *Sedative phenothiazines* (chlorpromazine, thioridazine) or *thioxanthenes* (chlorprothixene) combined with antidepressants like amitriptyline will achieve fair to good relief. According to the pathogenesis of pain, acetylsalicylic, metamizol, and indomethacin are effective analgesics. For intractable pain of reflex sympathetic dystrophy, cervicothoracic sympathetic blocks are highly effective. In addition a 2-week trial of *cortisone derivatives* is indicated prior to any narcotic administration.

The dull, compressing, tightening pain of lymphedema or solid tumor infiltration into nerve sheaths and blood and lymph vessels is difficult to treat. Repeated or continuous nerve blocks frequently decrease the edema and provide relief. Amitriptyline (30 to 75 mg/day) and levomepromazine (75 mg/day) are the most effective drugs in our experience. If inflammatory processes are present or only a short time has elapsed after radiation therapy, nonnarcotic analgesics with strong antiinflammatory properties will reduce this constant pain. Vasodilators and high-ceiling diuretics (e.g., furosomide) do not reduce edema or pain and should not be given.

Pain in and around inflamed and necrotizing tumor tissue is effectively treated with aspirin-like drugs and antibiotics. Narcotic analgesics are used only if other methods fail or cannot be used.

Neoplastic disease of the chest and brachial plexus is frequently accompanied by muscle hypertonicity and muscle spasms. In most cases this severe, dull pain is induced by positive feedback mechanisms associated with cancer pain and is not due to tumor infiltration of muscle tissue. Centrally acting relaxants (e.g., orphenadrine citrate) administered simultaneously with pharmacological doses of aspirin, paracetamol, or indometracin will control this muscular pain. Due to the interruption of motor reflex mechanisms nonmuscular pain is often reduced reflexly. If these prove ineffective, regional blocks should be used.

Many cancer patients develop a typical protective posture of the upper extremity and neck. This reflexly induces muscle-hypertonicity, muscular contraction, and typical dull, aching pain. As far as drug treatment is concerned, anxiolytic and sedative minor tranquilizers (e.g., diazepam), centrally acting muscle relaxants, and nonnarcotic analgesics are the drugs of choice.

Radiating, sharp pain in the thoracic region and upper extremity is most often considered to be due to tumor-induced nerve compression. Without careful examination many patients are started on narcotic analgesics, and the physician is awaiting total nerve compression. However, this radiating pain might be caused by muscular, ligamentous, or joint trigger-point syndromes with their pseudoradicular symptomatology. These can be most effectively relieved with infiltration of a local anesthetic into the trigger point. Depending on the patient's pain reaction, an anxiolytic phenothiazine (levomepromazine) or a more sedative drug (e.g., thioridazine) will enhance the effects of nonnarcotic analgesics and muscle relaxants.

In proven painful nerve compression, antiepileptics like carbamepazine (up to 800 mg/day) or phenytoin (diphenylhydantoin, up to 600 mg/day) and thioridazine (90 mg/day) will often reduce this sharp pain. In these patients we prefer a rapid increase in carbamepazine dosage to the normal, creeping administration. Until effective blood levels are attained nefopam, 90 to 120 mg, is given orally. If additional analgesics are required, a short-term application of phenylbutazone (600 to 800 mg/day) or nefopam (360 to 450 mg/day) is justified. With inadequate pain-relief the physician might have to fall back on tilidin (250 to 300 mg/day) or narcotic analgesics.

The dull, intrathoracic visceral pain associated with neoplastic disease of the esophagus and mediastinal structures can be controlled for a long period of time with metamizol.

The throbbing, boring, sometimes sharp pain of tumor invasion of bone and periosteum often becomes unbearable at night. Drug treatment consists of mood-elevating drugs and *sleep-inducing butyrophenones* (e.g., haloperidol 0.6 to 0.9 mg/day). Metamizol as a nonnarcotic analgesic often reduces pain to a tolerable degree. If a more potent analgesic has to be applied, tilidin is the most effective in this type of pain and has the advantage of long effective duration.

In my opinion, patients suffering from cancer pain of the chest and upper extremities should be carefully examined physically *and* psychologically. Severe cancer pain is often controlled by a combination of tricyclic antidepressant plus neuroleptic. It is a matter of course that nefopam, tilidin, and narcotic analgesics should be administered whenever other pain develops and other drug therapy is insufficient. We always give psychotropic medications with these potent drugs. Thus, we reduce the requirement for narcotics. In addition, we do rotate nefopam, tilidin, and narcotic analgesics administration every 3 weeks. It is our impression that with pain-relieving doses of each drug, the doses and adverse effects can be kept low.

Advances in Pain Research and Therapy, Vol. 2,
edited by J. J. Bonica and V. Ventafridda.
Raven Press, New York © 1979.

Role of Nerve Blocks in Pain Involving the Chest and Brachial Plexus

M. Swerdlow

Regional Pain Relief Centre, University of Manchester School of Medicine, Salford, M6 8HD, Lancashire, England

Patients with severe cancer pain in the thorax, with or without involvement of the brachial plexus, are frequently presented for treatment of the pain. Types of cancer causing the pain vary considerably.

Etiologic Factors

Thoracic-wall pain may result from pleuromesothelioma, pleurocarcinoma, or sarcoma of the spine. Chest-wall pain may also be due to pleural irritation or erosion of ribs and involvement of intercostal nerves, which causes severe, radiating pain along affected dermatomes. Sharp, localized, unilateral chest pain or dull, aching pain often results from extension of a tumor onto the chest wall. On the other hand pleural or pericardial fluid-formation due to carcinomatosis is not commonly associated with pain (14).

Cancer in the *mediastinum* can occur from direct spread of lung, breast, or esophageal cancer and thoracic nerves, pleura and the sympathetic chain may be involved. Mediastinal pain may also result from secondary involvement of mediastinal glands. It produces a dull, burning or boring, central, persistent pain. Tumors arising in the mediastinum are very common. Many are benign; of the malignant ones many are in lymph nodes (either reticuloses or secondary from carcinoma bronchus or esophagus) or from primaries outside the chest such as breast or stomach.

Slow-growing, space-occupying lesions within the thorax may reach a considerable size before producing any symptoms other than vague restosternal pressure, perhaps with discomfort in the back and between the shoulder blades; the advent of severe chest pain usually signifies invasion of the chest wall. Malignant deposits involving cervical nerve roots or the brachial plexus may cause severe, intractable pain in the arm of mysterious origin. Cancer of the lung and breast are the two commonest causes of involvement of cervical nerve roots and the brachial plexus. The first thoracic nerve is often involved secondary to vertebral involvement and is difficult to

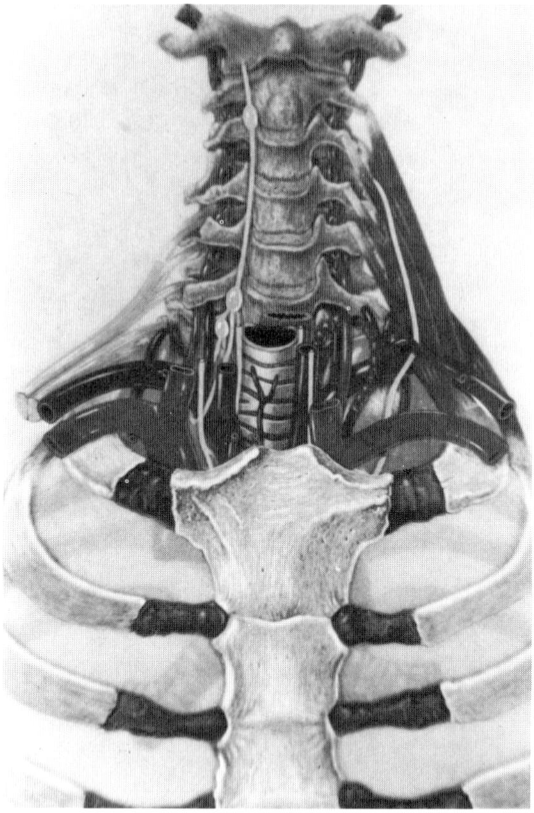

FIG. 1. Anatomy of cervico-axillary region.

visualize on X-ray; suggestive is a hard mass above clavicle together with a Horner's syndrome.

Tumors at the apex of the chest are commonly accompanied by Pancoast syndrome (the superior pulmonary sulcus syndrome)—unilateral pain in the upper chest, axilla, and arm, Horner's syndrome with some weakness of the arm. Study of the anatomy of the apex of the thorax demonstrates the large number of nerves which are at risk in this region (Fig. 1). Neuritic radiation is almost always at first in the distribution of the lower roots of the brachial plexus (16), sometimes limited to the ulnar nerve only. The cause is usually carcinoma bronchus, which as it spreads encroaches on the upper thoracic somatic and sympathetic nerves and on to the brachial plexus. Rarely the same syndrome can be caused by osteogenic sarcoma of the vertebrae or by upwardly extending mediastinal tumors.

Pain in the arm may also be caused by: (a) metastatic lesions of lower cervical or upper thoracic vertebrae or primary tumors of these vertebrae; (b) pressure on the brachial plexus, either supraclavicular, infraclavicular, or axillary; (c) pressure on large vessels by lesions in the axilla or root of neck.

Carcinoma Lung

The presenting symptoms and signs may have been present for 4 to 6 months with epidermoid cell tumor, which tends to cause local pulmonary symptoms and is the commonest cell type to cause the Pancoast syndrome. In contrast, small-cell carcinoma shows rapid growth and very early metastatic dissemination.

Lesions of the periphery of the lung which involve parietal pleura give rise to sharp neuralgia in the distribution of the intercostal nerves or dull, boring pain. If the central portion of diaphragmatic pleura is involved, pain is referred to the shoulder and neck. If sympathetic fibers are involved, there is diffuse, burning pain. Secondaries in the lungs most commonly originate from kidney, breast, thyroid, and prostate.

The median survival time after diagnosis is reported to be less than 6 months and the 5-year survival barely approaches 10% (16); however in the case of well-differentiated tumors the patient may live for many years.

Carcinoma Breast

Pain consequent to breast cancer usually results from bone metastases. According to Brennan (2), the amount of pain correlates with the rate of progression of the tumor rather than the extent of skeletal involvement.

Cancer of the breast is rarely the cause of local pain. However, advanced local breast cancer may be painful when inflammatory reaction distends the breast, when local infiltration of chest wall occurs, or if the tumor ulcerates. Secondaries in a rib or the sternum frequently cause intractable pain either from pressure on periosteum or on intercostal nerves or from pathologic fracture or involvement of pleura. Pain from such bone involvement may be alleviated by radiation.

Primary or secondary spread from breast cancer may reach the brachial plexus or major vessels of the arm causing edema, cyanosis, and burning pain in the limb. Stellate ganglion block will be necessary in addition to somatic block to provide pain-relief.

Development of bone pain in patients after mastectomy is difficult to attribute with certainty to metastases because osteoporosis and osteoarthritis are common in this age of patient; a bone scan may help in diagnosis (5). Local recurrence at the site of mastectomy may produce pain due to ulceration and secondary infection. Lymphedema of the arm may follow with severe shoulder-arm pain. The lymphatic spread to neighboring lymph nodes may also result in pressure on nerves and vessels.

Esophageal Cancer

Dysphagia is outstandingly the most common symptom in *esophageal* cancer. Carcinoma of the esophagus does however frequently cause retrosternal discomfort or aching pain in the back. Occasionally there is severe retrosternal pain, sharp or burning in nature, and usually only occurring on swallowing; it may radiate to the neck, shoulder, or between the scapulae. Occasionally also the vagus nerve may be involved, with pain referred to the ear or pharynx.

Skeletal Cancer

Pain from bone metastasis may be caused by stretching of periosteum, fracture of a rib, or collapse of a vertebral body. Primary or secondary cancer of the vertebrae produces pain which is at first localized but may spread to involve intervertebral nerves and produce root or girdle pain. Fibrosarcoma and chondrosarcoma of the upper ribs are uncommon causes of nerve involvement and pain. The development of back pain may be the first indication of metastasis to the spine. X-ray and bone scan may establish the diagnosis; if radicular pain is present it will help with localization. If no deposits are seen on X-ray, the pain should nevertheless be treated.

Spinal cord compression should be suspected in any patient with severe localized back or radicular pain especially if associated with sensory changes or motor weakness. Myelography should be carried out and, if necessary, urgent surgical or radiotherapeutic decompression of epidural metastases. Severe girdle-type back pain can result from extradural spinal metastases which can cause compression of the cord and spontaneous relief of pain.

TREATMENT

It will be clear from the above discussion that there are many different causes for thoracic pain in the cancer patient and a correspondingly wide range of treatments in relation to the nerves involved, the virulence of the growth, and the condition of the patient. In deciding on the type of pain treatment to be carried out the cell type and likely survival time will be important data. Needless to say the procedure must be carried out with full aseptic precautions, and the patient's informed consent should be obtained before commencing treatment. Pain sometimes becomes prominent at a time when the advent or existence of metastases is difficult to ascertain. Assuming that the state of the cancer coincides with the type and distribution of the pain and that possible coincidental causes for the pain (e.g., spondylolisthesis) are excluded, I believe it is reasonable to go ahead and treat the pain. To wait until it is proved beyond doubt that the pain is due to progress of the disease would often subject the patient to quite unnecessary suffering.

Pain of localized bone secondaries can often be easily controlled by radiation. Pain from nerve involvement however usually calls for relief by neurolytic methods, although it can sometimes be relieved by radiation, cytotoxic drugs, or antiinflammatory agents such as the corticosteroids (7) and the value of these various measures should be considered before proceeding to surgical or chemical neurolysis. The best treatment for pain from primary involvement of the chest wall is surgical excision as long as not more than two ribs are involved. Unfortunately Pancoast tumor is not amenable to palliative surgery.

The patient with thoracic pain should be referred as early as possible to an oncologist or radiotherapeutist if he has not already seen one. When the oncologists are unable to provide adequate pain-relief, some form of neural blockade may well provide the best possibility of relief. However, in a patient with a long life-expectancy (such as some patients with carcinoma of the breast) a cordotomy might well be the treatment of choice, or with localized pain a posterior rhizotomy. At the other extreme, a terminal patient with a very short survival expectancy might well be managed with appropriate analgesic and allied drugs if these can be made to provide adequate pain-relief. However, in patients with lung carcinoma, dyspnea may rule out cordotomy and may make narcotic drugs inadvisable; nerve blocking, with its minimal effect on respiration, will obviously then be advantageous.

Subarachnoid Neurolytic Blocks

In providing pain-relief by nerve blocking, by far the most useful measure in general is intrathecal neurolysis. In relation to the lower thoracic segments (i.e., caudad to T_5) this provides no real problems, and in fact this is the safest part of the cord to inject with little risk of producing bladder or limb paresis. Most workers report good results with the use of intrathecal neurolysis for the lower thoracic dermatomes. However, the spines of the vertebrae are very oblique in the mid-thoracic region, and the performance of spinal puncture can be very difficult; it is sometimes necessary to introduce the spinal needle at a technically easier spinal level (See Fig. 2) and then apply a corrective tilt of the operating table to "run" the solution towards the desired nerve root level; a somewhat larger volume of solution may be necessary (i.e., 1 to 1.5 ml).

When it comes to pain in the upper thoracic segments, particularly with Pancoast syndrome, the position is neither so simple nor so safe. The reason is by no means clear. There is a divergence of opinion on the value of subarachnoid neurolysis for pain in the upper chest and shoulder. Those who employ phenol or chlorocresol in glycerine find that the results in the cervical and upper thoracic levels are inferior to those obtained with these agents at lower spinal levels (13,15,18). On the other hand Kuzucu and his colleagues (10) and others who employ alcohol (8) report better results at high than at low spinal levels. This difference requires investigation.

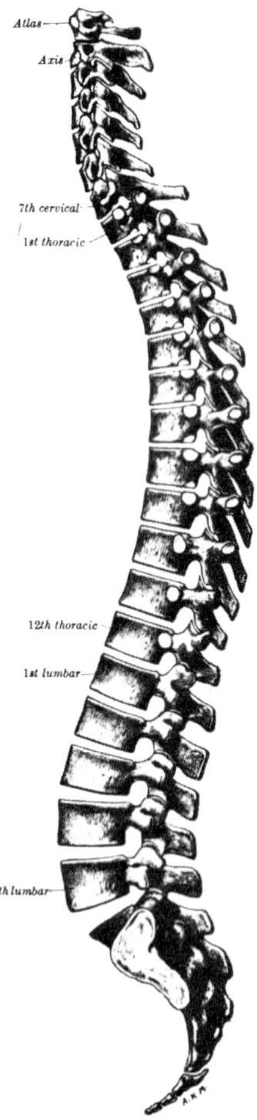

FIG. 2. Anatomy of spinal column.

Papo and Visca (15) found that of 21 patients with apical and upper chest pain, only 3 obtained good results and 9 fair; whereas of 17 patients with lower chest pain (caudad to T_6) 6 had good pain-relief and 5 obtained moderate pain-relief from intrathecal phenol. Kuzucu et al. (10) report that in 73% of their 322 patients pain was cervical or thoracic and results were very satisfactory. Katz (8) found that with intrathecal alcohol, thoracic pain was more easily treated than pelvic pain. Maher and Mehta (13) employed intrathecal 5% phenol or 2% chlorocresol in 235 cases of carcinoma shoulder, arm, lung, or breast and report that 72 were significantly relieved. Ventafridda and Martino (19) report "good" results in 71% with cancer pain in upper chest wall and in 56% with upper lung plus brachial plexus pain, but the duration of relief was only about 3 weeks.

Of the latest 140 cases in the author's series treated by intrathecal phenol or chlorocresol, 35 had pain in the thorax, of whom 15 had associated brachial plexus pain. Twenty-nine had lung cancer, 5 breast cancer, and 1 had a melanoma. Of the patients with lung cancer 15 had good or moderately good pain-relief up to death, but death occurred within a week in 4, within a month in 3 and within 3 months in 4 patients. The remaining 14 lung cancer patients obtained little or no relief from the subarachnoid neurolysis.

When there is widespread bilateral pain, it is worth trying the effects of intrathecal hypertonic saline which, however, frequently fails to give an adequate duration of relief. Papo and Visca (15) warn that "one stage bilateral phenolization should never be done at $T_{5\text{-}10}$ because of risk of hypotension."

In the event of unsuccessful intrathecal block, there are a number of alternative techniques which may be tried including subdural, extradural, and paravertebral blocks.

Subdural Blocks

Subdural injection is carried out with the aid of an image-intensifier. A spinal needle is inserted and advanced to the epidural space. It is gently advanced until it impinges on the dura and then pushed forward a fraction. Injection of a small amount of iophendylate will show when the tip of the needle is subdural; X-ray shows myodil in line between dura and arachnoid. One to three ml of 5 to 8% phenol in glycerine are now injected; injection is slightly resisted. The technique is not easy, and the relief is often of inadequate duration. The cervical nerve roots on both sides can be covered from a centrally placed needle, or the lower cervical plus upper thoracic nerve roots can be blocked at one session. Maher suggests that alternate injection of phenol and air will provide greater spread.

Extradural Blocks

Extradural injection of 5 to 10% phenol in glycerine may be employed in the upper thoracic and the cervical segments and has the advantage that there is no risk of its spreading beyond the foramen magnum and that severe headaches will not occur. The author has sometimes found extradural neurolytic block to give effective and lasting results. Others (11,12) report similar findings. Continuous or intermittent injection of local anesthetic via an indwelling extradural catheter should be considered in terminal cases.

Paravertebral Blocks

Paravertebral somatic nerve block is rarely used. As Bonica (14) points out, intrathecal or extradural block is preferable to paravertebral neurolysis because they act proximal to the site of the bony pressure on the nerve and because they spare the motor fibers of the nerve. *Intercostal* block is only useful for anterior and anterolateral metastases and, in my experience, neurolytic block of intercostal nerves usually does not last long enough. It can be used as an interim measure, while intrathecal, subdural, or rhizotomy/cordotomy is being planned. Intercostal neurolysis is useful in pathologic rib fractures; phenol or chlorocresol is injected between the fracture faces.

Pain in the distribution of the intercostal nerves due to invasion of the paravertebral chest wall may require paravertebral block not only of the affected roots but also of the adjacent ones caudal and cephalad. It is easier for the patient (and for the physician) to do an intrathecal rhizotomy of a number of posterior nerve roots. However, in some patients, pain in the shoulder from involvement of lower cervical roots can be effectively relieved by paravertebral block of the appropriate cervical nerve roots. The block is carried out at the tip of the transverse process(es), and it is advisable to perform a prognostic local anesthetic block before employing a neurolytic agent.

Brachial Plexus Blocks

When none of the above methods is satisfactory, Bonica (1) recommends that alcohol block of the brachial plexus should be performed if necessary. Brown (3) reports that when the brachial plexus is infiltrated with cancer cells, relief can be obtained "in a reasonable proportion of patients" by infiltrating the plexus with 1 or 2% aqueous phenol using not more than 20 ml of the solution. The procedure may cause severe pain for up to 48 hr after injection.

However, glandular infiltration in the supraclavicular region may make access to the brachial plexus (and to the stellate ganglion) difficult or impossible.

Sympathetic Block

Because of the invasive nature of many intrathoracic tumors, visceral fibers of the sympathetic nervous system may become involved. It is as well, therefore, in cases where somatic block does not produce complete pain-relief to try the effects of an appropriate sympathetic block with a local anesthetic solution such as bupivacaine or lignocaine. As an alternative to sympathetic nerve block, intravenous guanethidine may be tried for upper-limb pain (6).

Carcinoma of the breast is often accompanied by edema of the arm and severe, burning pain in the shoulder and arm. Stellate block may be helpful—it should be performed with local anesthetic first, before contemplating neurolytic block (17).

When treating pain due to carcinoma of the esophagus, thoracic sympathetic ganglion block of 2–5 T should be used for upper esophagus and block of 5–7 T ganglia for lower esophagus. If this doesn't relieve all the pain, vagus block should be performed just above the clavicle. A prognostic local anesthetic block should be performed prior to bilateral vagal section.

Invasion of the subclavian vessels will result in edema of the arm, which is objectively cool but subjectively has a burning sensation. These symptoms will be relieved by stellate ganglion block with local anesthetic, which should be tried before somatic block; as Challenger (4) points out, sympathetic block has the advantage of not producing paresis or sensory disturbance.

PAIN FOLLOWING ANTICANCER THERAPY

In addition to the pathological causes described above, the cancer patient may have pain in the thorax for a number of different reasons. Pain or discomfort in the chest and/or arm can occur as a result of surgical or radiation therapy.

Radiation fibrosis in the pectoral axillary area used to be a problem, but my colleagues at the Christie Cancer Hospital tell me that this rarely creates difficulties nowadays. However, irradiation therapy of carcinoma breast can cause brachial plexus neuropathies. Kiff (9) reports such a case successfully relieved by intravenous regional sympathetic block with guanethidine. However, frequently the pain of fibrosis of the brachial plexus requires neurosurgical pain-relieving operations.

Lymphedema in patients who have undergone axillary dissection can cause arm heaviness which may be accompanied by pain in the neck and shoulder region due to tissue traction by the weight of the arm. It is important to see to restoration of upper-limb function as well as reduction of lymphedema.

Pain in the scar of a mastectomy or lobectomy operation is not uncommon and may interfere with simple daily actions, such as washing. It may be a symbol of resentment of the scar itself and of the mastectomy, and this must be borne in mind when considering pain-relieving therapy.

Finally beware of post-herpetic neuralgia obscuring the onset of cancer pain. Cancer is one of the conditions which is thought to occasionally light up the dormant varicella virus. I have seen two patients with post-herpetic neuralgia which proved resistant to treatment, and in whom it became clear (fortunately without too much delay) that, in fact, cancer was causing pain in the same dermatomes as the herpetic rash.

REFERENCES

1. Bonica, J. J. (1953): *The Management of Pain.* Lea & Febiger, Philadelphia.
2. Brennan, M. J. (1973): In: *Cancer Medicine,* edited by J. F. Holland and E. Frei. Lea & Febiger, Philadelphia.
3. Brown, A. S. (1976): Pain relief in malignant disease. In: *Symposium on Malignant Disease.* Roy. Coll. Physicians Edinb. Publication No. 47.
4. Challenger, J. H. (1978): Sympathetic nervous system blocking in pain relief. In:

Relief of Intractable Pain, 2nd ed., edited by M. Swerdlow. Excerpta Medica, Amsterdam.
5. Creech, R. H. (1976): In: *Oncologic Medicine,* edited by A. I. Sutnick and P. F. Engstrom. University Park Press, Baltimore.
6. Holland, A. J. C., Davies, K. H., and Wallace, D. H. (1977): Sympathetic blockage of isolated limbs by intravenous guanethidine. *Can. Anaesthetists' Soc. J.,* Vol. 24.
7. Jackson, S. M. (1978): Radiotherapy, anticancer drugs and hormones. In: *Relief of Intractable Pain,* 2nd ed., edited by M. Swerdlow. Excerpta Medica, Amsterdam.
8. Katz, J. (1975): Subarachnoid alcohol injections for the management of chronic pain. In: *Recent Progress in Anaesthesiology and Resuscitation.* Excerpta Medica, Amsterdam.
9. Kiff, J. G. H. (1974): *Pain Relief.* Heinman, London.
10. Kuzucu, E. Y., Derric, W. S., and Wilber, S. A. (1966): Control of intractable pain with subarachnoid alcohol block. *JAMA,* 195:133.
11. Lourie, H., and Vanasupa, P. (1963): Comments on the use of intraspinal phenol-pantopaque for relief of pain and spasticity. *J. Neurosurg.,* 20:60.
12. Madrid, J. (1975): *Proceedings of Symposium on Cancer Pain.* Florence, Italy.
13. Maher, R., and Mehta, M. (1977): Spinal and extradural analgesia. In: *Persistent Pain,* edited by S. Lipton. Academic Press, London.
14. Olson, K. B., (1973): Pain. In: *Cancer Medicine,* edited by J. F. Holland, and E. Frei. Lea & Febiger, Philadelphia.
15. Papo, I., and Visca, E. (1976): Intrathecal phenol in the treatment of pain and spasticity. *Prog. Neurol. Surg.,* 7:56.
16. Selawry, O. S., and Hansen, H. H. (1973): Lung cancer. In: *Cancer Medicine,* edited by J. F. Holland and E. Frei. Lea & Febiger, Philadelphia.
17. Swerdlow, M. (1977): Peripheral nerve blocking in the relief of pain. In: *Persistent Pain,* edited by S. Lipton. Academic Press, London.
18. Swerdlow, M., editor (1978): *Relief of Intractable Pain,* 2nd ed. *Excerpta Medica,* Amsterdam.
19. Ventafridda, V., and Martino, G. (1976): Clinical evaluation of subarachnoid neurolytic blocks in intractable cancer pain. In: *Advances in Pain Research and Therapy, Vol. 1, Proceedings of the First World Congress on Pain,* edited by J. J. Bonica and D. Albe-Fessard, pp. 699–703. Raven Press, New York.

Advances in Pain Research and Therapy, Vol. 2,
edited by J. J. Bonica and V. Ventafridda.
Raven Press, New York © 1979.

Role of Neurosurgery in Pain Involving the Chest and Brachial Plexus

Donald E. Richardson

Department of Neurological Surgery, Louisiana State University School of Medicine, and Hotel Dieu Hospital Pain Rehabilitation Unit, New Orleans, Louisiana 70112

Carcinoma-induced pain involving the chest and brachial plexus can be one of the most rewarding types of pain for control by neurosurgical techniques. With rare exceptions, gratifying results can usually be obtained in a large number of patients and with minimal side effects and relatively low complication. The most common etiology of chest wall and brachial plexus pain in men is recurrent carcinoma of the lung, and it usually produces symptoms by invasion and contiguous spread. In women, the most common cause is recurrent carcinoma of the breast with either regional node metastasis or contiguous spread.

Pain in patients with recurrent carcinoma of the upper quadrant of the body may be caused by invasions of the pleura, the periosteum, or nerves involving the chest wall or brachial plexus. In addition to tumor invasion, however, benign causes of pain must be considered. Postsurgical changes, such as partial nerve injury, perineural scarring, loss of sensation with deafferentation pain, and occasionally radiation neuropathy are other causes for the pain which are not directly related to the patient's disease. One of the most common types of chest wall pain occurring in patients who have had thoracotomies for lung lesions is incisional pain or pain caused by damage to the intercostal nerves at the time of thoracotomy. This has been greatly reduced recently by the use of well-padded retractors or by the section of the intercostal nerves at the time of the primary surgery. Brachial plexus pain can be a difficult differential diagnosis in an occasional patient who has pain beginning a few weeks following surgery with dissection about his brachial plexus, either in the axilla or supraclavicular fossa. Fortunately for the neurosurgeon, the control of pain does not always require a specific diagnosis, except for the patient who continues to complain of pain that is primarily due to emotional factors and who is being treated for organic pain.

A rare cause of pain in the upper extremities and chest wall in patients with carcinoma is invasion of the spine itself with nerve root compression or localized bone pain. In these patients, the pain can be either midline or often bilateral, which not only produces a difficult pain syndrome to control surgically, but also may indicate impending spinal cord compression with paraplegia. Obviously, the prevention of spinal cord compression and paraplegia would be of primary importance, and the pain would have to be placed secondary in the line of treatment.

The two things that patients with terminal cancer fear the most are pain and loneliness. One must remember that, in patients with terminal disease, appropriate discussions with the patient regarding his treatment and his disease, a realistic but supportive attitude, psychiatric consultation, religious counseling, and a careful explanation to the patient and his family that pain-relieving procedures do not improve or retard the underlying disease process are a necessary part of treatment. The treatment of underlying depression and anxiety will greatly enhance the treatment of the pain problem itself and, at times, has provided enough pain-relief that the patient did not have to have a neurosurgical procedure carried out at all. The use of narcotics for the control of anxiety and depression can be misleading as an indication of the degree of the patient's pain.

TIME AND SELECTION OF THE PROCEDURE

In our clinic we consider pain-relieving neurosurgical procedures to be indicated when the patient has begun to require potent narcotic medications, that is, when the patient changes from codeine and propoxyphene to morphine, or other potent narcotics. The reason for this is that we believe tolerance to narcotics occurs fairly rapidly, making it necessary to increase the dosage to control the patient's pain. Moreover, in our experience, narcotics add to the anorexia, weight loss, and to the general debility of the patient with terminal cancer and often produce apathy, lethargy, and chronic depression.

Selection of procedures, of course, requires sophisticated consideration of the patient's problem. The most difficult consideration is the prognosis for life. Patients with very short life-expectancies can be adequately managed with nerve blocks or maintained on narcotics. Trying to provide an adequate prognosis on patients with terminal cancer is fraught with many problems and often is misleading. Our present recommendation is that, if the patient's life-expectancy is longer than 3 to 4 months, a neurosurgical pain-relieving procedure is indicated. In patients who have a very short life-expectancy, nerve blocks or large doses of narcotics or both are usually effective. If the patient's pain, however, is excruciating and cannot be controlled by nerve blocks, or is accompanied by much suffering and loss of emotional control, a saline lobotomy would be offered the patient with a prognosis of less than 3 to 4 months.

In patients with terminal cancer, there is always the question of how long one should wait for positive anticancer therapy, such as radiation or chemotherapy, to produce pain-relief before proceeding with neurosurgery. Waiting 3 to 5 weeks for a patient to respond to radiation therapy or chemotherapy is not an unrealistic consideration, but allowing continuation of pain and suffering while a series of chemotherapeutic agents are tried without considerations for the patient's comfort is without merit. It is our policy not to wait longer than 3 to 4 weeks following the termination of radiation therapy or a course of chemotherapy before offering the patient a pain-relieving procedure if his pain is not significantly improving at that time. It is unlikely that significant reduction of pain will occur later than 3 to 4 weeks following a course of such therapy.

PREOPERATIVE WORK-UP AND EVALUATION

The basic work-up required prior to pain-relieving neurosurgical procedures can be quite minimal. However, there are some specific indications and procedures that should be carried out in a reasonable attempt to ascertain whether the patient has a potentially complicating factor prior to surgery. In addition to the usual blood count, cardiogram, urinalysis, biochemical profile, and chest X-ray which are carried out on every patient, there are specific indications for further studies. Cervical and thoracic spine films should be obtained in patients if there is any reason to think that the patient may have spine invasion and potential spinal cord compression. In addition, isotope bone scans and soft tissue scans can be obtained to accurately delineate the degree of the patient's tumor recurrence and invasion. If there is significant question as to whether the patient has spinal cord invasion with potential spinal cord compression, a preoperative myelogram can be done without great difficulty. In patients with a large amount of pulmonary metastasis, postoperative pneumonectomy, radiation pneumonitis, or possible phrenic nerve palsy, pulmonary function studies and fluoroscopy of the diaphragms should be carried out before surgery to ascertain the potential for respiratory insufficiency, especially if a chordotomy or extensive rhizotomy is being planned.

In addition, in patients who have extensive tumor recurrence and who are to have general anesthesia, it is our policy to have a preoperative isotope blood volume carried out, because they often have a depleted blood volume and may need to have blood replacement with either whole blood or packed cells prior to any surgical procedure. In any patient with personality change that cannot be explained on the basis of medication or other central nervous system symptoms or manifestations, both isotope cerebral scans and computerized axial tomography are carried out to rule out the possibility of cerebral metastases. We have had 1 patient who had the diagnosis of cerebral metastasis made at the time of ventriculography before stereotaxic procedure for relief of his brachial plexus pain. Although this situation can usually be managed by use of large doses of steroids, it is obviously preferable to have a diagnosis prior to surgery and to avoid intercranial operations for pain-relief on patients with cerebral metastasis.

SELECTION OF THE SPECIFIC PROCEDURES

The selection of procedures for pain-relief are based on the location of the patient's pain, anticipated duration of life, and general condition of the patient. Obviously, an extensive rhizotomy with section of the sensory portions of the nerve roots involving the entire arm is not acceptable, since patients will not have the use of the extremity due to the loss of position sense and sensory feedback required for motor function of the extremity. An amputation of the extremity usually follows such ill-advised procedures. Time-consuming and extensive procedures on patients with only a few weeks to live are undesirable.

Below, are listed the procedures that we are using most commonly at the present time for pain involving the chest wall and brachial plexus in patients with recurrent cancer. This outline is then matched with the type of pain that each procedure can be used for in most cases. This outline does not take into consideration the longevity of the patient, which is discussed further in the discussion of each procedure, and leaves out some procedures that are rarely performed. Moreover, in each type of pain only one of these is indicated.

The procedures include: (A) sensory rhizotomy or neurectomy; (B) anterolateral cordotomy; (C) thalamotomy; (D) stimulation of periventricular gray; (E) hypophysectomy; (F) saline lobotomy.

Location of pain	*Procedures applicable*
Small area of chest pain	A, B
Large area of chest wall	B, C, D, E, (F)
Lower brachial plexus (and chest)	B, C, D, E, (F)
Upper brachial plexus (and neck)	C, D, (E), F
Bilateral chest and brachial plexus	C, D, (E), F

SPECIFIC PROCEDURES

Sensory Rhizotomy or Neurectomy

Use of spinal sensory rhizotomy can be extremely rewarding in patients with fairly well-localized chest wall pain. It is ideally suited for patients with postthoracotomy incisional pain due to damage to the intercostal nerves. In addition, relatively small areas of pain involving the chest wall can be quite adequately controlled with rhizotomy with minimal morbidity to the patient. It is one of the most easily tested procedures since, prior to operative rhizotomy, temporary paravertebral or intercostal nerve blocks can be carried out with relative ease with X-ray control. The diagnostic block helps to predict the amount of pain-relief the patient will derive from the surgery, allowing both the patient and the surgeon to be reasonably sure of his results prior to operation.

At the present time, we are using percutaneous X-ray controlled radiofrequency coagulation of nerve roots at the neural foramen. Stimulation of the nerve root can produce paresthesias in the area of the patient's pain. Once this is done, brief general anesthesia with intravenous Brevital® is given and the nerve root is then coagulated, either at 70°C or at 90°C. The 70°C coagulation is used in an attempt to differentially destroy the small, unmyelinated pain fibers and leave other sensation otherwise intact, and 90° coagulation for complete destruction of the nerve root. In patients with pain secondary to cancer, I have not attempted to do a differential rhizotomy, but have usually totally destroyed the nerve root. Usually, 1 min of coagulation at 90°C, if the electrode is well-placed against the nerve root, is sufficient for its complete lysis (9).

Anterolateral Cordotomy

Percutaneous, high cervical cordotomy is the procedure of choice in patients who have unilateral, lower brachial plexus and chest wall pain or a large area of chest wall pain that would require an extensive rhizotomy for control. Percutaneous, high cervical cordotomy between the lamina of C_1 and C_2 vertebrae carried out under local anesthesia has given excellent results if the patient is cooperative enough to allow the procedure to be done. Insertion of a small needle electrode into the anterior quadrant of the cord with stimulation followed by slowly increasing radiofrequency lesions will give good analgesia involving the lower brachial plexus and chest wall as well as the abdomen and leg if necessary. However, an attempt to raise the cordotomy to the upper brachial plexus or cervical plexus levels may cause extension of the lesion into the motor fibers of the spinal cord with contralateral weakness and can produce respiratory weakness or hemiparesis. In addition, in patients with bilateral pain, a bilateral cordotomy is considered highly dangerous owing to the production of sleep apnea with respiratory arrest.

In some patients, it is difficult to do a percutaneous cordotomy, either for anatomic reasons or because of poor cooperation on the patient's part. In these patients, we still use open high cervical cordotomy under general anesthesia. Our technique for this is quite simple and requires only 1 hr of operating time. A small, midline incision is made from the base of the skull to the C_3 spinous process, and the muscles are reflected unilaterally on the side opposite the pain so that the C_2 lamina is exposed on that side. A self-retaining retractor is placed between the lamina and against the muscles laterally, and when open, usually rotates the spine considerably. The C_2

lamina is then removed, and the dura is opened in a horseshoe-shaped fashion to hinge laterally and is sutured to the paraspinous muscles. The denticulate attachment is then sectioned, and the cord is rotated by grasping the dentate ligament. Low magnification with loops or the operating microscope can then be used with excellent visualization of the anterior quadrant of the spinal cord. Section of the anterior quadrant, beginning 1 or 2 mm anterior to the dentate ligament and carried to just medial to the exit of the ventral rootlets, is then carried out with ease.

In our experience, failures of pain control from chordotomy have been primarily due to late development of pain on the opposite side of the body or upward extension of tumors through the brachial plexus, reaching levels above the chordotomy sensory level. Thus, some consideration of the potential for further tumor invasion and spread of pain should be considered along with the other factors involving the selection of this procedure for pain control. In addition, chordotomy does not usually relieve disagreeable paresthesias and numbness. Careful discussion with the patient regarding the character of his discomfort and pain should be carried out, since some patients describe paresthesias and numbness as being painful (8), which is not relieved by chordotomy.

Thalamotomy

The advantages of radiofrequency-induced destruction of the medial thalamus are that the procedure can be carried out under local anesthesia, it carries minimal morbidity and mortality, it will control pain over the entire opposite side of the body, and it results in no detectable sensory loss.

On the other hand a disadvantage of thalamotomy is that pain-relief cannot be expected to be maintained for more than 6 months to 1 year. Most of the patients who have had thalamotomy for pain control have had excellent relief for at least 6 months but, between 6 months and 1 year, the pain recurs. In addition, an acutely painful experience, such as a pathologic fracture, may cause the previous chronic pain to return.

Lesions placed in the medial thalamus, including the centrum medianum, parafascicularis, and medial pulvinar will usually control contralateral pain quite well. Care should be taken with the placement of the lesion not to allow the destruction to extend laterally into the main sensory nucleus, since patients will complain bitterly of numbness and may have dysmetria following lateral extension of their lesion. Bilateral lesions can be carried out if carefully done for patients with bilateral pain with good results and no significant side effects. Patients who have thalamotomy for pain usually have a transient period of euphoria lasting a week to 10 days which then resolves (6).

This procedure can be very useful in patients with brachial plexus and upper chest wall pain who have had a previous pneumonectomy and have borderline pulmonary function and who might have further compromise of pulmonary function secondary to chordotomy or extensive rhizotomy.

Stimulation of Periventricular Gray

The technique of periventricular gray stimulation, while not widespread at this time, is very efficacious for relief of pain in any area of the body. The advantages of this procedure are that it can be carried out under local anesthesia, it does not produce a lesion of the nervous system with potential for complications from neural destruction, it is under the patient's control so that it can be used when needed, and it will control pain in any area of the body, including extensive unilateral pain or bilateral pain.

A detailed description of the procedure and its results are in a separate section of this volume ("Central Gray Stimulation for Control of Cancer Pain") (4,5). Briefly the procedure is carried out by stereotaxically inserting a stimulating electrode into the periventricular gray just anterior to the posterior commisure. Stimulation is then carried out using percutaneous leads until reassurance is obtained that the procedure is effective for relieving the patient's pain. Then, at a second procedure, the radiofrequency induction receiving device is placed under the skin and connected to the electrode pairs to be used for stimulation. The patient then uses a radiofrequency coupled transmitter to self-stimulate when necessary for pain control.

In most patients, continuous stimulation is not necessary, since intermittent stimulation may be effective for many hours. The secondary gain from this procedure is that patients who use ventricular gray stimulation seem to have an elevation of their mood with consequent relief of chronic depression. We have found that, with periventricular gray stimulation, some of the other side effects of tumor growth are not controlled. It will often control dysesthesias, paresthesias, and complaints of numbness associated with nerve destruction. However, in patients with burning pain secondary to deafferentation, the procedure may not be effective. Pressure sensation or discomfort secondary to tumor mass also is not relieved by these procedures and, if a patient is habituated to narcotics, it may not relieve the patient's pain completely.

Hypophysectomy

The usefulness of hypophysectomy for the control of carcinoma of the breast, prostate, and endometrium is widely recognized and is used extensively. Metastatic carcinoma of the prostate to the dorsal spine and ribs or cervical spine with secondary pain can be quite readily controlled with either a transnasal hypophysectomy, alcohol injections of the hypophysis, radiofrequency coagulation of the hypophysis, or transfrontal removal of the hypophysis. The results with carcinoma of the breast are somewhat less gratifying in that only about 50 to 60% of the patients have significant control of their disease with hypophysectomy. The use of hypophysectomy for endometrial carcinoma has been utilized in only a small number of cases in our experience, but excellent results were obtained by this procedure.

Hypophysectomy for pain of nonhormonal-dependent tumors has recently been utilized, and there is some early clinical evidence that control of pain from any cause can be relieved by hypophysectomy. The mechanism for control of pain by hypophysectomy is apparently by interference with an inhibitory mechanism for the endogenous opiate system. It has been well established that naloxone, a morphine antagonist, when given after hypophysectomy, causes immediate return of pain in patients who have received excellent pain-relief by this technique. At the present time, the selection of patients for hypophysectomy, the expected results, and the indications and contraindications for its use are not well established and will have to await further clinical trials (2,3).

Saline Lobotomy

The technique of saline lobotomy has not been utilized widely for pain control, though it is an excellent technique for relieving pain in patients who have a short life-expectancy of less than 4 months. It is also an excellent procedure in patients who have marked suffering and emotional stress associated with their illness and pain. The procedure can be easily done on patients who are quite ill and who have pain in any area of the body (chest, neck, brachial plexus, and bilaterally). The disadvantages of this procedure are that, if it has to be repeated over a period of time, as in cases where the patient has lived longer than anticipated, the patient will develop progressively more severe frontal lobe damage and personality changes that are undesirable from the point of view of maintenance of his personality and relationships with his family and friends. In patients with relatively short life-expectancy, however, the procedure gives excellent pain control with pain asymbolia and the alleviation of suffering with the ability to withdraw, or greatly reduce, large doses of narcotics rapidly with minimal side effects except physiological withdrawal symptoms.

This procedure, done under local anesthesia, entails placing bilateral trephines approximately 2 cm from the midline just anterior to the coronal suture line. A #20 spinal needle is then inserted into the frontal lobes bilaterally or, in most cases, unilaterally at the first injection; 8 to 10 cc of sterile saline are injected as the needle is slowly withdrawn from the frontal white matter. Usually, injections of 1 to 2 cc of saline every centimeter as the needle is removed produces an excellent result. The procedure can be titrated by talking to the patient during the injection and discontinuing the injection when there is an obvious change in the patient's affect or mood. It has been our experience that injections only on one side is all that is necessary at the initial time of treatment and, later, the second side may be added if necessary (1).

As the patient's pain begins to return, the procedure can be repeated percutaneously by simply inserting the #20 needle through the scalp over the burr holes after sterilizing the skin. Injections of saline, either unilaterally or bilaterally, can then be repeated as needed. Patients usually require injections at 6-week to 2-month intervals and, if no more than two or three injections are required, personality defects are relatively mild. However, the longer the patient survives, and the more injections required, the more permanent the frontal lobe effects become. At the present time, we reserve this procedure for patients who have a very short life-expectancy and who have severe pain and suffering not controlled with narcotics (7).

SUMMARY

An attempt has been made to present in a concise review the procedures that have been found to be efficacious and are currently in use in our clinic for the control of cancer pain in the area of the brachial plexus and chest. The development of newer procedures is continuing at a rapid pace at this time, and it is understood that these procedures will obviously be modified by newer techniques and by the experience of the surgeon involved. Emotional support for the patient and his family, as well as the recognition and treatment of underlying depression and anxiety regarding his disease and ultimate death are necessary for optimum control of the patient's pain. The procedures of sensory rhizotomy, anterolateral cordotomy, thalomotomy, periventricular gray stimulation, hypophysectomy, and saline lobotomy offer the neurosurgeon a wide armamentarium for the control of almost all types of pain involving the neck, arm, and chest wall. The indications for surgery at this time are pain that has not responded to radiation or chemotherapy and that has increased in severity to the point where the patient is requiring potent narcotics for pain-relief. The avoidance of narcotic tolerance, anorexia, weight loss, and suffering secondary to chronic pain, and the avoidance of the use of narcotics for a period of time longer than 3 to 4 months is thought to justify the performance of the procedures described.

REFERENCES

1. Bridges, T. J., and Liss, H. R. (1958): Saline lobotomy for relief of pain due to advanced cancer. *Cancer* (VI) 11:322.
2. Moricca, G. (1974): Chemical hypophysectomy for cancer pain. In: *Advances in Neurology Vol. 4, International Symposium on Pain,* edited by J. J. Bonica, pp. 707–714. Raven Press, New York.
3. Richardson, D. E. (1967): Recent advances in the neurosurgical control of pain. *So. Med. J.,* 60:1082–1086.
4. Richardson, D. E. (1974): Thalamotomy for control of chronic pain. *Acta Neurochir.,* [*Suppl.*], 21:77–88.
5. Richardson, D. E., and Akil, H. (1977): Long term results of periventricular gray self-stimulation. *Neurosurg.,* 1:199–202.
6. Richardson, D. E., and Akil, H. (1977): Pain reduction by electrical brain stimulation in man, Part 2: Chronic self administration in the periventricular gray matter. *J. Neurosurg.,* 47:184–194.

7. Rosomoff, H. L., Carroll, F., Brown, J., and Sheptak, P. (1965): Percutaneous radiofrequency cervical cordotomy: Techniques. *J. Neurosurg.,* 23:639–644.
8. Tindall, G. T., Nixon, D. W., Christy, J. H., and Neill, J. D. (1977): Pain relief in metastatic cancer other than breast and prostate gland following transsphenoidal hypophysectomy. *J. Neurosurg.,* 47:659–662.
9. Uematsu, S., Udvarhelyi, G. B., Benson, D. W., and Siebens, A. A. (1974): Percutaneous radiofrequency rhizotomy. *Surgical Neurol.,* 2:319–325.

Discussion

Part II. Management of Pain of Advanced Cancer: Pain Involving the Chest and Brachial Plexus

B. R. Fink (Moderator)

Questioner: Dr. Swerdlow, do you think that extradural neurolytic block is less harmful than subdural, and is it effective in relieving cervical pain?

Swerdlow (Manchester): Extradural block is certainly likely to cause less damage than intrathecal block, and in the cervical region it is certainly safer. Because so many of the patients we have treated have lived for a very short time, we found that very often extradural neurolytic block has been effective in this region. Elsewhere in the spinal cord we are less inclined to use it.

Questioner: How many milliliters of phenol do you use in performing extradural block?

Swerdlow: We usually use phenol aqueous solution and, of course, you have to be very careful indeed, ensuring that the tip of the needle is not within the theca. I use about 2 ml for each nerve segment that I want to block.

Sapio (Taranto): You mentioned three types of blocks: intrathecal or subarachnoid, extradural or peridural. What is the third type?

Swerdlow: The third type is subdural. That is to say, injection of the chemical between the dura and the arachnoid. There is a potential space between the dura and the arachnoid; and it is possible, using image-intensification and radio-opaque dye, to get the tip of the needle into this subdural space and then inject the phenol into the space. When this procedure is successful, it is very good because you can get a block of both sides with one injection and because it is very safe.

Rampulla (Urbino): I would like to know something about supraclavicular neurolysis of the brachial plexus.

Swerdlow: I should tell you that both alcohol and phenol when applied to the brachial plexus will give a period of 24 to 48 hr of agony to the patient, and it is important to give them sufficient analgesia medication. It depends on how infiltrated the area is. Of course, glandural infiltration in the supraclavicular region can sometimes make this procedure difficult; it can sometimes make cervical nerve blocks difficult.

Scalabrin (Padova): Dr. Brulé, you talked about the chemotherapic combination of neomicyn, *cis*-platinum, and vincristine. Do you have other data on the single or combined use of *cis*-platinum in the palliative or curative chemotherapy of thoracic neoplasia?

Brulé (Villejuif): I cannot give you any precise data yet. But we are studying *cis*-platinum as one of a small group of European chemotherapists, and we have made some screening. As you know, we already know that it is effective in testicular tumor and mainly on pulmonary metastasis of testicular tumor. But the action is very brief. You may have a complete disappearance of all metastatic lesions, but they will reappear in about 6 weeks to 2 or 3 months later. So the problem is to have a long remission. That is the reason why we are trying a combined therapy.

Graziussi (Napoli): Dr. Richardson, do you use local or general anesthesia in placing the cannula for percutaneous rhizotomy? And would you tell us the percentage of success in pain-relief according to your experience?

Richardson (New Orleans): We do it with local anesthesia. It should always be done with local anesthesia. We sometimes use intravenous Brevital,® which is a very ultra-short-acting barbiturate, during the period of coagulation to reduce the patient's discomfort. I cannot give you a percentage but, in general, we select rhizotomy for patients who have the least amount of pain, and our results have been excellent because we can always test for the effect of the rhizotomy by doing a temporary nerve block prior to the procedure. So our results are almost 100% successful, at least temporarily. We may have to do something else later if the patient's cancer spreads and involves a larger area.

Porges (Vienna): You did not mention the endoscopic thoracic sympathectomy for treatment of irradiation pain of the arm or of thoracic secondaries involving the sympathetic system.

Richardson: The main reason I did not mention it is that I have never done one. We do very few sympathectomies. We have sympathetic blocks done, and if the patient has good results, then we do sympathectomy. Most of the sympathectomies in my area are done by the transaxillary approach by the thoracic surgeons. I also find a very small number of patients who require sympathectomy.

Questioner: Dr. Swerdlow, do you have any experience with barbotage of spinal fluid in alleviation of cancer pain?

Swerdlow: It is by no means sure to produce any pain-relief, but it is pretty sure to produce a good headache.

Murri (Reggio Emilia): Dr. Gerbershagen, what are the advantages or disadvantages of tilidine in regard to morphine?

Gerbershagen (Mainz): The greatest advantage is that the effective duration is longer than that of morphine, about 6 to 8 hr on the average. As to addiction, dependence is no problem in cancer patients, otherwise I would say it is, in our experience, just about as addictive as morphine. In Germany it is not yet considered to be narcotic because of the structural formula, but I am pretty sure that in a couple of years it will be treated just as a narcotic.

Richardson: We have done hypophysectomy routinely, and we find it extremely effective for carcinoma of the prostate and moderately effective for carcinoma of the breast. And we are not trying to use hormone assays with tumor cell banning of estrogens to select patients for hypophysectomy of the breast. This has all been well established. My point was that hypophysectomy for non-hormonodependent tumors is still considered an experimental procedure. And I do not have reliable figures on efficacy, failure rate, and complication rate in non-hormonodependent tumors. We have a tremendous amount of data on patients with carcinoma of the breast and of the prostate. In my experience, hypophysectomy for carcinoma of the prostate with bone pain has been about 95% effective. With carcinoma of the breast, it has been about 50 to 60% effective.

Gerbershagen: In our Institute we have done over 400 hypophysectomies, and for 5 or 6 years we have not been doing them anymore or we are doing them very seldom—about 10 or 15 each year. That is due to better manipulating of medical hormonal treatment. At the very beginning, we did not have a good compound.

Advances in Pain Research and Therapy, Vol. 2,
edited by J. J. Bonica and V. Ventafridda.
Raven Press, New York © 1979.

Role of Analgesics and Related Drugs in Visceral and Perineal Pain

Raymond W. Houde

Department of Medicine, Memorial Sloan-Kettering Cancer Center, New York, New York 10021

Cancer involving the abdominal viscera and pelvis, and perineum, include a wide variety of neoplasms, both primary and metastatic, which can produce pain in a multiplicity of ways related either directly to the tumor itself or to complications of the disease or its treatment. Often the sources of pain are multiple and may involve both visceral and somatic afferent neural pathways for pain. The systemic analgesics, in particular the centrally acting drugs, are nonselective as to the site or source of pain, and thus provide an advantage over methods of controlling pain which rely upon precise identification of the involved pain pathways. This is especially true when both visceral and somatic structures are involved, or when the cause of the pain is in the midline or bilateral.

Centrally acting drugs such as the narcotics and their congeners are generally employed for the management of visceral and pelvic pain, although, contrary to popular opinion, the antiinflammatory-type analgesics are also effective and may be used to advantage in combination with other drugs. However, when there is gastrointestinal ulceration, bleeding, or the risk of perforation, salicylates and other antiinflammatory drugs are contraindicated. Since most nonnarcotics are also commonly administered by the oral route, they are obviously of little value when there is bowel obstruction or serious malabsorption.

The narcotic-type analgesics are also not without shortcomings, for most of these drugs will increase the tone of smooth muscle and of the sphincters; and they have hormonal effects, which can lead to urinary retention, obstipation, and fluid retention. Hepatic dysfunction can interfere with the metabolic disposition of most narcotics, although this does not commonly occur except in very far advanced disease of the liver. On the other hand, when hepatic function is intact and there is marked impairment of drug elimination by the kidney, active metabolites may accumulate and, as is the case with meperidine, lead to serious toxic reactions (1).

Most of the narcotic agonist-antagonists have effects similar to those of the narcotic agonists, to which they are most closely related. However, as partial agonists, these drugs tend to have ceiling effects, so that their effects may not be so intense as those of the typical narcotic agonist, particularly on the bowel.

The choice of an analgesic should be based on the nature and the quality of the pain and what is known of the extent of the disease. Pains may be dull and persistent, or intermittent and sharp, or cramp-like. If the patient is able to take medication by mouth, the combined administration of a narcotic and a nonnarcotic analgesic such as aspirin is generally indicated. For more severe pain, it may be necessary to employ parenteral medications but again, if it is not contraindicated, the concurrent administration of a simple analgesic by mouth may help to stay the too-rapid development of tolerance.

The indications of employing adjuvant drugs such as the anxiolytics, tranquilizers, and antidepressants are essentially the same as they would be in other clinical situations. With the exception of methotrimeprazine, there is no good substantial evidence that the phenothiazines or any of the other psychotropic drugs have any analgesic properties of their own, or that they are capable of enhancing the effect of standard analgesics in the absence of severe anxiety or depression, or symptoms contributing to suffering, such as nausea and vomiting. All of the narcotic analgesics increase the tone of smooth muscle including that of the intestine, and decrease peristalsis, so that one must be alert to the possibility of obstipation and obstruction. Commonly these patients do require stool softeners and cathartics to be taken on a fairly regular basis. The narcotic agonist-antagonists such as pentazocine have less of an effect on the bowel, but this drug is a somewhat shorter-acting drug than the morphine agonist analgesics, and there is a relatively high risk of psychotomimetic reactions. Methotrimeprazine, on the other hand, is a phenothiazine analgesic which has little effect on the bowel but can produce obstructive jaundice typical of the phenothiazines. Methotrimeprazine also has appreciable sedative and hypotensive actions, so that it is generally wise to start it at a lower dose than would be expected to be necessary for pain control. Methotrimeprazine may also be employed to supplement a narcotic analgesic, although there is an increased risk of precipitating both its hypotensive and sedative effects. Neither methotrimeprazine nor pentazocine will substitute for a narcotic in a narcotic-dependent patient, and, in fact, the pentazocine may precipitate abstinence.

In summary, the systemic analgesics and, in particular, the potent, centrally acting analgesics can play an important role in managing patients with intra-abdominal and pelvic pain. However, assessment for the possible causes of pain should always be done before prescribing any analgesic regimen, for many of these drugs may mask signs or symptoms which could delay the institution of definitive measures to prevent serious or life-threatening complications.

ACKNOWLEDGMENT

Supported in part by a Grant from the National Institute on Drug Abuse #DA 01707.

REFERENCE

1. Szeto, H. H., Inturrisi, C. E., Houde, R. W., Saal, S., Cheigh, J., and Reidenberg, M. M. (1977): Accumulation of normeperidine, an active metabolite of meperidine, in patients with renal failure or cancer. *Ann. Intern. Med.*, 86:738–741.

Advances in Pain Research and Therapy, Vol. 2,
edited by J. J. Bonica and V. Ventafridda.
Raven Press, New York © 1979.

Role of Nerve Block with Neurolytic Solutions for Pelvic Visceral Cancer Pain

Daniel C. Moore

The Mason Clinic, Seattle, Washington 98195

ANATOMICAL CONSIDERATIONS

Pain fibers from the pelvic viscera pass through the pelvic plexus, the hypogastric plexus, the aortic plexus, and the pelvic nerve. Pain fibers from the lower portion of the colon enter the spinal cord at the level of the first and second lumbar nerves and the second, third, and fourth sacral nerves. Those from the bladder enter at the level of the eleventh and twelfth thoracic and first lumbar nerves, as well as the second, third, and fourth sacral nerves. And those of the male and female reproductive systems enter at the tenth thoracic through the second lumbar nerves, as well as the second, third, and fourth sacral nerves (1).

The location of the plexuses prohibits safe, accurate placement of needles in or in close proximity to them. Therefore, block of the pain fibers from the pelvic viscera must be done where they, along with somatic nerves, enter the central nervous system—namely, paravertebrally or in the epidural or subarachnoid spaces (1,3,4,8,9,11,17,19,20). The injection of neurolytic solutions at these locations often results in incontinence of urine or feces and varying degrees of paralysis of the lower extremities.

An alternative method of eliminating pain, particularly when the male and female reproductive organs are its source, is ablation of the pituitary gland, which also has undesirable complications (2,10,12).

DIAGNOSTIC BLOCK

Seldom does cancer of the pelvic viscera remain within a single organ. Often it metastasizes to other intra-abdominal organs, and it frequently invades bone. These metastases exert pressure on somatic nerves, and this intensifies the pain. Therefore, prior to injection of a neurolytic solution for a lumbar sympathetic or epidural block, a diagnostic block using a long-acting local anesthetic drug—preferably 0.5% bupivacaine (Marcaine®) with 1:200,000 epinephrine—is advisable. However, diagnostic blocks are not used prior to ablation of the pituitary gland, where accurate needle placement presents problems initially and where a second placement would increase complications, or for subarachnoid block, where small quantities of local anesthetic drugs would not give a definitive result.

THERAPEUTIC BLOCKS

With the exception of lumbar sympathetic and unilateral subarachnoid block, the patient experiences intense, unbearable pain during administration of these blocks. Therefore, the patient must be anesthetized. During ablation of the pituitary, light general anesthesia or topical anesthesia with local infiltration usually suffices.

Lumbar Sympathetic Block

If pain is limited to the fundus of the bladder, bilateral block of the first through the third lumbar sympathetic ganglia with 5 ml of 50% to absolute alcohol or 6 to 7% phenol may give temporary pain-relief for 1 to 4 weeks, with no or minimal alteration in bladder, rectal, or lower extremity function. However, as the tumor grows and/or metastasizes and the pain recurs, final attempts to relieve pain with neurolytic drugs must involve more aggressive therapy—that is, placing of a neurolytic solution in the epidural or subarachnoid space.

Epidural Block (Lumbar or Caudal)

Weak solutions of alcohol, such as 30%, as well as 6% aqueous phenol, and volumes from 10 to 30 ml, have been injected with partial to complete relief of pain. The degree of dysfunction of the bladder, rectum, and lower extremities is usually proportionate to the volume and concentration employed. Relief from such an injection seldom has a prolonged duration.

Subarachnoid Block

Hypertonic saline. The neurolytic solution least likely to cause motor and sensory loss in the bladder, rectum, and lower extremities is hypertonic cold or partially frozen normal saline injected subarachnoidally (3,4,19,20). This technique involves removal of 30 to 60 ml of cerebrospinal fluid and replacement of it with 30 to 60 ml of partially frozen 7 to 15% normal saline. The higher volumes and the stronger concentrations result in the maximum pain-relief, the longest duration of action, and the most severe complications. The hazards of this technique range from reversible complications, such as severe pain during injection, hypotension, nausea and vomiting, and convulsions, to life-threatening or permanent ones, such as cardiac failure, pulmonary edema, incontinence of urine and feces, and paresis of the lower extremities.

Unilateral blocking of one to three dermatomes with alcohol or phenol. When the pain from the pelvic viscera is unilateral, blocking of one to three posterior spinal roots with 0.5 to 0.75 ml of absolute alcohol or 6 to 7% phenol (plain or in glycerine) may provide relief ranging from a few days to 2 to 3 weeks. Usually if more than two of the lumbar or sacral spinal roots are blocked unilaterally, weakness of the extremity can be expected, with or without incontinence of urine or feces. If bilateral block is attempted, one side should be done and then at least 24 hr should pass before the opposite side is blocked. Even if no complications result from the first injection, they are likely to occur following the second injection, particularly if more than two or three roots are blocked.

Transection of the spinal cord with alcohol. When the patient (a) is incontinent of urine and feces, (b) is not ambulatory, (c) has excruciating pain, or (d) preferably experiences all three, definitive treatment is subarachnoid injection and complete transection of the spinal cord with 10 to 15 ml of absolute alcohol at the first or second lumbar interspace (1,11). Prior to the injection of the alcohol, a similar amount of cerebrospinal fluid is withdrawn.

Pituitary Ablation with Alcohol

Certain primary cancers (male and female reproductive organs) and their metastases, which are susceptible to hormonal influence, can be treated with pituitary ablation employing 1.0 to 2.0 ml of absolute alcohol, depending on the size of sella (2,10,12). Pain-relief ranging from a few days to over 4 months results. The pain-relief varies from complete to partial in 70% of the patients, while the pain remains unchanged in 30% of the patients. Pain from other types of cancer has been treated with ablation of the pituitary with some success.

With this technique the bladder, rectum, and lower extremities are not affected, but rhinorrhea, nasal hemorrhage, leakage of cerebrospinal fluid, diplopia, hemianopia, and infection, as well as death from the injection, may occur. Also, as would be expected, diabetes insipidus, with or without hypopituitarism, ensues.

CONCLUSIONS

Treatment of cancer pain of the pelvic viscera with neurolytic drugs is a "trade-off" between pain-relief and complications—with or without pain-relief. Percutaneous or surgical cordotomy, myelotomy, and lobotomy usually are more accurate and effective (5,6,7,14,15,16,21). They are preferred to neurolytic, chemical sectioning techniques for they seldom require repeating, as is the rule with neurolytic drugs. However, these procedures too are associated with complications, such as lymphedema of the legs, partial to complete urinary and fecal incontinence, respiratory difficulties, and so forth; and they can be totally unsuccessful (13,14,18,21).

Block with a neurolytic drug should be done only when: (a) the patient and/or the family knows the consequences, (b) pain-relief, even for short periods of time, is desired, and (c) life-expectancy is limited.

The physician who does the block should: (a) have mastered the block technique, preferably learning it from an expert; (b) be skillful in its performance; (c) have the facilities and knowledge to cope with its complications; and (d) not become frustrated by less than optimal results—that is, partial to complete failures.

REFERENCES

1. Bonica, J. J. (1953): *The Management of Pain.* Lea & Febiger, Philadelphia.
2. Corssen, G., Holcomb, M. C., Moustapha, I., Langford, K., Vitek, J. J., and Ceballos, R. (1977): Alcohol-induced adenolysis of the pituitary gland: A new approach to control of intractable cancer pain. *Anesth. Analg.,* 56:414.
3. Hitchcock, E. (1967): Hypothermic subarachnoid irrigation for intractable pain. *Lancet,* 1:1133.
4. Hitchcock, E., and Prandini, M. N. (1973): Hypertonic saline management of intractable pain. *Lancet,* 1:310.
5. Lin, P. M., Gildenberg, P. L., and Polakoff, P. P. (1966): An anterior approach to percutaneous lower cervical cordotomy. *J. Neurosurg.,* 25:553.
6. Lipton, S. (1968): Percutaneous electrical cordotomy in relief of intractable pain. *Br. Med. J.,* 2:210.
7. Lipton, S., Dervin, E., and Heywood, O. B. (1974): A stereotactic approach to the anterior percutaneous electric cordotomy. *Adv. Neurol.,* 4:689.
8. Maher, R. M. (1955): Relief of pain in encurable cancer. *Lancet,* 1:18.
9. Mehta, M. (1973): *Intractable Pain.* W. B. Saunders Co., Ltd., London.
10. Miles, J., and Lipton, S. (1976): Mode of action by which pituitary alcohol injection relieves pain. In: *Advances in Pain Research and Therapy, Vol. 1: Proceedings of the First World Congress on Pain,* edited by J. J. Bonica and D. Albe-Fessard, p. 867. Raven Press, New York.
11. Moore, D. C. (1976): *Regional Block,* 4th ed. Charles C Thomas, Springfield, Ill.
12. Moricca, G. (1974): Chemical hypophysectomy for cancer pain. In: *Advances in Neurology, Vol. 4: International Symposium on Pain,* edited by J. J. Bonica, p. 707. Raven Press, New York.
13. Mulland, S., and Hosobuichi, Y. (1968): Respiratory hazards of high cervical percutaneous cordotomy. *J. Neurosurg.,* 22:291.
14. Rifkinson, N. (1978): Neurosurgery and pain control. *Anesthesiology News,* 4:11.
15. Rosomoff, H. L. (1969): Bilateral percutaneous cervical radiofrequency cordotomy. *J. Neurosurg.,* 31:41.
16. Rosomoff, H. L. (1974): Percutaneous radiofrequency cervical cordotomy for intractable pain. *Adv. Neurol.,* 4:683.
17. Stovner, J., and Endresen, R. (1972): Intrathecal phenol for cancer pain. *Acta Anesthesiol. Scand.,* 16:17.
18. Tenicela, F., Rosomoff, H. L., Feist, J., and Safar, P. (1968): Pulmonary function following percutaneous cervical cordotomy. *Anesthesiology,* 29:7.
19. Thompson, G. E. (1971): Pulmonary edema complicating intrathecal hypertonic saline injections for intractable pain. *Anesthesiology,* 35:425.
20. Ventafridda, V., and Spreafico, R. (1974): Subarachnoid saline perfusion. In: *Advances in Neurology, Vol. 4: International Symposium on Pain,* edited by J. J. Bonica, p. 477. Raven Press, New York.
21. White, J. C. (1965): Relief of terminal cancer pain. *Surg. Gynecol. Obstet.,* 120:115.

Advances in Pain Research and Therapy, Vol. 2,
edited by J. J. Bonica and V. Ventafridda.
Raven Press, New York © 1979.

Neurolytic Blocks in Perineal Pain

V. Ventafridda, C. Fochi, E. P. Sganzerla, and M. Tamburini

Department of Pain Therapy and Rehabilitation, National Cancer Institute, Milan, Italy; and Department of Anesthesiology, Universita degli Studi, 20133 Milan, Italy

Perineal pain due to neoplastic disease manifests itself as three different types of sensation which can be either separated or associated: a "burning sensation," tenesmus, and somatic pain without trigger points. In order to comprehend the intensity of this painful syndrome and the alteration which it can cause in the patient's personality, we report the results obtained from a study carried out in our Pain Therapy Department.

We have submitted two groups of patients affected by cancer of the rectum to a psychometric test (MMPI) (6): the first (control) group was composed of colostomy patients who were free from pain and disease; the second group consisted of 25 patients with perineal pain in an evolutionary stage. In the second group (Fig. 1) we observed a marked increase in all clinical personality scales; in particular 40% of such subjects (against the 12% of the patients in the first group) present a remarkable increase (scores superior to 70 T.) of the neurotic scales (hysteria, hypochondriasis, and depression) (Fig. 1).

Because these personality alterations cause a drop in the pain threshold, it is important to start therapy as soon as possible at the time the pain symptomatology is still localized and the usual nonnarcotic analgesic drugs are no longer sufficient. The simplest and most suitable treatment of these painful syndromes are neurolytic subarachnoid sacral blocks or chemical rhizotomy and peridural caudal block.

Neurolytic hyperbaric solutions offer some advantages over hypobaric solutions with alcohol, because it is easier technically to block the lower area affected by pain and it is less discomforting for the patient during the procedure.

Several authors have achieved good results with classic Maher's technique, which consists of performing subarachnoid infiltration with hyperbaric phenol in glycerine at the level of the L_5-S_1 interspace (9). Lifshitz et al. (8) reported that out of 90 patients with perineal pain due to gynecologic malignancy treated with one or more sacral phenol blocks, 77% of them derived satisfactory to excellent results. Using this technique, Stovner and Endresen (13) produced analgesia for almost 1 month for 83% of the patients affected by cancer of the rectum, anus, and external genitalia.

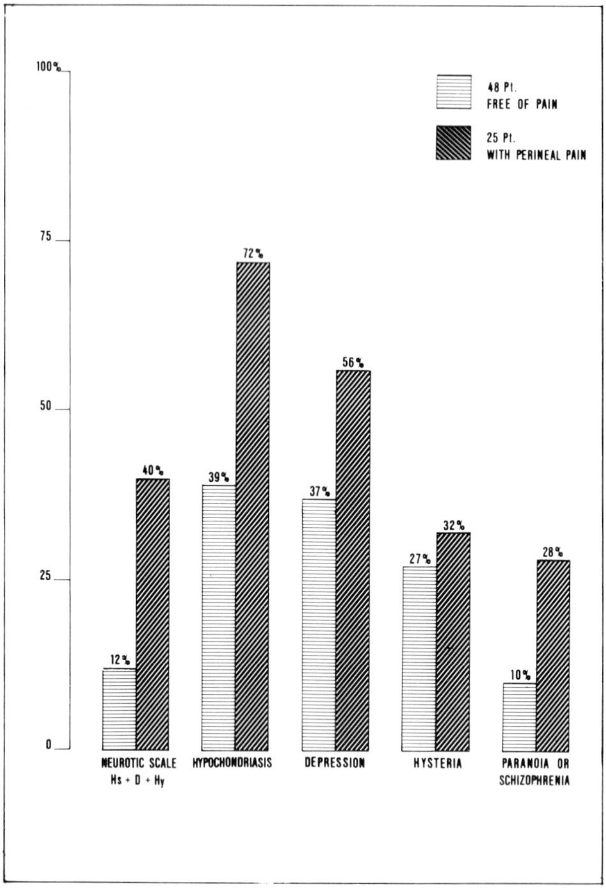

FIG. 1. MMPI significant percent scales with T > 70 on 73 ostomy patients.

Papo and Visca (11) also reported that 30 of 35 patients affected by cancer of the rectum derived good and fair pain-relief.

In 1975, Kuhner and Assmus (7) published the results of a study of 596 patients treated with hyperbaric phenol. They noted that the best results were obtained in patients with pain due to cancer of the rectum, 79% of whom derived complete relief and 13% partial relief of pain, and in patients with urogenital tumors of whom 67% obtained complete relief and 23% partial relief.

All of the authors who have reported on the technique mentioned bladder sphincter complications as being present in most patients.

In regard to perineal pain in patients treated with repeated peridural injection of bupivacaine, different authors reported prolonged analgesia in patients with nonmalignant pain (2,3,4,5). Furthermore, caudal blocks with bupivacaine and corticoid compounds have produced beneficial effects in patients with low back pain (1–14).

MATERIAL AND METHODS

We have treated 47 patients with pain caused by the following neoplastic primary tumors: 36 with cancer of the rectum; 4 with cancer of the uterus; 2 each with cancer of the vagina and prostate; 1 each with cancer of the vulva and sigmoid; and 1 with a cordoma. For these patients, two techniques were used: caudal blocks with local anesthetic and corticoids and chemical rhizotomy.

Technique of Caudal Epidural Block

The standard technique of caudal epidural block was used (Fig. 2A). Following placement of the needle into the sacral canal, 10 ml of 0.25% bupivacaine combined with 80 mg of methyl-prednisolone were injected. This procedure was repeated on an average of 6 times at intervals of 3 to 4 days.

Chemical Rhizotomy

The technique of chemical rhizotomy is as follows: With the patient in a sitting position, a 23-gauge needle was introduced through L_5-S_1 interspace (Fig. 2B) into the subarachnoid cavity. Once this was done, the point of the needle was carefully withdrawn posteriorly until CSF flow was reduced to a trickle in order to try to avoid the roots which lie more ventrally. A solution of 0.8 ml of 7.5% phenol in glycerine was injected slowly using two different positions:

1. *For bilateral pain,* the patient was in a sitting position, tilted backward at an angle of 15 to 30° to the edge of the table.
2. *For unilateral pain,* the patient was made to lie on the painful side with the head of the table raised 30°.

The patients kept these positions for 30 min.

An immediate indication of the extent of chemical rhizotomy was the appearance of an area of hypesthesia from S_2 to S_5 which was reduced to S_4-S_5 during the ensuing 48 hr. Each of these procedures was repeated as soon as the pain occurred.

The caudal epidural block with local anesthetic and corticoid was used when: (a) There was no clinical data indicating spread of the disease; (b) micturition was normal; (c) there was no skin erosion or trigger points; and (d) the patient was complaining of a burning sensation or tenesmus.

We used chemical rhizotomy when the patient affected by the perineal

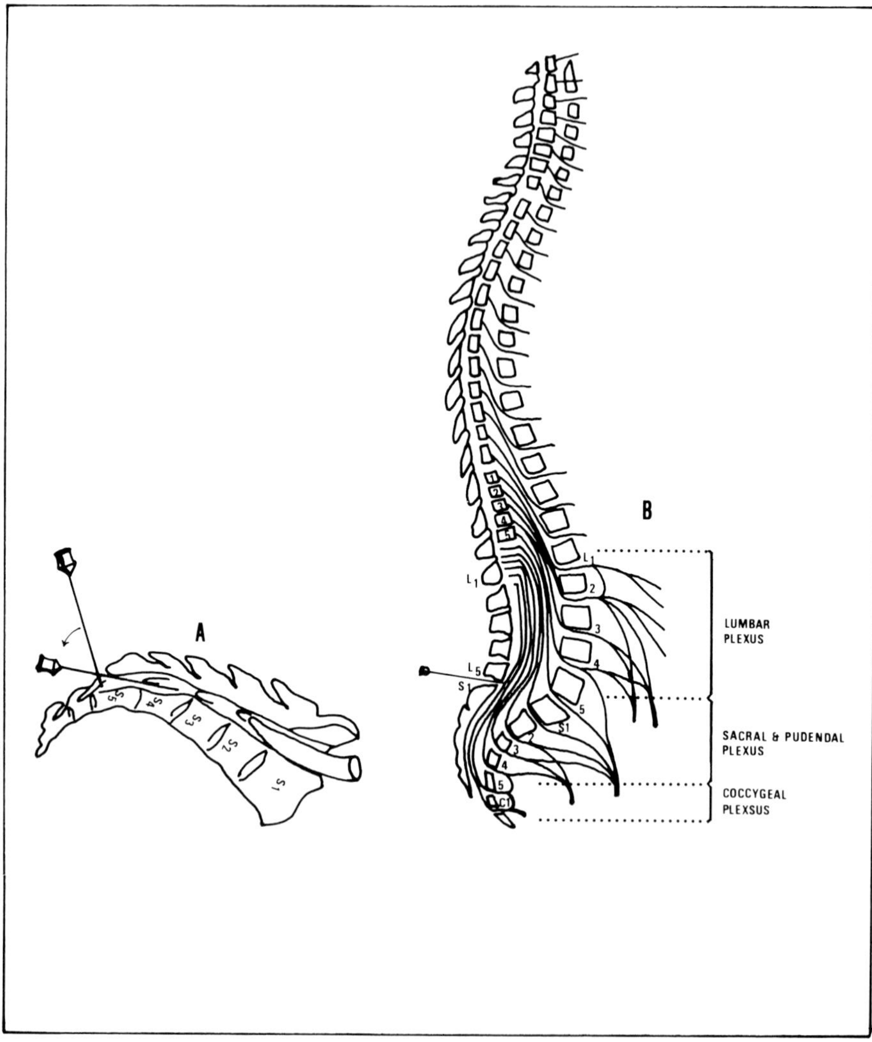

FIG. 2. A. Caudal-epidural blocks. **B.** Subarachnoid sacral blocks.

pain showed: (a) suspicious signs of recurrence of the disease; (b) macroscopic areas of vulvovaginal or pararectal erosions and evident "trigger points"; and (c) trouble with micturition or preexisting bladder dysfunction.

The follow-up of these patients was carried out every month until death of the patient or the further spreading of the pain. In addition, another group of 13 patients including 8 treated with caudal epidural blocks and 5 with chemical rhizotomy have been followed for 4 weeks using a weekly chart filled in by the patients and which included: (a) evaluation of pain intensity using the visual analogue of Scott and Huskisson (12); and (b) the total amount of time the patient spent standing, lying, sitting, and sleeping.

RESULTS

Of 47 patients affected by perineal pain due to neoplastic disease (Table 1), 39 have been treated with chemical rhizotomy. A total of 77 neurolytic blocks were performed for an average of 1.97 blocks for each patient. The average duration of pain-relief was 5.43 months. Bladder sphincter complication was noted in 19 patients (49%).

We carried out 48 caudal epidural blocks in 8 patients, averaging 6 blocks for each patient. In this group the average duration of pain-relief was 3.5 months.

The average time of pain-relief after chemical rhizotomy in 14 patients with trigger points was 5.92 months. In 14 patients with evident erosion areas, it was 8.35 months; and in 11 patients without trigger points or erosion areas but with pain spreading to $S_{2\text{-}3}$ areas, the pain-relief lasted only 1.09 months (Table 2).

Among the 5 patients who underwent chemical rhizotomy and were followed with the weekly pain charts, the visual analogue showed an average reduction of pain of 71.4%. The total number of hours the patient was up and about increased by 204%, while the time the patient spent sitting and lying down was diminished by 36%, and the total number of hours asleep were increased by 25%. Less favorable, though still-significant results were reported in 8 patients treated with caudal blocks: Pain was reduced by 47.4%, and the total hours the patient was active were increased by 37% (Fig. 3).

COMPLICATIONS

Prolonged muscle weakness in the lower limbs did not develop in any of our patients. We believe that this complication can be obviated with a correct technique.

Meningeal reactions and low pressure headaches may also be avoided with prophylactic measures such as the use of a fine spinal needle (21 to 23 gauge), bed rest, oral and parenteral administration of fluids (10).

TABLE 1. *Results with block therapy of perineal pain*

	Number of patients	Number of treatments	Mean N° of treatments	Mean analgesic time (months)	Bladder impairment
Caudal-epidural blocks	8	48	6	3.5	—
Chemical rhizotomy	39	77	1.97	5.4	19 (49%)

TABLE 2. *Duration of pain relief*

	N° of patients	Mean analgesic time (months)
With trigger points	14	5.9
With macroscopic ulcerations	14	8.35
Without trigger points or ulcerations with spreading	11	1.09

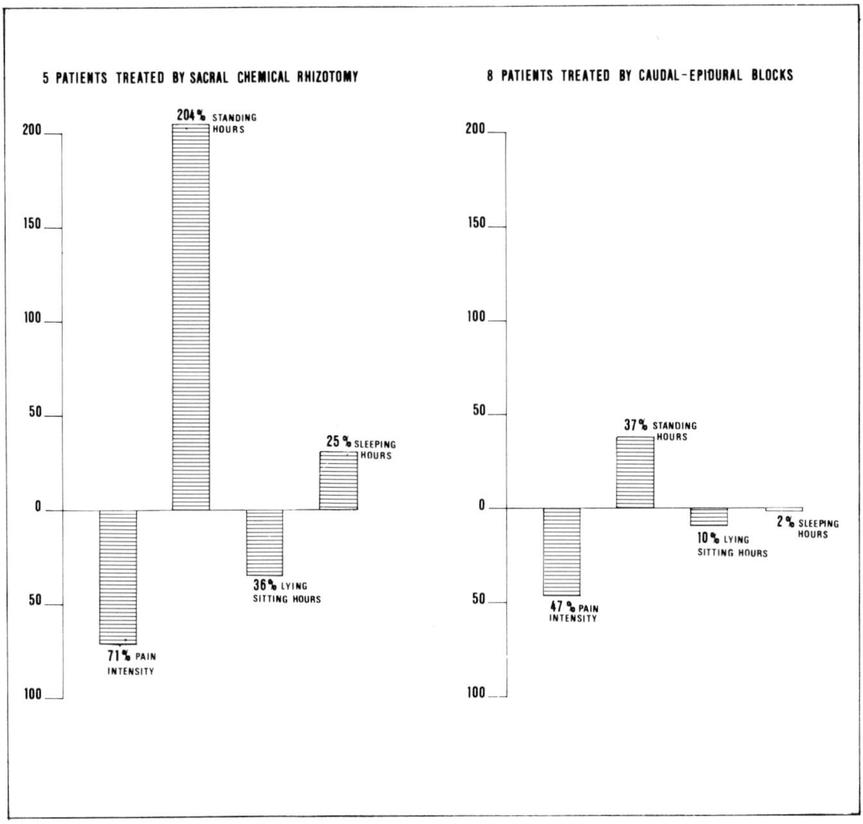

FIG. 3. Percent change of perineal pain intensity and some living activity data after one month on 13 patients affected by cancer of the rectum.

Problems concerning rectal dysfunction did not develop in our patients because 79% of them had a colostomy. Impotence, with loss of penile erection has also been reported after treatment in advanced cases (10). Bladder complications, such as incontinence or, more frequently, retention, are rather common, because among the roots affected by the chemical lesion are S_2-S_3-S_4, which contribute to the nervi erigentes and pudendal nerves with consequent relaxation of external and internal sphincters of the bladder. This kind of complication may be partially avoided when the pain is unilateral and the neurolytic block is performed with the patient lying on the painful side.

Of the group treated with chemical rhizotomy, 19 (49%) patients developed difficulties with micturition. A bladder rehabilitation, preceded by urodynamic tests, is important in such cases. Bladder retention, which often occurs, can be cured by inserting a urethral catheter right after the procedure. A few days later, the catheter is removed and the patient is encouraged to urinate at regular intervals by using manual suprapubic compression and by giving subcutaneous injections of 5 mg of urocoline for the first 5 days and the same dose orally for the following week.

CONCLUSIONS

Our experience and that of other writers (7,8,10,11,13) suggest that subarachnoid phenol block at level L_5-S_1 is useful, simple, and a very efficacious method in relieving perineal neoplastic pain. The best results are obtained in patients having tumors which involve peripheral nerve fibers. We noted the longest pain-relief in patients with trigger points, or perineal skin and mucous erosion, or necrosis due to neoplastic process or radiation therapy (tenesmus and burning sensation were partially relieved). Bladder dysfunction, the most common complication of neurolytic blocks, may be controlled by prompt rehabilitation.

Follow-up of patients must be performed at least monthly, and blocks must be repeated immediately as the pain develops in adjacent areas. In such instances, before undertaking cordotomy or an enlarged chemical rhizotomy, a scintigraphic study is useful to ascertain if there are further involved areas to treat with radiation therapy.

Pain control may be achieved for a significant period of time and in some patients it lasts until death. For those patients having perineal pain due to side effect of local radiation or surgical scar by Miles operation, the repeated caudal epidural anesthetic block is a practical tool free of complications in order to get a good and sometimes prolonged analgesia.

Our experiences lead us to conclude that pain-relief obtained by neurolytic block in perineal cancer pain improves the daily living activity of the patient and therefore, even for a short period, the quality of his life.

REFERENCES

1. Breivik, H., Hesla, P. E., Molnar, I., and Lind, B. (1976): Treatment of chronic low back pain and sciatica: Comparison of caudal epidural injections of bupivacaine and methyl prednisolone with bupivacaine followed by saline. In: *Advances in Pain Research and Therapy, Vol. 1, Proceedings of the First World Congress on Pain,* edited by J. J. Bonica and D. Albe-Fessard, pp. 927–932. Raven Press, New York.
2. Ciocatto, E. (1964): The management of pain. In: *International Anaesthesiology Clinics, Vol. 2.* Little, Brown, Boston.
3. Dogliotti, A. M., and Ciocatto, E. (1955): Method of differential block in pain relief. *Anesthesiology,* 16:623–626.
4. Defalque, R. J. (1974): Treatment of chronic pain with bupivacaine epidural block. *Anesth. Analg.,* 53:841–843.
5. Hannington-Kiff, J. G. (1971): Treatment of intractable pain by bupivacaine nerve block. *Lancet,* 2:1392–1394.
6. Hathaway, S. R., and McKinley, J. C. (1967): *Minnesota Multiphasic Personality Inventory: Manual for Administration and Scoring.* Psychological Corporation, New York.
7. Kuhner, A., and Assmus, H. (1975): Intrathecal application of phenol in the treat-

ment of intractable pain. In: *Brain Hypoxia-Pain: Advances in Neurosurgery, Vol. 2,* pp. 256–263. Springer-Verlag, Berlin, Heidelberg, New York.
8. Lifshitz, S., Debacker, L. J., Buchsbaum, H. J. (1976): Subarachnoid phenol block for pain relief in gynecologic malignancy. *Obstet. Gynecol. (N.Y.)*, 48:316–320.
9. Maher, R. M. (1966): Phenol for pain and spasticity. In: *Pain—Henry Ford Hospital International Symposium,* edited by R. S. Knighton and P. R. Dumke. Little, Brown, Boston.
10. Mehta, M. (1973): *Intractable Pain.* W. B. Saunders Company, Ltd., London, Philadelphia, Toronto.
11. Papo, I., and Visca, A. (1974): Phenol rhizotomy in the treatment of cancer pain. *Anesth. Analg.,* 53:993–997.
12. Scott, J., and Huskisson, E. C. (1976): Graphic representation of pain. *Pain,* 2:175–184.
13. Stovner, J., and Endresen, R. (1972): Intrathecal phenol for cancer pain. *Acta Anesth. Scand.,* 16:17–21.
14. Swerdlow, M., and Sayle Creer, W. (1970): A study of extradural medication in the relief of the lumbosciatic syndrome. *Anaesthesia,* 25:341–345.

Advances in Pain Research and Therapy, Vol. 2,
edited by J. J. Bonica and V. Ventafridda.
Raven Press, New York © 1979.

Role of Neurosurgery in Visceral and Perineal Pain

John D. Loeser

Department of Neurological Surgery, University of Washington, Seattle, Washington 98195

Neoplasms of the abdominal and pelvic viscera are not uncommon causes of chronic pain, although the actual incidence of pain associated with individual neoplasms is hard to determine. Those tumors which are locally invasive seem to be the more customary producers of visceral and perineal pain. It is also difficult to determine what percentage of cancer patients will endure chronic pain in the perineal or abdominal regions. Not only does the malignancy itself have the potential for causing pain, but the aftereffects of surgery and radiation therapy can also lead to chronic pain.

It may be very difficult in a particular patient to ascertain what the contribution of any one of these three may be to the patient's pain problem. We must also be aware of the possibility that a patient's complaint of pain may also be due to depression, fear, or feelings of isolation. While surgical measures are likely to alleviate pain due to noxious stimulation, cutting nerves is not a good way to relieve depression or fear. Careful patient-selection is clearly the single most important factor. Although much has been written on this topic, predictors of surgical outcome are still not well-established.

In general, the cancer patient is more likely to be relieved of pain by a surgical procedure than is a patient with chronic pain due to a nonmalignant disease process. It is ironic, then, that surgical relief of pain is often deferred far too long in the cancer patient and utilized far too quickly in the patient with a nonmalignant disease. The presence of narcotic addiction should not be a factor in determining who is offered neurosurgical relief of pain: If the operation is successful, it is not difficult to withdraw the patient from narcotics (8).

NEURECTOMY

A logical place to begin my discussion of neurosurgical therapy for visceral and perineal pain is in the periphery. Although neurectomies would appear to be a rational approach to discrete pain, they are rarely successful. The propensity of the neoplastic process to spread beyond the denervated zone is one reason not to consider peripheral neurectomy. To reach the involved nerve it may be necessary to operate through a previously irradiated field or traverse the neoplasm itself. In addition, visceral pain is notoriously diffuse. I can see almost no role for peripheral neurectomy in cancer pain.

DORSAL RHIZOTOMY

Pelvic and perineal pain may be alleviated by the appropriate dorsal rhizotomies (2,4,11,16,17,20,23,25,28,30). Midline pain requires bilateral rhizotomies; unilateral pain is often well-controlled by this procedure. The major problem with sacral dorsal rhizotomies for pelvic and perineal pain is the impairment of urinary and anal sphincters which follows extensive sacral denervation. Unilateral rhizotomies are usually well tolerated; bilateral rhizotomies will cause loss of voluntary control of bowel and bladder. This restricts bilateral sacral rhizotomies to patients who have already had a colostomy and a urinary diversionary procedure or a catheter (4).

Bilateral sacral rhizotomies are most easily performed via a midline incision from L_4 to S_2, a laminectomy of L_5, S_1, and S_2 and exposure of the dura at its caudal termination. The dura is opened and the roots identified by both morphology and the response to stimulation. All of the roots caudal to S_1 may be divided without compromising leg function. Unilateral rhizotomies may be done through the same incision or may be performed extradurally by exposing the roots through the sacral foramina. This procedure may also be accomplished with a radiofrequency probe passed percutaneously; reliable data on the efficacy of this method is not available.

If the pain involves segments higher than S_2, dorsal rhizotomy is likely to lead to significant difficulty with lower-extremity function. Although a single root of the lumbosacral plexus may be divided with impunity, one cannot totally denervate the extremity without causing paralysis and loss of protective reflexes. To the extent, therefore, that the pain involves the lumbar roots, dorsal rhizotomy is usually not a satisfactory mode of therapy. Since the origin of the pain is usually neoplastic involvement of nerves or viscera, the operative field for sacral rhizotomy is usually free of tumor. When the neoplasm has invaded the sacrum, dorsal rhizotomy is probably not a wise surgical choice.

The surgeon must be cognizant of the fact that pelvic and abdominal visceral pain may be transmitted via the autonomic nervous system and may not be relieved by sacral rhizotomy. Preoperative assessment with appropriate nerve blocks will indicate the sites of origin of the pain and the role of the autonomic and somatic afferent systems. Nerve blocks do not seem to be a reliable predictor of the long-term efficacy of a surgical procedure, however. Data on the efficacy of dorsal rhizotomy for visceral and perineal pain due to cancer are contained in Table 1.

TABLE 1. *Dorsal rhizotomy for visceral and perineal pain*

Author	Year	No.	% Success[b]
Barrash & Leavens (2)[a]	1973	71	70
Bohm & Franksson (3)	1958	7	100
Crue et al. (4)	1970	18	72
Loeser (11)[a]	1972	7	43
Onofrio & Campa (15)	1972	18	28
Paillas (17)[a]	1972	6	0
Ray (20)[a]	1943	?	?
Scoville (23)[a]	1966	2	100
Sindou et al. (25)	1974	12	75
White & Sweet (30)[a]	1969	35	58

[a] All patients had malignancies, percentage success for pain in this site uncertain.
[b] Pain-relief for 3 months or longer or until death if survival less than 3 months.

CORDOTOMY

Cordotomy is a particularly effective surgical therapy for visceral and perineal pain (5,7,10,12,15,19,21,23,28,29). There are many methods of sectioning the anterolateral quadrant of the spinal cord; common operative sites are upper thoracic and upper cervical. When the pain is midline, bilateral cordotomies will be required. Frequently, the patient reports unilateral pain; but, after a cordotomy, pain is found to be present on the other side as well. This is probably due to masking of a minor pain by a more severe one. When the major pain is relieved, the minor one becomes recognized.

A cordotomy will markedly reduce pain and temperature sensation on the contralateral side of the body. There is no nerve block which simulates this lesion, so preoperative testing of efficacy cannot be carried out. Unilateral cordotomies carry a low risk of bladder dysfunction; bilateral cordotomies will impair male sexual function and bladder control in either sex in about 10% of the patients. Leg weakness should be an uncommon complication. One of the major drawbacks of cordotomy is that the sensory loss and pain-relief may disappear months or years after the original operation. Repeat cordotomy is rarely effective. Of course, the short life-expectancy of most patients with pain due to cancer tends to reduce the likelihood of late cordotomy failure. Since the operation is performed in the cervical or thoracic regions, it is well removed from the neoplasm and radiation effect; wound healing is less likely to be compromised. Cordotomy is frequently the operation of choice for patients with visceral and perineal pain due to cancer (Table 2).

One of the most significant advances in the surgical management of pain due to cancer was the development of percutaneous techniques for cordotomy (10,15,21). These have made it possible to offer cordotomy to any

TABLE 2. *Anterolateral cordotomy for visceral and perineal pain*

Author	Year	Number	Type	Site	Mortality	Success[b]	Complications
Diemath et al. (5)	1961	50	0	C,T	8	82	~20
Frankel & Prokop (6)	1961	59	0	T	11	67	~20
French et al.	1966	103	0	C	0	96	~25
Lin et al. (10)[a]	1966	39	P	C	0	74	~ 5
Nathan (12)	1963	77	0	C,T	0?	77	~15
Nolan & Peyton (13)	1956	40	0	C,T	2.5	75	~10
Onofrio (16)[a]	1970	41	P	C	2	85	~ 5
Raskind (19)	1969	190	0	C,T	3	92	~15
Rosomoff (21)[a]	1974	1279	P	C	?	84	~ 5
Schwartz (22)	1960	73	0	C	12	70	~20
Simionescu (24)	1957	62	0	T	?	74	?
White & Sweet (29)[a]	1969a	271	0	T	8	77	~10
(29)[a]	1969b	28	0	C	?	75	~10

[a] Number of patients with visceral and perineal pain uncertain, all patients had cancer.
[b] Pain-relief for 3 months or longer or until death if survival is less than 3 months.

patient, regardless of cachexia or debilitation. A needle is placed in the cervical spinal cord under X-ray control, and its position verified by the responses to electrical stimulation; a lesion is made using radiofrequency current. Surgeons who utilize percutaneous cordotomy regularly have reported excellent relief of pain and few complications. The procedure is deceptively simple, and the inexperienced operator will have a significantly lower success rate and more complications.

Each neurosurgeon has his preferred site and method for performing a cordotomy. There seems to be no published evidence that one form of this operation is more likely to succeed than another or that one technique has fewer complications.

MYELOTOMY

Midline myelotomy is another surgical procedure that can be performed either open or percutaneously; a limited number of patients have been reported but pain-relief can be excellent. Most neurosurgeons have little experience with myelotomy, although this operation seems to be gaining popularity. It is designed to interrupt a multisynaptic, diffusely projecting system that is distinct from the spinothalamic pathways transected during a cordotomy (9,18,26,27). This can be accomplished in the thoracolumbar region on a segmental basis or in the high cervical region where more diffuse pain loss will ensue (9). Myelotomy seems to have a low complication rate and deserves further trial in patients with pain due to cancer. The available data on myelotomy are contained in Table 3.

TABLE 3. *Commissural myelotomy for visceral and perineal pain*

Author	Year	Number	Type[a]	Site[b]	Mortality	% Success[c]
Armour (1)	1927	1	O	TL	100	
Hitchcock (9)	1970	2	P	C	0	100
Papo & Luongo (18)	1976	4	O	C	0	25
Sourek (26)	1969	19	O	TL	0	100
Wertheimer (27)	1953	93	O	TL	7	65

[a] O = open; P = percutaneous.
[b] C = cervical; TL = thoracolumbar.
[c] Pain-relief for 3 months or longer or until death if survival is less than 3 months.

SYMPATHECTOMY

Sympathectomy can effectively relieve pain originating in thoracic and abdominal viscera (28). Nerve blocks are most helpful in delineating the exact structures involved in the transmission of noxious stimuli; neurolytic blocks are often superior to surgical resection. Splanchnectomy or ganglionectomy may be required to denervate the involved viscus. The vagus nerve may also carry afferents from the upper abdominal viscera (14). When a malignancy spreads from a viscus and involves parietal peritoneum or body wall, sympathectomy alone will not effectively relieve the pain. For this reason, cordotomy is usually superior to either dorsal rhizotomy or sympathectomy when visceral or perineal pain is due to cancer. No one procedure seems clearly superior. Meaningful contrasts between these operations are difficult because of unknown factors in patient-selection and differing criteria for pain-relief.

HYPOPHYSECTOMY

A few unfortunate patients with cancer have pain syndromes which are not amenable to any local denervating procedures. When prostatic carcinoma metastasizes widely to bone, for example, no local operation is likely to provide significant relief. Some of these neoplasms are responsive to hypophysectomy; both rate of tumor growth and pain are favorably altered (West, *this volume*). Of course, replacement hormone therapy is required. Nonetheless, excellent palliation can be obtained with some endocrine-sensitive neoplasms. The methods of destroying the pituitary gland are many; once again the surgeon's choice seems to be the relevant variable.

BRAIN OPERATIONS

Other patients with uncontrolled visceral and perineal pain may be candidates for *thalamotomy*. This stereotaxic procedure can effectively eliminate pain; unfortunately, the beneficial effects rarely last more than 1 year. A cancer patient with such a short life-expectancy might be a candidate for this operation, however. *Cingulumotomy* or selective mesial frontal lobotomy also has a place in the management of cancer pain. This operation markedly reduces the affective response to noxious stimulation without producing much change in actual sensory thresholds. It seems to be particularly valuable in the patient who is depressed and anxious as well as in pain. It is unfortunate that the furor about psychosurgery has limited so severely the availability of cingulumotomy for the small number of patients who have no other reasonable method of obtaining pain relief.

SUMMARY

Visceral and perineal pains due to cancer are often not well managed. Neurosurgical therapy is often delayed until after trials of chemotherapy, local surgery, and radiotherapy, all of which may be known to be of little value in the management of a particular neoplasm. Patients are placed on debilitating medications to control pain, because their physicians are unaware of the chronic effects of the drugs and the potential advantages of neurosurgical therapy. When survival for more than 3 months seems likely, pharmacotherapy is unlikely to be the optimal treatment modality. Prompt neurosurgical intervention can offer the patient complete relief of pain without the mind-clogging effects of narcotics. When survival is likely to be less than 3 months, percutaneous surgical or neurolytic techniques are usually superior. If survival is likely to be less than 1 month, pharmacotherapy is usually appropriate. Each patient's disease, personality, and environment must be carefully considered to plan optimal therapy.

REFERENCES

1. Armour, D. (1927): Lettsomian lecture on the surgery of the spinal cord and its membranes. *Lancet,* 1:691–697.
2. Barrash, J. M., and Leavens, M. E. (1973): Dorsal rhizotomy for the relief of intractable pain of malignant tumor origin. *J. Neurosurg.,* 38:755–757.
3. Bohm, E., and Franksson, C. (1958): Coccygodynia and sacral rhizotomy. *Acta Chir. Scand.,* 116:268–274.
4. Crue, B. L., Jr., Todd, E. M., Wright, G. H., and Maline, D. B. (1970): Sacral rhizotomy for pelvic pain. In: *Pain and Suffering,* edited by B. L. Crue, pp. 20–34. Charles C Thomas, Springfield, Ill.
5. Diemath, H. E., Heppner, F., and Walker, A. E. (1961): Anterolateral cordotomy for relief of pain. *Postgrad. Med.,* 29:485–495.
6. Frankel, S. A., and Prokop, J. D. (1961): Value of cordotomy for the relief of pain. *NEJM,* 264:971–974.
7. French, L. A., Chou, S. N., and Story, J. L. (1966): Cervical tractotomy: Technique and clinical usefulness. In: *Henry Ford Hospital International Symposium,* edited by R. Knighton, pp. 311–319. Charles C Thomas, Springfield, Ill.
8. Hall, T. C. (1970): Philosophy of pain control in cancer patients. *Postgrad. Med.,* 48:223–227.
9. Hitchcock, E. R. (1970): Stereotactic cervical myelotomy. *J. Neurol. Neurosurg. Psychiat.,* 33:224–230.
10. Lin, P. M., Gildenberg, P. L., and Polakoff, P. P. (1966): An anterior approach to percutaneous lower cervical cordotomy. *J. Neurosurg.,* 25:553–560.
11. Loeser, J. D. (1972): Dorsal rhizotomy for the relief of chronic pain. *J. Neurosurg.,* 36:745–750.
12. Nathan, P. W. (1963): Results of antero-lateral cordotomy for pain in cancer. *J. Neurol. Neurosurg. Psychiat.,* 26:353–362.
13. Nolan, Robert K., and Peyton, William T. (1956): Cordotomy for relief of pain in incurable squamous-cell carcinoma of the cervix uteri. *Am. J. Obstet. Gynecol.,* 71:790–792.
14. Oi, M., and Kobayashi, K. (1963): Vagotomy as a surgical procedure for relief of pain. *Am. J. Surg.,* 106:49–56.
15. Onofrio, B. M. (1970): Recent results with percutaneous cordotomy. *Mayo Clin. Proc.,* 45:689–694.
16. Onofrio, B., and Campa, H. K. (1972): Evaluation of rhizotomy. Review of 12 years' experience. *J. Neurosurg.,* 36:751–755.
17. Paillas, J. W., and Pellet, W. (1972): Dorsal nerve root section in the treatment of refractory peripheral pain. In: *Pain,* edited by R. Janzen et al., pp. 209–213. William & Wilkins, Baltimore.
18. Papo, I., and Luongo, A. (1976): High cervical commissural myelotomy in the treatment of pain. *J. Neurol. Neurosurg. Psychiat.,* 39:705–710.
19. Raskind, R. (1969): Analytical review of open cordotomy. *Int. Surg.,* 51:226–231.
20. Ray, B. S. (1943): The management of intractable pain by posterior rhizotomy. *Res. Publ. Assoc. Res. Nerv. Ment. Dis.,* 23:391–407.

21. Rosomoff, H. L. (1974): Percutaneous radiofrequency cervical cordotomy for intractable pain. *Adv. Neurol.,* 4:683–688.
22. Schwartz, H. G. (1960): High cervical cordotomy—technique and results. *Clin. Neurosurg.,* 8:282–293.
23. Scoville, W. B. (1966): Extradural spinal sensory rhizotomy. *J. Neurosurg.,* 25:94–95.
24. Simionescu, M. D. (1957): The management of pain due to pelvic malignancy: A follow-up of 122 cases. *Zlb. Neurochir.,* 17:284–287.
25. Sindou, M., Fischer, G., and Mansuy, L. (1976): Posterior spinal rhizotomy and selective posterior rhizidiotomy. *Prog. Neurol. Surg.,* 7:201–250.
26. Sourek, K. (1969): Commissural myelotomy. *J. Neurosurg.,* 31:524–527.
27. Wertheimer, P., and Lecuire, J. (1953): La myelotomie commissurale postérieure. *Acta Chir. Belg.,* 52:568–574.
28. White, J. C. (1968): Operations for the relief of pain in the torso and extremities: Evaluation of their effectiveness over long periods. In: *Pain,* edited by A. Souilairac et al., pp. 503–519. Academic Press, London.
29. White, J. C., and Sweet, W. H. (1969): *Pain and the Neurosurgeon,* pp. 678–767. Charles C Thomas, Springfield, Ill.
30. White, J. C., and Sweet, W. H. (1969): *Pain and the Neurosurgeon,* pp. 633–660. Charles C Thomas, Springfield, Ill.

Discussion

Part II. Management of Pain of Advanced Cancer: Viscereal and Perineal Pain

L. Gennari and J. Loeser (Moderators)

Frova (Milano): Dr. Houde, what do you think about drug treatment for visceral pain in children?

Houde (New York): At our Institution we apply the same rules to children that we do to adults. If they have pain that can be controlled with simple analgesics, those are the drugs that we employ. If they require more potent drugs, we go to more potent drugs, generally in combination with the simple analgesics, and more often than not by administering them by oral route. Our biggest problem, I think, in dealing with children is that doses have to be adjusted to their body size. Our biggest problem actually is in teenagers because they seem to be under the greatest psychological turmoil having pain and cancer. They tend to be the patients in whom we use the largest amounts of drugs including narcotics.

When we use narcotics and tranquilizers or the anxiolitic drugs, we frequently run into complications, and I think that we have generally found that the narcotics are actually good tranquilizers in themselves. Most people who misuse narcotics are those who try to combine them with other drugs.

Madrid (Madrid): Dr. Moore, could you describe your technique for spinal cord transection with absolute alcohol?

Moore (Seattle): The patient is placed in the jackknife position, the level of the injection is the second lumbar interspace, the level of the neurolysis is from the second lumbar interspace caudad, and the complications are those that you would expect; the block is not done unless the patient is incontinent of feces and urine and also has an involvement of the somatic nerves of the lower extremity with severe pain. It is a final and drastic procedure that is used to relieve pain.

Nicosia (Catania): Dr. Ventafridda, is the continuous epidural still an indication in pain treatment? Has anybody experienced a long-lasting continuous epidural by chronic infusion?

Ventafridda (Milano): The continuous epidural, the introduction of a foreign body for a long time, always gives a patient affected by a tumor some complications. The pain gets worse and is long-lasting. For this reason, we no longer use this technique. We have seen major cases of infection, and there is not anything worse than aggravating the condition of these patients.

Rampulla (Urbino): Dr. Moore, do you have experience of transsacral neurolysis with phenol in water? If you do, what are your impressions?

Moore: We have done a few cases of transsacral block. I assume that this is a question regarding the injection of the third sacral nerve at the foramina. They are, in our experience, not too effective. Furthermore, one cannot be selective in doing so, and, therefore, you may expect bladder, rectal and, to some extent, lower extremity involvement. So we have not used any technique of this nature in treating these patients.

Advances in Pain Research and Therapy, Vol. 2,
edited by J. J. Bonica and V. Ventafridda.
Raven Press, New York © 1979.

Overview of Analgesia

Robert G. Twycross

The Churchill Hospital, Headington, Oxford OX3 9EJ, England

A recent report has emphasized that many patients dying of cancer do so only after weeks or months of uncontrolled pain. Parkes (7) compared hospital-centered and home-centered terminal care by means of post-bereavement visits to the surviving spouse, and found that about 20% of the hospital patients died with their severe and mostly continuous pain unrelieved. A similar percentage of patients experienced pain of comparable intensity before admission to the hospital, which suggests that the hospital stay did not lead to improved relief. Of those who died at home, 10% had severe pain pre-terminally, but terminally the proportion rose to almost half. In contrast, following admission to St. Christopher's Hospice—a unit specializing in symptom control in far-advanced cancer—the percentage of patients with severe pain fell from 36% to 8%.

In the home-based patients, the main reason for poor pain control appeared to be a failure on the part of the general practitioner to ensure that regular doses of an appropriate analgesic were given in sufficient quantity to alleviate the pain. One man of 54 became totally demoralized and for several months spent much of the time crying. He was so frightened that he clung to his wife and became "hysterical" whenever she left the room. He received an injection each *week* and was not able to go into hospital as there was no bed available. Similar accounts given by other respondents suggested that neurotic exaggeration was not the explanation. Several patients put up with their pain without complaint on the supposition that nothing could be done to relieve it or that their chances of recovery would be enhanced if they refrained from taking powerful analgesics.

The medical profession has a lot to learn before it can confidently assure patients that severe pain in advanced cancer can be controlled. Reasons for inadequate relief are many, but more fundamental than the incorrect use of analgesics is the tendency for a doctor to cease to be systematic when confronted with a dying patient. Instead of carefully analysing the cause(s) of the patient's pain(s), the doctor prescribes a fixed dose of a standard preparation or, worse, underrates the intensity of a patient's discomfort and does nothing.

ASSESSMENT OF THE PAIN

Pain may be limited to one site or be multifocal. Each site where pain is felt should be recorded. The use of a body image to record the site(s) of pain is a great help. It acts as a base line for future reference, facilitates patient management in situations where several doctors are involved, and helps in the consideration of underlying mechanisms (Fig. 1). Descriptions of pain being "like raving toothache" and "stabbing, especially when I move" point to nerve compression and influence the course of treatment should analgesics alone fail to relieve (Table 1). A diagnosis of cancer does not, however, mean that the malignant process is necessarily the cause of the pain. As in other areas of medicine, diagnosis must precede treatment. Bedsores, constipation, peptic ulcer, cystitis, or musculoskeletal disorders may prove to be the cause, and are all conditions that benefit from specific treatment.

Intensity of pain is assessed not only by the patient's description but also

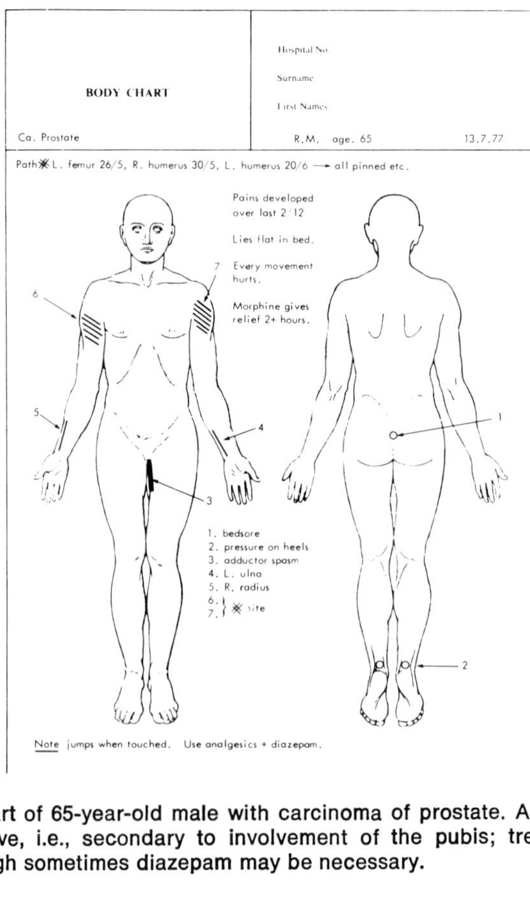

FIG. 1. Pain chart of 65-year-old male with carcinoma of prostate. Adductor spasm is usually protective, i.e., secondary to involvement of the pubis; treatment is as for bone pain, though sometimes diazepam may be necessary.

TABLE 1. *Treatment of pain in advanced cancer*

Mechanism		Analgesic adjuvants	Co-analgesic	Nondrug treatment		Other measures
Soft-tissue infiltration	morphine (severe) — codeine (moderate) — aspirin (mild)	laxative ? anxiolytic ? antiemetic			modification of lifestyle	diversion — heat — massage
Bone involvement			Aspirin	Radiotherapy		
Nerve compression			Prednisolone	Nerve block		
Raised cerebral pressure			Dexamethasone			
Lymphedema			Diuretic	Compression sleeve		
Abdominal visceral epigastric				Celiac axis ganglion block		
hypogastric				(Presacral block)[a]		
Ulceration—infection			antibiotic			
Constipation		Specific treatment				
Second pathology						

[a] The use of nerve blocks for lower abdominal pain is limited by probability of causing urinary retention.

TABLE 2. *Factors affecting pain threshold*

Discomfort Insomnia Fatigue Anxiety Fear Anger Sadness Depression Mental isolation Introversion (Past experience)	Threshold lowered ↓	Relief of symptoms Sleep Rest Sympathy Understanding Diversion Elevation of mood ——— Analgesics Tranquillizers Antidepressives	↑ Threshold raised

by discovering what drugs have failed to relieve, whether sleep is disturbed, and in what way activity is limited ("How long is it since you went out?", "What are you doing around the house?", etc.) In addition, the patient's spouse should be interviewed; generally speaking, one finds that the patient has made light of his suffering. A patient may be in severe pain without looking distressed. With an obviously distressed patient who says or implies, "It's all pain, doctor," detailed assessment is impossible. In this situation the pain is compounded by anxiety and fear, and the patient should be reviewed after an initial injection of diazepam and diamorphine or morphine. The dose will depend on the patient's previous medication and general condition, but 10 mg of each is usually not excessive in a young or middle-aged patient. In some patients, pain is minimal at rest but intolerable on movement.

A 4-year-old child with an inoperable pontine glioma experienced increasing pain in the head and occipital region. She lay flat all the time because elevation of the head caused a marked increase in pain. With this history it was necessary to postulate a local source of pain (possibly caused by postradiation meningeal adhesions) in addition to the diffuse headache of secondary hydrocephalus (which would have been helped by a more erect posture). The diffuse pain was relieved by small, regular doses of morphine, but not until she was transferred from a King's Fund to an Ellison bed (which elevates head, neck, and trunk in unison) was it possible for the child to sit up without pain. Subsequently, it became possible to transfer the child from bed to a high-backed reclining chair and, eventually, to lift her onto her mother's lap. This suggested that some of the pain had been caused by spasm of the neck muscles, and that the confidence engendered by the ability to sit up in bed allowed additional maneuvres to be undertaken without pain.

The probability of the initial prescription's being inadequate increases with the intensity of pain. Patients should, therefore, be reassessed within hours if the pain is overwhelming, or after 1 or 2 days if severe or moderate. If troublesome or unacceptable side effects result, treatment may need to be modified. In addition, the relief of the major pain may allow a second, less severe pain to become apparent.

An 85-year-old man with carcinoma of the prostate and pain in the right femur caused by a metastasis was treated with aspirin and morphine. Casual questioning the next day indicated that, although it was less severe, he was still in pain. Further questioning revealed that the site of pain was now retrosternal and epigastric; he had no femoral pain at all. The dose of morphine was, therefore, left unaltered, and the prescription of an antacid resulted in complete relief.

PAIN CONTROL

Relief of pain may be achieved by one or more of the following methods: (a) modification of the pathologic process; (b) elevation of the pain threshold; (c) interruption of pain pathways; and (d) immobilization.

Modification of Pathologic Process

Osseous metastasis is the main cause of pain in the majority of patients with carcinoma of the breast, bronchus, or prostate. Bone pain is also common in carcinomata of the kidney and thyroid and in multiple myeloma. Modification of the pathology by radiation, chemotherapy, or hormone treatment should always be considered even in far-advanced cancer, though it is important to ensure that the treatment is not worse than the disease. Moreover, because androgens or estrogens have been prescribed, this does not mean that analgesics should be withheld. A combined approach should be employed. If relief is obtained and there are no complaints of "breakthrough" pain, then the analgesic regimen can be modified—a less potent analgesic prescribed or the treatment withdrawn completely.

Radiation therapy gives partial or even complete relief in 90% of patients experiencing bone pain, and generally may be administered in a single, nonfractionated dose. A recent study showed that, although patients treated by a single dose commonly had more nausea and vomiting, many of those receiving fractionated treatment were exhausted by the end of the course (8). Fractionation is probably necessary only when there is a high risk of nausea and vomiting despite prophylactic anti-emetics, e.g., when irradiating in the region of L_1 and when treating half or more of the pelvis.

Elevation of Pain Threshold

Pain is a dual phenomenon, one part being the perception of the sensation and the other the patient's emotional reaction to it. This means that attention must be paid to nondrug factors that modulate pain threshold, such as anxiety and depression, as well as to the correct use of analgesics and other drugs (Table 2). Most patients fear the process of dying—"Will it hurt?", "Will I suffocate?"—and many fear death itself. Many of these fears remain unspoken unless the patient is given the opportunity to express them. The doctor needs to give time and opportunity for the patient to talk about his progress or lack of it. Tranquilizers have only a limited place in terminal cancer care. Patients who are markedly anxious or agitated usually need a combination of a tranquilizer and an analgesic; so does the patient with overwhelming pain.

Depression not only can, but frequently does, supervene in patients receiving so-called "euphoriant" drugs. The likelihood of this occurring increases the longer a patient is maintained on a narcotic analgesic (14). An antidepressant should be prescribed in these circumstances, starting with half the usual adult dose, as debilitated patients often become confused if a higher dose is given, particularly when other psychoactive drugs are being taken concurrently. Support and companionship are always necessary, particularly in cases where the depression is more properly described as sadness at the thought of leaving behind one's family, one's friends, and all that is familiar.

The use of analgesics is best seen as but one way—generally a powerful way—of elevating the pain threshold, though a failure to allow the patient to express his fears and anxieties can cause otherwise relievable pain to remain intractable.

Use of Analgesics

To allow pain to re-emerge before administering the next dose not only causes unnecessary suffering but encourages tolerance. "Four-hourly as required" or PRN medication has no place in the treatment of persistent pain; whatever its etiology, *continuous pain requires regular preventive therapy.* The aim is to titrate the dose of the analgesic against the patient's pain, *gradually increasing the dose until the patient is pain-free.* The next dose is given before the effect of the previous one has worn off and, therefore, before the patient may think it necessary. In this way it is possible to erase the memory and fear of pain. As patients do not like constantly taking tablets or receiving injections, a 4-hr interval between doses should be regarded as the norm though sometimes more frequent administration may be necessary. Many patients do not require a dose in the middle of the night though, if necessary, a patient should be awakened to take it (or set his alarm) rather than let him wake later complaining of pain.

The effective analgesic dose varies considerably from patient to patient; *the right dose of any analgesic is that which gives adequate relief for at least 3, preferably 4 or more hr.* "Maximum" or "recommended" doses, derived mainly from postoperative parenteral single-dose studies, are not applicable in advanced cancer. For example, the effective dose of *oral* morphine ranges from as little as 5 mg to more than 100 mg every 4 hr. Patients will usually accept two, sometimes three, analgesic tablets per administration, together with additional medication; four or more tablets of the same preparation are not often acceptable. Generally, if two tablets are not adequate, the patient should be transferred to a more potent alternative. Pain unrelieved by other measures, not short life-expectancy, is the primary criterion for prescription of morphine or other narcotic analgesics.

Anti-inflammatory Drugs

The importance of aspirin in the relief of bone pain has recently been reemphasized (13). Many osseous metastases produce or induce the production of a prostaglandin, probably PGE_2, which causes osteolysis (2) and also lowers the "peripheral pain threshold" by sensitizing free nerve endings (3). Aspirin (in high dosage) and other nonsteroidal anti-inflammatory drugs (NSAID) inhibit the synthesis of PGs and by so doing alleviate pain. This suggests that, compared with morphine, NSAID should be relatively more efficacious in bone pain than in pain caused by soft-tissue infiltration. Our experience in Oxford would support such a hypothesis (Fig. 2).

Response to PG inhibitors is, however, variable; a fact which can be explained if certain cancer-cell types synthesize osteolytic agents other than or in addition to PGE_2. It has been shown, for example, in patients with hypercalcemia in association with multiple myeloma or a reticulosis, that the urinary excretion of PG metabolites is normal and that bone resorption appears to be due to secretion of "osteoclast activating factor" by tumor cells (6). Other candidates include ectopic parathyroid hormone and active vitamin-D metabolites or related sterols.

Despite the variable response, it should now be regarded as a general rule that aspirin and other potent NSAID should be used either alone or in combination with a narcotic analgesic when seeking to relieve bone pain by pharmacologic means (13). Aspirin in a dose of between 3 and 6 g a day has much to commend it and is available in a variety of preparations. Phenylbutazone commonly causes fluid retention and, in the elderly and debilitated, indomethacin is prone to cause or exacerbate neuropsychiatric disturbances. Newer agents such as flurbiprofen and diflunisal appear promising, and it is possible that they may prove useful in patients who fail to respond to aspirin.

Corticosteroids

Corticosteroids prevent the release of PGs by exerting a "stabilizing" effect on cell membranes; they do not inhibit PG synthesis. They do, however, have an impact on elements of the inflammatory process not connected with PGs and commonly stimulate appetite and elevate mood (1). Even so, clinical impression suggests that corticosteroids are not so effective as aspirin in relieving bone pain, though they are probably more effective in alleviating

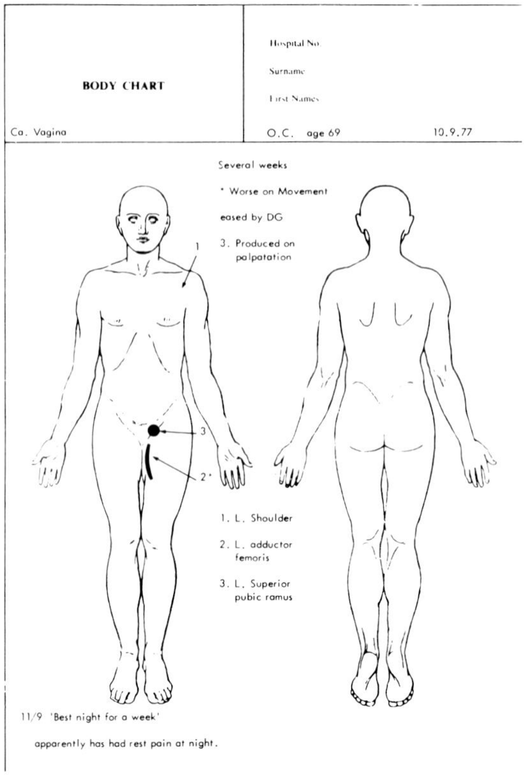
BODY CHART
Hospital No
Surname
First Names
Ca. Vagina
O.C. age 69
10.9.77
Several weeks
* Worse on Movement
eased by DG
3. Produced on palpatation
1
3
2*
1. L. Shoulder
2. L. adductor femoris
3. L. Superior pubic ramus
11/9 'Best night for a week'
apparently has had rest pain at night.

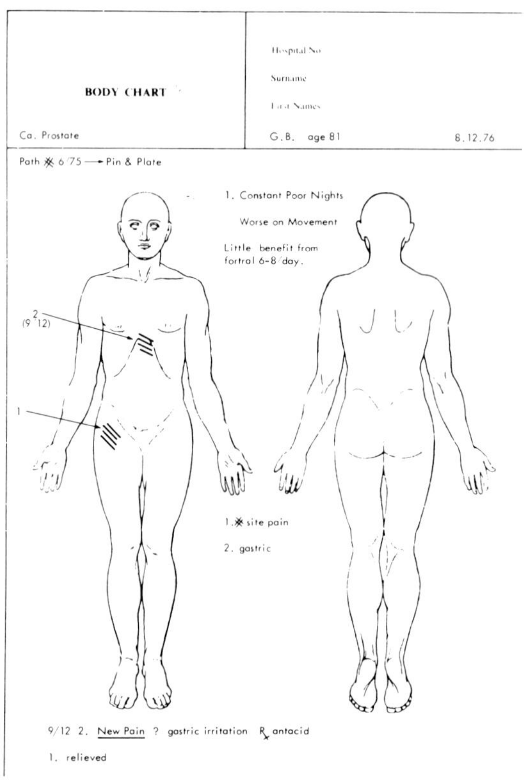
BODY CHART
Hospital No
Surname
First Names
Ca. Prostate
G.B. age 81
8.12.76
Path ※ 6/75 ⟶ Pin & Plate
1. Constant Poor Nights
Worse on Movement
Little benefit from fortral 6-8/day.
2 (9/12)
1
1.※ site pain
2. gastric
9/12 2. New Pain ? gastric irritation Rx antacid
1. relieved

pain associated with extensive soft-tissue infiltration in relatively circumscribed areas, e.g., head and neck cancers or pelvic malignancy and with massive hepatic metastases. Sometimes, particularly with pelvic malignancy, greater relief is obtained by using both aspirin and prednisolone in association with a narcotic analgesic.

The usual starting dose is prednisolone 10 mg t.i.d., reducing to 10 mg b.i.d. or 5 mg t.i.d. after a week. Prednisolone should also be used when pain is caused by nerve compression (*vide infra*). With headache caused by raised intracranial pressure, the more potent dexamethasone is often necessary, together with an analgesic. The usual starting dose is 4 mg t.i.d. reducing, if possible, to 2 mg t.i.d. or less when the headache has been controlled satisfactorily.

Narcotic Analgesics

When the nonnarcotic analgesics (aspirin and paracetamol/acetominophen) fail to relieve, a weak narcotic such as codeine or dihydrocodeine should be prescribed alone or with aspirin or paracetamol. Pentazocine, a partial agonist, has no place in the treatment of cancer pain. By mouth it is not a potent analgesic; 50 mg of pentazocine is less effective than two tablets of aspirin-codeine (Codis®) or of paracetamol-propoxyphene (Distalgesic®) (9). Moreover, the proportion of patients experiencing psychotomimetic side effects is unacceptably high and, although such side effects tend to be dose-related, they have been observed after even small doses by mouth. Similarly, orally administered pethidine/meperidine should not be regarded as a potent analgesic and, by injection, acts only for some 2 to 3 hr.

Papaveretum and dipipanone are useful intermediates between weak narcotics and morphine. Dipipanone is available only with cyclizine as Diconal®, though there is no evidence that it causes more nausea than other narcotics. Alternatively, aspirin and opium (Nepenthe®) may be used; each 1 ml of undiluted Nepenthe® contains about 10 mg of morphine and is usually supplied as a 10% (1 ml in 10) or 20% (2 ml in 10) solution in chloroform water. Precipitation occurs when stronger solutions are dispensed. Dextromoramide (Palfium® 5 and 10 mg) although potent is relatively short-acting; it is, however, useful as "top up" medication for patients who experience occasional exacerbations of pain but whose pain for the most part is well controlled.

The top of the analgesic ladder is not reached simply by prescribing morphine or diamorphine (diacetylmorphine, heroin). Both may be given in

---

←

FIG. 2. Pain charts of 2 patients with bone pain. Complete relief was obtained using morphine and aspirin. In both morphine was subsequently stopped without a return of pain, though after several weeks it became necessary to represcribe it. Virtually bedfast when admitted, both patients became fully mobile.

a wide range of oral doses, from 5 to 100 mg every 4 hr though, in fact, it is unusual to need more than 30 mg. By mouth, morphine and diamorphine have similar actions and unwanted effects but, owing to more complete absorption, oral diamorphine is about 1½ times more potent than oral morphine (12). Both opiates are commonly dispensed with cocaine in a vehicle containing alcohol and syrup ("The Brompton Cocktail"). Some patients, however, complain about the "sickliness" of such mixtures, while others dislike the alcoholic "bite." Moreover, the benefit of a small, fixed dose of cocaine is probably slight and has, on occasion, caused restlessness and hallucinations in the elderly. It is my practice, despite the recent inclusion of a convenient formulation in the British National Formulary, to dispense morphine in chloroform water alone, the patient adding blackcurrant juice or other flavoring as desired. If dispensed in combination with prochlorperazine or chlorpromazine, the incorporation of one of the flavored proprietary syrups usually circumvents the need for additional flavoring.

When regular injections are required I use diamorphine hydrochloride, available in ampoules as freeze-dried pellets. It is considerably more soluble than morphine sulphate—100 mg will dissolve in 0.2 ml. This means that the volume injected need never be large, an important consideration when repeated injections have to be given to a cachectic patient (Table 3). It should be emphasized that most patients can be maintained on oral medication. The main indication for parenteral administration, apart from the last few hours of life, is intractable nausea and vomiting despite the prescription of antiemetic.

The need for injections may sometimes be avoided by using morphine suppositories. Several strengths are available ranging from 10 to 60 mg Proladone® suppositories, which contain 30 mg of oxycodone pectinate are also available; after administration the oxycodone is slowly released from the pectin core over several hours. Thus one or two suppositories every 6 or 8 hr may be adequate. Fifteen mg of oxycodone is equivalent to 10 mg of morphine. Alternatively, round-the-clock relief may be maintained by using Duromorph®, a microcrystalline suspension of morphine, 2 or 3 times a day. It is available as an intramuscular preparation in capped vials each containing 70.4 mg of morphine base in 1.1 ml (64 mg/ml). The dose will depend on the patient's previous medication. For example, assuming a 1:3 oral to parenteral potency ratio for morphine, 32 mg of Duromorph® (0.5 ml) bd will probably substitute adequately for 30 mg of oral morphine 4-hourly.

Levorphanol (Dromoran® 1.5 mg) and phenazocine (Narphen® 5 mg) should be regarded as alternatives to morphine and diamorphine (Table 4). By mouth on a weight-for-weight basis, both are approximately 4 to 5 times more potent than morphine and have a longer duration of action. Methadone (Physeptone®) may also be useful in these circumstances but, because of its prolonged plasma half-time (15), should be used with care, if at all, in the elderly or extremely debilitated.

TABLE 3. *Injection volume of equi-analgesic doses of diamorphine and morphine*

Preparation	Solubility in water at 25°C (1 g in x ml)	Potency relative to diamorphine	Available ampoules (mg/ml)	Volume of equi-analgesic doses (ml)			
				30	60	90	120 mg
Diamorphine hydrochloride	1.6	1	(Freeze-dried)	0.1	0.1	0.15	0.2
Morphine sulphate	21	½	15[a]	4	4	12	16
			30[b]	2	4	6	8

[a] Maximum strength available in the United States
[b] Maximum strength available in the United Kingdom

TABLE 4. *Approximate oral analgesic equivalence of potent narcotics*

Analgesic	Tablet	Dose of diamorphine hydrochloride	Dose of morphine sulphate
Dipipanone (Diconal®)	10 mg (+30 mg cyclizine)	3 mg	5 mg
Papaveretum (Omnopon®)	10 mg	3 mg	5 mg
*Levorphanol (Dromoran®)	1.5 mg	5 mg	8 mg
*Phenazocine (Narphen®)	5 mg	15 mg	25 mg
Nepenthe (undiluted)	1 ml	8 mg	12 mg

Note: i. *Dextromoramide* (Palfium®)—single 5-mg dose is equivalent to diamorphine 10 mg/morphine 15 mg in terms of PEAK effect but acts only for 1–2 hr. Useful as an additional "as required" analgesic for intermittent, severe, breakthrough pain.
ii. **Methadone* (Physeptone®)—single 5 mg dose is equivalent to diamorphine 5 mg/morphine 7.5 mg. Has a prolonged plasma half-time, which leads to *accumulation* when given repeatedly. Thus, it is several times more potent when given *regularly.*
iii. *Often satisfactory 6-hourly.

Adjuvant Medication

Most patients with terminal cancer have more than one symptom. Nausea and vomiting are both common and the use of a narcotic analgesic tends to precipitate or exacerbate these symptoms, particularly if the patient is ambulant. Patients prescribed a narcotic analgesic should be questioned about nausea and vomiting and either have an antiemetic (e.g., prochlorperazine; metoclopramide, cyclizine) prescribed simultaneously or the need for one reviewed 2 or 3 days later. Constipation almost always occurs when a narcotic is taken regularly, but generally responds to the *regular* use of an appropriate aperient.

The value of diversional activity should not be forgotten. It ranges from back-rubs to craft work, talking books, access to radio and television, someone to talk to, and dayroom activities. Pain is worse when it occupies the patient's whole attention. Diversional activity does much more than just "pass the time;" it also diminishes the pain.

Narcotic Addiction and Tolerance

Although the term *drug addiction* has been replaced officially by *drug dependence,* unofficially it continues to be used. Drug dependence is currently defined as:

"A state, psychic and sometimes also physical, resulting from the interaction between a living organism and a drug, characterized by behavioural and other responses that always include a compulsion to take the drug on a continuous or periodic basis in order to experience its psychic effects, and sometimes to avoid the discomfort of its absence. Tolerance may or may not be present" (17).

This is a broader definition than that of 1964, which emphasized the need for both tolerance and an early development of physical dependence in addition to strong psychologic dependence (16). The term *drug dependence* now more closely approximates to the popular conception of addiction—a compulsion or overpowering drive to take the drug in order to experience its psychologic effects. Occasionally, a patient is admitted who appears to be addicted, demanding "an injection" every 2 or 3 hr. Typically such a patient has a long history of poor pain control and will for several weeks have been receiving fairly regular (4-hourly as required) but inadequate injections of one or more narcotic analgesics. Given time, it is usually possible to control the pain adequately, prevent clock-watching and demanding behavior, and, sometimes, transfer the patient to an oral preparation. But even here, it cannot be said that the patient is addicted, as he is not demanding the narcotic in order to experience its psychologic effect but to be relieved from pain for at least an hour or two.

Even so, many doctors are reluctant to use narcotic analgesics, particularly diamorphine or morphine, because they assume that tolerance will result in the medication's becoming ineffective. This is understandable as little information has been available concerning the long-term effects of narcotic analgesics when administered regularly to relieve persistent pain. The lack of data resulted in predictions being made on the basis of animal and human volunteer studies. However, in the studies using ex-addicts at the Addiction Research Center in Lexington, the emphasis has been on *inducing* tolerance and physical dependence as rapidly as possible by using maximum tolerated doses rather than administering the drugs in doses and at intervals comparable to a clinical regimen (5). Although such studies have been useful in predicting abuse liability, their relevance to clinical practice is questionable.

To allow predictions to be made on the basis of clinical experience, the notes of 500 patients admitted consecutively to St. Christopher's Hospice were reviewed (10). A total of 218 patients received diamorphine regularly for at least 1 week. By grouping the patients according to survival after commencing diamorphine, it was demonstrated that *the longer the duration of treatment the slower the rate of rise in dose*. In a second review (14), 115 patients who had received diamorphine regularly for at least 12 weeks were selected from approximately 3,000 patients admitted over 7 years. Dose-time charts were prepared. Visual analysis indicated that in many there was an initial phase when the dose was increased several times within 1 or 2 weeks followed by a prolonged phase when the dose was increased less often or not at all (Fig. 3). It was also clearly demonstrated that *the longer a patient survived after prescription of diamorphine, the greater the likelihood of a reduction in dose.*

Dose reductions were made on a trial and error basis in patients who had improved generally over a number of weeks and who had had no recent episodes of "breakthrough" pain. Reductions were also made after successful

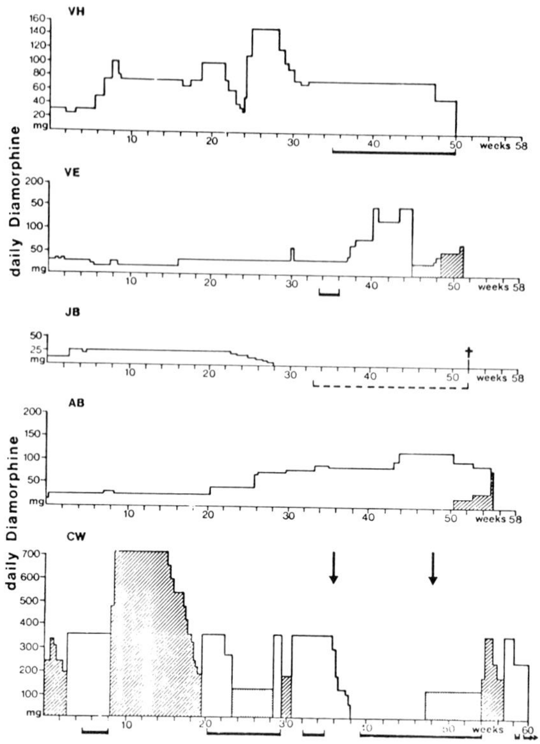

FIG. 3. Dose-time charts of 5 patients with advanced cancer (14). *Open areas,* diamorphine by mouth; *hatched areas,* diamorphine by injection; *dotted areas,* other narcotic analgesic (V. E., C. W.): *arrow,* phenol-in-glycerine nerve block; *horizontal bar,* time spent at home. V. H., V. E., and A. B. received diamorphine up to the time of death; C. W. is still alive.

intrathecal nerve blocks in 5 patients and after treatment with a cytotoxic agent or radiation in a number of others. A total of 9 patients stopped receiving diamorphine; 3 stopped taking diamorphine altogether; 4 patients stopped for more than 4 months; and 2 stopped for approximately 3 weeks.

It was concluded that, when used as part of a pattern of total care, diamorphine may be used for long periods without concern about tolerance. Moreover, although physical dependence probably develops in most patients after several weeks of continuous treatment this does not prevent the downward adjustment of dose when considered clinically feasible. Experience with methadone, levorphanol, and phenazocine suggests that the "natural history" of their long-term use in patients in pain is similar to that of diamorphine and morphine.

Interruption of Pain Pathways

The place of peripheral and intrathecal nerve blocks and neurosurgical procedures has been discussed elsewhere in this volume. It should be noted, however, that analgesics alone are often effective in relieving pain due to nerve compression. If the response is poor, however, the use of prednisolone 5 to 10 mg 3 times a day is recommended. By reducing inflammatory swelling around the growth, the effective tumor mass is reduced and the compression alleviated. In patients with a prognosis of only a few weeks, this may be sufficient to circumvent the need for chemical neurolysis. In those with a longer life-expectancy, the pain may return as the tumor continues to grow; in these a nerve block will be required. In patients whose morale is low or precarious, it is advisable to warn that a block may become necessary, in order to avoid loss of confidence should the pain return.

Modification of Lifestyle

Some patients continue to experience pain on movement despite analgesics, other drugs, radiotherapy, and nerve blocks. In these, the situation may be improved by suggesting commonsense modifications to daily activity. For example, a man may continue to struggle to stand when shaving unless the doctor suggests that sitting would be a good idea. Such a suggestion is accepted more readily if accompanied by a simple explanation of why weight-bearing precipitates or exacerbates the pain. Individually designed plaster or plastic supports for patients with multiple collapsed vertebrae or Thomas splints for femoral pain are occasionally necessary to overcome intolerable pain on movement in bedfast patients.

Internal fixation or the insertion of a prosthesis should be considered if a pathological fracture of a long-bone occurs, as these measures obviate the need for prolonged bed rest and pain is usually relieved. The decision whether or not to treat surgically depends on the patient's general condition; but, whereas in bronchial carcinoma or malignant melanoma pathological fracture often presages death, in breast cancer this is not generally so, particularly if the tumor is hormone-sensitive. The median survival after the first or only pathological fracture associated with breast cancer is about 6 months ranging from 2 months to 4 years (11).

EXPECTATIONS

A recent survey of patients with persistent pain suggested that patients' expectations in relation to relief are lower than they need be (4). However, whereas relief is obtained within 2 or 3 days in some patients, in others, particularly those whose pain is made worse by movement and in the very anxious and depressed, it may take 3 to 4 weeks of inpatient treatment to achieve satisfactory control. Even so, it should be possible to achieve some improvement within 24 to 48 hr in all patients. Although the ultimate aim is complete freedom from pain, we will be less disappointed but, paradoxically, more successful if in practice we aim at "graded relief." Further, as some pains respond more readily than others, improvement should be assessed in relation to each pain. The initial target should be a pain-free, sleep-full night. Many patients have not had a good night's rest for weeks or months and are exhausted and demoralized. To sleep through the night pain-free and wake refreshed is a boost to both the doctor's and the patient's morale. Next, one aims for relief at rest in bed or chair during the day; finally, for freedom from pain on movement. The former is always eventually possible; the latter is not. However, the encouragement that relief at night and when resting during the day brings, gives the patient new hope and incentive and enables him to begin to live again despite limited mobility. Freed from the day- and nightmare of constant pain, his last weeks or months take on a new look.

The doctor must be determined to succeed and be prepared to spend much time assessing and reassessing the patient's pain and other symptoms. Decisive action is needed to avoid the situation reported recently of a 90-year-old man, admitted to a London teaching hospital with bone pain, who died still in pain 3 months later (4). With cancer one is dealing with a progressive pathological process. This means that new pains may develop or old pains re-emerge. It should not be assumed that a fresh complaint of pain merely calls for an increase in a previously satisfactory analgesic regimen; it demands reassessment, an explanation to the patient and, only then, modification of drug therapy or other intervention.

ACKNOWLEDGMENTS

Tables 1 and 4 and Figs. 1 and 2 are reproduced by permission of Pitman Medical, Tunbridge Wells, England.

REFERENCES

1. Anonymous (1974): Corticosteroids in terminal cancer. *Drug Ther. Bull.*, 12:63–64.
2. Editorial (1976): Osteolytic metastases. *Lancet*, 2:1063–1064.
3. Ferreira, S. H. (1972): Prostaglandins, aspirin-like drugs and analgesia. *Nature New Biol.*, 240:200–203.
4. Hunt, J. M., Stollar, T. D., Littlejohns, D. W., Twycross, R. G., and Vere, D. W. (1977): Patients with protracted pain. *J. Med. Ethics*, 3:61–73.
5. Isbell, H. (1948): Methods & results of studying experimental human addiction to newer synthetic analgesics. *Ann. N.Y. Acad. Sci.*, 51:108–122.
6. Mundy, G. R., Raisz, L. G., Cooper, R. A., Schechter, G. P., and Salmon, S. E. (1974): Evidence for the secretion of an osteoclast stimulating factor in myeloma. *N. Engl. J. Med.*, 291:1041–1046.
7. Parkes, C. M. (1976): Home or hospital? Terminal care as seen by surviving spouses. *J. Roy. Coll. Gen. Pract.*, 28:19–30.
8. Penn, C. R. H. (1976): Single dose and fractionated palliative irradiation for osseous metastases. *Clin. Radiol.*, 27:405–408.
9. Robbie, D. S., and Samarasinghe, J. (1973): Comparison of aspirin-codeine and paracetamol-dextropropoxyphene compound tablets with pentazocine in relief of cancer pain. *J. Int. Med. Res.*, 1:246–252.
10. Twycross, R. G. (1974): Clinical experience with diamorphine in advanced malignant disease. *Int. J. Clin. Pharmacol.*, 9:184–198.

11. Twycross, R. G. (1977): Care of the terminal patient. In: *Breast Cancer Management—Early and Late,* edited by B. A. Stoll, pp. 157–163. Heinemann Medical Books Ltd., London.
12. Twycross, R. G. (1977): Choice of strong analgesic in terminal cancer: diamorphine or morphine? *Pain,* 3:93–104.
13. Twycross, R. G. (1978): Bone pain in advanced cancer. In: *Topics in Therapeutics 4,* edited by D. W. Vere, pp. 94–110. Pitman Medical, Tunbridge Wells.
14. Twycross, R. G., and Wald, S. J. (1976): Long-term use of diamorphine in advanced cancer. In: *Advances in Pain Research & Therapy, Vol. 1: Proceedings of the First World Congress on Pain,* edited by J. J. Bonica & Albe-Fessard, pp. 653–661. Raven Press, New York.
15. Verebely, K., Volavka, J., Mule, S., and Resnick, R. (1975): Methadone in man: Pharmacokinetics & excretion studies in acute & chronic treatment. *Clin. Pharmacol. Ther.,* 18:180–190.
16. World Health Organisation (1964): Expert Committee on Drug Dependence, 13th Report. *Technical Report Series,* No. 287.
17. World Health Organisation (1969): Expert Committee on Drug Dependence, 16th Report. *Technical Report Series,* No. 407.

Advances in Pain Research and Therapy, Vol. 2,
edited by J. J. Bonica and V. Ventafridda.
Raven Press, New York © 1979.

The Nature and Management of Terminal Pain and the Hospice Concept

Cicely Saunders

St. Christopher's Hospice, 51–53 Lawrie Park Road, Sydenham, S.E.26. 6DZ, England

Continuity of care for people suffering from persistent cancer aims to ensure that throughout the whole course of the disease they receive treatment appropriate to each stage and that, as far as possible, this is carried out in the place that accords best with their own way of life and its commitments. In this presentation I will consider this type of care as given at St. Christopher's Hospice.

We owe our patients the attempt to decide when our management has finally turned into care for their dying, even though this may be a difficult moment to identify. We define it as occurring when all active treatments only hold out diminishing returns coupled with increasing morbidity, when the incidence of side effects or the management required by the treatment itself serve only to isolate the patient from those around him and hinder him from completing life in his way.

Some may believe that both patient and doctor should fight for life until its end; but to talk of accepting death when its approach is inevitable is not mere resignation on the part of the patient, nor is it defeatism or neglect on the part of the doctor. For both of them it is the very opposite of doing nothing. If the doctor and his whole team play their part in managing pain and other problems, the patient will be given the opportunity to manage this part of his life himself. He may well make an intensely individual achievement of great importance to him and to his family.

It should never be said that *no* treatment is being offered. Much can be done in general management and in detailed medication, and at no time in the total care of a cancer patient is the awareness of him as a person of greater importance.

HOSPICE CARE

This phase of treatment and the attitude that should underlie it has recently attracted much professional and public interest and is frequently discussed under the title "Hospice Care." Although neither the traditional nor the modern hospices concern themselves exclusively with the needs of people

FIG. 1. "I am a scrap heap."—*E. S.*

with terminal malignancy, this has always been a major part of the work done in these facilities. The professional personnel in hospices set out to diagnose and treat what can often be termed *total pain,* for it includes physical, emotional, social (both interpersonal and financial), and spiritual aspects. In many such centers it has been impressively shown how this pain can almost always be relieved, while the patient remains alert until the disease process itself finally clouds his consciousness.

A series of pictures painted by St. Christopher's patients illustrate how they saw their terminal pain. They show the feeling of being impaled by a red-hot iron, of being totally isolated from the world by the encircling "muscles of tension," the sudden jab on movement, the implacable heaviness of pain, the conviction that one *is* a kind of scrap heap, the endless questions "Why?" and the fears of a lonely, threatening journey.

One woman, with a year's history of unrelenting pain from a carcinoma of the pancreas, drew it as a small rodent boring into the side of a tree trunk. A few traces of green at the top were described to me as, "My life, trying to get through." She was in St. Christopher's for 11 weeks and a friend wrote to me after her death:

> It was nothing short of a miracle. When I last visited her in a previous hospital she was like a demented animal—consumed with pain, incoherent of speech, and quite vicious. I was very frightened, not knowing how to cope, and felt unable to face another visit. Words cannot describe my reaction when I saw her in St. Christopher's—restored to the dignity of a calm, rational human being again. . . . From then on I was able to remain with her for hours at a time, instead of minutes, holding conversation and discussing things of interest dear to her heart. . . . By so doing, I too have gained in spiritual strength. I can only thank you for making my friend's last days bearable when once they were unendurable.

Vital signs in a ward specializing in the control of terminal pain include the hand steady enough to draw, the mind alert enough to write poems and to play cards, and above all the spirit to enjoy the family visits and spend the last weekends at home.

Incidence and Magnitude of Pain

Reports from several studies suggest that approximately half of those who die from various forms of cancer are likely to suffer terminal pain and that a great deal of this is not adequately relieved. Parkes (9) summarized the memories of more than 270 people 1 year after the death of a spouse from cancer in the area of St. Christopher's Hospice. Defining the terminal period as the time between the end of active treatment and death (average about 6 weeks), he divided his patients into home-, hospital-, or hospice-centered. Although the home-centered patients had less pain during the pre-terminal period (5% of some 130 patients), during the terminal period 28% of them were said to have had severe pain which remained unrelieved to the time of death. Of over 90 hospital-based patients 20% had pre-terminal pain, and this figure did not alter for the terminal period. In contrast, 36% of the 42 patients referred to the Hospice had unrelieved pre-terminal pain, but the figure dropped to 8% after admission. The amount of pain reported was the most significant finding of his study. All of these figures should, we hope, have been improved after 10 years of experience, and the survey is being repeated as part of the evaluation of the practice and teaching of St. Christopher's Hospice.

The following related case histories describe the pain suffered by 3 patients and illustrate their general management and the individual achievements and family reconciliations that were made possible:

Case 1. Mr. John G., aged 61, a self-employed retailer of wine-making supplies, came to St. Christopher's Hospice with a history from his doctor of 18 months of severe spinal pain from a carcinoma of bronchus unrelieved by laminectomy, radiotherapy, and increasing doses of morphine and chlorpromazine. He knew that he was terminally ill, and both he and his family were feeling exhausted and bitter after months of obviously intense suffering. His drugs were not altered for the first 48 hr because he began to respond immediately to the atmosphere of security and friendly activity in the ward.[1] After a few days a combination of anti-inflammatory drugs (prednisolone and phenylbutazone) produced a dramatic change in pain and mood. The 4-hourly dose of oral morphine was reduced from 150 mg to 120 mg, where it remained. Mr. G. took part fully in the life of the ward: he organized the raffle of a toy made by his sister and began occupational therapy. Two weeks later he was less well and was often drowsy and occasionally somewhat confused, but he continued to enjoy frequent visits from his family and

[1] "The importance of morale and sympathetic understanding in a unit devoted to the care of dying people cannot be over-emphasised, and added to this major contribution to their psychologic comfort may be an enhanced subjective effect of drugs. In assessing pharmacological efficacy in these circumstances the group effect should be considered." (4)

visits to the Hospice Bar. He was entirely clear-headed when he sent for his family and announced to them that he did not think he would be alive the next day. He handed over his raffle to another patient, thanked all the staff, and had farewell drinks with his family before he lapsed into unconsciousness and died peacefully 36 hr after he had called them in.

After his death his wife wrote to the ward: "I thank you from the bottom of my heart for the kindness, compassion and caring which you gave to my dear husband. The last month of his life was an unexpected bonus, which turned out to be pain-free, care-free and restored his faith—I would add—mine also. I will never forget. God bless you all."

His sister wrote to me:

". . . Please find money order. My wreath of flowers to my dear brother, John.

He had all his wreaths of flowers while at St. Christopher's through the very great kindness shown by the doctors and staff, so feel the money is more beneficent than flowers.

I experienced something wonderful during the month I visited John. Three men who had never met before got together as brothers. I used to call them the three Js, two Johns and a Joseph: They worked together side by side, helping each other and Joe sat by my brother's bed the whole day he was dying, fetching cloths as he needed them and talking to him.

Something else I witnessed that day also. During the early evening I saw John look straight ahead on two occasions and give the most wonderful smile; there was no one at the foot of the bed or opposite, for John H. had passed on a few hours before. . . .

If it hadn't been for St. Christopher's our family would never have had this last happy month together with our loved one.

Now the three Js have gone together in peace. May God bless your Christian belief and work always."

Case 2. Mr. John H., an accountant aged 56, was admitted a week after Mr. G. and died the day before him. His pain had also been persistent and poorly controlled ever since a laparotomy and colostomy had been performed 6 months before. At the time he was admitted neither dihydrocodeine by mouth more or less regularly nor pethidine by injection 3 times daily were relieving it. He was still hopeful that something might be done to close the colostomy. He also said he felt better immediately after he was welcomed into the ward community, but he never talked much about his illness. His unsatisfactory medication was immediately altered to a morphine mist every 4 hr with prochlorperazine by day (5 mg) and chlorpromazine at night (25 mg). The dose of morphine alternated between 20 and 30 mg during his 3-week stay as his pain occasionally broke through the constant level of control. During this time five injections of diamorphine (5 to 10 mg) were given with the phenothothiazine because of episodes of vomiting. He needed one injection of diamorphine 20 mg during the afternoon he died.

Mr. H. was able to complete some accountancy a few days after his admission; he joined his friends with occupational therapy and entertained his large family who came with him to Chapel and to other Hospice functions. Four days before he died he was still working, he celebrated his wedding anniversary with his family and came with Mr. G. and Mr. C. to the Hospice Pilgrim Club evening.

His family spent his last day at his side, and nine of them were present as he died. A staff nurse said prayers with them all (a St. Christopher's custom which is practically never refused by the family). Several of Mr. H's family came back to the Chapel for the Sunday morning service 2 days later.

His wife wrote to me: "For me, he kept a diary. . . . All my prayers were answered after my husband entered your hospice. He was completely without hope, yet he recovered to such an extent that he was able to enjoy happiness, friendship, and love for his fellow man."

Case 3. Mr. Joseph C., aged 68, a retired painter and decorator, was admitted to St. Christopher's Hospice with a history of several months' severe, left-sided and back pain from a metastatic carcinoma of kidney. He was loath to admit how much he had suffered during the months when he had been in and out of a local hospital until we had demonstrated that we could relieve his pain while he still remained alert and active. He was given a mist morphine 20 mg with prochlorpromazine 5 mg every 4 hr with almost complete pain control and, as he later told us, his first night's sleep for months. After 48 hr he allowed us to increase his dose of morphine, and it remained at 30 mg until his death 4 weeks later. He also was given prednisolone 5 mg and indomethacin 25 mg q.d.s. Soon after admission Mr. C. became active, performing surprisingly vigorous physio- and occupational therapy and completing a large number of mosaic trays. After 2 weeks he recorded a television interview for a National network in which he said that he felt that he and the Hospice were fighting his advanced cancer together, that he now no longer even thought of pain and hoped to have a little more life ahead.

As his two friends began to fail, he took charge of Mr. G's raffle, completed Mr. H's last mosaic tray and sat and talked with them and their families throughout their last day. He himself developed a chest infection during the 12 hr in which his two friends died, and he was very upset and grieved together with the staff at their loss. His condition deteriorated rapidly from then on; but his usual medication, now given by injection, controlled all physical distress, and he died peacefully in the middle of the night with his wife and her sister at his side. He had been in the Hospice for 5 weeks.

One of his friends wrote to me:

"In the early hours of this morning my friend Joe C's earthly sojourn ended. Joe was a down-to-earth man, a heart of gold, a comedian and often a "gor blimme" bloke. Please, will you and your ministering angels accept my heartfelt thanks for making the evening of his life a happy event, I repeat, A Very Happy Event. If there is another world, then Joe was living to go to it, an example I shall keep to the end—or my beginning."

These three men had a quiet, rather ill companion in their four-bed bay. Mr. M. watched their activities in a somewhat detached manner. He spoke little but obviously felt drawn to some extent into the ward "Club." He had expected the first two deaths but was more shocked when Mr. C also died. He told us that he missed them, but he was able to welcome two new patients with his usual quietness and at present is considerably better than on admission. All three families called back to see him.

These family groups made full use of the time given to them by the relief of the pain of terminal malignant disease. All three patients had suffered months of unrelieved distress, yet none of them presented physical problems that could not be tackled quickly and effectively by the specialist team of the Hospice. We could not take away the pain of parting; but the mental suffering of each patient was alleviated by the physical ease, which at the same time greatly decreased much of the exhaustion and anxiety of their families. Each of the three groups found new meaning in life and faith, and their spiritual pain was also comforted.

These patients lived and died in the small community of an open ward bay, part of the larger community of the Hospice. This way of sharing their experience made a major contribution to the control of pain and also to the support of the grieving families. The letters illustrate the nature of hospice care for terminal pain and provide reasons why the local registrar of deaths has stated that she can recognize by their peace the Hospice families in her waiting rooms.

Mr. G's family expressed what we must surely all feel, "Why could he not have had this help before?" Too many patients reach those who can offer them proper understanding and management of their pain late in its crippling course, or not at all. Their families are left with haunting memories, and from them comes the almost-universal public fear of the inevitability of pain in terminal malignant disease. We owe them better than this. Every hospice will have such stories, and in order to set them in context with ascertained facts concerning randomly selected families who have experience of hospice care, the reader is referred to the report of the Newhaven Hospice to the National Cancer Institutes on two years' experience (7) and to Parkes (9) report on some of his psychosocial studies at St. Christopher's.

Results of Comparative Study

Findings from a comparative study of 34 families of cancer patients who died at St. Christopher's Hospice matched with 34 families of patients who died elsewhere showed statistically significant differences favoring the group from the Hospice in ways which have already been illustrated in the story of the three men given above. The families of patients managed at the hospice recalled the following:

1. Greater mobility of the patient.
2. Less pain rated as severe (but not bought at the cost of greater drug-induced confusion).
3. Less anxiety among spouses during the period of terminal care with fewer somatic symptoms.
4. Spouses spent much more time at the patient's bedside and very much more time talking to staff, other patients, and visitors. They were more likely to have helped to care for the patient and more likely to know a doctor's name.
5. Doctors and nurses at St. Christopher's were less likely to be seen as "busy" or "very busy" than staff elsewhere.
6. Despite the fact that 2 or 3 patients died each week on each floor of the Hospice, only 6% were said to have been upset by the death of another patient. The same figure was given for those in other wards, none of which were for "terminal care."

In addition, 27 families from each setting completed a check-list which allowed them to agree or disagree with general statements regarding the hospital. The statement which best characterized St. Christopher's was, "The hospital is like a family," which was checked by 78% of the St. Christopher's families and only 11% of the rest. It was also shown that St. Christopher's families were no more likely to be active in their religion than the other families; but many recognized the existence of the Christian foundation, and all who did reacted positively to it.

Development of Hospices

St. Christopher's Hospice was established in 1967 to relieve suffering by developing methods of care, analyzing knowledge and carrying out research into the control of the physical, mental, and social distress of chronic and long-term illness. It has helped to establish a code of practice that can be shared with all those caring for patients with similar problems. Some patients will need the experienced and confident care of a separate, specialized unit, but for the majority this will not be an available option. Nor should it be necessary.

The attitudes and skills which are being developed have already been shown to be eminently transferable. From experience at St. Christopher's and elsewhere came the pioneering work of the Symptom Control Team of St. Luke's Hospital, New York, which has now been adapted by the Support Team of St. Thomas' Hospital, London. Similarly, the Continuing Care Units in the United Kingdom and the Palliative Care Unit and Service of the Royal Victoria Hospital, Montreal (also related to St. Christopher's) have already been replicated both in the U.S.A. and elsewhere. The Home Care Team in New Haven (Connecticut, U.S.A.) has roots in both St. Christopher's and St. Joseph's Hospices. Historically these are all related through the author's initial experience at St. Luke's Hospital, London which was developed during 7 year's work at St. Joseph's Hospice (10).

The Home Care and Symptom Control Teams have shown that the control of terminal pain does not have to be carried out in a geographically separate unit, though there are some patients and families who need the expertise and the space they should find there. A few such hospices will be needed for patients with intractable problems, for research, and for teaching in terminal care; but most patients will continue to die in general hospitals, cancer or geriatric centers or, best of all, in their own homes. The staff they will find there should be learning how to meet their needs.

GENERAL PRINCIPLES OF HOSPICE CARE

The following list of the essential components of terminal care is the fruit of years of working and visiting in different units and of discussions with others working and interested in this field (6,11). Above all, it is the outcome of the good fortune which gave me the opportunity of listening to patients and their families during the 30 years since a dying patient said to me that he wanted, "What is in your mind and in your heart."

Management by an Experienced Clinical Team

The team or unit for terminal care must carry out its practice in such a way as to earn the respect and cooperation of the doctors who refer their patients. A multidisciplinary medical approach is as important in the later stages of cancer management as in the earlier phases of the disease. Moreover, this concept applies to other patients who may present with terminal pain. Consultation will often be needed between physician, surgeon, radiotherapist, chemotherapist, and sometimes the psychiatrist and the clinician who runs the local Pain Clinic. It is no longer adequate medicine to try to cope alone with difficult decisions in terminal cancer management, even though the needs of many patients have been and still will be dealt with successfully by their own family doctors, single-handed.

A group of consultants in a unit or team may act merely as a resource while the patient remains in the care of his family doctor or of the specialist who was involved with his initial treatment. The team may, however, take over his care completely, particularly if there is some special need such as intractable pain and distress, which is still all too often most ineptly treated in acute care units as well as in the patient's own home. There should be no feeling of failure on the part of the doctor whose experience is other if transfer to a special ward or hospice is carefully discussed and planned. Whenever the original doctor keeps in touch, his visits are likely to have a special place in maintaining a patient's morale. Few patients expect miracles at this stage, but they are all prey to feelings of failure and rejection and respond to a gesture that implies continued concern.

Understanding Control of the Common Symptoms of Terminal Disease, Especially Pain in All Its Aspects

Doctors and nurses need to concentrate on the development of these skills and special units should initiate research and share their knowledge. Terminal pain is so different in character and meaning from most pain met in a teaching hospital that the methods of giving relief and the standards of comfort and alertness that should be expected are sometimes difficult to establish in a general ward. This has to be demonstrated to both doctors and nurses if their patients are to have adequate treatment for the many symptoms that often accompany this usually generalized disease.

Terminal care is being increasingly recognized as a facet of oncology, but it is not always recognized that symptom control and general support should accompany the chemotherapy of advanced disease.

Attention to this part of the patient's therapy brings staff of all kinds closer to the often isolated patient and brings him the personal support he may so greatly need. Once such an attitude and regime is established, it should then be easier to desist from inappropriate treatments.

Skilled and Experienced Team Nursing

These patients need the stability and continuity of an experienced nursing team built up of members with varied trainings and backgrounds. This demands confident leadership from the ward sister and close communication both among the nursing staff. Moreover, it requires close communication between the nurse and others who will be involved with their patients, including social workers, physiotherapists, occupational therapists and, of course, the doctors.

The flexible staffing pattern needed cannot always be established in a general ward, and lack of time is a constant problem. This can, however, be exaggerated: An attitude can be conveyed in a brief meeting or in the way in which procedures are carried out. Student and auxiliary nurses frequently bring a special contribution. Odd moments spent with the patients instead of in a Nurses' Station are an irreplaceable part of their care. The chaplain's place in the whole team may begin from his support of the nursing staff who, most of all, bear the daily burden of relationships with dying and sorrowful people.

A Full Interdisciplinary Staff

This is not the field for total individual involvement, which can be most unhelpful for both patient and staff member. It takes time to build the ways of working together but such teams are to be found in other specialized units, for example, those for Intensive Care or Renal Dialysis. They are particularly needed by staff members who are grappling with emotional as well as with practical demands. Psychiatrists and social workers have frequently been involved as support. Such a team, together with all its professional members, should be seen to include the ward orderlies, domestics, and porters, often the people to whom hospital patients turn to most easily. Their support should not be underestimated or ignored. Students of all kinds may also assume this role.

It is important that as many different members as possible should meet for frequent discussion. Though the clinician does not abrogate his clinical responsibility, each member should be ready to assume a degree of leadership concerning an individual patient or family. St. Christopher's has been open for less than 11 years and approximately one-third of the nursing staff have worked 5 years or more, one-third between 1 and 5 years and one-third are in their first year. There is very little unplanned turnover. All of the doctors, except for one rotating Junior Doctor, and most of the other staff and the volunteers have made a long-term commitment.

A Home Care Program

A Home Care Program involving all the different disciplines among the staff must be developed according to local circumstances and be integrated with the hospitals, the family practices of the area, and the inpatient unit. Patients can then be admitted at the moment of their choice and of accurately defined medical need, and they will also be able to move easily to and from the wards for periods varying from days to weeks or months as short-term improvements are fully exploited. The way home, like the way back to the "Acute Care System" must always remain open.

Relief of pain in itself may make possible unexpected progress in these directions. Confidence may enable a family to keep a patient at home, often confounding all predictions. Where patients have access to adequate nursing, a 24-hour on-call service and other support, which may well include good neighbours and volunteers, home is likely to remain their choice. Even so, many people who have said they would like to die in their own homes need inpatient care, if only for the last few days. Some families find much greater relief and unity in a professional milieu in the last hours, and others realize that they cannot face the thought of death at home after all. They must be enabled to accept the help of admission without feelings of guilt. Those who manage to the end have a great feeling of satisfaction to ease their bereavement but once again, this is only possible if pain is controlled. Half of St. Christopher's patients are being nursed in their own homes at any one time.

Recognition of the Patient and Family as the Unit of Care

Families should have every available option open to their choice and expect recognition of their cultural and individual needs. Once this has become part of the ethos of a ward it becomes largely self-perpetuating. Occasional visits by ward staff to a patient's home with a family doctor or a domiciliary team member will emphasize the importance of including the family in the care of any seriously ill person. Not everyone will have the time or the understanding to embark on long family discussions, but everyone can recognize the family by name and accept them as an integral part of the team caring for the patient.

We should aim to give the maximum privacy to those who need it for peace and for the expressions of tenderness which are inhibited in a general ward. Separate units usually have more opportunity to give a special welcome to the solitary, but I have often seen how nurses in a general ward are able to do this and to make the distinction between the lonely, who welcome their friendship and the isolate, to whom this may well be an intrusion.

Admission to a hospice does not mean the expectation of inevitable death, and some patients and families wish to maintain their denial of the likely outcome. The staff will accept this if it is a consistent choice but find that in most cases a more realistic sharing of the situation will develop. At St. Christopher's Hospice a sheet is kept in the notes for any member of staff to note relevant comments made by patients concerning their illness. Not all of these are used, as some patients just cannot discuss these matters and not all comments get recorded. Most of those that are completed (more than half of all patients) show a developing realization of the situation and acceptance of it.

A Mixed Group of Patients

Although the homes or hospices that welcome only dying patients have given superb care for many years and by doing so, have frequently outweighed any fear locally of a "death house," yet we do not believe that this should now be the ideal. A good community is usually a mixed one, as is pointed out by a letter from a patient in St. Christopher's Hospice with Motor Neurone Disease:

> I was very interested in the article about the death of Jane Zorza (February 25) but would like to say that the impression given, although accurate for the particular patient, does overstress the aspect of painless dying.
>
> As a patient who has been in a hospice for nearly 18 months my view is that this impression is far too narrow. The hospice is a caring community for anyone in need of total support, and provides the opportunity for patients to live in pleasant surroundings in the knowledge that every assistance will be given both to family and patient whenever and however it is required. Some, like Jane Zorza, are only helped to die painlessly but many live hopefully and often happily for long periods.
>
> As a patient I can give my own experience and also my observation of many other patients where the multi-sided care and treatment offered by the hospice have improved the quality and extended the length of life beyond any imaginable expectation. I have seen many patients enter the hospice, apparently near death and completely without hope, who have after a few weeks recovered to such an extent that they have been able to return home—in some cases for many months—to live happily with their families, knowing that they have the full support of the hospice home care team at all times.
>
> For those of us not able to be cared for outside the hospice there is an atmosphere of caring and living which is the point that needs to be stressed. We do not enter a hospice to die but to live what is left of our time as happily and fully as possible." (5)

St. Luke's Nursing Home Day Centre, Sheffield and most of the new Continuing Care Units include a proportion of patients with nonmalignant diseases of a longer-term nature. St. Christopher's Hospice has welcomed 10 to 20% of its ward patients from this group, and from the beginning there have been a number of elderly people who live in their own bedsitting rooms in a separate Wing. Transfers to and from the wards are fairly common, and there is no doubt that the Hospice will extend its longer-term accommodation when it becomes possible. The person with the prognosis of some 2 years has often more difficult problems to handle than the one with only a few months to live and may greatly need the support of a suitable community or a Home Care Team.

Bereavement Follow-up

Many hospitals make special arrangements for families who come to collect certificates and property, but our work should not end there. Family pain is part of terminal pain, and the family has to recover. A bereavement follow-up will identify and support those in special need, working in cooperation with the family doctor and any local services which can be involved. Many doctors give such support as part of their service to the families they have known over the years. Most of the bereaved are not so fortunate and a follow-up may fill this gap and ease the tragedy and long morbidity.

Social workers and chaplains have initiated such work from general hospitals, but normally a team, usually of volunteers, will be required to meet with all those in need, with a leader to train and support the visitors themselves. There is no doubt that many families suffer from the sudden break from a staff who have cared for the patient and who have perhaps for a long time been a great part of their lives. In a small unit the families will be recognized as they enter the door, and reception staff have a special role in this part of care for the bereaved. An informal welcome back may be all that is needed. It has been found that only a small proportion of the bereaved will remain dependent upon either this support or the more formal program for more than a few months.

Methodical Recording and Analysis

Detailed recording and analysis make possible the evaluation and monitoring of clinical experience and the establishment of soundly based practice. St. Christopher's Hospice now has nearly 6,000 detailed and analyzed records retrievable for its retrospective surveys.

Hinton's (3) important study of the physical and mental distress suffered by 102 patients in the general wards of a teaching hospital is a definitive work and essential reference point. From the enormous volume of writing now available we can still turn for enlightenment to the pioneer work of Worcester (12), who published the lectures he had been giving to the medical students of Harvard from his background of family practice. This classic is still in print (13), but gradually the anecdotal approach is being supplemented by the more analytical (8). This is a challenge to those who feel that "tender, loving care" is all that is needed. Nothing can take its place but terminal care of the 1970s developed from previous experience, but now it should not be the same as that of the 1900s or even the 1950s. "Efficient loving care" is our aim, and every resource of clinical and social medicine has to be exploited.

Teaching in All Aspects of Terminal Care

Teaching in this field is much in demand by students and graduates of all the disciplines concerned. This is being given in conferences and seminars, in rounds and visits, and in outside lectures by members of the staff. We find that lectures and ward rounds of this kind are likely to be overcrowded. Besides the encouraging comeback, often years later, of those who have attended only one session, there should be reinforcement of such teaching for medical and nursing students in their own hospital wards. One of many groups of medical students who visited the hospice at their own request wrote afterwards: "It was a relief to be able to discuss freely a subject which is usually actively avoided in a large teaching hospital." Another student said on a teaching round: "In our hospital the patients have to earn their morphine."

Much of the future growth must be more closely integrated with general teaching centers, and the development of specialist teams within them must be encouraged. Nevertheless, the special units are likely to maintain their role of stimulating initial interest and of organizing courses for those who will in their turn be moving into this field. This is no longer a discipline in which no past special experience need be required.

Imaginative Use of the Architecture Available

In planning and building these facilities it is essential to have rooms for families to visit in groups; windows for patients to look from, and opportunities for them to move around; room for staff to work easily and to relax and for anxious visitors to take time off or to brace themselves for a meeting. Beauty is healing, and a feeling of openness and access to the world outside are chief among the needs of a unit for terminal and long-term care. Some of us have been fortunate enough to plan purpose-built hospices; others have learned to adapt whatever they could find, and successful practice has often arisen from the imaginative use of structural peculiarities. Emphasis should be given to the need for rooms for private talk; these must be found, whatever the area offered.

The proportion of single rooms to bays or wards dictates the way a ward team handles the patient's last hours and the needs of his family at that time.

Some feel strongly that no patient should be expected to witness the death of another person dying in the same room or bay. Others, mainly those with fairly generous space, find that this can almost always be managed so that the reaction of most patients and their families is almost entirely positive (as in the case of the group of patients described above). The peaceful death of a patient who shows no distress in breathing or in any other way, who is not left alone and, above all, one who is not hidden behind screens and curtains, repeatedly enables other patients to feel more confident about their own end. A distressing death would indeed have the opposite effect, but those who are expert in such care should not let this occur. Families in the bays talk with each other and with other patients, and it is rare for them to return for the practical business of the next day without going to see those they have known to give thanks for the friendship that has comforted them all. A patient's widow wrote to us:

> One thought that I would like to pass on to you. I think one of the greatest aids I personally received from St. Christopher's was being able to watch other patients die peacefully and easily without being shuffled off behind curtains and so on. I think those experiences have been of great therapeutic value to me so that when the time came for Eric to die, I felt no panic or even great distress and consequently was able just to concentrate on sharing his last moments. My son and I have spoken of this, and he says that he felt exactly the same way.

Longer-stay patients play a special role in the life of a ward for they are part of its hospitality and support, although, like the staff, they will need a holiday from it at times. Patients admitted within a short time of death and certain others will require single rooms. As St. Christopher's Hospice enlarges from 6 single rooms in 54 beds to 18 single rooms in a total of 62 beds, it has these groups specially in mind.

An Efficient Administration

Efficiency is very comforting, and competence in administrative detail gives security to patients, families, and staff. It also eases the liaison with outside contacts that is so essential for the small, specialized unit.

What are the economics of the provision of such care? St. Christopher's Hospice has close links with the National Health Service and has contractual arrangements for the majority of its beds. This means that there is no financial barrier between any of its patients and their care, and it has been shown that the cost to the National Health Service of a hospice bed will be no more than 50 to 70% of the cost of a teaching hospital bed and 70 to 80% of a general hospital bed in the same area. Moreover, the modern hospice is likely to have at least half of its patients in their own homes. It offers specialist consultations and support on referral from the patients' own doctors, district nurses, and other community services.

The high nurse-patient ratio in a hospice is more than compensated for, not only by the less complex overhead costs of such a unit, wherever it is situated, but also by the omission of tests and treatments that are no longer appropriate. (The cost-effectiveness of hospice care is currently being studied by the National Cancer Institutes, U.S.A. which has contracts with three of the many hospice units opening in the United States.) Above all, the hospice movement sets out to ensure that every person who can no longer benefit from the increasing complexity of the general hospital will have the support he and his family need in the right place, whether it be in his own home (if he has one), his treatment hospital, a cottage or community hospital, or a hospice.

The Cost of Commitment and the Search for Meaning

Members of staff will at times become drained by the work of the wards and in other contacts with the families of patients, and some are at risk of developing what has been described as the "Staff Burn-out Syndrome" (2). Informal safety valves should arise spontaneously according to local personalities and surroundings, but care must be taken to see that regular discussions, off duty, study leaves, and extra time off are arranged before a crisis is reached. Staff members must be prevented from investing all their emotional commitment in their work.

The management of terminal pain in all its aspects will at times cause pain and bewilderment to all members of the staff. If they do not have the opportunity of sharing their griefs and their questions, they are likely to leave this field or find a method of hiding behind a professional mask. Those who commit themselves to remaining near the suffering of dependence and parting find they are impelled to develop a basic philosophy, part individual and part corporate. This grows out of the work undertaken together as the members find that they each have to search, often painfully, for some meaning in the most adverse circumstances and gain enough freedom from their own anxieties to listen to another's questions of distress.

Most of the early homes and hospices were Christian foundations, their members believing that if they continued faithfully with the work to which they felt called, help would reach their patients from God. Some of the traditional ways of expressing this faith are being interpreted afresh today, but there are also many people entering this field who have still to consider their own religious or philosophical commitment. This is not an optional extra; it has a fundamental bearing on the way the work is done.

In considering these essential components of terminal care, it is important to distinguish between the general principles being interpreted at St. Christopher's Hospice and its own peculiar characteristics, stemming from the personalities of its staff and, above all, from its Christian foundation. The seed from which the Hospice grew was a gift of £500 left by a man from the Warsaw Ghetto who died of cancer in a London hospital in 1948. His promise, "I'll be a window in your Home" was fulfilled 19 years later when the first patients were admitted. That phrase and his other request, "I want what is in your mind and in your heart," sum up the need of all patients for the skill combined with friendship that make up terminal care. The original gift of £500 had grown to £500,000 when the community of the Hospice was opened in 1967. Now, 11 years later, the need to extend further its research into the control of pain in all its aspects and the ever-increasing demands for teaching have grown far beyond its original ideas—but they have still to be balanced to the daily needs of each patient, family, and staff member.

The patients have always been the central members of the community. Every day they bring their pain and their feelings of anger, bitterness, and grief into the Hospice as they are admitted. Yet the overwhelming majority find the atmosphere is peaceful, welcoming, and often joyful, for their pain is relieved and most of these feelings are transformed. We believe this is the work of the spirit of the God who is in all men, however they may seek for truth.

It seems to us that only the belief that all men belong to the family of a God who shared and shares their death can bring an answer not only to those whom we try to help but to the millions of the deprived and wronged, above all to those who have never had any chance of finding either a worthwhile life *or* death. That all wrongs will be righted and all the comfortless comforted should be the perspective of the individual, personal care that is offered in a hospice.

This is also the perspective in which the St. Christopher's Hospice staff are able to say to those of different beliefs or of none who face the problems of terminal pain, together with the atheist doctor and the priest in Camus' novel *The Plague* "We're working side by side for something that unites us beyond blasphemy and prayers" (1).

REFERENCES

1. Camus, A. (1948): *The Plague.* Hamish Hamilton, London.
2. Freudenberger, H. J. (1975): *The Staff Burn-Out Syndrome.* Drug Abuse Council Inc., 1828 1st St., N.W., Washington, D.C.
3. Hinton, J. (1963): Mental and physical distress in the dying. *Q. J. Med.,* 32:1.
4. Hinton, J. (1964): Editorial problems in the care of the dying. *J. Chronic Dis.,* 17:201.
5. Holden, E. (1978): Letter in *The Guardian.* London, March, 1978.
6. Kastenbaum, R. (1976): Towards standards of care for the terminally ill. Part III. A few guiding principles. *Omega,* 7:191.
7. Lack, S. A., and Buckingham, R. (1977): *Final Report. A Continuing Care at Home Program for Patients with Terminal Cancer and Their Families.* Hospice, Inc., New Haven, Connecticut.
8. Mount, B. M. (1976): The problem of caring for the dying in a general hospital. The Palliative Care Unit as a possible solution. *Can. Med. Assoc. J.,* 115:119.
9. Parkes, C. M. (1977): Evaluation of family care in terminal illness. In: *The Family and Death,* edited by E. R. Pritchard et al. Columbia University Press, New York.

10. Saunders, C. M. (1967): *The Management of Terminal Illness.* Hospital Medicine Publications Ltd., London (Available from St. Christopher's Hospice).
11. Wald, F. (1976): Report of International Work Group in Death, Dying and Bereavement. "Proposed Standards for Terminal Care." *Personal communication.*
12. Worcester, A. (1935): *The Care of the Aged, the Dying and the Dead.* Charles C Thomas, Springfield, Ill.; Blackwells, Oxford (1961).
13. Worcester, A. (1977): *The Care of the Aged, the Dying and the Dead.* Re-printed by Arno Press, New York.

Advances in Pain Research and Therapy, Vol. 2,
edited by J. J. Bonica and V. Ventafridda.
Raven Press, New York © 1979.

Terminal Care from the Viewpoint of the National Health Service

Gillian Ford

Department of Health and Social Security, Alexander Fleming House, London SE1, England

This paper describes the management of the final stages of malignant disease within the context of the National Health Service (NHS) of Great Britain. This is not the place to embark on a detailed description of the vast organization for providing health care which is the British National Health Service. But there are one or two important points about it which need to be remembered. It differs from insurance-based systems in that it is not a mechanism for paying bills, or reimbursing bills paid by patients. It is a system which requires the Secretary of State to provide such services as he considers appropriate for the purpose of discharging duties laid upon him by various Acts of Parliament and to meet all reasonable requirements for hospital accommodation, medical and other professional services, the care of expectant mothers and young children, facilities for the prevention of illness, aftercare of those who have suffered illness and so on. The list is not quite endless but comprehensive enough to explain why more than 750,000 people are employed by the NHS in England, the total for Great Britain reaching over 900,000. Although the Secretary of State's responsibilities are thus far-reaching and comprehensive, he does not have the power to direct individuals who work within it to practice in any particular specialty or in any particular geographical area. His task is to make the service possible by providing the facilities, and employing staff—both of which are carried out through the health authorities to whom the Secretary of State delegates his powers.

Thus there are powers to provide services but not to direct individuals, either in the sense described (such as might occur in the armed forces) or as to the standard or type of clinical treatment provided. In this the members of the medical, nursing, and dental professions and physiotherapists are deemed to be the only arbiters. The concept of clinical freedom is zealously guarded both by those who practice within the NHS and those who administer it.

DEVELOPMENTS OUTSIDE THE NHS

In spite of the comprehensive nature of the NHS, some patients seek treatment as private individuals from privately-run institutions. A number of charitably-run homes supplement NHS or local authority accommodation for those who, because of age or disability, need a sheltered milieu. New developments in medical care often emerge from academic departments or research institutes, and generally such developments are absorbed into the NHS as their value is recognized; but occasionally the private/charitable sector makes a sustained contribution to care or treatment or both. Terminal care is an important example. Of the 40 or so special units for those with terminal malignant disease, only about 10 are wholly within the NHS although most of the others receive some financial support from health authority sources. The special units for terminal care have a unique approach to death and dying which does not deny the fact of death but sees that the troubles that precede it, whether these be of body, mind, or spirit, receive attention and care.

ESTIMATES OF NEED

A responsibility of those who are concerned with running and administering the NHS is to look at developments outside, in University Departments, or the private or charitable sectors, or in other countries and to try to assess the impact on the NHS. What, for example, is the population's need for kidney machines or for early detection of fetal abnormality? More particularly, what measures are there of the need for special facilities for the treatment of terminal malignant disease? In the U.K. details are, of course, collected for all deaths by diagnosis. Details are shown for 1973, in the following tables (5). (The large totals have been rounded.) Table 1 shows the total of all deaths by age group. Table 2 shows deaths in the same year from neoplastic disease in the same age groups and the percentage that these form of all deaths. Thus, totals are reached of about 120,000, or a fifth of all deaths, occurring from cancer. The majority of these take place in hospitals rather than at home—the proportion has been rising for cancer as it has for all causes. This is shown in Table 3. The proportion of deaths occurring in

TABLE 1. *Total deaths in the United Kingdom in 1973*

Sex	Age group 0–4	5–24	25–64	65+	Totals
Males	7,802	4,840	86,000	198,000	297,000
Females	5,704	2,324	50,000	233,000	291,000

TABLE 2. *Deaths from neoplastic diseases in the United Kingdom in 1973*

Deaths	Sex	Age groups 0–4	5–24	25–64	65+	Totals
Number of deaths from neoplastic disease	Male	172	642	24,000	41,000	65,000
	Female	124	438	21,000	35,000	56,000
Percent of total deaths due to neoplastic disease	Male	2%	11%	28%	21%	22%
	Female	2%	19%	41%	15%	19%

private institutions, which would include hospices outside the NHS, was 10% in 1974.

As far as sheer numbers are concerned, the tables show something of the problem. But illness, symptoms, distress, and pain are not revealed by such data. A recent article by Parkes (4) recounted a survey of 276 married patients under the age of 65 with cancer. Particular attention was paid to the amount and duration of pain, because this was the most prominent cause of distress. Of the sample, 60% of the patients died in hospitals, but the amount of time spent at home during the terminal stage was 3½ times that spent in the hospital by the sample as a whole. Table 4 shows the interviewer's assessment of two features of the final illness.

Since patients who had less pain *before* the terminal period were most likely to go home and remain there, the finding that a high proportion ultimately experienced severe to very-severe pain underlines the need for active treatment of pain in this group. The findings are not dissimilar from those of Cartwright and associates (2) who reported pain present in 66% of a stratified sample of 785 deaths from all causes studied by interview of relatives within 9 months. Pain was reported in 87% of those whose death was due to cancer, although the extent to which this remained unrelieved was not known.

TABLE 3. *Place where deaths occurred*

Year	All deaths: Home	Hospital[a]	Other	Cancer deaths: Home	Hospital[a]	Other
1965	38%	50%	12%	37%	60%	3%
1970	33%	54%	13%	33%	62%	5%
1974	31%	56%	13%	31%	64%	5%

[a] Non-psychiatric hospitals. Includes NHS and non-NHS facilities.

TABLE 4. *Interviewer's assessment of two features of the final illness*

	Home-centered (65 patients)	Hospital-centered (100 patients)
Mobility		
Confined to bed	6	45
Intermediate	45	43
Fully up	12	0
Pain		
None to mild	19	34
Moderate	13	32
Severe to very severe	29	19

Dr. Parkes also compared three groups of patients and the extent to which pain was relieved. The conclusions from this part of the study were that, of hospital-centered patients, 20% were said to have suffered severe and mostly unrelieved pain and this state did not change during the final phase of care in hospital. Those patients who were confined at home showed that pain became an increasing problem. Six percent experienced unrelieved pain prior to the final period, but this proportion rose to 42% during the final phase of care at home. Those patients admitted to St. Christopher's Hospice showed a reduction in severe and unrelieved pain from 36% in the pre-terminal period to 8% in the terminal phase. This clearly has implications for pain control irrespective of where the patient is being cared for.

SERVICES FOR PATIENTS WITH CANCER

There can be no doubt of the size of the problem. What is our capacity for tackling it?

The central core for the provision of medical and surgical services is the district general hospital. An urban population of 100,000 to 150,000 will almost certainly have such a general hospital, and there most treatment for cancer begins after referral from the patient's own general practitioner. But such a hospital is unlikely to have radiotherapy services or specialists in the use of cytotoxic therapy, or a clinical pharmacologist. These more specialized services are centralized within hospitals—often teaching hospitals—which serve a much bigger population than their immediate district. This means that some patients requiring prolonged treatment have to travel for radiotherapy or other cancer therapy. The annoyances of this have been partly eased in some places by building hostel-type accommodation so that patients can stay overnight without being admitted to a hospital bed. Treatment with cytotoxic drugs may be available in the same hospital as radiotherapy, but in only a few places are the cancer specialists grouped together in one unit for treatment of cancer as such. Only a few departments within hospitals and even fewer whole hospitals are designated for treatment of cancer alone. However, there is an increasing trend towards grouping together the various specialties concerned in it. In four NHS Regions experimental "Regional Cancer Organizations" have been established. These have the aim of providing high standards of diagnosis and coordinated treatment for all cancer patients throughout the Region. It is hoped that medical staff in other Regions will watch with interest the evaluation of this combined approach.

It has been shown that the majority of patients with cancer die in NHS hospitals in ordinary general wards. In some hospitals teams of specialists from different disciplines plan the management of the individual patient throughout the course of his or her illness. Most hospitals do not set aside a whole or part of a ward for those who are terminally ill. This may be a deliberate decision to avoid the stigma of the "death ward." It may be a deliberate decision by medical staffs, that they as individuals are each responsible for the total care of their own patients from beginning to end, even though other disciplines may be involved at intermediate stages. This may require a deliberate undertaking given to relatives or to the family doctor that admission to the acute ward is possible if symptoms or social conditions require it.

Community Services

Patients who are in their own homes will receive care from a number of sources; indeed, some patients will have reached hospitals because the community services will have provided screening procedures such as those for cancer of the cervix or lung cancer. More commonly, general practitioners dealing with patients who they regard as "at risk" because of their age, lifestyle, or symptoms will have initiated the sequence which leads to hospital treatment and continuing surveillance.

Both the community services of the health authority and those of the local authority will be involved in the care of patients in their own homes when hospital treatment has ceased. The objective of this care will be the sustaining both of the patient and the family. The family doctor is a key member in the organization of this. He may have a nurse working within his practice, or he may call upon the community staff or services run by health authorities, e.g., health visitors, home visits from occupational therapists or physiotherapists. Home helps provided by the local authority may be assisted by volunteers from the Womens' Royal Voluntary Service, who provide a service which delivers hot meals to patients' homes.

The social worker, also employed by the local authority, may assess the situation, which will include the need for practical services, walking aids, commodes and so on. This category of somewhat mundane objects and services may seem irrelevant to the pain of terminal malignant disease, but it must be remembered that the pain of a bedsore may be the most dominant feature in a patient's list of problems and maintenance of mobility is thus very important.

Care from the NHS primary health team comes from medical and district nursing staff, and health visitors. In addition there may be home visits from occupational therapists and physiotherapists. NHS staff may be supplemented by Marie Curie Foundation nurses and other helpers—some local authorities provide night sitters and laundry/incontinence services. The most sustained support comes from relatives and neighbours, and this has been described as "often remarkable" (6).

Teamwork

The teamwork of care at home is just as necessary as that within the hospital because of the multiple ills and sorrows which require attention. If symptoms are ignored, the problems of pain are likely to become worse—as later are those of bereavement. The advantages of teamwork in hospital and in the community are the mix of skills, personalities, and temperaments. The disadvantages are difficulties in establishing clear lines of communication and the diffusion of contacts which any one patient may have. If he feels that nobody is in charge, he is bound to experience *fear*. The hospital will offer an outpatient appointment—but it may be some weeks ahead. But if the family doctor has been kept fully in touch with the patient's progress and the plans for further treatment, if any, he has an invaluable role. Apart from mobilizing both health and social community services he may be the first person to whom the patient reveals the full extent of his pain, and he may need to consider more treatment deliberately aimed at pain, including further radiotherapy or changes or increases in analgesics.

Home, Hospital or Hospice?

Unfortunately, as we have seen, patients' needs for pain-relief are not always met. It is also clear that medical staff, hospital, and family doctors alike do not know the scope for pain control which is already available.

This is no fault of the NHS as a system of providing care. But the bigger the framework the more difficult for those operating within it to keep in touch and to know what the plan of management is, whether at home, in hospital or at home *and* hospital. The NHS provides community and specialist services in a unique way but combining the best elements of both takes patience and perseverance, as a general practitioner knows. Community care is not in itself necessarily better than hospital care. But because it is familiar to the patient it is believed to be what he would prefer, and so it will normally be until he sees his family using all their energies, and more, in looking after him. Hospital specialist services are not necessarily failing in their provision for terminal care, but the patient may not wish to be there.

A precise or absolute policy for terminal care is doomed to fail. It is a matter on which the patient's circumstances and preferences will have a profound influence. Certainly some staff feel that an acute general ward is not the ideal place to care for a dying patient, because its pace and atmosphere are geared for the acutely ill. The regular drug round may inadvertently be late because of an emergency admission. A 4-hour interval may be stretched to 6. Special arrangements for an evening at home or an outing to the "pub" consume staff time and may be trivial and burdensome to those who are responsible for order within the ward.

Patients too are often slow to bring their needs to staff busy with patients whose needs seem to be more pressing. Nevertheless, a patient may welcome a return to the ward where there are familiar faces and routine and, as the tables show, the majority of patients who die from cancer do so in ordinary general hospitals. Hospice care is often combined with a domiciliary team which provides experts who assist the general practitioner to care for patients in their own homes. This seems to provide the best answer in certain circumstances. Through the focused nature of their work, hospice staff became skilled at managing pain and other symptoms. Because hospices are small care given has a tailor-made quality, comforting to patient and family alike.

CONCLUSIONS

Future Developments Within the National Health Service

It goes without saying that ideally those who are experiencing their terminal illness should have no less attention and care paid to them than if there were a possibility of cure. But health services, insurance systems, and individuals have also to weigh the economic aspects of treatment. While "good health" may be the aim of a State for its population or a family for its members, a good death is not yet in the same category. In the light of the evidence of need, both measured and suspected, it is possible that there will be a conscious effort to include terminal care as one of the many priorities for NHS expenditure. Exactly how this will be accomplished is for health authorities to determine.

Hospice care is not cheap, but it appears to be considerably less expensive than care in a general hospital providing all acute services. Hospices for patients with terminal illness and with pain problems have tended to develop with substantial NHS support and sometimes even wholly within it. The National Society for Cancer Relief and the Marie Curie Memorial Foundation have also made very substantial contributions in this field. The NHS has looked to the hospices to pioneer developments in pain and symptom management, and they have became foci of excellence and a milieu for staff of all the different disciplines to receive training and to carry back to their own hospitals the essential features of hospice care.

Most staff working within the NHS will continue to be mainly occupied with primary care, or medical and surgical specialist services, or long-term care of the elderly, but many are realizing that the patient with terminal malignant disease, whether at home or in a hospital ward, has needs which should be met. Transfer to a special unit may not be possible or desirable, but the assurance of a hospice or hospital bed, when necessary, is an important factor in managing patients at home. For the future one looks at the following possibilities. The growth in the hospice movement suggests that most of the big centers of population in the U.K. may, by the next century, have such a development. In addition to the 40 or so already in existence, another 20 are planned. Ideally these would be closely associated with academic departments, that is, hospitals teaching undergraduates so that this subject may be taught in the early part of the curriculum, not left to postgraduate activities. It seems essential that such hospices should run or actively participate in home care schemes. These provide learning and teaching experience of care in the home and show clearly that it is not home care *versus* hospital/hospice care—the two are complementary.

Where care is being provided in a big general hospital a degree of skill may be acquired by a team of staff (the symptom control team) who provide the expertise within that hospital. Whether they have a part of the hospital, or part of a ward, solely for their own patients under their care is a matter for local agreement. It may be preferable to keep the patient in a ward with which he is familiar and use the team when and wherever they are needed. In the smaller hospitals outside the major conurbations the mixture of skills and specialties may not be diverse enough for it to be possible to set up such a team. For some particular types of pain the local hospital may provide a specialist service such as a pain clinic where nerve blocks and other surgical procedures may be carried out. These may be a small but very important part in the management of pain in the terminal and pre-terminal stages.

Patients living in towns or rural areas served by smaller hospitals may not have ready access to expert terminal care either while they are at home or when they are admitted to hospital. Fortunately there is not only an increasing interest in the subject, but also it is hoped that opportunities for postgraduate experience for medical and nursing staff, though few at the moment, will multiply as the number of units increase and more courses can be offered. Interested staff from a variety of disciplines are taking notice of developments and patients are benefiting as a result. But even so, a few informed professional staff scattered sparsely amongst a population of 100,000 to 200,000 people do not add up to a focus of skill and experience which can be recognized and drawn upon by doctors suddenly faced with problems of pain which appear insoluble. Patients are quick to realize when their medical advisors are becoming fearful that they will be unable to negotiate the next bend in the pain spiral. There is much anxiety about creation of addiction, of causing stupor alternating with pain. Since any family doctor will only have 4 or 5 patients a year who die of cancer, he is unlikely to become skilled at managing all the pain problems which may be present. But a very great deal can be done by frequent discussion in postgraduate medical centers (where hospital medical staff and general practitioners meet) and articles in the medical press. The Department of Health held a symposium in 1972, on Care of the Dying, and many helpful ideas were aired at that time (6).

Perhaps the most necessary adjunct at this stage, to patient-care and the continuing process of education, is the availability somewhere of expert advice when the doctor feels he has come to the end of his therapeutic armamentarium. The symptom control team of a big hospital may be miles away, the nearest hospice even further, but it is unlikely that they cannot be reached by telephone. Most of the hospices already offer this kind of advisory service for practitioners, and it is much appreciated and effective in instilling professional confidence.

A recent leading article in the *British Medical Journal* (1) concluded with a quotation from Hinton (3): "We emerge deserving of little credit; we who are capable of ignoring the conditions which make muted people suffer. The dissatisfied dead cannot noise abroad the negligence they have experienced." I would add that I believe that fear of inadequacy has caused professional staff to wear a mask of indifference and that this fear is unnecessary. Many have now demonstrated that though the home or the hospital may be far from ideal, it is possible to cope with patients' pain. It does not require a million pounds, or magic, but confidence that pain control is possible, with detailed attention to a variety of therapeutic measures coupled with that attitude which accepts the whole patient and his needs but sees him as a person.

REFERENCES

1. *Br. Med. J.* (1978): Pain and the dissatisfied dead. 25:459–460.
2. Cartwright, A., Hockey, L., and Anderson, J. L. (1973): *Life Before Death.* Routledge and Kegan Paul, London, Boston.
3. Hinton, J. (1972): *Dying,* 2nd ed. Penguin Books Ltd., Harmandsworth, Middlesex, Baltimore.
4. Parkes, C. M. (1978): Home or hospital? Terminal care as seen by surviving spouses. *J. R. Coll. Gen. Pract.,* 28:19–30.
5. *Registrar General's Statistical Review of England and Wales Tables (Medical)* (1973): Her Majesty's Stationery Office, London.
6. Silver, C. P. (1976): Terminal care. *Br. J. Hosp. Med.,* 16:579–584.

Discussion

Part II. Management of Pain of Advanced Cancer: Continuing and Terminal Care

Questioner: Dr. Ford, what is the cost of patients managed in hospices compared to those patients managed in general hospitals?

Ford (London): It is considerably cheaper to provide care in a separate unit than in an acute hospital providing the full range of special services.

Questioner: Dr. Saunders, do you think that respiratory depression due to high doses of narcotics necessary to control severe pain of a terminal cancer patient makes it impossible to use them for adequate pain-relief?

Saunders (London): I have had 30 years experience with such patients and have found that side effects of narcotics are very much less when these drugs are given to control severe cancer pain than when they are given to normal volunteers. We do not find that the respiratory depression is a clinically difficult problem to handle. Remember that as tolerance to analgesia increases so does their tolerance to side effects.

Twycross (Oxford): I'd go along with that. In practice when morphine is given by mouth there is no problem with respiratory depression. Indeed we sometimes use morphine purposely to lower the respiratory rate in some of our patients who have respiratory distress, and this can be of great benefit to the patient.

Questioner: Dr. Saunders, what are the psychologic reactions of the medical and paramedical staff to the continuous and exclusive contact with patients who suffer and die?

Saunders: The nurse that I showed you with the patient near the end showed a degree of grief and affection for that patient. Like many of us she moved into this field because of knowing personally the problem of pain and bereavement in her own family. She is able to see that patient relieved of the pain and making something creative out of his time. That is totally different from walking up and down at the end of a bed and seeing a patient with unrelieved pain and despair. Even so the staff grieve when a patient who has become very much a part of the ward dies. And I'll certainly never stop feeling sad when I see a family member walking alone out of the house.

Questioner: Dr. Saunders, are the patients dismissed from St. Christopher's with antalgic therapy followed by the Hospice's staff? What relationship is there between the Hospice's staff and the family doctor?

Saunders: Our work is integrated with that of the ordinary community services. We keep in constant communication with the family doctors who have the responsibility of the patient. We work alongside. We will have made recommendations and give support in prescribing, and be ready for consultation and may be called to the home, but not need to bring the patient into the Hospice.

Iacono (Ragusa): Dr. Saunders, what is the numerical ratio between patients and medical and paramedical staff in the Hospice?

Saunders: We have at the moment 54 beds, and we are going to increase this to 62 leaving aside the wing for old people. At any time we will also have about 60 patients at home. For this patient population of about 120 we have 40 doctor's sessions a week, that is 20 half-days of which 12 are at least taken in straight teaching. We are going to increase our doctor coverage as the number of beds increase. We also have one whole-time-equivalent nurse in the establishment for each patient bed. That means day duty, night duty, study leave, and all the rest of it. For example, if we have an 18-bed ward we will have 7 or 8 nurses on duty in the morning, 4 or 5 in the afternoon, with an overlap for discussions, and 2 or 3 on duty at night. Roughly one-half of our nurses are trained and one-half untrained. Our tendency is to move to having more trained nurses in proportion.

Lipton (Liverpool): Dr. Ford, why do you believe that pain-control methods cannot be spread throughout the British hospital service?

Ford: What I said was that I believe there would be centers where some highly specialized procedures for controlling pain were carried out but that it would be up to the local hospital staff to acquire the knowledge which will permit them to refer patients for specific procedures. I emphasized the need for treatment to be available locally, because the nature of terminal care is such that patients usually are unwilling to remain away from their families and friends for very long. The onus then is on the medical staff to provide the best personal care and the best pain-relief. Doctors used to know which patients might benefit from nerve block, neurosurgery, or other modalities and to refer them to the right facility. I did not say that pain control would not spread because of the nature of National Health Service, but rather because of the nature of terminal care, which precludes that these procedures would be on everybody's door step.

Questioner: Dr. Twycross, are not oral preparations of morphine in the homes of patients easily obtained by addicts who have ready access to such patients?

Twycross: As far as I know no solution of morphine in any home in Britain has ever fallen into the hands of an addict. We do not have a big addict problem fortunately, and certainly we have had no alarms on this score.

Ford: I should add that a dilute solution of morphine is not going to be of very great interest to an addict.

Twycross: That is right. The solution of morphine is generally not stronger than 10 mg. It may be weaker but usually not stronger in the majority of patients.

Bonica (Seattle): Dr. Saunders, how many hospices are there in Britain?

Saunders: Between 38 and 40, but the impact these hospices are having is very much greater and more widespread than the number of patients managed in them would suggest.

Bonica: Dr. Saunders, what percentage of patients with advanced cancer are managed in hospices?

Saunders: Very small number because we have 600 admissions a year in this 60-bed facility. Altogether, there are something like 800 beds in hospices, so that if we use St. Christopher's data a total of about 8,000 patients are managed in hospices. This is a very small percentage of the 820,000 patients with cancer, but the effect of what we are doing, although difficult to assess accurately, involves many more patients. Many family doctors in our area, after having shared care of a patient with us once or twice will then take care of patients themselves and call us only if we are needed for special consultation.

Bonica: Dr. Saunders, what percentage of patients outside hospices are managed properly with pain-relief?

Saunders: I think that Dr. Parkes' figures give us the feeling that roughly 50% of patients who die of cancer are likely to experience moderate to severe pain. And if we take Dr. Parkes' figures which are more optimistic than Dr. Cartwright's, we can expect that half of those are going to die with unrelieved pain. In other words, 25% of cancer patients continue to have pain which remains unrelieved until they die. I am afraid we are not doing well and have a long way to go to provide good pain-relief to terminal cancer patients.

Fink (Bethesda): In the United States of America, there has been some interest in the hospice concept for several years, and there has been a fostering of the development of hospices by the National Cancer Institute, which is the primary agency of our Federal Government responsible for cancer research and therapy. However, recently, through the interest of our President, Mr. Jimmy Carter, and his medical advisor, Dr. Peter Bourne, and much interest on the part of our media, newspaper, television, and public interest groups, there is a rising awareness of the kinds of concepts which have been discussed and relate to hospice. At the current time, hospices or organizations called hospices are springing up all over the U.S. In some instances the hospice concepts are much as has been discussed by Saunders and colleagues. In others these are simply names used for the typical nursing homes which exist in our country. From the point of view of the Federal Government we are most interested in evaluating the hospice in the U.S. to determine its efficiency and effectiveness in dealing with the type of symptoms that have been discussed by our colleagues of the United Kingdom. It is also fair to point out, however, that in the United States the practice of medicine is generally a private practice. Therefore, before laws become firm we must ascertain how the hospice concepts will be handled in the United States.

Fontanella (Milano): Dr. Twycross, have you ever encountered a patient with such severe pain that it could not be relieved? If you have, and his life-expectancy was very short, do you think it would be better for him to live or to die early?

Twycross: We approach pain control on a sort of graded scale. First of all, we set out to achieve freedom from pain at night and assure the patient of a good night's rest, and that we achieve with 99.5% of our patients. We then try to produce ample pain-relief during the day, with the patient at rest, sitting or lying. The round figures from several institutions including St. Christopher's would be 98%. In other words, we are highly successful in producing pain-relief at rest during the day. The third stage is pain-relief on movement during the day. This is where we have to compromise a bit, and the figure is probably about 80% success. But even in those who do not get complete relief on movement during the day, the pain is reduced. Moreover, we introduce what I call "modification of lifestyle" or relative immobilization to help reduce pain on movement from an intolerable to an acceptable level. There have been 1 or 2 patients where we have really been in trouble; those have been patients with paraplegia due to spinal cord compression and nerve root infiltration. The situation was resolved by doing a spinal cord transection. On occasion it is necessary to reduce the level of consciousness in order to achieve good pain-relief. Just what percentage of patients require this I can't say, but these constitute a small number of patients. I emphasize a small number of patients in whom a combination of physical, spiritual, and psychologic factors prevent us from producing ample pain-relief without reducing the level of consciousness. Of course when that happens, one is hastening the development of terminal hypostatic pneumonia, but this is a very small percentage of our patients.

Saunders: I think that the question being asked is really, "Do we think that there does come a time for any number of terminal cancer patients when it would be better to kill them rather than to go on trying?" And it is some form of legalized euthanasia that is perhaps in his mind. I would like to say that in the very great number of years that I now have known these patients, the number who have consistently asked to be permitted to die is very small indeed, and their reason has not been pain, but despair or just anger in a person who has had previous emotional problems. I am not saying that we can absolutely produce complete pain-relief while the patient is alert; I would say that we can always relieve pain at the expense of some alertness. But I would like to add one more thought about this. If, because of previous treatment the patient's pain is very difficult or impossible to control, and the patient asks you to kill him, you are going to be in a very difficult position, and you are going to need to call in the expert. Let us suppose for the moment that active euthanasia is part of the law in one of our countries, and consequently some patients will demand it and say this is a personal freedom they should have, but it would take away the right of every other patient on long-term care. But we are offering a positive alternative of producing ample pain-relief. We should be reaching the stage at which nobody needs to make the desperate request for death, and I believe we can.

Moricca (Rome): With regard to euthanasia I would like to remind all of us that we are not responsible for the disease. We are responsible for the therapy. Therefore we must not kill, but we must fight pain and effectively relieve it. And there are many possibilities against pain. Some are offered during the terminal phase of the disease, others are those that have been discussed and explained during this symposium. I therefore think that the problem of euthanasia doesn't exist and should not exist.

Panel: Future Needs, Goals, and Directions

J. Bonica and V. Ventafridda (Moderators)

Bonica (Seattle): Ladies and Gentlemen, after 3½ days of long and extensive discussions on almost every aspect of pain of advanced cancer, we have reached the focal point of this international symposium: consideration of future goals. We must set a direction and consider actions we must take to improve the control of pain of advanced cancer. For this portion of this program we have gathered an outstanding panel of experts. I regret that Prof. Veronesi was unable to remain for this session because, as current President of the International Union Against Cancer (UICC), he has been in a position of making suggestions in setting goals for the management of pain of cancer patients everywhere. Fortunately, Prof. Pietro Bucalossi, President of the Italian League Against Cancer and former Director of the Milan Cancer Institute, has graciously agreed to give his thoughts about this problem. Moreover, we are fortunate in having Professor Emilio D'Ambrogio, representing the Minister of Health of Italy, and Dr. Diane Fink, Director of the Division of Cancer Control and Rehabilitation of the National Cancer Institute of the United States. Both will be able to present the current and future position of the governments of these two countries regarding this problem of cancer pain.

Prof. Loeser will discuss the neurosurgical aspects, Prof. Bond will represent psychology and psychiatry, Profs. Houde and Twycross will consider future needs regarding systemic drugs, Professors Pannuti and Gennari will discuss the needs in anticancer modalities, while Prof. Ventafridda as co-Chairman of this panel will make the closing remarks. It is hoped that each member of the panel will consider future goals, directions, and needs within the framework of the current status of each area, particularly regarding the deficiencies which exist.

I will start the discussion by making certain general observations and remarks. The presentations made in this symposium have substantiated and confirmed my conviction about the current deficiencies that exist in the management of patients with pain of advanced cancer. As I have listened to each speaker and the informal discussions of the panels, certain points have emerged which impressively emphasize the critical need for much greater research and educational efforts, and consequently improvement in the control of pain of cancer.

In regard to research, I wish to stress my strong conviction that one of the first orders of business is to carry out comprehensive national and regional epidemiologic studies to ascertain the incidence and magnitude of pain in cancer in general, and the incidence, severity, and duration of pain with each specific type of tumor in particular. Data presented here has confirmed the suspicion of many of us that pain develops much more frequently in cancer patients than most people believe. Moreover, it is clear that in most instances it is not effectively relieved. I believe we have reached the consensus that the multidisciplinary approach for team management of the pain of cancer, which I have suggested for many years, is one of the most effective, if not the most effective way, of dealing with this serious health problem.

Another area of research that needs to be done urgently, is to study the basic biochemical, neurologic, and psychologic mechanisms of cancer pain. Why and how do large tumors pressing on major nerves or plexuses produce pain? Is it stimulation of axons, lowering of nociceptor thresholds, or increased sensitivity to norepinephrine as occurs with other types of peripheral nerve injuries, or is it due to production of pain-producing substances? What role does block of large fibers with consequent loss of their pain-inhibitory action play in this type of pain? Why and how do bone tumors produce pain which is usually excruciating? How does infiltration of cancer cells in perineural, perivascular, and perilymphangetic tissue cause pain? Is it a biochemical, neurologic, or pathologic process?

Does ischemia consequent to obstruction of large arteries by tumors really produce pain by producing asphyxia, cellular breakdown with the liberation of pain-producing substances? Is the pain of venous engorgement edema caused by compression of large veins due to primarily mechanical or biochemical nociceptor stimulation? How does fibrosis of the brachial plexus or the lumbosacral plexus that follows cancer therapy produce pain?

What role do the recently discovered endorphins play in cancer pain and its relief? How can we manipulate them to achieve maximum analgesia? I am convinced that once we obtain answers to these basic questions, we have the science and technology to produce agents or techniques, or both, with which we'll be able to exert exquisitely specific anti-pain action to produce relief.

Still another extremely important area of research is in the psychologic, psychosocial, and behavioral aspects of cancer pain. Although hundreds of studies have been directed to the problem of cancer per se, very few have looked at the impact of the pain. What influence does the pain of cancer have on the emotional and behavioral condition of the cancer patient and conversely, what impact do psychologic, personality, environmental, and psychosocial factors have on the pain experienced by the cancer patient. I hope Prof. Bond will suggest future activities in this area.

In my introduction to this symposium I emphasized, and indeed almost belabored, the critical need to improve the education of medical, dental, nursing, and psychology students, and students from other health professions to become involved in the management of patients with cancer. Equally important is the education or reeducation of graduate physicians and other health professionals in the basic principles of cancer pain diagnosis and therapy. All members of the oncology team should become appreciative of the importance of optimal cancer-pain control. By the same token, pain therapists who become involved in managing cancer pain must also become fully acquainted with the other aspects of oncologic process. In other words, we must develop well-integrated multidisciplinary teams, each member of which knows "all of the plays" of the game and not just his or her field.

Although during this symposium we have achieved greater interaction and communication among participants from various disciplines than has been the case heretofore, it is clear that we still have some way to go before we have the optimal integrator approach. For example, in discussing the application of various therapeutic modalities, there is still a tendency to consider each by itself and not as part of a combined pain therapy. Moreover, with some exceptions, there was the tendency to extol the virtues and the advantages of each technique while its disadvantages, limitations, and complications were not given due emphasis. These are reflective of the tubular vision I spoke about in my introductory remarks.

Now for a few comments on particular topics. In regard to the anticancer modalities I was pleased to learn of the comprehensive data on the incidence and magnitude of pain of cancer presented by Foley and Pannuti. I hope other oncologists follow their example and collect and publish data on the problem of pain as well as other aspects of cancer treatment.

In regard to the systemic analgesics there is an obvious need for well-controlled studies of large doses of aspirin and other nonnarcotic analgesics in a sufficiently large number of cancer patients in order to more accurately define their efficacy and limitations. Moreover, in view of the significant incidence of depression, it is surprising to note the very meager amount of data from control studies of psychotropic drugs. Similarly, in view of the significant role played by psychologic factors in chronic pain, it is surprising that there are virtually no data on large numbers of patients managed with hypnosis, biofeedback, and/or behavioral modification techniques for cancer pain.

Although nerve blocks and neurosurgical procedures have been used extensively in patients with cancer pain, there have been very few controlled clinical trials on sufficient numbers of patients to permit us to define the role of each of these techniques in managing cancer pain. In addition to the use of these techniques in a sufficiently large number of patients, it is essential to apply the basic principle of the controlled clinical trial in evaluating each of the methods for the type or types of cancer pain for which the specific technique is indicated. Only with these types of data will it be possible for us to define more precisely the indication and advantages, as well as limitations and disadvantages and complications of each procedure for each type of pain (i.e., considering the mechanism, intensity, site, degree of spread, and other characteristics of the pain).

These are some of the many factors which must be considered in the future. And now, let me call upon Prof. Bucalossi to make some general comments on the symposium and some suggestions for future goals and activities.

Hon. Prof. Pietro Bucalossi

President, Italian League Against Cancer; Vice-President, House of Representatives of the Republic of Italy

When Professor Bonica asked me to take part in this meeting I think he did so because of my 30 years' experience at the Milano National Cancer Institute—the second such facility created in the world (after the one in Leningrad) for the specific treatment of cancer. I was sent to this Institute, then a place for terminal patients, from a general surgery hospital and it was quite different from today.

I often remember the terrible screams of a poor woman who was suffering from cancer of the pelvis with excruciating pains. At the time there was a solid obstacle that did not permit the use of the drugs and other modalities that have been rightly emphasized at this symposium. Then pain was considered from a religious point of view, an instrument for the spiritual life of the individual. Therefore, the use of drugs was banned, because it was believed that it accelerated the death of the patients. These notions were discounted in part by the late Pope Pius XII in the early 1950s.[1] Subsequently, this first battle was won, and the result was that by eliminating or reducing pain in those patients, it was possible to lengthen their lives and permit them to live more comfortably until their deaths. Since then there has been an impressive evolution in the specific treatment of pain in cancer. In these patients tragic factors, such as unbearable pain, together with the physical disability caused by the tumor or the anticancer therapy, produce a progressive deterioration of the personality.

The first experiences in our Institute (I say "our" fondly, but I am no longer part of the Institute) were directed toward neurosurgery applied to pain. The Department that is now directed by my friend, Ventafridda, with competence and passion, and to whom much is owed for the success of this meeting, was created in our Institute.

This symposium is a very special one and has the entirely new characteristic of having gathered here physicians and scientists of different disciplines: Oncologists are meeting and interacting with physiologists, neurologists, pharmacologists, anesthesiologists, and those of other disciplines and comparing their experiences with those of investigators. I have had this type of experience, and I wish to make a consideration regarding a certain attitude that I had towards cancerology. I have heard my colleague, Bonica, who is

---

[1] See p. xxix in Introduction.

the most prominent person in the organization of this symposium, point out the necessity of an interdisciplinary character of our medical and paramedical knowledge. I agree wholeheartedly on this point if it means that from these meetings questions are posed and ideas emerge which stimulate more and better research by those who are qualified in investigation, and hopefully this will produce new knowledge which then can be applied to the care of patients with cancer pain.

I would have some doubts, and I say this quite frankly, if the decision of the application of such knowledge for the care of patients were to be made by an assembly of this kind. And this goes for all problems connected with cancerology where we have seen and still see the prominence of technical factors over clinical ones. My dear departed friend, D'Argent, Professor of Clinical Oncology in Lyon, France, in his lessons said something regarding cancerology and cancer pain treatment with which I completely agree. That is: At a certain point a decision must be made regarding the patient, and this decision can be made only by the person who knows the possibilities of treatment the particular form of cancer requires. He further stated that the oncologist must be like a conductor who knows perfectly well what the violin, the brass, and the drums can produce and who is able to harmonize these sounds and to use them to create a concert that is the expression of perfect harmony. I believe in the treatment of cancer pain this consideration has its importance, because in the treatment of pain in cancer we have to deal not only with the pain and the associated psychologic effects present in all kinds of illnesses, but must consider that elements which are both curative and exclusively palliative intertwine. Obviously, the doctor who must prescribe the therapy must be fully aware of the advantages, disadvantages, limitations, and complications of a large number of interventions proposed to him so he can judge and decide, based on his own experience and the information provided by consultants, the application of the most effective therapy at the right time and in the right sequence so as to provide optimal pain-relief.

I agree with what Dr. Ford said about the creation of special centers qualified to give information regarding what should be done, because it is impossible to have in each and every hospital one or more persons who can solve these problems promptly and effectively.

I would like to end my short discourse by emphasizing that the Floriani Foundation has taken the initiative on this very important topic and has had great success which is due not only to its generosity but to the intelligence with which this initiative has been realized. I think that when we ask what should and can be done in the future, I think that this Foundation could represent a standard of reference for this type of meeting and the notions presented that there should be continuous interaction of researchers of various disciplines in order to conduct a strategy of the fight against cancer pain. So, in the future let's not leave it a dream but make it become a reality by creating these centers for the study and treatment of cancer pain from which indications of the strategy that is to be applied can be diffused out.

Bonica: I very much appreciate the comments made by my esteemed colleague, Professor Bucalossi, not only because he is one of the great pioneers of cancerology and has had vast experience in this field, but also because of his sustained interest and the national and international prestige and influence he has acquired. The doubt he expressed about who should make the final decision about the most appropriate therapy for each patient is both of theoretical and clinical importance. Professor Bucalossi, perhaps you are not aware that in conceiving and espousing the multidisciplinary approach to the management of chronic pain (including cancer pain) during the past three decades, one of the crucial points I've made is that no matter how many other physicians and health professionals are included in the decision-making process about mechanisms of diagnosis and therapy, each patient must have one and *only one* physician whom I have called "the manager." It is the responsibility of the managing physician not only to carry out the basic principles of diagnosis and therapy inherent in medical practice, but also to coordinate in an exquisite manner the consultations and to collect the information which will permit him to decide what is the correct diagnosis and what is the most appropriate therapeutic strategy. In the case of patients with cancer, it is the oncologist who should assume this responsibility. In order to "orchestrate" the actions of various consultants and put their ideas together so as to produce a "concert," it is essential for the oncologist not only to know all about the disease (tumor) but also to know well the mechanisms of the pain associated with cancer and to know all about the various modalities available for its relief, i.e., indications, advantages, limitations, complications, and contraindications. Unfortunately, in the past, with the exception of you and a few of your colleagues working in cancer who have had the precocious foresight and perspicacity, most oncologists have neglected the problem of pain or at least given it low priority in their consideration of the problem as a whole. Earlier, I presented evidence that in the past and even currently, cancer pain is usually badly managed and many patients continue to suffer moderate to severe pain until they die.

I have also presented the various reasons for this sad state of affairs and these need reemphasis here. For one thing, in virtually all of the exhaustive studies on virtually every aspect of cancer, the pain has received little or no attention. For another, with the exception of persons in some comprehensive cancer centers, oncologists have not interacted with neurologists, physiologists, pharmacologists, anesthesiologists, and all of the other people who could provide expert advice to permit the oncologist to make the right decision as to what is the most effective therapy for the pain (in contrast to the cancer). Because unfortunately no one person can have all of the knowledge, skills, and expertise to know all about each of the many therapeutic modalities and apply them effectively, it is essential for the oncologist to consult these various individuals and to obtain and collate the information they provide him and then make the right decision as to which therapy will be most effective for a particular patient. I hope that this symposium will serve as a stimulus for oncologists to collaborate and work in "concert" with other health professionals who have expertise in pain management so that in the future *all* cancer patients will be provided with maximum relief of their pain and suffering.

I now call upon Dr. Diane Fink, Director of the Division of Cancer Control and Rehabilitation of the National Cancer Institute of the United States, to tell us about the plans of the American Government to help solve the serious problem of cancer pain.

Diane Fink

National Cancer Institute, Bethesda, Maryland

My remarks will be divided into three major areas: (a) general areas of concern in the U.S.; (b) specific areas of concern of the National Institutes of Health (NIH); and (c) areas of concern and future directions for the National Cancer Institute (NCI).

In my comments during the discussion of terminal care I mentioned that there is a great interest in the U.S. in the problems of chronic pain and suffering and death and dying not only in cancer but in all of the major diseases. This interest is at the highest legislative level from our President, Mr. Jimmy Carter, to many of our congressional leaders within the Congress of the United States. In addition, we are seeing a great deal of interest manifested by the general public of our country as reflected by activities of many groups representing consumer interests, the news media, and by the many articles and discussions about the critical need to improve the care of patients with chronic pain and the problem of suffering. And quite amazingly much interest in improvement in the care of the dying patient.

Based on these kinds of interests and others, Dr. Donald Fredrikson, Director of the National Institutes of Health, has organized a study team composed of representatives from all governmental agencies that might be involved in the areas that I have mentioned and specifically in pain research. The purpose of this study team is to coordinate the federal government's approach to the problems of pain and suffering. This group plans to make a number of recommendations to Dr. Fredrikson, who will then make determinations along with the heads of other agencies within our government as to directions and future support, primarily for pain research but also for improving patient-care. The recommendation will include greater support for pain research and other needs for experimental studies in the area of pain.

I won't go into specific detail because I am really quite amazed, John, that as you went through your list of future goals and needs, the thinking of the NIH team is along these lines. In addition to pain research there will also be recommendations regarding needs for studies in the problems of terminal care and the need for demonstration programs in terminal care. And perhaps most importantly, programs to facilitate research in pain in its broadest sense. These considerations will include the very important allocations of funding and the development of specifically related study sections which we use to judge applications that will be concerned with pain research. Recommendations will also include greater needs in training of scientists for pain research and of physicians in the proper care of patients with cancer pain. I am speaking in rather broad terms.

We will also recommend centers for pain research and therapy whether these be in Comprehensive Cancer Centers, as described by Dr. Bonica, or perhaps in other institutions which have the kinds of expertise that would be necessary to deal with pain problems. And then also procedures to allow the rapid development and clinical experimental use of investigations of new drugs that might fall under what we call "Schedule One" of our narcotic laws, so that we can allow the proper pharmacologic and clinical studies to be undertaken of such agents. These recommendations will be presented to Dr. Fredrikson within the next several weeks. The Pain Study groups have been meeting every week since last fall, and since I serve on many of them I know that we hope to have our work finished in the very near future. Now from this we expect to hold a national conference in the U.S. on issues of pain and suffering, to look not only at research and demonstration needs but also health-care-delivery type issues. We have found that such National Conferences to raise awareness are exceedingly important to stimulate the various members of our scientific community to areas of importance found by groups such as Dr. Fredrikson's study group.

With regard to the National Cancer Institute, which is part of the NIH, we have the major responsibility for cancer research and demonstration, but the overall view of needs by the NIH in all areas of pain research we feel is exceedingly important for cancer pain, because these will help to elucidate certain basic mechanisms of pain. Whether this is done in the categorical institutes such as ours, or these discoveries come from institutes like the National Institute for Neurological and Communicative Disease and Stroke, or the National Institute of General Medical Sciences, does not matter, as long as it has applicability to the cancer patient. We consider this cross-fertilization among the various institutes and among the many parts of the government exceedingly important. As Dr. Bonica has mentioned, my own Division of Cancer Control and Rehabilitation has supported the majority of cancer-related pain research, psychological research and terminal-care activities of the National Cancer Institute. However, the Division of Cancer Treatment Research is becoming increasingly involved in the problems of pain research, and through its drug development program it can deal with our problems of assessing new analgesic drugs. It can also set the stage for development of new drugs and the kind of pharmacologic studies that will be required. In addition it has a large network of investigators throughout the U.S. that have dealt with oncologic treatment, and currently it is seeking ways of including pain research and clinical trials into this network. This division has at its disposal a large hospital service in the Washington, D.C. area. With regard to our own activities our primary responsibility is dealing with that large percentage of cancer patients who are seen in community hospitals. In addition to the research we have described, our major activity has been in attempting to set up a hospice program, not necessarily of the type of St. Christopher's because of the difference in medical practice, economic factors, and other considerations in the United States. However, we plan to set up a program that can be evaluated in a scientific way so that eventually we will know what it will take to deal with terminal care in a hospice-like atmosphere.

In addition we are quite concerned about the problems Dr. Bonica has talked about, such as how is cancer pain handled by the average practitioner in the U.S. and the so-called patterns of cancer care for pain. We are exceedingly interested in the epidemiologic studies dealing with the incidence, severity, and magnitude of cancer pain as national and regional health problems and its psychologic, physiologic, sociologic, and economic impact on the patient, the family, and society. The continuing education of physicians, nurses, and other health professionals is an important task ahead; but perhaps most importantly it is conferences of this type that make the interest of our federal government in an area as broad as chronic pain research known to the people and to the biomedical community. You can help us disseminate the word that there is great interest within the U.S. federal government of the development of good, solid, scientific studies that deal with cancer pain.

Bonica: Dr. Loeser, What can be done in the future to improve the area of neurosurgical approach to the management of cancer pain?

John Loeser

Department of Neurological Surgery, University of Washington, Seattle, Washington

I think that the primary problem in the use of neurosurgical procedures for the relief of cancer pain is careful selection of patients. Any surgeon who contemplates destructive or even stimulating neurosurgical procedure must know the process of the diseases that the patient has, must have the necessary technical skills, but most importantly, must have more than just a technical approach to human disease and human suffering. It is very difficult to evaluate the results of surgical procedures for pain-relief because there are much fewer of them done than nerve blocks, for example; and because all too often they are the last step in the treatment road, and the patient has already become a very different human being from what he or she was at the beginning of the illness.

Bonica: Dr. Loeser, Should all neurosurgeons be taught how to do all of the common techniques for cancer pain, or should we develop special centers where patients can be referred for particularly highly specialized techniques?

Loeser: Most of the stimulation techniques, and particularly the intracranial procedures, are experimental, and therefore their use should be restricted to major centers wherein surgeons will do enough cases to acquire extensive experience. However, I think that every neurosurgeon should be capable of performing cordotomies, dorsal rhizotomy, myelotomy, and the analogous procedures on the trigeminal and glossopharyngeal nerve. The number of centers needed is a function of the transportation and communication system that a community has. It is a lot cheaper to move patients to doctors than to try to put a neurosurgical center in every town.

Bonica: Dr. Bond, What needs to be done in the future regarding the role of psychiatrists and psychologists in the management of cancer pain?

Michael Bond

Department of Psychological Medicine, University of Glasgow, Glasgow, U.K.

My remarks must be interpreted against my background belief that cancer pain controlled by psychologic means is part of a psychosomatic attitude. That is one that takes account of psychologic, biological, and social aspects of the person's illness. I say this because in my view the balance is not right in medicine at the moment. The biomedical model or that part of medicine based on basic sciences far outweighs in terms of interest and resources the behavioral aspects of the disease. This needs to be corrected so that the two aspects can be brought into line with each other. Failure to treat cancer pain successfully is due in part to this tendency to use the unilateral (biomedical) approach to patients. The first goal or step to achieve this is to change the attitudes of graduate and postgraduate doctors and the general public towards illness in general and cancer in particular. Secondly, I believe it is clear to everyone here that no one person can deal with a cancer patient and his or her family. We have to have a team, the composition of which inevitably varies depending on the local resources. From a psychiatrist's point of view, and I think I speak for psychologists too, we need to extend our current methods of assessing the behavioral aspects of the pain of cancer and with that develop further contributions toward its control. One of the things we need to know a good deal more about is the pattern of psychologic changes which occur with different forms of cancer and with different treatments. We need to know not only what happens when the person is in pain, we need to know what happened before and what happens after treatment. Often people tend to be neglected in this phase. If we follow the model set by St.

Christopher's Hospice we can't go wrong. The reason for wanting to know more about the pattern of psychologic and social changes that occur is that this should enable us to identify people who are at risk in terms of their ultimate pain level and the behavior they exhibit when in pain. As psychiatrists and psychologists we are concerned not only with trying to lower the level of pain but we must also be involved in trying to help people come to terms with their disability, to cope with their pain if it cannot be completely relieved which is quite often the case. We need to look at these different age groups to find out what the patterns are.

In regard to the use of psychotropic drugs the literature is not sufficiently precise to allow their use with confidence. We need to be more precise about the indications for their use, and we also need to know more about the metabolism of these drugs in people who are in states of cachexia, or who are receiving potent drugs and who have a variety of physical problems including vomiting, and diarrhea, which may alter the normal metabolism of these drugs.

Finally, coming to psychologic treatments, my own view, like Dr. Saunders, is that psychiatrists usually are not there to treat cancer patients but are more likely to be involved in helping the doctors, nurses, and others who do the day-to-day treatments by counseling them and dealing with their own psychologic needs. One of the problems is that very few psychiatrists and psychologists will participate in this kind of work because the patients are very difficult to handle, and traditional training in psychiatry and psychology tends not to expose trainees to these types of problems. Therefore, we need to rectify this deficiency in our teaching program so that in the future psychiatrists and psychologists will play a more active role in managing patients with cancer pain. We also need to assess more extensively and precisely the therapies including individual psychotherapy, group therapy, family therapy, behavior modification, and biofeedback.

Bonica: Drs. Houde and Twycross, I would like you to discuss the proper use of systemic drugs for cancer pain, what new and better drugs might be developed and what else might be done for the better application of this general method of cancer pain control.

Raymond Houde

Department of Medicine, Memorial Sloan-Kettering Cancer Center, New York

I was glad to hear what Dr. Fink said about drugs, because most of the research that has been sponsored by the United States government has been supported by those agencies that have been concerned with drug abuse. In fact this is where we get most of our support. In terms of what we should do in the future, these fall into the three broad categories everyone has mentioned: education, training, and research. With respect to education it is quite obvious that there is a critical need to teach students and doctors how to use these drugs most effectively. Unfortunately, our international treaties have imposed a variety of constraints which have impaired the proper use of narcotics for cancer pain. The over-concern with the illicit traffic of drugs, for example, has had a serious impact on medical practice. We have to look at both sides of the coin: These drugs have particular pharmacologic properties which can be applied much more effectively to control pain in cancer. I agree with Dr. Saunders that we can control all pain of cancer with narcotics if we are willing to decrease consciousness. What we should be able to do is to achieve pain-relief but keep the patient as functional as possible within the capabilities of the consequences of their disease. This is what we should aim to do and this involves a lot more than just using analgesic drugs. Although our concern is with pain-relief, there are many other factors that impact on this, and the doctor must consider them in the total care of the patient. Narcotics don't just act on pain; they have other pharmacologic effects that must be considered. Moreover, the doctor may have to use adjuvant drugs in order to provide the patient with the most benefit.

Is there a need for new drugs? Obviously there is. We need new drugs that have different pharmacologic spectra. Not all patients are the same. There are some patients who tolerate one spectrum of pharmacologic activities of drugs and not another. For example, narcotic analgesics have many disadvantages in terms of some of their side effects; they produce constipation, but if the patient has diarrhea that is not a disadvantage but beneficial. In addition to their pain some cancer patients have intractable cough, which can be suppressed with narcotics. But then there are other patients who have different kinds of effects of their disease, and there you may need drugs of different spectra of activity.

Of the new drugs unrelated to narcotics, the new nonsteroidal anti-inflammatory drugs are extremely promising. What we do need to do is to look at them objectively. We have to design studies to look at them by methods scientifically acceptable and to make our decisions as to which drugs we wish to promote for the relief of pain on that kind of basis. Finally, we must acquire a better understanding of how drugs act in the body, of the physiology of pain, of drugs such as endorphins and to understand how best we can elaborate these endogenous antipain mechanisms.

Robert G. Twycross

The Churchill Hospital, Oxford, U.K.

I wish to discuss the problem of drugs for pain-relief under three headings: teaching, research, and political action. I will begin with political action. We are part of the International Association for the Study of Pain, which has helped us to come together and exchange information. We should help each other to make sure that in every country there are at least aspirin, codeine, and morphine available and the latter should be available for use both by mouth and by injection. Moreover, for patients who have some idiosyncratic disability we should have available at least one alternative to these three basic analgesics.

In regard to research, I agree with Dr. Houde. In teaching we must select the most important aspects of what we have been discussing. It is far more important that every nurse and every doctor should really understand that pain is a psychobiologic phenomenon or experience which is modulated by mood, meaning, culture, and many other factors. If the doctor and nurse appreciate these aspects of pain, he or she can do more for the patient in pain than if he or she is familiar with the latest information about A-delta and C-fibers, or the latest information about prostaglandins and endorphins. I am not against science, but we must give priority to those aspects that enable the doctor or nurse to help the patient most. The other point that should come out about teaching is that we cannot wait for all the clinical trials to be completed before we begin to use drugs. We know and can agree that certain drugs are better than others. We are agreed, for example, that partial agonists, like pentazozine, have little or no place in advanced cancer pain-relief. Broader aspects of teaching should also include that it is just as much a medical success to help a patient die in comfort as it is to cure him and see him walk out through the hospital door. The medical ethic, as I understand it, is not to preserve life at all costs but to sustain life when, from a biologic point of view, it is sustainable and worthwhile. Therefore the application of acute medical support systems and interventions with radical palliative methods that prolong the distress of dying rather than adding useful, worthwhile life should not be considered.

Bonica: Now I call upon Dr. Pannuti to comment about future needs and goals in oncology with emphasis on pain control.

F. Pannuti

Division of Oncology, Marcello Malpighi Hospital, Bologna, Italy

I am an oncologist, so I would like to give my point of view about some essential facts. First, what does the oncologist want in the future from society? We oncologists are looking for structures in which there are also present centers specializing in pain therapy. I want to make myself clear: I believe that in Pain Centers the oncologist is as important as the pain therapist in the management of pain of cancer. Oncologic structures mean a greater financial support from the government and society as a whole. We have to build schools for oncologists and pain therapists, and the wealthier nations have, in my opinion, to give this cultural heritage and make available the information presented at this conference and similar types of meetings, to underdeveloped countries.

Secondly, also we should want something new at the nurses' level. I believe that nurses should be good interpreters of the medical act, but to do this they must also develop their own role in their relationship with the patient. In this regard, I believe Rogers' description of the role of nurse is useful and I agree with it. Indeed we have already carried it out in Bologna, where nurses have become more cognizant of what they are doing and more autonomous toward the individual patient.

Another area where we oncologists can develop something new is in pharmacology. We must realize the difference between the pharmacology of analgesic drugs and the pharmacology of antitumoral drugs. I believe we should promote more extensive studies in stage 3, i.e., a precise check on new analgesic drugs compared with the traditional ones, in order to eliminate all those drugs that are not useful and to identify which new drugs are better than the traditional aspirin, codeine, and morphine. New and old antitumoral drugs constitute another important topic. As for the new ones, we oncologists should again require them to be studied preclinically, i.e., on animals not only to see whether or not they reduce tumor mass, but also to study their effectiveness in relieving pain. For example, currently we are testing MAP and comparing it with prostaglandins. We agree with Bonica that in addition to evaluating their anticancer efficacy the oncologic therapist should also monitor the signal symptoms such as pain and anorexia.

Still another level where something new can be foreseen is the one concerning the physician, but here the job is more complex. The physician should work in close relationship with the psychologist in order to be advised about the patient. After the oncologist has been at his job for many years he needs psychologic support for reasons given by Drs. Saunders and Bond. I believe the psychologist is important for modulating the physician-patient relationship. In regard to the patient-physician relationship we can act at two different levels: The first one is to ask ourselves whether or not we should tell the patient the truth about his or her disease. This will be determined by many considerations including the patient's personality, culture, traditional and social conditions. In my opinion, we must inform the patient whenever these considerations suggest it is to the best interest of the patient and family. The second important level is that physicians together with nurses must more and more keep the patient informed of what is happening. The last important point is that the physician must devise a therapeutic approach based on a comparison of other patients in a controlled way, i.e., by means of protocols and a data bank. In closing, I propose that Bonica and Ventafridda repeat this type of conference regularly every 2 or 3 years. Moreover, between each conference a permanent multidisciplinary commission should operate to get the proceedings published and to establish guidelines for interdisciplinary and international programs intended to improve the care of patients with cancer pain.

Leandro Gennari

Istituto Nazionale per lo Studio e la Cura Tumori, Milan, Italy

What can we do for the future? As regards the traditional therapies, I would say we cannot do more than what has been done already. Surgery has achieved its highest possibilities, if you take into account that to treat cancer and to avoid recurrence of the disease and pain, operations such as "hemicorporectomy" have been done. As for radiotherapy, we still have chances for the future. There is a lead that should be followed, which is further and more extensive radioimmunologic studies. The investigation of those antigenic substances, which are secreted by the tumor and found in the organism, are capable of giving signs that will make possible a very early diagnosis of the disease. This means that an early diagnosis allows not only a more appropriate and earlier surgical or radiation therapy, but equally important it means discovering the recurrence of the neoplastic process several months earlier than has been possible heretofore. Therefore, we can intervene with other methods to avoid the pain of advanced cancer.

As for chemotherapy, we are confronted by a great obstacle: that the lack of selectivity of the drugs at our disposal does not allow us to destroy the diseased cells and save the healthy tissue. We hope we can find a drug that has this selectivity or more drugs, so that we can study the best combination of drugs. Finally, I must say that chemotherapy can make a significant contribution not only in pain therapy but also in avoiding the development of pain when it is administered prophylactically after surgical removal of the tumor. There are documented cases of prolonged survival and of longer periods free from disease after surgical treatment of breast cancer or amputation of a limb for osteosarcoma followed by complementary chemotherapy.

Vittorio Ventafridda

Istituto Nazionale per lo Studio e la Cura Tumori, Milan, Italy

The struggle against pain can be carried out successfully provided that the oncologist also becomes involved in the treatment of pain. He or she becomes appropriately involved when he or she appreciates that pain is one of the most important aspects of cancer and assesses and collects it as one of the kinds of data that must be kept in the therapeutic files. I have seen dozens of protocols in the treatment of cancer, but pain is never taken into account or included in the protocol. Only when he or she has a quantitative dimension of the pain can he or she improve the strategy for its effective control.

Qualified persons must be trained for this task. The neurooncologists are among the most qualified persons to diagnose the pain and to help develop the most appropriate therapeutic strategy. Foley is a neurooncologist in a large cancer center, and she has shown us in a simple way the possibilities of achieving results. Those who work in pain therapy, whether anesthesiologists, neurosurgeons, or pharmacologists, must also be oncologists. There cannot be an anesthesiologist who does pain therapy in oncology, just because he does blocks. He must also know oncology!

Another important point is the development of rehabilitation programs: The physical disability is a very important factor which contributes to the patient's pain and suffering, and rehabilitation therapy gives wonderful results in these patients.

Clinical trials to evaluate analgesic agents must be controlled and carried out by well-established conditions and criteria. We also must develop pain-control departments or teams in cancer centers and institutes which are able to effectively treat all types of cancer pain. The team should include persons with experience and expertise to carry out the various therapeutic modalities which we have discussed here. In these centers, it should also be possible to administer narcotics to outpatients as well as inpatients under controlled conditions. This will require support from social workers and other health professionals.

Finally, such centers should carry out studies of new systemic analgesics which provide maximum relief with few or no side effects. There is a special need for the availability of an effective oral narcotic preparation in Italy.

John Bonica

Department of Anesthesiology, University of Washington, Seattle, Washington

It is clear that much needs to be done to improve the care of patients with pain of advanced cancer. I hope that the discussions and interactions of the past 4 days will help all of us to improve the care of these patients. Moreover, the publication of these proceedings should also help many other health professionals who could not attend and who have the serious responsibility of pain control and total management of patients with advanced cancer.

I hope I reflect the opinion of many, if not most of you, when I state that the goals and objectives of this symposium as enunciated at the beginning have been achieved. Indeed, the success of this conference is beyond my most optimistic expectations. For this I wish to express my sincerest thanks and appreciation, as well as those of the Scientific Program Committee, the Local Arrangements Committee, and the Floriani Foundation, to all the speakers and participants. Much of the success of the symposium has also been due to the interest, attentiveness, patience, and persistence of the audience. Despite the unique tourist attractions of Venice, most of the registrants have remained in attendance until the very end of each session.

I wish to thank again Cardinal Luciani and the various governmental officials for their moral support; special thanks are also due to the five agencies that auspiced this symposium.

Finally, I cannot adequately express the thanks and appreciation and indeed gratitude to the Floriani Foundation on behalf of all the participants and speakers and especially the millions of patients with cancer pain throughout the world who are suffering needlessly and hopefully will be helped by the information presented here. The foresight and generosity and warm friendship of Ing. and Mrs. Virgilio Floriani have made possible this highly successful symposium, this uniquely outstanding meeting facility, and the very elegant social activities that have been sponsored by Mr. and Mrs. Floriani. In this regard I thank them also on behalf of the wives of the speakers as well as others who took advantage of the opportunity to participate in these social activities.

Ing. and Mrs. Floriani have initiated what I believe will prove to be a long-range movement which will have a major impact on the care of patients with pain of advanced cancer. I hope that this highly successful international, multidisciplinary cancer pain symposium will be the first of many such meetings that will continue to provide a forum for the exchange of new information that eventually will have a beneficial effect on these patients.

I hope that in the near and remote future, federal, provincial, and municipal governmental agencies will support more research, better education, and better patient care. Moreover, we hope that this symposium will stimulate physicians and other health professionals, but especially oncologists to include the teaching of students and graduate doctors in providing optimal cancer pain control. The ultimate goal of these efforts is to provide people everywhere with better health care in the prevention and treatment of cancer and the associated pain.

I hope that the torch lighted by Ing. and Mrs. Floriani will be readily taken over and carried in the future not only by federal agencies but also private foundations in making possible this type of intense multidisciplinary international meeting on the subject of cancer pain.

Subject Index

24/81
36/81
37/81